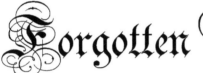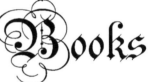

ISBN 978-1-5284-4195-7
PIBN 10918417

1 MONTH OF
FREE
READING

at
www.ForgottenBooks.com

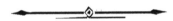

By purchasing this book you are eligible for one month membership to ForgottenBooks.com, giving you unlimited access to our entire collection of over 1,000,000 titles via our web site and mobile apps.

To claim your free month visit:
www.forgottenbooks.com/free918417

English
Français
Deutsche
Italiano
Español
Português

www.forgottenbooks.com

Mythology Photography **Fiction**
Fishing Christianity **Art** Cooking
Essays Buddhism Freemasonry
Medicine **Biology** Music **Ancient**
Egypt Evolution Carpentry Physics
Dance Geology **Mathematics** Fitness
Shakespeare **Folklore** Yoga Marketing
Confidence Immortality Biographies
Poetry **Psychology** Witchcraft
Electronics Chemistry History **Law**
Accounting **Philosophy** Anthropology
Alchemy Drama Quantum Mechanics
Atheism Sexual Health **Ancient History**
Entrepreneurship Languages Sport
Paleontology Needlework Islam
Metaphysics Investment Archaeology
Parenting Statistics Criminology
Motivational

The JOURNAL

of the

Iowa State Medical Society

INDEX

Volume XXIV, January to December

1934

Editor: RALPH R. SIMMONS, M.D., Des Moines

Some Causes of Professional Unrest
R. G. Leland, M.D., Chicago, Illinois..................603

Southeastern Surgical Congress Meets in Nashville.........118

Speakers Bureau Activities............................
........33, 111, 161, 216, 257, 302, 346, 457, 497, 534, 593, 638
Special Lectures at the Mayo Clinic....................110
Standard for Industrial Medicine, A.......................494
Standardized Serology in Syphilis.........................634
State Department of Health
Walter L. Bierring, M.D., Des Moines
....21, 103, 155, 209, 252, 296, 341, 450, 492, 529, 587, 631
State Society of Iowa Medical Women......................181
Study of Neonatal Deaths at the University Hospital, A
John H. Randall, M.D., Iowa City.....................477
Surgeons View Sickness Insurance Plans..................453
Surgical Clinics
Verne C. Hunt, M.D., Los Angeles, California.........469
Syphilis, Standardized Serology in........................634

Systolic Apical Murmurs, The Significance of
E. L. Wurtzer, M.D., Clear Lake......................626

T

Test of Organized Medicine, The
Oliver J. Fay, M.D., Des Moines......................205
Thorium Dioxide Sol, Roentgen Visualization of the Liver and
Spleen with
L. G. Ericksen, M.D., Dubuque.......................438
Thorotrast, Demonstration of Liver Metastases by Means of
L. G. Ericksen, M.D., Dubuque.......................101
Thymic Disturbances in Children
G. E. Harrison, M.D., Mason City.....................188
Thyroid Surgery, Indications for
T. E. Davidson, M.D., Mason City.....................440
Tic Douloureux, Clinical Observations in
Frank A. Ely, M.D., Des Moines...................... 81
Tinted Lenses a Fad..531
Tobacco Smoking, Hyperglycemia a Result of..............344
Toxoid in Diphtheria Prevention   .
Bennett A. Melgaard, M.D., Sioux City................ 14
Transactions, House of Delegates, Iowa State Medical Society,
Eighty-third Annual Session............................350
Traumatic Rupture of the Intestine
F. P. McNamara, M.D., Dubuque.......................292
Treatment of Burns
N. M. Whitehill, M.D., Boone.........................481
Treatment of Functional Menstrual Irregularities of Young
Women, The
Della G. Drips, M.D., Rochester, Minnesota............. 1
Trigeminal Neuralgia, The Diagnosis and Treatment of
Walter D. Abbott, M.D., Des Moines...................193
Trudeau, Dr. Edward Livingston.........................636
Tuberculosis in Infancy
Arnold M. Smythe, M.D., Des Moines..................200
Tuberculosis of the Knee Joint
Donald C. Conzett, M.D., Dubuque.....................202
Tuberculosis, The Industrialized Community and..........455
Tuberculous Patients, Increased Hospital Beds for.........345
Turkish Licensure Regulations.......................... 42
Two Distinguished Scientists Die—Roux and Calmette........ 30

U

Unilateral Fused Kidney
Otto N. Glesne, M.D., Fort Dodge.....................291
University Hospital, The................................ 26
Unusual Congenital Anomaly, An: Case Report
William O. Purdy, M.D., and B. E. Stofer, M.D., Des
Moines 527
Urinary Findings in Nephritis, The Significance of
F. P. McNamara, M.D., Dubuque.......................614
Uterine Cancer, Additional Data on
Robert M. Collins, M.D., Iowa City................... 71

V

Vaginal Hemorrhage in the Newborn
Henry E. Kleinberg, M.D., Des Moines.................286
Value of Resection of the Presacral Nerve, The
Walter D. Abbott, M.D., Des Moines..................607
Venereal Disease Information............................210

W

Warning 221, 263, 586
What is the Basic Science Law?..........................531
Who Are Graduates in Medicine?
Charles B. Taylor, M.D., Ottumwa....................269
Why Are We Here and Where Are We Going?
Gordon F. Harkness, M.D., Davenport.................271
Why Does Iowa Need the Basic Science Law?.............590
Winneshiek County, Inter-professional Association in........ 40
Woman's Auxiliary, Iowa State Medical Society...........181
Woman's Auxiliary News................................
.........34, 112, 162, 217, 258, 303, 347, 457, 498, 536, 594, 640
Women Physicians, History of........................... 29

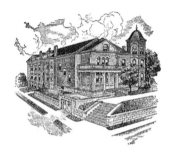
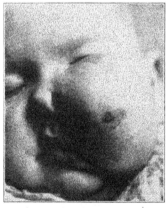
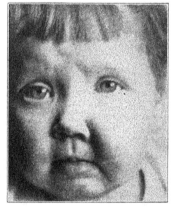

The JOURNAL

of the

Iowa State Medical Society

| V͏ᵒ͏ᶦ· XXIV | Des Moines, Iowa, January, 1934 | No. 1 |

THE TREATMENT OF FUNCTIONAL MENSTRUAL IRREGULARITIES OF YOUNG WOMEN*

Della G. Drips, M.D.,
Division of Medicine, The Mayo Clinic,
Rochester, Minnesota

A young woman who menstruates irregularly may speak of missed periods or periods of less duration or amount; these conditions are considered as of the amenorrheic type of menstruation. On the other hand, she may complain of having too frequent, too prolonged or too profuse menses; these are irregularities of the metrorrhagic type. Essentially, irregularity of menstruation is a deviation from what the woman considers normal for her. A marked disturbance of the rhythm of the cycle is sometimes the characteristic feature of the irregularity, long or short periods of flowing following long or short intervals between the flow. From a description of the irregularity only it may be difficult to classify such cases in either group.

Functional menstrual irregularities differ in no essentials from those dependent on organic causes. If the irregularity has been present intermittently since the onset of menstruation, or has followed abortion or parturition, it is more likely to be due to a physiologic disturbance of function of the organs involved in the production of regular normal menstruation than to lesions in these organs which usually precipitate irregular menstruation rather abruptly on a formerly regular course.

Secondary menstrual irregularity due to general systemic disease must likewise not be confused with the functional types; here the cause lies outside of the glands involved in menstruation. Local pelvic lesions, such as tumors and inflammation, which are usually the cause of irregular menstruation, also must be carefully ruled out.

The treatment of such amenorrheic and metrorrhagic types of functional menstrual irregularity has been put on a much more logical basis in recent years as a result of clinical and laboratory investi-

* Presented before the Eighty-second Annual Session. Iowa State Medical Society, Des Moines, May 10, 11, 12, 1933.

gations, made in an effort to determine just which of the glands involved are at fault. Gynecologists have been concerned largely with the anterior lobe of the pituitary gland, the ovaries and the uterus. Studies relative to the thyroid gland and the suprarenal glands which have been carried on have aided greatly in an understanding of the complexity of menstrual phenomena.

The greatest aid in locating the seat of the trouble has been the investigations made for the purpose of determining the amounts of ovarian estrogenic and pituitary anterior lobe hormones in the blood, urine and feces of normally and abnormally menstruating women over considerable periods of time representing a number of cycles and during pregnancy and lactation. As yet one is hampered by knowing almost nothing about the amount of ovarian luteal hormone which is secreted, since it has not been recovered outside of the corpus luteum. The result of such studies, together with the information gained by comparing clinical histories, physical types, basal metabolic rates, and by noting the response of patients to treatment made as specific as possible, have made it possible to distinguish certain clinical groups in which a given form of treatment applies. It is now believed that the amenorrheic type of case represents hypofunction of one or more of the glands involved, and these cases have been divided accordingly into four groups, by Mazer and others.

1. The hypopituitary group comprises probably three-fourths of all the cases. There is a tendency to obesity with the periods of amenorrhea, the obesity being confined to the hips and thighs, shoulders and breasts. The severe form of pituitary failure is exemplified in Frölich's syndrome, or adiposogenital dystrophy. I have seen few such cases. Frequently the distribution of hair is of the male type. The patients usually have few symptoms aside from menstrual irregularity and the consequent associated sterility. Severe dysmenorrhea, menstrual molimina and vasomotor disturbances, particularly hot flashes, are not common. The metabolic rate is normal or somewhat

lowered, often around minus 15. Little if any ovarian estrogenic hormone and pituitary anterior lobe hormone are found in the blood and urine.

2. The hypo-ovarian group comprises about a fourth or less of the cases of amenorrhea. The patients are usually of normal weight or below, often tall and slender. They complain of dysmenorrhea before the onset, with the onset, and frequently during the period of short, scant flow. Menstrual molimina such as headache, nervousness and dizziness are common, and hot flashes during the periods of amenorrhea often occur. The basal metabolic rate is usually within normal limits. Little if any ovarian estrogenic hormone is found in the blood and urine and the pituitary anterior lobe hormone is normal or is in excess in the blood and urine. With complete ovarian failure, the pituitary follicle ripening hormone tends to appear in excess for a period of several months.

3. This group is designated as the hypothyroid group although the syndrome is in no way similar to myxedema. It comprises a small group of cases in which the patients have low basal metabolic rates, around minus 25 to minus 32, who are of normal habitus and usually are of normal weight or underweight. If they are overweight, the weight is normally distributed. The onset of the amenorrhea in the cases I have observed has been associated with severe fatigue and often loss of appetite. After a period of severe exhaustion, the amenorrhea develops and in its wake, a train of symptoms appears, such as headache, nervousness, dizziness, intolerance to cold, and often nausea and vomiting akin to the anorexia nervosa syndrome. In such cases the patient may die in spite of all treatment. The hormones of the ovary and the pituitary gland are low or absent from the blood and urine in this group.

4. The hypo-uterine group comprises a small group of cases in which it is felt that the uterus is in some way at fault. The women apparently are normal, except for periods of amenorrhea. The uterus is often normal in size, and the patients complain of cyclic discomfort in the pelvis; they may become pregnant without menstruating. The hormones are found in normal amounts in the blood and urine. At times, there is an excess of ovarian estrogenic hormone in the urine while there is the normal amount in the blood, leading to the belief that a low renal threshold for the hormone may be responsible for the amenorrhea. It would hardly seem that the integrity of the uterus could be thus maintained sufficiently to keep its normal size and allow normal nidation of the ovum.

As yet, it seems impossible to distinguish functional metrorrhagia on a pituitary or ovarian basis.

Study of the hormones in the blood and urine in these cases so far has revealed in a considerable number an excess of the ovarian estrogenic hormone, especially just before and during the periods of bleeding. Frank[5] and Zondek[14] have reported a number of such incidents. This is especially true in the cases of so-called bleeding of puberty. It was consequently assumed at first that this condition was due to overstimulation of the ovaries by an overactive pituitary gland during the period of growth, and represented hyperfunction of the ovaries. If so, it seems that the anterior pituitary hormone should also be in excess in the blood and urine, but it has usually been found in normal amount. Because the uterus and endometrium in these bleeding cases resemble that of the castrated animal, given injections of large doses of estrogenic hormone only, it is assumed that the luteal hormone is not being secreted in amounts necessary to balance the effect of the estrogenic hormone. Smith and Smith[11] have shown experimentally that the ovarian luteal hormone, progestin, promotes the urinary excretion of the estrogenic hormone and thereby a physiologic balance is maintained. Whether this lack of luteal hormone is the result of a pituitary or ovarian failure is unknown. Slight cystic degeneration without corpora lutea is a common finding in the ovaries in these cases, but such a condition may not be inherent in the ovaries; it may be due to insufficient stimulation to luteinization from the pituitary anterior lobe.

These women usually are of normal habitus and normal weight with a normal metabolism. However, some are of the obese pituitary type with a somewhat lowered metabolism, and some are of the underweight asthenic type with a low metabolism. These patients, especially those of normal habitus, do not complain of dysmenorrhea, menstrual molimina or hot flashes. Some gynecologists have attributed this to the presence of excess ovarian estrogenic hormone. The women are sterile almost as frequently as those of the amenorrheic type. Of seventy-seven married women of this type, 44 per cent were sterile after an average of six and nine-tenths years of married life, and the average number of pregnancies in the other group was 1.6. Of 144 women of the amenorrheic type, 53 per cent were sterile after six and one-tenth years of married life, and the average number of pregnancies in the other group was 1.4. The women with metrorrhagic tendencies are much more incapacitated than the others, because of the prolonged and at times profuse bleeding with the consequent secondary anemia.

Certain principles of treatment have been established in these cases of functional menstrual irregularities. Treatment is instituted both to alleviate associated disagreeable symptoms and to attempt to reëstablish regular normal menses. In this paper I shall refer only to patients treated in an attempt to bring on and regulate the menses. The improvement noted in Tables I and II means then, improvement in the regularity of the periods and not merely in subjective symptoms or general health. Doubtful cases were omitted as were cases in which treatment was not conducted for sufficient time to obtain results. With the exception of one case in which there was insufflation and a few cases in which treatment was given for cervicitis, no other treatment for sterility was instituted beyond the attempt to regulate the menses. The male factor could not be ruled out in most cases as the patients came to the clinic without their husbands. It has not seemed reasonable to try to affect the regularity of the cycle of a woman aged more than thirty-four years; hence treatment for this purpose has been confined to the younger women. The average age in the group of amenorrheic women treated was twenty-four and nine-tenths years; in the metrorrhagic group, twenty-five and six-tenths years. It was found that the younger the patient, and the shorter the duration and the less the degree of irregularity, the more satisfactory was the response to treatment, proving that it is best to institute treatment early.

For the amenorrheic type of patient it seems best to begin treatment after three months of amenorrhea, and treatment should be given to women who do not menstruate oftener than four times a year, particularly if the intervals are tending to become longer or the flow scantier, and if the woman is anxious to have children. The treatment for both types of cases, at best, is still very unsatisfactory even with the newer hormone preparations. In fact, the disappointing results in many cases in which the new hormones alone have been tried, have proved that there is still much more to be learned about the physiology of the secretory glands involved. Emphasis must be placed on the necessity for continuing study of hormones in the blood and urine, and of gathering data on response to well-directed treatment.

Various gynecologists have mentioned cures of patients who have been observed for a few months. It would seem safer to designate these as improved only, since so many patients return after a lapse of months or a few years, complaining of the original trouble. Many young girls are apparently cured of irregularities that have not been too long continued or pronounced, by simple means, but the more severe types are very difficult to cure with any treatment now available, and one can usually only hope to alleviate symptoms or to bring about regular periods of menstruation long enough to allow conception to take place.

The first consideration of treatment should be attention to the general hygiene, especially in regard to food and exercise. Diets high in vitamins and protein have proved efficacious for the amenorrheic patient. Adding yeast to the diet often helps. For the metrorrhagic patient diets high in

Table I
RESULTS OF TREATMENT OF AMENORRHEA

Treatment	Patients				Improved after 1 year				Patients not improved				Pregnancies occurring within 1 year after treatment			
	January 1927 to October 1928	October 1928 to January 1930	1930	1931	January 1927 to October 1928	October 1928 to January 1930	1930	1931	January 1927 to October 1928	October 1928 to January 1930	1930	1931	January 1927 to October 1928	October 1928 to January 1930	1930	1931
Ovarian extracts (not standardized)	32	42	26	19	23	24	19	13	9	18	7	6	3		1	2
Ovarian and anterior lobe hormone (standardized)		6	6	11		5	5	7		1	1	4				2
Thyroid (desiccated extract)	3	2	2	5	1		2	1	2	2		4				
Thyroid and ovarian preparations	7	2	2	4	6	2	1	3	1		1	1	1			
Low dosage irradiation of ovaries and pituitary gland	10	5	19	7	7	3	12	5	3	2	7	2	3	1	4	
Low dosage irradiation and ovarian or thyroid extract	10	2	1	1	6	2	1	1	4				1			
Instructions in general hygiene only		6	4	10		3	1	3	.	3	3	7			1*	1
Total	62	65	60	57	43	41	41	33	19	26	19	24				
Grand Total	244				156 (63+per cent)				88				20†			

* This patient had an insufflation also.

† The pregnancies occurred among 86 married women whose conditions were improved by treatment, and two single women who were married shortly after treatment.

fat and high in calcium, with the addition of cod liver oil, have proved beneficial. In prescribing a diet, the normal weight of the patient should always be approximated. The next consideration should be the basal metabolism. Desiccated thyroid gland even in small amounts, has proved valuable even when the basal metabolic rate is normal. If the metabolism is definitely below normal, it has seemed best to administer sufficient thyroid gland extract to bring the patient to a normal rate and to keep the rate there for two or three months before other specific treatment is started. Raising the basal metabolic rate may be sufficient to correct the irregularity; usually it is not. The administration of some reliable non-standardized form of ovarian extract often is sufficient for the young woman with a mild degree of amenorrhea. Table I shows the number of women who improved following this treatment alone.

In cases in which considerable uterine atrophy is present, and the amenorrhea has existed for six to twelve months or longer, it has been necessary to resort to the standardized hormone preparations, or to low dosage irradiation of the ovaries and pituitary gland. If the expense of the hormone treatment does not make it prohibitive it is given a trial before irradiation is advised; it is a rule in The Mayo Clinic not to use irradiation unless medical treatment has failed.

Whenever uterine atrophy is marked, one can assume without making tests that the ovarian estrogenic hormone is low or absent from the urine. I believe it is reasonable to consider giving this hormone first in an attempt to bring the uterus back to the normal interval condition in normally menstruating women. It can more easily respond to the hormone from the ovaries when these are stimulated. Werner has recently reported giving large doses of theelin to castrated women and bringing the atrophic uterus with its endometrium back to the normal interval condition.

Siebke[10] has shown that normally menstruating women excrete as much as 2,000 mouse units of ovarian estrogenic hormone in the urine and feces during a cycle. It is evident, then, that when only a small amount, or no ovarian estrogenic hormone can be recovered from the urine of an amenorrheic woman over a three-day period, the administration of small doses of this hormone usually will have no effect. The dosage should be adequate. In the normal physiologic cycle Frank found this hormone to be increased in the blood during the premenstrual period. This can be imitated by increasing the dosage during the time that corresponds to the third and fourth week of the cycle. In imitation of a physiologic cycle, the hormone should be administered for three weeks, omitted for a

week and repeated. This should be continued for three months at least. The week of omission is considered as the menstrual time, or first week of the cycle. This does not mean that the hormone is always absent during menstruation but when present it is usually found in only small amounts. The ovarian estrogenic hormone can be given intramuscularly or orally. The preparations of the pure hormone have been obtained from the urine of pregnant women and pregnant mares. Theelin is a common intramuscular preparation and theelol the oral form. Amniotin is available for intramuscular injection and is put up in oil for oral administration. When the hormone is given orally, four times the amount prescribed for intramuscular injection should be given. Oral administration permits the administration of divided doses at more frequent intervals, thus keeping some hormone continuously in the circulation, less being excreted.

It is known that the ovarian luteal hormone is secreted, in addition to the estrogenic hormone, during at least the fourth week of the cycle; and again in imitation of the physiologic process, it should be added during this time. It has been clearly shown by Knaus[8] that the true premenstrual or pregravid secreting decidual endometrium cannot be produced in the castrated rabbit without the addition of the active ovarian luteal hormone, which evidently initiates the secretion phase in the endometrial gland cells, thus providing the one essential for successful nidation of the ovum. There is no standardized luteal hormone on the market in this country; Corner's progestin would be the ideal substitute if it were available. Consequently, we apparently have not had as much success in bringing on true menstruation as German physicians seem to have had in adding Knaus' luteogan to the estrogenic hormone. Kaufmann[6] has reported the production of true menstrual bleeding, the shedding of a real decidua menstrualis in women after surgical castration by the administration of both ovarian hormones. He found, as Werner[18] did, that the quantities of hormones necessary to produce menstrual changes in the uterine mucosa of castrated women are much larger than those heretofore employed in treatment with ovarian hormones. The only luteal preparation available in this country is sistomensin. This contains both a standardized amount of the estrogenic hormone and a non-standardized amount of the luteal hormone. I believe it should be given until a better preparation is available. Some gynecologists have had better results using a combination of the ovarian estrogenic hormone with an extract of the whole ovary. Progynon is such a preparation. There seems to be a feeling prevalent in Europe that the pure ovarian estrogenic hormone, especially that derived from the urine, needs the presence of some other ovarian substance to allow it to act on the uterus.

As a result of the treatment described here, menstruation may ensue. It will probably not continue without the substitution treatment unless concomitant treatment of the glands primarily responsible for the amenorrhea is also given. This means that after the uterus has been primed, treatment must be given which will stimulate the hypofunctioning glands. If it cannot be decided whether the pituitary gland or the ovary is at fault, both should be treated. A hormone which directly stimulates the pituitary gland is not available, but low dosage roentgen rays seem to stimulate pituitary activity.

A considerable number of so-called anterior lobe hormone preparations are in use for stimulation of the ovaries. Most of those on the market are made from the urine of pregnant women. Emmenin made from the placenta also seems to activate the ovaries, or low dosage roentgen rays can be used over the ovaries. I have had little experience, and so far no success, in starting the menstrual flow with the so-called anterior pituitary hormone preparations made from the urine. I believe that a potent extract made from the anterior lobe of the pituitary gland which will do this will soon be on the market. I have used emmenin alone with some success in cases of amenorrhea of not more

Table II
LOW DOSAGE X-RAY 1927 TO 1931 INCLUSIVE

Patients	66*
Fields covered	
Ovarian	47
Pituitary	5
Ovarian and pituitary	17
Single women treated	29
Menses reestablished for 3 months at least	21
Menses not improved	8
Menses continued fairly regular for from 1½ to 6 years	17
Women married and pregnant since	2†
Married women treated	37
Average number of years married	6.4
Patients who had been pregnant	16
Patients who had had one pregnancy	13
Patients not heard from	2
Incorrect diagnosis (1 patient died with pituitary tumor; 1 was pregnant)	2
Married women whose menses were reestablished for 3 months at least	20
Married women not improved	13
Women becoming pregnant directly after irradiation	9
Women still menstruating with fair regularity 1½ to 6 years after treatment	14

* Three patients had two treatments
† In one case, second irradiation in 1932 after marriage; pregnancy followed immediately.

than six months' duration and in which there was not much uterine atrophy. This was the emmenin complex which contains some estrin.

Thus far, I have had the greatest degree of success in the more severe types of amenorrhea with low dosage irradiation. Table II gives an analysis of the cases in which this treatment was used during the years 1927 to 1931, inclusive. It was at the suggestion of Dr. Frances A. Ford, who studied this group of cases with me and prescribed the amount of irradiation to be given that this treatment alone be used until some definite conclusion was reached as to its effect. As a consequence, additional treatment was given in a few cases only. Our success in reestablishing menstruation and fertility up to 1927 in the same type of case which later was selected for irradiation, had been practically nil. Ford began cautiously to irradiate only over one ovary. The technic has been described.[1] The second patient treated was obese (pituitary type), weighing 213 pounds. She was thirty-two years of age, had never been married seventeen years, had never been pregnant, and had not menstruated for two years. She was given irradiation over the left ovary only. Menstrual periods were reestablished, and she became pregnant within three months. The first child died at birth, apparently from trauma. The menses recurred and she again became pregnant, and gave birth to a healthy child. Her periods were very irregular again after the last childbirth, but at present she is menstruating regularly and hoping to have another child. This case illustrates the success occasionally obtained with treatment that does not inconvenience the patient, and is inexpensive. The longest period of amenorrhea prior to the institution of treatment with irradiation was three years. There is no excuse with the Friedman test available, for irradiating any pregnant woman. It was formerly, indeed, frequently difficult to decide about early pregnancy because of the marked irregularity of menses. In our one case the irradiation was given over the pituitary gland and had no apparent ill effect. There have been no ill effects noted in any cases of our series. Several women have had two irradiations over the ovaries, with normal pregnancies following. Because of severe dysmenorrhea, Ford repeated low dosage irradiation over the ovaries as many as six times in one case over a period of six years, and the patient is still having regular and normal menstrual periods. She was warned that the menopause might be induced, but because of the incapacitating effects of the dysmenorrhea and because the roentgen rays helped after many other measures had failed, including several surgical procedures, she wished to take the risk.

From our experimental studies on the effects of roentgen rays on the ovaries of the white rat, Ford and I concluded that low dosage irradiation over the ovaries produces only temporary hyperemia.[2] Just what happens in the human ovary as a result of this hyperemia is not known, but apparently it increases the activity of the secretory cells in the ovaries, and as a result, a follicle must mature and rupture or become luteinized. I have been told that diathermy over the ovaries will bring on the cycle in the same way. I have had no experience with this treatment.

Undoubtedly the results of treatment of amenorrhea will be greatly improved during the next few years. It has been noted in the clinic that low dosage of roentgen rays can be used without injury to the gland and that it does stimulate activity. I am trying to improve the results by giving a second irradiation after three to six months if the regularity of the menses lapses again. The addition of thyroid gland extract, if only in small amounts, seems to aid in the treatment. I believe that more patients will respond to the new hormone preparations who have not responded to the old non-standardized preparations, and many may respond to a combination of hormone preparations and irradiation when they have been resistant to either alone.

The usual treatment of the metrorrhagic patient is shown in Table III. The younger patients are placed first on sistomensin and calcium (recently calcium gluconate and viosterol have been used) to check the amount and shorten the periods of bleeding. If the bleeding persists and the patient is anemic or partially incapacitated by the metrorrhagia, curettage usually is next considered and following this a small amount of radium is applied within the uterus, the amount depending on the age of the patient. For a patient eighteen years of age, a dose of 150 mg. hrs. is used; for a woman thirty years of age, 350 mg. hrs. Stacy and Mussey[12] reported a series of these cases in 1929. They advised that the initial dose be small enough to preclude any possible injury to the ovary and be repeated several months later if necessary. The effect of the radium may not be apparent until at least six weeks after application. After six weeks, menstruation usually ceases for two or three months, during which time the patient regains her strength and overcomes the anemia. When the menstrual periods return, they tend to be more regular and the duration and amount of flow are more normal. Other methods of treatment have been tried, but none has proved more effective. Recently, antuitrin "S" has been tried in large doses. This certainly checks the bleeding but the expense of the drug, and the discomfort of injecting 2 or 3 c.c. doses intramuscularly relegates it to an emergency procedure only. Before long, Corner's progestin may be on the market in some

Table III
RESULTS OF TREATMENT OF METRORRHAGIA

Treatment	Patients				Improved after 1 year				Not improved			
	January 1927 to October 1928	October 1928 to January 1930	1930	1931	January 1927 to October 1928	October 1928 to January 1930	1930	1931	January 1927 to October 1928	October 1928 to January 1930	1930	1931
Sistomensin and calcium	15	26	29	24	14	16	23	14	1	10	6	10
Thyroid only	2				1				1			
Thyroid in addition to organotherapy	1	1		1	1			1	1			
Ovarian estrogenic hormone (theelin)				1				1				
Attention to diet and general hygiene only		2	4	6		1	1	2		1	3	4
Curettage and sistomensin and calcium	11	12	7	6	8	9	6	4	3	3	1	2
Curettage only	6	13	8	4	3	10	6	4	3	3	2	
Curettage and small dose intra-uterine radium		3	6	5		3	4	5			2	
Curettage, radium and organotherapy	2	1			2	1						
Radium and organotherapy	4	1		2	4	1		2				
Low dosage x-ray over ovaries and pituitary gland	1	1		2	1			2		1		
Sufficient x-ray over ovaries temporarily to suppress function	2				1				1			
Resection of ovaries	1		1	2	1		1					2
Total	45	60	55	53	34	42	41	35	9	20	14	18
Grand Total	213				152 (71 per cent)				61			

form that can be given by mouth, and this will probably constitute the best substitution treatment in these cases. Kaufmann, in 1932[7], reported twelve cases of severe uterine menorrhages treated with corpus luteum hormone in which the bleeding was controlled within a few days. Other treatment had been employed without avail. I have tried low dosage roentgen rays over the ovaries and pituitary glands in only four cases of this type, fearing that the increased blood supply or hyperemia might increase the bleeding. Three patients were definitely benefited and one continued to bleed. I am not inclined to urge this type of treatment in these cases, as I prefer the small doses of radium within the uterus.

SUMMARY

Functional menstrual irregularities are divided according to the predominant symptom, into two groups: amenorrhea and metrorrhagia. The clinical and laboratory features characteristic of each group are presented.

The results of treatment in 244 cases of the amenorrheic type, observed for one year, are evaluated. Low dosage irradiation of the ovaries and hypophysis has proved to be the most valuable therapeutic agent in reestablishing the menses, and thus making pregnancy possible in the more severe cases in which organotherapy has failed. Results in a follow-up study of cases in which treatment was given during the years 1927 to 1931, inclusive, are recorded.

In the metrorrhagic group, a study of the results of treatment in a series of 213 cases, observed for one year, has proved that small doses of radium within the uterus constitute the most effective treatment in the more intractable cases in which organotherapy fails.

BIBLIOGRAPHY

1. Drips, Della G. and Ford, Frances A.: Irradiation of the ovaries and hypophysis in disturbances of menstruation. Jour. Am. Med. Assn., xci:1358-1364 (November 3) 1928.
2. Drips, Della G. and Ford, Frances A.: Study of the effects of roentgen rays on the estrual cycle and the ovaries of the white rat. Surg., Gynec. and Obst., xv:596-606 (November) 1932.
3. Ford, Frances A.: Roentgen-ray treatment in cases of dysmenorrhea. Proc. Staff Meetings of Mayo Clinic., v:142-143 (May 21) 1930.
4. Frank, R. T.: The role of the female sex hormone. Jour. Am. Med. Assn., xcvii:1852-1857 (December 19) 1931.
5. Frank, R. T.: Frank, Marie-Louise, Gustavson, R. G. and Weyerts, W. W.: Demonstration of the female sex hormone in the circulating blood. I. Preliminary report. Jour. Am. Med. Assn., lxxxv:510 (August 15) 1925.
6. Kaufmann, Carl: Echte menstruelle Blutung bei Kastrierten Frauen nach Zufuhr von Follikel und Corpus luteum-Hormon. Klin. Wchnsch., xii:217-218 (February 11) 1933.
7. Kaufmann, C. and Bickel, L.: Uber die Behandlung genitaller Blutungen mit Corpus luteum-Hormon. Zentralbl. f. Gynak., lvi:1329-1333, 1932.
8. Knaus, Hermann: Der biologische Test fur des Corpus luteum Hormon. Klin. Wchnschr., x:742-743 (April 18) 1931.
9. Mazer, Charles and Goldstein, Leopold: Clinical Endocrinology of the Female, page 519, W. B. Saunders Company, Philadelphia, 1932.
10. Siebke, Harald: Ergebnisse von Mangenbestimmungen des Sexualhormons. 4. Sexualhormon im Harm und Kot bei regelmassigem mensuellem Zyklus, Zyklusstorrungen und bei Hormontherapie. Zentralbl. f. Gynak., liv:1734-1747 (July) 1930.
11. Smith, G. V. S. and Smith, O. W.: The role of progestin in the female reproductive cycle. Jour. Am. Med. Assn., xcvii: 1857-1859 (December 19) 1931.
12. Stacy, Leda J. and Mussey, R. D.: Radium in the treatment of menorrhagia of adolescence and of the menopause. Am. Jour. Obst. and Gynec., xvii:502-508 (April) 1929.
13. Werner, A. A. and Collier, W. D.: The effect of theelin injections on the castrated woman., Jour. Am Med Assn., c:636-640 (March 4) 1933.
14. Zondek, Bernhard: Die Hormone des Ovariums und des Hypophysen Vorderlapens, page 343, J. Spriner, Berlin, 1933.

DIABETES AND ITS COMPLICATIONS

EDWIN B. WINNETT, M.D., Des Moines

The complications of diabetes offer the most serious obstacle in the treatment of the disease. The treatment of a diabetic patient with no complication is only a matter of prescribing the correct amount of insulin necessary to burn up the excess glucose, and regulating the diet in such a way that complications do not arise. To treat this condition successfully, then, it is essential that a careful study be made of the more common complications, to the end that if they cannot be prevented altogether, they can at least be treated intelligently and properly.

In this paper, I wish to discuss the complications found in one thousand cases of diabetes which have been under my care during the last ten years of private practice. All patients included in this series belong to the insulin therapy period, or the period described by Joslin as "The Banting Era." The study was made from case records taken from the files in regular order. Reports of patients, for whom records were not complete, or those in which the patients did not remain under observation, have been omitted. Since I have included in this series the case records of some patients who were treated before insulin had become generally available, we cannot regard this study as a fair example of what can be accomplished by insulin therapy. Only a small amount of H-5 and H-10 Iletin (Lilly) could be procured, and it was given only to those patients who had the most severe type of diabetes. For example, one patient entered the hospital in a deep coma. The forty units of H-10 Iletin, which she was given, had no evident effect on the diabetic coma. The same patient today would receive two or three hundred units.

All patients who lived and are included in this study, received the usual instructions in diabetic management, including the figuring and weighing of the diet in grams, the proper use and timing of insulin, the care of infections, and the thorough treatment of diabetes. The various complications were demonstrated to them by allowing them to mingle with other patients.

There does not seem to be any appreciable difference in the frequency of diabetes in males and females. Figures obtained from this series credit females with 505, or 50.5 per cent, and males with

495, or 49.5, a difference of only one per cent. The incidence reaches its peak in both sexes between the ages of sixty and seventy years.

This group of patients represents 1,354 hospital admissions. It was necessary for every third patient to return to the hospital to relearn a lesson which had been forgotten. Although the diabetic patient leaves the hospital, firmly determined to follow the simple rules insisted upon by his physician so that he may avoid complications or death, he very often is led astray by his general feeling of well-being. When the ordinary individual feels well, he does not think of health or health problems. The diabetic patient tends either to break his diet, or to discontinue the insulin, or both. As a result, complications may occur, or infection may develop, which disturb the balance to which the patient has been adjusted. Infection is a two-edged menace; first, because it always increases the severity of the diabetic condition, and second, because the infection itself is a complication which must be treated.

Any disorder associated wtih diabetes should be classed as a complication. The condition existing in a diabetic patient is that the pancreatic island hormone is either not secreted in sufficient amount to burn the food necessary for bodily needs, or the patient has some unknown substance which inactivates the already existing insulin. The task for the physician, then, is to supply the necessary amount of insulin from the same island cells of the pancreas of animals. If this is accomplished, the majority of complications will be avoided, providing, of course, that the patient's diet is being regulated. The personal element of the patient enters into the picture, because many patients cannot be taught the dangers of complications, and will not control the appetite even when they are allowed a large selection of foods.

Any complication in the diabetic patient deserves the most careful attention on the part of the physician and patient, because the most trivial one may become serious. An added strain on the patient's tolerance may drive it so low that even after the complicating condition has been relieved, the tolerance may not return to its previous level. The removal of a slight complication may change the severe type of diabetes to a mild type; it may change a patient requiring a large amount of insulin into one requiring none. This transition is best illustrated by one of my patients who had had diabetes for four years. She required 75 units of insulin daily, and her diet consisted of 90 grams of carbohydrate, 60 grams of protein, and 150 grams of fat. After the removal of tonsils, which showed so little infection that much persua-

sion was necessary before the surgical consultant would remove them, her diet consisted of 125 grams of carbohydrate, 60 grams of protein, and 150 grams of fat, and she required no insulin to maintain a normal urine and blood sugar.

Of the one thousand cases in this series, 304 were uncomplicated cases when first examined, and 696 had one or more conditions to treat. One hundred forty-one, or 28.5 per cent of the males, and 122, or 24.1 per cent of the females, died during the ten-year period under discussion. If the patients are studied in age groups it will be noticed that the complications increase with each decade. The peak for the male reaches its highest point between sixty and seventy years of age, while the peak for the female reaches its highest point between fifty-five and sixty years of age. In my series the youngest female was fifteen months of age and the youngest male was fourteen months of age, although in consultation I have seen a boy eight months of age and a girl seven months of age. The pediatrician informed me that they were both living and well in September, 1933.

The following conditions were diagnosed in the 696 complicated cases: arteriosclerosis, 454; diabetic coma, 167; surgical conditions, 145; gangrene, 97; pneumonia, 25; syphilis, 23; pregnancy, 21; tuberculosis, nine; encephalitis, three; hemachromatosis, two; and mixed diabetes, two.

Arteriosclerosis. The large number of patients who developed arteriosclerosis testifies to the urgent need for comprehensive study of its etiology and a means of control. The majority of the deaths, as well as the complications, were caused directly or indirectly by arterial changes. A diagnosis of arteriosclerosis was made when the general clinical picture showed that arterial changes and symptoms were already present. It is probably true that arterial changes begin shortly after birth and continue in all of us until death, so that everyone has some degree of arteriosclerosis. Patients included in this series as having arteriosclerotic complications were those with several signs and symptoms, such as palpable arteries, mental changes, signs of cardiac or renal involvement, intermittent claudication or gangrene. Symptoms of sclerosis were present in 454 or 45.4 per cent of the entire series. Of this number, 193 or 42.5 per cent are dead; 102 were males and 91 were females. The reason that so many more females, who developed this condition, are still alive over a ten-year period is the better arterial hazard in women then in men. Men are more prone to accidents and are less careful with their diets than women. Since men must support their families, they are subject to more risks. Men in certain occupations must travel, and thus find it very difficult to regulate their diets.

The decade between sixty and seventy years of age is the one in which arteriosclerosis is most common, and in which the majority of deaths occur. It is interesting to note that these diabetic patients with arteriosclerotic involvement also had the following additional complications: gangrene, ninety-seven; cerebral arterial changes, thirty-five; apoplexy, thirty-five; coma, twenty-two; pneumonia eighteen (only four lived); coronary disease, seventeen; cataracts, twenty-one; nephritis, thirteen; syphilis, ten; angina pectoris, nine; cancer, six; prostatic operation, six; pulmonary tuberculosis, three; pernicious anemia, three; hemachromatosis, two; gall stone operation, two; and appendicitis, one. I cannot say whether the arterial changes are a result of the diabetes or a result of the manner in which diabetic patients are fed; but I can say that arteriosclerosis and diabetes seem to go hand in hand.

Coma. This condition is such a frequent and unnecessary complication of diabetes that it deserves the utmost consideration. That it occurs frequently is evidenced by the fact that 167 of the one thousand cases were seen in coma. A diagnosis of coma was made when the patient had the classic symptoms, including air hunger. No carbon dioxide tests were made, but a diagnosis of coma is so simple that only a few laboratory tests are necessary. The clinical picture and the history of the patient, with positive sugar and diacetic acid tests are all that are required. The results of the mortality encountered are illustrated by the following figures:

	Alive	Dead	Total
Treated between 1923-1927	57	49	106
Treated between 1927-1933	42	19	61

The table shows that during the last five years the death rate has decreased 37.1 per cent. It is also apparent that the actual number of coma cases has decreased. This fact indicates that physicians in Iowa have treated diabetes more successfully during the last six years than during the first four years. Diabetic coma occurred most frequently between the ages of thirty and forty years in females and between the ages of ten and twenty years in males, as illustrated in the accompanying graph; furthermore, most of the deaths in coma occurred during the second and third decades of life. Deaths in coma are far too frequent in this series, and some comment is required to explain why such an unnecessary complication should be the cause of so many deaths. Many patients were first seen in coma; many had traveled long distances in an ambulance, or on a cot in a train,

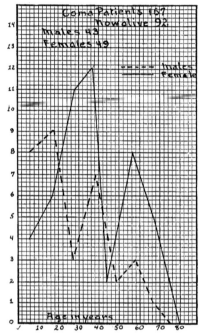

Coma Patients 167 now alive 92
Males 43
Females 49
----- males
Female
Age in years

without having received even one dose of insulin before they left home, or while they were on their way to the hospital. Early diagnosis and early treatment spells the difference between a diabetic coma patient who will live and one who will die.

After a diagnosis of coma has been made, insulin is the first requisite. The earlier the first dose is given, the better is the patient's chance of recovery. Of course, other measures such as enemas, rest, warmth, and administration of fluids, are necessary, but insulin, and insulin in large doses, is the prime essential. To make an early diagnosis of coma or impending coma, one must take a careful history, and make a thorough examination of the patient. Nausea or vomiting, respirations that are increased or deeper than normal, and nervousness or restlessness with thirst, combined with a urine containing sugar, acetone, and diacetic acid, are the very early signs. A few doses of insulin at this stage will prevent the patient from going into a diabetic coma. A delay of twenty-four hours, and in some patients of even two hours, may be the cause of a patient entering into this deep coma state, presenting the symptoms with which we are so familiar. Not one of this group of patients developed coma without evident cause; sixty-four were untreated diabetic patients; thirty-seven had discontinued the use of insulin; thirty-five developed influenza; ten, pyogenic infections; six, pneumonia.; five, gangrene; two, osteomyelitis; two, goiter; and one each, encephalitis, alcoholism, ether and a fractured hip, an accident, pyelitis, and acromegaly.

The fact that forty-four of these patients developed coma while taking insulin, indicates that one out of every three patients had not been sufficiently instructed, or that they failed to use the knowledge they possessed. The usual story from friends or relatives of the patients is that they felt sick, did not care to eat, insulin was omitted, and soon vomiting began. So many of these patients developed coma in this way that I cannot refrain from repeating Dr. Joslin's seven rules, which are set forth with a clarity that cannot be improved upon.

Rule 1. Call a doctor
Rule 2. Secure someone to care for you
Rule 3. Go to bed
Rule 4. Drink a cupful of liquid every hour
Rule 5. Take an enema
Rule 6. Keep warm
Rule 7. Be sure to continue the use of insulin

These rules are very important, but many times they are unobserved. Rule No. 1 does not always prove to be an aid, because a few of the doctors give the patient other medicines rather than insulin and fluids, until it is too late to help the unconscious patient who is gasping to get his breath.

A patient who is taking insulin may develop the unconsciousness of hypoglycemia due to an overdosage of insulin, ill-timed doses of insulin, emesis of food, diarrhea, or indigestion. The differential diagnosis between an insulin reaction and the unconsciousness of a diabetic coma is not difficult. The following comparisons may be of some value in questionable cases:

DIABETIC COMA

1. Comes on slowly   .
2. Patient dehydrated
3. Pulse rapid and weak
4. Nausea or vomiting precedes
5. Movements coordinated
6. Blood sugar high
7. History of thirst preceding
8. Normal vision
9. Urinary sugar, acetone, and diacetic acid present

INSULIN REACTION

1. Comes on quickly
2. Patient covered with sweat
3. Pulse strong
4. Nausea or vomiting rare
5. Movements not coordinated
6. Blood sugar low
7. No history of thirst preceding
8. Usually double vision
9. No urinary sugar, acetone, or diacetic acid present

A trace of sugar may be found, which is retained in the bladder from the previous meal.

Surgery. During recent years, surgical conditions have assumed an important place in the complications of diabetes, because first, the life span of the diabetic patient has been increased, which makes him liable to more surgical procedures; second, by the use of insulin, he is able to enter more useful occupations, and is, therefore, subjected to the same industrial hazards as the non-diabetic person; and third, he is much more liable to arterial changes and the possibilities of gangrenous conditions arising. Most of the surgery is necessary during the arteriosclerotic zone of life, and for this reason diabetic patients are much greater surgical risks. However, as our knowledge of insulin increases, it may be possible to eliminate many of the surgical complications that were found to be present in the pre-insulin days. One extremely important fact should be emphasized; namely, that the surgical diabetic patient requires constant attention so that any irregularities may be noted immediately and appropriate measures instituted to prevent disastrous results.

In this series, not one case of coma developed after surgery. The following conditions were noted in the 182 patients operated upon, some for more than one cause; thigh amputation, thirty-eight; drainage of abscess, thirty-five; cataract, twenty-one; amputation below the knee, nineteen; toe amputation, fifteen; goiter, twelve; cholecystectomy, ten; tonsillectomy, eight; carbuncle requiring a general anesthetic, eight; cancer of the stomach, six; prostate, six; hysterectomy, six; appendectomy, four; arm amputation, three; open fracture reduction, three; two each of mastoid operation, cancer of the colon, cancer of the rectum, cancer of the breast, curettage, drainage requiring anesthetic; and one each of orbital abscess, anal fistula, ascites, hernia, ishiorectal abscess, hemorrhoids, ovarian cyst, cancer of the pancreas, cancer of the lung (tissue removed for examination), cancer of the esophagus, and cancer of the kidney.

The following table shows the age groups of those patients who were operated upon under a general anesthetic.

Age	ALIVE		DEAD	
	Male	Female	Male	Female
Under 10	0	1	0	0
10 to 20	0	0	1	1
20 to 30	7	5	0	0
30 to 40	0	9	1	0
40 to 50	4	10	2	5
50 to 60	11	20	2	3
60 to 70	15	16	4	9
70 to 80	8	2	7	2
Total ...	45	63	17	20

Gangrene. Ninety-seven patients, or 9.7 per cent of this series, developed gangrene. Of this number, forty-eight are still alive and forty-nine are dead. Gangrene may occur in any part of the body. In one patient, gangrene involved the entire abdominal wall following an appendectomy. Gangrene affected the toes, legs, feet, buttocks, nose, neck, hard and soft palate, including the face, scrotum, penis and fingers. Eight patients had both legs amputated above the knee. Of these, three are living and are able to earn a living. Gangrene is, in many instances, a preventable complication. Patients who are in the arteriosclerotic zone of life should be instructed in the proper care of the feet and skin, the value of exercise, and the treatment of simple infections involving the skin. The high carbohydrate diet and low fat diet have not been used long enough to establish any conclusive proof that they are of value in preventing arterial changes. It is my practice to avoid either the high carbohydrate diet or the low carbohydrate diet, and to allow the patient enough food to make a palatable diet, with restrictions on the calories to avoid obesity. The following table shows the age groups of the patients who developed gangrene.

Age	ALIVE		DEAD	
	Male	Female	Male	Female
Under 10	0	0	0	0
10 to 20	0	0	0	0
20 to 30	0	0	1	0
30 to 40	0	0	0	0
40 to 50	1	2	2	1
50 to 60	8	10	3	5
60 to 70	8	17	13	13
70 to 80	2	0	9	2
Total	19	29	28	21

Pneumonia. The occurrence of this disease as a complication of diabetes is relatively infrequent. It is, however, more common than one glance at these statistics would indicate, because a diabetic patient with an infection often develops coma. This is especially true when the infection is as severe as pneumonia, and death is then attributed to coma rather than pneumonia. A pneumonia patient can be protected against coma if he is carefully watched, and if insulin is given in large enough doses. The insulin must be buffered with food and fluids. In this series, twenty-five patients developed pneumonia; ten are still living and fifteen are dead. The following table shows the age groups.

Age	ALIVE		DEAD	
	Male	Female	Male	Female
Under 10	0	0	0	0
10 to 20	0	0	0	1
20 to 30	0	0	0	0
30 to 40	1	0	1	1
40 to 50	2	0	1	1
50 to 60	2	0	0	2
60 to 70	4	0	5	2
70 to 80	1	0	1	0
Total	10	0	8	7

Syphilis. Another infrequent complication of diabetes is syphilis. Only twenty-three patients, or 2.3 per cent, had positive Kahn or Wassermann reactions, or other evidences of syphilis which could be elicited by physical examination. When syphilis is found as a complication, the diabetes is usually of the mild type, and many patients can omit the use of insulin after antisyphilitic treatment has been received for from three months to a year. Of the twenty-three patients whose conditions were complicated by the presence of syphilis, only four had a severe type of diabetes. Eleven are dead; two committed suicide; four developed general paresis; and two developed gangrene of the leg.

Pregnancy. In this series there were twenty-one patients whose conditions were complicated by pregnancy; that is, either a diabetic woman became pregnant, or diabetes made its appearance during the course of a pregnancy. The diagnosis of diabetes was made in these patients by the finding of sugar in the urine, by finding sugar that would ferment, by a blood sugar test that was above normal fasting, and by one or more symptoms in the patient. Many pregnant women show a reduction of copper in the test solution, and yet do not have diabetes. The diabetic pregnant woman needs much more careful attention than the non-diabetic woman. Insulin was required for thirteen of the patients; seventeen delivered full term babies; ten delivered full term babies and received insulin throughout the pregnancy; five aborted more than once, and one is now·five months pregnant.

Hemachromatosis. This condition was found to exist in two patients. Both died, and the diagnoses were confirmed at autopsy.

Insulin Refractory Diabetes. In this series, only one insulin refractory patient could be listed. In every other instance when the insulin did not produce the expected results, some hidden infection was found to be causing the trouble. A few experienced some difficulty in timing their doses of insulin, and it was necessary for a few to have insulin at midnight. One patient, a girl eight years of age, required insulin as soon as school was over in the afternoon. Insulin.given at any other time would either not desugarize the patient, or would produce an unsatisfactory reaction.

CONCLUSIONS

1. This paper is an analysis of the complications in one thousand patients with diabetes, seen in private practice.

2. Arteriosclerosis is by far the most common complication.

3. Coma is much more frequent than necessary, and causes far too many deaths.

4. Complications in diabetic patients should (a) be avoided if possible, and (b) be recognized early and treated immediately.

5. Only the intelligence of the patient can avoid many complications. The patient can be "diabetically intelligent" only when he is "taught diabetes."

RHEUMATIC HEART INFECTION IN
CHILDHOOD*

ROLAND STAHR, M.D., Fort Dodge

In the months just passed many of you have again been faced with the unpleasant experience of caring for children with rheumatic infection. Rheumatic heart infection is too large a subject to be considered in detail in the short time allotted. The gaps in the knowledge of this disease are wide. The controversies about many of its phases are numerous. It is the purpose in this discussion to stress present conceptions regarding the recognition and treatment of rheumatic infection of the heart in childhood.

For all practical purposes rheumatic infection and rheumatic cardiac infection are synonymous. The opinions are in accord that cardiac involvement occurs in most cases of rheumatic infection. White[1] stated, "The rheumatic infection usually or always involves the heart." Swift[2] said, "The

*Presented before the Eighty-second Annual Session, Iowa State Medical Society, Des Moines, May 10, 11, 12, 1933.

infection in childhood leads more frequently to cardiac sequelae; indeed it is often questionable whether the first tissue to be attacked by the virus in the early years of life is not that of the heart." Wilson, et al.,[3] stated, "The heart is probably always affected at the onset of this (rheumatic fever) disease."

A child with signs of rheumatic cardiac damage presents an entirely different problem than does the adult having the same physical signs. The difficulty in the adult is chiefly mechanical. Heart muscle reserve must be balanced against heart damage and bodily activity. In the child the problem is infection. The search for and the treatment of the infection is far more important than the making of a fine diagnosis regarding the site of cardiac damage. It is known that clinical signs of heart damage may appear as late as six to twelve months after the rheumatic onset.

You are more or less familiar with the clinical picture of rheumatic infections. The manifestations, acute rheumatic fever or true arthritis, chorea, pancarditis and rheumatic nodules are easily recognized by all. Bear in mind, however, that the diagnosis of a low grade rheumatic infection may depend on the correct interpretation of such manifestations and laboratory findings as are tabulated below:

1. Joint and muscle pains.
2. Recurrent nose and throat infections.
3. Low grade fever.
4. Rapid pulse without apparent cause.
5. Anemia and unexplained attacks of pallor.
6. Nose bleeds.
7. Unexplained weight loss.
8. Unexplained chest and abdominal pain.
9. Various forms of skin eruptions.
10. Easy fatigue and poor appetite.
11. Vomiting.
12. Leukocytosis.
13. Prolongation of auriculoventricular conduction time by electrocardiogram.
14. Increased sedimentation rate of red blood cells.

You will recognize that the manifestations of rheumatic infection are variable. You have learned to look upon tuberculosis or lues as active or inactive, needing prolonged care and observation. Even so, you must recognize rheumatic infection in the heart or elsewhere as being either active or inactive, needing care and observation through the years. Upon this recognition hinge the efforts of treatment.

TREATMENT

There is no specific drug or serum known to be curative in rheumatic infection. Although the treatment of rheumatic infection is often difficult and disappointing, much good can be accomplished by efficient treatment, especially in the early stages. It has been learned by bitter experience that the prognosis in the majority of cases depends on the efficiency of treatment.

Rest. The most valuable weapon in the treatment is bed rest. Complete and prolonged rest in bed until all evidence of rheumatic infection has gone offers the greatest surety of limiting the process. Stated in other words, bed rest gives the best assurance of holding heart damage to a minimum. The child with rheumatic infection who is allowed freedom and activity may in a short time suffer irreparable heart damage. In cases where cardiac damage is evident, the rest should certainly be of no less than six months duration, often longer, depending on the findings at repeated and thorough examinations. It is much better to keep a child in bed for a year too long than to let him up too soon. Much has been said and written regarding the patient becoming over-anxious of his heart; in other words developing a cardiophobia. No child need ever be told that he has "heart trouble." To me there is a crime worse than that; it is the neglect to treat rheumatic cardiac disease. Many years of invalidism or greatly shortened life are still not preferable to a year or more of bed rest. Contrary to the lay opinion of children being weakened by bed rest, it is known that rheumatic children thrive and bloom nutritionally under such therapy.

Salicylates. During the acute stage, symptomatic treatment adds greatly to the comfort of the child. Sodium salicylate with sodium bicarbonate or amidopyrine given in adequate dosage has a favorable effect on the pain and fever. While still without statistical proof, many clinicians believe that prolonged or intermittent use of salicylates is helpful in preventing recurrence of rheumatic infection.

Nutrition. Maintenance and improvement of nutrition by a rational diet together with adequate fluids and satisfactory elimination is important as in every infection. As with all normal children cod liver oil should be considered a food.

Digitalis. Digitalis is never indicated in acute rheumatic carditis without insufficiency. Opinions vary on the use of digitalis in cardiac insufficiency. Albutt[4] advised against digitalis in the acute stage. Schwartz[5] concluded that digitalis is contraindicated in children with rheumatic fever and signs of cardiac insufficiency. Sutton and Wyckoff[6] on the other hand concluded that digitalis is of value in the treatment of children with heart failure

that it is effective in the presence of active cardiac infection and that it is effective in doses comparable to those required by adults without necessarily producing intoxication.

Focal Infection. Probably no phase of treatment has been so controversial as that of focal infection, tonsillectomy in particular. Kaiser[7] interpreting his observations of six hundred rheumatic children over a period of ten years stated, "The first attack of rheumatic fever and rheumatic heart disease occurred thirty-three per cent less commonly in tonsillectomized children. Chorea and recurrent attacks were not influenced by removal of tonsils." This work suggests that the tonsil bears a close relation to the initial infection. Fraser[8] demonstrated rheumatic nodules in the pharyngeal lymphoid tissue of two recurrent and two early cases of rheumatic fever. In three of these cases there was no clinical evidence of such lesions causing symptoms or complaint of throat trouble. The last word relating to focal infection in rheumatic disease has not been spoken.

Despite statistical evidence and pessimistic views regarding the failure of tonsillectomy in preventing rheumatic recurrence, its value in treating a septic focus can not be denied or over-estimated. In my limited experience, no bad effects have been noted from tonsillectomy in the early subacute stage of rheumatic infection. To the contrary, striking improvement in the rheumatic condition has often followed. One must also bear in mind that the lymphoid tissue, which often is incompletely removed, is not the only site in the upper respiratory tract that may harbor infection. Paranasal sinuses may be infected and alveolar abscesses may occur.

Vaccine Treatment. On the basis of rheumatic infection being caused by a streptococcus; vaccines, antisera and soluble antigens have been prepared. At present it is hoped that some of these may prove helpful in treatment. They should not be made commercially available until adequate proof is presented from controlled use.

After Care. When the child has recovered from the first acute rheumatic attack, remember that the disease is chronic. Respiratory infections must be guarded against by avoiding exposure and fatigue and by maintaining normal nutrition. Every new respiratory infection, every break in nutrition as expressed by loss of weight, anemia, etc., may demand radical changes in the regime. Any new manifestation may be followed by recurrent cardiac involvement. Careful periodic examination and supervision is a definite part of the treatment.

SUMMARY

1. For practical purposes rheumatic infection and rheumatic cardiac infection are synonymous in childhood.

2. Rheumatic manifestations may be mild and difficult to diagnose, but, nevertheless they are extremely important.

3. There is no specific curative drug or serum for rheumatic cardiac infection known at present.

4. Bed rest is the most valuable procedure in treatment.

5. Further treatment includes good nursing care; salicylates for pain; rational means of maintaining and improving nutrition; eradication of foci of infection by surgical or medical means, and possibly the use of digitalis in cardiac insufficiency.

6. Prolonged observation and supervision are as important in the rheumatic child as in the tubercular or luetic child.

REFERENCES

1. White, P. D.: Heart Disease, Macmillan Company, New York City, 1931.
2. Swift, H. F.: Oxford Medicine, Vol. 11-38, Oxford University Press, New York, 1921.
3. Wilson, M. G.; Lingg, C.; and Croxford, G.: Statistical studies bearing on problems in classification of heart disease; heart disease in children. Am. Heart Jour., iv:164-196 (December) 1928.
4. Albutt, Sir Clifford: Diseases of Arteries, Macmillan Company, London, 1915.
5. Schwartz, S. P.: Digitalis studies on children with heart disease: auricular fibrillation in children with early toxic digitalis manifestation. Am. Jour. Dis. Child., xxxix, 549-559 (March) 1930.
6. Sutton, L. P., and Wyckoff, J.: Digitalis; its value in treatment of children with rheumatic heart disease. Am. Jour. Dis. Child., xli:801-815 (April) 1931.
7. Kaiser, A. D.: Relations of tonsils and adenoids to infections in children, based on control study of 4,400 children over a ten year period. Am. Jour. Dis. Child., xli:568-581 (March) 1931.
8. Fraser, A. D.: Lesions of pharynx in acute rheumatism. Arch. Dis. Child., vii:181-190 (August) 1932.

TOXOID IN DIPHTHERIA PREVENTION*

B. A. MELGAARD, M.D., Sioux City

The use of toxin-antitoxin and the revolutionary results it produced in the control of diphtheria has no parallel in the history of medicine. The ability to give a simple painless series of inoculations to a child, and to give the parents the assurance that they may cease fearing diphtheria, has been one of the greatest joys which has come to those of us who but a few years ago had no such blessing to offer our patients.

When toxin-antitoxin first made its appearance, and it had been definitely established that it would prevent diphtheria in nearly all children, physicians were enthusiastic in pushing its use. A great many children were inoculated, and so great was our faith that we neglected to insist on the patient's return after a few months for a Schick test in order to make sure that the prophylaxis had been effective. Small wonder it is then that for the first

*Presented before the Eighty-second Annual Session, Iowa State Medical Society, Des Moines, May 10, 11, 12, 1933.

two or three years after the advent of toxin-antitoxin some of us were negligent in performing a post Schick test. The result was that after immunizing hundreds of these little patients, a few of them developed diphtheria. In my own experience there were three of these, all of the laryngeal type. Since the cases were of the severe type, antitoxin was given without delay and severe serum reactions resulted in all three patients.

I am aware that some writers tell us that the serum reaction is negligible, but I am inclined to think these observers have done their work in orphanages where the parent is out of the picture. In private practice serum reactions are decidedly embarrassing.

In many instances after selling the idea of toxin-antitoxin to parents, they are disappointed that immunity is not forthcoming at once, but that they must wait for it a number of months. Members of the human race have never appreciated the medical profession and are unreasonable in their demands. They want immunity for their children; they want it to be immediate, they want it to be painless, and they are often unwilling to pay the price. The medical profession is, of course, anxious to go as far as it can in meeting these demands, in the interest of science and the welfare of children. Therefore, painstaking experiments have been conducted to meet the two chief objections to the toxin-antitoxin method of immunization; namely severe serum reactions and delayed immunity. In these few moments allotted to me I cannot review the history of the experimentation carried forward to accomplish this purpose. Suffice it to say that in diphtheria toxoid we not only have a more quickly developed immunity with the danger of sensitization eliminated, but we also obtain a higher percentage of immune patients.

In order to appreciate the reason for the different action of the two methods of diphtheria immunization we have but to recall that in the one we are dealing with a serum while in the other we have the toxin only Whenever we use a serum, our patient potentially becomes subject to a serum reaction some time later. Serum is used in toxin-antitoxin as a safeguard against the diphtheria toxin. This delays the action of the toxin and extends the time during which the patient will react positively to the Schick test.

In diphtheria toxoid there is no serum that may sensitize the patient; also it is not there to buffer the toxin, and consequently a reaction at the time, or shortly thereafter is possible. Conversely, there being no neutralizing agent, the processes that bring about immunity are not hindered, with the result that it is brought about more quickly.

Diphtheria toxoid is at present prepared from a virulent strain of diphtheria bacilli which have grown for a week. The broth on which the bacilli are grown is filtered and the filtrate treated with formalin. It is then incubated at 40 degrees Centigrade until the standardized strength is obtained. The standard unit is contained in the one c.c. dose and represents the amount necessary to protect 80 per cent of guinea pigs that have received five fatal doses of diphtheria toxin. It is a more stable product and the danger from freezing is not so great as that of toxin-antitoxin.

Virtually the only objection one hears to the use of toxoid in comparison to toxin-antitoxin is that a reaction may be expected in a certain percentage of the children thus immunized. All experimentation and clinical evidence point conclusively to the superiority of toxoid over toxin-antitoxin, in the higher percentage of immunity obtained and the lessened time required to produce it. The child reacts negatively to the Schick test several weeks earlier when toxoid is used, probably because there is no resistance of antitoxin as in the toxin-antitoxin mixture.

In children under six years of age there is almost never any reaction to toxoid administration. This is the period of life when the child is most susceptible to the disease and is, therefore, the period in which we should endeavor to immunize the majority of children. If we stress the fact that toxoid should be given to children under six, we eliminate, to a great extent, the risk of reactions. Another advantage is that the toxoid is usually given in two doses only. In some of the literature, we read that three doses are still being used by some men, but it has been determined that two will do as well. We, therefore, eliminate one visit of the child to the office, and the consequent fear of the hypodermic injection is lessened to that extent.

In older children there may be varying degrees of reaction with fever, headache and anorexia for two or three days. I see no reason why this should deter us from using toxoid. After all, we are doing this work in order to immunize the child. The method which will accomplish this with the greatest degree of certainty and speed is naturally the one of choice. To be sure, we do not need to fear the serum reaction which occurred before goat's serum was used in making toxin-antitoxin. Many of you no doubt had an occasional embarrassment from that source; nevertheless toxoid has the advantage of containing no serum, so that objection is eliminated.

Toxin-antitoxin may be used when large numbers of older children are being immunized. In this way the first dose serves as a modified Schick test and will eliminate the necessity of giving the two following doses to the children having a negative Schick reaction. It stands to reason that if you are going to immunize a large number of older school children with toxoid, there might be a number of reactions that would mitigate against the good feeling we want the laity to have toward immunization. Therefore, when large numbers of older school children are to be immunized, it is well to use the toxin-antitoxin method. If one wishes to avoid any possibility of a reaction in giving toxoid to older children, they may be tested for "reactors" with minute intradermal doses of toxoid, as you would in a tuberculin test. Reactors may then be given toxin-antoxin.

It is well known that parents habitually postpone diphtheria immunization because of neglect, fear caused by misinformation, or because of the criminal propaganda of certain cults. When these folks hear of a death from diphtheria, possibly in the school their child attends, they come rushing to the physician for toxin-antitoxin, only to be told that it will not give immediate immunity. Of course, toxoid will not do so either, but it will do it more quickly and more certainly.

SUMMARY

1. Diphtheria toxoid gives immunity several weeks earlier than does toxin-antitoxin.

2. It produces a higher percentage of immune patients.

3. There is no reaction in children under six; the years in which we ought to be immunizing the children.

4. Older children may be tested for reactors, and positives may be given toxin-antitoxin.

5. Where large numbers of older children are given toxin-antitoxin, the first dose serves as a modified Schick test.

6. Do not fail to do a post Schick test in all cases.

NON-DIPHTHERITIC LARYNGITIS*

DENNIS H. KELLY, M.D., Des Moines

I wish to present this eight months' old boy who when four months of age was seen at home with a mild croup. The usual therapeutic measures were instituted and the next day he was better. That evening the croup again recurred and persisted during the night. The following morning he had a temperature of 101° and moderate dyspnea was present. There was some stridor, although the crying voice was normal; the color

*Presented before the Eighty-second Annual Session, Iowa State Medical Society, Des Moines, May 10, 11, 12, 1933.

was good, and the babe was smiling and happy. However, it was considered advisable to hospitalize because the facilities at home were not adequate and the baby's condition was not improving.

Within three hours after admission to the hospital and despite constant steaming the condition rapidly became worse. The temperature rose to 103°, the pulse became very rapid, restlessness developed, the respirations became labored and accompanied by stridor, suprasternal and epigastric retraction occurred, a grayish pallor developed, and the finger tips became cyanotic. A direct examination of the larynx revealed no membrane. The voice was good. The ventricular bands or false cords were red and swollen. The true cords appeared practically normal. The mucosa of the trachea in the subglottic region was swollen, producing an obstruction.

An immediate tracheotomy was performed. On incising the trachea a thick brownish mucus was expelled. A number one tube was inserted with difficulty because of the small lumen. Breathing was free after tracheotomy. Following the tracheotomy the patient had rather a stormy course. Thick, tenacious secretions formed so rapidly that it was necessary to aspirate the trachea every fifteen or twenty minutes. At intervals breathing became very labored and examination of the chest would reveal that air was not entering one or the other lung. Suction would remove a dried plug of secretion from the bronchus and breathing would again become normal. During the entire course of the illness a diffuse bronchitis was present. Extubation was finally accomplished eight weeks after intubation.

This little fellow shows nothing in particular except his tracheotomy scar. He still has a tracheitis and spasmodic cough, but since he has finally learned how to cough, he gets along very well and we are rather proud of him.

This case is typical of acute laryngotracheobronchitis. The unusual aspects of the case are: (1) The age of the patient. The youngest reported case in the literature is nine months. The small size of the trachea predisposes to obstruction. (2) X-ray revealed an enlarged thymus which may have contributed to the obstruction.

I wish to report another similar case in a fourteen months' old girl, who developed obstruction to breathing six days after the onset of an upper respiratory infection. Laryngoscopy revealed findings identical with those described in the last case, an obstruction in the subglottic region of the trachea. Intubation afforded no relief and tracheotomy was performed.

Following tracheotomy, dry, tenacious secretions formed rapidly and frequent suction was necessary. Plugs of dried exudate formed at the bifurcation of the trachea and in the bronchi. Bronchoscopy was done twice and the dried exudate removed. Death occurred thirteen days after the onset of the disease. This child died from cardiac failure. She became extremely restless, dyspnea was marked, the color was not cyanotic but a characteristic grayish pallor, the pulse became extremely rapid and weak, and she succumbed not from suffocation but from complete exhaustion resulting from the effort to obtain air. In the last year we have seen four similar cases, not as severe and not requiring tracheotomy. They were hospitalized and given constant steaming.

Acute laryngotracheobronchitis is a distinct clinical entity of childhood and is one of the most critical conditions with which we are confronted. It occurs as a complication of a simple respiratory infection and has been described in epidemic form. It is a not uncommon complication of measles. It is usually due to the streptococcus or staphylococcus. The characteristic pathology is an inflammation in the subglottic region of the trachea. There is marked swelling and the production of a viscid secretion. The small size of the subglottic chink, the loose attachment of the mucosa and the rich lymphatic supply predispose to the condition. Bronchitis is invariable and bronchopneumonia is common. The symptoms at the onset are those of an upper respiratory infection with croup. The temperature is usually over 101° and may be 105°, and the child seems more ill than a patient with simple croup. Symptoms of obstruction may occur in a few hours or after several days.

Since it is the obstruction that presents the serious problem it is important that the early symptoms be recognized and early treatment instituted. The patient becomes restless and tosses about, the breathing becomes labored and is accompanied by suprasternal and epigastric retraction. Stridor is present but in contrast to diphtheria the crying voice is usually normal. The pulse becomes rapid and a characteristic grayish pallor develops, the patient is not cyanotic but pale. If an air way is not established the patient succumbs from exhaustion and cardiac failure. Direct laryngoscopy reveals a diffuse redness and swelling of the ventricular bands. The glottis shows but little involvement. The mucosa of the trachea is swollen and a thick secretion is seen between the cords. Examination of the chest reveals the presence of many sibilant rales, and not infrequently evidence of a bronchopneumonia.

The treatment we have employed is constant steaming. Toxemia is combated by the oral and

parenteral administration of fluids. When symp‑
toms of obstruction develop, early tracheotomy is
conservative treatment. After treatment with
suction to remove the dried exudate is most im‑
portant. Bronchoscopy may be necessary. Some
of these patients are more comfortable under
oxygen.

The prognosis should be guarded. Gittins of
Sioux City who has reported fifteen cases requir‑
ing tracheotomy had a mortality of 54 per cent.
Recurrent obstruction in the trachea and broncho‑
pneumonia frequently cause a fatal termination.

After seeing a few of these cases it is easy to
become panicky over a case of croup. A child with
a persistent croup and a temperature over 101°
should be hospitalized so that proper treatment
may be instituted if the emergency arises. The
patient should be isolated and proper precautions
taken until laryngeal diphtheria is eliminated as a
possibility. If there is any question about the
diagnosis, diphtheria antitoxin should be adminis‑
tered. However, complete reliance must not be
placed in antitoxin, and surgical treatment must
not be delayed so long that a fatal termination re‑
sults. Direct examination of the larynx will settle
the diagnosis. Catarrhal laryngitis usually begins
suddenly in the evening, is relieved by steam and
by ipecac, and recurs the next night. The tempera‑
ture is rarely over 101°. A foreign body in the
larynx may be differentiated by laryngoscopy and
x-ray. The aspiration of vegetable substances fre‑
quently produces a similar picture. Retropharyn‑
geal abscess, edema of the larynx, congenital laryn‑
geal stridor, glottic spasm, enlarged thymus, etc.,
should not present any particular difficulty if the
case is analyzed carefully and thorough examina‑
tion made.

DIVERTICULUM OF THE GALLBLADDER

Albert L. Pertl, M.D.,

Windom, Minnesota

Anomalies of the gallbladder are rare, and only
a few references to such cases can be found in the
literature.

Careful search of the literature reveals but
nine references to cases of this nature. Of these
nine reports those by Abbott, Nadeau and Ross
are of particular interest. In the case reported
by Abbott the diverticulum was near the fundus,
no stones were present, nor was the gallbladder
highly pathologic. Nadeau's report was undoubt‑
edly of a·congenital anomaly for there was no evi‑
dence of severe inflammation nor injury found in
this region. In the case reported by Ross a pouch

near the fundus, was located; it was examined
microscopically and proved that only one side
of the pouch thought to be that which corresponds
with the interior of the gallbladder proper. No
such appearance was seen on the opposite side, so
from these findings, as well as from the gross
appearance, the pouch was not congenital, but
rather an acquired type.

Anomalous gallbladder of the type and compli‑
cation, which I wish to call to your attention has
never been reported. The specimen was not ex‑
amined microscopically, so I cannot say definitely
whether or not it was a congenital pouch; but at

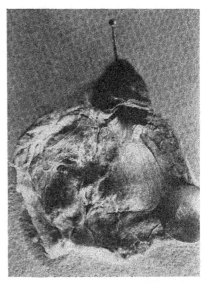

Illustrating the diverticulum at the fundus of the bladder.

the time of operation the communication between
the pouch and the gallbladder proper was only one
millimeter.

The patient was a young married woman,
twenty-seven years of age, who had always been
well before her marriage in 1927. Her weight at
that time was 140 pounds, and showed a gradual
increase up to 150 pounds during the three fol‑
lowing years. In 1929, the patient noticed dis‑
tress after eating oranges, but other foods gave no
trouble. During the patient's first pregnancy,
which took place in August, 1930, she suffered
much from nausea, vomiting and belching during
the entire period of gestation. Seven days after

delivery, in June, 1931, she suffered a severe attack of belching, nausea and pain throughout the entire right abdomen and extending through to the right scapular region. Similar attacks of variable duration and severity occurred following extreme fatigue or the eating of fatty foods, pastry and meats. In July 1932, the patient complained of constipation and mentioned her inability to eat celery. At this time she was slightly jaundiced.

I was called to see the patient at 2:00 a. m. November 2, 1932, because of another severe abdominal pain extending through to the back on the right, with vomiting and nervousness. Temperature, pulse and respiration were normal and the pain was relieved by hypodermic injections of morphine gr. ¼. I was told that the pain had been present for the past week and had gradually become more acute. By afternoon of the same day the vomiting had persisted without change in the previous findings, but a slight jaundice of the skin and sclera was noticed. The blood pressure was 120/60 and the white blood count was 9,000. The patient was taken to the hospital at once and given 3,000 c.c. normal salt solution subcutaneously and four sodium amytal capsules per rectum. The following day the subcutaneous injection was repeated, and three tablespoonfuls of citro-carbonate of sodium and 500 cc. of water were given every five hours per rectum. The following day a five per cent glucose solution was administered subcutaneously and ten per cent of the same solution intravaneously. The patient was able to leave the hospital November 7 and improvement continued until November 17, when a similar attack occurred, and the patient returned to the hospital for operation. Preceding the operation three sodium amytal capsules were given per rectum and two hours later one cc. pituitrin subcutaneosly. This was followed by operation under ether anesthesia some twenty minutes later.

An upper right rectus incision was made and upon opening the abdomen a few adhesions in the region of the gallbladder and liver were found. The tip of the gallbladder was adherent to the jejunum and when freed, a diverticulum of the gallbladder was found to have perforated the wall of the bowel. The opening in the bowel was sutured at once and upon further inspection the gallbladder wall was found to be slightly thicker and more congested than normal. In the cystic duct was a stone three-fourths of an inch in diameter which was milked back into the bladder before the duct was tied and the gallbladder removed. The appendix appeared to be subacutely inflamed and was therefore removed. Drain was inserted lateral to the incision.

Fluids were given subcutaneously and per rectum following the operation until liquids could be taken by mouth and the recovery was uneventful. The accompanying illustration is a photograph of the removed gallbladder showing the diverticulum at the fundus of the bladder.

REFERENCES

1. Kremer, A.: Cholecystography in diverticulum. Bratisl. lekár. listy., xii:315-317 (June) 1932.

2. Csillag, M.: Diverticulum of the gallbladder. Orvosi betil., lxxiv:85-89 (January 31) 1930.

3. Barsony, T., and von Friedrich, L.: Divertikal der Gallenblase. (Durch Cholecystektomie verifiziert). Klin. Wchnschr., vii:216-217 (January 29) 1928.

4. Sebening, W., and Schöndube, W.: Large diverticulum of the gallbladder with stenosis of the pylorus. Arch. of klin. Chir., cxxxvii:308-314, 1925.

5. Abbott, G. K.: Diverticulitis of the gallbladder. Surg. Gynec. Obst., xxxvi:466-467 (April) 1923.

6. Nadeau, O. E.: Diverticulum of the gallbladder perforating the liver. Med. and Surg., i:73 (March) 1917.

7. Ross, George C.: Pseudo-diverticulum of gallbladder. Ann. Surg., lxiii:627-629 (May) 1916.

8. Michalski, J.: Blindsackbildung der Gallenblase. Schweiz. Med. Wchnschr. Basel, i:492, 1920.

9. Kammerer, Frederic: Diverticulum of the gallbladder. Ann. Surg., lv:320 (January) 1912.

THE FINLEY HOSPITAL CLINICO-PATHOLOGIC CONFERENCE

AORTIC STENOSIS WITH CALCIFICATION

LAURENCE E. COOLEY, M.D., Dubuque

Aortic stenosis with calcification has received little attention in the literature. Two cases of this clinical entity are presented.

CASE I

The patient, an unmarried female musician, sixty-four years of age, was first seen March 9, 1933. Her chief complaint was shortness of breath. This appeared for the first time about eight years previously. Five years ago it became more noticeable. At frequent intervals during the last five years she had had a feeling of faintness which lasted for several minutes. There had been no definite loss of consciousness during these attacks. One year before consulting me the patient had all of her teeth removed. After that she had not felt at all well. Three months before the first examination the patient noticed a slight cough and a swelling of the ankles. She was unable to walk more than a few steps without shortness of breath.

Past History. The patient had scarlet fever during childhood. Three years ago the patient had arthritis. There was no history of rheumatic fever or tonsillitis. There had been an occasional sore throat.

Family History. The grandfather died of "heart trouble" at the age of sixty-seven and the father had valvular heart disease. He died at the age of sixty-four. The mother was ninety-one years old and was in good health. The anamnesis by systems revealed no additional relevant facts.

Physical Examination. The patient was a thin, elderly female, sixty-four years of age, who appeared in obvious distress. She was unable to talk without considerable dyspnea. The pupils were equal and regular and reacted to light and accommodation. The arteries in the fundus were tortuous. The lips were cyanotic. The throat was reddened. The tonsils were present and appeared atrophic. The neck vessels were engorged. There were many fine moist rales in both

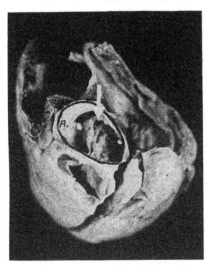

Fig. 1. View of the heart looking down into aorta (a) (outlined in ink) and showing the nodular calcification of the cusps. The arrow points to the slit-like opening into the left ventricle.

lung bases. Otherwise the lungs were normal. The left heart border was three centimeters to the left of the mid-clavicular line in the fifth interspace. The right heart border was three centimeters to the right of the sternal margin in the fourth interspace. There were no thrills. A rough systolic murmur and a softer blowing diastolic murmur were heard over the entire precordium. The systolic murmur was transmitted to the axilla. The point of maximum intensity of these murmurs was at the left sternal margin at the junction of the fifth rib. This point did not vary with the change of position of the patient. The heart rate was 110 per minute. Every fourth to tenth beat was an extrasystole. The blood pressure was 184 systolic and 110 diastolic. The liver was tender and extended three fingers below the costal margin.

There was a pitting edema of the extremities. The electrocardiogram showed (a) T wave in lead I low voltage, diphasic, (b) extreme left axis deviation, (c) idioventricular extrasystoles. On fluoroscopic examination the heart was found to be enlarged to the left as well as in the region of the left auricle, suggesting a combined mitral and hypertension or aortic heart. The urine was negative.

The patient was put to bed and given 1½ grains of the powdered leaf of digitalis four times daily. During the next week the heart rate decreased to 82 beats per minute and the blood pressure rose to 207 systolic and 104 diastolic. The congestion in the lung bases, the dyspnea and edema all improved. The patient made no further improvement during the next seven weeks, evidences of slight congestive failure being constantly present. Attacks of nocturnal dyspnea began to occur gradually. The edema increased and signs of fluid developed in the right chest. The blood pressure dropped to 150 systolic and 88 diastolic. Ammonium chloride and salrygan were given at frequent intervals to relieve the edema. On June 8, the temperature began to rise. The patient became comatose and the respirations were of the Cheyne-Stokes type. A catheterized specimen of urine showed many granular and hyaline casts, three plus albumin and many red and white blood cells. On June 11, the temperature reached 103° Fahrenheit. By June 14 the temperature was normal and the patient was conscious again. Her condition remained the same for the next ten days. The blood pressure on June 23 was 136 systolic and 84 diastolic. The next day the patient became unconscious again and a paralysis of the left arm and leg was noted. The patient died four days later. The clinical diagnoses were (1) mitral stenosis and regurgitation, (2) possible tricuspid stenosis and regurgitation, (3) essential hypertension, (4) cardiac decompensation, (5) acute endocarditis with embolic infarction of the kidneys and brain (hemiplegia). Autopsy of the trunk was obtained.

Necropsy. The summary of the laboratory findings were: "The heart was dilated in all chambers but particularly on the right. The right auricle contained an organized thrombus. There were a few verrucose vegetations on the edges of the mitral cusps. The aortic cusps presented an unusual picture. The leaflets were thickened and adherent so that only a small slit measuring ten millimeters in length and averaging two millimeters in width remained. Over the superior surfaces of the cusps there were a few fresh verrucose vegetations as well as many calcified nodules so that each formed a rigid mass. (See figure 1.)

The aorta showed only a few atheromatous plaques and except for the hypertrophy of the left ventricle and auricle the heart was otherwise unremarkable. The other important findings were fresh infarcts of the lungs and old and recent infarcts of the spleen and kidneys. There were 500 cc. of a seropurulent fluid in the right pleural cavity. The gallbladder was thickened and contained several irregular stones. The viscera showed passive congestion.

"Anatomic Diagnosis;

Primary;

Chronic aortic endocarditis (calcification, stenosis, and regurgitation) ; subacute mitral endocarditis; cardiac hypertrophy and dilatation; organized thrombus of the right auricle; infarcts of the lungs; spleen and kidneys; right fibrinopurulent pleurisy; chronic passive congestion of the viscera.

Subsidiary;

Moderate arteriosclerosis; chronic cholecystitis and cholelithiasis."

Comment. Calcification of the aortic valves was not suspected in this case until autopsy. The location of the murmur led to the mistaken diagnosis of tricuspid valvular disease. There was no thrill, a point that does not coincide with the accepted clinical picture of aortic stenosis. It is possible that a thrill might have been present if the patient had been seen when fully compensated. The high blood pressure is another finding that does not fit in with the usual aortic stenosis.

CASE II

The patient, a male laborer, forty-eight years of age, was first seen August 18, 1933. During the preceding year he had had a pain across the forehead and a numbness of his hands on severe physical exertion. He had considerable shortness of breath on exertion for about the same length of time. There had been some palpitation on exertion and an occasional slight pain in the region of the left nipple.

Past History. The father died at the age of sixty-nine of a "glandular disease". The mother died of "heart trouble" at the age of seventy-five. The wife was in good health and had had no miscarriages or stillbirths. There were seven children living and well.

By Systems. There had been no hemoptysis or hematemesis. The appetite was good. The bowels were regular and there were no genito-urinary symptoms. The patient denied any venereal infection.

Physical Examination. The patient was a well developed, well nourished, thick chested male about forty-five years of age who did not appear to be acutely ill. The pupils were equal and regular and reacted to light and accommodation. The throat was slightly injected and the tonsils were removed well. The lungs were negative. The left heart border was in the fifth interspace in the mid-clavicular line by percussion. There were no thrills. In the third left interspace there was a distant murmur, systolic in time and rough in character. This murmur was much louder when the patient bent forward. The heart was regular and the rate was 64 per minute. The pulse rose slowly and was sustained. The blood pressure was 116 systolic and 86 diastolic. On deep inspiration the liver descended one finger below the costal margin. It was not tender. There was no pitting edema of the extremities. The electrocardiogram showed a large Q wave in lead III and a left axis deviation. The urine was negative. The fluoroscopic examination of the heart showed a "boot shaped heart of rather marked degree". The patient was re-examined fluoroscopically for the possibility of calcified aortic valves. The report reads: "A density was seen in the region of the aortic valves which was thought to be calcified leaflets. This seemed to move with the contractions of the heart. Films were taken in various directions but it was not possible to project this shadow".

The clinical diagnoses were: (1) cardiac enlargement, (2) beginning calcified aortic stenosis.

The patient was given 1½ grains of the powdered leaf of digitalis once daily and was told to limit his activity. He has been seen several times since then. His symptoms have been controlled by these measures.

Comment. This is a case of cardiac enlargement due to disease of the aortic valve. There was no history of rheumatic fever or hypertension to account for the cardiac enlargement. Fluoroscopic examination of the heart revealed a density in the region of the aortic valve. If it were a calcified gland one should be able to demonstrate calcification on a film. This case illustrates the inadequacy of percussion in determining the size of the heart in the thick chested individual. Without x-ray examination the shape of the heart might easily have been overlooked. The pain in the head and the numbness of the hands are regarded as being due to inadequate blood supply to these parts when the patient exerted himself considerably.

LITERATURE

While calcification of the aortic cusps has been well known to pathologists for some time, it was not a well recognized clinical entity until recently. In 1931 Christian[1] reported a series of twenty-three cases and since that time several others [2, 3 and 4]. have discussed various phases of the disease. Christian emphasized the physical signs and symptoms and stated that the condition should be recognized clinically more frequently than it has been. The reader is referred to Christian's article for a full discussion of aortic stenosis with calcification.

SUMMARY

Two cases of calcified aortic stenosis are presented, one case with autopsy. The clinical findings of these cases are described and discussed briefly.

BIBLIOGRAPHY

1. Christian, H. A.: Aortic stenosis with calcification of cusps; distinct clinical entity. Jour. Am. Med. Assn., xcvii: 158-161 (July 18) 1931.

2. Margolis, H. M.: Ziellessen, F. O., and Barnes, A. R.: Calcareous aortic valvular disease. Am. Heart Jour. vi: 349-374 (February) 1931.

3. Cabot, R. C.: Facts of the Heart, p. 206. W. B. Saunders Company, Philadelphia, 1926.

4. Sosman, Merrill C., and Wosika, Paul H.: Calcification in aortic and mitral valves, with a report of twenty-three cases demonstrated in vivo by the Roentgen ray. Am. Jour. Roentgenol. and Radium Therap., xxx:328-348 (September) 1933.

STATE DEPARTMENT OF HEALTH

A YEAR AHEAD

We took long strides forward in the promotion of public health activities in 1933, and we can look forward with assurance of further progress during the coming year. With the cooperation of an energetic medical profession, a county-wide prevention program will be instituted which will go far to lessen the incidence of diphtheria, scarlet fever, smallpox and other infectious diseases. The importance of a pure public water and milk supply, as well as the significance of the carrier problem, is being more widely recognized by the general public. Industrial diseases and accidents, nutritive disorders such as diabetes and pernicious anemia, and the continued spread of cancer are now regarded as public health problems, and will require the concerted effort of the profession and the public to bring them under better control.

With the efficient help of the Speakers Bureau of the Iowa State Medical Society the achievements of modern medicine will become a part of public knowledge and this information will promote a better appreciation of the needs of the highest standards of medical licensure.

The Department of Health is fortunate in the personnel of its administrative staff, representing as it does the highest type of scientific efficiency, which promises well for the work of 1934.

Walter L. Bierring, M.D.

COUNTY-WIDE PREVENTIVE PROGRAMS

An outline of the policies governing the State Department of Health in the organization and conduct of county-wide preventive programs has been prepared. The department proposes to follow a plan approved by organized medicine, whenever the group method of immunization is employed.

At a recent meeting of the committee on Child Health and Protection of the Iowa State Medical Society, the proposal to submit such a plan to the Council of that society was made. Although the action taken by the Council as a whole is not known, preliminary reports from H. A. Spilman, M.D., chairman, indicate that a majority of the Council favor the adoption of the plan which follows:

The State Department of Health shall:

I. Refer the sponsoring agency to committee on Child Health and Protection, or to the officers of the county medical society.

II. Require sponsoring agency to furnish satisfactory evidence to the effect that:

A. A majority of the county medical society or the local medical practitioners acting as a group has approved the principles of such a program and the plan of organization and conduct.

B. The literature used has been reviewed and approved either by the local county medical society or the committee on Child Health and Protection of the Iowa State Medical Society.

C. The physicians will be paid for their services.

D. The sponsoring agency has arranged to provide for—

1. Nurses, whenever possible, to assist with the treatment of children.
2. Clerical help.
3. Payment of physicians' fees, cost of materials, etc.
4. Treatment of under privileged and privileged children.
5. Treatment stations.
6. Transportation of children, whenever necessary, to and from treatment stations.
7. An accurate record of the names, addresses and the ages of the children treated.
8. An intensive educational program.
9. Treatment of children of preschool age.
10. Written consent of the parents.
11. Adequate follow-up work.

III. Provide without cost—

A. Diphtheria preventive agents in an amount sufficient to treat completely 20 per cent of children availing themselves of this opportunity, provided an accurate record of the names, addresses and the ages of the children treated is submitted to the department by the sponsoring agency.

B. Literature which has been approved either by the committee on Child Health and Protection of the Iowa State Medical Society or a majority of the membership of the local county medical society or group of local medical practitioners.

C. Consent slips.
D. Records of the occurrence of diphtheria in the past years whenever available.

The Local County Medical Society shall:
I. Offer a plan in which the members of the county society will administer the necessary treatments to groups of children at a given place on designated dates for a fee.
II. Determine
A. The preventive agent to be used.
B. The methods employed.
C. The allocation of physicians to districts.

If a preventive program is to be organized and conducted only on a township, city or town, or rural school district basis, the same principles as outlined for county-wide programs will be adhered to by the department except that when the plan and procedure has been approved by a majority of the medical practitioners residing in that governmental unit, approval of the plan and procedure by the county medical society will not be considered necessary.

County-wide preventive programs can be organized and conducted successfully only if the constituent county medical societies will prepare a plan which provides for the treatment of groups of children at a given place on designated dates for a fee. If all the county medical societies submitted such a plan to the State Department of Health, that organization could advise intelligently the lay organizations seeking to sponsor preventive programs in any given county.

C. H. Kinnaman, M.D.

THE PREVENTION OF SCARLET FEVER

Scarlet fever, although not as virulent in this country as formerly, is as prevalent as ever. In 1930, 2,836 cases were reported to the State Department of Health for the state, and there were 3,086 cases in the following year. Reports in 1932 numbered 1,917. For the first eleven months of 1933, reports of 1,640 cases were received.

The Dick Test—The Dick test to determine susceptibility to scarlet fever is of much value and should be a preliminary step to other procedures. In 1929 Dr. and Mrs. Geo. F. Dick reported results of tests carried out on 32,400 persons. Of this number 20,856 or 64 per cent were negative, and 11,544 or 36 per cent were positive.

Active Immunization Against Scarlet Fever— Views regarding scarlet fever and immunization or protection against the disease, have been widely divergent. Some physicians have experienced rather severe reactions following treatments; others have reported the occurrence of scarlet fever in children, after protective treatments had been administered. Platou reported six cases of scarlet fever in a group of 366 individuals, following three treatments with Larson's (ricinoleated) antigen. On the other hand, no cases of the disease occurred in a group of 70 persons following a course of five treatments with scarlet fever toxin. It is apparent that more enduring protection results from the five-treatment method. Melnick discusses transient reactions such as head-

ache, fever, nausea, vomiting, abdominal distress and rash, which may be associated with the use of scarlet fever toxin. He observed one or more of the above symptoms in from four to nine per cent of those treated. To obviate reactions, he advises that two tablespoonfuls of milk of magnesia be given the evening before and that little food be taken on the day of treatment. Milk products are best avoided, food being limited to thin cereals, toast and fruit juices. Inoculations may be given toward evening and preferably on Friday or Saturday. Since the chief purpose in using graduated doses of scarlet fever toxin, is to prevent the disease and its unfortunate complications, transient reactions which now and then occur, might be overlooked. The usual procedure is to perform another Dick test about two weeks after the fifth treatment to make certain that immunity has been established.

Scarlet Fever Toxoid—The chief disadvantage associated with the Dick method of building up protection against scarlet fever is that so many treatments are required—including the preliminary Dick test to determine susceptibility and the subsequent repetition of the test to certify immunity, seven different treatments are involved. This number of injections might appear small to a diabetic patient who is in the habit of receiving numerous injections of insulin, but it is nevertheless large from the standpoint of the average healthy child. In a recent number of *Public Health Reports* (May 26, 1933), Veldee describes scarlet fever toxoid, the method of preparation and its use in developing immunity in susceptible persons. Following three treatments at three-week intervals, administered to a group of 1,700 individuals, he found that 83 per cent were Dick negative. Constitutional reactions occurred but rarely. In the diphtheria preventive work, newer preparations of diphtheria toxoid have reduced the number of treatments necessary to establish immunity. When a similar product can be made available to prevent scarlet fever, this will mark a significant advance and prove a boon to the many children and adults, now susceptible and in need of measures which build up a high and fairly permanent degree of resistance to a treacherous infection.

Carl F. Jordan, M.D.

PUBLICATION OF CANCER SURVEY

At a recent meeting of the Council of the Iowa State Medical Society, William Jepson, M.D., Sioux City, Iowa, State Chairman of the American Society for the Control of Cancer, requested the assistance of the Commissioner of Health in regard to the publication of the findings of a cancer survey of Iowa made by Frank Leslie Rector, M.D., Field Representative of the American Society for the Control of Cancer. This survey was made in 1932, upon the request and with the approval of the Council of the Iowa State Medical Society. When the report of this survey was submitted to the Iowa State Medical Society the cost of publication prevented that organization from making its findings available to the physicians of the state. Fortunately the State Department of

Health was able to cooperate with the State Society and is publishing the report in a special bulletin. A copy of this bulletin will be mailed to every physician licensed to practice medicine in the state of Iowa. The Department of Health is pleased to play this small part in helping to inform the physicians of Iowa in regard to this major cause of death.

UNDULANT FEVER CASE RECORDS IN IOWA

During 1933 cases of undulant fever, reported to the State Department of Health by attending physicians and through laboratory reports numbered 151. The following analysis of 112 cases is based entirely on information contained on case record forms forwarded to physicians from the Division of Communicable Diseases of the State Department of Health. Acknowledgment is here made to the many physicians (numbering nearly 100) whose fine help and generous cooperation made possible this consideration of the subject of undulant fever in Iowa.

Distribution According to Age and Sex—Information taken from 112 undulant fever case records received from physicians during the year 1933, shows the following distribution of cases according to sex and age groups:

TABLE I

Age Groups		Male	Female	Total
1- 4 years		0	1	1
5- 9 "		4	2	6
10-19 "		12	5	17
20-29 "		26	9	35
30-39		20	3	23
40-49		10	4	14
50-59		8	2	10
60-69 "		1	2	3
70 years and over		0	0	0
Age not stated		3	0	3
Total		84	82	112

As indicated in Table I, 84 males represented 75 per cent of the patients in this series of cases, outnumbering females three to one. Patients of both sexes, included in the age groups 10 to 49, numbered 89, or 79 per cent of the total number.

Distribution According to Counties—The counties in which indulant fever occurred have been arranged according to number of cases reported, and insofar as possible, alphabetically, as follows: Pottawattamie, thirty-three cases; Jones, five; Black Hawk, four; Kossuth, four; Plymouth, four; Polk, four; Jasper, three; Sioux, three, and Wapello, three. Two cases each occurred in Carroll, Cherokee, Clinton, Dubuque, Fremont, Henry, Humboldt, Pocahontas, and Shelby counties. Additional counties reporting one case were: Adair, Benton, Buena Vista, Calhoun, Cass, Cerro Gordo, Clay, Dickinson, Fayette, Floyd, Grundy, Hancock, Hardin, Iowa Jefferson, Linn, Lyon, Mahaska, Marion, Marshall, Montgomery, O'Brien, Page, Taylor, Webster, Winnebago and Woodbury making a total of 112 cases.

A significant fact in the above list of counties, in all but one instance, is the sporadic nature of the occurrence of undulant fever, as many as forty-six counties being represented in this group of cases. Another outstanding fact, the one exception to the foregoing statement, was the occurrence in Council Bluffs (Pottawattamie county) of a milk-borne epidemic of undulant fever, affecting thirty-one persons. The source of infection in all but several of these cases was definitely traceable to raw milk distributed by one of the dairies. Blood cultures obtained from a number of the patients yielded Brucella melitensis (variety suis). The same type of organism was isolated through guinea pig inoculation, from cream samples obtained from infected cows in the dairy herd concerned.

Seasonal Distribution of Cases.—In the series of 112 case records, onset of symptoms in one case was in 1931, and in nine more cases, in 1932 (last months of the year). Of the remaining 102 cases, onset of symptoms occurred during the months of 1933, as follows: January, six cases; February, fourteen cases; March, twenty-six; April, twenty; May, twelve; June, thirteen; July, four; August, five, and September one. Case records are not available at this time for patients, whose onset of illness occurred later than September 1st. Although in rare instances diagnosis and report are made within two weeks following onset of symptoms, the interval between onset and report is often one or several months, due largely to the insidious type of onset, and consequent delay in seeking medical care.

Occupation.—Table II shows six types of occupation in their order of frequency:

TABLE II

Occupation	No. of Cases	Per Cent of Total
Farm work	50	45
School—urban	17	15
Housewife—urban	11	10
Packing house employee—urban	8	7
Store or office work—urban	6	5
Housework—rural	4	4
Other occupations (chiefly urban*)	16	14
Total	112	100

*These include two preschool children (urban), a live-stock dealer, a blacksmith, a superintendent of a county home, a merchant and a laboratory worker.

Symptoms.—The case records, coming from so many sources, show a striking agreement with reference to the main symptoms. The ten chief symptoms and the frequency with which these received mention were: fever, seventy-nine; pains, aching or soreness, fifty-five; chills, thirty-nine; headache, thirty-five; sweats, thirty-four; weakness, thirty-four; malaise, twenty-one; tired feeling, fourteen; anorexia, nine, and loss of weight, five. Other symptoms mentioned were: vomiting, four; dizziness, three; cough or bronchitis, three; constipation, three; insomnia, two; lassitude, two; nausea, one; neck stiffness, one, and sore throat, one.

Probable Source of Infection.

A. Raw dairy products.

One hundred three or 92 per cent of the 112 patients used raw milk, cream or home churned butter. In addition to the thirty-one patients concerned in the milk-borne epidemic, ten others were urban dwellers who gave no history of contact with animals and apparently acquired infection through the ingestion of raw dairy products. On farms the use of raw dairy products is likewise of importance in causing infection although the factor of contact with farm animals looms large, as evidenced by the preponderance of males over females.

B. Contact with animals or their tissues.

1. Packing house workers.

Eight of the patients were packing house employees, all of whom had direct contact with hogs. Five of these men used pasteurized milk and two of the remaining three, raw milk wholly or in part. The factor of raw dairy products is therefore out of consideration in the majority of this group of persons.

2. Other types of contact in urban residents.

A laboratory worker who used only pasteurized milk, apparently acquired illness from exposure to blood specimens from hogs. An urban housewife who used but little raw milk, developed symptoms two weeks after butchering a hog. A blacksmith who drank no milk and whose only contact with animals was in the shoeing of horses, suffered a moderately severe attack of undulant fever.

3. Types of contact on the farm.

Those engaged in farm work have special types of contact with cows and hogs, in milking, butchering, marketing, ringing, handling of little pigs, feeding, etc. Some of the case records indicated that onset of illness occurred shortly after one or more of these special types of contact. Contact with sheep was mentioned only three times in this series of 112 case records, and contact with goats not at all.

Further Study Necessary.—It is highly desirable that the investigation of cases of undulant fever be continued, so as to determine more accurately the source of infection, whether in hogs or cows. Blood cultures, taken at the height of the disease, give valuable information whenever Brucella melitensis, variety abortus and variety suis, are isolated. From the economic viewpoint as well as the health standpoint, farmers and dairymen should be urged to have their cows and hogs tested by veterinarians as an initial step in eradicating infectious abortion.

Prevention of Undulant Fever.

1. Carefully controlled pasteurization of all dairy products in cities and towns is essential to the prevention of undulant fever acquired through ingestion.

2. The prevention of cases of undulant fever resulting from exposure to infected animals, animal products or contaminated surfaces, is closely related to the task of eradicating Bang's disease in cattle and hogs. In addition the contact factor should be reduced to a minimum.

3. Specific prevention.

Specific and other forms of treatment of the disease have certain limitations similar to those in typhoid fever. The prophylactic use of vaccine would seem indicated, in order to increase individual resistance to undulant fever infection through the development of an active immunity. Such preventive measures would be largely confined to groups in which the hazard of exposure is greatest (farmers, packing house workers), and to farm households having contagious abortion in the immediate environment.

Carl F. Jordan, M.D.

PRENATAL LETTER SERVICE

Recently the Division of Child Health and Health Education directed a communication dealing with the subject of the method of distribution of prenatal letters to the secretary of each county medical society. The pertinent facts contained in this letter were:

"As you know the letters are available upon request only of a physician. In the past the only method used for the distribution of the letters has been as follows: When a request card signed by a physician was received by the department, the letters were mailed by the department to the expectant mother at intervals so that the last letter reached her prior to the eighth month of her period of waiting. Physicians may still mail request cards to the department and the letters will be mailed to the mother. If any physician desires, he may obtain the letters by requesting a supply either from the department or from the secretary of his local county medical society. The physician can then give or mail the letters to the expectant mother under his care.

"It is the hope of the Commissioner that every physician will avail himself of the prenatal letter service. The letters have been reviewed recently by the Committee on Child Health and Protection of the Iowa State Medical Society and in the very near future another revision of these letters will be made by the department in conjunction with that committee."

PREVALENCE OF DISEASE

	Nov. '33	Oct. '33	Nov. '32	Most Cases Reported from
Diphtheria	81	82	72	Pottawattamie, Polk
Scarlet Fever	358	272	152	Polk, Taylor
Typhoid Fever	4	16	2	(For State)
Smallpox	40	4	85	Monona, Woodbury
Measles	11	6	9	Harrison, Woodbury
Whooping Cough	71	96	47	Black Hawk, Dubuque
Cerebrospinal Meningitis	4	1	3	Woodbury
Chickenpox	325	80	498	Woodbury, Dubuque
Mumps	22	10	82	Woodbury
Poliomyelitis	4	13	2	(For State)
Epidemic Encephalitis	6	13	1	(For State)
Tuberculosis	29	39	37	Linn, Pottawattamie
Undulant Fever	10	4	4	(For State)
Syphilis	179	130	177	(For State)
Gonorrhea	183	185	186	(For State)

The JOURNAL of the
Iowa State Medical Society

ISSUED MONTHLY

RALPH R. SIMMONS, Editor..................Des Moines
PUBLICATION COMMITTEE
RALPH R. SIMMONS, Editor..................Des Moines
ROBERT L. PARKER, Secretary..................Des Moines
OLIVER J. FAY, Trustee..................Des Moines
JOHN I. MARKER, Trustee..................Davenport
EDWARD M. MYERS, Trustee..................Boone

SUBSCRIPTION $3.00 PER YEAR

*Address all communications to the Editor of the Journal,
1122 Bankers Trust Building, Des Moines*

OFFICE OF PUBLICATION, DES MOINES, IOWA

Vol. XIV   JANUARY, 1934   No. 1

A NEW PURE FOOD, DRUG AND COSMETIC LAW

To the veteran health crusader, the late Dr. Harvey B. Wiley, the great but gullible American public owe thanks for the passage of the pioneer food and drug act of 1906. This act, emasculated by amendments before its passage, remains on our statute book today in practically the same form and wording of the original law. Despite the fact that each successive chief food and drug administrator for the past ten or fifteen years has openly and publicly declared the shortcomings of the law, the American public, with child-like confidence, has imagined that the term "Pure Food and Drug Act" was in itself a guarantee that all foods and drugs would be pure and unadulterated.

Donning the discarded mantle of Dr. Wiley, modern crusaders will again besiege Congress when it convenes in January in an effort to enact an entirely new and completely rewritten Pure Food, Drug, and Cosmetic Law. To do this a peacefully sleeping public must be awakened to their danger. Much of this campaign to enlighten the public must be carried on by the medical profession, and it is to them that an appeal is made to weigh carefully the shortcomings of the old law and the remedial proposals of the new law, and upon a basis of their investigation, to work not only for the bill, but to enlighten their friends and patients so that they may also use their influence for its passage.

At the direction of the President, Dr. Rexford Tugwell, Assistant Secretary of Agriculture, collaborating with Mr. Walter G. Campbell, chief of the food and drug administration, and Senator Royal S. Copeland of New York, has prepared a bill known as the Copeland Bill (S. 1944), which if passed in its present form will greatly strengthen and materially increase the scope of usefulness of our Food and Drug Acts. The bill is designed to insure the sale only of pure foods and drugs; to inform the public of the composition of medicines; to insure against fraudulent claims made to promote their sales; and to demand that cosmetics be made only from pure and harmless ingredients. The most marked innovation in the Copeland Bill, and the one which will motivate much of the opposition to the bill is the inclusion of cosmetics along with foods and drugs. Cosmetics as such were but little in vogue at the time of the passage of the original Federal Food and Drug Act. Today the industry is reckoned in the billion dollar class, and the compounding of cosmetics with dangerous ingredients has become a health problem affecting every American home.

Much attention has been directed recently to the use of thallium acetate in depilatory creams, aniline dyes in hair and eyelash stain, lead compounds in hair tonics and restorers, and mercury salts in skin bleachers. Under the existing law the cosmetic manufacturer is not restricted, and at present may prey upon the public until judgment from damage suits forces him out of business. The new law defines cosmetics as "all substances and preparations intended for the cleansing or altering of or promoting the attractiveness of the person." This wording will include not only such substances as powder, lipstick, eyebrow pencils, and the like aids to feminine charms ordinarily included in the term cosmetic, but also soaps, toothpastes, shaving creams, face lotions and other generally used preparations. A wail of protest, second only to that registered by the manufacturers of worthless patent medicines, will be heard from many "gyp" cosmetic manufacturers, who realize that if only the truth is told of their products (and this truth must appear not only on the trade package, but also in newspaper and magazine advertising, and over the radio) their products cannot be sold in competition with those more reliable manufacturers whose products will bear public scrutiny. Legislation always has and always will be governed to a very considerable extent by its effects upon trade and commerce, but the hope for the inclusion of cosmetics in this bill lies in the fact that the legitimate, honest and sincere manufacturer of cosmetics has nothing to conceal, and is now willing to represent truthfully the virtues and shortcomings of his products. Furthermore, he will favor the passage of a bill which will require the unscrupulous, "gyp" manufacturer to either conform to standards that are honest and honorable, or receive not only federal censure, but also rather drastic federal punishment.

Under the present Food and Drug Act, misrepresentation is forbidden insofar as it affects food and drugs, and only if the misrepresentation appears on the label of the trade package. To prove, however, that a manufacturer is in violation of this act, it must be proved not only that the product is not what it is claimed to be, but that the maker knows that it is not, and that he has made his claims with deliberate intentions to deceive and defraud. Is it surprising that convictions are not, and cannot be obtained under the old law? The new law defines as automatically false "any advertisement of a drug representing directly or by ambiguity or inference to have any effect in the treatment" of a long list of diseases, mentioning specifically blood poisoning, cancer, diabetes, paralysis, dropsy, "sex weakness," tuberculosis and tumors—conditions for which drug-vending quacks have long supplied popular remedies. It further states, "if in any particular it [the advertisement of food, drugs or cosmetics] is untrue, or by ambiguity or inference creates a misleading impression regarding such food, drug or cosmetic," the manufacturer is guilty of misrepresentation.

To strengthen the provisions concerning food and food products the bill provides for the establishment of standards for all food products which must be met by manufacturers and packers; and best of all, provides real and severe penalties for all violators of any provision of the bill.

It is significant that the new law broadens, as it justly should, the avenues of misrepresentation to include not only the printed word on the label of the trade package, but any representation of the preparation which may appear in any printed or spoken form sponsored by the manufacturer. This phase is of particular importance as it pertains to the misrepresentation of foods, drugs and cosmetics by radio broadcasting. It has been estimated that there are now in operation between fourteen and twenty million radio receiving sets in the United States. The entertainment broadcast for the reception of these millions of sets is paid for by manufacturers seeking to advertise their products. In the early stages of the development of the various broadcasting systems great scrutiny was directed to the character of the representations made by the broadcaster, and broadcasting stations generally held themselves rigidly aloof from patent medicine advertising. In more recent times they have considered their duty to the listening public fully discharged when they announce that the period of broadcast is paid for and sponsored by a particular manufacturing concern. The result is that the listeners receive a terrific verbal barrage of extravagant, unscientific and unwarranted claims for various products, from breakfast food and mouth wash to cancer cures

and medicines for the restoration of sexual vigor—and such drivel and rot as one hears! Superlatives and extravagant claims are so universally present that one wonders how sickness, disease and death can ever occur except to that limited group of non-believers who fail to use the sovereign preparation which pays the orchestra and prepares the speech for the announcer.

Get the bill and study it. Be informed!

THE UNIVERSITY HOSPITAL

Confronted by the allegation that because of an over-crowded condition, more than 5,000 Iowa residents were being denied care at the University of Iowa hospitals, the Forty-fifth General Assembly early last spring appointed a committee of nine[1] distinguished physicians and laymen "to seek the cause or causes of at least one of Iowa's present misfortunes, viz., unprovided for sick and suffering," and to submit "such recommendations as to the committee seem fit and proper." Organized with Dr. E. E. Munger as chairman and Dr. A. W. Erskine as secretary the committee under date of April 1, 1933, submitted a preliminary report[2] to the Governor. Agreeable to a final recommendation in the preliminary report that "your committee respectfully requests that it be not discharged" the activities of the committee were continued under authority for report at the special session of the General Assembly, which convened in December.

Pursuant to its instructions the committee continued the investigations, culminating its work by a "Report of Interim Committee named to Investigate Indigent Patient Problem"[3] included in the Iowa State Senate Journal of November 21, 1933 (page 122). Most significant of the committee's nine recommendations were:

1. That half the basic cost of hospitalizing indigents be charged to the county of their residence.

2. That investigation to determine indigency be made under the direction of the County Board of Supervisors.

Of the nine members of the committee only seven signed this report[4] and two of these signers

1. Appointed by the Senate.
    Dr. Morris Moore of Walnut
    Ed Hicklin of Wapello
    G. W. Patterson of Burt
  Appointed by the House:
    Paul L. Millhone of Clarinda
    John Speidel of Washington
    Dr. E. E. Munger of Spencer
  Appointed by the Governor:
    Dr. Arthur W. Erskine of Cedar Rapids
    Dr. Oliver J. Fay of Des Moines
    Dr. W. A. Sternberg of Mt. Pleasant
2. Reported in The Journal, April, 1933, page 221. Ibid, July 1933, page 408.
3. Full text of report given in this issue of The Journal, page 47.
4. Oliver J. Fay, W. A. Sternberg, A. W. Erskine, E. R. Hicklin, M. Moore, Paul L. Millhone, John Speidel.

did so with reservations.[5] Supporting the present operating plan of the University Hospitals three members of the committee submitted a supplemental report[6] to the Governor endorsing the action and plan of the State Board of Education and recommending that the County Quota Plan should be given a further trial." This recommendation was written into the bill as submitted to the Senate as Sec. 8. Later Senator Moore offered an amendment substituting the County Part Payment Plan for Sec. 8 of the bill. This amendment, if passed, would restore the bill to its original form as submitted by the Committee in its final report.

Chairman Munger and member Patterson of the committee being out of harmony with the final report of the majority, submitted a minority report[7] to the Governor under date of December 14, 1933. The most outstanding and perhaps the most radical of the recommendations of the minority was to "provide for the repeal of the adult indigent law . . . restore the Perkins law to its original status and take necessary steps to establish the last two or three years of the State University of Iowa Medical College in the city of Des Moines," or if the city of Des Moines "is not in a receptive mood . . . then give only the first or first and second years of medicine at Iowa City and let the last two or three be taken elsewhere."

From a review of the various reports of the investigating committee and other interested persons it becomes immediately apparent that "an emergency exists wherein more than 5,000 residents of the state of Iowa—men, women and children—are clamoring for admission to the State University Hospitals." It is further apparent that to relieve "this distressing situation" and to remove the "humiliation that is ours with the publication of these facts to the world," an earnest and sincere effort has been made by the committee to discharge its duties, but unfortunately the entire committee has been unable to agree upon a single plan of operation. Indicative of the probable action of the General Assembly, the bill as submitted by the committee including the "Quota Plan" for admission of patients to the State University Hospital, passed the House by the overwhelming vote of 96 to 2. If this very decisive action is followed by like approval of the Senate, a new and untried program will be adopted by the University in administering hospital and medical care to the indigent of the state.

Regardless of the form which this bill may assume in its final passage, one cannot escape the conviction that a change in the existing law is demanded and that the problem is one intimately

affecting not only every physician, but every citizen and taxpayer in the state. Because of these several vital factors the Journal has considered the matter of sufficient importance to reproduce in their entirety the several resolutions and comments from the committee.

5. Representative Speidel signed the majority report, with reservations respecting recommendations Nos. 1 and 4. Senator Moore signed the minority report, with the reservation that he would except the words "who shall attend the physician who is to attend him" in recommendation No. 3.
6. Full text of Supplemental Report and signers given in this issue of the Journal, page 51.
7. Full text of Minority Report given in this issue of the Journal, page 54.

HENRY JAMES PRENTISS MEMORIAL*

Geo. C. Albright, M.D., '14
Iowa City

Mr. Chairman, Ladies and Gentlemen:

The Alumni Association of the College of Medicine today finds itself in the grip of varied emotions. We are grateful to the Alumni Association of the University for the prominence given to us and our project in this Homecoming. We are happy to welcome all Alumni at this board—Dutch treat—though it must perforce be. As an Association, we rejoice in the goal achieved, which makes possible this commemorative occasion. We are thankful to have known the man whose memory we meet to honor. Through all our joy, however, there runs a minor note, one of sadness and regret, sadness for one who has gone, regret that this slight token of our esteem and affection might not have been shown while he was yet with us. We are anxious that you who are not Alumni of the College of Medicine, may regard us as one with you in a devotion to a common purpose—a still better University of Iowa.

It seems altogether fitting that we digress for just a few moments to render clear the motives which animate us as a small group within the larger University family. True to biblical precedent the Association was "conceived in sorrow" and "brought forth in great travail of spirit." Born a little over six years ago when the very foundations of our school appeared to be shaken, the hope of its parents was that it might prove, if not the Moses, to lead the way into the promised land, at least the Aaron and Hur, who might sustain the upraised hands of Moses until Justice and Right might prevail over the sinister forces of Amalek that threatened disruption of the school, and nullification of two decades of painful progress.

The Constitution of the Association sets out two main objectives. The first is to cooperate with

* Delivered at presentation of bronze portrait of Dr. Prentiss to the University of Iowa, October 21, 1933.

the authorities of the University in every legitimate way possible in the solution of the grave questions facing them. This cooperation was, and is, intended to work within the University family, on the campus, to aid in any way possible to make their work easier and more effective; but going further, this cooperation was proffered to promote better and more amicable relations between that university family and the great mass of the medical profession of the state. Hopes were, and are maintained, to be able to change

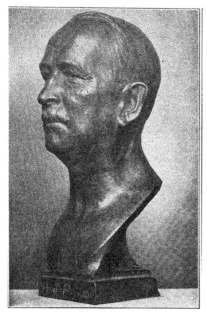

Bronze bust of Henry James Prentiss

adverse critics and lukewarm supporters of the Medical School into loyal, ardent, enthusiastic supporters of the Medical Faculty in the great service they are striving to render the people of Iowa.

The second objective is to seek to render tribute to, and to perpetuate the memory of those men within the College of Medicine whose labors have so nobly advanced the prestige of the school, whose labors have made a great school possible. We earnestly desired, and do desire to bring to them that need of love, loyalty, and honor which is the highest compensation of those true teachers who

build character into men while imparting knowledge to them.

Rebuffed in their proffers of cooperation upon the campus, the Association has gone steadily forward in its efforts to promote better feeling through better understanding. It has fostered more cordial and more amicable relationships between the College of Medicine and the profession of the state. Upon the continuation of these cordial, amicable relationships the present and future success of that College unequivocally depends.

The initial fruit of the second main objective of the Association—that of rendering honor to those loyal men who have served Iowa well, is being gathered today. It is the cause of our assembling here. We are met today to render belated homage to, and to honor the memory of, a man who spent the best years of his life in tireless, ceaseless effort, striving always to increase the prestige of this, his adopted school. For twenty-seven years, from 1904 until the time of his premature passing away, there was one man who came into direct personal contact with every freshman of the College of Medicine. It is significant that those contacts were so frequently, and so intimately preserved throughout the four or five years those men were upon the campus. It is significant, yet not at all mysterious, nor hard of comprehension, for the subject he taught, he impressed upon all, was the very foundation, the Alpha and Omega of all medical practice. Henry James Prentiss made the surgeon and internist, as well as the veriest beginners, constant attendants at his tables of knowledge, those of the anatomic laboratory.

Further than this, not only did he strive to make his laboratories the Mecca of the men within the school, but his avowed purpose was to make those laboratories of direct personal service to any physician in the state who wished to come there for either general or specific information. To the value of this opportunity many of us physicians who are here today, can bear silent though eloquent testimony. It is not at all unlikely, that there are some here who are not physicians, but were patients, who are more deeply indebted to this phase of Dr. Prentiss' philosophy of service than they realize. The results of this policy are well known to the medical faculty, to his colleagues here in the city, and to the medical profession of the entire state. His unselfish interest in every problem brought to him by any physician of the state made of that physician an ardent supporter for life. One illustration of the results of this philosophy of service will suffice. Several years ago the anatomic laboratories were seriously short of material for the students. Dr. Prentiss asked the local medical society to elect him delegate to the state society. This they did. At the state meeting, he told the physicians there of this shortage and asked their support in overcoming it. Within a year the shortage had disappeared and from that time on, in spite of increased enrollment in the medical school, anatomic material has been adequate.

This is no time for fullsome eulogy. Such would be a work of supererogation. Encomiums are useless, for he needs none. To those of us who were privileged to be his friends, comes the knowledge that could he hear, such pronouncements would be repugnant to him. One eulogy only need be made. When the proposal was made to honor some man who had labored through the years for the good of Iowa—there was a singular unanimity of opinion as to who that man should be. It was hoped that this memorial, as we must now regard it, might be a recognition during his lifetime. This hope was doomed to early disappointment, for the work had barely started when came the news of his untimely passing. It is the sincere hope of the Association that the members of his family, those who are here today, and those who are unable to be here, may take added satisfaction in this knowledge; which their father unfortunately cannot share. We are happy to have them know again of the place their father held in the esteem, affection and love of us, his former students, colleagues and friends.

It is the wish of the Association that this portrait of our friend and teacher, may find its final place within the walls of that college with which he was so long associated, and in those buildings in which he so tirelessly labored, the medical laboratories.* We cherish the hope that there it may continue to remind the students of coming years of the man who was so largely responsible for their anatomic opportunities. We hope that they may know something of the ideals for which he stood, restless, searching after truth, never to be satisfied with theories when facts were available, and above all, his striving to realize the ideal which he expressed in his presidential address before Sigma XI, "To reach that stage of ethical thinking when you become your own severest critic seeking not to satisfy the judgment of others, but the mandates of your own intellectual conscience."

In his association with students and colleagues,

* The memorial now rests in the Medical Library of the University. It was placed there November 6, 1933.

he proved himself worthy of the fine tributes which Sir Andrew McPhail paid to the great pathologist poet of McGill, John McCrae, the author of the greatest poem of the World War, "In Flanders Fields." Of him, he said, "His philosophy of life was expressed in the religion of his everyday living. 'What I spent, I had, what I saved, I lost, what I gave, I have.'"

One of the finest attributes of character which he possessed—one that impressed friend and non-friend, admirers and critics alike, was his indomitable moral courage. Faced in one short year with the loss of his beloved wife, and the eldest of his two sons to whom he was passionately devoted, he accepted the inevitable with a fortitude that amazed even those who knew him best. Not one of his innermost circle of friends was ever asked for consolation, nor did that circle ever hear one word of rebellion against his lot, or any Job-like cries of self-pity.

His last days were as he often wished they would be—days of activity to the very end. He must have felt as did Silas Weir Mitchell, the poet-neurologist of Philadelphia, for Dr. Mitchell wrote:

"I know the night is near at hand,
    The mist hangs low on hill and bay,
    The autumn sheaves are dewless dry,
But I have had the day.

"Yes, I have had, O Lord, the day
    When at thy call I have the night,
    Brief be the twilight, as I pass,
From light to dark, from dark to light."

Mr. President, on behalf of the Alumni Association of the College of Medicine, may we present to the University of Iowa, this bronze portrait of our former teacher and friend. May we also transmit to you this pedestal—the gift of three close friends; physicians, though not Alumni, N. G. Alcock, Verne C. Hunt, and C. J. Rowan. It is our sincere hope that the memory of Dr. Prentiss may be as imperishable as is the bronze from which the portrait is cast.

HISTORY OF WOMEN PHYSICIANS

Dr. Kate Campbell Mead, of Haddam, Connecticut, is writing a history of medical women in the United States. All physicians in Iowa, who have known women physicians practicing in this state, are requested to send such information to Dr. Nelle S. Noble, 1107 Bankers Trust Building, Des Moines, Iowa, who is compiling the Iowa section for Dr. Mead.

Two Distinguished Scientists Die
Roux and Calmette

Within a few days interval the illustrious Institute Pasteur of Paris lost two of its most distinguished leaders. On October 29, Dr. Albert Calmette died at the age of seventy years, and on November 3, Dr. Emile Roux, Director of the Institute, died at the age of seventy-nine years. In addition to their leadership in the medical sciences, they represented two interesting personalities of rare charm and creative genius, quite apart from that of other mortals.

As a student of the Pasteur Institute in Paris in 1894, the writer first came under the inspiring influence of Doctor Roux. It was an eventful period in the practical application of the basic truths developed by the great Master Louis Pasteur. Roux and Yersin had discovered diphtheria toxin in 1887. During the spring and summer of

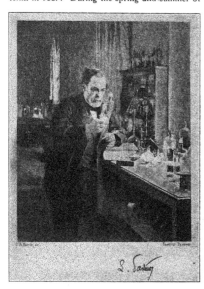

A' Monsieur Bierring en Souvenir de son
sejour a' l'Institut Pasteur,
20 Juillet 1894
Dr. Roux.

1894, Roux with his co-workers Martin, Borrel and Chamberlin demonstrated successfully the preventive and therapeutic use of diphtheria antitoxin in the first large series of cases reported

(three hundred). There was available for comparison of results a similar number of diphtheria patients in an adjoining hospital in which diphtheria antitoxin was not used. Pasteur was still

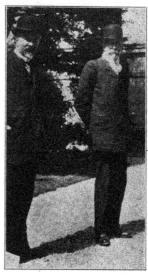

Dr. Calmette   Dr. Roux
Pasteur Institute, Paris, July, 1919

among the living, and it was through Doctor Roux's gracious introduction that the writer was privileged to have an audience with the founder of bacteriology. The accompanying photograph, inscribed by Dr. Roux, is commemorative of this visit. As an assistant of Pasteur during his early labors, and being closely associated with the triumphs of maturity particularly in the control of rabies, Doctor Roux then and for a period of forty years after Pasteur's death vivified the spirit and work of the master. Although universally recognized as one of the world's foremost savants, Roux was the essence of modesty. A bachelor, he lived in modest quarters of very simple furnishing in the garden of the Institute, which served him as office and living room. He was a man of frugal habits, never owned an automobile, and it is said always refused the salary to which he was entitled as director of the Institute. Science and hard work were to him the two most important things of life. He spoke only French, but had an excellent memory for names and faces. At each succeeding visit it was the same hearty greeting "A 'monsieur Bierring (Barang) comment-' allez-vous". During a visit in 1919 the photograph of· Calmette and Roux was taken in the garden of the Institute.

His distinguished colleague who preceded him in death by a few days, presented a somewhat different type of personality. Of distinguished appearance, modest and quiet manner, he too seemed to exist solely for the interests of science and the welfare of humanity. Always tactful and polite, he represented that type of French gentleman rarely encountered by foreigners, and which always left an impression of something worthy of reverence. Calmette gave the world antivenin serum, tetanus antitoxin, and in his later years succeeded in developing a method which re-aroused world interest in the eradication of tuberculosis. The World War brought its tragedies close to Calmette. In July 1914, his brother, the brilliant editor of Le Figaro, leading newspaper of Paris, was shot in his office by Mme. Caillaux. During the entire German occupation of Lille between 1914 and 1918, Calmette was director of the Pasteur Institute in that city. Although frequently-threatened with arrest he was allowed to pursue his medical investigations undisturbed on condition that he did not leave the city. By command of the German commander, however, Mme. Calmette was carried away to a distant prison camp at Hanover as a hostage. During a visit to the Institute in July, 1919, Calmette spoke with emotion of the untimely death of his brother, and of the ordeal during his four years confinement in Lille when he was not allowed to communicate with his imprisoned wife or his officer son, who fought at the front with the French artillery. In more recent years he was deeply affected by the tragedy at Lubek in which more than seventy children died following vaccination with a contaminated Bilie Calmette Guérin vaccine, said to have come from Calmette's laboratory, but subsequently adjudged by the Superior Court at Leipzig to have been ill prepared by the German bacteriologists at Lubeck.

Roux and Calmette were worthy disciples of Pasteur. Each discovery formed the basis of a new truth to follow. It is difficult to estimate to what extent the era of Pasteur influenced human events. Both will always remain a source of inspiration to all those who were privileged to know them as scientist, master or friend.

WALTER L. BIERRING, M.D.

CLIMATE INFLUENCES HEALTH

At the recent annual meeting of the American Society for Tropical Medicine several important observations regarding the influence of climate upon health were presented. Particularly noteworthy are the observations presented by Dr. Clarence A. Mills of the University of Cincinnati. He points out that southerners who migrate to the north are more susceptible than northerners to arteriosclerosis. "The great influx of southerners, both white and colored, into the manufacturing cities· of the North during the last fifteen years has presented us some important health problems quite aside from those of sanitation and personal hygiene."

This observation is in keeping with those reported from other sources that the average blood pressure of the inhabitants of the south is appreciably lower than that of the inhabitants of the north. Since Dr. Mills presents no adequate explanation for this observation, it appears that his report should open a productive line of research. Certainly the factor of climate alone is insufficient to explain this variation in average blood pressure.

Curiously Dr. Mills' observations not only revealed an increased susceptibility to arteriosclerosis, but also a greater prevalence of acute respiratory diseases, such as pneumonia, sinusitis and colds, and also an increased incidence of toxic goiter and diabetes. Various types of asthenia with nervous exhaustion are particularly prominent among these migrants from the south.

Not only are these observations of provocative interest to workers in medical research, but they should also prove of the greatest importance to industrialists employing such migrants. If Dr. Mills' observations are correct, they would suggest by inference that a southern or even tropical climate might be beneficial in the treatment of the several conditions mentioned. Such a postulate would require long· and painstaking observations for its proof, but is perhaps worthy of such an investigation.

INTERSTATE POST-GRADUATE ELECTS DOCTOR MAYO

Dr. Charles H. Mayo, Rochester, was chosen president-elect of the Interstate Post-Graduate Medical Association of North America at the annual meeting in Cleveland, October 16-21. Dr. John M. T. Finney, Baltimore, became president.

THE OPEN FORUM

THE UNIVERSITY HOSPITAL*

To the Editor:

President Robert Maynard Hutchins recently spoke before an assembly of some 2,000 students and faculty members of his own school on the proposed merger of Chicago and Northwestern universities. Some of his statements should challenge the attention of every thinking person interested in problems of education and state economics.

In summing up aspects of duplication and imitation in the educational field, he said that they are engendered by "the casual interest of donors, and the ambitions of faculties, graduates, trustees and presidents."

In commenting upon proposals for federal aid to public education, he spoke even more forcefully: "Any such arrangement would perpetuate all the weakness and waste of the present system, and that is what most educators want. They do not want to be disturbed, or improved, or changed; they want to be supported."

The financial situation of which President Hutchins takes frank cognizance is unfortunately one with which the citizens of Iowa have become all too familiar. The attitude of "faculties, graduates, trustees and presidents" is also one which we have had every opportunity to observe.

It seems difficult for those whose personal ambitions and interests are bound up with a certain school, let us say, to see the educational problems of that school from any other angle, or to consider dispassionately the financial aspects of a situation even when that situation becomes a critical one.

During boom times we in America learned to spend riotously, to consider many luxuries as necessities, and we find it hard to unlearn this attitude. Yet such fine disregard for adjusting our expenditures to our income and our needs still persists in the educational field.

It is particularly unpardonable in the case of educational institutions supported by public funds, since the taxpayer has a right to demand that such institutions consider public needs and depleted public coffers.

The state of Iowa can absorb some 50 new physicians a year, to replace those lost by death, through removal from the state, and to meet any emergency and a possible though undemonstrated increasing need.

The training of more physicians at state expense is indefensible, yet authorities of our state university would have us increase the more than one million dollars spent annually for the university hospital in order to provide teaching material for this unneeded number of medical students—some 90 instead of 50 graduates yearly.

* Reprinted from The Des Moines Register, December 28, 1933.

It is true that the university hospital serves a twofold purpose in that it is not only a teaching institution but also provides free medical care for certain classes of indigents.

Insofar as such indigents afford teaching material needed for the training of an adequate number of physicians, their transportation to the university hospital at state expense, and their maintenance there at a cost materially greater than that which would be incurred in caring for them locally, is right and proper.

When these increased expenditures of public funds represent the training of a larger number of physicians than our state can possibly use, when they serve only to gratify "the ambitions of faculties, graduates, trustees and presidents," then it is high time that our legislators, who are at least theoretically the guardians of our treasury, should call a halt.

The pending bill (S. F. 81 and H. F. 112) to provide for the clinical needs of the hospital and care for the indigent sick effectively guards against any possible crippling of the medical college through a lack of suitable teaching material, and at the same time provides for the care of indigents without the long delays which in the past have often entailed mental and physical suffering.

It thus not only effectively meets the two cardinal demands but it also provides needed safeguards for the public treasury. By placing the responsibility for determining the question of indigency with the county board of supervisors, with whom the care of county indigents already rests under our Iowa laws, willful abuse of the law would be prevented in most cases, and a means for correcting possible slips would be provided.

The proposed amendment, charging half of the actual cost of hospital care back to the county (the state would continue to pay for transportation and other special expenses) would not add to the cost to the counties, as has been alleged; funds expended by the state come from the taxpayer just as surely as those expended by the county.

It would result in a more equitable division of the expense, and result in a lessened cost to the 70 counties that now send less than their share of patients to the university hospital.

One cannot long escape the conviction that the chief point at issue is the continued provision of something over a million dollars to be spent as those in charge of the university hospital see fit.

It is as though a state institution of learning, instead of assuming the dignity of the position of helpmate, willingly and helpfully sharing vicissitudes and lessened income, were, like a mistress, wantonly to insist upon being maintained in the luxury and even profligacy to which she had become accustomed during boom times.—DR. OLIVER J. FAY, Des Moines.

SPEAKERS BUREAU ACTIVITIES

WHAT IS A GOOD MEDICAL MEETING?*

Man is so constituted that he can do better work and enjoy his labor more when he works in groups than as an individual. This is the reason for the existence the world over of a legion of human associations. This is the reason for the existence of organized medicine. However, human groups, like human individuals, are prone to stray away from the straight and narrow path that leadeth to more abundant life. Therefore, it becomes necessary for each member of an association, and especially the officers, to have clearly in mind what the ideal goal for the society really is in order that they may steer the society persistently and consistently on the right course.

Since our existence as a medical profession is justified only by our success in preventing and curing disease and in the alleviation of suffering from disease, it is obvious that the goal of any medical society is to make its members excellent physicians. This goal may be accomplished by:

1. Keeping its members abreast of medical progress.

2. Inspiring them to live up to the high ideals of medicine.

3. Obtaining for its members the joy of living which comes from the friendships of their colleagues.

The prime need of keeping its members well informed in medicine is recognized by every association of physicians the world over. Various types of programs are presented to fill this need. Some societies have their programs given by experts from afar. Others resort to what might be called the "wheel-horse" method, whereby all programs are presented by the same few members. Still others obtain their scientific programs from as large a percentage of their own members as possible.

It is generally conceded that the scientific standards of an individual society are highest where the last mentioned variety of program prevails. Real stimulation can after all come only from within the society. A medical society is active to the degree to which each individual member takes an active part in its functioning. Not all members can take an official part in the society's activities but each one can participate in the program. Medical meetings planned on this basis build for the society and for the individual doctor in the following ways:

1. A discussion given by any member, whether it

*This article was prepared for the Blackhawk County "Voice" but the message seems so appropriate at this time for every society that it is being printed here also.

deals with his original observations or with his own views on a phase of medicine can never fail to interest and instruct the listeners, provided that the individual has put his very best into his theme.

2. Such a presentation never fails to produce in the minds of the rest of the members the desire to go forth and do likewise.

3. Any doctor who has done his very best in presenting his subject is himself the greatest beneficiary since such an effort never fails to make him a better physician.

Religious leaders have always been cognizant of the fact that the zeal and good works of their flocks could be maintained only through constant inspiration of some kind. This applies equally well to medicine. A medical meeting that fails to leave in each member a desire to go forth and become a better doctor is not an ideal meeting.

Medical meetings might be varied by occasionally inviting a guest speaker of outstanding ability in medicine. These men by their own achievement, by their personality and by their technic of presentation have a powerful revivifying influence on the society. The excessive use of such talent, however, leads to the stagnation and decay of the society.

A good medical meeting is the most potent means for the promotion of good fellowship among the individual members of a society. In the stress of life in the professional competition of one's colleague's, irritating traits will occasionally crop out and cause resentment among his professional brethren. It seems to be the easiest thing in the world for the offending brother to make a mountain out of each molehill of this kind to the great detriment not alone of the offender and the offended but to the entire medical profession. Frequent medical meetings at which each doctor expresses his own medical views and hears and discusses the views of his colleagues, make it impossible for the injustices produced by petty jealousies, small indiscreet acts and other minor defects to distort the evaluation of a colleague in this way. It is also impossible, as Dr. McManus has often said, "to break bread together at frequent intervals and keep from admiring and respecting your professional associates."

Frequent medical meetings of the type outlined are doing wonders all over the state in uniting the medical profession into one solid body of intelligent, friendly physicians working together and enjoying working together for the benefit of the sick. When that day comes, our present annoyances, quacks, social injustices and detrimental legislation will have ceased to exist, for "seek ye first to become ideal physicians and all other things will be added unto you."

D. J. Glomset, M.D., Chairman,
Speakers Bureau Committee.

WOMAN'S AUXILIARY NEWS

Edited by the Press and Publicity Committee

MRS. OLIVER J. FAY, *Chairman*, 10 Thirty-fifth Street, Des Moines

*The Officiary of the Woman's Auxiliary to the Iowa
State Medical Society extends to every Auxiliary member sincere wishes for a happy and prosperous new year.*

HINTS FOR AUXILIARY ACTIVITIES

The following excerpts are round table discussions, held at the Tenth Annual Meeting of the Woman's Auxiliary to the Kentucky State Medical Association. They are reproduced here in the hope that the field of activities thus described may inspire our members to enlarge their scope of usefulness.

Educational

"Education: Our debt from present to future generations."

For the new organization I would plan first the study of our "State Health Laws" and the bulletins as they are issued by the State Board of Health of Kentucky, for "The public health is the foundation upon which rests the happiness of the people and the welfare of the nation."

The study of public health should be the first duty of each of us.

The study envelopes of the Auxiliary to the American Medical Association revised to date, may be secured from the chairman of public instruction. Copies of it are available at this meeting and we urge all county officers to procure them.

County program chairmen should write for the catalog published by the American Medical Association, located at 535 North Dearborn Street, Chicago, Illinois, from which may be selected pamphlets that will be very helpful to them.

The American Medical Association requests that county auxiliaries use and push the sale of *Hygeia* for educational purposes. This magazine should be in every school.

Programs in some of our most active auxiliaries have been composed of articles found in *Hygeia*.

Philanthropic

Under this heading we find auxiliaries doing the following work:

Visiting charity wards in hospitals, taking fruits, flowers, jellies, jams, etc.

Visiting children's hospitals, taking books, toys and providing story hours for convalescents.

Assisting the public health nurse by furnishing layettes for needy mothers.

Showers of linen and clothing for baby or charity hospitals.

Making surgical dressings and aprons for physicians and nurses in their charity work; gowns and bed-jackets for tuberculosis patients.

Visiting institutions for the aged, furnishing diversion and entertainment for them.

Soldiers old and young provided with entertainment.

Donating Christmas trees and entertainment to charity institutions.

Providing milk for under-nourished children.

Preparing school lunches at a minimum cost.

Giving first aid tents to Boy Scout Camps and rest tents for Salvation Army Camps.

Sending baskets of fruit, jellies and jams to orphan homes at Christmas.

Filling stockings for the "Empty Stocking Crusade" at Christmas.

Donating to Community Chests.

Making loans to needy physicians or their families.

Each auxiliary should find the greatest need in their county and under direction of the Advisory Board do all in their power to alleviate that need.

Do not undertake too much at first but finish what you undertake. Nothing succeeds like success.

Mills County

The Woman's Auxiliary to the Mills County Medical Society met in conjunction with that society, in Glenwood, December 7, and elected the following officers to serve during 1934: Mrs. I. U. Parsons of Malvern, president; Mrs. M. S. Campbell of Malvern, vice president; and Mrs. J. M. Donelan of Glenwood, secretary and treasurer.

Monroe County

Mrs. T. A. Moran of Melrose, was elected president of the Woman's Auxiliary to the Monroe County Medical Society, at a meeting held in Albia, Thursday, December 14. Other officers are: Mrs. C. N. Hyatt of Albia, vice president; Miss Mabel Gray of Albia, secretary and treasurer; Mrs. J. F. Stafford of Lovilia, parliamentarian; and Mrs. T. R. Castles and Mrs. Burke Powell, both of Albia, advisors.

SOCIETY PROCEEDINGS

Audubon County Annual Meeting

Newly elected officers of the Audubon County Medical Society are: Dr. R. H. Payne of Exira president; Dr. W. R. Koob of Brayton, vice president; Dr. P. E. James of Elk Horn, secretary and treasurer; and Dr. L. E. Jensen of Audubon, delegate. The meeting was held in Audubon, Wednesday, December 6.

Black Hawk County Annual Meeting

Tuesday, December 19, members of the Black Hawk County Medical Society met for the regular annual election of officers. Dr. A. A. Hoffmann of Waterloo, was named president elect. New officers for 1934 are: Dr. J. R. Thompson, president; Dr. R. E. Russell, vice president; Dr. F. Harold Entz, secretary; Dr. George C. Murphy, treasurer; Dr. Thomas F. Thornton, delegate; and Dr. T. U. Mc-Manus, alternate delegate.

The following resolutions were unanimously passed:

Whereas, the present law of Iowa pertaining to the indigent sick (Perkins, Haskell-Klaus Law) seems to be inequitable, wasteful to society and the cause of considerable embarrassment to the indigent patients seeking relief;

Therefore, be it resolved, that the Black Hawk County Medical Society endorses paragraphs 1, 2 and 3 as recommended in the majority report of the Committee of Nine, which are as follows:

1. That half the basic cost of hospitalizing indigents be charged to the counties of their residence.

2. That investigation to determine indigency be made under the direction of the County Board of Supervisors.

3. That if an indigent person who can probably be benefited can be received at the University Hospitals within thirty days, except in obstetric and orthopedic cases, the court shall order him committed. If he cannot be received, the court shall order the county to provide immediate care at home or in a hospital.

Be it further resolved, that the remaining paragraphs of such report, involving purely economic questions, be omitted from our endorsement.

Eugene Smith, M.D., Secretary.

Bremer County Annual Meeting

The annual meeting of the Bremer County Medical Society was held Thursday, December 14, at the Mercy Hospital in Waverly. Arthur W. Erskine, M.D., of Cedar Rapids, delivered the address of the evening, speaking on the subject, Fractures of the Wrist. At the business meeting the following officers were elected to serve during 1934; Dr. F. J. Epen-

eter of Denver, president; Dr. L. D. Jay of Waverly, vice president; Dr. J. E. Whitmire of Sumner, secretary and treasurer; Dr. L. C. Kern of Waverly, delegate; and Dr. F. R. Sparks of Waverly, alternate delegate.

Buchanan County Annual Meeting

Members of the Buchanan County Medical Society enjoyed a six-thirty dinner at the Hotel Gedney in Independence, Thursday, December 7, followed by a program, at which James E. Whitmire, M.D., of Sumner, spoke on Appendicitis. Officers elected for the ensuing year are: Dr. J. W. Barrett of Independence, president; Dr. John F. Loeck of Aurora, vice president; Dr. M. C. Melrose of Independence, secretary and treasurer; Dr. H. A. Householder of Winthrop, delegate; and Dr. F. F. Agnew of Independence, alternate delegate.

Buena Vista County Annual Meeting

Results of the annual meeting of the Buena Vista County Medical Society, held in Storm Lake, Monday, December 11, are as follows: Dr. M. A. Armstrong of Newell, president; Dr. W. C. Porath of Storm Lake, vice president; and Dr. J. H. O'Donoghue of Storm Lake, secretary and treasurer.

Carroll County Annual Meeting

Wednesday, December 6, the Carroll County Medical Society held its annual meeting at St. Anthony's Hospital in Carroll. The scientific program was as follows: Birth Injuries, R. E. Crowder, M.D., of Sioux City; and Diseases of the Newborn, Robert H. McBride, M.D., also of Sioux City. At the business session, it was unanimously agreed to re-elect the present officers for the coming year. They are: Dr. D. H. Hopkins of Glidden, president; Dr. V. T. Lindsay of Glidden, vice president; Dr. Walter A. Anneberg of Carroll, secretary and treasurer; Dr. L. W. Chain of Dedham, delegate; and Dr. W. M. Shirley of Carroll, alternate delegate.

Walter A. Anneberg, M.D., Secretary.

Cerro Gordo County Annual Meeting

Dr. T. E. Davidson of Mason City, was elected president of the Cerro Gordo County Medical Society, at the annual meeting of that organization, held in Mason City, Tuesday, December 19. Dr. C. M. Franchere was named vice president, and Dr. William C. Egloff, was re-elected secretary and treasurer.

Cherokee County Annual Meeting

The Cherokee County Medical Society met in regular session in Cherokee, Tuesday, December 5, and elected the following officers to serve during 1934; Dr. John M. Pope of Cherokee, president; Dr.

Charles H. Swift, Jr., of Marcus, vice president; and Dr. Gerald D. Tipton of Cherokee, secretary and treasurer.

Clinton County Annual Meeting

At the annual meeting of the Clinton County Medical Society held at the Lafayette Hotel in Clinton, the following officers were elected: Dr. Ralph F. Luse, president; Dr. W. H. Foster, vice president; and Dr. Eugene V. Donlan, secretary and treasurer. At the close of the business meeting, a buffet luncheon was served, and a social time was enjoyed by the members present who represented a majority of the society.

A mis-statement appeared in last month's write-up of the Clinton county meeting, in regard to Dr. Starr's advice for the treatment of pernicious anemia. The explanation should be, "He told us that a blood count should be taken every month, even when the patient apparently felt well, gauging the maintenance dose on the laboratory finding only."

Ralph F. Luse, M.D., Secretary.

Crawford County Annual Meeting

Officers elected for the Crawford County Medical Society at the annual meeting held in Denison, December 12, are as follows: Dr. W. A. Garner of Kiron, president; Dr. C. L. Sievers of Denison, vice president; Dr. J. James Duffy of Denison, secretary and treasurer; Dr. H. W. Clasen of Denison, delegate; and Dr. Edward M. Mark of Manilla, alternate delegate.

Davis County Annual Meeting

The Davis County Medical Society met Friday, December 15, and elected Dr. C. D. Fenton of Bloomfield, president for the ensuing year. Dr. E. R. Newland of Drakesville was named vice president; and Dr. H. C. Young of Bloomfield was re-elected secretary and treasurer.

Decatur County Meetings

Friday, November 10, members of the Decatur County Medical Society met in Leon, and the scientific program was furnished by two Des Moines essayists. Douglas N. Gibson, M.D., presented a paper on Colles' Fracture, and Walter D. Abbott, M.D., spoke on Brain Injuries. Both addresses were illustrated with lantern slides, and both excellent papers were discussed by nearly everyone present. The evening's entertainment was opened by a sumptuous dinner furnished by the hospital trustees to the doctors of this county and their guests. This was followed by a short welcoming address, given by the superintendent, Miss Eva Green, on behalf of the hospital trustees. The meeting adjourned at a late hour with an inspection trip through the hospital by all the visiting physicians present.

The annual election of officers was held Friday, December 15, with the following results: Dr. J. W. Wailes of Davis City, president; Dr. C. A. Conklin of Garden Grove, vice president; Dr. J. E. McFarland of Leon, secretary and treasurer; Dr. G. P. Reed of Davis City, delegate; and Dr. Fred A. Bowman of Leon, alternate delegate. The society went on record as being unanimously in favor of the majority report of the committee investigating the University Hospitals.

M. W. Rogers, M.D., Secretary.

Dickinson County Annual Meeting

The annual meeting of the Dickinson County Medical Society was held in Spirit Lake at the Antlers Hotel, Thursday, December 7. Continuing the heart program outlined by the society at the beginning of the year, the topics for discussion were as follows: Mitral Valvular Disease, A. H. Schooley, M.D., of Terril; Treatment of Decompensation, W. E. Bullock, M.D., of Lake Park; Arteriosclerosis and Hypertension, F. J. Smith, M.D., of Milford; and Syphilis of the Heart, Q. C. Fuller, M. D., of Milford. The following officers were elected for 1934: Dr. Don E. Rodewig, president; Dr. C. S. Shultz, secretary and treasurer; Dr. C. G. Nicholson, delegate; and Dr. P. G. Grimm, alternate delegate. All officers are of Spirit Lake.

An invitation from the Emmet County Medical Society to hold joint meetings monthly during 1934, meeting alternately at Estherville and Spirit Lake, was unanimously accepted. The first of the joint meetings will be held at Estherville, Thursday, January 18.

C. S. Shultz, M.D., Secretary.

Dubuque County Annual Meeting

Dr. L. H. Fritz of Dubuque was named president of the Dubuque County Medical Society for the year 1934, at the annual meeting held at Leiser's, Sageville, Tuesday, December 12. Other officers are: Dr. F. P. McNamara, first vice president; Dr. R. C. Sherman of Farley, second vice president; Dr. D. F. Ward, secretary; Dr. F. W. Meyers, treasurer; Dr. Donald C. Conzett, delegate; and Dr. McNamara, alternate delegate.

Emmet County Annual Meeting

At the business meeting of the Emmet County Medical Society held in Estherville, Tuesday, December 5, the following officers were elected for the coming year: Dr. W. E. Bradley of Estherville, president; Dr. J. B. Knipe of Armstrong, vice president; Dr. Smith C. Kirkegaard of Ringsted, secretary and treasurer; Dr. Herbert D. Mereness of Dolliver, delegate; and Dr. C. E. Birney of Estherville, alternate delegate.

Floyd County

L. W. Clark, M.D., of Chester, and Thomas S. Walker, M.D., of Riceville, were guests and speakers at the scientific program of the Floyd County Medical Society and the Cedar Valley Hospital Clinical Society, presented at the Y. M. C. A., Tuesday, November 28. Dr. Clark spoke on Internal Hemorrhoids and· Their Treatment by Injection Methods, and Dr. Walker presented a paper on Varicose Veins of the Extremities.

Henry County Annual Meeting

The Henry County Medical Society held its regular monthly meeting at the Harlan Hotel in Mt. Pleasant, Tuesday, December 19, and elected the following officers for 1934: Dr. E. C. Allen of Wayland, president; Dr. Byron D. Hartley of Salem, vice president; Dr. J. W. Laird of Mt. Pleasant, secretary and treasurer; Dr. W. A. Sternberg of Mt. Pleasant, delegate; and Dr. Hartley, alternate delegate.

J. W. Laird, M.D., Secretary.

Iowa County Annual Meeting

Members of the Iowa County Medical Society met in Marengo, Friday, November 24. The scientific program consisted of a paper ·on Deafness from the Standpoint of the General Practitioner, by Carl A. Noe, M.D., of Amana, and an address on Nephritis in Children, by Morgan J. Foster, M.D., of Cedar Rapids. Officers elected at the business session are: Dr. C. H. Hermann of Amana, president; Dr. Thomas D. Clark of Victor, vice president; Dr. I. J. Sinn of Williamsburg, secretary and treasurer; Dr. C. F. Watts of Williamsburg, delegate; and Dr. J. L. Augustine of Ladora, alternate delegate.

Iowa County Annual Meeting

Dr. E. A. McMurray of Newton was re-elected president of the Jasper County Medical Society, when that organization met in Newton, Tuesday, December 5, for the annual election. Other officers are: Dr. H. W. Canfield of Baxter, vice president; and Dr. S. E. Hinshaw of Newton, secretary and treasurer.

Johnson County Annual Meeting

O. H. Plant, M.D., of Iowa City, furnished the scientific program when the Johnson County Medical Society met in Iowa City, Wednesday, December 6. Dr. Plant presented an illustrated lecture on The Effect of Opium and Its Derivatives on the Muscular Activities of the Alimentary Canal. Officers elected at the business session are: Dr. Matt Ware of West Branch, president; Dr. H. Dabney Kerr of Iowa City, vice president; Dr. H. M. Korns of Iowa City, secretary and treasurer; Dr. Ewen M. MacEwen of Iowa City, and Dr. George C. Albright of Iowa City, delegates; and Dr. E. D. Plass of Iowa City, and Dr. Milford E. Barnes of Iowa City, alternate delegates.

Lee County Annual Meeting

Thursday, December 21, members of the Lee County Medical Society met in Fort Madison for the annual election of officers. Results are: Dr. Frank R. Richmond of Fort Madison, president; Dr. A. A. Johnstone of Keokuk, vice president; Dr. Blinn Dorsey of Keokuk, secretary and treasurer; Dr. B. J. Dierker of Fort Madison, delegate; and Dr. Frank M. Fuller of Keokuk, alternate delegate.

Linn County Meetings

The December 21 meeting of the Linn County Medical Society was attended by about 250 physicians from various parts of the state. Following a six-thirty dinner at the Hotel Montrose, Frank H. Lahey, M.D., of Boston, gave an excellent presentation of The Treatment of Thyroid Disease and Associated Conditions. His address was discussed by Drs. O. J. Fay of Des Moines, W. A. Rohlf of Waverly, F. R. Peterson of Iowa City, and Charles Krause of Cedar Rapids. Roy K. Keech, M.D., of Cedar Rapids, read a paper on Fractures of the Elbow and Complications.

On Thursday, January 11, Walter A. Fansler, M.D., of Minneapolis, will conduct an operative clinic at St. Luke's Hospital at 3:00 P. M. Following a dinner at the Hotel Roosevelt, Dr. Fansler will deliver an address on What the Doctor Should Tell His Patient When He Presents Himself with Carcinoma of the Rectum.

T. F. Hersch, M.D., Secretary.

Marion County Annual Meeting

The Marion County Medical Society met Thursday, December 21, in Knoxville for a dinner and business session. The program included the president's annual address, which was delivered by Dr. Frank P. Ralston, retiring president, and a paper on The Relationship of the Board of Supervisors and the County Medical Society, read by Mrs. M. D. Twitty, county social worker. Newly elected officers for 1934 are: Dr. E. P. Bell of Pleasantville, president; Dr. A. E. Reiter of Melcher, vice president; Dr. C. S. Cornell of Knoxville, secretary and treasurer. Dr. E. C. McClure of Bussey, delegate; and Dr. H. L. Bridgeman of Knoxville, alternate delegate.

Marshall County Annual Meeting

Dr. A. R. Lynn of Marshalltown was named president of the Marshall County Medical Society at a meeting held Thursday, December 14. Other officers are: Dr. L. E. Noble of Rhodes, vice president; Dr. G. E. Hermence of Marshalltown, secretary and treasurer; Dr. A. D. Woods of State Center, delegate; and Dr. J. J. Noonan of Marshalltown, alternate delegate. Otis R. Wolfe, M.D., of Marshalltown, presented an illustrated lecture on Spain, and explained new methods of removing cataract.

Mills County Annual Meeting

The annual meeting of the Mills County Medical Society was held at the state institution in Glenwood, Thursday, December 7. George M. Agan, M.D., of Glenwood, delivered a paper on Current Medical Economics, which was generally discussed. An interesting addition to the planned program was an extemporaneous address by George Mogridge, M.D., of Glenwood, on Eugenic Sterilization. At the business meeting it was unanimously voted to re-elect the present officers to serve during 1934. They are: Dr. H. B. Dye of Glenwood, president; Dr. J. M. Donelan of Glenwood, secretary and treasurer; Dr. I. U. Parsons of Malvern, delegate; and Dr. Donelan, alternate delegate.

J. M. Donelan, M.D., Secretary.

Monroe County Annual Meeting

Thursday, December 14, the Monroe County Medical Society met in Albia for the annual election of officers which resulted as follows: Dr. S. T. Gray of Albia, president; Dr. J. F. Stafford of Lovilia, vice president; Dr. T. A. Moran of Melrose, secretary and treasurer.

Muscatine County Annual Meeting

The Muscatine County Medical Society held a meeting Wednesday, December 15, and elected officers for the coming year as follows: Dr. B. E. Eversmeyer, president; Dr. C. P. Phillips, vice president; Dr. R. R. Goad, secretary and treasurer; Dr. L. C. Howe, delegate; and Dr. T. I. Wigim, alternate delegate. All officers are of Muscatine.

C. P. Phillips, M.D., Secretary.

O'Brien County Annual Meeting

Dr. W. R. Brock of Sheldon was elected president of the O'Brien County Medical Society for 1934, at a meeting held in Primghar, Tuesday, December 12. Other officers are: Dr. LeRoy Avery of Primghar, vice president; Dr. J. W. Myers of Sheldon, secretary and treasurer; Dr. Avery, delegate; and Dr. T. D. Kas of Sutherland, alternate delegate.

Polk County Annual Meeting

The annual meeting of the Des Moines Academy of Medicine and Polk County Medical Society was held at the Hotel Fort Des Moines, Tuesday, December 19, at which time Dr. Fred Moore took office as president of the organization. Dr. George A. May was named president-elect, and Dr. Leonard A. West was elected secretary and treasurer.

Pottawattamie County Annual Meeting

Dr. C. F. Baumeister of Avoca was elected president of the Pottawattamie County Medical Society at its meeting Thursday, December 14. Other officers are: Dr. Raymond M. Rice of Council Bluffs, vice president; Dr. Arnold L. Jensen of Council Bluffs, secretary and treasurer; Dr. F. Earl Bellinger of Council Bluffs, delegate; and Dr. Gerald V. Caughlan of Council Bluffs, alternate delegate.

Poweshiek County Annual Meeting

Tuesday, December 5, the Poweshiek County Medical Society met at the Community Hospital in Grinnell. A short business meeting was held at which the following officers were elected: Dr. E. J. Ringena of Brooklyn, president; Dr. C. D. Busby of Brooklyn, vice president; Dr. C. V. Lawton of Grinnell, secretary; Dr. J. T. Padgham of Grinnell, treasurer; Dr. E. B. Williams of Montezuma, delegate; and Dr. Busby, alternate delegate. The scientific program consisted of a paper on Water Homeostasis, read by John Parish, M.D., of Grinnell. Dr. Charles B. Taylor of Ottumwa, president of the State Society was a guest of the society, and spoke briefly of plans for the annual session.

C. V. Lawton, M.D., Secretary.

Scott County

James G. Carr, M.D., professor of medicine, Northwestern University, Chicago, was the speaker of the evening when the Scott County Medical Society met in Davenport, Tuesday, December 5. Following the six-thirty dinner, Dr. Carr delivered his address on Cardiovascular Diseases and Cardiac Pain.

Story County Annual Meeting

Following a joint meeting of the Boone and Story County Medical Societies, at Ames, Tuesday, December 19, the Story county group held a business session at which officers for 1934 were elected. They are: Dr. H. W. Bowers of Nevada, president; Dr. G. E. McFarland of Ames, vice president; Dr. W. B. Sperow of Nevada, secretary and treasurer; Dr. E. B. Bush of Ames, delegate; and Dr. W. B. Armstrong of Ames, alternate delegate.

Wapello County Meetings

Tuesday, November 21, the Wapello County Medical Society and Sunnyslope Sanatorium were hosts to the Ninth Councilor District, and physicians from Washington, Henry, Jefferson, and Van Buren counties. The program was presented as printed in last month's JOURNAL, with the exception of the toastmaster. Because of Dr. Peck's inability to attend the meeting, Dr. Daniel J. Glomset, of Des Moines, kindly consented to assume this responsibility. His performance was perfect. The two hour social dinner was resplendent with many witty and appreciative toasts.

Tuesday, December 5, the annual meeting of the Wapello County Medical Society was held at the St. Joseph Hospital in Ottumwa. Dr. J. C. Kepler of Kirkville was elected president; Dr. L. H. Prewitt of Ottumwa was named vice president; Dr. Evon Walker of Ottumwa was re-elected secretary and treasurer; Dr. F. L. Nelson of Ottumwa was re-elected delegate; and Dr. E. B. Howell of Ottumwa was named alternate delegate. The scientific program was furnished by E. B. Howell, M.D., of Ottumwa, who read a paper on Biliary Infections; the discussion was led by W. C. Newell, M.D., of Ottumwa.

The next outstanding program of the Wapello County Medical Society will be on Tuesday, January 16, when Frank Smithies, M.D., professor of medicine, University of Illinois, Chicago, will deliver an illustrated lecture on Newer Knowledge Concerned with the Diagnosis, Prognosis and Treatment of Peptic Ulcers. Dr. Smithies will conduct a medical clinic at the St. Joseph Hospital at 10:00 A. M. There will be a cover charge for the dinner meeting, and anyone wishing to attend will be very welcome. However, they should notify the secretary of their intentions to do so, in order that ample provisions may be made for all who attend.

Evon Walker, M.D., Secretary.

Washington County Annual Meeting

The election of officers for the Washington County Medical Society which took place Tuesday, December

12, resulted as follows: Dr. A. L. Braden of Wellman, president; Dr. W. L. Alcorn of Washington, vice president; Dr. W. S. Kyle of Washington, secretary and treasurer; Dr. Alcorn, delegate; and Dr. E. E. Stutsman of Washington, alternate delegate.

Webster County Annual Meeting
Dr. L. L. Leighton of Fort Dodge was elected to head the Webster County Medical Society during 1934, at the annual election of that organization held Friday, December 8. Other officers are: Dr. H. M. Kiesling of Lehigh, vice president; Dr. John C. Shrader of Fort Dodge, secretary and treasurer; Dr. Roland Stahr of Fort Dodge, delegate; and Dr. J. H. Bruce of Fort Dodge, alternate delegate.

Woodbury County Annual Meeting
The Woodbury County Medical Society conducted its regular monthly meeting Tuesday, December 19, at the Martin Hotel in Sioux City. The following officers were elected: Dr. L. R. Tripp, president; Dr. R. H. McBride, vice president; Dr. Lawrence E. Pierson, secretary and treasurer; Dr. T. R. Gittins, delegate; and Dr. Roy E. Crowder, alternate delegate. After the election a smoker and social evening was enjoyed by the members.

L. E. Pierson, M.D., Secretary.

Four County District Medical Society
The regular winter meeting of the Four County District Medical Society, comprised of members from Buena Vista, Cherokee, Ida and Plymouth counties, was held in Cherokee, Thursday, December 14. After the six-thirty dinner, the following program was presented: Present Day Knowledge of Strabismus and Its Treatment, J. E. Dvorak, M.D., Sioux City; Treatment of Acute Middle Ear Disease, M. J. Joynt, M.D., of LeMars; Ante Partum Hemorrhage, T. R. Campbell, M.D., of Sioux Rapids; and Toxemia in Pregnancy, R. B. Armstrong, M.D., of Ida Grove.

Iowa Academy of Ophthalmology and Otolaryngology
The fourth annual meeting of the Iowa Academy of Ophthalmology and Otolaryngology was held in Des Moines, Tuesday, December 5. At the business session the following officers were elected for 1934: Dr. W. F. Boiler of Iowa City, president; Dr. Dean M. Lierle of Iowa City, vice president; and Dr. L. A. Taylor of Ottumwa, secretary and treasurer.

Sixth Councilor District Meeting
Members of the Hardin County Medical Society were hosts to physicians in the Sixth Councilor District when that organization met in Eldora, Tuesday, December 5. Mr. E. H. Mulock, state director of the federal relief administration was a guest, and addressed the group on the civil works program, its aims and objectives. Thomas A. Burcham, M.D., of Des Moines, chairman of the committee on public policy and legislation, spoke on Legislative Activities of the State Society; and Robert L. Parker, M.D., of Des Moines, secretary of the state society, discussed Society Membership.

Southwest Iowa Postgraduate Medical Society
Dr. Benjamin S. Barnes of Shenandoah was named president of the Southwest Iowa Postgraduate Medical Society at the meeting held in Atlantic. Monday, November 27. Dr. J. F. Aldrich, also of Shenandoah, was elected secretary and treasurer.

INTERESTING NEWS
In Brief
A new tasteless quinine has been recently prepared synthetically.

The present enrollment of the medical school at Iowa City is quoted as 329. Of this number only 18 are residents from outside the state.

The 1933 meeting of the American Association for the Advancement of Science was held in Boston from Wednesday, December 27 to Tuesday, January 2.

Recent international statistics on mortality for diabetes place the United States at the top of the list with a rate of 26.3 for each 100,000 persons in 1932.

British Red Cross chapters have been organized and are now training detachments for air ambulance service, fully instructing each member in first aid work and in litter bearing.

A successful attempt to treat bichloride of mercury poisoning has been announced by the United States National Institute of Health employing formaldehyde sulfoxylate.

Sixty-eight physicians, members of the Scott County Medical Society, were awarded the contract for the care of the county poor for the ensuing year at a figure said to be $25,752.

A new chemical preparation designated as 3-5 diiodothyronine has been successfully used in the treatment of myxedema by a group of English scientists. The preparation is administered orally.

A new universal growth-promoting acid, termed pantothenic acid, has recently been described. Its discoverers state "that it is more widely distributed in nature than any known physiologically potent substance."

The Annual Convention of Phi Beta Pi, a national medical fraternity, held in Iowa City December 26 to 30, was attended by representatives from forty-four chapters located in class A medical colleges throughout the United States.

Employing the sound recording device used in motion picture work, a London neurologist is studying irregularities of speech, particularly that of disseminated sclerosis. His observations so far indicate that this method is of value in differential diagnosis of this and like conditions.

An acid prepared from paprika and designated as "paprika acid" has been used successfully in Denmark for the treatment of scurvy. It is likely that paprika acid is identical to ascorbic acid, which is generally thought to be identical with Vitamin C.

The Board of Supervisors of Winneshiek county and Webster county have each advertised for bids for the medical and surgical care of the poor within the respective counties. This work for the past year in Winneshiek county has been carried on under a contract drawn with the Winneshiek County Medical Society.

Observations made in the Michigan Department of Health where bacteriophage has been employed in the treatment of a number of bacterial diseases for the past several years, would indicate that bacteriophage is not a toxin and is not itself an antitoxin, but it produces or stimulates the production of antitoxin in the body.

X-ray in the treatment of cancerous disease is now employed for as long as twenty hours out of the twenty-four, the x-ray being used with low voltage and remote from the patient. "Experience with this method in 134 cases over a period of two years indicates that it is a valuable addition to the treatment of several radio-sensitive tumor processes."

PERSONAL MENTION

Dr. Draper Long of Mason City spoke before members of the Phalanx fraternity, Wednesday, December 20, on the subject, "Anesthetics."

Dr. J. N. Kenefick of Algona addressed the local Rotary Club, Monday, December 18, on "The Progress of Medical Science."

Dr. R. A. Stewart of Independence, addressed the Clarksville Lions Club, Monday, December 4. He spoke on "Mental Hygiene and Insanity."

Dr. Thomas W. McMeans, who was graduated from the State University of Iowa College of Medicine in 1931, has located for practice in Davenport with offices at 1027 Davenport Bank Building. After finishing a year's internship at the United States Marine Hospital in San Francisco, Dr. McMeans became a ship's surgeon for the McCormick Steamship Lines.

Dr. F. L. Knowles of Fort Dodge, addressed the American Academy of Orthopedic Surgeons, at a meeting held in Chicago, January 7, 8, and 9. Dr. Knowles spoke on "Hip Fractures," and illustrated his paper with moving pictures.

Dr. C. A. Henry of Farson, who has been ill for several weeks, is now showing some improvement.

Dr. R. O. Hughes, pediatrician of Ottumwa, was recently operated upon for appendicitis. He recovered nicely, and is back to work now.

Dr. Charles Obermann of Clarinda spoke before the local Hi-Y Club, Thursday, November 23, on "Mental Hygiene."

Dr. Grant D. Bullock, formerly of Calumet, has opened an office in Washta for the practice of medicine.

Dr. D. J. Keating, formerly of Dubuque, has opened an office in Ottumwa for the practice of medicine.

MARRIAGES

Friday, December 28, the marriage of Miss Eleanor Cherney of Independence and Dr. Keith W. Woodhouse of Van Horne, took place at the bride's home in Independence. The bridegroom is a son of Dr. and Mrs. G. R. Woodhouse of Vinton, and was graduated from the State University of Iowa College of Medicine in 1932. The young couple will make their home in Van Horne, where Dr. Woodhouse is practicing medicine.

The marriage of Miss Edith Robinson of New York to Dr. Hyman M. Hurevitz of Iowa City, took place at the St. George Hotel in New York City, Sunday, November 12. After a short honeymoon at Atlantic City, Dr. and Mrs. Hurevitz returned to Iowa City, where the bridegroom is a staff member of the faculty at the College of Medicine.

DEATH NOTICES

Dilley, Harry Horace, of Des Moines, aged forty-one, died December 13, as a result of uremic poisoning. He was graduated in 1917 from Rush Medical College, and at the time of his death was a member of the Polk County Medical Society.

Singleton, Eustace, of Marshalltown, aged sixty-nine, died November 29, following a short illness. He was graduated in 1891 from Northwestern University Medical School, and at the time of his death was a member of the Marshall County Medical Society.

INTER-PROFESSIONAL ASSOCIATION IN WINNESHIEK COUNTY

The Winneshiek County Inter-professional Health Association was organized at a meeting held in Decorah, Thursday, December 14. Officers elected were: Dr. T. N. Stabo, president; Dr. G. R. Luce, first vice president; Mr. Roy Darling, second vice president; Miss Thompson, R.N., third vice president; Dr. W. L. Strunk, secretary; and Dr. C. P. Wilson, treasurer. A code and by-laws were adopted, providing for three meetings a year. The purpose of the association is to promote health matters in the county by the intelligent cooperation of physicians, dentists, pharmacists, nurses, veterinarians, and others interested in public welfare.

HISTORY OF MEDICINE IN IOWA

Edited by the Historical Committee

DR. HENRY B. YOUNG, Burlington
DR. FRANK M. FULLER, Keokuk
DR. JOHN T. McCbhrison, Iowa City

DR. TOM. B. THROCKMORTON, Des Moines
DR. WALTER L. BIERRING, Des Moines

An Historic Paper
Relation of Micro-organisms to Disease

Presented before the Polk County Medical Society,
May, 1866

A. G. FIELD, M.D.,
Des Moines

The conjecture that micro-organisms are in some way concerned in the causation of disease is of very early date. In our own country, early in the present century, Dr. Holland wrote upon the subject after, as he states, having had it under consideration and observation for a period of over thirty years. Dr. Holland does not appear to have attempted to bring the microscope into use in the course of his observations, and any verification by cultivation and inoculation was then unthought of. His treatment of the subject is confined entirely to logical sequences observed in the phenomena and clinical history of disease. From these he concluded that some of these invisible organisms had means of aerial migration, regardless of courses of atmospheric currents, and he therefore believed that they were both animal and vegetable. The logical sequence and its phenomena led him to believe that cholera was due to an animal parasite instead of bacillus or vegetable, as later claimed by Dr. Koch.

As far back as the twelfth century we find evidence of a belief among medical men that some sort of poison was peculiar to or had a constant abode or habitat in particular localities which they called "genius epidemicus."

Diodorus in attempting to account for a virulent outbreak of the plague is recorded as having said that great multitudes of people streamed into the city from all quarters, and being cramped for room, breathed corrupted air.

Sanitary regulations were also instituted in the early civilizations which implies a belief in disease poisons which were self propagating under sanitary conditions, moisture, filth and neglected habitations.

In the fourteenth century black death, the most virulent of all pestilences of history, decimated whole districts and paralyzed the energies of nearly the whole civilized world.

As far back as the Roman Empire, Vairo and Columetta attributed malarious fevers to low organisms supposed to have found entrance into the blood.

The mere conjecture derived some support shortly after, when, with such rude microscopes as had then been constructed, minute forms of both animal and vegetable life were first brought to view. The discovery of the animal-like forms of spermatozoa by Lewenhoeck in 1677 was accepted as evidence that animals infested the human body, not only in disease, but in health also; and from this the notion became prevalent that in hideous forms and variegated colors the air was filled with the minute organisms whose business it was to shake off the shackles of human life whenever they should find access to the human body. Among the sanitary reforms one writer recommended the sounding of trumpets during prevailing epidemics, to drive away the pestilence. The extravagant claims of the advocates, unsupported by scarcely any unequivocal demonstration of truth, soon brought ridicule and silence; but there was still the belief in the minds of thinking men that some extraneous and foreign agencies, living or otherwise, by finding entrance into the body, caused disease and that as a germ it slumbered through the vicissitudes.

In the meantime, the phenomena of fermentation and its analogy to the progressive history of disease began to be regarded with favor. Stahl in 1831 arrived at the conclusion that fermentation and putrefaction were at least analogous processes; and soon followed a recognition of the striking analogies between both of these processes and that of epidemic and endemic diseases. Asteir in 1813, acting upon an already recognized fact that fermentation was something more than mere chemical action, proposed to use as remedies in the treatment of diseases such agencies as arrested fermentation, the phenomena of which had been announced to be a propagation and growth of minute organisms. This doctrine met with but little opposition until about 1840, when Liebig, who had already begun to be acknowledged as an authority, combatted the doctrine of the whole germ theory, not even acknowledging the existence of the yeast cell or other similar factors. From his standpoint all pathological changes were purely chemical, and his argument was so convincing that his followers were numerous. Hence arose the two sects, the humorists after Liebig, and the advocates of the germ theory after Schwann.

The perfection of microscopes and the multiplication of evidences has left for the humoral side of the problem, as advocated by Liebig, but little, if any support, and the means of verification found in cultivation and inoculation, as introduced about the middle of the present century by Needham of London and Spaldanzani of Italy, sustained the other side of the controversy. The studies and methods of Pasteur are familiar to all, but without detracting from the great service he has done the world as a biologist and sagacious philosopher, it is apparent that in the role of plain pathologist and medical man, with hydrophobia as his subject, he has been a failure.

Bastian followed Liebig with advocacy of molecular motion, passing over into vital forms constituting spontaneous generation.

Schroeder, in 1854, had found that floating atmospherical germs could be collected, and Schwann's and Pasteur's labors led to the idea of antiseptic surgery, of which Lister became the leading exponent; and, influenced by him, the system was adopted in all of the leading hospitals of Europe.

Without taking further time to refer to the history of the theory to which Rindflesch contributed, by finding micro-organisms in the tissues of traumatic diseases, as well as Hirschfield in finding micro-organisms in the pus cell incident to the first appearance of pyaemia, it is sufficient to say that among converts were Thiersch, Lister, Billroth, Virchow, Klebs and others.

Against this array of high authority it is proper to say that Beal has been an opponent of the theory, regarding the microbes found as the degraded offspring of broken-down tissues; and Dr. B. F. Richardson of London had much the same views.

The following may be summed up as representing the present state of medical opinion:

1st. That bacteria do exist in the air we breathe, the food we eat, in the secretions of the mouth and mucous membrane, etc.

2d. That of the many forms, but few are poisonous or in any manner concerned in the causation of disease.

3d. That all persons are not equally susceptible to poisons, nor the same person at all times equally so.

4th. That as there is a difference in the susceptibility of different individuals to any given kind of poison bacteria, so there is a still greater difference between the different kinds of animals as to susceptibility, rendering the experiments by inoculation uncertain.

5th. That it is the life products or life waste rather than the bodies of bacteria themselves that embody the poison, and that by cleanliness and antiseptics the poisons are diminished, regardless of the presence of the parasites.

6th. That while the presumption is strong that all infectious and contagious diseases, including endemics, are due either directly or indirectly to specific forms of germ poison, there are as yet but a few in which the poison has been satisfactorily identified.

COMMENT

Dr. Archelaus G. Field was one of the most interesting men in Iowa medicine. His biography has been published in Fairchild's History of Medicine in Iowa. The above paper was included in a small monograph of collected papers under the title "Foot Prints Made in the Dark" issued by Dr. Field in 1910. Dr. Field served as Secretary of the Iowa State Medical Society from 1869 to 1872 and was elected President in 1872. He died in 1924 at the age of ninety-five years.

W. L. B.

TURKISH LICENSURE REGULATIONS

In order to become a practicing physician in Turkey, the doctor must now become a citizen of the country and after that it is necessary to comply with some very rigid restrictions. A foreign doctor holding a teaching position in a government institution is not permitted to engage in any private practice, but he may be called for consultation.

The History of Medicine in Lucas County

Tom Morford Throckmorton, A.M., M.D.,
Chariton

Tom Bentley Throckmorton, B.Sc., M.D.,
Des Moines

(Continued from last month)

PHYSICIANS WHO HAVE PRACTICED IN LUCAS

The town of Lucas came into existence May 9, 1868. Two years previous the Burlington and Missouri River Railroad Company, predecessors of the Chicago, Burlington and Quincy Railroad, had constructed its road through Lucas County and had located a station named Lucas in Jackson township. Accordingly, H. S. Russell, who platted the town of Russell, likewise laid out and platted the town of Lucas. It consisted of twelve blocks and contained one hundred and eight lots. It was not until the discovery of coal in the vicinity, in 1876, that the town began to grow. For many years the mining of coal was the principal industry of the community. Consequently a large number of the inhabitants of the town were miners. That they should receive adequate medical and surgical care was important; hence many of the physicians who located in the new town became contract surgeons for the various companies which operated the local mines.

Dr. W. A. Sawyer

The first physician, of whom we have any record, to locate in Lucas, was Dr. W. A. Sawyer. He came from the Empire state, New York, to Iowa, in 1870. Just where the doctor had received his medical education and training is unknown; nor do we know where he first located when he came to Iowa. He became a resident of the town of Lucas in 1876. Two years later he moved to a farm in English township. Where he went after his removal to the farm is not a matter of record.

Dr. S. G. Wright

Dr. S. G. Wright was a graduate of the Bennett Medical College, Chicago, Illinois, in the class of 1874. He was located in Lucas in 1876. There is no record of when he came to the town or when he departed from it.

Dr. R. M. DeWitt

Dr. R. M. DeWitt, the third physician to locate in Lucas, was a native of New York. He was born November 8, 1849. At the age of fourteen years he enlisted in Company C. Ninth New York Heavy Artillery and served with it for ten months. He was with General Sheridan in all the engagements of his army in the Shenandoah Valley

region; he also took part in the Petersburg engagement. He rode as an orderly for Sheridan and was present at the final capitulation of General Lee at Appomattox. He was honorably discharged from the army in July, 1865; after which he went to Michigan. Sometime later he came to Iowa, where he was engaged in teaching school and in reading medicine. He attended medical lectures in the College of Physicians and Surgeons, at Keokuk, and was graduated in the class of 1877. He at once located in Lucas and began the practice of medicine. He was soon the leading physician in that thriving village and also the owner of a drugstore. The doctor moved to Des Moines, Polk County, about 1885.

Dr. D. W. Williams

Dr. D. W. Williams was a native of South Wales, England. He was born October 15, 1838. He began the study of medicine before coming to America, having attended medical lectures at St. Thomas Medical College in London, in 1856. In 1857 he came to the United States and went to New Orleans, where he entered the Louisiana Medical College from which institution he was graduated in 1859. He then began the practice of medicine in New Orleans. In 1862 he went to Wisconsin, where he joined the colors and was appointed Assistant Surgeon in the Seventeenth Wisconsin Infantry. He served in that capacity until he was mustered out of the service in August, 1865. During the Civil War, Dr. Williams witnessed the bloody fields of Shiloh, Corinth, and those of other engagements. He was with General Sherman's army on its "march to the sea." During that campaign he was captured, July 22, 1864; and later was taken to Andersonville prison. Fortunately he was exchanged the following October, after which he immediately joined his old command. He received an honorable discharge at the close of the war.

Dr. Williams came to Lucas in 1879. He soon gained the respect of the community and became a successful physician. He was married twice. His first wife was a Miss Means. By this union he had three children; Carrie M., Ida M., and David Hayes. His second wife was Miss Emily Kitto, a daughter of John Kitto, a native of England, who came to Lucas County and was for many years, as a resident of Lucas, interested in the mining industry. Dr. Williams and Miss Kitto were married in Lucas, December 22, 1880. There were no children by this union. The doctor died at his home in Lucas and his body was buried in the country cemetery a few miles from the town.

Dr. Thomas Croston

Perhaps one of the most colorful physicians ever to practice in Lucas was the late Thomas Croston. He was a son of Henry and Ellen (Williams) Croston of Manchester, England. He was born in Wigau, England, December 12, 1846. He came to Iowa in 1879 and immediately located in Lucas. While in England, he had received some instruction under Dr. John Skelton, the

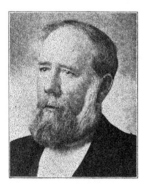

Thomas Croston, M.D.
1846-1922

author of some medical works of the eclectic school of medicine. After coming to Lucas the doctor became connected with the operating of the coal mines about the town; especially in treating the miners and their families. He bought good medical books, of the regular school of medicine, and became quite proficient in treating the ills and ailments of the people. He was popular as a citizen and was elected to positions of honor and trust. He was a member of the board of education for many years, and he served on the city council for six years. He was the local health officer for four years, and filled the office of mayor for several terms. The doctor belonged to the Masonic Order; also to the Independent Order of Odd Fellows. Dr. Croston was married in England to Miss Eliza Fletcher, in 1868. This union was blessed by three children; Ellen Ernest

and George. The doctor died from the effect of a strangulated hernia, August 12, 1922. His body was interred in the Lucas cemetery.

Dr. George Colville Croston

Dr. George Colville Croston was the son of Dr. Thomas and Eliza (Fletcher) Croston. He was born in Bolton, England, December 11, 1877. He came with his parents to Lucas in 1879. Here he grew up with the town and attended its schools. He was married to Ina Belle Clouse, of Troy, Iowa, September 20, 1899. He began the study of medicine in his father's office and later matriculated in the Medical Department of Northwestern University, Chicago, Illinois, from which institution he received his doctor's degree in the class of 1905. Following his graduation he returned to Lucas, where he was associated with his father for a few years. He then moved to Sapulpa, Oklahoma, where he has continued in the practice of his chosen profession.

Dr. George Warrette Dosh

Dr. George Warrette Dosh was born in Albany, New York, in 1853. There is no record as to the time he came to Iowa. He attended Grinnell College at Grinnell, Iowa, and was graduated from that institution in 1872. He later attended medical lectures in Chicago, and received his doctor of medicine degree from Rush Medical College of that city, in 1879. Evidently the doctor still continued in search of more knowledge, for he became a student in the Des Moines School of Pharmacy and was graduated from it in 1883. He then located in Lucas and divided his time between the practice of medicine and the drug business. After a stay of about five years in the town, the doctor moved to Brighton, Washington County, Iowa. Here he resided for many years. Dr. Dosh was married to Miss Mary Wineman of Malcolm, Iowa. He died in Brighton, about 1930.

Dr. Charles Herman DeWitt

Dr. Charles Herman DeWitt, a brother of Dr. R. M. DeWitt, was born in New York in 1859. Evidently he migrated westward, perhaps stimulated by the suggestion of Horace Greeley "Go West, young man," for he enrolled as a student in the College of Physicians and Surgeons in Chicago, and was graduated from that school in March, 1883. Four years later he located in Lucas, where he became one of the leading physicians of that community. He afterwards moved to Glenwood, Mills County, Iowa, where he continued to practice for many years. The doctor died in Glenwood, October 13, 1931, at the age of seventy-two years.

(To be continued next month)

THE JOURNAL BOOK SHELF

BOOKS RECEIVED

SURGICAL CLINICS OF NORTH AMERICA—Volume xiii, No. 4, Mayo Clinic Number, August, 1933. Per clinic year, February, 1933, to December, 1933. Octavo of 215 pages with 65 illustrations. W. B. Saunders Company, 1933. Price, paper, $12.00; cloth, $16.00.

THE SURGICAL CLINICS OF NORTH AMERICA—Volume xiii, No. 5, Chicago Number, October, 1933. Per clinic year, February, 1933, to December, 1933. OctaVo of 254 pages with 93 illustrations. W. B. Saunders Company, Philadelphia and London. Price, paper, $12.00; cloth, $16.00.

A TEXTBOOK OF PHYSIOLOGY ... Ph.D., M.D., Sc.D., LL.D., Emeritus Professor of Physiology in the Johns Hopkins University, Baltimore, Maryland. Twelfth Edition, thoroughly revised. 1132 pages with 308 illustrations. W. B. Saunders Company, Philadelphia and London, 1933. Price, $7.00.

THE YEAR BOOK OF GENERAL MEDICINE, 1933. Edited by George F. Dick, M.D., Lawrason Brown, M.D., George R. Minot, M.D., William B. Castle, M.D., William D. Stroud, M.D., and George B. Eusterman, M.D. The Year Book Publishers, Chicago. Price, $3.00.

BOOK REVIEWS

ANNUAL REPORT OF THE ROCKEFELLER FOUNDATION FOR 1932

Including the reports of the secretary and treasurer, the director of the International Health Division, and the directors for the medical sciences, natural sciences, social sciences, and humanities. Printed by The Rockefeller Foundation, 49 West 49th Street, New York City.

This Annual Report covers the work of the Foundation in the medical, natural and social sciences, and the humanities in the International Health Division. Advances in the control of yellow fever, malaria, and hookworm disease are presented in considerable detail. Researches in public health, particularly those directed toward the study of the common cold, undulant fever, yaws and tuberculosis are reviewed in a comprehensive fashion.

The Report presents a very interesting study of the expenditure of some $13,000,000 by the Foundation in the advancement of its many projects.

LIFE BEGINS AT FORTY

By Walter B. Pitkin, professor in journalism, Columbia University. McGraw-Hill Book Company, New York and London, 1932. Price, $1.50.

The author of this book, an educator of national distinction, is apparently an advanced psychologist and a close observer of human traits. In this book he successfully defends his predication that life after forty is fuller and more abounding in the worthwhile things than that under this period.

The author achieves his aim without resort to flimsy, "Pollyanna" methods. His discourse is logical and apparently accurate. "Bacteria, insects, mice and fools die young. The superior man barely strikes his pace at an age when the inferior passes his prime."

Written in a wholesome, easy to read style, this volume will appeal to physician and layman alike, and is especially recommended to those individuals who feel that all of life's work and ambition should be crowded in its accomplishment into those early years immediately following his entrance into the business or professional life.

Dr. Pitkin's book, a direct challenge to the gloom of advancing years, should find a place in the library of the physician particularly, since he perhaps, because of his own observations with the vicissitudes of life, often needs the buoyant encouragement which this volume offers.

MAYO FOUNDATION LECTURES ON THE HISTORY OF MEDICINE

A series of lectures at the Mayo Foundation and at the Universities of Minnesota, Wisconsin, Iowa, Northwestern, and the Des Moines Academy of Medicine, given between 1926 and 1932. Octavo of 516 pages with 26 illustrations. W. B. Saunders Company, Philadelphia and London, 1933. Price, $5.00.

Between the years of 1926 and 1932 a series of lectures dealing with the history of medicine were delivered under the auspices of the Mayo Foundation and a group of other scientific bodies in Minnesota, Iowa, and Wisconsin. In Iowa the Des Moines Academy of Medicine and the Medical School of the University at Iowa City each subscribed to the course.

To those members of these Iowa bodies who had the privilege of personally hearing one or more of these lectures, this volume will need no recommendation. To those unacquainted with the series it may be stated that the lectures were not planned with the thought of completely or systematically covering the field of medical history. The several distinguished speakers were invited to prepare addresses and were allowed complete freedom in the selection of their various themes. The results, as compiled in this volume, offer the reader a survey of many of the outstanding characters and developments in medical history, each complete in itself and presented in a most fascinating style.

As an inspirational, educational and informative volume, this collection of addresses is outstanding and richly merits the careful attention of every physician.

THE YEAR BOOK OF RADIOLOGY

Edited by Charles A. Waters, M.D., associate in roentgenology, Johns Hopkins University, and Ira I. Kaplan, M.D., director, division of cancer, Department of Hospitals, City of New York. The Year Book Publishers, Chicago, Illinois, 1933. Price, $7.00.

The Year Book Publishers now present the second annual edition of the Year Book of Radiology, a newcomer to the line of long established Year Books offered by these publishers to the medical profession. Apparently the reception accorded the 1932 Year Book of Radiology encouraged the publishers in continuing this valuable work, although the project has not yet become a financially profitable one.

The volume is divided into two sections, the one dealing with radiologic diagnosis, and the second with radiotherapeutics. In the former the year's advances in diagnostic radiology are discussed by systems with concluding chapters on technic. In the section on radiotherapeutics, the theory, biology and physics of radiation are presented followed by chapters dealing with the employment of this therapy in lesions of the various sections of the body such as the bones, skin, breasts, pelvic organs, etc. A final chapter in this section deals with "Injuries in Radiation Therapy."

Except for the specialist who is able to study carefully the voluminous literature in this specialty, such a condensation and compilation as that offered in this publication seems invaluable. To those thousands of physicians who employ the x-ray as an adjunct to diagnosis or treatment, but who because of the press of other matters cannot keep abreast with the current literature, this book will be indeed welcome.

THE STORY OF CHILDBIRTH

By Palmer Findley, M.D., Omaha, Nebraska. 376 pages with 124 illustrations. Doubleday, Doran & Company, Garden City, New York, 1933. Price, $3.00.

The Story of Childbirth, as presented by Dr. Palmer Findley, should have an especial appeal to Iowans, because the author is an Iowan by birth, and because he has attained preeminence in the dual specialty of obstetrics and gynecology.

The development of obstetric knowledge is followed down through the centuries, as superstition gradually gave way to the scientific approach, culminating in the fundamental achievements of Simpson and Semmelweis. Folk superstitions and the taboos of aboriginal peoples are interestingly discussed in their relations to menstruation, childbearing, and fertility, and are linked to customs and practices which still persist in certain parts of our country.

The author has written for the lay public and has introduced short chapters on venereal disease and on the physiology of childbearing, which combine clarity with brevity in an admirable fashion. Exception might be taken to certain statements, as, for example, that syphilis causes abortion and miscarriage, and that fertility is greatest in the few days just preceding the onset of menstruation, but in general the facts are well chosen and have the authority of majority opinion.

"Martyred Mothers" is the title of a chapter on prenatal care, in which an appeal is made for a more determined campaign against the preventable causes of maternal death. The unfavorable position of the United States in this connection is emphasized, and it is stated that: "Well directed prenatal care will reduce the hazards of childbearing to less than half." Dr. Findley points out again that the opportunities for obstetric training in the United States are not adequate and that more successful obstetric practice can only be hoped for when medical education has met the challenge.

"The Lost Art of Obstetrics" gives the author an opportunity to point out the fallacies and dangers in the recent tendency to interfere with the normal process of labor in order to appease the demands of the modern woman for a shorter and less painful parturition. He emphasizes the fact that cesarean section is, even in the best hands, a dangerous abdominal operation that should be undertaken only for well-defined indications.

The author in discussing birth control says "there is too much indiscriminate breeding among the thoughtless masses and too little discriminate breeding among the more favored classes," and then points to the ancient Maori as having "properly regulated reproduction" by selecting for that purpose only the "physically perfect." Data are presented to show that 10,000,000 among the 45,000,000 individuals in the United States under eighteen years of age, are "handicapped by physical disabilities, by social restrictions, by mental deficiencies, and by poverty," and the author then asks, "How much more profitable would it be if this loss could be prevented rather than accepted as inevitable?" Doctor Findley evidently believes that contraceptive information should be given only for strictly medical reasons, although he feels that wider dissemination of birth control methods would have no serious effect on sexual morality.

The illustrations throughout the volume are drawn from many sources and serve effectively to emphasize certain facts.

The book should be well received by the laity whose interest in the subjects covered has recently been stimulated. So many older books on these problems have faced the issues in such a biased fashion that a straight-forward, non-emotional exposition of facts should be appreciated.   E. D. P.

Reports and

Recommendations

of

Committee for the Investigation

of the

Indigent Patient Problem

Appointed Under House Joint Resolution No. 7 of the Forty-fifth General Assembly

---

NO. 1. REPORT OF INTERIM COMMITTEE NAMED TO IN-
VESTIGATE INDIGENT PATIENT PROBLEM

To His EXCELLENCY, the Governor of the State of
Iowa and to the Members of the Forty-fifth
General Assembly:

The undersigned committee, appointed pursuant
to the provisions of House Joint Resolution No. 7
adopted by the Forty-fifth General Assembly, begs
leave to submit a majority report supplementing
and completing the preliminary report previously
submitted.

According to House Joint Resolution No. 7:
"The sole purpose of this committee shall be to
seek the cause or causes of at least one of Iowa's
present misfortunes, viz., unprovided for sick and
suffering, and report back to the Forty-fifth General Assembly at the earliest possible moment the
result of their consultations and conferences with
such recommendations as to the committee seem
fit and proper for the deliberate consideration of
the Governor, the Senate and the House of Representatives, and for further action by them as
circumstances warrant." In considering the problem of the unprovided for sick and suffering of the
state as set forth in this resolution, the waiting list
of indigent patients committed to the University
Hospitals presented itself to your committee as of
paramount importance. On March 1st, the records of the hospitals disclosed a waiting list of
5,434 persons, a number which was, however, only
approximately accurate since many of the persons
originally committed to the hospitals may have
died or received treatment elsewhere during the
prolonged period of waiting necessitated by so long
a list. It has recently been reported that the waiting list has been reduced to less than three thousand. If this be the case, it is to be assumed that
this list has been revised with the elimination of
those patients who for one of the reasons set forth
are no longer waiting to receive care at the University Hospitals, since there has been no change
in the basic conditions affecting the problem of the
indigent sick.

The statutes of the state of Iowa place the primary responsibility for the care of indigents,
whether sick or well, upon the board of supervisors
of the county in which they reside. The Perkins-
Haskell-Klaus laws modified this responsibility by
providing for the state care of the indigent sick
with certain limitations, not primarily with the intent of relieving the counties of their humanitarian
duty, but rather for the purpose of supplying adequate clinical material for the instruction of students of the College of Medicine. Any solution
of the problem of providing adequate care for the

sick must also safeguard the supply of clinical
material for the teaching needs of the College of
Medicine, and must also take into account the
necessity for avoiding all unnecessary expense
during this time of unusual stringency. In other
words, while humane care of the sick is our first
duty, it should be so provided as to meet every need
for clinical instruction at the University Hospitals,
and at the same time not work any unnecessary
hardships on the already overburdened taxpayer.

Elimination of the Waiting List: A waiting
list of five thousand, three thousand, or even one
thousand obviously falls short of standards of
humane care since in most cases of illness, waiting
works a real hardship even if it does not actually
endanger life. A waiting list was not anticipated
when our laws providing for the commitment of
patients to the University Hospitals were passed.
The number of patients seeking admission to the
hospitals has been increased far beyond the anticipated number and the needs of the College of
Medicine because of the depression, unemployment,
bank failures, and the general uncertainty of
agriculture, and because certain abuses have been
possible under our laws, such as misinterpretation
of emergency, misrepresentation of the degree of
indigency, incomplete investigation of cases of
alleged indigency, and the unnecessary commitment of cases which have no value for teaching
purposes. It is not only essential that the waiting
list be reduced, but that there should be a selective
reduction which shall not cripple the College of
Medicine nor prevent or delay the admission of
such cases as can best be treated there.

The Quota Plan: There is no reason to believe
that the quota plan, under which patients are now
being admitted to the University Hospitals, will
in any way lessen the waiting list. It provides
that committed patients be admitted to the hospitals in proportion to the population of counties
of their residence instead of as the laws seem to
contemplate in proportion to the number of commitments. It may be considered more equable
from the standpoint of the taxpayers of those
counties which have received less service than the
taxes which they paid into the state fund would
seem to entitle them, but it can have no possible
effect upon the long waiting list except such reduction at the source as would follow full cooperation
on the part of all counties, which can hardly be
expected. When a patient has once been committed to the University Hospitals, the county may
be under the expense of providing local care pending his admission, but no final disposition can well
be made of his case because of the uncertainty as
to the time when he can be admitted. Your Com-

mittee believes that the quota plan will eventually seriously interfere with the primary function of the Perkins, Haskell-Klaus laws of providing adequate material for the instruction of medical students, since the Boards of Supervisors might preserve their quotas by committing patients requiring long and expensive care, and provide for the treatment of accident and obstetrical cases, and those of acute illness in their home commun ities. It has been proposed by the hospital authorities that those counties desiring to commit patients beyond their allotted quotas would pay for the overflow at the same rates charged the state. Your committee believes that the counties cannot and will not pay so much when they can get some kind of hospital service for less at home.

The County Whole Payment Plan: The suggestion has been made that careful investigation of the question of indigency, and of the advisability of hospitalization in the University Hospitals might best be insured by the county whole payment plan, charging back to the county the entire cost of hospitalization, but a majority of your committee believes that this suggestion should be rejected since its adoption would jeopardize the flow of patients necessary for clinical instruction in the College of Medicine. Without some help from the State, it is believed that the counties would feel that they cannot afford to send their sick and crippled indigents long distances and pay for their entire care, but would instead provide for hospital service at home at less cost.

The County Part Payment Plan: Reduction of the waiting list should be made *at the source,* in the first instance, by elimination of those cases which are not truly indigent through adequate investigation of the individual case. This should be primarily the duty of the Board of Supervisors, who are charged with the fundamental duty of caring for the indigent residents of the county, and who should accordingly be conversant with existing indigency. Adequate medical examination will eliminate those patients who have no value for teaching purposes and for whom a stay in the University Hospitals promises neither improvement nor cure. Provision can and should be made for the local care of such patients, affording them any possible immediate and adequate relief, thus releasing hospital beds needed for other patients. It is possible that the number of hospital beds may be still further increased by effecting certain economies in hospital administration which, while maintaining the present high standards of medical care, may seem justified by the lowered standards of living imposed upon the

population as a whole by the existing economic conditions. Your committee is convinced that adequate investigation and exclusion of non-indigents would be insured by the county part payment plan, and that this plan, with adequate safeguards, would not jeopardize the clinical material needed by the University Hospitals, but would on the contrary, make possible effective selection of the type of material needed. The selection of cases at the source with the elimination of those without teaching value and for whom no benefits from such hospitalization are to be anticipated, would at the same time effect material savings. To insure reasonably prompt care of the sick your committee believes that it should be made mandatory that the patient be sent to the hospital or otherwise cared for within thirty days but the provision of a thirty day threshold in all cases except in obstetrical cases, cases of crippled children and those in which such delay does not endanger the patient, and the submission of all commitments to the admitting physician of the University Hospitals for his acceptance or rejection, not only insures clinical material in sufficient numbers but also permits the selection of the type of patients needed for the instruction of medical students, and insures the inclusion of a sufficient number of obstetrical patients and patients with acute diseases. Both obstetrical and crippled patients would be exempt from the thirty day limitation of the waiting period.

Limitation of the Number of Medical Students: As indicated in its preliminary report and the exhibits attached thereto, to which your attention is directed, your committee is unanimous in the opinion that the present yearly average of 95 graduates of the Medical College of our State University is at least twenty more than is required to supply the medical needs of the state and to replace the annual loss to the medical profession through death, retirement, and removal from the State. Since the number of practicing physicians in the United States also apparently greatly exceeds the need of the country as a whole, there is no reason to fear any unusual loss through migration to other parts of our country, nor to feel any altruistic urge to train physicians for other parts of the country that might be less well supplied. If the number of students in the Medical College should be limited so as to provide only such additions to the medical profession as are needed, the quantity of clinical material for the teaching of the lesser number of students could be correspondingly reduced.

During the year ended June 20, 1932, there were 8,719 patients admitted to the University

Hospitals. The average period of hospitalization for these patients during the same time was 17.7 days. The average daily number of patients, therefore, at the hospitals was 492.6, a number which would be considerably in excess of the teaching needs of a College of Medicine large enough to supply the medical needs of Iowa. It therefore follows that some other means must be employed in order to care for the indigent sick of the state than the law as contained in Chapter 199, Code of Iowa, 1931, as presently administered, in order to obviate unnecessary delays and unwarranted expense.

Since the need is not for more, but rather for less and better trained physicians, we should be primarily concerned with limitation of the number of students through selection of those best qualified to profit by the training they are to receive, and with better training for those thus selected. It is, therefore, the conclusion of your committee, and it so recommends, that the Legislature authorize the State Board of Education to adopt standards of admittance on a competitive basis to the medical school which would keep the student body of the College of Medicine within such limits as would produce for the last two years thereof an average of approximately 75 members for each of said years and would also raise the standard of the type of student which is admitted to and graduated from the College; subject to the same limitations under the existing regulations whereby Iowa citizens are preferred.

Economic Considerations: While measurably prompt and adequate relief for sick and suffering indigents and an adequate supply of clinical material for the instruction of the students in the College of Medicine of our State University, as envisaged in the Perkins, Haskell-Klaus laws, must be the primary consideration in the formulation of any plan for the care of the indigent sick of the State, it is also essential that when the obligations to relieve suffering and to supply needed clinical material for the University Hospitals have been met, the economic method of meeting these obligations should be given consideration. This factor has been briefly touched upon in considering methods for eliminating the long waiting list of committed patients, but the problem involved is so important that it merits further consideration.

The elimination of those patients not entitled to be classed as indigents, and of those not needed for clinical instruction and for whom a stay at the University Hospitals promises little or no benefit would not only do away with the suffering and loss incident to a long waiting list, but would also result in material savings to the tax-payer.

Since the state would still meet the expense of commitment, transportation, and escort, there would be no geographic discrimination against any county, and since one-half of the costs of hospitalization would be charged back to the county, greater care in investigating alleged indigency should be insured. The cost to the county of the hospitalization of an indigent would remain a debt due the county from the patient or those legally responsible for his care, to be collected if and when it becomes collectible, thus providing further safeguards against pseudo-indigency, possible only where the financial responsibility is placed on local agencies. Moreover, as the laws now operate, there is a marked inequality of distribution of service and costs among the counties, about one-third of which receive more hospital service than their populations, or the taxes they pay into the state funds would seem to entitle them to receive, while the remaining two-thirds of the counties receive less than they pay for. Charging one-half the cost of caring for committed patients back to the county of their residence would tend to correct this injustice, equalizing the distribution of service and costs, because those counties sending many patients would pay more, those sending few would pay less. It would also lift from the counties a part of the burden of providing local care for indigents now on the waiting list. Last year more than $1,000,000.00 was spent for medical and hospital care within the counties of the state as compared with $450,000.00 expended in 1928. Making the County Boards of Supervisors responsible for the care of sick indigents not needed for clinical instruction at the University Hospitals and for whom hospitalization in this hospital promises no special benefit, would have the added economic advantage of giving needed financial support to many smaller hospitals which, while performing a valuable function in the community particularly in times of epidemics and emergencies, find it difficult to keep open their doors. In most cases such care can also be provided locally at less expense than that incurred in transporting the patient to and from the University Hospitals, caring for him there, and in many instances providing an escort to and from the hospital.

Lesser savings can also be effected by reducing the fee allowed the examining physician from $5.00 to $3.00, and the per diem charge of the escort when such is needed, from $3.00 to $2.00. In all cases in which the escort is a member of the patient's family or a close relative, no fee is allowed.

Because of the facts set forth in the foregoing

report, and as a result of its study of the problem of the elimination of the waiting list, your committee respectfully makes the following recommendations:

1. That half the basic cost of hospitalizing indigents be charged to the counties of their residence.

2. That investigation to determine indigency be made under the direction of the County Board of Supervisors.

3. That if an indigent person who can probably be benefited can be received at the University Hospitals within thirty days, except in obstetrical and orthopedic cases, the Court shall order him committed. If he cannot be received, the Court shall order the County to provide immediate care at home or in a hospital, and shall designate the physician who is to attend him.

4. That the size of the Medical College be reduced by suitable entrance requirements, so that the average number of graduates will not exceed seventy-five per year.

5. That the physician's examination fee of $5.00 be reduced to $3.00.

6. That escorts' wages of $3.00 per day be reduced to $2.00 per day.

7. That all purchases of supplies and materials for the University Hospitals be made upon open competitive bidding.

8. That the cost to the county of hospitalization of an indigent shall be a debt due the county from the patient or those legally responsible for his care, and that it be collected if and when it becomes collectible.

9. That before receiving other than committed indigent patients, that is, cost, pay and private patients, the hospital authorities shall collect the estimated cost of their hospital care.

No. 2. SUPPLEMENTAL REPORT

To HIS EXCELLENCY, the Governor of the State of Iowa, and to the Members of the Forty-fifth General Assembly:

We, the undersigned, members of the committee, appointed in accordance with the Provisions of House Joint Resolution No. 7, adopted by the Forty-fifth General Assembly, beg leave to submit the following Supplemental Report:

That since the signing of the Majority Report, that we have investigated the County Quota Plan, which the State Board of Education made effective on the admission of patients at the University Hospitals, starting August 1, 1933, and find that it has reduced the waiting list of patients to a considerable extent, and provides for a more equable division of indigent patients of all the counties of the State, and feel that it should be

given a further trial, and we recommend that with a suitable legal authorization, it be continued at least for awhile.   E. R. HICKLIN,
PAUL L. MILLHONE,   JOHN SPEIDEL.

NO. 3. THE BILL. SENATE FILE NO. 81

Public Health.   November 21, 1933.   By Hicklin (Millhone and Speidel).

A bill for an act to amend chapter one hundred ninety-nine (199) of the Code of Iowa, 1931, by inserting after section four thousand eighteen (4018) a new section to be known as four thousand eighteen-f (4018-f); to amend sections four thousand twenty-five (4025), four thousand twenty-six (4026) and four thousand twenty-eight (4028); and to repeal sections four thousand ten (4010), four thousand twelve (4012), four thousand sixteen (4016), four thousand seventeen (4017), and four thousand twenty-one (4021) of the Code of Iowa, 1931, and to enact substitutes therefor, all relating to the treatment of indigent persons.

Be It Enacted by the General Assembly of the State of Iowa:

Section 1. That section four thousand ten (4010) be repealed and the following substituted therefor: "When such complaint is filed, the clerk shall furnish the county attorney and board of supervisors with a copy thereof and said board shall, by the overseer of the poor or such other agent as it may select, make a thorough investigation of facts as to the legal residence of the patient, and the ability of the patient or others chargeable with his support to pay the expense of such treatment and care; and shall file a report of such investigation in the office of the clerk, at or before the time of hearing."

Sec. 2. That section four thousand twelve (4012), Code, 1931, be repealed and the following substituted therefor: "The county attorney and the overseer of the poor, or other agent of the board of supervisors of the county where the hearing is held, shall appear thereat. The complainant, the county attorney, the overseer of the poor or other agent of the board of supervisors, and the patient, or any person representing him, or her, may introduce evidence and be heard. If the court finds that said patient is a legal resident of Iowa and is pregnant or is suffering from a malady or deformity which can probably be improved or cured or advantageously treated by medical or surgical treatment or hospital care, and that neither the patient nor any person legally chargeable with his or her support is able to pay the expenses thereof, then the clerk of court, except in obstetrical cases and cases of crippled children, shall immediately ascertain from the admitting physician at the university hospital whether such person can be received as a patient within a period of thirty days, and if the patient can be so received, the court shall then enter an order directing that said patient be sent to the university hospital for proper medical and surgical treatment and hospital care. If the court ascertain, excepting in obstetrical cases and orthopedic cases, that a person of the age or sex of the patient, or afflicted by the complaint, disease or deformity with which such person is affected cannot be received as a patient at the said university hospital within the period of thirty days, then he shall enter an order directing the board of supervisors of the county to provide adequate treatment at county expense for said patient at home or in a hospital. Obstetrical cases and orthopedic cases may be committed to the university hospital without regard to the limiting period of thirty days hereinbefore stated.

"In any case of emergency the court without previous inquiry may at its discretion order the patient to be immediately taken to and accepted by the university hospital for the necessary care as provided in section four thousand fourteen (4014) herein, but if such a patient cannot be immediately accepted at the university hospital as ascertained by telephone if necessary, the court may enter an order as in certain cases above set forth directing the board of supervisors to provide adequate treatment at county expense for the said patient at home or in a hospital.

"On the date this act becomes effective the commitments of all persons then waiting for treatment at the university hospital are hereby cancelled. Should commitments be applied for on behalf of any of those said patients within six months thereafter, they may be committed without regard to the thirty day provision of the preceding paragraph and they shall have preference as to sixty (60) per cent of the beds of the university hospital available for the use of indigent patients."

Sec. 3. That section four thousand sixteen (4016), Code, 1931, be repealed and the following substituted therefor: "If the physician appointed to examine the patient shall certify that an attendant to accompany the patient to the said hospital · is necessary, and the university hospital attendant and ambulance service is not available, then the court or judge may appoint an attendant who shall receive not exceeding two dollars ($2.00) per day for the time thus necessarily employed and actual necessary traveling expenses by the most feasible route to said hospital whether by ambulance, train or automobile; but

if such appointee is a relative of the patient or a member of his immediate family, or receives a salary or other compensation from the public for his services, no such per diem compensation shall be paid him. The physician appointed by the court to make the examination and report shall receive therefor three dollars ($3.00) for each examination and report so made and his actual necessary expenses incurred in making such examination, but if such physician receives a salary or other compensation from the public for his full time services, then no such examination fee shall be paid. The actual, necessary expenses of transporting and caring for the patient shall be paid as hereinafter provided."

Sec. 4. That section four thousand seventeen (4017), Code, 1931, be repealed and the following substituted therefor: "An itemized, verified statement of all charges provided for in the preceding section and in section four thousand twelve (4012), in cases where the patient is admitted or accepted for treatment at the university hospital shall be filed with the superintendent of the university hospital, and upon his recommendation, when approved by the judge under whose order the same were incurred, they shall be charged on the regular bill for the maintenance, transportation and treatment of the patient, and be audited and paid in the manner as hereinafter provided."

Sec. 5. That section four thousand twenty-one (4021), Code, 1931, be repealed and the following substituted therefor: "Treatment of other patients. The university hospital authorities may at their discretion receive into the hospital for medical, obstetrical or surgical treatment or hospital care, patients not committed thereto under the provisions of this chapter; but the treatment or care of such patients shall not in any way interfere with the proper medical or surgical treatment or hospital care of committed patients.

All of the provisions of this chapter except as to commitment of patients shall apply to such patients. The university hospital authorities shall collect from the person or persons liable for the support of such patients reasonable charges for hospital care and service and deposit the same with the treasurer of the university for the use and benefit of the university hospital. Earnings of the hospital whether from private patients, cost patients, or indigents shall be administered so as to increase as much as possible the service available for indigents."

Sec. 6. That section four thousand twenty-five (4025), Code, 1931, be amended by adding after the period in line six (6) thereof the following: "If the physician, surgeon or nurse is not in the regular employ of the state board of education, his or her compensation shall be paid by the county upon approval of the board of supervisors."

Sec. 7. Amend section four thousand twenty-six (4026), Code of Iowa, 1931, by striking out all of the same following the period in line seven (7) and inserting in lieu thereof the following: "But he shall render separate bills showing the actual cost ot all appliances, instruments, x-ray and other special services used in connection with such treatment, commitments, and transportation to and from the said university hospital, including the expenses of attendants and escorts.

All purchases of materials, appliances, instruments and supplies by said university hospital, in cases where more than one hundred dollars ($100.00) is to be expended and where the price of the commodity or commodities to be purchased are subject to competition, shall be upon open competitive quotations, and all contracts therefor shall be subject to the provisions of chapter sixty-two (62), Code of Iowa, 1931."

Sec. 8. That chapter one hundred ninety-nine (199) of the Code of Iowa, 1931, is hereby amended by inserting after section four thousand eighteen (4018) thereof, a section to be known as section four thousand eighteen-f (4018-f), and reading and providing as follows:

"County Quotas. Subject to subsequent qualifications in this section, there shall be treated at the university hospital during each fiscal year a number of committed indigent patients from each county which shall bear the same relation to the total number of committed indigent patients admitted during the year as the population of such county shall bear to the total population of the state according to the last preceding census. This standard shall apply to indigent patients, the expenses of whose commitment, transportation, care and treatment shall be borne by appropriated funds and shall not govern the admission of either obstetrical or orthopedic patients. If the number of patients admitted from any county shall exceed by more than ten per cent of the county quota as fixed and ascertained under the first sentence of this section, the charges and expenses of the care and treatment of such patients in excess of ten per cent of the quota shall be paid from the funds of such county at actual cost; but if the number of excess patients from any county shall not exceed ten per cent, all costs, expenses, and charges incurred in their behalf shall be paid from the appropriation for the support of the hospital."

Sec. 9. That section four thousand twenty-eight (4028), Code of Iowa, 1931, be amended by adding at the end thereof the following: "The

superintendent of the said university hospital shall certify to the auditor of state on the first day of January, April, July and October of each year, the amount as herein provided not previously certified by him due the state from the several counties having patients chargeable thereto, and the auditor of state shall thereupon charge the same to the county so owing. A duplicate certificate shall also be mailed to the auditor of each county having patients chargeable thereto.

"The county auditor, upon receipt of such certificate, shall thereupon enter the same to the credit of the state in his ledger of state accounts, and at once issue a notice to his county treasurer authorizing him to transfer the amount from the poor or county fund to the general state revenue, which notice shall be filed by the treasurer as his authority for making such transfer; and he shall include the amount so transferred in his next remittance of state taxes to the treasurer of state, designating the fund to which it belongs.

"The state auditor shall certify the total cost of commitment, transportation and caring for such indigent patient under the terms of this statute to the county auditor of such patient's legal residence, and such certificate shall be preserved by the county auditor and shall be a debt due from the patient or the persons legally responsible for his or her care, maintenance or support; and whenever in the judgment of the board of supervisors the same or any part thereof shall be collectible, the same board may in its own name collect the same and is hereby authorized to institute suits for such purpose; and after deducting the county's share of such cost shall cause the balance to be paid into the state treasury."

Sec. 10. This act being deemed of immediate importance shall be in force and effect from and after its passage and publication in Avoca Journal Herald, a newspaper published at Avoca, Iowa, and in the Morning Sun News-Herald, a newspaper published at Morning Sun, Iowa.

NO. 4. AMENDMENT BY SENATOR MOORE TO
SENATE FILE 81

Amend Senate File No. 81 by striking all of Section eight (8), and substituting in lieu thereof the following:

"Sec. 8. Amend section four thousand twenty-seven (4027), Code of Iowa, 1931, by adding at the end of said section the following: 'The cost of all medicine, care, x-ray, laboratory and maintenance furnished to such patients, shall be paid one-half by the state and one-half by the county of each patient's legal residence. The cost of the commitment, transportation, attendants and other special appliances and treatments of all patients admitted or accepted for treatment at the University Hospital shall be paid by the state.

"'The Auditor of State shall make a quarterly estimate of the per diem charge for medicine, care, x-ray, laboratory, and maintenance based upon such reports and audits as he shall require, and in the final quarter of each year he shall provide for an audit to determine the said per diem charge for medicine, care and maintenance, and upon the basis of the same adjust any and all irregularities and errors found to exist as the result of the quarterly estimates.'"

MORRIS MOORE, M.D.

NO. 5. MINORITY REPORT OF THE COMMITTEE ACTING
UNDER HOUSE JOINT RESOLUTION NO. 7, OF THE
45TH GENERAL ASSEMBLY, REGULAR SESSION

His Excellency the Governor, the Lieutenant Governor, the Speaker of the House, Members of the Forty-fifth General Assembly in Extraordinary Session:

Pursuant to the provisions of House Joint Resolution No. 7 and the request that your committee be not discharged, which was attached to their preliminary report, the undersigned, the minority of the committee, not entirely agreeing with the committee report, desire to express their views on a subject of vital importance to every man, woman and child now living or soon or hereafter to be born in Iowa, if not in the United States; and of great economic importance to the taxpayers and to those who still harbor the hope that they, too, sometime may add to Iowa's income, if not to that of the United States.

House Joint Resolution No. 7 made it incumbent upon the committee to report back to the 45th General Assembly at the earliest possible moment the results of their consultations and conferences, with such recommendations as to the committee seem fit and proper, for the deliberate consideration of the Governor, the Senate and the House of Representatives and for such further action by them as circumstances warrant.

The committee having been duly organized, a sub-committee of three was appointed to "hold a consultation with the faculty, or with individual members of the faculty of the State University of Iowa Medical College and with the staff or with members of the staff of the State University Hospital;" they were also to "confer with the State Board of Education or members thereof and with the president of the State University and with any or all agencies having knowledge of conditions and being in a position to offer suggestions as to remedies."

At the organization meeting in Des Moines, March 7, 1933, the chairman of your committee "in order to obtain information for the use of the committee," was requested "to interview and consult with such individuals and agencies outside the State of Iowa as may have a vital interest in the university hospitals." This gave your chairman carte blanche to go outside the state in an effort to solve the riddle of the adult indigent law. He has been asked by no one to give an account of his activities at the expense of the State of Iowa, and he feels that now, before stating the objections of the minority to the committee report, he should briefly detail his itinerary and invite attention to the results of his consultations and conferences, which will follow in the minority report.

On March 12th, 1933, he arrived in Chicago; on Monday, the 13th, discussed with Drs. Olin West and Wm. D. Cutter Iowa's predicament and made an appointment with Dr. H. S. Houghton; Tuesday, the 14th, a long conference with Drs. Cutter and Houghton at the office of the Council on Medical Education and Hospitals of the American Medical Association; Wednesday, the 15th, luncheon and conference with Dr. Houghton at the University of Chicago Clinics, at which time Dr. Houghton kindly consented to give your chairman a note of introduction to Dr. Allen Gregg, Secretary of the General Education Board, Rockefeller Foundation; Thursday and Friday, the 16th and 17th, correspondence; Saturday and Sunday, the 18th and 19th, Chicago to Washington; Monday, the 20th, Department of Agriculture—desired to see Secretary Wallace but Under-Secretary C. W. Ackerson, with much diplomacy, said, "Sorry, but impossible"; no difficulty experienced in getting an appointment with the office of the Bureau of Agricultural Economics, although the chief, Dr. Galpin, was not there; Tuesday, the 21st, called at the offices of Iowa's Senators and Congressmen; Wednesday, the 22nd, Bureau of Agricultural Economics, then Surgeon General's office, Dr. C. E. Waller; Thursday, the 23rd, New York Academy of Medicine; phoned Dr. Nathan E. Van Etten, who suggested seeing Dr. E. H. L. Corwin for further appointments; Friday, the 24th, conference with Dr. Willard C. Rappleye, Dean of Columbia University, director of the study made by the Commission on Medical Education; luncheon with Dr. and Mrs. Van Etten at their home; conference lasted all afternoon; Saturday, the 24th, conference at offices of Commonwealth Fund with Mr. H. J. Southmayd and Dr. L. J. Evans; then to the Rockefeller Foundation to meet Dr. Allen Gregg; Dr. H. S. Houghton of Chicago, former Dean of the State University of Iowa College of Medicine, was present; Dr. Frederick F. Russell, M.D., director of the International Health Board, and Dr. W. A. McIntosh were called into the conference, which lasted long after closing time in New York City.

From this conference the chairman of your committee brings to the 45th General Assembly in Extraordinary Session, direct from the lips of Dr. Allen Gregg, whose countenance radiates probity, these words: "The gift to Iowa was an outright gift with no strings attached—there were no commitments, gentlemen's agreements or understandings of any kind." Your chairman came away with the impression, although no one said so, that the Rockefeller people were as badly disappointed with their investment as the state of Iowa is with theirs.

The chairman of your committee expresses the hope that at some future time, not too far distant, a conference may be held to further discuss the important subjects of the conversations with Drs. Russell and McIntosh, and Dr. Waller of the Surgeon General's office.

Monday, the 27th, to Baltimore to keep appointment at Johns-Hopkins Hospital with Dr. Dean Lewis, President of the American Medical Association. Wednesday, the 29th, again at the Bureau of Agricultural Economics in Washington.

The preliminary report stated that the chairman of your committee "consulted with the officials of the Brookings Institution in Washington, D. C." He did spend a pleasant social hour with Mr. H. P. Seidemann at the institution. Iowa's troublesome problem was mentioned, but not discussed. Thursday, the 30th, Chicago; Friday, the 31st, arrived Des Moines and went to the office of Dr. Oliver J. Fay, where the report of the committee was read. The chairman of your committee concurred in Senator Hicklin's dissent and dictated the letter of transmittal, making the report preliminary. He then signed both the report and the letter.

Having come now to the committee report, recent events cause the minority to wonder whether there is enough left of it to either subscribe or object to. While the minority were endeavoring to prepare their report objecting to and agreeing with parts of the committee report which had already been delivered to the Speaker of the House and released to the press, the Des Moines *Register*, Saturday, Nov. 18th, carried a report that "pressure from non-members" had caused members of the interim committee of nine to change their minds. The *Register* stated someone "wished to have members of the committee hear the University's attitude on the committee's previous recommendations."

The minority worked away as best they could, the chairman being confined to his hotel for more than a week, in the belief that when a committee report was delivered to the assembly, it had at last

found a place of refuge. The committee had notified the press there would be a minority report, and not able to resist the temptation, released, from carbon copies sent to each member of the committee prior to its last meeting, what they assured the public would be among the minority's recommendations.

The minority were laboring under the impression that the majority, after they had substituted nearly everything the University had requested for what they (the majority) had incorporated in the preliminary draft, had been fairly faithful in hearing the "University's attitude" "on the committee's previous recommendations." In fact, from the mass material presented at committee meetings, the minority believed the matter had been given exhaustive study. Somehow, perhaps by reason of the provisions of House Joint Resolution No. 7, the minority had gotten the idea that inasmuch as the University Medical College, Hospitals, etc., was an institution of some dimensions, belonging to the State of Iowa, the committee was going to make a report to the 45th General Assembly and permit them, along with the Governor, to give the whole matter "deliberate consideration" and take such "action as circumstances warrant."

If the adult indigent law is to remain in the statutes of Iowa, the minority stand just where they did when they signed the preliminary report. However, the minority challenges the statement of the majority that "the Perkins-Haskell-Klaus law was for the purpose of supplying adequate clinical material for the instruction of students of the College of Medicine." The minority grants that may have been the purpose of the promoters, but it is not so stated in the law, and they would not presume to assume the function of the Supreme Court of Iowa.

A little while before the recent muddle the Brookings report appeared in the press with "recommendations suggested in Appendix C, on medical care of the indigent sick in the hospitals of the State University of Iowa." Any country doctor who reads the history under I, A, B, C, D, II, III, IV, V, then turns the covers back and gently palpates the abdomen, will tell your honorable body that it is a dangerous appendix and prompt removal offers the only hope for the patient. Their recommendations follow:

I. They would not have the Perkins-Haskell-Klaus law modified—only minor modifications.

A. "That the county auditor, or in counties with trained social workers, those agents should investigate indigency instead of the county attorney." This is at variance with the committee recommendation, who would place that duty under the direction of the county Board of Supervisors; with this the minority agree.

B. Both the Brookings Institution and the committee agree the physician's examination fee should be reduced from five dollars to three dollars. Neither states why it should be made three dollars instead of two as recommended by all members of the committee of nine in their preliminary report. Without reason, the minority cannot be so fickle.

C. "The patient's escort's fee should be reduced from three dollars to two dollars a day." All members of the committee of nine subscribed to this in their preliminary report.

D. "Section 4021 of the code of Iowa, 1931, should be amended to conform with practice." The minority believe that would establish a bad precedent.

II. "Appropriations for the indigent service at the University hospitals should be increased sufficiently to run those hospitals to capacity." The first selective recommendation of the minority report ought to satisfy the most voracious appetite for indigents.

III. "The law should be amended to authorize the state board of education to establish and enforce locally as far as is practical a county patient quota plan, to apportion annually as equitably as possible the available services." The minority believe, after some thought, that this does qualify as a "minor modification" for the reason that while it proposes to put teeth in the law they can be only false teeth and are sure to rattle and fall out. As to the impracticability of the "county patient quota plan," both the majority and the minority were in complete accord.

IV. "A hospital field agent is necessary to link the hospitals with the service in local communities, to establish a better understanding of the service and constantly to check on the operation of the law from the point of view of the people." That is a high sounding phrase, but the minority respectfully suggests, that if the adult indigent law is to remain in the statutes, a much more important function for the field agent would be for him to be on the alert to locate those who die enroute to the hospital or soon after arrival, and assist in getting them back to the family undertaker.

V. "Local county provisions for medical aid to the indigent sick should be reconstructed along lines suggested above: (1) Filling the county's quota intelligently; (2) supplementing that quota with such local service as will put the medical and

hospital service to indigents upon an acceptable level in co-operation with the local medical society." The minority pleads inability to comment on this paragraph without the aid of an interpreter.

The minority is in complete accord with recommendation I of the Brookings Report that "the Perkins-Haskell-Klaus law should not be modified." It should be repealed, the Perkins law restored to its original status and the adult indigent law forever scrapped. It is an abominable law—made up of incongruities, inconsistencies and impossibilities, incompatible with common sense. It makes possible, if it does not encourage and compel the perpetration of fraud; fraud upon the indigent and the tax payers, fraud upon the sick and well, fraud upon the reputable faculty of the college of medicine, fraud upon the medical students, fraud upon the reputable medical profession of the state, fraud upon the patient with heart disease, who runs after advertised remedy, when he should be at home, quiet in bed; fraud upon the severely injured, especially skull fractures, whose lives are jeopardized or lost by reason of the long haul; fraud upon the aged and decrepit, who should be encouraged to die at home among comforting friends. Iowa's adult indigent law is the alpha and omega of all that is bad in legislation providing for the state care of sick indigents. There is no law in the United States to compare with it.

The majority, having completed the committee report, debated how best to present it to the 45th General Assembly. They looked around for a mild-eyed broncho, named her Iowa, and saddled her with their study of the situation; they put under the saddle a blanket woven out of the "elimination of the waiting list," "the quota plan," "the county whole-payment plan," "the county part-payment plan," "the limitation of the number of medical students," "economic considerations" and nine recommendations. They decorated the flaps of the blanket with "forms of proposed laws to carry out the recommendations." These "proposed laws" had been drafted largely in accordance with the wishes of the university authorities.

The minority felt that their report was a bit more humane and constructive than that of the committee and argued that the adult indigent law was a lump in a woman's breast, that it was malignant and that delay in advising radical measures was unjustifiable on any grounds. But when minority is told to go back and sit down, discretion suggests compliance—at least for a time.

The committee led their pony to the capital and

found a stall for her; there was a little sign, hardly legible, on the saddle which read "Ride her, Cowboy, ride her." University folks knew about it, so it wasn't long before a couple of tenderfeet came over and took a look at "Iowa." Then a few got together and held a rump caucus—someone called it a committee meeting. The university fully looked at the saddle, and said "It isn't on straight, needs adjustment." So they loosened up the girth and took some of the blanket out and put other pieces in. Being connected with the university instead of a veterinary college, they didn't know very much about ponies and when they tightened the belly-band, they put it quite a little farther back than the pony was accustomed to. So long as she was riderless it did not matter. They little dreamed that those additions were full-grown cockleburs between the saddle and a very thin blanket. These novices went home and someone told the newspapers about what had happened. Next day Erskine and Sternberg heard about the "committee meeting" and through Verne Marshall in the Cedar Rapids *Gazette* of Friday, November 17th, they had a lot to say. They had gone the limit in keeping inviolate whatever understandings there may have been between the majority and university authorities. For this example of fidelity the minority had only praise. The minority had no entanglements. Monkeying with the saddle on their "Iowa" was too much; it was a thrust below the belt. It wounded them in that tender professional spot known as ethics and the wound was not made by confreres, but by intruders.

All this newspaper dope was ground up, some of it sprinkled with gentian, to add to her oats and hay, some of it mixed with fluid extract of ginger, to add to the pony's drinking water—a real tonic. The date for the Rodeo is not yet set. When this important event is announced, Dr. Thos. Burcham, on invitation, may be available to assist with the mounts.

Returning to the Brookings Institution "program for long time and immediate development of state and county governments," the minority timidly inquires: Since when did the Brookings Institution become the Brookings Health Institute? Who are the physicians and surgeons in that establishment who have driven all over Iowa, night and day, in mud to the hub, horses on their knees while the tires sparkled and flashed like emery wheels sharpening the plow-shares? If no physicians are on the faculty, why be so liberal with advice and demands in matters medical? From whom do they take advice or orders?

What business is it of the Brookings Institution where the State Medical Library is located? The medical profession of Iowa, the 38th General Assembly and Governor Harding settled that in 1919. They propose the establishment of a state Board of Public Welfare, with a lot more swivel chairs; they would re-make the State Board of Health with still more chairs and white collars. They even suggest "in the re-organization of the state department, provision should, if possible, be made for additional or other adequate quarters for the State Health Department." All of which means more taxes and more indigents, Iowa needs no imported sociological phantasmagoria.

Suppose one of these philosophers gets sick on his plantation along the Potomac, can his wife notify his philosopher neighbors and right away have thirty of them come over to his place, husk thirty acres of philosophy, which would spoil if not taken care of, wash their hands and faces, feet—if need be—in the watering tank, go in to a big feed and call it a grand time? The philosopher says it is not according to the modern concept of sociology. No? But it is human; it is the kind of neighborly concern for the other fellow that grows straight up with the tall corn and is the warp and woof of Iowa's social fabric. Why adulterate it with colorful shoddy?

To introduce these philosophic ideas into a state which rapidly is evolving its own medico-social program, is like adding another great toe to each foot; with nails polished and painted they may be highly ornamental, but at best they can only impede progress. What would the Brookings Institution philosophers say if a doctor of chiropody stepped in and told them what changes ought to have been made in state and county administration? The Chairman of your committee, not knowing what part of the thirty thousand dollars it cost to get the socialized medicine recommendations, makes bold to say that in his opinion they are not worth a nickel a ream.

If the Brookings Institution philosophers are still here, they are cordially invited to meet the minority at the foot of the Grand Stairway—grand is only feebly descriptive—fix their eyes upon "Westward" as they solemnly ascend; consider the progress that has been and is Iowa's. Let them lift their eyes to the mosaics in the balcony over the stairway, note "Defense", "Charity", the "Executive", the "Legislative", the "Judiciary", "Education", and imagine "Health" soon to find a niche; look around the rotunda, note the lunettes: "Hunting", "Herding", "Agriculture", "the Forge", "Commerce", "Education", "Science", and "Art"; if no heart disease, go on to the gallery by way of the winding stair, it gives a little time for reflection; turn their eyes to the West and read these words:

"The ideal state—that in which an injury done to the least of its citizens is an injury done to all."—Solon.

Since the committee report was filed a supplemental report appeared in the Senate Journal, Tuesday, November 21, 1933. It was signed by three members of the committee of nine. They had investigated the county quota plan and found "that it has reduced the waiting list of patients to a considerable extent, and provides for a more equable division of indigent patients of all the counties of the state, and feel that it should be given a further trial, and recommend that with a suitable legal authorization, it be continued at least for a while." No explanation of how the quota plan brought about this reduction in the waiting list is offered. "Suitable legal authorization" appears in House File No. 112 and Senate File No. 81. In part it reads: "On the date this act becomes effective the commitments of all persons then waiting for treatment at the university hospital are hereby cancelled. Should commitments be applied for on behalf of any of those said patients within six months thereafter, they may be committed without regard to the thirty day provision of the preceding paragraph and they shall have preference as to sixty (60) per cent of the beds of the university hospital available for the use of indigent patients."

All the minority can say for Sec. 4018-f1— County Quotas—is that it is the superlative of confusion confounded. Is it any worse to suggest the repeal of such an inhuman law than it is to propose such merciless statutory disregard for "unprovided for sick and suffering?" Does anyone believe that such legislation is not cockle-burs under the saddle of the pony called Iowa? Does anyone think she will not dislodge the rider when weight is put on the saddle?

Forget for the moment, "unprovided for sick and suffering," and find any consideration for the taxpayer in either the committee report or the Brookings Institution socialized medicine recommendations, except on page 123 of the Senate Journal, Tuesday, November 21, 1933, where the former says "Any solution of the problem of providing adequate care for the sick must also safeguard the supply of clinical material for the teaching needs of the College of Medicine, and must also take into account the necessity for avoiding all unnecessary expense during this time of unusual stringency. In other words, while humane care of the sick is our first duty, it should be so provided as to meet every need for clinical instruction at the University hospitals, and at the same

time not work any unnecessary hardship on the already overburdened taxpayer."

The committee in their report already have advised the people of Iowa, through the press, of the minority's intention to have for one of its selective recommendations the repeal of the adult indigent law, the restoration of the Perkins law to its original status and take necessary steps to establish the clinical years of medicine in the city of Des Moines. The people were correctly informed by the committee.

It is at once argued that such change is impossible because the constitution says all departments of the University must forever be at Iowa City. Is there anything in the constitution that requires the taxpayers of this state to stand on their heads, with their pockets turned inside out, in order that their feet may support a great university medical center until Gabriel blows his trumpet? If there is, it ought to be amended or repealed or prayer offered that the sound of that instrument soon may be heard. It is not proposed to move the Department of Medicine; it should remain at Iowa City. The proposal is to give the clinical years at Des Moines where many emergency cases fresh from the street make the hospitalized clinic material of much better quality and the number of out patients, so necessary for the teaching and training of medical students, is so much greater that the minority wonders why the reputable faculty does not request the change. Much of the clinical material at Iowa City is second, third or fourth hand often gathered from the discard and of little or no value for clinical teaching purposes. If legal advice is to the effect that change in the constitution is necessary to save the state one million dollars ($1,000,000.00) a year and make a better medical school by salvaging a much better quality and quantity of clinical teaching material than is now provided, surely someone will initiate the steps necessary to effect the change.

Is it not time that someone suggested diplomatic negotiations on the part of the State of Iowa with the County of Polk and the City of Des Moines with a view to determining what reciprocal relations might be established that would save the state a million or more dollars a year, lift a part of the load from Polk County which would be reflected to every other county in the state and be the salvation of the State University of Iowa Medical College?

The attention of your Honorable Body is invited to the following comparative tabulation of clinical teaching material at Broadlawns Polk County General Hospital with 100 beds and at the University Hospital at Iowa City with 954 beds.

BROADLAWNS GENERAL DEPARTMENT—FIGURES FROM ANNUAL REPORTS

Year—	No. Out Patients Treated	No. In Patients Treated	Total No. Pts. Treated	No. of Out Patient Visits	Hospital Days Care Rendered	Average Length of Stay in Hos.	Daily Average	Tuberculosis Department No. of Patients Admitted	Tuberculosis Department No. of Days Care Rendered	Contagious Department No. Patients Adm'd	Contagious Department Days Care Rend.
1928	3,632	2,600	6,232	19,791	32,899	12 +	90 +	180	25,251	· 266	4,544
1929	4,896	2,589	7,485	19,261	31,352	12 +	86—	171	27,693	370	8,033
1930	6,208	3,004	9,212	30,370	34,758	11 +	95 +	176	26,380	336	5,540
1931	14,699	3,313	18,012	40,714	36,722	11 +	100 +	172	25,225	237	3,705
1932	18,818	4,076	22,894	51,576	37,669	9 +	103 +	143	23,797	251	4,320
For 10 Months 1933	24,886	3,657	28,543	67,998	32,140	· 9 — ·	88 +				

NUMBER INDIVIDUALS TREATED AT UNIVERSITY HOSPITAL

Taken from Report of the Committee on Medical Education and
Hospitals—Handbook for the House of Delegates—
May 10, 11, 12, 1933.

	No. Out Patients Treated	No. In Patients Treated	Total No. Pts. Treated
1928-1929	1,407	5,662	7,069
1929-1930	1,263	6,957	8,220
1930-1931	2,064	7,551	9,615
1931-1932	2,225 ·	8,719	10,944

For detailed reports see Addenda A. 1.

DELIVERIES—BROADLAWNS GENERAL HOSPITAL

1928	288
1929	202
1930	232
1931	339
1932	394
1933, for first ten months as shown below	417
January	50
February	47
March	43
April	40
May	41
June	42
July	42
August	35
September	32
October	45
	417

CLINIC VISITS—OBSTETRICAL PATIENTS 1933

	Prenatal Patients	Prenatal Visits	Postnatal Patients	Postnatal Visits
January	104	217	18	22
February	92	154	11	14
March	98	184	19	30
April	96	194	23	39
May	119	191	16	20
June	99	151	17	20
July	89	148	17	23
August	81	139	18	24
September	91	178	12	14
October	94	171	9	15
	963	1,727	· 160	221

In passing let the chairman of the committee of nine say, that in all his conferences with able, informed persons, professional and non-professional, no more constructive and statesman-like statement has been heard than that made by Dr. Charles H. Sprague, Superintendent of Broadlawns Polk County Public Hospital, only a few days ago: He "believes the state should maintain a medical college, when and where there is sufficient clinical teaching material to enable it to maintain a Class A standard, large enough to graduate each year a number of physicians sufficient to comply with the law of supply and demand. In return for what the state has done for the students, the state should require that the graduates give two years of service as internes in the hospitals of the state." Why is the state engaged in the business of medical education unless it is to have some return from its investment?

Just as the minority were about to call their report finished, here came House Joint Resolution No. 2, November 24, 1933, reciting a lot of old stuff. (See exhibit D.) It calls to mind a conversation of the chairman of your committee with Dr. H. S. Houghton at the office of Secretary W. D. Cutter, on March 14th, 1933, at which time Dr. Houghton said about all the words that are in H. J. R. No. 2 and added as nearly as it is possible to quote conversation, "The county payment plan will close the institution. It is unthinkable, but we may have to open the hospital to citizens of the state without restrictions." There was considerable more conversation, which need not be repeated at this time.

Suppose now the 45th General Assembly in extraordinary session drop from the picture, for the time being, the State Board of Education and administrative officers, they are not licensed to practice medicine in Iowa. Call the faculty of the College of Medicine, ask them how they would like to get out from under lay domination.

Call Dr. Oliver J. Fay and Dr. E. D. Plass, ask either one if Dr. Fay did not say he "had no desire to interfere with the flow of clinical material which is necessary for you to properly instruct your students in obstetrics and gynaecology;" also that he had no "desire to interfere in any way with the teaching of medicine at the State University of Iowa;" ask if he did not propose to "lean over backwards to help anywhere that he could to keep the medical department of the State University of Iowa on its present high level." See Exhibit L.

Just how entangled must the reputable profession of Iowa become to satisfy the greed of Iowa's imported octopus? Didn't Dr. Fay, along with Drs. Erskine and Sternberg, go to about the limit of human endeavor to be on the square?

Call in the Drs. Mayo, widely known and justly famous; ask them what they think of the long haul for acutely sick and injured; ask them what they think of Iowa's clinical teaching facilities?

Call in Dr. Rappleye, although that is hardly necessary, for you have his book, marked Exhibit M. Dr. Walter L. Bierring, State Commissioner of Health, was a member of that commission and will, no doubt, be glad to explain any of the more technical medical education discussions.

Call in your family physicians, who ushered most of you into the world and who will be the medical court of last appeal for you before the final summons. Ask them how the adult indigent law functions.

Call Wm. D. Cutter, Secretary of the Council on Medical Education and Hospitals, or better, call the Council; Dr. Cutter has not been Secretary very long. Ask them when the last inspection of the State University of Iowa Medical College was made for rating purposes. Ask if it wasn't November 14, 1919?

Call in A. M. Schwitalla, S.J., Ph.D., President of the American Catholic Hospital Association, just to get the reaction of an eminent priest.

Refer to exhibit N; read for yourselves digests of all the laws in the United States having even the slightest similarity to Iowa's adult indigent law. Read letters, commitment blanks, etc., from the Deans of University Medical Colleges.

While you are asking questions, ask someone how it happened that in the laws of 1919; 86 Ch. 76, Section 1 read as follows: "Whenever it shall appear to any physician, county supervisor, township trustee, public health nurse, overseer of the poor, policemen, priest or minister, that there is any legal resident of his or her county, etc." was changed by reason of Code Commissioner's Bill No. 92 which provided for amendments "for the purpose of remedying defects in the statutes, discovered in their practical application." Section 2 says "it shall be the duty of physicians, public health nurses, members of boards of supervisors and township trustees, overseers of the poor, sheriffs, policemen, and public school teachers, having knowledge of persons suffering from such malady or deformity, to file or cause such complaint to be filed." What was the defect that made it necessary to drop out "priest or minister?" See exhibit O.

No question mark was ever placed after S. U. I. Medical College in the days of Doctor W. F. Peck, he with the Civil War middle finger; Pappy Farnsworth with his little dog trot, but who knew his materia medica and therapeutics; Dr. J. C. Schrader with his leather manikin and mulato leather baby, with which he taught pretty good obstetrics, especially in his remarks about meddlesome midwifery; Dr. C. M. Hobby, austere, but able, who knew his eyes and ears; Dr. Elmer F. Clapp, the eminent anatomist and the Chauncey DePew of the faculty; Dr. Wm. D. Middleton, the perfect gentleman-surgeon, with no personal pronouns in his vocabulary; Dr. L. W. Littig, gruff, but a one hundred percenter; Dr. J. R. Guthrie, physiology; Dr. Woods Hutchinson, the gifted anatomist, the scholarly gentleman, later of *Saturday Evening Post* fame; Dr. Charles S. Chase, loquacious, but brilliant and honest; Dr. James W. Dalby, ophthalmology and otology; Dr. Walter L. Bierring, pathology and bacteriology; Dr. A. C. Peters, laryngology and rhinology; F. S. Aby, normal histology; E. McClain, medical jurisprudence; Dr. Gershom H. Hill, psychiatry; E. L. Boerner, pharmacy; Dr. J. W. Harriman, anatomy; W. T. Barlow, chemistry; W. R. Whiteis, pathology and bacteriology; Albert M. Barrett, histology; Dr. W. E. Robinson, anatomy; Frank Carroll, chemistry; Billy Green, anatomist par excellence; Elbert R. Rockwood, comparable to Dr. Walter S. Haines—shades and shadows of them all, look at us now!

Iowa's adult indigent law is a smoldering fire, every now and then bursting into blaze. It will burn to the first, second or third degree, those who play about it, just in proportion to the zeal and zest with which the moth flies into the flame. It will put toxines in the professional blood, albumin in the professional renal secretion; it will make professional dizziness, headache and nausea; it may blight, if it does not blast, what, in a normal environment, might become eminent professional careers.

The adult indigent law, in its operation, keeps highminded, competent, ethical men constantly between Scilla and Charbidus, and when out of that channel they find themselves between the devil and the deep sea. Again, the chairman of the committee of nine asserts it is an abominable law and he speaks with knowledge.

Coming soon to the minority report proper, let a moment be taken to recall a little history. The speaker of the house, along with sixteen other representatives and fifteen senators must have had some rare kind of foresight which public hindsight is just beginning to see, when in the 40th General Assembly they voted No on both the donation and appropriation. They were:

Senators—15

Brookhart, Brookins, Browne, Cessna, Eithel, Fulton, Johnson, McIntosh, Nelson, Price, Romkey, Shinn, Snook, Thurston, Tuck.

Representatives—17

Aiken, Anderson, Berry, Blume, Dooley, Fackler, Frahn, Huff, Leonard, Miller, Napier, Orr,

Rewolt Scott of Appanoose, Smith of Lucas, Stookesberry, Ulsted.

Nobody ever sold them the Brooklyn Bridge, the Chicago Art Museum or an heirship to a Dr-eam estate.

When, during supposedly prosperous times, the state of Iowa enlarged its medical education program, it did just what many of its citizens did in various fields of industry, it invested heavily and grievously encumbered itself with tax obligations, giving little thought to a day of reckoning.

In May, 1929, at the annual meeting of the Iowa State Medical Society the House of Delegates, on the recommendation of the Committee on Public Policy and Legislation, passed a resolution authorizing the Council to appoint a Committee on Medical Education and Hospitals. Their duty was: "(1) to collect information relative to the medical care of the indigent sick in Iowa; (2) to secure information as to the costs of such care in Iowa as compared with the costs in other states of relatively equal and like population; (3) to collect information as to the operation of the Perkins-Klaus Laws as they pertain to the commitment of indigent persons to the University Hospital and the cost to the state of the same; (4) to determine to what extent the operation of these laws supplies the Medical Department of the State University with proper clinical material for teaching purposes, and to collect such other information relative to medical education and hospitals as may be of value to the profession of the state."

The members of this committee were Drs. B. L. Eiker, Chairman, Leon, Arthur W. Erskine, Cedar Rapids, A. V. Hennessy, Council Bluffs and Mr. Vernon D. Blank, Executive Secretary. Their report was made at a special meeting of the House of Delegates held in Des Moines, December 17, 1930, in its foreword the committees said:

"It is the purpose of this report to present a careful study of the various economic, social, educational and medical problems connected with the care of the indigent sick in Iowa.

"The public, the tax payers, the legislators, the courts, the College of Medicine and hospital authorities, the medical profession and the indigents of Iowa each have separate and distinct relations, and separate and distinct reactions to this problem.

"That there has been criticism and dissatisfaction is evidenced by the fact that in both the Forty-second and Forty-third General Assemblies there was introduced legislation intended to modify the laws governing the operation of the University

Hospitals and the commitment of indigent patients thereto. Discussion in connection with these proposed changes made it apparent that there was a lack of factual evidence upon which to base sound judgments."

The following excerpts are from the report:

"The laws of the State of Iowa direct the Boards of Supervisors to provide medical care for the indigent sick within their respective jurisdictions. The usual means of providing such care are employed in Iowa by the Board of Supervisors, either directly or through their representatives, the over-seers of the poor, are:

1. Medical care rendered on individual fee basis.

2. Contract with individual physicians.

3. Contract with County Medical Societies.

4. Provision for hospital care by county owned and operated hospitals.

"The amount of money spent by the various counties in the state during 1928, through their Boards of Supervisors, for the care of the indigent sick is set forth in Table I, page 8, the total amounting to $446,970.78. The amount of money spent from State funds in the operation of the Perkins, Haskell-Klaus Law for the period ending December 31, 1928 was $903,835.78. The grand total spent by the State of Iowa for its care of the indigent sick through the two sources previously referred to was $1,350,806.56 for the calendar year 1928. (The distribution according to counties of the state funds expended under the Perkins-Haskell-Klaus Law during the year ending June 30, 1930, is shown in Table II, pages 10 and 11.)"

For the year 1931 the amount expended by the various counties through the Boards of Supervisors, for the care of the sick indigent was $648,470.64. The amount appropriated from state funds, in the operation of the Perkins, Haskell-Klaus Law for the year ending June 30, 1931 was $1,000,000.00, a total of $1,648,470.64. For the year 1932 supervisors spent approximately $1,000,000.00 and the state through its indigent hospital, another $1,000,000.00. If to this amount were added the money spent by various charitable organizations and by individuals for the relief of the sick indigent in Iowa the total would be augmented by thousands of dollars; if to this sum were added the value of the services of physicians, surgeons and hospitals in Iowa, donated to the indigent and to a great number of deserving poor, this total would be increased by many more thousands of dollars, and if to this total were added the value of services rendered by physicians, surgeons, hospitals and nurses to dead-beats, who deliberately contracted the obligations, with no thought or intent of paying for same, the whole sum would stagger right minded persons and put to shame, if not silence, the sharpest and most subtle critic of the reputable medical profession.

Chapter 199 of the 1924 Code of Iowa provides for medical and surgical treatment of indigent persons as follows:

4005—COMPLAINT. Any. adult resident of the state may file a complaint in the office of the clerk of any juvenile court, charging that any legal resident of Iowa residing in the county where the complaint is filed is suffering from some malady or deformity that can probably be improved or cured by medical or surgical treatment or hospital care, and that neither such person nor persons legally chargeable with his support are able to pay therefor.

4006 — DUTY OF PUBLIC OFFICERS AND OTHERS. It shall be the duty of physicians, public health nurses, members of boards of supervisors and township trustees, over-seers of the poor, sheriffs, policemen, and public school teachers, having knowledge of persons suffering from any such malady or deformity, to file or cause such complaint to be filed.

4007—"PATIENT" DEFINED. The word "patient" as used in this chapter means the person against whom the complaint is filed.

4021—TREATMENT OF OTHER CHILDREN. The hospital authorities may in their discretion receive into the hospital for medical or surgical treatment or hospital care, patients under sixteen years of age not committed thereto under the provisions of this chapter; but the treatment or care of such patients shall not in any way interfere with the proper medical or surgical treatment or hospital care of committed patients.

All of the provisions of this chapter except as to commitment of patients shall apply to such patients. The hospital authorities shall collect from the person or persons liable for the support of such patients, the cost of such care and treatment, determined as in this chapter provided, and shall deposit it to the credit of the hospital fund.

"This section provides for cost patients under sixteen years of age, and is a remnant of the original Perkins law which applies to the Orthopedic Hospital. However, the same principle of procedure has been applied by the hospital administration to the general hospital."

4025—TREATMENT GRATUITOUS. No physician, surgeon, or nurse who shall treat or care for such patient shall charge or receive any compensation therefor except the salary or compensation fixed by the state board of education to be paid from the hospital funds.

"The four classes of patients admitted to the hospital are defined as follows:

"1. STATE. Those patients admitted under the Perkins, Haskell-Klaus law. The expenses of these patients are paid by the state from the appropriation.

"2. COST. Those patients referred by practicing physicians outside the hospital, and recommended as worthy of hospital care but unable to pay professional fees, and who therefore pay only the basic hospital costs. In order to be admitted to such service a physician must sign a form setting forth the above facts.

"3. PAY. Those patients who are admitted to the private wards and who pay all fees, including professional, but who are receiving treatment in departments which are on a full time basis. These fees are placed by the Treasurer of the University in a special fund which may be used only for the scientific work of the department concerned, upon the approval of the President and Dean.

"4. PRIVATE. These patients are the same as (3) above except that these are receiving treatment in departments which are on a part time basis, so that the professional fee goes to the individual faculty member."

According to table VIII on page 21 of the report for the year ending June 30, 1930, hospital earnings from private patients were $100,317.83; cost patients, $64,018.23; staff patients, $11,-539.50; out patients, $55,903.88; total, $231,-779.44. Total hospital receipts, $1,231,845.11.

The committee further reported: "The increasing number of patients waiting for treatment at the University Hospitals (at that time 1,934) is becoming a matter of grave concern to the patients themselves, the physicians attending them, and the university authorities." It pointed out some of the reasons for the large waiting list as follows: Increase in indigency, abuse of the law, misinterpretation of emergency, misrepresentation of degree of indigency, commitment of unnecessary cases, incomplete investigation, improved facilities of transportation, expenses paid from state funds and limitation of beds." To these may be added, quoting from another source, "It is one of the weaknesses of human nature which some people find hard to resist, to want to get something for nothing."

There are those who think the most important reason for the constantly increasing number of adult sick indigents, seeking treatment at the University Hospital, is the adult indigent law itself, exacting an annual toll of $1,000,000.00, apportioned to the ninety-nine counties in sums varying between $5,000.00 and $58,000.00, and definitely, if not completely, blocking attempts at the solution of the sick indigent problem in the community, where, in part, it originates and where, ultimately, it must be solved. This state appropriation not only interferes with the solution of the community sick indigent problem, but also with the solution of the health and economic problems of both the sick and well tax payer. The enlargement of the medical school, of which the hospital is an integral part, was conceived with the noble idea of providing a "comprehensive system of taking care of the poor of the state." How well it has fulfilled its purpose can best be answered by surveys of your own communities.

The full report of the committee on Medical Education and Hospitals, replete with information concerning the operation of Iowa's Indigent law, is submitted herewith, marked exhibit A and made a part of the minority supplemental report.

Much as the minority desires so to do, they find it difficult to deal with the community sick indigent problem, including the ever increasing waiting list, and avoid reference to the College of Medicine. The enlarged University Medical College and Hospital program contemplated a school of 500 students. In 1920-21 the enrollment was 169 with 46 graduates; in 1929-30, there were 490 enrolled, 98 graduates.

Below is a comparative tabulation of population of cities where university medical colleges are located, number of students, graduates and teachers of 15 University Medical Colleges with state supported hospitals. Session, 1932-33.

Arbor, near Detroit with its one and one-half million population; Virginia with only 247 students, 59 graduates; Wisconsin, 313 students, 50 graduates. In California the work of the first year is given at Berkeley, the last three at San Francisco; in Indiana, the first year is given at Bloomington, the last three at Indianapolis; Kansas gives the clinical courses at Kansas City.

There are 77 class A, or approved, medical colleges in the United States. Six state university medical colleges, and two others give only the first two years of the medical course, the last two years being taken at the college of the student's choice; they are Alabama, Missouri, New Hampshire (not university), North Carolina (one university, one other), North Dakota, South Dakota, Utah and West Virginia. There are 41 "university" medical colleges, some state, some private, and 13 whose names do not include "university". All of these function without state supported hospitals. Of the entire list only 8 exceeded in enrollment (1932-1933) the goal set for Iowa, viz. 500; these are Georgetown University, Washington, D. C., registrants 591, graduates 132; Northwestern University, Chicago, R. 550, G. 124; University Illinois, Chicago, R. 637, G. 118; Harvard University, Boston, R. 519, G. 129; St. Louis University, R. 532, G. 115; New York University, University and Bellevue Hospital Medical College, R. 511, G. 122; Jefferson Medical College, Philadelphia, R. 572, G. 140; University of Pennsylvania, Philadelphia, R. 522, G. 138. Besides these only thirteen exceeded Iowa's enrollment of 373 with 93 graduates for the session 1932-33; these are: College of Medical Evangelist, Loma Linda—Los Angeles, Registered, 389, graduates, 68; Loyola

STATISTICS OF APPROVED OR CLASS A MEDICAL COLLEGES*

State University Medical College** with state supported hospitals	Population of city where college is located	Number of students registered 1932-1933	Graduated since July 1, 1932	Teachers
Berkeley (82,109)				
California...............San Francisco	634,394	231	54	379
Colorado...............Denver	287,861	220	47	187
Illinois................Chicago 3,376,438	637	118	293
Bloomington (18,227)				
Indiana.................Indianapolis	364,161	459	102	270
Iowa...................Iowa City	15,340	373	93	109
Lawrence (13,726)				
Kansas.................Kansas City	121,857	288	61	176
Louisiana..............New Orleans***...................	458,762	171	..	149
Maryland...............Baltimore	804,874	406	85	231
Michigan...............Ann Arbor	26,944	485	132	219
Minnesota..............Minneapolis	464,356	470	125	303
Nebraska...............Omaha	214,006	338	74	122
Ohio...................Columbus	290,564	365	86	129
Oklahoma..............Oklahoma City	185,389	255	56	138
Virginia...............Charlottesville	15,245	247	59	69
Wisconsin.............Madison	57,899	313	50	131

*From Educational Number Journal Medical Association August 26, 1933.
**For complete medical college data see Exhibit B.
***Louisiana State University Medical Center; recent.

It will be noted that the above State University Medical Colleges and Medical Center are located in large cities, except Iowa, Michigan, at Ann

University School of Medicine, Chicago, R. 450, G. 114; Indiana University, Indianapolis, R. 459, G. 102; Tulane University of Louisiana School of

Medicine, New Orleans, R. 474, G. 104; University of Maryland School of Medicine and College of Physicians and Surgeons, Baltimore, R. 406, G. 85, Tufts College Medical School, Boston, R. 462, G. 117; University of Michigan, Ann Arbor, R. 485, G. 132; University of Minnesota, Minneapolis, R. 446, G. 138; Long Island College of Medicine, Brooklyn, R. 424, G. 99; Columbia University, New York, R. 378, G. 116; Hahnemann Medical College and Hospital, Philadelphia, R. 469, G. 108; Temple University School of Medicine, Philadelphia, R. 449, G. 125; University of Tennessee, College of Medicine, Memphis, R. 401, G. 109.

The next table compares the number of beds, average patients and patients admitted to the state supported hospitals connected wtih university medical schools in table above.

bring them into more satisfactory relationships with the newer conceptions and methods of university education, on the one hand, and with the needs of present-day society, on the other. It was believed that such a study would assist the efforts to develop a program adapted particularly to the educational, economic and social conditions in this country."

Quoting from this report it was pointed out in your committee's preliminary report that the supply of physicians in this country probably exceeds the need by at least 25,000, and it was recommended that the number of registrants at the state university of Iowa college of medicine be kept "within such limits as would produce for the last two years an average of 75 members for each of these years," and that the quantity of clinical material be correspondingly reduced. The average

STATE UNIVERSITY HOSPITAL DATA*

State University Hospitals	Pop. of City Where Hospital Is Located	Beds*** Rated Capacity	Average Patients	Patients Admitted
California—San Francisco	634,394	255	162	5,329
Colorado—Denver	287,861	158	128	2,965
Illinois—Chicago—Research and Educational Hospital	3,376,438	355	227	5,128
Indiana—Indianapolis	364,161			
Robt. W. Long Hosp. (Affil.)		167	105	2,231
James Whitcomb Riley Hos. for Children (Affil.)		270	211	3,582
William H. Coleman Hosp. for Women (Affil.)		68	63	2,795
Iowa—Iowa City	15,340	954	608	12,937
(Beds used for Indigents, 550)				
Kansas—Kansas City (Bell Memorial Hospital)	121,857	230	152	4,166
Louisiana—New-Orleans Charity Hospital**	458,762	1,756	2,102	45,483
Maryland—Baltimore	804,874	250	250	5,343
Michigan—Ann Arbor	26,944	1,251	1,112	22,207
Minnesota—Minneapolis	464,356	420	332	6,452
Nebraska—Omaha	214,006	215	178	3,472
Ohio—Columbus	290,564	251	183	4,933
Oklahoma—Oklahoma City	185,389	440	445	6,346
Virginia—Charlottsville	15,245	289	194	6,994
Wisconsin—Madison	57,899	630	604	8,708

*From Hospital Number Journal American Medical Association, March 25, 1933. For complete hospital data see exhibit C.
**Established 1786. "No direct official connection between the Louisiana Medical Center and the Charity Hospital." (Personal letter.)
***Many of the state university medical colleges make use of beds in other hospitals for teaching purposes.

It will be noted that the number of hospital beds at Iowa's University Hospital is exceeded only by Michigan. Just why the state of Iowa should be ambitious in the field of medical education and research, with only indigents, taxes and a few pay patients for support, has not been made clear to the minority.

In 1932 two significant volumes were published dealing with medical problems, the Final Report of the Commission on Medical Education, Willard C. Rappleye, M.D., Director of Study, and the Report of the Committee on the Costs of Medical Care, Harry H. Moore, Ph.D., Director of Study. The following excerpts are from the former:

"The Commission on Medical Education was organized in 1925 by the Association of American Medical Colleges to make a study of the educational principles involved in medical education and licensure, and to make suggestions which would

number of graduates for all medical colleges in the United States for 1933 was 73; average registrants 291. It is worth while in discussing Iowa's sick indigent problem and the waiting list in connection with a tax supported university hospital and medical college, which legislation had insured "an increase in hospital facilities and provided a comprehensive system for taking care of the poor of the state," to inquire what becomes of its graduates. Table 19, page 115, of the Commission's Report, shows "the extent to which recent graduates enter directly into the specialties":

SPECIALIZATION AMONG RECENT GRADUATES BY SCHOOLS

All Medical Colleges.................................... 36.1%
Albany Medical College................................ 41.8
University of Buffalo School of Medicine.............. 26.2
Columbia University College of Physicians and Surgeons.. 39.1
Hahnemann Medical College of Philadelphia............ 14.7
Harvard University Medical School.................... 64.1
Howard University College of Medicine................ 4.6
University of Illinois College of Medicine............ 31.1
State University of Iowa College of Medicine......... 48.9

Jefferson Medical College of Philadelphia................. 26.0
Johns Hopkins University School of Medicine.'........ 75.1
Long Island College of Medicine......................... 17.8
University of Michigan Medical School................... 43.5
University and Bellevue Hospital Medical College........ 25.3
University of Pennsylvania School of Medicine......... 39.4
University of Chicago, Rush Medical College............ 44.5
Stanford University of School of Medicine.............. 55.8
University of Toronto Faculty of Medicine............... 56.0
Tufts College Medical School........................... 27.5
Tulane University School of Medicine................... 36.1
University of Virginia Department of Medicine........... 61.5

The commission comments: "It is well established that the percentage of specialists in the larger cities is much higher than in smaller communities. In such typical states as Wisconsin, Indiana and Louisiana twenty to thirty per cent of all practitioners in cities of 50,000 or more restrict themselves to a limited field, whereas in communities of 10,000 or less the proportion is about three per cent and in those of 5,000 or less, about two' per cent." (See tabulation in preliminary report.)

"Not only is there a concentration of physicians in the larger cities, particularly of recent graduates, but a large proportion of them limit their practices to a specialty, often without a sufficiently broad clinical experience."

Table 37, page 283 of the report shows the source and amount of income of 63 schools for 1926-27. "A large but not readily isolated fraction of the total was for research work, which, in some instances, is conducted quite independently of the teaching program."

INCOME OF MEDICAL SCHOOLS

Students' fees	$ 4,057,304
Endowment income	2,784,527
State or City	2,574,973
Other sources	2,567,069
	$11,983,873

"The average cost of maintaining the medical schools was approximately $794 per year per student for 1926-27. The average of the students' fees paid was $254. These are only averages and in some of the medical schools the cost is now above $3,000 per student per year."

The per capita cost of medical education to Iowa for 1929-30 has been given as $665.00. If to the regular budget for medicine, less the receipts from tuition and fees, is added the appropriations for the university hospitals as integral units of the college of medicine, the per capita cost will be somewhat greater; if the per capita cost per annum of the 373 medical students is compared with that of the 6,373 students in all other departments, Iowa's generosity to medical education will be apparent.

Concluding the Commission's report on the cost of medical education is found the following comment: "It is highly important and desirable that some schools which can obtain liberal support should develop programs of research and the training of personnel, particularly for the scientific and teaching field, but it is neither necessary nor desirable that the large budgets of this group of schools should become the standard for all . . . The large expenditures of some medical schools should not be regarded as the standard for all because medical students can be well trained in schools which have modest budgets."

Coming now to the Majority Report of the Committee on the Costs of Medical Care it may be quickly, and sanity suggests finally, dismissed by presenting what it had to offer to once rural states like Iowa. One suggestion was that a "university medical service may be expanded and developed to meet wider needs"; another that "In the rural areas our problems are more difficult. We will probably have to think there in terms of 'medical stations' rather than elaborate hospital centers, of places where patients can come and doctors can go and where such facilities as are possible can be provided. With the present state of agriculture, particularly in the southern states, it does not seem likely that any adequate form of rural medical care can be carried out without support from the state or elsewhere. There is not enough in the way of resources." Where does the state's money come from, with which to expand its university medical service and leave to the tax payer a "medical station". Is Iowa's goal an ever increasing flow of indigents to its University Medical Center, or is it NO INDIGENCY IN IOWA? The fact of the matter is, Iowa is no longer rural; good roads have made every farmer a suburban resident of and much nearer to his county seat or nearest large town than are residents of cities living like distances out, by reason of less traffic and fewer stop signals.

The minority report of that committee has been summarized by Dr. Nathan B. Van Etten, in part, as follows: "The minority objects to the large medical center as projected by the majority on the ground of exclusion of many physicians, of oppressive competition, of big business technique erecting machinery which eliminates personality and destroys personal relations by factory form. Mere bigness is often a liability.

"The minority recognizes the practicability of centering medical service in small places where there are only one or two hospitals where all of the physicians of the community are permitted to use all of the facilities of the hospitals in a true community spirit, the institution being supported by taxation or by gifts."

Dr. Dean Lewis, President of the American Medical Association, recently said: "The medical profession should take an active interest in hospitalization. Hospital planning should be undertaken. A city or town of 15,000 people should not have three hospitals. One good hospital could take care of the needs of such a community. Better have one hospital that is full and active than three partially filled. The partially filled hospital has an enormous overhead." Presumably, in a state like Iowa with few cities of 15,000, the county would be considered a community.

In 1926 the U. S. Department of Agriculture published a pamphlet, "Rural Hospitals", by Wayne C. Nason, Assistant Economic Analyst, Bureau of Agricultural Economics, Farmer's Bulletin No. 1485. In it may be found the following:

"More and more President (Theodore) Roosevelt's expressed desire for country people, 'a good kind of life on the farm' is being realized. . Modern schools, less denominational rivalry with resultant better rural churches, community building, little country theatres, country parks and playgrounds, country visiting nurses, cooperative farm business enterprises, improved roads, telephone, the radio, electric equipment, and modern home conveniences are accomplishing notable results. They are bringing to farm people more contentment and to the Nation a more enduring agriculture. And now rural hospitals are being erected, in fulfillment of a long-known need, to give added satisfaction to rural life."

What has happened in Iowa and in the United States since 1926 is common knowledge.

Comes now President Franklin D. Roosevelt, addressing the American Legion, in Chicago, October 2, 1933:

"There are many veterans of our wars to whom disability and sickness unconnected with war service has come. To them the federal government owes the application of the same rule which it has laid down for the relief of other cases of involuntary want or destitution.

"In other words, if the individual affected can afford to pay for his own treatment he cannot call on any form of government aid. If he has not the wherewithal to take care of himself, it is first of all the duty of his community to take care of him and next the duty of his state. Only if under these circumstances his own community and his own state are unable, after reasonable effort, to care for him, then, and then only, should the federal government offer him hospitalization and care."

How is the community to provide for the disabled veteran's hospitalization in many places? What about the veteran's family, the tax payer and his family, indigents on the waiting list; and many whose lives are jeopardized or lost by long distance transportation?

A recent newspaper report of the meeting of the American College of Surgeons quoted a speaker as saying: "In Chicago 62 of your 85 hospitals are on the approved list." In Iowa, 39 of 128 hospitals are on the approved list and these are located in 22 cities. According to the Medical Directory of the American Medical Association, 1931, there are 120 Fellows of the American College of Surgeons in Iowa; 89 of these are located in 20 of the 22 cities having approved hospitals in which to work.

Is it any wonder that Dr. Dean Lewis says "Hospital planning should be undertaken"? Perhaps, because of the relation of sickness, accidents, physicians, surgeons and hospitals to both intra and interstate traffic, President Roosevelt may note a reason for interesting the Public Works Administration in offering inducement to counties or communities, not already supplied, to make suitable hospital provision for such care of medical and surgical cases as can there properly be given and where will be assured a standardized equipment and service that will enable competent, honest consultation, in serious cases, to properly function. The government's interest and activities in the field of public health and its efforts to establish county public health services could well be correlated with hospital planning. In any such undertaking, due consideration must be given to existing hospitals whose control is now either church, community, county, independent, or, in some cases, private.

In December, 1928, Dr. Thomas A. Burcham, chairman, made a report of the legislative committee of the Iowa State Medical Society before the Conference of Secretaries and Deputy Councilors. This report dealt with conferences in 1927 between Dean Houghton, President Jessup, Department Heads of the University Medical College, and the Legislative Committee and officers of the State Medical Society. Two problems remained unsettled after these conferences: "First, the extent to which the new University Hospital should be used for private patients; second, methods of meeting the demand of those who supported proposed changes in the Perkins, Haskell-Klaus laws without curtailing the supply of clinical material at the University Hospital." Proposed changes and the reasons therefore were detailed and the decision of the Board of Education given, with the following comment: "After a careful analysis of the resolution from the Board of Education, one is convinced that the Board does not feel inclined to use its influence in any way to have the present

Perkins, Haskell-Klaus laws changed in any manner. Although they agree that certain changes should be made they are unwilling to consent to such changes being made in the law but desire that the changes be a policy of the board."

The full report (1928) of the Legislative Committee of the Iowa State Medical Society, is submitted herewith marked exhibit D and made a part of the minority's supplemental report.

As has been mentioned, there were introduced in both the Forty-second and Forty-third General Assemblies, bills for legislation intended to modify the laws governing the operation of the University Hospital and the commitment of indigent patients thereto. Such bills will continue to be introduced indefinitely unless now the Forty-fifth General Assembly in extraordinary session gives consideration to the tax payer as well as the tax eater.

Operating under House Joint Resolution No. 7, your committee, through its sub-committee, has held several conferences with hospital authorities in the hope that bills which, in a measure, might be satisfactory to all concerned could be agreed upon, to be presented to the special session of the Forty-fifth General Assembly. Before the supplemental report of your committee had been agreed upon or even drafted, the Des Moines Register, September 17, 1933, carried a front page news article from Iowa City detailing opposition on the part of hospital authorities to measures submitted with its preliminary report. This opposition in part was said to have been based on "the Brookings Institution report on state finances and management, although the committee of nine has been refused a copy of the Brookings report on hospital management." The Des Moines Register article is submitted herewith, marked exhibit E.

Copy of a letter written by the chairman of your committee under date of March 16, 1933, and addressed to Dean H. S. Houghton, University Clinics, University of Chicago, Chicago, Ill., to which no reply has been received, together with an editorial from the Mason City Globe Gazette of April 6, 1933, is submitted herewith, marked Exhibit F and made a part of the minority report.

Copy of the Spencer Reporter, February 5, 1931, containing an article based upon the searching, fact finding report of the Committee on Hospitals and Education of the Iowa State Medical Society, illustrated with a map of Iowa showing pertinent facts relative to hospitals and indigents, is submitted herewith, marked Exhibit G.

A Questionnaire sent to Iowa district judges together with replies are submitted herewith, without comment, and marked exhibit H.

In order that the Forty-fifth General Assembly may be informed concerning the promotion of Iowa's enlarged medical college and hospital program, certain literature, much of it "Not to be released until December 27," 1922 just prior to the convening of the Fortieth General Assembly, is submitted herewith, without comment, and marked Exhibit I.

Newspaper clippings, reprints, and unsolicited letters, dealing with the operation of the adult indigent law, are submitted herewith, without comment, marked exhibit J.

In conclusion, it appears from the Des Moines Register article (Exhibit E) that no matter what proposals your committee or the committee of the Iowa State Medical Society may have made or make, "Like the state board of education, university heads and the hospital staff feel there is no need for legislation" and opposition to any proposed reforms has been promised. There comes a time when patience is exhausted in endeavors to square a circle. The mere fact that Iowa has a capital investment of $5,000,000.00 or $6,000,000.00 in an enlarged medical college and hospital plant, with an overhead of approximately $1,500,000.00 per annum, not including interest on the investment, is no reason for carrying on at any cost, even if that were possible for a little while longer. The state's relation to its investment is comparable to that of some farmers and their once inflated land values and to that of all farmers with products for which there is no reasonable market; interest and taxes have helped to eat them out of house and home. Big business has had to suffer because of questionable promotion and for other reasons; small business, the industries, the professions and labor have been engulfed or overwhelmed in the debacle, and all realize we are living in a changing world.

The minority would direct your attention to the fact that every year enough clinical material, for teaching purposes, goes to waste, in the city of Des Moines, to furnish a much needed variety and a sufficient number for the instruction of all the new doctors there is need for each year in Iowa. It is not primarily essential that the state university medical college should be at Iowa City, except, perhaps, because of a constitutional provision, any more than that Nebraska should be at Lincoln, Indiana at Bloomington, or Kansas at Lawrence. At Des Moines it would be as much the university of Iowa medical college as are those at Omaha, Indianapolis and Kansas City, Kansas, the university medical colleges of their states. As a matter of fact, a similar condition is found at Rush and the University of California. Laws have been repealed, constitutions have been amended, and amendments, both state and national, have been or are being repealed. To whom does the Iowa State University Medical College and Hospital belong?

The state of Iowa having invested heavily in medical education, the minority directs your attention to one of the "Essentials of an Acceptable Medical College" required by the Council on Medical Education and Hospitals: "At least fifteen maternity cases should be provided for each senior student, who should have actual charge of these cases, under the supervision of the clinical instructor." Prior to February 12, 1933, the requirement was ten maternity cases. "During the calendar year of 1929 there was a total of 285 deliveries, while from January 1, 1930, to Sept. 29, 1930, 284 patients were delivered." Great and earnest effort is made to secure the needed number of obstetrical cases—1,500 for a graduating class of 100, 48 per cent of whom are said to have recently engaged in the various specialties. In 1929 there were 828 births in Des Moines hospitals and two other institutions; including these, the total for Des Moines was 2,823 births; in Polk county, outside Des Moines, 208, total for Polk county, 3,031. For the same year there were 524 births in Iowa City (See A. addenda) including births at university hospital; Johnson county, outside Iowa City, 186, total 710. For the year 1932, the number of births at the University Hospital reached a total of 713. What part of Polk county's 3,000 or more births may have been available for clinical teaching is not definitely given, but the number must have been and is considerable. It is good public policy even to endeavor to collect from all over the state the required number of obstetrical cases, legitimate and illegitimate, on or near the campus of the state university?

There were 5,238 on the waiting list for free treatment at the University Hospital on Feb. 7, 1933; many had waited for years, some had suffered and died enroute or while they waited and others are still waiting, notwithstanding other Iowa hospitals have had their beds only about 60 per cent filled, and churches, independent organizations and a few counties have struggled on against tremendous odds to keep their hospitals from putting out the sign "Closed for want of funds." What might it mean to Polk county if it could economically spend its $58,750.00, less $5,767.60 for special fees at Iowa City, presuming these would be similar anywhere—$52,982.44, within its own borders? The latter sum was spent (July 1, 1930-June 30, 1931) as follows: Board and room, $31,020.50; railroad fare, $4,020.19; bus,

taxi and ambulance, $674.36; hotel, meals and telephone, $339.49; escorts, $415.50; doctors examination fees, $1,070.00; a total of $37,540.04, which with the special fees, makes $43,307.70 as the cost of all the inclusive service to 379 Polk county sick indigents that year; adding to this the excess charged to Polk county for which it received no service, makes the total $58,750.00. Proportionate amounts can be applied to 59 of the 99 counties, and it may be seriously questioned whether very many of the other 40, whose contribution is less than their total cost of service, really struck a bargain by taking advantage of the provisions of the adult indigent law. What would it mean if all this money could circulate in the various communities? Isn't this something for the P. W. A. to think about?

How did the other 172,458 inhabitants of Iowa's most important bailiwick, some of whom paid this indigent bill, manage to get along with the ministrations of their local physicians? What of its year-round floating population? True, for various and sufficient reasons, an occasional patient may have gone to Chicago, Rochester, Omaha, Minneapolis, St. Paul, St. Louis, Kansas City, New York, Philadelphia, Baltimore and other noted medical centers; may be some to Sioux City, Davenport, Cedar Rapids, Waterloo, Council Bluffs, Dubuque, Mason City, Marshalltown and smaller cities; to make up for all this migration they went from everywhere to Des Moines, and believe it or not, it has happened that some have gone back to the country doctor, the old family physician, to inquire what it was all about. That was and is their right. How did the remaining 2,288,616 Iowa people manage to keep afloat? Many of them did not; they sank, and Iowa City, with its "comprehensive system of taking care of the poor," "dedicated to the service of the Iowa people," suggested neither life preserver nor attempt at rescue. The reputable physicians and surgeons and the existing hospital set up of this state, insufficient and inequitably distributed as it is, did and do a much better job of taking care of the "sick poor of the state." Let it be understood here and now that the minority disavows any thought of reflection upon the eminent ability of members of the faculty of the State University Medical College. They deal with an immensely important social problem with four sides; the sick and injured, the reputable medical profession, the depleted tax payer and the humanities. Along with these and intimately associated with each is an urgent economic problem.

As long ago as 1923 or 1924 Dr. Olin West, addressing a state medical society, said: "The one great outstanding problem before the medical profession today is that involved in the delivery of adequate, scientific medical service to all the people, rich and poor, at a cost which can be reasonably met by them in their respective stations in life." Presumably, in their own communities, where reasonable and intelligent cooperation on the part of the public with the reputable medical profession is an essential part of the problem. He did not say the one great problem was to maintain a great university medical center at any cost.

One of the distressing features of Iowa's adult indigent law is that the truly indigent citizen, well to do a short while ago, poor today, in need of medical care, must first become "a ward of the state" and surrender what would appear to be a very important right, the right to have, if possible, the physician of his choice. That right is preserved to him in his own county by the board of supervisors and its contract with physicians for the care of the sick poor. To deny the patient the stimulation of his confidence in his own physician works a great injustice. Another most annoying feature of the sick indigent law is the demand, by those who "want to get something for nothing," that they be sent to Iowa City whether any real need exists or not, firm in the belief that some physician will acquiesce. The effect upon the community morale is bad. Of the many bad features of Iowa's adult indigent law, one is most repugnant, one which no lawyer, priest or minister would have tolerated for even the few years that reputable physicians have stood aghast, viz'., A patient against whom complaint has been filed for no other reason than that he is poor and in need of medical care, must waive his right of privileged communication and the physician is compelled to violate his obligation to hold as a trust matters of delicacy and secrecy and hang the whole story on the line in the office of the clerk of the district court. The adult indigent law is wrong in principle and in application.

If it is admitted by your honorable body that indigency, in some or all of its phases, is primarily and largely a community problem, and that sickness of the indigent is very distinctly a community problem, this very large hospital plant belongs to your great commonwealth and it is up to you as its representatives—the trustees of its interests—to determine, in the light of experience, the practicability of the huge undertaking of Iowa City with its immense capital investment and enormous overhead.

Having been promised, in the press of the state, opposition on the part of university and hospital authorities to recommendations and proposed

amendments to Chapter 199, Code of Iowa, 1931, in its preliminary report, which purported to be an approach to a square deal for the sick indigents, the reputable medical profession, the taxpayers and the state university medical college of Iowa, the minority now deems it fit and proper to submit, for the deliberate consideration of the Governor, the Senate and the House of Representatives, the following selective recommendations, reasons and requests for such further action by your honorable selves as circumstances warrant:

1. Increase the appropriation for the university hospital by an indeterminate amount, but sufficient to fill unoccupied beds, provide more beds for the waiting list, whose chief characteristic is growth, and still more beds for those who insist upon free treatment and care at the hands of the state; or

2. Limit the students to a lesser number than that recommended in the preliminary report, limit indigent patients to the number required for the teaching of the smaller number of students and charge the entire cost for their care and treatment to each county according to service received; or

3. Provide for the repeal of the adult indigent law to become effective at a future time, giving due consideration to certain involved principles and relationships, restore the Perkins law to its original status and take necessary steps to establish the last two or three years of the State University of Iowa Medical College in the city of Des Moines, thereby relieving Iowa of a frequently whispered doubt, first openly expressed at a meeting of the Board of Education and found on page 18 of the Report of the Iowa State Board of Education for the biennial period ending June 30, 1928. Part of the letter follows as exhibit F of that report.

"EXHIBIT F"

"On February 20, 1928, a called meeting of the Board of Education was held at Iowa City. Part of a letter from Dr. H. S. Houghton, Dean of the College of Medicine, was read, as follows:

" '(1) The Medical College has approximately two hundred (191) students registered in the two final years of the medical course. Their studies are almost entirely clinical, and to a great extent, depend on the use of patients. To take medicine as a typical example, it appears that the department has 400 hours teaching, all of which require the use of ward patients; this excludes the hours devoted to physical diagnosis, clinical laboratory and therapeutics. It likewise takes no account of such allied subjects as pediatrics and neurology, which in this institution are independent departments. It is manifestly impossible to give two hundred students four hundred hours of exercises in practical medicine with a daily census of sixty patients. One scarcely needs to press the question further, but it may be added that the minimum called for by the council of Medical Education of the A. M. A. as far back as 1910 was 100 beds for the use of combined classes numbering 200. Any institution falling below this requirement failed of recognition as a Class A College. In other words, it may be questioned whether this college at the present moment would qualify either under the Council of the American Medical Association or of the American Association of Medical Colleges as an approved and acceptable institution. What I have indicated with regard to the Department of Medicine is equally true of other departments, with the possible exception of orthopedics and otolaryngology, but these departments are under special pressure for the care of indigent patients, particularly sick and crippled children.

" 'A comparison of six of the large Class A Medical colleges, three of which are state institutions and three private, makes apparent the deficiency to which I have directed your attention in the preceding paragraph:

University	Hours of Clinical Instruction Requiring Students Ward Patients		Beds under Hospital Faculty Control
	3 Yr.	4 Yr.	Med.	Surg.	
Minnesota 100	100	300	217	1,000
		288	432	
Harvard 134	184	432	288	2,000
Hopkins 71	77	330	297	1,000
Michigan 118	116	324	250	1,162
Western Reserve.. 59	36	48?	600	2,000
Iowa 91	100	408	338	346
" '(2)				
" '(3)				

" 'I submit, in the light of the foregoing facts that the critical condition of the teaching and medical service responsibilities entrusted to the University of the State, should promptly be made known to the members of the Board of Education and that they be asked to deal with the difficulties involved, all of which are outside of the province or powers of the Medical Faculty.

Yours sincerely,

(Signed) HENRY S. HOUGHTON,
Dean' "

(See Exhibit P.)

The minority earnestly petitions your honorable body to give serious consideration to this recommendation in order that Iowa may regain and hold her proud position among American medical schools, and accomplish the purpose of the Board of Education and the administration of the university . . . "namely, to put this institution in the front rank of medical colleges in the United States and keep it there." You are reminded that propaganda, landscaping, Gothic or Renaissance architecture and size do not determine RANK among medical colleges.

The minority further recommends that, if this third proposal appeals to your deliberate judgment as a possible or probable solution of the vexing problems that confront and confuse "The public, the taxpayers, the legislators, the courts, the College of Medicine and hospital authorities, the medical profession and the indigents of Iowa", due consideration be given to members of the faculty of the State University of Iowa Medical College, who have labored under the most trying circumstances. You are again reminded that they did not enact the impracticable adult indigent law, nor did they match the philanthropic gifts of the Rockefeller Foundation and the General Education Board. The good faith and beneficient intent of the Thirty-eighth and Fortieth General Assemblies is not doubted, but a mistake was made, and the minority expresses the hope that you may be able to correct it in the best possible way. There is no occasion for tears; correction may hurt a little, but restoration to a place in the sun will compensate for that. The medical college can yet be made the pride of its alumni, the joy of its faculty, the delight of its students, a somnificacient for the President of the University, a sedative for the State Board of Education, a cerebral stimulant for the uninformed and a very real asset to the state of Iowa.

4. As provided in No. 3, except if the city of Des Moines, notwithstanding its relativity, is not in a receptive mood and does not care to be approached with a proposal which would add to its assets as well as to those of the State, then give only the first or first and second years of medicine at Iowa City and let the last two or three be taken elsewhere, for the reason that no city in the state of Iowa, other than Des Moines, has the environment essential to the clinical years of a Class A medical college. Located at Iowa City and Des Moines, it can be put just where the Board of Education and the administration of the University would have it, not large, but meritorious, and be somewhere "in the front rank of medical colleges in the United States."

Signed this 29th day of November, 1933, in the city of Des Moines.

By the minority,
E. E. MUNGER, M.D.
G. W. PATTERSON

The JOURNAL

of the

Iowa State Medical Society

Vol. XXIV   Des Moines, Iowa, February, 1934.   No. 2

ADDITIONAL DATA ON UTERINE CANCER

R. M. Collins, M.D., Iowa City

Department of Obstetrics and Gynecology, State University of Iowa, College of Medicine

In March, 1933, Miller[1] recorded certain data obtained from a study of 219 consecutive cases of carcinoma of the female generative organs admitted to the University Hospitals from 1917 to November 1, 1927. From the latter date until June 30, 1933, 395 additional new cases were admitted to the clinic. The histories of these patients have been studied after the manner adopted by Miller so that certain facts in the two series may be compared to determine whether the state-wide effort at cancer control has wrought any significant changes.

TABLE I

Region Involved	Miller's Series No.	Pct.	New Series No.	Pct.	Combined No.	Pct.
Cervix	167	76	231	58.5	398	64.5
Fundus	24	11	70	17.7	94	15.3
Ovary	16	7.5	53	13.4*	69	11.3
Vulva	8	4	17	4.3	25	4.1
Vagina	3	1	13	3.3	16	2.7
Tube	1	0.5	2	0.5	3	0.5
Clitoris	0	0.0	2	0.5	2	0.4
Site unknown	0	0.0	7	1.8	7	1.2
Total	219	100.0	395	100.0	614	100.0

*The relatively high percentage of ovarian carcinoma in this series is worthy of note.

Table I shows that there has been a considerably altered distribution of the cancer patients sent to the gynecologic clinic. Cancer of the cervix represents only 58 per cent of cancer admissions during the past five and one-half years as against 76 per cent in the earlier series. This difference is compensated for by increases in the proportion of cancers of the fundus, ovary, and vagina, and in those far advanced cases where it was impossible to determine the original site of the malignant change. The reduced number of admissions for cervical carcinoma may be due to (1) more patients in this group being treated in their home communities by locally owned radium and x-ray, or (2) an actual decrease in the number of patients with cancer of the cervix due to better care after

parturition. When it is considered that our records show an increase in admissions for all pelvic malignancies commonly treated by operative extirpation, we are inclined to believe that more patients with carcinoma of the cervix are being treated with radiation therapy by their own physicians.

Following Miller's scheme, the cases of cervical and fundus carcinoma have been analyzed regarding certain significant clinical facts which can be obtained from the histories. No attention has been paid to the pathologic grouping of the tumors, nor to their extent, except as it indicates operability. It is obviously too early to report the results of therapy. In general, cancer of the cervix has been treated by radiation, and cancer of the fundus by extirpation of the entire uterus whenever it was possible.

CANCER OF THE CERVIX

Parity. Cancer of the cervix more commonly occurs in women who have borne children but is not confined exclusively to that group. Table II shows that the percentages of nulliparas in the two series are remarkably constant. It is, however, significant that 14 per cent of the entire group had never been pregnant. The average number of children among the parous women in the two series has remained stationary and probably represents the average of the state.

TABLE II

Cancer of the Cervix in relation to parity.

	Miller's Series No.	Pct.	New Series No.	Pct.	Combined No.	Pct.
Nullipara	22	14	28	12	50	13
Multipara	141	86	200	88	341	87
Parity not stated	4	—	3	—	7	—
Total	167		231		398	
Average number of children in the parous group	4		4		4	

Operability. It is recognized that the term "operability" is subject to such individual interpretation as to be almost valueless. To overcome this objection, all patients showing no palpable infiltration of the parametria (Schmitz Groups I and II) have been arbitrarily classified as "operable." On this basis, the number of operable (early) cases is seen (Table III) to have risen from 18 per cent to 28 per cent, largely because the medical profession is paying more attention to abnormal uterine bleeding, as is emphasized later when the causes for delay in securing adequate treatment are considered.

TABLE III

Cancer of the Cervix

Operability—Schmitz Groups I and II

	Miller's Series		New Series		Combined	
	No.	Pct.	No.	Pct.	No.	Pct.
Operable	30	18	63	28	93	23
Inoperable	137	82	166	72	303	77
Not stated	0	—	2	—	2	—

The fact that even now 72 per cent of our cases of cervical cancer are "inoperable" when admitted indicates that cancer education must be continued unabated. It will be shown later that the physician's responsibility for the delay has been materially lessened, but that little progress has been made with the laity. Education has made the public "appendix conscious" and education can in time make for general cancer consciousness. Abnormal vaginal bleeding, especially continued or repeated intermenstrual bleeding which is aggravated by exertion or contact, must be stressed, since "spotting" is the earliest symptom in three-fourths of all cases.

Diagnosis Before Admission. Correct diagnosis is essential to proper treatment and it is encouraging to find that the number of patients with cervical cancer coming to the clinic with correct diagnoses has increased from 56 per cent to 77 per cent. On the other hand it should be noted that 15 patients (7 per cent) in the recent series had not been examined vaginally before admission. There can be no excuse for not examining patients with abnormal vaginal bleeding, when this symptom so often indicates malignancy.

TABLE IV

Cancer of the Cervix ·

Diagnosis before admission.

	Miller's Series		New Series		Combined	
	No.	Pct.	No.	Pct.	No.	Pct.
Correctly diagnosed	71	56	162	77	233	69
Incorrectly diagnosed	55	44	48	23	103	31
Not examined	4		15		19	
History indefinite	41		21		62	

The fact that the percentage of cases correctly diagnosed before admission (77 per cent) agrees so closely with the proportion of advanced cases (73 per cent) suggests that late "textbook" cases are generally diagnosed, while the earlier lesions escape recognition. The differentiation of early cervical cancer from non-malignant inflammatory lesions of the cervix is difficult but yet essential, since the possibility of cure is largely limited to those cases which fall in groups I and II of the Schmitz classification. In any doubtful case it is imperative that material be removed by biopsy for microscopic examination by a competent pathologist. It is far better that ten, twenty, or fifty such biopsies show only benign lesions than that one early carcinoma be missed by failure to remove tissue for examination. In this connection it should also be emphasized that biopsy should always, especially after the menopause, be accompanied by dilatation and curettage.

Postmenopausal Bleeding. In 167 (42 per cent), of the total of 398 cases of cervical carcinoma, the first symptom (bleeding) appeared after the menopause—six months subsequent to the last vaginal bleeding that could be looked upon as menstrual in character. That the significance of postmenopausal bleeding is being better appreciated is attested by the fact (see Table V) that 82 per cent of these cases in the new series were correctly diagnosed before admission as against 64 per cent in the earlier series and 77 per cent for all cases in the recent group (Table IV). Even in the recent series seven patients in this group were not examined before admission.

TABLE V

Cancer of the Cervix

First symptom after the menopause.

	Miller's Series		New Series		Combined	
	No.	Pct.	No.	Pct.	No.	Pct.
History definite....	64		103		167	
History indefinite..	29		13		42	
Total	93		116		209	
Correctly diagnosed	41	64	84	82	125	75
Incorrectly diagnosed	23	36	19	18	42	25
Total	64	100	103	100	167	100
Not examined	1		7		8	

Responsibility for Delay. Delay in securing adequate treatment for cancer patients rests with the *patients* who do not report to their physicians promptly on the appearance of symptoms, and with the *physicians* who do not examine the patients vaginally, or, if they do, cannot appreciate the character of the lesion and the need for prompt therapy.

There is a widespread belief that vaginal manipulations should not be carried out in the presence of bleeding, and this idea, common alike to the laity and the profession, frequently leads to unjustifiable postponement of an examination which might conduce to earlier diagnosis. Bimanual palpation is demanded by the occurrence of persistent bleeding, and nothing should be allowed to interfere with its performance.

The practice of treating uterine bleeding with

oxytocic agents before accurate diagnosis has been made is perhaps the most common professional error in such cases, but in other instances there is unwarranted persistence in local treatments—tampons, medicinal applications and cauterizations—without the evidence offered by biopsy that the lesion is not malignant.

In doubtful cases, digital examination and inspection alone cannot with certainty make the diagnosis, and it is questionable whether the various accessory diagnostic methods, other than biopsy, can be relied upon. The probe test of Chrobak (a fine silver probe pressed strongly against a carcinomatous cervix penetrates easily into the underlying malignant tissue with the production of bright bleeding) is useful, but may also be positive in certain non-malignant conditions, such as syphilis of the cervix. When Lugol's solution is applied to a suspicious cervix (Schiller's test), the normal tissue takes a brown stain, while malignant tissue remains pink; but again there may be difficulties of interpretation, especially in early cases, where the diagnosis is really in doubt. Biopsy remains the only reliable test for the presence or absence of malignancy.

Delay on the part of the patient is due to the fact that menstrual disorders are common and that unusual bleeding is likely to be looked upon merely as an "irregularity," or, after the menopause, as a "return of the periods." Popular educational programs must insist that unusual bleeding is abnormal and should be investigated no matter what the age or condition of the patient.

Table VI
Cancer of the Cervix
Responsibility for delay in securing treatment.

	Average time wasted		
Miller's Series	Days	Weeks	Mos.
Time from first symptom to first examination 175		25	6.2
Time from first examination to first treatment 168		24	6
AVERAGE TOTAL TIME LOST—1 YEAR			

New Series			
Time from first symptom to first examination 196		28	7
Time from first examination to first treatment 63		9	2.25
AVERAGE TOTAL TIME LOST—9¼ MONTHS			

Combined			
Time from first symptom to first examination 184		26.3	6.6
Time from first examination to first treatment 112		16	4
AVERAGE TOTAL TIME LOST—10½ MONTHS			

According to Table VI, Miller found that the average delay in cervical carcinoma was one year, with the responsibility divided equally between the patient and the physician, whereas in the recent series the total time loss was reduced to nine months with the medical profession responsible for only one-quarter of the time wasted. No doubt, the marked improvement from the professional point of view can be attributed directly to the cancer campaign which has been waged by state and national organizations. The Iowa Section of the American Society for the Control of Cancer was organized in 1927 with Dr. William Jepson, of Sioux City, as director, and to it must go considerable credit for stimulating a greater interest in the earlier recognition of cancer. On the other hand, it is obvious that our efforts in the direction of lay education have been, according to the evidence here presented, of no avail. If it were possible to reduce the time of the patient's delay in proportion to that of the physician's delay, the death rate from cervical cancer should show a decided drop, since there is no doubt that adequate treatment of early malignancy does lead to "cure" in a reasonable percentage of cases.

CANCER OF THE UTERINE FUNDUS

Although carcinoma of the uterine body is, according to our statistics, only about one-fourth as common as cervical cancer, it represents the second largest group of genital malignancies in the female.

Parity. Among the 70 cases of fundus cancer in the present series there were 21 nulliparous women, 30 per cent, as compared with 13 per cent in Miller's series (see Table VII). For the combined groups, the incidence of multiparity is 26 per cent, a value more consonant with other reported statistics and supporting the usual conception that women who have never borne children are more susceptible to fundus than to cervical carcinoma.

Table VII
Cancer of the Uterine Fundus
Relation to parity.

	Miller's Series		New Series		Combined	
	No.	Pct.	No.	Pct.	No.	Pct.
Nulliparas	3	13	21	30	24	26
Multiparas	19	87	48	70	67	74
Parity not stated	2		1		3	
Total	24		70		94	
Average number of children in parous group	3		3		3	

Operability. The proportion of operable cases increased from 71 per cent in Miller's report, to 81 per cent in the new series.

Table VIII
Cancer of the Uterine Fundus
Operability.

	Miller's Series		New Series		Combined	
	No.	Pct.	No.	Pct.	No.	Pct.
Operable	17	71	57	81	74	79
Inoperable	7	29	13	19	20	21
Total	24		70		94	

Corpus cancer is usually slow-growing and remains operable for months and even years, whereas the more invasive cervical carcinoma may be inoperable when the first symptom is noted. With complete hysterectomy, the accepted treatment for corpus cancer, the high percentage of operable cases explains the relatively favorable prognosis in this type of malignancy. Moreover, operative attack clearly establishes the significance of the term "operable" by denoting an absence of extension beyond the uterus.

Diagnosis Before Admission. There has been a slight increase in the number of correct diagnoses before admission.

Table IX

Cancer of the Uterine Fundus

Diagnosis before admission.

	Miller's Series No.	Pct.	New Series No.	Pct.	Combined No.	Pct.
Correctly diagnosed	10	55	34	67	44	64
Incorrectly diagnosed	8	45	17	33	25	36
Not examined	2		3		5	
History indefinite	4		16		20	
Total	24		70		94	

In many instances, the "correct diagnosis" was little more than an intelligent surmise, since diagnostic curettage had not been done. Cancer of the body of the uterus cannot be diagnosed by bimanual palpation and inspection, since there are no characteristic findings, but the history of irregular bleeding and watery discharge in a woman at or past the menopause always arouses the suspicion of corpus cancer. If the uterus is found to be slightly but symmetrically enlarged, and particularly if the passage of a uterine sound is followed by a trickle of bright blood, the suspicion is greatly strengthened. Final diagnosis must, however, rest upon the gross and microscopic examination of material obtained from the uterine cavity by the curette. In any suspected case, dilatation and curettage are demanded at the earliest possible moment.

Postmenopausal Bleeding. Vaginal bleeding after the menopause (more than six months after the last bleeding that could be of a menstrual character) must be considered prima facie evidence of genital malignancy. Approximately two-thirds of all patients with postmenopausal bleeding have malignancies somewhere in the genital tract,[2] more commonly in the cervix or the body of the uterus.

Table X

Cancer of the Uterine Fundus

First symptom after the menopause.

	Miller's Series No.	Pct.	New Series No.	Pct.	Combined No.	Pct.
Correctly diagnosed	6	50	31	67	37	64
Incorrectly diagnosed	6	50	15	33	21	36
Not examined	2		3		5	
Total	14		49		63	

The fact that the percentage of correct diagnoses has risen from 50 per cent in the earlier series to 67 per cent in this group indicates that physicians are becoming more aware of the relation of postmenopausal bleeding to genital malignancy. However, the present percentage of correct diagnoses corresponds exactly with the percentage of malignancies in a large group of patients with postmenopausal bleeding. If one may hazard a diagnosis of malignancy in two out of every three cases of postmenopausal bleeding without the formality of an examination, it would seem that after physical examination and bimanual palpation the percentage of correct diagnoses should be much higher. From the standpoint of practical medicine, it is better to make a provisional diagnosis of malignancy and to have the lesion proved benign after curettage, than to err in the opposite direction:

Responsibility for delay. In Miller's series the average total delay in securing adequate treatment for cancer of the fundus was more than two years from the appearance of the first symptom, while in this compilation the average was slightly more than twelve months. The delay on the part of the patient was reduced from 16 months to 9 months, while the physician's delay was lowered from 9½ to 4 months.

Table XI

Cancer of the uterine fundus—Responsibility for delay in securing treatment.

		Average time wasted Days	Weeks	Mos.
Miller's Series				
Time from first symptom to first examination		448	64	16
Time from first examination to first treatment		266	38	9.5
AVERAGE TOTAL TIME LOST—OVER 2 YEARS				
New Series				
Time from first symptom to first examination		250	35.6	8.9
Time from first examination to first treatment		103	14.7	3.8
AVERAGE TOTAL TIME WASTED—12.7 MONTHS				
Combined				
Time from first symptom to first examination		312	44.6	11.1
Time from first examination to first treatment		157	22.3	5.6
AVERAGE TOTAL TIME LOST—16.7 MONTHS				

Such figures indicate that there has been a marked improvement in the patient, as well as in the professional attitude toward the significance of continued slight vaginal bleeding in women near the menopause. Doubtless this is reflected in an improved recovery rate from corpus cancer but sufficient time has not yet elapsed to permit the compilation of such statistics.

DISCUSSION

The comparison of certain data on cervical and fundus cancer here presented offers considerable encouragement to those who are advancing the program of cancer education and to all who are interested in the problem of cancer control. As contrasted with the 11 year period up to November, 1927, the 5½ year interval from that date to June 30, 1933, shows marked improvement in that:

1. The percentage of operable cases is significantly increased.

2. The percentage of correct diagnoses before admission is much higher in both the premenopausal and postmenopausal groups.

3. The time lost by the physician in securing adequate treatment for his cancer patients has been reduced by more than one-half.

4. The time wasted by the patient before she consults her physician has been considerably reduced in cases of fundus cancer, even though no improvement has been noted in this connection in cervical malignancies.

The reverse of the picture is, however, still dark, and points clearly to the need for continuing and expanding our efforts at professional and lay education. The 72 per cent of advanced (inoperable) cancers of the cervix and the 19 per cent of inoperable fundus carcinomata constitute a challenge, as does the total average time wasted before adequate treatment is secured—nine months in cancer of the cervix and more than one year in cancer of the body of the uterus.

REFERENCES
1. Miller, Norman F.: Some data on uterine cancer. Jour. Iowa State Med. Soc., xxiii:132-135 (March) 1933.
2. Brown, Preston T.: Postmenopausal vaginal bleeding. Jour. Iowa State Med. Soc., xxiii:261-262 (May) 1933.

AGRANULOCYTOSIS*

FREDERICK H. LAMB, M.D.†
Davenport

Eleven years ago, under the title of "Different Throat Infections," Werner Schultz[1] reported six cases of a disease, which he designated "angina agranulocytica." The patients were all middle-aged women, in whom the illness was characterized by marked prostration, fever, severe progressive oral sepsis, jaundice, a decided reduction in or absence of circulating granulocytes, and a rapidly fatal termination. The following year Friedemann[2] used the term "agranulocytosis" in a report of similar cases. Although other instances of the disease had been observed before 1922, as for example, that reported by Brown[3] in 1902 and by Türk[4] in 1907, recognition by Schultz of the symptom complex stimulated a widespread interest in all leukopenic conditions reflecting a decrease in the neutrophilic leukocytes.

It is the consensus among writers on this sub-

ject that the term agranulocytosis is ambiguous, and moreover, that angina is not a constant or specific manifestation of the disease. Idiopathic or pernicious neutropenia are terms more in keeping with hematologic terminology, and altogether more appropriate. Just as one refers to the Addison-Biermer type of pernicious anemia, so might one designate the Schultz syndrome in pernicious neutropenia, thus commemorating the value of Schultz's contribution.

It is a question whether this disease should be considered as a separate and distinct clinical entity as held by Schultz, by Friedemann, by Leon[5], and more recently by Kracke and Roberts[6], or whether the available facts do not justify this conception. In favor of the view of a disease entity is the important observation that bone marrow dysfunction, even though initiated by an unknown agent, and lacking uniformity, is the primary and fundamental pathologic change which antedates all other manifestations. It is generally agreed that oral sepsis and ulcerative processes elsewhere are not only sequelae, but the direct result of the loss of a defensive mechanism to which the granulocytes normally contribute.

On the other hand, Hartwich[7] concludes that neutropenia simply mirrors a constitutional inferiority of the bone marrow. Rose and Hauser[8] contend that so-called agranulocytosis is nothing more specific than a type of reaction on the part of the leukopoietic system, "to an infection so overwhelming as to destroy the neutrophiles and paralyze their centers of production." They cite the neutropenia of overwhelming sepsis and lobar pneumonia; the absence of a constant etiologic agent; failure of experimental reproduction; lack of epidemicity, and the general character of leukopenic reactions as being against the view of a specific pathologic entity.

The more one studies the literature, particularly detailed case reports, the more one is impressed with the necessity of classifying cases of neutropenia on a basis of symptoms and pathology. Some such grouping as the following might serve until further progress has been made in etiologic studies. At least two major types may be recognized. The pernicious or malignant group comprises those cases in which the symptom complex adheres closely to Schultz's own sharp definition: an acute febrile disease with angina, prostration and jaundice, a normal red blood picture, extreme leukopenia with nearly or quite complete absence of granulocytes, a normal number of blood platelets with absence of any tendency to hemorrhage, and an invariably fatal ending. Although there is some virtue in the concise and trite char-

* Presented before the Eighty-second Annual Session, Iowa State Medical Society, Des Moines, May 10, 11, 12, 1933.
† From the Laboratory Department, St. Luke's Hospital, Davenport.

acter of this definition, it would simplify the classification for practical purposes to include in this group, cases without jaundice, with ulcerative processes other than angina or altogether absent, a moderate degree of anemia, a chronic as well as an acute course, cases of recovery, and finally those with relapse or recurrence.

The second major group should then include those cases characterized by a neutropenic state, a persistent leukopenia, the white cells remaining well below 5,000. As observed clinically, there are two or three types of reaction on the part of the patient in this group. In some, a leukocyte count totaling between 2,500 and 5,000 does not seem to be incompatible with good health. When intercurrent pyogenic infections intervene, a normal adequate leukocytosis develops promptly. It is Doan's[9] view that the rhythm of delivery of white cells to the circulation is normal, and in these individuals a satisfactory hemopoietic equilibrium obtains, except that it operates at a level somewhat below that of normal individuals. Other patients who show a chronic leukopenia of similar grade are definitely not in good health. Roberts and Kracke[6] have attempted to describe a clinical syndrome embracing the most commonly observed symptoms, which are weakness, tendency to fatigue and chronic exhaustion. From a study of 8,000 records they show that the majority of these patients are women between the ages of forty and sixty years. Doan[9] frequently finds in this type of patient, a relative lymphocytosis, and an absolute neutropenia with moderate left shift in the nuclear pattern of those neutrophiles which are present. There seems to be a persistently low reserve of cells of the myelocytic series. Any unusual demand on the bone marrow, even that of a minor infection, may precipitate a more severe leukopenia. Stated simply, they have a lowered resistance, but as a group tend to recover spontaneously. In one such case studied by Doan[9] there were transitory minimal responses on the part of the granulocytes to adenine sulphate, epinephrine, and nucleotide. The possibilities of grave insufficiency in these patients are imminent; they are candidates, as it were, for the more severe reactions.

Cases of chronic, regularly recurring, periodic neutropenia have been reported, and constitute still another sub-group, although the phenomenon may not be strictly of bone marrow origin. It illustrates another type of the neutropenic state for which the name recurrent neutropenic habitus has been proposed.

Notwithstanding this subdivision and enhancement of the symptom complex as defined by Schultz, to a point possibly beyond the reasonable confines of a specific pathologic entity, the disease shades off, nevertheless, into a variety of other conditions which closely simulate, but cannot be definitely included in the concept of agranulocytosis. Other hematologic terms such as, irradiation granulopenia, anemic granulopenia, thrombopenic granulopenia, infectious and chemical granulopenia, more adequately designate these conditions. The more important of these are the panmyelopathies that sometimes occur during the use of the arsphenamines, bismuth or mercury, and also in cases of industrial benzene poisoning. Cases of malignant neutropenia have been held to pass over into the aleukia stage of acute lymphatic leukemia. It is doubtful whether this really happens, or whether the resemblance is so close that they are readily confused. Until something more definite is known about the etiology of agranulocytosis, confusion will persist, and no classification will be wholly satisfactory.

To summarize at this point, there is evidence that neutropenia is a more important biologic state, and much more widespread blood condition than is indicated in the concept of Schultz. Although typical cases are unmistakable, some provision must be made in a comprehensive classification for the large number of less typical cases in which the essential neutropenia is a persistent factor (and probably the only one) even though it varies in degree. Neutropenia then may be acute, chronic or recurrent, severe or mild, with a variety of clinical symptoms, both in kind and degree, with fatal outcome, or followed by complete recovery, much depending on the extent to which the granular cells are reduced. The agranulocytosis of Schultz and earlier observers represents only the extreme state with fatal sepsis.

The following condensed case reports are intentionally brief, and offered chiefly to illustrate the foregoing classification:

Case No. 1—Mrs. D. R., forty-one years of age, was admitted to St. Anthony's Hospital, Rock Island, Illinois, August 5, 1930, with a diagnosis of follicular tonsillitis. Three days before admission she became ill with fever, marked prostration, headache, and sore throat. Her physician noted pus oozing from both faucial tonsils, and considerable cervical adenopathy involving the glands along the borders of both sternomastoid muscles. Her temperature ranged from 103° to 106°, her pulse gradually rose from 92 to 160, and her respirations varied from 18 to 32. Six leukocyte counts made during the eight hospital days varied from 2,500 on the first day to 500 on the day of her death. Two differential counts failed to reveal any granulocytes. Erythrocytes numbered 3,240,000 and the hemoglobin was 60 per cent (Dare) on the first hospital day. After consultation

August 7, with her physician, I transfused this patient with 750 c. c. of whole blood, following which she had a severe reaction. The next (fourth hospital) day the red cells and hemoglobin were recorded, 3,960,000 and 70 per cent. A slight icteric tint noticeable from the first became a well marked jaundice on the fifth hospital day (eighth day of acute illness), and bile in the urine was first noted. Becoming progressively weaker with excessive nausea and vomiting, irrational at times, and with generalized convulsions, profuse diaphoresis and singultus, the patient expired on the eleventh day of her illness.

Case No. 2—Mrs. M. L., sixty-three years of age, was admitted March 1, 1931, to St. Anthony's Hospital, Rock Island, Illinois. Her physician has kindly permitted me to make this report. The patient first became ill February 15, with chills, fever, and general bodily aching. After three days in bed, she seemed to be convalescent for two days, when the fever and prostration returned, accompanied by an acute exacerbation of chronic cystitis. Coryza, cough, constant headache, severe backache, restlessness, and insomnia marked the second five day period after onset of symptoms. The clinical picture suggested influenza. On February 25, ten days after onset, the patient developed diarrhea with from ten to fifteen stools containing mucus and dark clotted blood, in twenty-four hours. The next day she complained of a sore mouth. Previous to this time daily examination of the oral and throat mucosae revealed no evidence of irritation. March 1, the day of admission, jaundice of the skin and sclerae was first noted. Several large purpuric nodules appeared on the upper back and neck. During the five hospital days the temperature ranged from 102.6° to 106°, the pulse from 108 to 130, and respirations from 26 to 38. The blood count the first day was: red blood count, 3,420,000; white blood count, 500; hemoglobin, 60 per cent (Dare). The subsequent daily leukocyte counts were 600, 300, and 350; all were lymphocytes; no granulocytes were found at any time. A urine specimen March 2, contained albumin 1+, bile pigment 3+, granular casts 2+, specific gravity, 1.012. The last five days of illness were characterized by a rapid decline, pharyngitis, jaundice, diarrhea, vomiting, irrational periods, localized muscular twitchings, restlessness, and dyspnea. A 500 c. c. transfusion of citrated blood, and one x-ray treatment seemed to be without effect. The patient expired on March 4, 1931, twenty days after onset of illness.

Case No. 3—Miss M. S., thirty-five years of age, a visiting nurse, was first seen on November 23, 1932, and her physician has also kindly permitted this report. She was on duty at the time, but because of a severe headache and a temperature of 101.6° was advised to go home. The next morning her temperature was 105.8°; she had a sore throat with red edematous pillars, fetid breath, severe backache, and prostration. There was a marked bilateral cervical adenopathy. She was admitted to Mercy hospital, Clinton, Iowa, profoundly ill, restless and cyanotic. Her blood count is recorded: red blood count, 3,910,-

000; white blood count, 1,325, with 78 per cent lymphocytes, 12 per cent mononuclears, and no granulocytes. My own examination of blood films from this patient revealed no granular leukocytes. A 310 c.c. blood transfusion was without effect. The patient expired the following day, the fifth day of illness.

These three cases illustrate the first group of pernicious neutropenias. Case No. 1 conforms most closely to Schultz's own definition, although there was a moderate degree of anemia present; it did not, however, progress. Case No. 2 with an onset simulating influenza developed a diarrhea with bloody mucus on the tenth day, pharyngitis on the twelfth day, and jaundice with purpuric nodules on the thirteenth day. Since there was no blood count prior to the hospital admission, it might be doubted that neutropenia existed from the first. Yet, the initial count included a white blood count of 500, and it is more than likely that some degree of neutropenia antedated this count. Case No. 3 represents the acute fulminant type with a total duration of symptoms of but five days.

Case No. 4—Mr. S., a farm boy, eighteen years of age, was admitted to the Hammond Hospital, Geneseo, Illinois, April 15, 1922. He had become ill five days previously with headache, backache, fever, weakness, and restlessness. The day before entrance to the hospital the gingivae and oral mucosa became swollen, purplish red and tender. Blood oozed from around the teeth, both anterior and posterior nares and from both auditory canals. Oral and pharyngeal sepsis rapidly became worse. The second hospital day the red cells numbered 4,600,000, white cells 850, and hemoglobin was 65 per cent. No platelet count was made, but the bleeding time was more than thirty minutes, and the tourniquet test was positive. After consultation with his physician, I transfused this patient with 800 c. c. of citrated blood, following which the oozing of blood ceased for two days, and the patient improved. A second transfusion on the fifth hospital day was also of temporary benefit. The oozing of blood returned, this time with melena. A leukocyte count on the seventh day in the hospital by Dr. F. M. Smith of Iowa City, who saw the patient was 200. Death occurred two days later.

This case illustrates the shading off, previously referred to, or combination of malignant neutropenia with another element, namely thrombopenia, and in hematologic terms should be designated as thrombopenic neutropenia.

PATHOLOGY

In the acute fulminant cases and the chronic severe cases of malignant neutropenia, the pathologic findings vary widely, depending on whether or not the infection has become generalized. Necrotic orificial lesions of the mouth, rectum, and vagina are characterized by edema, necrosis and an absence of a surrounding inflammatory infiltration, since the neutrophiles are not available to supply it. The lungs frequently show sub-pleural hemorrhages with areas of fibrinous exudate over the pleurae. The digestive tract may show ulcerations throughout. The heart, liver, and kidneys show changes associated with bacterial toxins, including areas of cloudy swelling, fatty degeneration, and focal necrosis with gangrene. Extensive bacterial emboli, fibrin nets, and necrosis of arterioles and venules have been described. Throughout the body there may be focal or diffuse collections of lymphocytes, clumps of fused red cells, and plasma cells accompanied by fluid, but without granulocytes.

It is held that that portion in the peripheral circulation of the life cycle of the granular leukocytes is probably of not more than four or five days' duration. If delivery of neutrophiles to the circulation is cut off sharply, either through a sudden arrest of maturation of the young cells in the marrow, or a complete failure of development, the neutrophilic count should fall rapidly. There is abundant evidence clinically that one or the other does happen, as shown by the complete disappearance of neutrophiles from the blood stream within a few days.

Until recently, reports of the condition of the bone marrow have stressed the fatty, hypoplastic, liquefied state of marrow, with an absence of myeloblastic cells. Erythrocytic regeneration has been noted repeatedly, but such remarks as "an astonishing scarcity of myeloid cells," and "complete myelocytic destruction" have been encountered frequently. Last year, Fitz-Hugh and Krumbhaar[10] raised an objection to the current hypothesis of granulocytic aplasia as constituting the primary pathologic mechanism of the disease. On the basis of a critical study of rib and femoral marrow in one fatal case, and confirmed to some extent in two other fatal cases, they found that about 20 per cent of the marrow cells were myelocytes, promyelocytes, and myeloblasts. There had been no roentgen ray stimulation of the marrow to account for the increased presence of progenitors of the granular cells, and in the five days' illness the patient's white cell count dropped from less than 1,000 to 200 (all lymphocytes) the day of death. These authors offer an interesting explanation of this profound peripheral neutropenia, while at the same time the leukopoietic centers for granulocytes were supplied with parent-cells. They suggest that a maturation factor acts either to arrest development of the granular leukocytes, or to induce degenerative changes in them before there is sufficient development for normal migration into the blood stream. Viewed from this

standpoint, the analogies between the relapsing type of neutropenia and pernicious anemia are obvious. Both diseases are, as yet, idiopathic, exhibit remissions, one with a maturation arrest factor in the granular series of blood cells, the other in the red cell series. Untreated, pernicious anemia may terminate in an aplastic stage similar to the granulocytic aplasia, which characterizes many of the pernicious neutropenias. Fitz-Hugh and Comroe[11] in a paper published last month (April, 1933) state that in more than half the cases studied by them there has been a plentiful supply of leukopoietic centers in the marrow, further strengthening the hypothesis of a maturation arrest. Baldridge and Needles[12] observed an instance in 1930 of myelocytic and myeloblastic overgrowth, "almost as marked as in myelogenous leukaemia." Dameshek and Ingall[13] and R. W. Buck[14] have reported similar findings.

Thus the bone marrow changes at necropsy may exhibit aplasia or hyperplasia of the granular cell progenitors. The operation of a hypothetical maturation arrest factor in the hyperplastic marrow may explain the peripheral leukopenia, and it is not impossible that the cases of terminal aplasia may have passed through a transitory hyperplastic stage. It is reasonable to conclude that in a disease with as many variants as neutropenia, the underlying pathology is not uniform. The acute fulminant case dead in from four to six days after the onset of symptoms, and the case of a mild chronic neutropenic habitus are poles apart clinically, and no doubt, to a great extent pathologically. About the only common demoninator is in the diminished number of neutrophiles, and that a matter of degree.

DIAGNOSIS

The most important single factor in the early diagnosis of neutropenia is to have the condition in mind, and the next is the leukocyte count. Progressive oral sepsis with prostration and fever should promptly warrant an enumeration of the white cells, and a study of the blood film. Finding a reduction in granulocytes is of paramount diagnostic importance. So far as I know the conditions offering the greatest difficulty in differential diagnosis are the febrile cases of mononucleosis with mebraneous angina[17], and the aleukia stage of lymphatic leukemia with angina. Both combinations are rather rare.

On the other hand, the many infectious processes affecting the oral, nasopharyngeal and gingival mucosae may be segregated from malignant neutropenia on the basis of normal or increased numbers of granulocytes. Of the very common disorders, Vincent's angina, influenza, and the common cold with sore throat simulate most closely malignant neutropenia in the early stages. Diagnosis of the neutropenic state requires a series of several differential counts with due consideration for variations in the daily rhythm of delivery of cells to the circulation, amounting at times to as much as one hundred per cent.[18]

TREATMENT

Even a cursory review of the substances which have been reported in the therapy of this disease reveals a long list including sodium cacodylate, yeast, cod liver oil, sodium thiosulphate, calcium gluconate, quinine, various dyes intravenously, turpentine intramuscularly and many others. So far as I can learn, none of these has been considered particularly meritorious. Indeed, it is very difficult to evaluate any form of treatment since spontaneous recovery occurs in some cases, while others prove rapidly fatal in the face of any and all treatment. Aside from symptomatic treatment, only three remedies deserve consideration at the moment; they will probably be used in conjunction with each other, or independently until something better is offered.

Blood transfusion is probably the least effective of the three, yet it may have a place for two reasons. First, it may be helpful in tiding a patient over a two or three day period until another remedy can become effective. Second, in those cases shading off into aplastic anemia, or thrombopenic neutropenia, repeated blood transfusions may prolong life.

The use of roentgen therapy dates from Friedemann's first communication in 1927. Burgheim[15] exposed the long bones of healthy individuals to one-twentieth the erythema dose; in each case he observed a slight but definite rise in the granulocyte count, often within two hours. Thoma gave roentgen treatments to typhoid patients with a marked leukopenia and observed a rise of from 1,000 to 3,000 in the leukocyte count. Taussig and Schnoebelen[16] reported four cases treated with minimal doses of x-ray, two of whom recovered and two died. It was noted that there was a temporary response following treatment in each of the four cases, but after a relapse in two, there was no further response to the x-ray. In 1928 Friedemann reported six of ten patients (60 per cent) recovered after x-ray treatment. In 1930 Friedemann and Elkeles[19] reported a total of forty-three cases with recovery in 13 (30 per cent). However, they point out that twenty-three of these patients had sepsis or pneumonia; therefore, x-ray therapy in their uncomplicated cases produced a

recovery rate of 65 per cent. Unfortunately, it is no more effectual in the serious malignant type of case, than is blood transfusion.

The third method of treatment to receive any considerable trial is the purine or nucleotide therapy. In 1924 Henry Jackson, Jr.,[20] demonstrated for the first time the existence in the normal human blood of pentose nucleotides. It has been shown that neucleic acid and its decomposition products have a stimulating effect on white blood cell formation. Jackson and his associates[21] in 1931, reported twenty cases of malignant neutropenia in which treatment with the unbroken pentose nucleotides ("neucleotide K 96," Smith, Kline and French Company), had been given adequate trial. "Of these twenty cases thirteen were typical agranulocytic angina; five patients had marked leukopenia and extreme lowering of granulocytes in the presence of various infections, and two had extreme neutropenia and anemia secondary to benzene poisoning." Of the thirteen cases usually referred to as agranulocytosis, seven of the thirteen recovered; of the entire group of twenty cases, fourteen recovered. Clinical and hematologic improvement occurred quite consistently about five days after treatment was begun. Lately Jackson has collected sixty-nine nucleotide treated cases with a mortality rate of 26 per cent.[22]

It should be noted, that while pentose necleotide may be used either intravenously or intramuscularly, extremely severe reactions are apt to follow intravenous administration. Indeed, alarming reactions may follow intramuscular use, as exemplified in a very recent experience. The administration of 0.4 c.c. doses of adrenalin modified the severity of these reactions considerably.

A young physician suffering from agranulocytosis was probably the first patient to be treated with the salt of a purine base. As reported by Paul Reznikoff[23] on December 20, 1928, this patient was given adenine sulphate intravenously and promptly recovered. Recently the same author[24] has reported that of fifteen uncomplicated cases of agranulocytosis treated with adenine sulphate, eleven patients, or 70 per cent, recovered. The dose suggested is one gram boiled in 35 or 40 c.c of physiologic saline administered intravenously, sufficiently warm to prevent precipitation, three times a day, for at least three days. In most patients a favorable response was noted in forty-eight hours, frequently within twenty-four hours. As much as 10.4 grams have been given to a patient within 24 hours. This substance has been obtained from the Eastman Kodak Company.

Although a mortality of 25 to 30 per cent leaves

much to be desired from a therapeutic standpoint, it seems that purine base and nucleotide therapy may be credited with noteworthy reduction in fatalities from the disease, and for the present is the treatment of choice. Both substances should be available for immediate use in cases where their neutropenic character is recognized.

INCIDENCE AND PROGNOSIS

In a recent review of the reported cases of neutropenia in the United States, Canada and Great Britain, Kracke[22] has tabulated the incidence of case reports since 1924. In the past nine years, this tabulation year by year is as follows: 1924, one case; 1925, two; 1926, two; 1927, twelve; 1928, twenty-nine; 1929, thirty-six; 1930, seventy; 1931, one hundred seventy-two; and 1932, forty-seven. Incidentally, only two cases were reported from Great Britain. The mortality rate for the entire series was 63 per cent. These figures lead to speculation as to why the incidence is so much higher in this country, also whether it is actually occurring more frequently, whether it is being recognized more frequently, or both.

I know of no disease in which the clinical course from day to day, and the ultimate outlook are more uncertain. A segregation of those cases characterized by a chronic neutropenic state from the maglignant neutropenia group may be helpful in this way: patients with a persistently low white count may be warned of the danger, and until it is definitely assured that their leukocytes function normally, except at a lower than normal level, they should be kept under observation. The acute fulminant type of. case, so far as present forms of treatment are concerned is probably hopeless from the beginning. The more chronic and subacute cases tend to recurrence and relapse, so that a guarded prognosis is in order, even though the patient may seem to have fully recovered.

REFERENCES
1. Schultz, Werner: Ueber eigenartige Hulserkankungen. Deutche Med. Wchnschr., xlviii: 1495 (November 3) 1922.
2. Friedemann, U.: Ueber angina agranulocytica. Med. Klin., xix: 1357 (October 14) 1923.
3. Brown, P. K.: A fatal case of primary acute infectious pharyngitis with extreme leukopenia. Am. Med., iii: 649-651, 1902.
4. Turk, W.: Septic diseases with destruction of granulocytes. Wein. Klin. Wchnschr., xx: 157, 1907.
5. Leon, A.: Agranulocytosis, Deutiche Arch. of Klin. Med., cxliii: 118, 1923.
6. Roberts, S. R., and Kracke, R. R.: Agranulocytosis: Its classification. Ann. Int. Med., v: 40, 1931.
7. Hartwich, A.: Das Krankheitsbild der agranulocytose. Ergebu. A. inn. Med. u. Kruderh., xli: 202, 1931.
8. Rose, E., and Hauser, K. M.: The identity of so-called agranulocytic angina. Arch. Int. Med., xliii: 533, (April) 1929.
9. Doan, C. A.: The neutropenic state. Jour. Am. Med. Assn., xcix: 194-202 (July 16) 1932.
10. Fitz-Hugh, Jr., T., and Krumbhaar, E. B.: Myeloid cell hyperplasia of the bone marrow in agranulocytic angina. Am. Jour. Med. Sc., clxxxiii: 104 (January) 1932.
11. Fitz-Hugh, Jr., T., and Comroe, B. I.: Agranulocytic angina (pernicious leukopenia). A study based on eighteen cases with nine necropsies. Am. Jour. Med. Sc., clxxxv: 552 (April) 1933.
12. Baldridge, C. W., and Needles, R. J.: Idiopathic neutropenia. Am. Jour. Med. Sc., clxxxi: 533 (April) 1931.
13. Damashek, W., and Ingall, M.: Agranulocytosis (malignant neutropenia). Am. Jour. Med. Sc., clxxxi: 502 (April) 1931.
14. Buck, R. W.: Agranulocytosis associated with anal ulcer. Jour. Am. Med. Assn., xciii: 1468 (November 9) 1929.
15. Burgheim, F.: Zur Rontgentherapie der Agranulozytose. Shrahlentherapie, xxxviii: 152-156, 1930.
16. Taussig, A. E., and Schnoebelen, P. G.: Roentgen treatment of agranulocytosis. Jour. Am. Med. Assn., xcvii: 1757, (December 12) 1931.
17. Baldridge, C. W., Rohner, F. J. and Hansmann, G. H., Glandular fever (infectious mononucleosis). Arch. Int. Med., xxxviii: 413 (October) 1926.
18. Lamb, F. H.: The blood picture and certain related clinical implications. Jour. Iowa State Med. Soc., xxiii: 59 (February) 1933.
19. Friedemann, U., and Elkeles, A.: Die Roentgenbehandlung der Agranulozytose. Deutsche Med. Wchnschr., lvi: 947-950 (June 6) 1930.
20. Jackson, Henry, Jr.: Studies in nuclein metabolism; isolation of a nucleotide from human blood. Jour. Biol. Chem. lix: 529-534 (April) 1924.
21. Jackson, Henry, Jr., Parker, F., Rinehart. J. F., and Taylor, F. H. L.: Studies of diseases of the lymphoid and myeloid tissues. Jour. Am. Med. Assn., xcvii: 1436-1440 (November 14) 1931.
22. Kracke, R. R.: Personal communication to the author and unpublished data. April 3, 1933.
23. Reznikoff, P.: Nucleotide therapy in agranulocytosis. J. Clin. Investigation. ix: 381, 1930.
24. Reznikoff, P.: The treatment of agranulocytosis with Adenine sulphate. J. Clin. Investigation, xii: 45-53, (January) 1933.

Discussion

Dr. Benjamin F. Wolverton, Cedar Rapids: This paper by Dr. Lamb is one that should be read as well as heard. I hope that everyone here will watch for this paper when it appears in the Journal and will read it carefully. It represents an unusually fine summary of the literature up to date on the agranulocytic or neutropenic syndrome.

It seems to me, without any question, that the original concept of the disease as laid down by Schultz is obsolete and much too narrow. Schultz stated that the disease occurred only in middle-aged women, and that the disease was uniformly fatal. As Dr. Lamb has brought out, the disease occurs at almost any age. It has been reported in children and in males, and the mortality is not 100 per cent.

For my own purposes I prefer to think of the condition, not as a disease entity but as a syndrome, representing a bone marrow deficiency on the part of the granulopoietic function in response to infection, until a better concept appears. My experience with this syndrome is limited to only two cases, neither of which conforms to the original concept of Schultz. Both of these cases were seen before the advent of nucleotide therapy.

The first case was in a woman twenty-six years of age, who had pin-point ulcers in her throat and very slight redness. She was extremely sick. It seems to me that the characteristic feature of this syndrome is the fact that the patient is sicker than can be accounted for on the basis of any objective lesion that can be found, and that a careful study of the blood is therefore indicated.

This patient had a total leukocyte count of 1,400 on the first count, and no granulocytes, or polymorphonuclear cells, were found. The blood picture varied from day to day, but until recovery was definitely under way, the maximum percentage of granulocytes was 19.

Strangely enough, her clinical improvement was

coincident with the advent of serum sickness. Streptococci had been cultivated from the throat, and antistreptococcic serum was given, not with the hope of doing any particular good but there seemed to be nothing else to do. The patient went along in a very sick state until a late serum reaction occurred, with all the typical manifestations. The patient recovered and is still living. The blood picture since recovery has not shown a neutropenia, the chronic neutropenic state such as described by Doan.

The other case was a woman fifty-three years of age, who also did not exhibit any particular throat or mucous membrane ulcerative lesions but who had simply a very severe toxemia with high fever, and a toxic psychotic state. She was treated with leukocytic extract, with no apparent result whatever. I do not know just what leukocytic extract contains, but it would be reasonable to suppose that it does contain some nucleic acid derivatives. However, in this instance, in spite of large doses, there was no response, and the patient died. Since autopsy was refused, no opportunity was given for a study of the bone marrow.

It seems to me that the important, practical point to be gained from Dr. Lamb's paper is that the disease should be constantly borne in mind, and whenever we see a patient who is acutely ill, with insufficient findings to explain the severity of the condition, a careful study of the blood should be made. If an acute neutropenic state is found, energetic treatment with the nucleotide, as advocated by Jackson, should be carried out.

I want to urge you to read this paper because I believe you will get more out of it by reading it than you can by listening to it.

CLINICAL OBSERVATIONS IN TIC DOULOUREUX

Frank A. Ely, M.D., Des Moines

Tic douloureux, or trifacial neuralgia, as it is better known, presents many interesting clinical features. It has been my privilege, during the past fifteen years, to treat by the alcohol injection method, over one hundred patients who have suffered from this painful malady, and I am here setting forth some of the pertinent observations afforded by this experience.

As far as I am able to ascertain from the literature, the etiology of this disease is not definitely known. Attempts have been made to account for it on the assumptions of ganglionitis, congenital anomalies of the foramina from which the divisions of the trifacial nerve emerge from the skull, infected teeth, intracranial arteriosclerotic changes, etc., but the real cause is still open to question. It is never a good thing to become dogmatic concerning a subject of this kind, yet our failure to explain things satisfactorily should not dampen our investigative ardor. From my own observa-

tions, one thing is conspicuous; that trifacial neuralgia is essentially a disease of the involution period, notwithstanding the fact that children and young adults have been known to suffer from it. Well recognizable signs of generalized arteriosclerosis are present in most patients. The youngest person coming under my observation was twenty-eight years of age when she first experienced her typical facial pains. Odd as it may seem, I have no knowledge of a single trifacial neuralgia patient dying from cerebral hemorrhage. In my list of patients, without an exception, all have had teeth extracted in a hopeless search for relief, and I do not know of a single one who received any benefit from dental surgery. The slaughter of teeth has been appalling. There is no question but that there is some seasonal predilection for the recurrence of the periods of pain. The changeable atmospheric and barometric conditions of early spring and late fall seem to precipitate recurrence of the painful attacks.

Tic douloureux is a definite disease or clinical entity, and for want of a better term, may be called an essential neuralgia. Of recent years, glossopharyngeal and occipital neuralgia have also been recognized as belonging to the classification of essential neuralgias. There should be no excuse for a wrong diagnosis in cases of trifacial neuralgia if the following diagnostic symptoms are held in mind. The pains are abrupt, terrific, and relatively short in duration. They are felt in the upper lip and wing of the nose, the lower jaw, and just below the angle of the mouth, or just above the eye with radiation to the vertex. True tic douloureux pains are never constant. In contradistinction to symtomatic facial neuralgia, there will usually be found what are known as "trigger zones." By this is meant localized areas where stimulation will bring on a paroxysm. When the lower or mandibular division is involved, chewing, swallowing, or rubbing the under lip will produce a painful explosion. When both middle and lower divisions participate in the painful orgies, the pain may be started by almost any irritant applied to the side of the face. Early in my experience of treating this disease, I was mystified when a patient complained of pain referable to the middle division of the nerve, yet continued to do so when I had successfully blocked it with an alcohol injection. After a time I learned to block the inferior division as well, and in almost every instance the pain was immediately relieved. This indicates that the trigger zone for one division may be elsewhere than in the location naturally expected.

Pain of trifacial neuralgia is usually pain of the

waking hours. Patients who sleep soundly are seldom awakened by it, but if they are aroused from sleep by other causes, the paroxysms are in evidence. Persons who develop tic douloureux most frequently experience the first pain in the distribution of the middle division of the trifacial nerve. I have several patients whom I have injected at intervals for many years who have never experienced pain in any except the middle division. Supra-orbital pain is rare. Bilateral involvement is quite infrequent; personally I have never observed it. As has been intimated, tic douloureux is subject to spontaneous remissions, which may last for months and even years, but the prompt relief observed after alcohol injections is so obvious that their efficacy cannot be discounted, because the pains occasionally subside with no treatment at all.

It is now generally known by the medical profession that there are only two methods of treating trifacial neuralgia. One is that of blocking the involved division of the nerve external to the cranial cavity, and the other, resection of the sensory root of the gasserian ganglion within the skull on the homolateral side. All other attempts at relief are unsuccessful. Selection of the form of treatment depends upon the mental attitude of the patient; his or her familiarity with the permancy of relief to be expected; treatment hazards; and the age of the sufferer. There are many surgical and medical procedures which, though scientifically correct, are not always expedient. Many experienced brain surgeons have found that it is often unsatisfactory to perform a ganglion root section on persons who have recently developed tic douloureux. The reason for this is very simple. Few persons relish having a complete, permanent obliteration of sensation in one side of the face, and even though forewarned, many who have had a ganglion operation early in the course of their trouble, have complained bitterly of the resultant facial analgesia. Since there are psychologic reasons for not resorting early to ganglion operations, alcohol injections into the nerve trunks have come to be a very satisfactory palliative treatment. It has the following advantages. It usually affords prompt, temporary relief without loss of time or prolonged hospitalization; the procedure is relatively safe and is not unbearably painful; the sensibility of the blocked areas returns after a few months; and it accustoms patients to the facial sensory changes which must be permanent if they later submit to the ganglion operation. The one outstanding disadvantage is a lack of permanent relief from pain. In my own series of cases, freedom from pain after alcohol blocking, has ranged

from six months to eight years, the average being between nine and twelve months. It is not at all unusual, after an effective blocking, to have a patient free from pain for two or three years.

For the enlightenment of physicians especially interested in this subject, it may be well to discuss in detail some phases of the alcohol injection method. The trifacial divisions take their origin in the gasserian ganglia on the anterior surfaces of the petrous portions of the temporal bones. Each ganglion has a motor and sensory root, the latter being the one cut in modern ganglion operations. The terminal portions of the superior divisions of the trifacial nerves emerge from the skull at the supra-orbital foramina. The middle divisions emerge from the skull via the foramina rotunda, pass across the sphenomaxillary fossae, through the superior maxillae, and out upon the face through the infra-orbital foramina. The inferior divisions emerge from the skull via the foramina ovale and their terminal portions pass out of the mental foramina in the lower jaw. There are two methods of injecting the middle and lower divisions. In one, a needle is passed through the cheek in such a manner as to reach these trunks when they emerge from the skull proper. The chief landmarks for making these injections are the zygomatic notch in the molar bone and the pterygoid process of the sphenoid. If a long calibrated needle is passed through the cheek at a right angle to the plane of the cheek with its point of entrance at the zygomatic notch on the lower margin of the molar bone, the needle, at a depth of four centimeters will impinge upon the pterygoid process of the sphenoid. It may be observed on a skull that the foramen ovale is about one-half centimeter posterior to the base of the pterygoid process and that the sphenomaxillary fossa through which the middle division of the trifacial nerve passes, is about the same distance anterior. In injecting the inferior or mandibular nerve, after having located the pterygoid process, the needle is withdrawn two or three centimeters and the direction changed in such a manner as to direct the point one-half centimeter posteriorly and a little upward. The needle is then advanced to a depth of from four to four and one-half centimeters. When the nerve is engaged the patient, if not anesthetized, will complain bitterly of pain in the lower jaw and in the angle of the mouth. This reaction is a good indication that the needle is on or in the nerve. At this point a syringe should be fitted to the needle and suction made to be sure no blood vessel has been entered. Following this, from one to three c.c.'s of 80 per cent alcohol may be injected. I have found by experience that if the alcohol goes in without resistance, the injection will not be uniformly successful. The local pain reaction manifested by the conscious patient and resistance to the plunger of the syringe upon injection are two valuable signs that the right spot has been reached. In making an injection into the middle division of the trifacial nerve, the preliminary steps are the same, but after the pterygoid process has been located, the needle is partially withdrawn and directed slightly upward and one-half centimeter forward. The depth at which the foramen rotundum is reached in the sphenomaxillary fossa is approximately five centimeters. In this injection, the pain reaction of the patient and resistance to the injected alcohol holds good, but the pain will be experienced in the upper lip, wing of the nose, and upper jaw.

The supra-orbital nerve is difficult to reach anywhere except at the supra-orbital foramen or just above it. In the beginning, I attempted to transfix this nerve by pushing a small hypodermic needle directly into the nerve from the front, but by this method, I often failed. Knowing that this nerve lies on the periosteum of the skull, just beneath the scalp, I adopted the method of locating the supra-orbital foramen. This having been done, I introduced a long, slender needle directly down upon the skull, a centimeter to one side, then directed it parallel with the contour of the frontal bone in such a manner as to go under the nerve, often pushing the needle an inch or so along the supra-orbital ridge. Then, as the needle was withdrawn, from one to two c.c.'s of 80 per cent alcohol were distributed in the needle's path. In this manner the nerve was almost certainly blocked.

Injecting alcohol near the base of the cranium might seem to be a dangerous procedure. Experience has shown that very few harmful results have been produced. In injecting the inferior division of the fifth nerve by the deep method two things may happen. The eustachian tube may be injured or the alcohol may pass back along the tract of the needle and cause a partial ankylosis of the jaw. I have never observed an instance in which the latter disability was extensive or seriously disabling. Deep injections of the middle division of the fifth nerve have, in a few instances, resulted in temporary paralysis of some of the extrinsic muscles of the eye. These untoward results have been caused by pointing the needle too high in the sphenomaxillary fossa. Because of the possibility of the above mentioned unpleasant complications, I began many years ago to inject the three divisions of the fifth nerve at their points of emergence on the face. I found that the mid-

dle division is easily reached at the intra-orbital foramen. The mouth of this foramen is directed downward, forward, and outward, and is reached with the needle point just below the lower margin of the orbit, a little to the nasal side of its vertical midline. A fine inch and a quarter needle is introduced through the cheek with its point of entrance two centimeters below the foramen and directed upward, backward, and slightly inward. With a little gentle feeling around, the needle point will be felt to enter the foramen. When the location is established, about two c.c.'s of 80 per cent alcohol are injected. The results should be a decided analgesia of the homolateral ala of the nose and upper lip. Peripheral injections of the inferior divisions at the mental foramina of the lower jaw are attended with some uncertainty because of the variation in the location of these bony apertures. These foramina are usually located opposite the bases of the first bicuspid teeth or a little posterior. In aged people whose teeth have been extracted, absorption of the aveolar bone brings this foramen into a relatively higher position. I have found that the best approach to this foramen is through the cheek at, or just anterior to, the angle of the mouth. If the bicuspid teeth are present, and the aveolar process not absorbed, a little feeling around will locate the foramen, but in many instances the treatment has to be repeated two or three times before results are obtained. It may be of interest to state that if a perpendicular line is dropped from the supra-orbital foramen in such a manner as to pass over the infra-orbital aperture, a continuation of the line will pass directly to, or over, the foramen in the lower jaw, if the jaws are lightly closed.

It is well to state that the possible untoward effects of the peripheral injections are few and infrequent, yet they should be borne in mind. Alcohol is a tissue divitalizer or it would not temporarily stop the functioning of the nerve trunks we attempt to reach. After peripheral injections, there is considerable swelling of the soft tissues of the face, and at times discoloration. As a rule, this subsides in about seven days with no ill effect. In five of my patients, there were more serious complications with which to deal. In three patients there was a necrotic ulceration with a slight sequestration of the alveolar process, accompanied by the loss of a tooth or two. In one instance, a patient experienced a skin necrosis of the side of the nose which resulted in a slight nicking of the right nostril, and in one instance a small necrotic ulcer occurred at the point where the needle was introduced. The unusual thing about these unfortunate accidents is that without exception, the healing process was remarkable. An attempt has been made to determine why these incidents occurred. I have come to the conclusion that where alveolar sequestration has taken place, an osteomyelitis about an abscessed tooth must have been present. This has led to radiographic studies of the teeth before treatment. Just why one patient had a skin necrosis on the side of her nose, I have not determined. In self-justification it may be said that an honest search for errors in technic or in compounding the solution injected, was made without any enlightenment.

Section of the sensory root of the gasserian ganglion is the only permanent relief for tic douloureux. The operation, in the hands of a trained brain surgeon, carries a very low mortality rate. The operation should not be performed until the operative prospect has been trained by alcohol injections to experience the resultant numbness of the face. Persons suffering from tic douloureux can be kept very comfortable for many years by occasional alcohol injections, but it is incumbent upon physicians who inject these people to see that they are fully informed concerning the ganglion operation before they reach such an advanced age as to render them poor operative risks.

In recent months, neurosurgeons have reported some good results in trifacial neuralgia from cervical sympathectomy, but this form of treatment cannot be advised until more experience has been acquired.

RENAL ANEURYSM*
JOHN E. BRINKMAN, M.D., Waterloo

The literature on renal aneurysm as compared with that of any other subject which enters into the equasion of medicine and surgery, is practically nil, there being approximately only seventy published articles, many of which are in a foreign language.†

The first authentic record of this condition was given the profession by Dr. Daniel Nebel in 1718. Fate had decreed that the first case reported occurred in a physician. In the 182 years between 1718 and 1900, thirteen cases were reported. Since 1900 forty-four cases have been added. The case herein described is the forty-fifth, making the total number of individual cases on record since 1718, fifty-eight. The discrepancy in the articles published and the actual number of cases reported is due to the fact that in several instances the same case had been reported by more than one individual. To substantiate the claim of its relative infre-

*Presented before the Eighty-second Annual Session, Iowa State Medical Society, Des Moines, May 10, 11, 12, 1933.
†A complete bibliography of pertinent literature will be found in the author's reprints.

quency I have but to cite the report of a series of over 67,000 autopsies done throughout the world. In this large group only nine cases of renal aneurysm were found. In the traumatic aneurysms incident to the World War, none is reported as having involved the renal artery.

These reports include all types of renal aneurysms; those which were unruptured and were disclosed incident to autopsy but could not be listed as the cause of death, and those which had progressed to the final stage in which a rupture had occurred. Is it not possible, however, that the medical profession has not had its attention called to this subject often enough to emphasize the possibility of its occurrence, and that as a result, there may have been numerous unreported cases of ruptured renal aneurysms with a fatality in which the real cause of death was not recognized?

As you know, the renal arteries are short vessels which arise from the sides of the abdominal aorta, each artery before reaching the hilum dividing into three to five branches, which enter into the substance of the kidney independently at the hilum. It is only natural to assume that a rupture of this vessel would be accompanied by a rather rapid loss of blood from the arterial system, simulating some of the other types of concealed hemorrhage with a syndrome difficult of interpretation. In commenting on the difficulty of correct diagnoses in this condition, Mathé* says: "Aneurysm of the renal artery is exceedingly difficult to diagnose, only seven of the reported cases having been detected prior to the time of operation or death." Therefore, this case is apparently the eighth on record in which a correct preoperative diagnosis has been made. However, I am frank to admit the inefficiency of my diagnostic ability in this connection, and as a result this case was subjected to two operations, the second of which would have been unnecessary had I been able to evaluate properly the symptom complex. I wish at this time to give credit to Dr. Allan B. Knavel of Chicago for having aided me in making the diagnosis. Fortunately, Dr. Knavel was in Waterloo for an address before the Waterloo Medical Society. In talking over the problems of this case he said: "I am of the impression that you are dealing with a very rare condition, viz., a renal aneurysm which has ruptured."

It is my hope and endeavor in this brief discussion to call your attention to the fact that renal aneurysms do occur; that because of their apparent infrequency they are likely to be unrecognized, or at least not recognized early enough to permit the

*Mathé, C. P.: Aneurism of the Renal Artery. Jour. Urology, xxvii:607-636 (June) 1932.

use of surgery for relief; and that a renal aneurysm may rupture and in some instances, at least, show little or no change in the urinary findings.

CASE REPORT

The patient was Mrs. C. R. H., a housewife, twenty-seven years of age. Her family history was irrelevant. She had always enjoyed good health. In 1923, an appendectomy had been performed, but there was no history of other serious illness.

Symptoms and Onset. On January 31, 1928, about 6:00 P. M., while getting off a street car, she had a sudden, intense, stab-like pain in the left upper abdomen, followed by vomiting. At the time of my first visit her body was flexed so that her chest practically rested on her knees. The pulse was 80, regular and of good quality. The only symptom at this time was the excruciating pain. I gave her morphine, grains ¼, atropine, grains 1/150, and sufficient chloroform to relieve the intensity of her suffering until the opiate took effect. The relief was only temporary and in an hour and a half I gave her an injection of H.M.C. No. 1, following which she became comparatively comfortable. She vomited four or five times during the night. On going to the bathroom the next morning she collapsed. Upon my arrival I made a diagnosis of a pronounced concealed hemorrhage, evidenced by distinct pallor, air hunger, and a rapid, thready pulse. She was immediately taken to the hospital. The blood picture revealed the following figures: red blood count, 2,100,000; leukocytes, 14,000; hemoglobin, 40 per cent; polymorphonuclears, 80 per cent; lymphocytes, 15 per cent, and large mononuclears, 5 per cent. There were no abnormal red cells. The Wassermann reaction was negative. Urinary findings were: Color, amber; odor, characteristic; specific gravity, 1025; sediment, none; albumin, negative; sugar, negative; indican, present; bile, negative; acetone, negative; diacetic acid, negative; casts, negative; blood, negative; and pus cells, a few. In this connection it might be of interest to know that the urine remained negative throughout her entire stay in the hospital.

General Physical Examination. Examination showed a fairly well nourished female, with pronounced pallor, a rapid feeble pulse, respiration 26, temperature 100.6°. There was evidence of free fluid in the peritoneal cavity with some dullness and moderate muscular rigidity in the left renal region, extending forward and involving a portion of the left abdominal wall.

Let me stop just a moment. We doctors pride ourselves on being close observers. During the tenseness of this particular moment, when we were typing the individual, preliminary to transfusion, I ordered a dose of fibrogen. I presume you have all given it. I had a nurse who was unusually intelligent. She came to me and said, "Doctor you ordered fibrogen. Have you read the directions on the box?" She called my attention to this printed warning: "Do not use before transfusion. Transfusions and the use of antitoxins and sera *should be avoided while fibrogen*

is in effect." That rather forcibly brought to my attention the fact that some time ago one of the men reported a case of hemorrhage. In the history he said he had given her large doses of fibrogen; he transfused her, and she almost died. He transfused her again, and she did die. Was the administration of the fibrogen contraindicated? Do these people put this on the package to limit the sale of it, or is it a real contraindication? The label reads: "Avoid while fibrogen is in effect." Who knows how long it is effective. I am sure that I do not. I am just throwing this hint out for what it may be worth. Maybe there is nothing to it, but I would not want to be transfused when those who manufacture fibrogen caution against its use under certain conditions, yet I dare say that nine-tenths of the physicians in this room have used this preparation, but have never noticed this caution.

Treatment. The patient was given a transfusion of 425 c.c. of citrated blood and two hours later under novocaine, with an occasional whiff of ethelyne, an exploratory laparotomy was performed. Upon exposure the peritoneum appeared dark and edematous. The peritoneal cavity contained a considerable quantity of bloody looking fluid. There were no clots. There was a marked extravasation of blood covering the entire descending colon and its mesentery from the splenic flexure to the sigmoidal juncture. In fact, there was a marked discoloration of both the visceral and parietal peritoneum, covering practically its entire surface. That the hemorrhage was retroperitoneal was evident, but we could not determine its origin. Nothing further was done. She made an uneventful convalescence and was discharged from the hospital February 18 with a blood picture of: red blood count, 3,420,000; leukocytes, 8,400 and hemoglobin, 60 per cent. So far, so good, but just six days after leaving the hospital she had a recurrence of the pain and again showed marked indications of another hemorrhage. She was readmitted into the hospital. At this time her red blood count was 1,850,000; leukocytes, 12,400; and hemoglobin, 48 per cent. The urinary findings were: albumin, present; sugar, negative; indican, negative; bile, negative; acetone, negative; diacetic acid, negative; no epithelial casts, no granular casts, and four or five hyaline casts to a field; a few small cuboidal epithelial cells, occasional blood cells and a few pus cells.

She was immediately given another transfusion, this time 500 c.c. after which there was considerable improvement in her general condition, although there was a constant pain in her left side. On February 27 (three days after entering the hospital) the pain radiated into the left leg and hip, which required the daily administration of opiates to relieve. There was no evidence of a phlebitis. On March 3, after having rested easily the previous night, she complained of pain in the cardiac region and had an emesis of bright red blood. There was no recurrence of the vomiting and the chest pain disappeared during the day. She had a fair night. The following morning there was a marked change for the worse. Her pulse rose from 90 to 140. The pallor became more marked and her general condition was most·critical. It was on the previous evening that Dr. Knavel gave me the clue which enabled me to make the diagnosis of a "ruptured renal aneurysm." Her urinary findings at this time were: marked evidence of albumin; sugar, negative; indican, present; bile, negative; marked trace of acetone; diacetic acid, negative; a few hyaline casts, no epithelial casts, a few granular casts; a few small cuboidal epithelial cells, occasional blood cells, and occasional pus cells.

She received another transfusion of 500 c.c. at 11:00 A. M., and was taken into the operating room at 2:00 P. M. We were unable at this time to count her pulse because of the increasing rate and its extremely thready quality. Under novocaine and a small amount of nitrous oxide, a left nephrectomy was performed. The kidney was practically embedded in a huge blood clot. While we were removing this clot the lower part of the kidney literally broke off. The renal artery and ureter were ligated en masse and the remaining portion of the kidney was removed. Two soft rubber drains were inserted and the wound was closed. Upon her return to the room she was given normal saline by hypodermoclysis and glucose, intravenously. She made an uneventful recovery and was discharged from the hospital March 18.

SUMMARY

1. There is very little literature on this subject.

2. The condition is relatively infrequent in its occurrence.

3. It is exceedingly difficult to diagnose.

4. The majority of cases are not recognized early enough to save the life of the individual.

5. It may occur in the absence of decided change in the urinary findings.

6. In any case of a sudden onset and intense pain, followed by symptoms of a concealed hemorrhage, the possibility of a ruptured renal aneurysm should be given due consideration.

7. Surgery offers the only hope for relief.

I am deeply grateful to the personnel of the Iowa State Medical Library for their hearty cooperation in supplying me with literature for the preparation of this paper, and particularly to Dr. Jeannette Dean Throckmorton for her deep interest and assistance which has made it possible for me to give the medical profession a bibliography of practically all the literature pertaining to the subject of renal aneurysm.

I now have the pleasure of presenting to you in person, Mrs. C. R. H., the fifty-eighth case of renal aneurysm on record, and the eighth reported case in which a correct preoperative diagnosis was made.

ASPECTS OF LOWERED RESISTANCE AND TUBERCULOSIS AS A FOUNDATION FOR COMPENSATION UNDER WORKMEN'S COMPENSATION ACTS

Kurt Grave, M.D.,

Member of the California Bar, Los Angeles

Aetna Life Insurance Company v. Graham, et al.,[1] was a proceeding under the Texas Workmen's Compensation Act. The evidence tended to prove that the employee, daughter of claimants, died from tuberculosis, claimed to have been caused or superinduced while in the employment of defendant Thompson company, a manufacturer of shoe polish. The shoe polish, composed of various chemicals, was manufactured by mixing them in barrels and adding different kinds of powders so as to produce the desired colors. During the process of mixing the deceased was required to stand over the barrel, thus necessarily inhaling the fumes. When she began work two years prior to her disease, she was a healthy girl, but gradually she developed tuberculosis and had to quit, continuing to grow worse steadily until she died. It was claimants' theory that the fumes from the liquid, an alcoholic mixture, passing into the lungs caused an irritation of their membranes, and that because of such irritation tuberculosis germs had fastened themselves upon the irritated area leading to active tuberculosis. It seems that this theory was supported by the testimony of a physician as an expert witness. The Court of Civil Appeals of Texas held this to be an injury compensable under the Workmen's Compensation Act. "If the fumes incident to the mixture of chemicals in making shoe polish, inhaled by Artie Graham," said the Court, "produced and kept the membranes of her nose, throat, and lungs in an irritated condition, then this was an 'injury' to the physical structure of her body, and if, on account of or by reason of said irritated condition, tubercular germs seized upon said injured parts and developed into tuberculosis, then, we think, said disease 'naturally resulted from said injury.' It is not necessary that said injury should have resulted from an accident. Any injury sustained by the employee in the course of his employment is insured against, whether it is accidental or not. We think it is immaterial whether such injury and its resultant disease developed suddenly or at once, or whether it developed gradually and imperceptibly. We also think it is immaterial that the employee is unable to state the date on which such injury is received. Our Workmen's Compensation Law contemplates that all injuries received by the employee in the course of his employment, with certain exceptions, shall be compensated, whether such injuries were proximately caused by some act or omission on the part of the employer or not, and that in case of death of the employee from a disease which resulted from said injury as the exciting and efficient cause, the beneficiaries are entitled to compensation, although they are unable to prove that such death was proximately caused by the injury received, as the term 'proximate cause' is used in the law of negligence. If the evidence as a whole was sufficient to show that the inhalation by Artie Graham of the fumes above referred to was the exciting cause of tuberculosis which resulted in her death, then it must be held that her death was caused by an 'injury' or 'personal injury' as those terms are defined by the statute."

This is a most liberal construction of the Workmen's Compensation Act in favor of the employee. Has such a construction been followed by other courts? Some aspects of lowered resistance and tuberculosis as foundations for compensation under workmen's compensation acts may throw light upon this question in the coming discussion.

THE ISSUES OF LOWERED VITALITY AND RESISTANCE

The bulk of workmen's compensation cases in which tuberculosis is claimed to have caused the employee's disability, is founded upon lowered vitality and the reactivation of living, through dormant tubercle bacilli which have become awakened to activity by reason of prior injuries due to the nature of the employment. The state of lowered resistance may be brought into existence by reason of three different situations:

1. By a sudden attack of a sufficiently strong industrial vulnerating force such as a blow, fall, etc.

2. Gradually through the slow development of impairment of the employee's health. The industrial vulnerating force in such a case is usually dust, fumes, or other noxious gases and air, under the traumatic influence of which the employee has been working for his master over a long period of time.

3. By the combination of a first gradual, and then sudden exposure to vulnerating forces, causing a gradual and then a sudden decline of the resisting powers.

Railroad Water and Coal Handling Company v. Industrial Commission, et al.,[2] represents the first of these situations. A bridge worker, who prior to his accident had worked steadily at hard labor without visible effect, and who had been an apparently healthy man previously, sustained injuries to his back, and three ribs of the right side were broken. Four months later he was found to be suffering from tuberculosis of the right lung. There was medical testimony that, if the workman had a latent tuberculosis at the time of the accident, the injury and the shock incident to the accident would tend to arouse the tubercular germs to activity. It was held that the claimant was entitled to compensation for his tuberculosis. As an example of the second type, the case of *Simmons v. Etowah Monument Company*[3] may be mentioned. In this case the employee was engaged in operating in a closed room an air hose through which sand was blown on marble, thereby creating considerable amounts of sand and marble dust in the room. By reason of faulty construction and adjustment of the mask furnished to the workman to prevent the inhalation of such sand and marble dust, and also by reason of improper and insufficient ventilation, the employee contracted silicosis, which resulted in tuberculosis. The court held that no recovery could be had under the workmen's compensation act, since "the mere lodging of the particles of dust and sand in defendant's lungs constituted in itself no injury or accident to the employee in the sense of the act," and that "the diseases of the lungs which resulted therefrom were not, for this reason, caused by any injury or accident to the employee."

The third class of cases would consist of a combination of circumstances such as found in the two above given instances.

MEDICAL EXPERT TESTIMONY

Several problems for the medical expert arise out of the application of workmen's compensation acts in connection with tuberculosis as a cause of disability or death, when claimed by the workman or his dependents, to have been caused by the nature of the employment. Where there is a pre-existing "open tuberculosis," no claim can be made that the tuberculosis had been caused directly by the injuries due to the employment. The only question remaining is that of acceleration or aggravation to its final termination by reason of the employment. In such a case it would appear that a concurrence of the opinions of medical experts inter sese and with the commission could be easily enough obtained. However, this is not always so.

In the case of *Jefferson, et al. v. District Court of Ramsey County, et al.,*[4] the employee sustained injuries while in the defendant's employ. The workman was crushed by, and under, a load of lumber so that he suffered several broken ribs and other lesser injuries. From the time of his accident until his death he was confined to his bed. An autopsy disclosed that he had had pulmonary tuberculosis in such an advanced stage that one lung had been entirely destroyed and the other one to a considerable extent. There were also other diseases, not described in the decision. The defendant called three physicians who testified that, in their professional opinions, the employee's death had been caused solely by his pulmonary tuberculosis. and that the injuries sustained had not been sufficient either to cause or to hasten his death. On the side of the dependent claimant, however, it was proved that the employee had apparently been in good health prior to his accident, that he had worked continuously at hard labor, and that he had never been able to leave the bed after the accident. Compensation in favor of the dependent claimant was awarded and affirmed by the higher court. It is not an easy matter to trace the reasoning of the three medical experts in testifying as they did, since the record is devoid of any details in this respect. Possibly the injuries were such as would not have caused or hastened death in a healthy person, but can one be so certain that they did not contribute to, or hasten, the death of this employee? It would seem that the commission was correct in its conclusion; and it thus appears that medical expert testimony must not only be true, but must also appear true and in accord with common knowledge and experience in order to find a willing ear before the triers of facts.

How medical experts are led away from their original medical theories to one in favor of the party opponent is best shown in the case of *Osage Coal Company v. State Industrial Commission, et al.,*[5] where the employee received an injury to his chest, rendering him unconscious for six hours and keeping him in bed for three weeks thereafter. He was unable to leave the house for six months after the accident. On appeal from an order of the commission granting an award in favor of the injured employee, the appellant employer relied upon testimony of certain medical experts to the effect that "there was no such thing as traumatic pulmonary tuberculosis or tuberculosis caused from injury." It was, therefore, contended that the injuries did not cause the employee's tuberculosis. The following questions were asked of one of the medical experts on direct examination:

Q. "Doctor, would a blow on the chest aggravate or accelerate tubercular germs that were there?"

A. "If I understand your question, I would like to say that the authorities state that trauma on the side of tuberculosis may precipitate a tuberculous action, that is, bring it about. In my own observation I have never seen a case in which I

would figure that trauma had the least effect on it."

On cross-examination the same doctor testified as follows:

Q. "Dr. McCarley, a great many people have tubercle bacilli in their lungs, do they not?"

A. "Yes, sir."

Q. "And the greater quantities of people throw it off, don't they?"

A. "No, they don't."

Q. "They are dormant, then, you might say?"

A. "Yes."

Q. "And anything that lowers a man's vitality might precipitate or cause it to become active, the tubercle bacilli?"

A. "Anything that lowers a man's vitality might contribute to the tuberculosis becoming active."

Q. "In other words, a man in good health would be more likely to develop tuberculosis, and the tuberculosis would be more likely to become active if his vitality were lowered either by an injury or by disease?"

A. "Yes, that is correct."

It may be conceded that "all human beings are susceptible to tuberculosis," that "the disease is always found where an opportunity for infection is present," and that "the very widespread dissemination of the disease throughout the world and the frequency with which tuberculosis is found in necropsies indicate that natural immunity probably does not exist." "Since living bacilli have been found in calcified foci it is highly probable that complete destruction of all tubercle bacilli even in a small isolated lymph gland is the exception rather than the rule, and may never occur at all, we are unable to destroy the invading enemy, but we may protect ourselves against his multiplication and further invasion and against superinfection." Since "not all human beings, however, become infected with tubercle bacilli," and "probably five to ten per cent escape insofar as finding evidence of the disease after death is concerned, and especially in necropsies of individuals living in the rural districts,"[6] medical testimony necessarily carries in itself a certain, although comparatively small, amount of speculation as to possible prior tuberculous infection. However, in regard to injured workmen from rural districts it might well be urged that medical testimony as to reactivation of a latent, encapsulated tuberculosis be more guarded than where the injured employee has been, or is, a city dweller.

The question of certainty and sufficiency of medical expert testimony is another problem, most vexing to both attorneys and medical experts.

How much value has the medical expert's opinion in the eyes of the commissions and reviewing courts? Two situations present themselves. When the medical expert testimony is such as to form the exclusive basis upon which the trier of facts bases his decision, a greater amount of certainty is required than when other facts, extraneous to medical testimony are available. On the other hand, where extraneous matters satisfy the requirements of a reasonably sound conclusion, the medical expert testimony may be more reserved without being impaired in its value. The Supreme Court of Errors of Connecticut has discussed this subject in *Madore v. New Departure Manufacturing Company.*[7]

"If upon the facts the medical expert is merely willing to testify that the disease might have, or was likely to have, resulted from the employment, or the conditions under which it was carried on, but is unwilling to go further and testify that, in his opinion, taking into consideration all of the facts presented and considering every other hypothesis suggested, it was reasonably probable that the disease resulted from the employment, and therefore the employment was its direct cause, the commissioner or court should not conclude that the disease did result from the employment, unless the facts outside this medical testimony fairly warrant that conclusion." This court adds: "We do not intend by this to exclude from consideration the testimony of the medical witness who merely states that the accident or disease might have resulted from the employment, or the conditions under which it was carried on; it may be invaluable, as an expression of a cautious opinion, in corroboration of other testimony. What we do intend is that the trier cannot himself reach a definite conclusion when he has nothing to rely upon but the opinion of the medical witness who is unable with all of his professional learning and experience, to reach the definite conclusion which the court is required to reach upon the same facts in making an award."

EVIDENTIARY FACTS OF RECORD

CONTRASTING "MEDICAL" AND "JUDICIAL" PSYCHOLOGY

There are a number of evidentiary facts by which commissions and courts are guided in their decisions, even though such facts might mean little or nothing to the medical expert. For instance, the fact of apparent good health prior to the injury and to the development of manifestations of tuberculosis thereafter, tends to prove either latency of, or freedom from, tuberculosis to the judicial mind,

while to the medical man the same evidentiary fact has little, if any, weight at all. Often the age of the injured employee is given by courts in their decisions, as though tuberculosis is a disease peculiar to certain periods of life. Strong suspicion is cast upon an accident and the subsequent lowered resistance, where the tuberculous condition becomes manifest immediately, or within a reasonably short time, after the accident. Even this circumstance may not be very persuasive to a medical man. The judiciary will ask why these two events should be mere coincidences. Furthermore, when the injured employee does not return to his former state of health within a normal period for the recovery from the accidental injuries, commissions will attribute this fact to the accident, while a physician may be very much more skeptical in this respect. Thus, it may appear that the medical expert is likely to show a much greater reserve in assisting the court in arriving at a sound conclusion than is expected by it of the doctor; and yet, while in the opinion of the medical expert, the outcome of the litigation may not be in accord with his medical views, the evidentiary facts of apparently previous good health, when coupled with that of an accident, an industrial vulnerating force, an injury, a lowered vitality and a poor, or no, recovery, all taken together, have a most persuasive influence upon the lay mind, any medical theory to the contrary. In *Industrial Commission v. Rice*,[8] the evidence showed that the "plaintiff, prior to the alleged injury, was in good health and free from tuberculosis and that on the date of the injury he was forced to breathe heated gas and fumes from oil burned in defendant's furnace, when trapped and incarcerated therein for a period of about three minutes, in consequence of which the workman became incapacitated by reason of tuberculosis." That judgment was rendered in favor of the employee permits of little doubt. The record showed that at the time of the accident the servant had been an able-bodied man, about thirty-two years of age, in good health, who had never received an injury of any kind, and that the injury to the chest rendered him unconscious for about six hours and kept him in bed for three weeks, whereafter he was unable to leave his home for another six months. There was also ample evidence to sustain an award for tuberculosis, reactivated by the injury to the chest caused by his employment.[9] One should here evaluate the evidentiary fact of the man's age, i. e., thirty-two years of age. One may imagine how the layman is inclined to visualize a young man in the prime of his manhood, young, healthy, strong, in full possession of all his faculties, and one can easily judge the effect which such a mental picture must have upon the judicial mind.

In *Kelly v. Watson Coal Company, et al.,*[10] the employee was winding a crab when the crank flew out of his hand, struck him on the hand and at a point on the left side of his abdomen near the waistline, and knocked him down. Five days later he complained of soreness in the region of his left testicle, which upon physical examination was found to be swollen, inflamed and tender. About a month later the testicle was removed and found infected with tubercle bacilli. Further complications set in, so that the patient died from tuberculous peritonitis about eight months after the accident. Medical men testified that there was a direct connection between trauma, injury, and the tubercular condition, basing their opinions upon the theory that shock after the accident and the consequently lowered resistance had rendered the injured man particularly subject to the quick development of the disease, and that such disease and its development was, in all probability, due to the assigned causes. This quick development of the disease after the accident seems to be a circumstance which courts favor in their decisions when upholding awards made by the commissions in favor of the claimant. In an Iowa case, *Fraze v. McClelland, et al.,*[11] the claimant, a woodworker, while moving a heavy oaken door toward the elevator for the purpose of transporting it to another floor, was squeezed by its weight against a wall, when the door tipped. The happening was momentary. The door was immediately righted, and the operation proceeded. Immediately thereafter the employee sought a bench where he laid down and felt quite sick and helpless for the time being. He resumed his work later and engaged in his usual occupation for the three succeeding days, after which he reported to the company doctor. The patient developed fever soon, an abscess of one lung developed which finally resulted in tuberculosis. The defendant produced as medical experts some very distinguished medical specialists, whose testimony was to the effect that trauma could not produce tuberculosis, but who admitted by implication that tuberculosis might be lighted up or accelerated. They denied, however, that the claimant's injury was sufficiently adequate for such an acceleration. Compensation in favor of the claimant was upheld by the Supreme Court. The court said in its decision: "It appears without dispute that up to the time of his injury the plaintiff weighed from 165 to 170 pounds, and that immediately following such injury he lost weight rapidly, until he was reduced to 135 pounds. It further appears that he had always been an apparently

healthy man, and was not aware of any infirmity, and that he had never lost a day's work because of illness, except some years previous, during an influenza epidemic, of which he also was a victim. Taking this fact in connection with the further fact that plaintiff's disability began with the day of the accident, and that its development was rapid, and much more rapid than the normal progress of tuberculosis under ordinary conditions, we think it is highly probative in its character."

On the other hand, a relatively considerable lapse of time between the accident and the manifestations of the subsequent tuberculosis, unless filled in by signs of tuberculous development, will greatly weaken the judicial inference of causal connection between employment, injury, and tuberculosis. This rule seems to bring medical experts and judicial officers more closely into accord than most of the other evidentiary facts usually a duced. This idea is clearly expressed in another Iowa case, *Guthrie, et al., v. Iowa Gas and Electric Company, et al.,*[12] where it was held that the evidence was insufficient to show causal connection between employment and tuberculosis. The workman had received an injury to his knee, caused by a blow from a hod of brick. There was some pain at the immediate time of this injury, but after a short rest the employee resumed his duties, continued his work, and remained with the company at his employment regularly for approximately two months, when the employment terminated. Thereafter he was employed by a coal company to haul coal, and worked for this company for some time. The rest of the history is seen in the following portion of the decision of the Supreme Court which reversed an award in favor of the workman. "We therefore have a situation," said the Court, "where it appears that the injury complained of did not result in immediate serious inconvenience to the workman. He suffered some pain at the time, but not sufficient to interfere with the continuing of his employment thereafter and for two months following. It was two years after the injury before the condition developed in the knee requiring the services of a physician, and a year later before the diagnosis of tubercular infection was made. Can it be said that there is sufficient 'competent evidence' to show causal connection between injury and the tubercular condition that was ultimately discovered therein?" The Guthrie case had been commented on by the Supreme Court in the Fraze case. Speaking of the Guthrie case the court said: "In that case, no alleged disability therefrom was asserted until six years thereafter. The question was whether the tuberculous infection of August,

1919, was attributable to a comparatively light blow received March 1, 1917. We held that evidence to that effect was wanting. In the case at bar, we deem the evidence materially stronger, and as sufficient to sustain the finding below."

However, when the injuries are severe, and the interval of time between injuries and the appearance of tuberculosis, contains indications of development of anything suggestive of tuberculosis, the probability of reactivation of tubercle bacilli will not be excluded by judicial officers. In *Maurer v. South Pennsylvania Collieries Company, et al.,*[13] claimant, a coal miner, fell down a manway and was severely injured. Three months thereafter he was able to accomplish some light duties, but he had to change to lighter ones, until a year and a half after the accident he was totally incapacitated. A medical expert in answer to a question stating in effect, "Having treated him for three months in which no diagnosis was made of tuberculosis (the patient had gone back to work and worked for a period of thirteen months and then developed tuberculosis) do you believe it is a reasonable proposition that the injury which occurred in February, 1925, lit up the present condition?" replied in the affirmative, adding that tuberculosis was simply a progressive systemic condition hastened by the injury. "We cannot say," added the court of last resort on appeal, "that this testimony was not sufficient to sustain the award." This medical testimony is not unreasonable, although it appears boldly unqualified, considering the medical history of this patient. In the Guthrie case it is mentioned that after the accident the workman intermittently suffered some pain in his knee, and that a doctor treated him later for synovitis and arthritis until the diagnosis of tuberculosis was made. One cannot help wondering if this intermittent pain and the synovitis and arthritis were not in fact symptoms of tuberculosis, even though below the threshhold of medical diagnosis. The perusal of the case as a whole leaves a certain dissatisfaction with the outcome thereof in the mind of a fair, but somewhat critically inclined reviewer. One may ask, whether or not it is really necessary that the injuries are obviously severe at the time of the accident in order to warrant compensation after a considerable lapse of time?

THE DECISION OF THE AETNA CASE DOES NOT GO UNCHALLENGED

The decision of *Aetna Life Insurance Company v. Graham, et al.,* our opening case does not go unchallenged. What is the intent of workmen's compensation acts? Do they insure the employee's life and health at the expense of the employer? Clearly, if by insuring is meant that any and every disability of the employee, whether due to the employment or not, is to be compensated out of workmen's compensation funds, the employer would be deprived of his property without due process of law. However, there is another aspect of life and health insurance. The disability arises out of the employment and includes the wear and tear, the physical depreciation of the employee's body due to his work, its surrounding conditions, and the risks incident thereto. It even comprises the after-effects of such wear and tear even though remote in time. In this sense a workmen's compensation act could become a health and life insurance. It is at this point that uniformity of decisions becomes lacking. This is due partly to the wording of the diverse acts, and partly to the different interpretations which courts of last resort have given to it. Elements of the old law of master and servant are preserved in many of the decisions. Thus, why should it not be held that the servant by engaging in his calling assume the risks incident to his employment, or consents to the wrongful act or omission of his employer?

In a New York case, *Wager v. White Star Candy Company,*[14] tuberculosis resulted from working in a damp, unsanitary, and unventilated cellar. The employee failed in her action. "The plaintiff," said the court on appeal, "was fully aware of the condition under which she worked, and continued in the employment from June to December in spite of such knowledge. It is from her testimony that we learn that the walls of the cellar were wet to touch; that a cesspool backed up liquids which wet the floor; that the cellar was devoid of windows to light or air it; that dead rats were left about; that odors were vile; that no fires were kept in the upstairs room; that the plaintiff worked in a drafty place; that the upstairs room was damp. It is common knowledge that such conditions are deleterious to health. The plaintiff is chargeable with such knowledge. We think that the plaintiff, as a matter of law, assumed the risk attendant upon her remaining in the employment, and that recovery may not stand. The judgment and order should be reversed on law, with costs, and the complaint dismissed. All concur." Such a judgment was possible in the year of our Lord nineteen hundred and twenty-six, in the age of social hygiene and laborers' welfare. How much more humane is the Aetna decision in this respect? Some statutes require the showing of some accidental happening, i. e., of an event occurring suddenly, violently, unexpectedly, and unforeseen, caused by improper and unnatural force. In such jurisdictions the plaintiff in the Aetna case would have his remedy, as a rule, only in a civil action before a court, possibly with a jury, subjecting the patient to heavy expenses and all the delays, uncertainties, and legal technicalities, incident to such action. Thus, in *Depre v. Pacific Coast Forge Company*,[15] the employer operated a galvanizing plant in connection with his general business. The injured employee was in charge of this plant. A part of the plant consisted of a large tank, into which was poured a mixture of muriatic acid, sulphuric acid, and water. The mixture was then heated almost to the boiling point. Adequate ventilation to carry away the gases which arose from this mixture was not provided. The employee developed tuberculosis. The court held that this did not constitute an accidental injury, but that the employee might sue for violation of the Factory Act at law, and that the assumption of risk by the employee was no defense in such an action. The Aetna decision expressly brings such cases within the jurisdiction of the commission, and thereby places the workman under the workmen's compensation law with its informal, speedy and inexpensive procedure.

Still more liberal are the courts which are subject to the pure "injury" clause in the acts, although some of them require that elements of accidental happening be shown. In this respect the Aetna decision proves that the Texas courts have aligned themselves with the courts not requiring any earmarks of accident. The Aetna case continues: "Our Workmen's Compensation Act contemplates that all injuries received by the employee in the course of his employment shall be compensated * * * and that in case of death of the employee from a disease which resulted from said injury as the exciting and efficient cause, the beneficiaries are entitled to compensation, though they are unable to prove that such death was proximately caused by the injury received, as the term 'proximate cause' is used in the law of evidence." These utterances would seem to shock many an orthodox lawyer; and yet, it may be that in regard to tuberculosis there is a certain justification for such court action.

Three possibilities arise out of a case such as the Aetna decision represents:

1. The employee was affected, prior to entering upon his employment, with a latent, "encapsulated" tuberculous infection. No germs from the outside entered the chain of events which led to the active tuberculosis. The disease is "lit up" by the type of employment.

2. The employee was not affected by tuberculosis when he entered upon his duties, but the tubercle bacilli entered the chain of events as an active causative agency from the outside after the condition of lowered vitality by reason of the gradual decline was caused by the employment.

3. The employee was suffering from a pre-existing "encapsulated" tuberculosis, and during the course of his employment and by reason of his lowered resistance due thereto, outside tubercle bacilli entered his system.

However, these possibilities are mere medical hypotheses and who can tell which is correct? The third one is most likely. The picture of the pathologic process as it might go on in the employee's body is then one in which one army, the resisting powers of the body, is encircled by two parts of the enemy army, the tubercle bacilli. On one front they are in reserve. On the other battle line there is much activity. The resisting powers are constantly bombarded by molecules of noxious gases. Finally, the lines of vitality must give way, but which part of the army of the tubercle bacilli will first set into motion the course of the active tuberculosis? If the "encapsulated" army does so first, the tuberculosis develops by reason of some intrinsic infirmity of the employee, for which, as a rule, the master is liable. If the outside germs prevail, some extraneous matter entered the body of the employee. Suppose an employee suffered a concededly industrial accident by sudden trauma, in consequence of which he is hospitalized, and that, while in the hospital, he contracts measles, the employer would not be held liable for the latter disease, even though it may be proved by medical expert testimony that the patient would not have contracted measles, had his resisting powers not been impaired by reason of the preceding injuries. In legal psychology the chain of events was not an uninterrupted line. There was an independent intervening cause, which broke the original chain of causation. The employment was the proximate cause of the compensable injuries and of all their after-effects which intrinsically developed by reason thereof, but it was not an efficient cause of the measles.[16] However, measles and tuberculosis are not the same in cases of injuries to the lungs. There is a fine difference of affinity. It is this and the uncertainty of medical testimony which creates a position in which courts have to form their own opinions and have to decide one way or the other. Because workmen's compensation acts are to be construed liberally in favor of the employee, the latter has a good chance to win over the employer in such a contest. It would seem, however, that the Court of Texas would award compensation, even though outside germs had caused the course of active tuberculosis quite independently of the "encapsulated" bacilli in the inside of the employee's body. Finally, a gradual lowering of resisting powers of the employee's body, when caused by the employment, is usually connected with the concepts of occupational diseases or such as are in the nature thereof. There are jurisdictions under the "injury" acts which exclude occupational diseases from the reach of workmen's compensation acts. The Aetna decision is seemingly indicative of an intention to the contrary.

The Iowa Workmen's Compensation Act provides for compensation for "injuries." What the Supreme Court of Iowa, when faced with a like or similar problem, has decided, or is likely to decide, is unknown to the writer. It is to be expected that this Court, known from other decisions to be open-minded and liberal, will lend a willing ear to the pros and cons of the problem discussed, when the opportunity should arise in a case of first impression.

2008 West Seventh Street.

CITATIONS

1. Tex. Civ. App. —, 279 S. W. 923 (1926); rehearing denied 1926.
2. 334 Ill. 52, 165 N. E. 225 (1929).
3. 42 G. A. 633, 157 S. E. 260 (1931).
4. 138 Minn. 334, 164 N. W. 1012 (1917).
5. 128 Okla. 191, 261 Pac. 933 (1927).
6. "Infection, Immunity, and Biologic Therapy," by Kolmer, 3rd edit. p. 1042, (W. B. Saunders Company, 1924).
7. 104 Conn. 709, 134 Atl. 259 (1926).
8. 26 Ohio App. 497, 160 N. E. 484 (1927).
9. Osage Coal Co. v. State Industrial·Commission, et al., 128 Okla. 191, 261 Pac. 933 (1927) see 5.
10. 272 Pa. 39, 115 Atl. 885 (1922).
11. 200 Iowa 944, 205 N. W. 737 (1925).
12. 200 Iowa 150, 204 N. W. 371 (1925).
13. 295 Pa. 69, 144 Atl. 822 (1929).
14. 227 App. Div. 316, 217 N. Y. S. 173 (1926).
15. 151 Wash. 430, 276 Pac. 89 (1929).
16. Mossop v. Mossop, 108 Conn. 148, 142 Atl. 739 (1929).

PROPHYLAXIS AND TREATMENT OF GAS GANGRENE*

T. J. IRISH, M.D., Forest City

Gas gangrene is one of the more rare conditions seen in the average civil practice, but when once encountered the picture is so striking that it leaves a lasting impression on the minds of all connected with the case. First described in 1853, it was not until the World War that its importance became evident. In the American Expeditionary Forces alone in 128,265 wounds of the soft parts there were 1,389 who developed gas gangrene. Of this number, 674 died. Statistics are not readily available from civil practice but Millar in 1932 was able to collect 607 cases from the literature with a mortality of 49.7 per cent. In my small series of nine cases there have been three deaths.

* Presented before the Austin Flint-Cedar Valley Medical Society, Cedar Falls, June 20, 1933.

ETIOLOGY

The infection has been associated with a variety of cases. It has been reported with spontaneous gangrene from diabetes and vascular causes, from hypodermic injections, fistula in ano, perforated peptic ulcer, appendicitis, infected abortion, and other causes. However it is particularly common in traumatic wounds with gross contamination, the best examples of which are the compound fractures, and it is with this group alone that this paper deals.

A number of organisms may cause gas gangrene. All are anaerobes and are commonly present in cultivated soils and highways. The most important are the B. aerogenes capsulatus, of Welch or perfringens, the vibrion septique, and the B. of malignant edema. The Welch bacillus is the most common and is found in about 75 per cent of the cases. However, in 50 per cent, more than one organism is found. Symbiosis with streptococci or staphlococci is common. With the single exception of the B. histolyticus all of the group has as a characteristic, the saccrolytic decomposition of tissue with the formation of gas. Muscle furnishes a readily available source of glycogen, and the presence of devitalized muscle forms the most essential predisposing factor in the development of gas gangrene. Compound fractures are so commonly associated that it is believed the liberation of calcium salts from the disintegration of bone exerts a favorable factor in its development. Although the same conditions are favorable to the development of tetanus I have been unable to find a report of the double infection, possibly due to the fact that the patient with gas gangrene often dies before there has been time for the tetanus to develop. It is probable that not only may different organisms cause the disease but that there are different strains of the same one with wide differences in virulence. This would help account for the delayed onset and milder course sometimes seen.

SYMPTOMS AND PATHOLOGY

The period of incubation is from one to four days although in rare cases because of the decreased virulence of the organism or conditions less favorable to its development, it may be longer. There is good reason to believe that bacilli may remain dormant and then result in a fulminating infection at some later date as has been seen in delayed operations for non-union. The longest incubation period in my series was six days. This was a compound fracture of the forearm where the bone had barely penetrated the skin. There was not a great deal of traumatism and the parents for some reason did not take the child to a physician until she became desperately ill. These cases must be borne in mind but for all practical purposes a case under observation which shows no signs of gas bacillus infection at the end of five or six days can be considered past the stage of danger. The vast majority will appear within forty-eight hours, usually within eighteen to twenty-four.

The initial symptom is pain or an increase in pre-existing pain, with the complaint that the dressings are too tight. Locally an increase in the swelling is seen. The skin becomes tense and pale and the distal portions of the limb become cold and mottled. There is no redness of the surface nor is there an increase in the temperature of the part. The discharge from the wound is serous in nature, a dirty brown in color and with the foul sickly odor of putrescent meat. As gas is formed the skin takes on a bronzed appearance which is characteristic. The swelling is firm and tense and does not pit on pressure. Blebs form on the extremity and with the death of tissue the pain is somewhat relieved. When the infection is due to the B. of malignant edema the swelling spreads with great rapidity and may cover the entire body in a few hours. The first case I saw was of this type and followed a compound fracture of the hip. Eighteen hours after the injury, edema of the scrotum was noted. Two and one-half hours later death occurred from suffocation. The first pathologic change noted is the outpouring of serum which advances rapidly along the neurovascular spaces. When seen at the higher levels above the active process this is perfectly clear and seldom contains organisms. By its pressure it aids in mechanically blocking the circulation. Thrombosis is due to the toxins liberated and the mechanical pressure occurs with early death of tissue. The process originating in devitalized muscles spreads by muscle planes rather than between muscles and in the earlier stages may be confined to one group. The serous surfaces as the joints, the peritoneum and the pleura seem to possess a peculiar resistance and are seldom affected. The toxins produced cause a marked destruction of red corpuscles, and may cause early death by paralysis of the medullary centers.

Gas formation begins in the deepest portion of the wound or where devitalized muscle is most abundant. It does not occur at the very earliest part of the infection and the presence of gas bubbles in the discharge from the wound is not seen until the process is well advanced. Its early detection is made by auscultatory percussion, later simple percussion gives a tympanitic note and the characteristic crepitation is felt. X-ray examination will show at first a few dark streaks along the course of the muscle and later a definite mottled appearance. It is often possible to detect the pres-ence of gas by the x-ray earlier than by any other method. The gas itself is not toxic but by its pressure dissects its way in advance of the infection proper, blocking the circulation and making new channels for the infection to follow. One appreciates the pressue generated from the experiment of Taylor who attached an autoclave gauge to a tube containing a culture of B. Welchii in dextrose broth. Within two hours the pressure began to rise and at six hours the gauge blew off at twenty-three pounds. Death occurs either from the toxemia and the products of proteolytic disintegration, or as in the case mentioned, from edema of the glottis.

The constitutional symptoms are in keeping with the changes described and represent an overwhelming infection against which the patient musters little resistance. There is no or only moderate leukocytosis, and the temperature shows only a moderate elevation. From the onset the pulse becomes very rapid and is easily compressible. In comparison with the flushed cheeks of the ordinary pyogenic infection the patient shows a striking pallor. If not rapidly fatal icterus develops as the result of hemolysis. The patient is restless, often unusually bright, but coma usually precedes death. Blood cultures may be positive. The blood picture is in keeping with the anemia.

The diagnosis is of course easily made. Crepitation as seen in subcutaneous emphysema and occasionally in a hematoma is distinguished by the associated symptoms and findings. The circulatory collapse and the pallor may suggest a concealed hemorrhage, but hemorrhage if not otherwise ruled out does not lead to gas formation.

PROPHYLACTIC TREATMENT

Treatment is firstly prophylactic and secondly curative. When proper prophylactic measures are taken, gas gangrene is a condition which should rarely occur. Prevention depends entirely upon the early management of the injury, and can be considered under two headings; first the surgical, and second the use of antitoxin.

So much has been written about the treatment of compound fractures and other mutilating injuries of the extremities that it is unnecessary to go into any detail at this time. Briefly the principles are as follows:

A. Immediate immobilization of fractures to prevent further trauma.

B. The treatment of shock.

C. The careful surgical treatment of the wound. Devitalized muscle must be carefully excised until muscle tissue is reached which is normal in color, bleeds when cut and contracts when pinched. All foreign bodies and clots must be removed and the wound irrigated with Dakin's solution. Loose fragments of bone which cannot be utilized must be removed. Careful hemostasis must be secured. As to whether or not primary closure can be secured depends upon the operator's judgment in the individual case. Where there is any question about the thoroughness with which devitalized tissue has been removed it is better to leave the wound wide open, lay in loosely gauze, soaked in Dakin's solution, and put irrigating tubes in place. Secondary closure may be accomplished at any later date which seems fit. In most cases associated with fracture this step is not necessary since the wound heals as soon if not sooner than bony union is complete, and convalescence is not prolonged. Other solutions may be used in the place of Dakin's solution but it is still our most practical means for the handling of contaminated wounds. One point is not commonly mentioned in connection with its use. Plain catgut does not stand up well when bathed in Dakin's solution and the slipping of ligatures may result. Where its use is contemplated it is better to use chromic catgut for the more important bleeders. I have seen one very serious case of delayed hemorrhage where this was the cause. With our modern tendency to conserve tissue one wonders if we do not sometimes err on the side of being too conservative, and if more immediate amputations of badly mangled limbs are not justified.

The use of antitoxin in the prevention or treatment of gas gangrene first came into use during the latter part of the World War. In a condition which can be produced by several organisms any antitoxin to be practical must necessarily be of a polyvalent nature. At present none of our manufacturers of biologicals produce a prophylactic package including more than two; all of them include the B. Welchii, and most of them the vibrion septique. These are combined in a single ampule with the customary 1500 units of tetanus. It is easily administered intramuscularly, of course, after the usual precautions for sensitization have been taken. Reactions are somewhat more common than after the straight tetanus antitoxin. I have seen one patient develop a gas bacillus infection after the use of antitoxin, and this was a mild infection, coming on after five days, and recovering after incision alone. I believe that the combined antitoxin should be used as a routine in those cases where the nature of the injury presents conditions favorable to the development of gas gangrene. However, it must not in any sense be used as a substitute for thorough surgical treatment of the wound, but rather as an added and valuable precaution.

CURATIVE TREATMENT

The treatment of a patient who has developed a gas bacillus infection is a major problem. It can be considered under three headings, all of which are interdependent for their effectiveness.

1. *The use of antitoxin.* With the first appearance of symptoms the patient is given antitoxin intravenously. This is now conveniently supplied in an ampule containing 10,000 units perfringens, 10,000 units vibrion septique, 200 units B. of malignant edema, 200 units sordelli, 25 units B. histolyticus. The serum must be given slowly, five minutes for the first c.c., although the remainder of the dose may be given somewhat more rapidly. As a precaution one c.c. of adrenalin is given subcutaneously at the start of the injection and repeated as necessary. The serum is given at body temperature. Some advise diluting the concentrated serum as supplied with 100 c.c. of normal saline and claim that reactions are minimized by this method. If the condition of the patient does not show definite improvement in six hours the dose is repeated. In any event it is repeated every twenty-four hours until convalescence is obvious. The later doses may be given intramuscularly; from 30,000 to 70,000 units are required in the average case. Serotherapy is mentioned first because it may be begun while preparations are being made for surgical treatment. Secondly in the cases where some delay is justified it may cause such improvement that operative treatment can be much less radical.

2. *Surgical treatment.* The established surgical treatment consists of early amputation above the level of infection. Obviously it is often impossible to get above the level of edema and crepitation. This should not prevent one from amputating when we remember that gas and serum precede the actual infection by several inches. Often the tissue of the groin or the axilla will crepitate and gas and serum will escape after the amputation, but the tissues will be vital and recovery may take place. Under such circumstances free incisions should be made above the level of amputation. The type of operation can be made to fit the individual case. In general it should be as simply and quickly performed as possible. In the thigh at least some attempt at flap formation is justified. Only in the most favorable cases should the wound be loosely closed over rubber tissue drains. In the majority of cases it is better to leave the stump wide open. Many solutions have been used locally, most of them based upon the assumption of supplying oxygen to the affected area. None of them has proved of the least value unless other treatment was used in conjunction. Hydrogen peroxide is

the most commonly used for irrigation of the stump and areas opened by incision. I have used it in my few cases but cannot state just what effect it had upon the course. Dressings should not be permitted to become dry and hard but should be changed several times daily.

One will see, and it is hoped with increasing relative frequency, patients in whom the process is comparatively mild, due to the use of prophylactic antitoxin or some factor which diminishes the virulence. Where there is no evidence of actual gangrene of the limb and the constitutional symptoms are not so severe, incisions which will permit the escape of gas and serum will often suffice. At least one is justified in trying this before an immediate amputation is performed. Patients have recovered under this procedure alone but certainly the therapeutic use of antitoxin is indicated.

Kelley has recently reported a series of twelve cases in which x-ray therapy was used in conjunction with serotherapy and surgery. He feels that it exerted a very favorable influence. Perhaps some of you have had experience with this form of treatment but I have not.

3. *Supportive treatment.* The supportive treatment is that of any acute infection. For the profound anemia due to the hemolytic toxins, repeated transfusions are of benefit. Fluids must be given freely either by mouth or intravenously. Any theoretical objections that may be attached to the use of glucose intravenously are more than offset by its values. Rest must be secured by the free use of morphine.

SUMMARY

1. Gas bacillus infections although comparatively rare, are always a potential danger in contaminated wounds, and are particularly common in compound fractures. The presence of devitalized muscle is the most important predisposing factor.

2. Various degrees of virulence are seen. A typical case unless promptly treated sets up a vicious cycle which is one of the most rapidly fatal of all infections.

3. The treatment is first of all prophylactic and consists of proper surgical care of the wound and the use of prophylactic antitoxin. The treatment of the actual infection is surgical together with the use of antitoxin. The antitoxin is of definite value in the control of the process and often makes the more radical operative steps unnecessary.

INFANTILE ECZEMA*

H. C. WILLETT, M.D., Des Moines

There is no such disease as infantile eczema, *per se.* Infants have a skin eruption that we have been calling eczema, but it is no different from the so-called eczema of the adolescent or adult. The histologic and pathologic changes in the skin are the same, whatever the age may be. The only difference is possibly an etiologic one, and that is due largely to the immaturity of the skin in the infant. The corneous layer of the epidermis is not so well developed, hence the delicate structures beneath this layer are more easily reached by an irritant. This irritant causes a mild or severe inflammatory reaction and increases the permeability of the cell. This permeability of the cell is occasionally increased by some endogenous toxin which aggravates the dermatitis. While in a great many instances it is very difficult to find the external irritant, it generally can be done if we search earnestly and carefully. When this is done the endogenous element as a rule takes care of itself.

Eczema is a term which has long been and is still, too commonly applied to any inflammatory condition of the skin, the cause or nature of which the observer is ignorant. It is almost literally translated by the word eruption, which means to boil over or burst out. The skin responds to irritation just as any other organ, by hyperemia and exudation. The amount of this response depends on the degree and type of the irritant, and the susceptibility of the individual. The less one knows of skin diseases, the more likely he is to call all skin eruptions eczema. The longer one investigates skin conditions and the different types of skin, the more likely he is to identify in certain cases, either a definite recognizable cause, or a definite sequence of events, which will permit the arrangement of certain skin diseases under more instructive headings. Most all eruptive diseases at some period of their history have been called eczema. This is true of the common diseases such as scabies, impetigo, psoriasis, the ringworm infections, lichen planus and many more itching and scaling dermatoses. These diseases in many ways resemble so-called eczema and it is only the identification of their causes which has lead us to their separation from that chaotic conglomeration.

The word eczema has kept the medical profession ignorant and in darkness of actual dermatologic conditions more than any other term. In other words, to use a slang parlance, "It is a shot in the arm" that has had such a soothing effect that we stop thinking of other possible conditions.

The older members of the profession well re-

*Presented before the Eighty-second Annual Session, Iowa State Medical Society, Des Moines, May 10, 11, 12, 1933.

member that if anything happened in the upper three-fourths of the abdominal cavity it was called inflammation of the bowels. At the present time the diseases of that cavity are well catalogued. The term inflammation of the bowels is almost forgotten, as I hope the term eczema will be in a short time. I wish to quote from my old professor, Dr. James Nevins Hyde, who spoke thus a number of years ago before his death. "Is it not clear that the word eczema has outworn its usefulness? The word eczema in the mouth of the expert has become a feature of the man in the street, of the advertiser, of the charlatan; the doom of the word is probably written. It will survive where it belongs and with no greater repute than attacks in general to the outworn and discredited." Such are the words of one of the keenest and most cultured dermatologists that I have ever had the pleasure to meet.

As already mentioned there is no difference in the pathology in a dermatitis, whether it occurs in an infant or an adult, or whether it is caused by poison ivy, wool, soap or face powder. There is a difference in degree of inflammatory reaction depending on the type of irritant; the strength of the irritant and the resistance of the skin. Any type of skin will succumb if the irritating agent is strong enough or if its application is sufficiently prolonged.

The type or severity of a dermatitis depends entirely upon the individual and the etiologic factor in a particular case. As this paper should necessarily deal with the dermatitis occurring in infancy we will confine our remarks to the more probable causes at this age, remembering that all the causes producing an inflammatory condition of the skin in adults is more potent in infancy but because of the early age they are not so frequently exposed. An example of this is occupational dermatitis.

Heredity is an important factor. If we obtain a careful family history we will usually find some or several members that have had allergic diseases; namely, various kinds of dermatitis, urticaria, angioneurotic edema, hay fever, asthma, chronic bronchitis, rhinitis, colitis, migraine and several other conditions not found so frequently. These allergic diseases are distinctly hereditary. Duke says that allergy is the most prominent of all hereditary conditions. Biologically it may be either a dominant or recessive characteristic. In some families almost all the members have some allergic disease; in others it only occasionally occurs. There is no way of curing allergy except by proper mating. Civilization has not reached the stage of accepting this idea. We use far more intelligence in the proper mating of our domestic

animals and pets than we do with our children. Allergy, roughly speaking, is a manifestation of an unstable autonomic nervous system, the end result of which is an unstable cell. The permeability of the cells is increased. Certain proteins in various articles of food increase this, then certain external irritants come in contact with the skin and we have what is generally called eczema or dermatitis.

The type of skin is an etiologic factor in the production of a dermatitis. The seborrheic skin is much more easily irritated than the normal skin. The dry and icthyotic skin is also more easily affected by external agents. If you will review your anatomy of the skin you will find that it is composed of three layers; namely, the subcutaneous, the corium and epidermis. The corium has two layers and the epidermis four layers. The most important of these, as far as protection to the delicate structures beneath, is the outer corneous layer. This consists of several layers of stratified epithelium which contain a substance called keratin. This prevents the entrance, in a large measure, of any substance or fluid into the skin. However, this armor is weakened to some extent by the hair follicle coil and sebaceous ducts. These ducts have only one or two layers of cells containing keratin, and if the individual is sensitive to certain substances these spaces are the points of entrance.

Since the skin of the infant is not fully matured, and because the corneous layer is thinner and contains less keratin, it is much more easily irritated than that of the adult. You have all noticed that you see very few of these scaling or weeping skins after the child has reached the age of two or three years. You can now feed him the food that you formerly thought caused his early eczema and he will have no eruption. By what magic has he been cured of his allergic skin reaction? Is it not more logical and reasonable to think that his skin has developed and as keratinization has developed it is more resistant to external irritants? Of course these individuals will have numerous attacks of various kinds of dermatitis later in life. Then you will diagnose their conditions as ivy dermatitis, primrose dermatitis, soap dermatitis, trade or occupational dermatitis, or what not, and hundreds of other kinds with the proper qualifying adjective. We advise these patients to avoid these external irritants; when they are infants we try to feed them away from them.

The manner in which an infant is cared for when first born is an important etiologic factor in producing this disease. An infant that is born with an allergic family history should receive extra preventive care in regard to external irritants both chemical and physical. The obstetrician and the pediatrician if called immediately should obtain the history and take measures to prevent this aggravating and distressing condition. The fetus has been developing for nine months in the mother's uterus at the same temperature, surrounded by the amniotic fluid and nourished by the mother's blood. The mother may be allergic, she may have had a dermatitis, part or the whole time of her pregnancy, she has eaten all kinds of foods and when the child is born, it has no eczema. At least I have attended personally over one thousand women in confinement and have never seen a child born with eczema. I have also asked a number of other physicians who have had a large obstetric practice and they have not noted this disease at birth. I cannot remember of seeing one reported in the literature. We have seen a rash appear twenty-four or forty-eight hours after birth, but this can always be attributed to too much or ill advised care. If infantile dermatitis is caused by a toxic protein from food there should be some slight manifestation in the skin occasionally at birth.

There are many things in the early life of the infant, which it can and does come in contact with, that will produce a dermatitis. If the infant has an allergic family history there may be a number of things. For first consideration let us speak of water. Water is the most widely distributed substance in nature. It may almost be called the universal solvent, disintegrator and dissociator. Light, heat and water are the instigators of all molecular or electric activities; number and concentration of ions govern their intensity. Distilled water is acid, tap and well water are usually alkaline, owing to the presence of carbonates and other salts. In a sense water is the most common single injurious agent acting on the skin. Dirt, which is matter in the wrong place, may be found on the skin without harmful effect; but not so in the presence of water. Against it, the skin's greatest defense is the secretion of the sebaceous glands. A prolonged soaking of the hands will demonstrate this in a convincing manner, because the palms and soles do not contain these glands. Maceration soon takes place because these portions lack this protection that is found on other parts of the body. On a sore or wound, water, if isotonic, is non-irritating. Distilled water being hypotonic dessicates the cells; if it contains a sufficient quantity of and added soluble though inert salt it becomes hypertonic, and is irritating. As the fluid dries off from a salt solution it becomes stronger, and any tendency which the basic or acid radical possesses to injure, becomes intensified. Hard water is always objectionable for bathing purposes; as it

evaporates its alkalinity or acidity is accentuated. If there is predisposition to a dermatitis in an infant, a few baths may cause the condition and will certainly much aggravate it if present. The time is much too short for a detailed discussion of all skin irritants that may cause an eruption on an infant's skin. Almost everything about the home and nursery has to be considered. The most common of these irritants are all soaps, regardless of make, wool, silk, rayon, houseplants, toys especially those made of rubber, dolls with dyed hair, toy animals stuffed with kapok, the mother's or nurse's cosmetics, the fluid used in waving the hair of either for they contain flaxseed or orris root, feathers in the pillows and about the bed, animal pets about the house, and any other irritants with which they are occasionally brought into contact.

Time will not allow me to go into detail in describing the action of these many irritating substances. Consideration of water as an irritant has been gone into more in detail because it is universal and it has too infrequently been taken into consideration as a prevocative in a dermatitis, although it has long been recognized as an aggravator after the eruption has appeared.

In conclusion we wish to state that we do not want to give the impression that there is no endogenous factor responsible for eczema, because in some cases it does play a more or less important rôle. We do wish to infer that the exogenous factor is far more important, and to stress the fact that this should be searched for intensively and in a systematic manner, if we wish to give the quickest relief to these little sufferers.

ACUTE PERFORATION OF DUODENAL ULCER

WITH REPORT OF NINE CASES*

M. J. McGRANE, M.D., New Hampton

Acute perforation of duodenal ulcer occurs with sufficient frequency and is such a serious abdominal emergency that prompt recognition and early interference is imperative. A grave responsibility falls upon the one who is first called, and as this is usually the family physician or general practitioner it is well for him to be familiar with the symptoms and the serious consequences, if operation is not performed at the earliest possible hour.

SYMPTOMS AND DIAGNOSIS

The onset usually occurs with lightning-like rapidity. There is sudden, severe, agonizing pain in the upper abdomen which may be referred to the chest or right shoulder. If the victim is in an

*Presented before the Austin Flint-Cedar Valley Medical Society, Cedar Falls, June 20, 1933.

upright position, he may fall. There is nausea but vomiting is not prominent; rather, there is an earnest effort to suppress the vomiting act. The face is pale and anxious; the skin is moist and cool; respirations are rapid, shallow and thoracic because of a fixed diaphragm; the abdomen is retracted, and rigidity is generalized and board-like. Often the hands are clasped together in a protective gesture over the upper abdomen. Almost invariably the patient occupies a recumbent position with his knees flexed. He begs for relief but pleads with the physician not to move him for examination or other purpose. As a rule, the pulse, blood pressure and temperature are unchanged previous to the onset of peritonitis.

A history of indigestion over a long or short period may or may not be obtained. In fact, any statement on the part of the patient is often of little value. He is not so concerned in any preceding events as he is in immediate relief. This was exemplified in a recent case. There was the usual sudden onset of severe upper abdominal pain about three hours preceding admission. The abdomen was board-like, the face was pale and anxious, the skin moist and cool, the knees flexed, the hands clasped over the abdomen, respirations shallow, rapid and thoracic. The patient had received morphine gr. ¼ hypodermically, but this afforded little or no relief. He denied previous stomach trouble but had had two operations for appendicitis. We allowed the scar in the lower right quadrant to influence our diagnosis of high obstruction. At operation, which was not delayed, a perforation of the duodenum in the anterior wall was found. By the time the patient was returned to his room, his wife had arrived, and from her a clear-cut, three-year history of duodenal ulcer was obtained.

The diagnosis should not be difficult if the patient is seen early. A careful history of possible digestive disturbance is most important and is more reliable if obtained from a close relative or friend, and is of value only if it is positive. The location and agonizing character of the pain are typical of this condition. It is frequently referred to the chest and Oehlecker[1] has found it referred to the right shoulder in 90 per cent of cases. If, in addition, there is generalized board-like rigidity with little or no change in pulse, temperature or blood pressure, a tentative diagnosis of perforation can with limitations be made at the bedside. After the patient has been removed to the hospital, fluoroscopic examination in the prone or left lateral position may show pneumoperitoneum. Vaughan and Singer[2] found pneumoperitoneum in 85 per cent of sixty-three cases.

DIFFERENTIAL DIAGNOSIS

They rely upon the presence or absence of pneumoperitoneum to differentiate between frank perforation and the "forme fruste" type. Acute pancreatitis, which is relatively infrequent, is perhaps the most difficult condition to rule out. According to Moynihan[3], "pain is the chief symptom, and is, of all the pains the human body can suffer, the worst." It is epigastric and referred with intensity to the back and loins. Profound collapse occurs early. The pulse is rapid and of low volume. There is an early fall in blood pressure, while in perforation, the pulse rate, volume and pressure remain practically unchanged. Vomiting in pancreatitis is early and frequent, while in perforation, vomiting is not prominent. Generalized board-like rigidity is not characteristic in pancreatitis.

Acute perforation of duodenal ulcer has frequently been mimicked by acute appendicitis. Competent surgeons have opened the abdomen through muscle splitting incisions for removal of the appendix only to find, when the peritoneum was incised, a normal appendix and free fluid gravitating downward from above. This possibility should be kept in mind and where any doubt exists, a rectus incision will avoid embarrassment.

Acute perforation of the duodenum may be confused with acute embolism or thrombosis of the mesenteric vessels. Quoting Moynihan[4], "The patient is usually middle aged and obese. He may have arteriosclerosis, chronic valvular disease or an operation may have been recently performed." The onset is sudden with intense colicky pain in the abdomen which later becomes continuous. Nausea, vomiting and collapse occur early. Either diarrhea or constipation may be present; if diarrhea, the stools are blood stained. The abdomen soon becomes distended from obstruction, and the pulse rapid and poor in quality. The temperature is often subnormal.

A history of missed menstruation, sudden, severe, knife-like pain in the lower abdomen, rapid, thready pulse, air hunger, cold, clammy skin, low blood pressure and a bloody vaginal discharge will be interpreted as tubal rupture or abortion rather than duodenal perforation.

In intestinal obstruction, the intermittent, colicky character of the pain, distention of the bowel above the point of obstruction, possible visible peristalsis, absence of generalized board-like rigidity and early profuse vomiting in high obstruction, should be sufficient to differentiate this condition from perforation of the duodenum.

In renal colic, the contortions and restlessness contrast strikingly with the anxious, almost motionless attitude in perforation. The unilateral, knife-like pain with its characteristic radiation differs definitely from the constant agonizing epigastric pain of perforation.

Coronary occlusion, which is frequently manifested by abdominal symptoms, may be mistaken for duodenal perforation. Relief from morphine, amytal nitrite or nitroglycerine, and absence of generalized board-like rigidity may prevent an unnecessary laparotomy.

TREATMENT

Treatment can be summarized in a few words; early diagnosis, immediate operation, rapid and minimal surgery under ethylene anesthesia, if possible. Dineen[5] has shown by his statistics that seven per cent die when operated upon before the sixth hour following perforation, 31 per cent if operated on between the sixth and twenty-second hour, and 81 per cent if operated on after twenty-two hours. It is generally conceded by American surgeons, Dineen[5], Corvese[6], Shelley[7], White and Patterson[8], Brenner[9], Stewart and Barber[10], that simple closure of the perforation meets the indication in the majority of cases. Among foreign surgeons who favor the simplest procedure are Kotzareff[11], Schmidt[12], Williams and Walsh[18], and especially Urrutia[14]. Urrutia, who has performed over five hundred radical resections for gastric and duodenal ulcers, is positively opposed to more than simple closure in perforation unless there is a definite duodenal or pyloric stenosis, the effect of closure of the perforation or contraction from previous scar tissue.

The question of drainage I believe should be decided in each individual case. If operation has been performed in the early hours following perforation and peritoneal soiling has not been extensive, no drain should be necessary. When several hours have elapsed and extensive leakage has caused damage to the peritoneum, it may be advisable to place a Penrose drain under the liver and possibly a second drain in the pelvis through a suprapubic stab incision.

After operation, sufficient morphine or pantopon should be employed to subdue pain and lessen peristalsis, for forty-eight to seventy-two hours. All liquids and foods should be withheld and 2,000 to 4,000 c.c. glucose in normal saline should be administered intravenously and subcutaneously. After the third day, liquids and soft foods may be given gradually. Sippy management should be carried out for six to twelve months. Better cooperation will be obtained from the patient if he understands that perforation is more likely to recur if he does not faithfully carry out instructions. Secondary

gastro-enterostomy, pyloroplasty or resection should be performed only if unfavorable symptoms persist after thorough medical management has failed.

CASE REPORTS

Case 1. Sept. 18, 1923. Male, age 72. Retired farmer. Admitted four and a half hours after perforation. Had had attacks of pain and indigestion for twenty years. Perforation was in the anterior duodenal wall. Abdomen contained abundant free fluid. Perforation excised and closed. Lumen of duodenum was constricted. Primary anterior gastro-enterostomy was performed. Recovery was satisfactory except for infected wound. Drains were used. He is still active and free from symptoms.

Case 2. Nov. 4, 1923. Male, age 48. Blacksmith. Ulcer symptoms and some treatment for twelve years. Admitted within one hour following onset. Perforation found in anterior duodenal wall. Lumen constricted. Ulcer excised and closed. Primary gastro-enterostomy performed. Recovery was uneventful and there have been no symptoms since.

Case 3. July 29, 1925. Male, age 60. Retired farmer. Definite ulcer symtoms for two years. Admitted one hour after onset. A perforation admitting finger tip was found in anterior duodenal wall. The abdomen contained a large amount of bloody fluid. Perforation was sutured and primary gastro-enterostomy performed. Convalescence was satisfactory. Four years later he had a sudden severe hemorrhage but has since been free from symptoms.

Case 4. July 24, 1926. Male, age 75. Admitted thirty-six hours after acute onset presenting positive evidence of peritonitis. Had history of long standing indigestion. Examination at Mayo Clinic four years previously and duodenal obstruction diagnosed but operation not accepted. Abdomen opened and generalized peritonitis found as result of perforation in anterior duodenal wall. Perforation was closed and abdomen drained. He died within forty-eight hours following operation.

Case 5. Dec. 11, 1931. Male, age 42. Farmer. Recurrent attacks of indigestion for fifteen years. Admitted four hours after acute onset. Perforation was in anterior duodenal wall. There was moderate discharge. Lumen not constricted. Only simple closure of perforation was done. His recovery was uneventful and he has been free of symptoms since.

Case 6. March 16, 1932. Female, age 82. Had had stomach trouble for thirty years. For past three months frequent pain required opiates for relief. Admitted five hours after onset of severe epigastric pain and collapse. Consent for operation not obtained from relatives until seven hours more had elapsed. When abdomen was opened a moderate amount of free fluid was found. There was a perforation in the anterior duodenal wall which was excised and closed. The gallbladder contained two stones about the size of ordinary dice, one of which was in the cystic duct. These were removed and gallbladder drained. Gastro-enterostomy was indicated but postponed because of patient's unsatisfactory condition. Two months later gastro-enterostomy became necessary and she recovered without unfavorable incident.

Case 7. May 5, 1932. Male, age 15. No history of indigestion. He was awakened at 12:30 A. M. with severe epigastric pain. When I saw him, one hour later, the clinical picture was that of perforation. Because of his youth and the absence of positive history my diagnosis was that of acute appendicitis. A high right rectus incision disclosed free greyish fluid and a perforation in the anterior duodenal wall. Simple closure of the perforation was done. Convalescence was uneventful. He pays no attention to dietetic instruction but is perfectly well.

Case 8. Oct. 30, 1932. Farmer, age 38. Attacks of pain and indigestion in the spring and fall for the past two years. Present illness began four days before admission with sudden epigastric pain, so severe that he says he fell to the ground. About thirty-six hours later he was taken to the hospital by his physician. The stomach was lavaged because of vomiting. Pituitrin and enemata were given for distension and absence of evacuation. When I saw him he was markedly dehydrated, cyanotic and the abdomen very distended. No peristalsis could be heard. The pulse and temperature however did not indicate generalized peritonitis. The abdomen was opened through a right rectus incision opposite the umbilicus. The abdominal wall immediately collapsed from the escape of gas. The intestines were collapsed. About one-half pint of pus was found in the culdesac. The appendix was not involved. The incision was extended upward and a partially walled-off abscess was found under the liver. There was a perforation in the anterior duodenal wall. The perforation was closed. A No. 20 F catheter was placed in the ileum about thirty inches above the iliocecal valve. Penrose drains were placed under the liver and into the pelvis. He drained for about three months. He has regained his former weight and not only pays no attention to dietetic instruction but has done all his farm work since spring.

Case 9. April 19, 1933. Male, age 41. Has been previously referred to. Simple closure of the perforation resulted in an uneventful convalescence.

Three of the above cases have been reported through the courtesy of my associate, Dr. N. Schilling.

CONCLUSIONS

1. Acute perforation of duodenal ulcer requires early recognition and immediate operation.

2. Simple closure meets the indication in the majority of cases.

3. Primary gastro-enterostomy should be performed only when closure of the perforation or previous scar tissue causes pyloric or duodenal stenosis.

4. Secondary gastro-enterostomy, resection or plastic operation should be performed only after thorough medical management has failed to relieve symptoms.

REFERENCES

1. Oehlecker, F.: Pain referred to right shoulder in acute perforation of duodenal ulcer. Arch. f. klin Chir. cxxvii:344-356, 1923 (illus.) ; ab. Jour. Am. Med. Assn., lxxxi:2155 (December 29) 1923.
2. Vaughan, R. T. and H. A. Singer: Value of radiology in diagnosis of perforated peptic ulcer. Surg. Gynec. Obst., xlix:593-599 (November) 1929.
3. Moynihan, B.: Acute pancreatitis. Abdominal Operations, Moynihan, fourth edition, ii:454.
4. Moynihan, B.: Embolism and Thrombosis of the vessels of the mesentery. Abdominal Operations, Moynihan, fourth edition, ii:160.
5. Dineen, Paul: Acute perforated ulcers of stomach and duodenum. Ann. Surg., xc:1027-1034 (December) 1929.
6. Corvese, A.: Acute perforated peptic ulcer. New England Jour. Med., ccvii:390-392 (September 1) 1932.
7. Shelley, Harold J.: Perforated peptic ulcer. Amer. Jour. Surg., xv:277-303 (February) 1932.
8. White, W. C, and H. A. Patterson: Late results of simple suture in acute perforation of duodenal ulcer. Ann. Surg., xciv:242-255 (August) 1931.
9. Brenner, Edward: Perforated ulcer of the duodenum. Ann. Surg., lxxxvi:393-400 (September) 1927.
10. Stewart, George D., and Wm. H. Barber: Acute perforated ulcer of stomach or duodenum. Ann. Surg., lxxv:349-355 (March) 1922.
11. Kotzareff, A.: Perforation of gastroduodenal ulcers and their surgical treatment. Lyon chir., xix:158-170 (March-April) 1922; ab. Jour. Am. Med. Assn., lxxix:590 (August 12) 1922.
12. Schmidt, E. R.: Perforation of gastric and duodenal ulcers Acta. Chir. Scandinav., lv:313-342, 1922 (in English) ; ab. Jour. Am. Med. Assn. lxxx:591 (February 24) 1923.
13. Williams, H. and Chas. H. Walsh: Treatment of perforated peptic ulcer. Lancet, i:9-12 (January 4) 1930.
14. Urrutia, Louis: Late results in perforated gastro-duodenal ulcer. Ann. Surg., xc:73-78 (July) 1929.

THE FINLEY HOSPITAL CLINICO-PATHOLOGIC CONFERENCE

DEMONSTRATION OF LIVER METASTASES BY MEANS OF THOROTRAST

L. G. ERICKSEN, M.D., Dubuque

The case to be presented illustrates the value of thorotrast in diagnosing metastases in the liver and spleen.

CASE REPORT

A white man, fifty-two years of age, was admitted to the Finley Hospital July 20, 1933, with a complaint of "loss of weight and strength of four months' duration." The past and family histories were unimportant. The physical examination showed the patient to be in fair condition with slight pallor but no jaundice. The edge of the liver was palpable but no abdominal masses could be felt. A gastro-intestinal x-ray examination made outside the hospital had revealed a scirrhous carcinoma involving the pyloric portion of the stomach which was apparently resectable. The hemoglobin was 55 per cent, and the red blood count was 3,990,000. The urine was negative. Blood grouping was done along with other work preparatory to surgery. It was then decided to investigate the possibility of metastases in the liver. The patient was given a total of 75 c.c. of thorotrast intravenously in three doses on successive days without any reaction whatever. A roentgenogram of the abdomen taken twenty-four hours after the last injection showed multiple metastases to the liver (Fig. 1). As the condition was obviously hopeless the patient was· discharged from the hospital without surgery.

COMMENT

·In 1929, Radt published his work on the visualization of the liver and spleen with a 25 per cent colloidal suspension of thorium dioxide (now marketed under the trade name of thorotrast) injected intravenously. Until Radt's work, our methods for examining the liver and spleen were limited to very gross means of determining its size through indirect methods, such as palpation, roentgen examination of the colon and pneumoperitoneum. We had no means of demonstrating structural changes within these organs. The thorium particles which are opaque to x-rays are carried through the venous sinuses of the liver and spleen and are picked up by the reticulo-endothe-

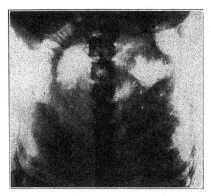

lial cells of these organs. How long the thorium particles remain here has not been accurately determined as yet. Elimination is very slow, however, and probably occurs through the intestines and lungs.

One can readily see the number of conditions to which this procedure is applicable where hitherto we have been severely handicapped in making an accurate diagnosis. Perhaps foremost in value is its application to the preoperative diagnosis of. metastasis to the liver. It is a well known fact that carcinoma of the stomach, rectum, etc., metastasize to the liver very early and we have all opened abdomens which appeared to contain operable lesions,

only to have to close up again because of liver metastasis. In the department of surgery at the University Hospital, University of Minnesota, this procedure is now routine in all preoperative cases of malignancy ·of the gastro-intestinal tract, and in other primary malignancies when indicated. The diagnosis of primary tumors, cysts and abscesses of the liver and spleen, the origin of abdominal masses and cirrhosis of the liver are all facilitated by the use of this procedure. In experienced hands there should not be over a five per cent error.

The patient is given a total dose of 0.8 c.c. of thorotrast per kilogram of body weight when a very diagnostic detailed shadow of the liver and spleen is wanted. This is given intravenously, undiluted, in three doses on successive days. Films of the abdomen taken before injection, and twenty-four hours after injection, are compared. For a more detailed account of. technic, diagnosis, etc., the reader is referred to a previous publication in the *Journal of the American Medical Association* for June 3, 1933.

As far as we can determine up to the present time, thorotrast produces no damaging effects when used in doses necessary for diagnostic visualization. It has not been proved, however, that this procedure is entirely harmless; only time can settle this question. Therefore, until sufficient time has elapsed we believe it should be used only· on patients of advanced years, and mainly for the diagnosis of those diseases of the liver and spleen in which the eventual mortality rate is very high whether the procedure is used or not. When it is used to determine the outline of the liver and spleen, it is only necessary to use one-third to one-fourth the average dose, and we do not believe this could cause any harm.

AMERICAN PUBLIC HEALTH ASSOCIATION

The American Public Health Association announces that its sixty-third annual meeting will be held in Pasadena, California, September 3-6, 1934. The Western Branch of the American Public Health Association, with a membership of more than 1,200 from eleven western states, will hold its fifth annual meeting at the same time.

. Dr. J. D. Dunshee, health officer of Pasadena, has been appointed chairman of the local committee on arrangements. He will be assisted by Dr. John L. Pomeroy, president, and Dr. W. P. Shepard, secretary of the Western Branch, and other prominent public health authorities on the west coast.

STATE DEPARTMENT OF HEALTH

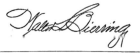

DEPRESSION AND PUBLIC HEALTH

In times of adversity preventive measures should be uppermost in all human activities. As history records the last three years of economic depression, to the eternal glory of medical men and women, it will be said that at no time did they relax their efforts and devotion to relieve the sick and prevent the spread of disease. There is danger that administrative agencies may not have the same concept of guarding against the inroads of disease in the future. The medical profession can do much to arouse an enlightened citizenship to a keener appreciation of its responsibilities in this regard.

COUNTY-WIDE PREVENTIVE PROGRAMS

The policies governing the organization and conduct of county-wide preventive programs outlined by the Committee on Child Health and Protection and the State Department of Health have been approved by the Council of the Iowa State Medical Society. Reports received from several county medical societies indicate that, either the plan has already been considered favorably or will be acted upon in the near future. Counties from which such reports have come include Appanoose, Buchanan, Cerro Gordo, Harrison, Linn and Mahaska.

The following two questions have been raised in regard to payment of the physicians' fee: How much will the doctor be paid for giving preventive treatments? Who will pay the doctor? The answers to both of these questions should be determined by a majority of the membership of the local county medical society.

The department offers the suggestions which follow to direct attention to some of the problems involved.

  I. How much will the doctor be paid for giving preventive treatments?

  A. Possible solutions:

    1. Determine an amount which each child treated shall pay predicated on:

    a. A flat fee basis, arbitrarily chosen.

    b. The ability of the parents to pay.

    2. Charge for the work of each physician on an hourly basis.

    3. Contract as a society to render certain services for a lump sum.

  B. Comment on alternatives suggested:

    1. The problem of "fee scaling" is encountered.

When the group method of immunization is employed the physician's fee is usually less than the established fee for such treatments when given to individuals in the office. The possibility that the public will consider the *reduced fee* as the *usual fee* for such work must always be remembered.

    2. Provide adequate compensation for services rendered.

The hourly rate for physicians' services may be set sufficiently high to compensate adequately for their work, the time taken from their practices and the incidental expenditures involved (mileage, etc.). What is equally important, the practice of "fee scaling" is avoided.

    3. Disadvantages may outweigh apparent advantages.

    a. Disadvantages include: Inadequate compensation for individual physicians, establishment of a group practice precedent, etc.

    b. Advantages include: Direction and execution of program by organized medicine, obvious community benefits, etc.

 II. Who will pay the doctor?

  A. Possible solutions:

    1. Privileged (paying) group bears the expense of treating the underprivileged (non-paying) group.

Children whose parents are able to pay are required to pay a certain sum. The amount which each privileged child pays may be determined by dividing the total expenses of the program by the total number of privileged children treated.

    2. Privileged (paying) group pays a certain fee determined by the medical profession and the underprivileged (non-paying) group does not pay.

    a. Children whose parents are able to pay bring an amount determined by the medical profession.

b. Children whose parents are unable to pay are not required to pay a fee, but the physicians are paid for treating these children from a fund provided by the sponsoring agency.

B. Sources of money:

1. From organizations.
   a. Official or tax levying bodies, including boards of education and city or county officials.
   b. Non-official groups, including local Red Cross chapters, seal sale funds, civic organizations, etc.
2. From individuals.
   a. See II A—1.
   b. See II A—2.

MILD CASES OF SCARLET FEVER

Attention is called to the mild character of certain cases of illness, which have in a few localities been regarded as "24-hour measles." It is hoped that some of the milder cases of scarlet fever will not be confused with other conditions. Much of the increased prevalence of scarlet fever during the past weeks has doubtless resulted from failure to call the attending physician. It is, however, a matter of importance that all cases of scarlet fever, even though mild in character, be reported as such and quarantined.

MEASLES OUTBREAK EXPECTED

An epidemic of measles affecting many areas in the state, is expected to occur during the early months of 1934. This statement is based on the periodicity of the disease, major outbreaks occurring about once in three years. The following table shows the number of cases and deaths from measles in Iowa from 1924 to and including 1933:

MEASLES IN IOWA 1924-1933

Year	Cases	Deaths	Case-fatality Rate
1924	3,701	262	7.1
1925	247	13	5.3
1926	4,495	63	1.4
1927	10,604	230	2.2
1928	895	14	1.6
1929	2,154	39	1.8
1930	9,894	199	2.0
1931	904	5	0.6
1932	156	5	3.2
1933	894	5*	0.6*

*First eleven months.

From the above table it is apparent that the years 1924, 1927 and 1930 were measles years in Iowa. Increased prevalence of the disease was expected in 1933, but this developed in only a few localities, notably in southwestern Iowa. During the past ten years, the largest number of cases have been reported

in March, with February, April and May taking second, third and fourth places.

A special article entitled "Convalescent Blood and Serum in the Control of Measles," by the late Dr. Howard A. Lanpher, M.P.H., and Dr. Fred Moore[1], appeared in the February, 1930, issue of the JOURNAL. Physicians will do well to re-read this article, which was carefully prepared and is as applicable at this time as it was four years ago. Of special interest in this article is the report of the use of parental whole blood in modifying the attack of measles in a group of children.

Kaiser[2] has recently reported favorable results with the use of immune adult blood, in attenuating measles in infants and young children who have been exposed. The procedure can be carried out readily in the home. Ten c. c. of blood are withdrawn from an arm vein of one of the parents and injected at once into the gluteal muscles of the child. As a rule, a Wassermann test need not be made. The injection is given from the third to the seventh day after exposure, preferably on the fourth day. Some advise the injection of a larger amount of whole blood (20 c.c.). Treatment during the first few days after exposure will prevent an attack, which may be desirable in infants or children with lowered resistance. Disease in attenuated form after exposure, is preferable in healthy children, because an active, permanent immunity is conferred.

Stallybrass[3] stresses the fact that the fatality rate in measles is highest during the first two years and minimal after five years of age.

As shown in the above table, there were 262 deaths from measles in 1924. In 1927, deaths numbered 230 and in 1930, the number was 199. The problem of lessening the number of deaths from measles, presents a distinct opportunity and challenge to the medical profession. The fact that the blood of one or both parents contains immune bodies which may be life-saving to one or more children in the home, is truly remarkable. Many physicians will want to avail themselves of this method of preventing or attenuating measles, inform parents of the facts and keep careful records of the results.

REFERENCES

1. Lanpher, Howard A., and Fred Moore: Jour. Iowa State Med. Society, xx:78-79, (February) 1930.
2. Kaiser, Albert D.: New York State Jour. Med., xxxiii:521 (April 15) 1933.
3. Stallybrass, C. O.: Jour. Royal Sanitary Institute, liv:388-396, (January) 1934.

PREVALENCE OF DISEASE

	Dec., 1933	Nov., 1933	Dec., 1932	Most Cases Reported from
Diphtheria	56	81	90	Polk, Pottawattamie
Scarlet Fever	350	358	185	Polk, Pottawattamie
Typhoid Fever	16	4	2	Dubuque, Wayne
Smallpox	20	40	155	Monona, Ida
Measles	143	11	8	Fremont
Whooping Cough	71	71	32	Blackhawk, Dubuque
Cerebrospinal Meningitis	4	4	4	(For State)
Chickenpox	347	325	452	Woodbury, Dubuque
Mumps	100	22	85	Woodbury
Poliomyelitis	2	4	2	Floyd, Polk
Epidemic Encephalitis	4	6	0	(For State)
Tuberculosis	18	29	25	(For State)
Undulant Fever	5	10	4	Wayne
Gonorrhea	183	183	137	(For State)
Syphilis	129	179	149	(For State)

The JOURNAL of the
Iowa State Medical Society

ISSUED MONTHLY

RALPH R. SIMMONS, Editor.....................Des Moines
PUBLICATION COMMITTEE
RALPH R. SIMMONS, Editor.....................Des Moines
ROBERT L. PARKER, Secretary..................Des Moines
GEORGE T. ~~~~~, ~~~~~~~ ....Des Moines
JOHN I. MARKER, Trustee......................Davenport
EDWARD M. MYERS, Trustee.........................Boone

SUBSCRIPTION $3.00 PER YEAR

*Address all communications to the Editor of the Journal,
1122 Bankers Trust Building, Des Moines*

OFFICE OF PUBLICATION, DES MOINES, IOWA

Vol. XXIV   FEBRUARY, 1934   No. 2

THE NEW DEAL AND THE PHYSICIAN

We have all heard considerable discussion regarding the New Deal. To the unemployed it has meant employment; to the manufacturer it has meant a market for his products; to the farmer it has assured a living return for his labors; to the financier it has guaranteed values; but so far, the net results to the practicing physician have not been apparent. We repeat that these results have not been apparent, since little doubt is entertained but that the medical profession will ultimately be swept to greater prosperity on the new tide. To some, relief is imminent; but to others the prospects of financial return approaching or equalling that of a decade ago are remote.

Some see relief in the several paternalistic adventures of the federal government into the field of medical care; others see only disaster in this plan. Some see relief in the program of federal aid to indigents guaranteeing medical fees. The county contract plan for the care of the indigent has already brought some remuneration to physicians in many communities for services which formerly were gratuitous. The CWA extending government compensation for injuries and illnesses to a group of some two million workers has brought at least temporary financial relief to physicians in many communities. With the resumption of work, privately sponsored, industrial physicians and those engaged in compensation work have become transfused with new life.

One cannot but wonder, however, if these factors, to which reference has already been made, are not, after all, minor items in the general consideration of the problem of a New Deal for physicians. They all contribute to the solution but in themselves are insufficient. A recent survey indicates that of the 142,000 physicians now practicing in the United States, only about 21,000 are connected with medical institutions, and per-

haps an equal number are privately engaged in industrial or contract work. Accepting these figures as roughly correct, some 100,000 physicians will receive little, if any, permanent benefit through the various avenues previously cited. If physicians in general are to receive relief, and surely they will, this relief must be accomplished by other means. We believe that the New Deal will bring the long sought relief to physicians only when it has readjusted the economic machinery of the country, and men in all avenues of life feel its magnetic influence.

One is tempted to repeat the story now going the rounds in several forms, having to do with Mrs. A who bought a coat from shopkeeper B and paid cash because her husband had benefited by the federal relief program. B in turn purchased an automobile from C and paid cash, and C bought a diamond from D and paid cash, and D paid his doctor. With more money in circulation, with more people with purchasing power, with a revival of optimism regarding the future, and with a will to spend, the physician will prosper. We are informed that these conditions are already operating in some of the eastern states, and that physicians are enjoying better returns for their services. In the middle western states however, the change is not yet apparent. Better times are ahead, and those who accept this fact overwhelmingly outnumber those who deny it. If we possess no other assurance of a business revival for physicians than this indisputable vote of optimism, that alone would suffice since it is perhaps the safest index of business health.

Some would have us believe that the only way by which physicians can enjoy a New Deal is to relinquish our birthright to free and untrammeled practice and to permit laymen, untrained in medicine, to arrange our affairs. Our colleagues across the sea have had much experience with such plans to their sorrow. Let us foster no "noble experiment" insofar as vital matters of health are concerned, but keep steadily before us the unfailing signs of the times which point to greater prosperity for the profession in the not too distant future.

Appreciating the significance of these forecasting shadows we believe that the medical profession, through its organized society, should persevere in maintaining medical practice as a free and independent enterprise, unhampered by lay or federal control, with the assurance that the physician of tomorrow can and will occupy that enviable position of respect and plenty which has so signally marked the life of the physician throughout the ages.

THE OPPOSITION TO THE FOOD, DRUG AND COSMETIC BILL

A bill to provide a new Pure Food, Drug and Cosmetic Law (S. 1944) now pending in Congress, was discussed editorially in last month's JOURNAL. This editorial outlined the outstanding provisions of the new act and compared it with the present Pure Food and Drug law, stressing particularly the inclusion of cosmetics in the proposed bill, the requirement for truth in advertising, and the sections designed to enable the enforcement of penalties for violation of the act. As predicted in this article a storm of opposition greeted the bill, and if one interprets newspaper reports correctly, much money and time is being expended by opponents of the bill to insure its defeat or, if this seems impossible, to divest it of its power. It has been both interesting and instructive to analyze the shortcomings of the bill as represented by its opponents.

Paul Hayward, writing in *The Nation's Business* for January, 1934, presents the opponents' viewpoint in the following paragraph: "They do not contend that the bill cannot accomplish its announced and desirable purposes. Indeed, it is so broadly and comprehensively drawn that it is a well-nigh perfect instrument so far as enforcement is concerned. The rub, opponents point out, comes in the fact that it is so broadly drawn that it can go far beyond those purposes. Further, they declare, it includes ambiguous phrases, confers dictatorial powers on the Secretary of Agriculture and his agents, might ban secret formulae, give rise to many practical difficulties, impose penalties disproportionate to offenses, handicap advertising, make possible organization of a vast political army of 'supervisors' whose salaries industry would have to pay, and so on."

As one attempts to analyze Mr. Hayward's summary of the bill's defects only three objections seem important. First, they see in the bill a threat of bureaucracy. Whether we know it or whether we believe in it, the fact remains that the various bureaus of the federal government are endowed with more powers, and are operating more independently of Congress than ever before in the history of the nation. If departmental authority to push forward accomplishments and to meet emergencies as they arise constitute bureaucracy, then bureaucracy we have at the present time. It may be contended that this law by granting regulatory power to the Department of Agriculture would be permanently projected into the future, whereas the enlarged scope of authority now accorded the various other departments is a temporary measure and would be set aside when this economic emergency is past. Perhaps this is so, but it is a common observation that it is much-easier to give than it is to take away. If bureaucracy can deliver a more wholesome and harmonious working of the federal government, then the system will not be set aside.

The objections to the requirement for truth in advertising is, in our humble opinion, a much larger fly in the ointment. As one goes about his daily living he is surrounded by "untruthful advertising, by ambiguity, delusion or inferences created to mislead." The radio, now carrying advertising to twenty million or more homes in these United States, is so flagrantly misusing its privilege by permitting misleading or untrue representation that it seems obvious that the manufacturers consider the listening public as devoid of the ability to reason. If this were not true, it would surely seem that a frankly truthful representation of value would be used from choice. How ridiculous this advertising becomes when during the course of an evening's entertainment one will hear a half dozen remedies advertised, all by inference or statement certain to prevent the common cold. If these statements were true the news, for news it would certainly be, could not be suppressed. However, do not assume that the pill vendors are the only manufacturers whose enthusiasm exceeds their veracity. Other groups of advertisers, even of such staple articles as gasoline, breakfast foods or coffee, all claim such superiority and employ such superlatives that even a child realizes their absurdity.

It is not only the radio with time "on the air" to sell that taxes our credulity and assails our judgment. In a paper or magazine our eyes are greeted with the same brands of bunkum, hokum or just plain lying, as you may wish to designate. Is it possible that the truth will not sell a useful and honestly made product? At any rate it appears that newspaper and magazine publishers have joined very wholeheartedly with radio operators in the opposition of this bill on the assumption that if truth were required in advertising, advertising would be killed. One publisher is quoted as saying that should this bill become a law his excellent line of publications would become bankrupt. Are we to assume that this publisher maintains his several publications by permitting advertising, which by "ambiguity or inference," or by direct untruth, upholds products unworthy of such commendation? Does he assume that advertising in order to be effective and therefore command a price must be of such a blatant and extravagant character that it constitutes fraud? If these viewpoints are valid, it would appear that merchandising in this country has fallen to a very low level indeed. Certainly we cannot subscribe to such a view. We believe that American manufacturers are for the most part just as anxious as the buying public for their products to be advertised truthfully. Competitive sales methods have in our opinion stretched the already elastic truth until now one may look and look again before discerning the proverbial grain of truth. Let us not deceive ourselves. The requirement that the manufacturer cannot lie about his product will not prohibit advertising of legitimate products. Manufacturers cannot stop advertising and stay in business, and they know it. They must go on with it even at the cost of being truthful.

Finally, it is pointed out that if "fully informative labeling of foods and drugs" is required, secret, expensive formulae would be lost to competitors. Perhaps we do not understand the full situation insofar as foods and cosmetics are concerned, but certainly in the field of medicine where fully informative labeling is now done by choice by many high-grade manufacturers, no instances of losses have come to our attention. Fully informative labeling does not contemplate the publishing of trade secrets or non-essentials. It does contemplate, however, the publishing of such essential information that the purchaser may not be deceived in his purchase. If a remedy contains poison the purchaser should be warned. If the food contains a harmful preservative the consumer should know it. If a cosmetic contains a drug which may produce constitutional disease, this should not be considered a trade secret. For persons possessing idiosyncrasies such as are seen to quinine, phenophthalein, cascara, etc., a statement on a trade package may prevent a serious accident. Again, informative labeling is essentially a matter of honesty and fair dealing in merchandising.

The opposition to the new Food, Drug and Cosmetic bill insofar as the manufacturers are concerned, seems largely confined to three distinct groups. The first group, fortunately small, opposes any legislation designed to bring any form of legal control to their industry, because it sees in such control a loss of opportunity to exploit the public for financial gain. A second group sincerely believes that the provisions of the bill are too inclusive and might handicap the orderly and honest pursuit of business. The third group in the opposition apparently misunderstands the significance of the proposed law, and views with suspicion that which it does not comprehend. With information many of this large group of opponents would become proponents of the bill.

Because of the far-reaching effect of the proposed bill upon public health and public welfare it seems clearly the duty of physicians to disseminate information whenever and wherever possible

regarding this measure. To discuss the bill intelligently demands a full knowledge of its provisions. If you are not familiar with the proposal in its entirety, get the bill and study it. Nothing goes farther in combating unwarranted opposition than a sound conviction supported by facts.

OBSERVATIONS ON SEX CONTROL

A short time ago Dr. F. Unterberger of Königsberg, Germany, announced methods which in his hands had been successful in controlling the sex of unborn offspring. He stated that an acid condition of the fluids surrounding the germ cell at the time of conception favors the production of female offspring, while an alkaline condition favors the birth of males. He advised, when a boy was wanted, that the mother render the vaginal canal alkaline by washings with a weak solution of sodium bicarbonate and, where a female child was desired, that the genital tract be bathed in a weak solution of lactic acid.

According to the German physician, this method had proved uniformly successful. The method is too new and untried in this country to warrant conclusions, and the first critical and controlled investigations of the possibilities of this method are incorporated in a recent report of experiments carried on with swine at the Wisconsin Agricultural Experiment Station at Madison. Here Prof. L. J. Cole and Dr. Ivar Johansson, of the Genetics Department of the University, selected two groups of brood sows of similar characteristics for observation. In the first group of thirty-two animals they treated the vaginal tract with a sodium bicarbonate solution before the animal was bred, following the procedure described by Dr. Unterberger. In a second group of similar animals no treatment was involved. When the respective litters were born it was found that the relative number of males and females among the offsprings were identical in the two groups.

While it is recognized that other factors may be present in swine which do not pertain in the human, the results of Doctors Cole and Johansson strongly suggest that perhaps the method of sex control prescribed by Dr. Unterberger is not as infallible as his observations would lead one to believe, and that these methods require much additional observation before they can be unequivocally recommended.

This issue contains an announcement of special interest to members of the county medical society auxiliaries. See Woman's Auxiliary News, page 112.

MEDICAL CARE OF CWA WORKMEN

As a corollary to the federal emergency relief program, the government is forced to provide medical care for the "civilian employees of the government for disability or death resulting from personal injuries, including diseases proximately caused by the employment, sustained while in the performance of their duties, except when the injury or death is caused by the wilful misconduct of the employee or by the employee's intention to bring about the injury or death of himself or of another or when the use of intoxicating liquors or drugs is the proximate cause of injury or death."

Insofar as possible medical treatment will be furnished at governmental medical establishments, but where such facilities are not available public medical facilities, either state, county or municipal, will be utilized. In the absence of these public medical facilities the local civil works administrators are authorized to arrange for medical care by reputable physicians. "This does not include the use of osteopaths or chiropractors unless treatment by such practitioners is recommended by the government or designated physician."

In Special Bulletin No. 2 the local administrators received definite instructions from the government to consult the officers of their county or district medical society to establish avenues of medical aid where government medical establishments are unavailable or inadequate to furnish the service required. Not only does the act provide for "reasonable medical and hospital services and supplies," but it further provides for the use of specialists in consultation "where the assistance of another physician would be beneficial to the prompt recovery of the injured workman." To further this plan the state civil works administrator has appointed the following advisors to assist him in the designated sections of the State:

"In the eastern zone, all counties east of Howard County on the north and Van Buren County on the south, should counsel and advise with Dr. Peter A. Bendixen, American Bank Building, Davenport. In all counties from Mitchell County on the north and Davis County on the south, to and including Emmet County on the north and Taylor County on the south, physicians should counsel and advise with Dr. Oliver J. Fay, 1215 Bankers Trust Building, Des Moines. From Dickinson County on the north to Crawford County on the south, to and including Monona County, physicians should counsel and advise with Dr. Arch F. O'Donoghue, Trimble Building Sioux City. In the area of Harrison County on the north to Page and Fremont counties on the south, physicians should consult Dr. Matt Tinley, 520 Third Street, Council Bluffs."

For services rendered by designated or private physicians and hospitals the commission "will settle all reasonable charges for fees not in excess of those charged patients in the same income class as the injured person." As with all government works, correct and proper forms must be submitted in reporting the treatment and care of all workers, and proper payment vouchers must be submitted before settlement can be expected. Full instructions in the use of report forms can be secured by a review of "Rules and Regulations No. 5" of the Federal Civil Works Administration as revised under date of December 12, 1933, or Special Bulletin No. 2, or by directing your inquiry to L. J. Cowen, Comp. Claim Dept., State Civil Works Administration, Federal Office Building, Des Moines, Iowa; or to the central office of the Iowa State Medical Society at 1122 Bankers Trust Building, Des Moines.

THE OPEN FORUM

Viewpoints and opinions expressed in this section are those of the individual contributor and not necessarily those of the Journal.

A REORGANIZED MEDICAL PROFESSION

Editor Iowa State Medical Journal:

In the past two decades, so many changes have taken place in the economic, medical and political world that the reorganization promulgated by the A.M.A., some thirty years ago, has become well-nigh archaic. Entirely new conditions have to be met.

It is of small moment now that a few of us then protested the semi-unionization in the scheme, as inadequate for the ends (most of them) in view; or that my twenty years of isolation (outside the pale of organized medicine) was, in itself, proof that the medical man, seriously and honestly disposed, did not need the organization as much as the organization needed him. That's ancient history.

The fact remains that the profession has not thereby been unified—too much "go as you please" in matters of policy; and unity is the crying need of today, if we would not see ourselves so exploited that there would be little inducement for greater knowledge or better service. It's no less—in fact rather more, a case of "united we stand, etc.," as preached these thirty years; but to get this united stand we must have something more than the A.M.A., as now constituted. It never was—

could not be, logical to assume that every licensed regular practitioner had an inherent right to membership in a scientific body. That license simply makes him eligible in proportion as he demonstrates his fitness for it, by tangible evidence that he could, and would, become a worker in it; and not use it for selfish ends. In plain words, this assumption, cleverly presented and amusingly swallowed, was a subterfuge to get an enrollment for purposes other than scientific. Thus, the organization shield had *science* on the obverse and *politics* on the reverse and we should not have to be reminded of the warning against the mixture of incompatibles. We need to think only of the fifty-five years of struggle to get medical legislation adequate, alike, for the protection of the public and the doctor—and still unattained, to realize that the day of divided interests is past; likewise that the day has come for a bill of divorcement between the scientific and political purposes of our national and state organizations.

To a degree, this has already been recognized in the organization of the Physicians and Allied Professions' Political League (in the East); but in the A.M.A. and state associations we have a better set up, if we choose to make use of it, as we should.

For the present, the scientific work, now featured in these bodies, can be relegated to the background, perhaps eliminated; because it could be carried on just as well in sectional gatherings under the auspices of the parent organizations. For good measure, there are the national associations of specialists; College of Physicians, College of Surgeons, Academy of Ophthalmology and Otolaryngology, Society of Obstetrics and Gynecology, etc. What more natural then to think of the A.M.A. and state associations as particularly adapted to the consideration, solely, of Medical Economics? With the present record of $630,000,000 of free medical care annually, and 66 per cent of the available hospital beds under governmental (national, state, county and municipal) control, which means management by laymen, there will be no dearth of problems to be solved.

In an association constituted for the study of medical economics, with its congener, administrative medicine, the inherent right of every licensed regular practitioner to membership is beyond question. More than that, the membership of all such should be compulsory, under pain of ostracism. Sounds like trade unionism, doesn't it? Well, like it or not, that's the least of the degredations' impending. Hanging together, in every sense, is better than hanging separately; and trade unionism has shown how hanging together may be assured. Its rules of conduct, formulated by the majority, carry stiff penalties for infractions; and therein is the recognition of the fact that "moral suasion" has its limitations—a fact that the medical profession has apparently overlooked.

Results speak for themselves. People don't make a practice of "putting one over" on a trade union.

These are not the vaporings of a "radical." On the contrary, they are the unhappy conclusions of a dyed-in-the-wool "conservative," that through organized (?) medicine's persistent misinterpretation of "lay" psychology the triumphs of modern medicine have lost much of their appeal; and that it is high time for every practitioner to be aroused to the necessity of changing front.

As a basis for this change of front, it should be remembered that while medicine has changed, from year to year, the average sick man is much the same that he was a thousand years ago. Not actually irrational—in its usual sense, he is still, by reason of bodily distress, lacking in discrimination. For any reason but the right one, authentic information touching the doctor's character and attainments, he calls in Dr. X; and if Dr. X displays a bit of "hooey" he—well, isn't there a bit of mystery about everyone who does things?

To make a long story short, two oft quoted injunctions need only be added:

(1) Put yourself in his place; and

(2) Cast not your pearls before swine, lest they turn again and rend you.

Nobody has suffered more from their disregard than the medical profession. For the "other fellow" has seen in medical legislation an attempt to create a monopoly; and in medical publicity a jealousy of the cults.

How much better it would have been to have "sawed wood," and let the other fellow do the talking.

H. B. Young, M.D., Burlington

REFLECTED VALUES

Editor Iowa State Medical JOURNAL:

In the academic sense, your argument under the above caption is unanswerable. But it is equally true that "circumstances alter cases." The practical aspect of a conceded doctrine; and the conditions which have led to altered consideration of membership in the State Society are, in many instances, a cause of deep concern. When one realizes that the payment of the $10 annual dues means still more in a retrenchment in other essentials—already cut to the bone—he begins to look up details of little former interest. Mayhap, he meets an Illinois doctor, and learns that said Illinois doctor can have the same facilities for $7.50. Why, therefore, has the Iowa organization concluded that $10 is a fair charge? Then it may occur to him to peruse the annual statement; and when he sees that there is a reserve fund of some $40,000* (to which he may have contributed) he wonders what better its purpose than to meet the drafts (likewise draughts) of "the rainy day."

Curtailment of expenditures, particularly those of the Committee on Legislation, comes next into the picture. The returns have been so small, mostly negative at the capitol, for the outlay. The ordinary purchaser must in these days, be tempted with extra values; and doctors, reluctantly perhaps, are coming to believe that what is "sauce for the goose is sauce for the gander."

That my sympathies are with the malcontent must be manifest from my votes, as delegate, at the 1932 and 1933 meetings. It may be that I have lived too long to become enthusiastic over a splurge in medical activities to prevent my neighbor from employing such cultist (directly established by our, not mine, appeal to law) as he wishes; but I do not see that, with all the advances in our knowledge of disease, and facilities in handling it, the doctor's lot has been made materially happier, or the dignity of his calling enhanced as they should have been.

Such a result in the business world would be set down to bad management; and we can look back to jealousies, both intramural and extramural, and the worship of false gods, increasingly in the sixty years since I began practice.

That the cultist should tax himself $15 for the creation of a propaganda fund (legislative in particular) is no reason for our taxing ourselves $10 for a similar purpose. Propaganda is his stock in trade, and let alone will soon grow stale. It's also indisputable that "a knock's a boost."

H. B. Young, M.D., Burlington

*Editor's Note: This figure does not represent a reserve fund, but is the approximate net worth of the society.

SPECIAL LECTURES AT THE MAYO CLINIC

A special program of lectures and demonstrations in medicine will be held under the direction of the Mayo Foundation from March 5 to 9, inclusive. Mornings will be devoted to surgery, demonstrations of oxygen therapy and of intravenous therapy, and consideration of postoperative complications. In the afternoons medical subjects, including gastro-enterology, dermatology and syphilis, will be discussed, and a symposium on dyspnea will be held. In the evenings clinicopathologic conferences will be conducted.

While this program is arranged primarily for the Fellows of the Foundation, visiting physicians are invited to attend.

"DOCTORS ONLY" BILLS

Physicians and medical societies throughout the United States, no matter which side they take on such a highly controversial subject, are watching with interest proposed legislation before the Seventy-third Congress calling for amendment of the present federal birth control laws. These amendments, commonly known as the "Doctors Only" bills, are Senate Bill 1842, sponsored by Senator D. O. Hastings of Delaware, and House Bill No. 5978, introduced by Representative Walter Pierce of Oregon. This proposed legislation would amend the existing federal restrictions so as to legalize the sending or receiving of contraceptive information, instruments and medicines between physicians and their patients, medical colleges and hospitals and from physician supply houses and manufacturers. Under the present statutes, penalties of heavy fines and imprisonment may be inflicted for transporting any article intended for the prevention of conception or for receiving for distribution to others any such article that has been transported interstate or by the government mails.

NORTHWEST REGIONAL CONFERENCE MEETS FEBRUARY 25, 1934

The Northwest Regional Conference will hold its annual meeting, Sunday, February 25, 1934, at the Lowry Hotel in St. Paul, with Dr. Benjamin F. Bailey, president, presiding. The following program is scheduled to be given: Informal discussion of Interstate Radio Broadcasting Health Programs, and State Office Organization, E. A. Meyerding, secretary of the Minnesota State Medical Association, Robert L. Parker, Secretary of the Iowa State Medical Society, and H. M. Camp, secretary of the Illinois State Medical Society; County Medical Societies Can Conduct Their Own Clinics, Philip H. Kreuscher, president of the Illinois State Medical Society; Common Abuses in Committing Mental Cases to State Hospitals, W. H. Hengstler, St. Paul; Medical Care of the Indigent in Wisconsin, Mr. George Crownhart, executive secretary of the Wisconsin State Medical Society; Problems Connected with Compensation Insurance, Roy Fouts, Omaha; The Test of Organized Medicine, Oliver J. Fay, chairman, Board of Trustees, Iowa State Medical Society, Des Moines; Medical Problems Resulting from Recent Federal Legislation, Charles B. Wright, trustee, American Medical Association, Minneapolis; Economic Trends and Their Influence on Medical Economics, R. K. Packard, chairman of the Council, Illinois State Medical Society, and Albert W. Skelsey, secretary of the North Dakota State Medical Association.

SPEAKERS BUREAU ACTIVITIES

HEALTH ESSAY CONTEST

The Woman's Auxiliary of the Iowa State Medical Society is sponsoring a Health Essay Contest in the high schools throughout the state. They are offering several prizes to those high school students who write the best essays on the subject: "Health— Our Greatest Asset—And How To Maintain It." Any student in the ninth, tenth, eleventh or twelfth grades of the public schools in Iowa is eligible to enter this contest.

The Speakers Bureau is cooperating with the Woman's Auxiliary in promoting this contest, which is probably one of the biggest health education projects ever launched in the state of Iowa. The State Department of Public Instruction has heartily endorsed and approved this plan and is urging the county superintendents to cooperate in it. The only way to build a healthy nation is to start with the young people. If they can be made to reflect on the value and importance of health, they will be much more inclined to follow the rules of health.

Letters have been sent to all city and county superintendents in the state, explaining the contest and enclosing a copy of the rules. It is hoped that every high school in the state will enter this contest. The members of the Iowa State Medical Society can be of great help in boosting it. Turn to the Woman's Auxiliary page in this issue of the JOURNAL and familiarize yourself with the rules of the contest. Then talk to the superintendent of schools in your town and urge him to have the students of his high school enter the Health Essay Contest. Your county medical society could make the contest even more interesting by offering a prize to the student writing the best essay in your county. This added incentive should induce a larger number of students to write essays.

This project of the Woman's Auxiliary is essentially worthwhile and deserves our support. Whatever you or your county society do to help should be done immediately. The contest opened February 1 but it does not close until March 15, so if the schools in your county have not already entered it, there is still time for them to do so.

HERE AND THERE

Every month the Speakers Bureau receives many complimentary reports on the various speakers sent out or in regard to the radio broadcasts or some other phase of the Bureau's activities. We cannot attempt to publish all of them but believe that a few of the more unusual reports should be of interest.

One doctor was asked to address a Lions Club in another town. Since he was a member of the Lions Club in his own town several of his fellow members accompanied him and attended the meeting at which he talked. After the doctor had finished his interesting health talk, his son, who had also accompanied him, provided musical entertainment for the remainder of the program on his violin. The club was enthusiastic in its appreciation of this varied and delightful program.

Among the requests received for copies of our recent radio broadcasts, was one from Dr. Charles H. Mayo, of the Mayo Clinic for "The Greatest Gifts," broadcast Thursday, December 21, from WSUI, Iowa City, and Friday, December 22, from WOI, Ames.

A minister in the northern part of Iowa wrote in for a copy of the radio talk on "Whooping Cough." He stated that they had lost their only child from this disease and that they wanted to print the talk in their local newspaper in order that other parents might read it and benefit from the information given.

These reports give a fair indication of the type of work the Bureau is doing in health education, the variety of people it reaches and the far-reaching results of its health education program.

RADIO TALKS

WSUI—Thursdays, 8:00 p.m.

WOI—Fridays, 4:00 p.m.

February   2—The Sneezing Sickness—T. E. Davidson, M.D.

February   9—Heart Pains—John C. Parsons, M.D.

February 16—Improving the Complexion—H. C. Willett, M.D.

February 23—Vaccines—F. P. McNamara, M.D.

March   2—Diseases Transmitted by Food—Carl F. Jordan, M.D.

March   9—Sinus Trouble—J. B. Naftzger, M.D.

WOMAN'S AUXILIARY NEWS

Edited by the Press and Publicity Committee
Mrs. Oliver J. Fay, *Chairman*, 10 Thirty-fifth Street, Des Moines

HEALTH ESSAY CONTEST

The Health Essay Contest being sponsored by the Woman's Auxiliary to the Iowa State Medical Society is now under way. In the November Journal, this page carried an announcement of the decision of the Auxiliary Board members to sponsor such a contest. Since that time the Education-Program Committee has completed the plans and with the cooperation of the Speakers Bureau of the Iowa State Medical Society, has sent letters to all county and city superintendents in the state suggesting that their high school students enter the contest.

Each auxiliary member can do her part in making this project a success. Urge your superintendent to have his high school take part in the contest. Immediate action is imperative as the contest opened February 1 and closes March 15. The State Department of Public Instruction has enthusiastically approved the plans of this contest and is urging the cooperation of the county superintendents.

A copy of the rules of the contest appears below. Familiarize yourself with them and then do all that you can to boost this worthwhile health education program.

RULES OF THE CONTEST

1. Subject: Health—Our Greatest Asset—and How To Maintain It.

2. Length of essay: 800 to 1,000 words.

3. Participants: Any student in the 9th, 10th, 11th or 12th grades of the public schools of Iowa.

4. Dates of contest: Begins February 1 and closes March 15, 1934. This means that all essays must be in the Contest Office, 1122 Bankers Trust Building, Des Moines, by March 15, 1934.

5. Elimination: The three best essays from each school may be submitted. These essays should be typewritten. Student's name should not appear anywhere on the essay, but the student's name, town, county, grade and superintendent's name should be typed on a small piece of paper and clipped to the essay. Each essay received at the Contest Office will be given a number and no judge shall know to which student that number has been assigned.

6. Prizes: First prize, $15.00; second prize, $10.00; third prize, $5.00; and twenty $1.00 prizes to the next twenty highest ranking essays. The Speakers Bureau is cooperating in this contest and offers an additional prize to the winner of first place of a trip to radio station WOI, at Ames, or WSUI, at Iowa City, to present the winning essay over the radio.

7. Judges: Preliminary eliminations will be made by members of the Woman's Auxiliary. The final judges will be:

   a. A member of the State Department of Public Instruction.

   b. A member of the State Department of Health.

   c. A member of the Iowa State Medical Society.

   d. Two members of the Woman's Auxiliary to the Iowa State Medical Society.

8. Basis for judging essay: Originality, composition, evidence of study.

9. The decision of the judges is to be final.

10. No essays are to be returned to their authors.

SOCIETY PROCEEDINGS

Black Hawk County

Edwin P. Sloan, M.D., head surgeon of the Sloan Clinic at Bloomington, Illinois, presented an illustrated lecture on Subnormalics from Hypothyroidism, before the Black Hawk County Medical Society, Tuesday, January 16. Dr. Sloan's paper was discussed by Charles H. Arnold, M.D., of Lincoln, Nebraska; H. W. Rathe, M.D., of Waverly; J. L. Kestel, M.D., and J. E. O'Keefe, M.D., both of Waterloo; and R. L. Benjamin, M.D., of Kankakee, Illinois.

Boone-Story Society

Members of the Boone and Story County Medical Societies met in Boone, Tuesday, January 16, for their regular joint meeting. A symposium on Acute Abdominal Conditions was presented by Bush Houston, M.D., of Ames and A. I. Haugen, M.D., also of Ames. Discussion of the two papers was led by Dr. A. B. Deering of Boone.

Calhoun County Annual Meeting

Thursday, December 21, the Calhoun County Medical Society met for the regular annual election of officers. Results are: Dr. F. W. Hobart of Lake City, president; Dr. W. W. Weber of Pomeroy, vice president; Dr. W. W. Stevenson of Rockwell City, secretary and treasurer; Dr. D. J. Townsend of Lohrville, delegate; and Dr. P. W. Van-Metre of Rockwell City, alternate delegate.

W. W. Stevenson, M.D., Secretary.

Cerro Gordo County

On Tuesday, January 16, the Cerro Gordo County Medical Society held its regular monthly meeting at the Hanford Hotel in Mason City. Thirty-five members were present and discussed various activities which will be carried out during the coming year.

A financial budget was adopted, a portion of which will be used to obtain speakers to address the society; thus affording the advantages of a postgraduate course. It was decided to issue a monthly bulletin, which will carry reports of the activities of the Cerro Gordo County Medical Society to the members and doctors of the surrounding territory. The subject of organizations and clubs requesting service and talks by physicians was freely discussed. All requests are to be referred to the county society, and the members will cooperate gladly with such organizations.

The next meeting will be held in Mason City, Tuesday, February 20.

W. E. Long, M.D.

Clinton County

The first regular meeting of the Clinton County Medical Society for the new year was held Thursday, January 4, at the Lafayette Hotel in Clinton. A strictly business session was held, and such subjects as caring for the county indigent, plans for solicitations, and the arranging of scientific programs for the ensuing year, were discussed at length by the members. Two new physicians in the county were elected to active membership; Dr. R. C. King and Dr. A. K. Meyer, both of Clinton. Following the business meeting a luncheon was very much enjoyed by all present.

E. V. Donlan, M.D., Secretary.

Dallas-Guthrie Society

The Dallas-Guthrie Medical Society met at Adel, Thursday, January 18, for the regular monthly meeting. After a noon luncheon the following program was presented: President's Address, George McMahon, M.D., of Waukee; Botulism, E. J. Butterfield, M.D., of Dallas Center; and Lantern Slide Lecture on Skin Diseases, J. W. Bailey, M.D., of Des Moines.

S. J. Brown, M.D., Secretary.

Davis County

Dr. R. M. Sorenson, formerly of Cumberland, and now stationed with the Citizens Conservation Camp at Drakesville, entertained the members of the Davis County Medical Society recently at a six-thirty dinner. A scientific program was held with the following speakers: Injection of Varicose Veins, G. W. Gilfillan, M.D., of Bloomfield; The Doctor and the Dentist, E. R. McClurg, D.D.S., of Bloomfield; and Clean Milk, J. C. Conner, D.V.M., of Bloomfield.

H. C. Young, M.D., Secretary.

Des Moines County Annual Meeting

A. A. Eggleston, M.D., of Burlington, furnished the program for members of the Des Moines County Medical Society who met in Burlington, Tuesday, January 9. Dr. Eggleston read a paper on Colitis and Pseudocolitis. Officers elected at the annual business meeting are: Dr. C. J. Lohmann, president; Dr. J. N. Patterson, vice president; Dr. F. H. Aid, secretary and treasurer; Dr. J. T. Hanna, delegate; and Dr. C. E. Kauffman, alternate.

Floyd County Annual Meeting

Officers elected at the annual meeting of the Floyd County Medical Society held in Charles City, Tuesday, January 2, include: Dr. A. F. Kober of Charles City, president; Dr. H. W. Kruse of Rockford, vice president; and Dr. J. B. Miner, Jr., of Charles City, secretary and treasurer.

Fremont County Annual Meeting

At a meeting held in Hamburg, Friday, January 19, the Fremont County Medical Society elected the following officers to serve during 1934: Dr. H. P. Cole of Thurman, president; Dr. G. L. Roark of Tabor, vice president; and Dr. A. E. Wanamaker of Hamburg, secretary and treasurer. Dr. Wanamaker has held this position for twenty-five years.

Jackson County Annual Meeting

Dr. John W. Jordan of Maquoketa has been named to head the Jackson County Medical Society during 1934, at the recent election held in Maquoketa, Friday, January 12. Other officers are: Dr. J. C. Dennison of Bellevue, vice president; Dr. William Lowder of Maquoketa, secretary and treasurer; Dr. F. J. Swift of Des Moines, but a member of the Jackson County Society, delegate; and Dr. E. L. Lampe of Bellevue, alternate delegate. Miss Ruth Walker, public health nurse for Jackson County, discussed tuberculosis prevention work, and members of the society participated in a round table discussion on The Physician and Charity.

Jasper County

Members of the Jasper County Medical Society were hosts to members of the Jasper County Dental Society, at a dinner meeting held in Newton, Tuesday, January 2. After a short business session, S. E. Hinshaw, M.D., of Newton, read a paper on Sarcoma of the Mouth, which was discussed by R. W. Wood, M.D., J. C. Hill, M.D., and H. R. Gustafson, D.D.S., all of Newton.

Johnson County

At the regular monthly meeting of the Johnson County Medical Society, Wednesday, January 3, C. Gregory Barer, M.D., spoke on Some Aspects of Epidemic Encephalitis, and William Malamud, M.D., discussed The Diagnostic Significance of Cerebral Spinal Fluid Examination.

Dr. J. T. McClintock, the retiring president, presented the incoming president, Dr. Matt Ware, with a gavel made from some of the Northern white pine which formed the original eaves of Old Capitol. This wood came from trees which had been standing for more than a hundred years when they were sacrificed in 1840 to furnish material for the building of Old Capitol.

Dr. George C. Albright read an obituary of H. V. Scarborough, M.D.

Horace M. Korns, M.D., Secretary.

Jones County Annual Meeting

The Jones County Medical Society met at the John McDonald Hospital in Monticello recently, and elected the following officers for 1934: Dr. C. R. Smith of Onslow, president; Dr. H. F. Dolan of Anamosa, secretary and treasurer; Dr. Dolan, delegate; and Dr. Earl H. DeShaw of Monticello, alternate delegate.

The officers of the county enjoyed the dinner given by Dr. Arthur Erskine in Cedar Rapids on January 24. Fifty officers from the nine counties in this district were guests of the councilor, who stressed the necessity of the medical profession uniting and rendering efficient service in the CWA program. Dr.

Erskine's hospitality was enjoyed by all, and the officers pledged him their support.

H. F. Dolan, M.D., Secretary.

Kossuth County Annual Meeting

Dr. Robert L. Williams of Lakota was again named president of the Kossuth County Medical Society at the annual election of that organization held in Burt, Thursday, January 11. Dr. Pierre Sartor of Titonka, was also re-elected secretary and treasurer. Dr. James Mueller, who recently located at Fenton, was elected into membership.

Linn County Meetings

Thursday, February 8, Clarence Van Epps, M.D., professor of neurology, University of Iowa College of Medicine, presented a neurologic clinic with patients from his own department at the University, for the members of the Linn County Medical Society.

The society will have as its guest, Thursday, March 8, Morris Fishbein, M.D., of Chicago, speaking on Current Trends in Medical Practice. Physicians from surrounding counties are cordially invited to attend this meeting, and it is hoped that a considerable number will avail themselves of this opportunity.

T. F. Hersch, M.D., Secretary.

Louisa County

Two physicians from Burlington furnished the scientific program for members of the Louisa County Medical Society, at a meeting held in Wapello, Thursday, January 11. The subject, Empyema in Children, was discussed from a medical viewpoint by John McKitterick, M.D., and from a surgical viewpoint by A. A. Eggleston, M.D. A. R. Morledge of Wapello, superintendent of schools, addressed the group on The Relation of the Parent-Teachers Association to the Medical Profession.

Lucas County Annual Meeting

At the annual meeting of the Lucas County Medical Society, held in Chariton, Tuesday, January 9, the following officers were elected: Dr. R. A. Hills of Russell, president; Dr. L. Throckmorton of Chariton, vice president; and Dr. H. D. Jarvis of Chariton, secretary and treasurer.

Mahaska County Annual Meeting

Dr. E. M. Williams was re-elected president of the Mahaska County Medical Society at the meeting held in New Sharon, Wednesday, January 3. Other officers are: Dr. E. B. Wilcox, vice president; Dr. L. F. Catterson, secretary; Dr. L. A. Rodgers, treasurer; Dr. B. G. Williams, delegate; and Dr. George H. Clark, alternate delegate. All officers are of Oskaloosa.

Marshall County

Members of the Marshall County Medical Society met Tuesday, January 9, at the Hotel Tallcorn in Marshalltown, when W. E. Sanders, M.D., of Des Moines, spoke on The Cancer Problem.

Mitchell County Annual Meeting

Tuesday, January 30, members of the Mitchell County Medical Society elected the following officers for 1934: Dr. J. O. Eiel of Osage, president; Dr. George Krepelka of Stacyville, vice _president; and Dr. T. G. Walker of Riceville, secretary and treasurer.

T. G. Walker, M.D., Secretary.

Pottawattamie County

C. W. Poynter, M.D., Dean of the University of Nebraska College of Medicine, was the guest speaker for the Pottawattamie County Medical Society, at a meeting held Thursday, February 1, in Council Bluffs. Dr. Poynter spoke on The Modern Trend of Medical Education.

A. L. Jensen, M.D., Secretary.

Sac County Annual Meeting

The Sac County Medical Society met at the Hotel Park in Sac City, Friday, January 26, for a dinner and business session. With one exception, every eligible physician in the county was present. Dr. G. H. Bassett, a new arrival in Sac City, was present, and we also had the pleasure of having Dr. A. Groman present. Dr. Groman concluded fifty years of practice some years ago. Election of officers resulted in Dr. Henry L. Fobes of Auburn being elected president, and Dr. J. R. Dewey of Schaller being re-elected secretary and treasurer.

J. R. Dewey, M.D., Secretary.

Scott County

The regular meeting of the Scott County Medical Society was held Tuesday, January 9, in Davenport. Following a six o'clock dinner, the speaker of the evening, C. C. Maher, M.D., assistant professor of medicine, Northwestern University, Chicago, addressed the group on Heart Disease.

Tama County Annual Meeting

Friday, December 29, members of the Tama County Medical Society met at Garwin for the annual election of officers. Results are: Dr. C. S. Stoakes of Dysart, president; Dr. B. F. McNeil of Clutier, vice president; Dr. F. W. Gessner of Dysart, secretary and treasurer; Dr. F. T. Launder of Garwin, delegate; and Dr. A. A. Pace of Toledo, alternate delegate.

Van Buren County Annual Meeting

Dr. L. A. Coffin of Farmington was named president of the Van Buren County Medical Society, at a recent meeting held in Keosauqua. Other officers are: Dr. H. E. Woods of Birmingham, vice president; Dr. C. N. Stephenson of Milton, secretary and treasurer; Dr. Coffin, delegate; and Dr. J. W. Webb of Bonaparte, alternate delegate.

Wapello County Meetings

Tuesday, February 6, H. W. Vinson, M.D., of Ottumwa, addressed members of the Wapello County Medical Society on The Care of Expectant Mothers.

E. G. Barton, M.D., also of Ottumwa, led the discussion.

Another local talent program will be presented Tuesday, February 20, when L. H. Prewitt, M.D., of Ottumwa will speak on Bronchiectasis, and E. B. Hoeven, M.D., of Ottumwa will lead the discussion.

Tuesday, March 6, another dinner meeting will be held, with Fred M. Smith, M.D., of Iowa City, as the guest speaker. His subject will be The Diagnosis of Arteriosclerotic Heart Disease.

Wayne County Annual Meeting

The Wayne County Medical Society met Thursday, December 7, in regular session at Corydon and elected the following physicians to serve as officers for the society during 1934: Dr. C. N. Hyatt of Humeston, president; Dr. T. D. Englehorn of Lineville, secretary and treasurer; Dr. J. H. McCall of Allerton, delegate; and Dr. B. S. Walker of Corydon, alternate delegate. The program was furnished by S. W. Corbin, M.D., of Millerton, who read a paper on The Treatment of Gonorrhea, and C. N. Hyatt, M.D., of Humeston, who spoke on Encephalitis.

T. D. Englehorn, M.D., Secretary.

Second Councilor District Meeting

A joint meeting of physicians in the second councilor district and members of the Hancock-Winnebago Medical Society was held Thursday, January 25 at Forest City. After a delightful dinner served by the Lutheran Ladies Aid Society, the following program was presented: Edema, William C. Egloff, M.D., of Mason City; Fractures of the Vertebrae, Ivan T. Schultz, M.D., of Humboldt; and Rheumatic Fever, C. V. Hamilton, M.D., of Garner. The papers were very ably presented and elicited a great deal of discussion. There were twenty-eight doctors in attendance at the meeting in spite of unfavorable weather.

Physicians in the second district have five meetings a year. Four of the meetings are similar to the one just reported; that is, joint meetings with one of the county medical societies in the district, with scientific programs presented by men within the district. The fifth meeting is a picnic to which all the doctors and their families are invited. The next meeting is scheduled to occur sometime during March.

L. R. Woodward, M.D., Councilor.

Sioux Valley Eye and Ear Academy

The annual meeting of the Sioux Valley Eye and Ear Academy was held at the Warrior Hotel in Sioux City, Tuesday, January 23. Two papers were read during the morning session: Fundus Changes in Arteriosclerosis, Hypertensive Disease and Nephritis, with lantern slides and fundus photographs, William H. Stokes, M.D., of Omaha; and Oral Leukoplakia, Leo P. Coakley, D.D.S., of Omaha. After the noon luncheon, members convened for the following afternoon program: Acute Laryngotracheobronchitis, S. D. Maiden, M.D., of Council Bluffs; Biochemistry in Rhinolaryngology, T. R. Gittins, M.D., of Sioux City; A Preliminary Report on the Ocular Effects due to Thallium Acetate Poisoning, C. M. Swab, M.D., and

H. F. Gerald, M.D., both of Omaha; and Benign Tumors of Eyelids, E. P. Weih, M.D., of Clinton. The session closed with a six-thirty banquet at the Hotel Warrior. Present officers of the organization are: Dr. C. L. Chambers of Des Moines, president; Dr. J. J. Hompes of Lincoln, Nebraska, vice president; and Dr. F. H. Roost of Sioux City, secretary and treasurer.

Upper Des Moines Medical Society

The regular winter meeting of the Upper Des Moines Medical Society was held at the Hotel Kermoore in Emmetsburg, Tuesday, January 23. The afternoon session consisted of the following papers: Congenital Pyloric Stenosis, J. P. Clarke, M.D., of Estherville; Acute Pancreatitis, Don Rodewig, M.D., of Spirit Lake; Serum Therapy in Pediatrics, Peter P. Fransco, M.D., of Ruthven; and Consideration of the Acute Abdomen, Dean King, M.D., of Spencer. After dinner addresses were made by Fred C. Knowles, M.D., of Fort Dodge, speaking on Reduction of Fractures of the Neck of the Femur—Double Pin Method, illustrated with motion pictures, and Joseph B. Priestley, M.D., of Des Moines, who discussed The Surgical Management of Peptic Ulcer. Officers were elected for the coming year as follows: Dr. J. M. Sokol of Spencer, president; Dr. J. B. Knipe of Armstrong, vice president; and Dr. George H. Keeney of Mallard, secretary and treasurer.

INTERESTING NEWS
In Brief

The fact that artificial fractures in rats show quick repair after irradiation of the thymus suggests the use of a comparable treatment in human cases.

Observations made in Guatemala suggest that the average blood pressure of the South American is notably lower than that of the North American.

As protection against fraud and substitution the University of Sydney has decided to use thumbprints as well as signatures for identification on its diplomas.

The Committee on Medical Ethics of the Wayne County Medical Society, Detroit, Michigan, has ruled that all bold face type for directory listings of physicians is unethical.

The Board of Midwifery Education of China, a national institution, has established a central midwifery school in Nanking, with an enrollment limited to thirty students.

Dr. J. Dewey Bisgard, formerly of Harlan, Iowa, has been appointed to the department of surgery in the division of fractures, at the University of Nebraska College of Medicine.

Ruling that a physician's automobile is one of the "tools or instruments" of his profession, the Louisiana Court of Appeals recently held that a physician's automobile could not be seized by a creditor.

In Great Britain and France there is one physician to 1,500 of the population; in Germany, one to 1,200; in Norway, one to 1,600; in Sweden, one to 2,600; compared to one in 785 in the United States.

Dr. Richard Lucke, formerly of Jefferson, Iowa, has resigned from the Department of Internal Medicine, University of Nebraska, to enter the Research Department of the Abbott Company in Chicago.

Statistics collected by the United States National Institute of Health indicate that about 1,000 persons in the United States contracted tularemia during the past year from skinning or dressing wild rabbits.

A new universal growth-promoting acid, termed pantothenic acid, has recently been described. Its discoverers state "that it is more widely distributed in nature than any known physiologically potent substance."

In recognition of his outstanding work in the treatment of pernicious anemia, Professor G. R. Minot of Harvard Medical College, has been awarded the Moxon Gold Medal of the Royal College of Physicians of London.

Susceptibility or immunity to common colds has been demonstrated at Western Reserve University as an inconstant factor for an individual, these qualities varying markedly in a survey of the students conducted from year to year.

A statistical study of homicide rates conducted by the Metropolitan Life Insurance Company indicates that Nevada had the highest rate among white people for the years 1929 to 1931, while Missouri led the list among colored people for the same period.

A British member of the International Committee for the Prevention of Tuberculosis has recently advanced a theory that tubercle bacilli may change from the bovine type to the human type in the body. He cites a case in which he believes this has occurred.

Scientists working at the National Institute of Health in Washington and at the Rockefeller Institute for Medical Research in New York City, have discovered that encephalitis patients apparently develop immune bodies in their blood which give resistance to the disease.

Said to measure anesthetic risk with mathematical accuracy a new heart load formula has been devised, combining the systolic and diastolic blood pressure readings, and multiplying the sum by the pulse rate. The more nearly this figure approaches 14,400, the more standard the risk.

Pointed out as highly significant as a causative factor in the alarming increase in diabetes in this country, it has been determined that during the past century the average person in the United States has increased the amount of sugar consumed from 10 pounds to 105 pounds per year.

Experimenting with 213 children, Dr. P. C. Jeans of the Pediatrics Department at Iowa State University, advances the theory that night blindness results from a deficiency in Vitamin A, and that the condition may be promptly relieved by supplying an adequate amount of Vitamin A to the diet.

Lester J. (Old Doc) Tilton of Clinton lost his second legal battle in two years when a federal district court jury in Davenport recently decided that he had violated the pure food and drug act by selling as "cure-alls" a liquid which contained 98 per cent water and an ointment which was 96.3 per cent vaseline.

Federal Relief Administrator Harry Hopkins has recently announced that there are six million children in the United States without enough to eat because their parents are "taking the licking in this depression." The Federal Relief Administration has provided funds for the examination of these children.

In recogniton of his meritorious work in researches on trichomonas vaginalis vaginitis, Dr. Henry C. Hesseltine, formerly of Iowa City, and now instructor in obstetrics and gynecology at the University of Chicago, was awarded the annual prize offered by the Central Association of Obstetricians and Gynecologists.

An observer in the eye clinic of the University of Basel, Switzerland, observes that rabbits fed on naphthalene develop cataract, and at the same time Vitamin C disappears from the aqueous humor of the eye. Based upon this observation he advances the theory that cataract may be due to a lack of Vitamin C.

Contributing to the sum total of our knowledge regarding the chemistry of cancer, Dr. Leslie J. Harris of the Nutritional Laboratory, Cambridge, England, has recently announced a dichlorophenoliodophenol dye reducing or oxidizing substance found in cancerous tissues, resembling Vitamin C, to which he gives the name "reducytin."

Recent observations made by the United States Public Health Service indicate that in spite of the depression "there is substantially no change in the weight of boys and a slight increase in the number of underweight girls during the last few years of the economic depression." The observations upon which this statement was based were made among the elementary school children of Hagerstown, Maryland.

PERSONAL MENTION

Dr. F. L. Knowles of Fort Dodge, attended the recent meeting of the American Orthopedic Academy in Chicago, where he presented a paper on "Fractures of the Neck of the Femur."

Dr. Taylor R. Jackson of Chariton, in an effort to recover from a serious illness has left for a two months' vacation trip through the South. During his absence, Dr. George F. Niblock of Derby, will take care of Dr. Jackson's practice.

Dr. John Kenefick of Algona, was the guest speaker for the local Rotary Club, Monday, December 18, when he discussed "The Discovery of Bacteria and the Use of Serum."

Dr. Herman J. Smith announces the opening of offices at 1102 Equitable Building in Des Moines. Dr. Smith was graduated from the University of Iowa College of Medicine in 1931, and has spent the past two years at the Michael Reese Hospital in Chicago.

Dr. Arthur Steindler of Iowa City, delivered an illustrated lecture on orthopedic hospitals in Germany and Italy, at the Iowa City Lions Club luncheon, Wednesday, January 24.

Dr. C. W. Baldridge of Iowa City, was elected supreme vice archon of Phi Beta Pi medical fraternity in the final business session of the national convention held recently at Iowa City.

Dr. Donald G. Mackie, who located a few months ago in Vinton, has accepted a commission of three months' duration with the Citizens Conservation organization, and will be located in Little Rock, Arkansas. At the end of that time, he expects to return to Vinton.

Dr. Lester Leserman has announced the opening of an office in Rolfe. Dr. Leserman comes direct from Chicago, where he has been connected with the Michael Reese Hospital, since his graduation from Rush Medical School.

Dr. Frank Ely of Des Moines, addressed the Corydon Parent-Teachers Association, Monday, January 15, on the subject, "The Value of Social Restraint."

Dr. Zella White Stewart of Iowa City, left recently for a four months' cruise through the southern hemisphere. She will visit the Hawaiian Islands, the South Sea Islands, New Zealand, Australia, New Guinea, the Dutch East Indies, the Malay states, India, and Barbados, returning to New York about June 1.

Dr. A. H. Lazere, a native of Sioux City, has returned to his home city to begin the practice of medicine. Dr. Lazere was graduated from the University of Illinois College of Medicine, Chicago, and has completed his internship at Michael Reese Hospital, also in Chicago.

Dr. R. F. Neilson of Cedar Falls, spoke before the Cedar Falls Hi-Y, Thursday, January 11, on "Prevention of Diseases."

MARRIAGES

The wedding of Miss Betty Groeger of Omaha, and Dr. Eugene Smith of Waterloo, took place Sunday, February 7, at St. Mary Magdalene's Church in Omaha. After a short wedding trip the couple will return to Waterloo, where Dr. Smith has been practicing for some time.

DEATH NOTICES

Brown, Cecil W., of Clinton, aged fifty-seven, died January 8, following a long illness. He was graduated in 1906 from the University of Western Ontario Medical School, and had long been a member of the Clinton County Medical Society.

Grimes, Eli, of Des Moines, aged sixty-six, died January 14, as a result of cancer of the pancreas. He was graduated in 1897 from the University of Iowa College of Medicine, and at the time of his death was a member of the Polk County Medical Society. (A more extended obituary will be found in the History of Medicine Section of this issue.)

McCray, Frank Herbert, of Schaller, aged sixty-seven, died January 14, following an extended illness. He was graduated in 1896 from the Sioux City College of Medicine, and at the time of his death was a member of the Sac County Medical Society.

Schmidt, Arthur Albert, of Postville, aged fifty-two, died January 22, after a short illness with a throat infection. We was graduated in 1893 from Keokuk Medical College, and at the time of his death was a member of the Allamakee County Medical Society.

Smith, John Christopher, of Stacyville, aged forty-five, died suddenly on December 28. He was graduated in 1915 from the St. Louis University School of Medicine and at the time of his death was a member of the Mitchell County Medical Society.

Svebakken, Otto O., of Decorah, aged fifty-nine, died January 12, as the result of automobile injuries received in an accident near Gainesville, Florida, where he had gone for a short winter holiday. He was graduated in 1906 from the Chicago College of Medicine and Surgery, and at the time of his death was a member of the Winneshiek County Medical Society.

SOUTHEASTERN SURGICAL CONGRESS MEETS IN NASHVILLE

The Southeastern Surgical Congress will hold its fifth annual assembly in Nashville, Tennessee, March 5, 6 and 7. The Andrew Jackson Hotel will be hotel headquarters and the lectures and exhibits will be in the War Memorial Building.

The following doctors will occupy places on the program: Fred H. Albee, New York; W. Wayne Babcock, Philadelphia; Vilray P. Blair, St. Louis; J. B. Brown, St. Louis; George W. Crile, Cleveland; John F. Erdmann, New York; M. S. Henderson, Rochester, Minn.; Arthur E. Hertzler, Halstead, Kansas; Chevalier Jackson, Philadelphia; Dean Lewis, Baltimore; Joseph F. McCarthy, New York; C. Jeff Miller, New Orleans; John J. Moorhead, New York; George H. Semken, New York; Arthur M. Shipley, Baltimore; and Waitman F. Zinn, Baltimore.

For information write Dr. B. T. Beasley, 1019 Doctors Building, Atlanta, Georgia.

AMERICAN ASSOCIATION FOR THE STUDY OF GOITER ESSAY CONTEST

The American Association for the Study of Goiter, for the fifth time, offers Three Hundred Dollars ($300.00) as a first award, and two honorable mentions for the best essays based upon original research work on any phase of goiter presented at their annual meeting in Cleveland, Ohio, June 7th, 8th and 9th, 1934. It is hoped that this contest will stimulate valuable research work, especially in regard to the basic cause of goiter.

Competing manuscripts must be in English, and submitted to the Corresponding Secretary, J. R. Yung, M.D., 670 Cherry St., Terre Haute, Indiana, not later than April 1, 1934.

LAY PUBLICATION DISCUSSES MEDICAL COSTS

The difficult and complex problem of providing adequate medical care for rich and poor alike, at a cost which can reasonably be met, has been widely discussed for the past several months. Articles, editorials, and newspaper stories on the subject have appeared in such a quantity that it is neither possible nor desirable to read all the remarks and opinions of the various solutions for this important problem. Of the worth-while articles on this topic, we would call your attention to a discussion appearing in the August, 1933, issue of *The Rotarian*. With the title, "Cutting Medical Costs," a question, "Is the Group Plan the Best Remedy?", is asked and answered in the affirmative and in the negative by two prominent physicians. The discussion of both sides of the question appeals to us as being a fair presentation of the advantages and disadvantages of the group plan in operation.

HISTORY OF MEDICINE IN IOWA

Edited by the Historical Committee

DR. HENRY B. YOUNG, Burlington   DR. TOM. B. THROCKMORTON, Des Moines
DR. FRANK M. FULLER, Keokuk   DR. WALTER L. BIERRING, Des Moines
DR. JOHN T. McCLINTOCK, Iowa City

The History of Medicine in Lucas County

TOM MORFORD THROCKMORTON, A.M., M.D.,
Chariton

TOM BENTLEY THROCKMORTON, B.Sc., M.D.,
Des Moines

(Continued from last month)

PHYSICIANS WHO HAVE PRACTICED IN LUCAS

Dr. William Sanford Carpenter

Dr. William Sanford Carpenter was born in Lucas County in 1871. He received his medical education in the University of Louisville, Louisville, Kentucky, and was graduated from that institution in the class of 1894. The doctor then located in Lucas, where he practiced his profession for several years. He afterwards located in Des Moines. At present he is living in Atloona, Polk County, Iowa, and is serving the county in the capacity of coroner.

Dr. William M. Bain

Dr. William M. Bain was born in Ohio. He was a graduate of the Ensworth Medical College, St. Joseph, Missouri, in 1886. The doctor came to Lucas from Mahaska County, Iowa, in 1890. Just how long he remained in Lucas, and for what region he departed, we do not know.

Dr. William Boone Bullard

Dr. William Boone Bullard was born in Missouri. Like his predecessor, Dr. Bain, he was a graduate of the Ensworth Medical College, St. Joseph, Missouri, but was a member of the class of 1893. Dr. Bullard came to Lucas from Des Moines, Iowa, in 1897. There is no record of the length of time the doctor remained in Lucas or to what locality he moved when he left the town.

Dr. Mary Caroline Reed

Dr. Mary Caroline Reed was a native of Wisconsin. She received her medical education in the Woman's Medical School, University of Chicago, Chicago, Illinois, and was graduated from that institution in the class of 1893. She practiced for a

time in Mitchellville, Polk County, Iowa, from which place she came to Lucas in 1900. There are no records available concerning the doctor's activities after she left Lucas, or as to where she may have relocated.

Dr. J. A. Wilson

Dr. J. A. Wilson came to Lucas in 1886. He was a graduate of the Kentucky School of Medicine, Louisville, Kentucky, being a member of the class of 1881. After two or three years' stay in the town he moved away.

Dr. A. S. Davidson

Dr. A. S. Davidson was a graduate of the St. Louis Eclectic Medical College, St. Louis, Missouri, in the class of 1877. He was located in Lucas in 1886 or 1887. We have no further knowledge of his activities.

Dr. D. W. Jones

Dr. D. W. Jones was a graduate of the Medical Department of the Iowa State University, Iowa City, Iowa, in the class of 1885. He came to Lucas about the year 1886. No further records concerning him are available.

Dr. Robert S. Gray

Dr. Robert S. Gray was born in England. His certificate to practice medicine was issued by the state in May, 1887, since he had practiced seven years in Iowa. The certificate was filed in the county May 12, 1887. We have no date of his leaving the town.

Dr. Thomas Clarkson

Dr. Thomas Clarkson came from Winterset, Madison County, Iowa, to Lucas, in 1887. He was born in Scotland in 1834. The doctor was licensed in 1887 by the State Board of Medical Examiners, because of fourteen years of practice in Iowa. We have no further record concerning him.

Dr. L. W. Morley

Dr. L. W. Morley was born in Michigan. He was licensed by the state in 1886, by virtue of his ten years of practice in Iowa. The doctor came from What Cheer, Keokuk County, Iowa, to Lucas, in 1890. We have no further history of him.

Dr. Leverne A. Badger

Dr. Leverne A. Badger came from Clinton, Clinton County, Iowa, to Lucas, March 14, 1891. He was a native of Pennsylvania, and was graduated from the University of Buffalo, Buffalo, New York, February 23, 1875. We have no record of when the doctor left Lucas, or where he may have relocated.

Dr. Phillips Daniel Carper

Dr. Phillips Daniel Carper, a native of Iowa, came from Colfax, Jasper County, Iowa, to Lucas, in 1894. He was graduated from the Medical Department of the Iowa State University, Iowa City, Iowa, March 7, 1888. We have no record of when he left Lucas, or where he may have relocated.

Dr. Jonathan Henry Baker

Dr. Jonathan Henry Baker, a native of Maryland, came from Sioux City, Woodbury County, Iowa, to Lucas, in 1897. He was a graduate of the Physio-Medical Institution, Chicago, Illinois, having received his diploma from that institution, March 14, 1888. We have no further record of him.

Dr. Albert Alexander Potterf

Dr. Albert Alexander Potterf, a native of Ohio, came from Kansas City, Missouri, to Lucas, March 20, 1901. He was graduated from the Homeopathic Medical College, St. Louis, Missouri, March 14, 1898. The doctor remained in Lucas only a short time.

Dr. Harry Alonzo McChesney

Dr. Harry Alonzo McChesney was born in the state of New York. He came from Audubon, Audubon County, Iowa, to Lucas, in March, 1897. He was graduated from the Homeopathic Medical College, St. Louis, Missouri, March 14, 1889. He remained in Lucas only a short time.

Dr. John William Starr

Dr. John William Starr came from Avery, Monroe County, Iowa, to Lucas in March, 1897. He was a native of Missouri. The county records

show that a certificate was issued to him by the State Board of Medical Examiners, bearing the date, November 3, 1889. There is no further record.

Dr. James Muir

Dr. James Muir was in Lucas County for two or three months, some thirty odd years ago. We have no further record of him.

Dr. Mary A. Stratton

Dr. Mary A. Stratton located in Cleveland, Lucas County, in 1904. The towns of Lucas and Cleveland, Mines No. 3, were adjacent mining towns in Jackson township. We have no further record of the doctor's activities.

Dr. John C. Bell

The writer has purposely left Dr. John C. Bell for the last in his consideration of the medical men and women who have served the town of Lucas and its surrounding territory. The inference should not be drawn that Dr. Bell is, by any means, the least of those personages, for he is not. It is the writer's fortune to have known the good doctor for many years, during which time he always found him to be an honest, upright man, and a good physician. Dr. Bell was born in Antioch, Monroe County, Ohio, November 21, 1856. He was graduated from the College of Physicians and Surgeons, Keokuk, Iowa, in the class of 1883. After receiving his diploma, the doctor returned to his native state and began the practice of medicine in Stafford, Monroe County. Here he remained for seven years; after which time he came to Lucas, where he has continued to practice. For years he has been the only available physician in the town.

The following names of physicians, who have been located in Lucas, were given to the writer by an old time settler in the town.

Dr. Wilson was located in Lucas between the years 1880 and 1884. He moved to Kansas. Dr. Hicks and Dr. Boney were in the town about that same time. Dr. W. S. Church was in Lucas in 1876. The doctor's death occurred while he was a resident of the town.

PHYSICIANS WHO HAVE PRACTICED IN DERBY

In all probability the village of Derby would never have existed if it had not been for the construction of the branch railroad from Chariton to Saint Joseph, Missouri. When the road was built through Union township, it missed by several miles the little village of Freedom which was situated in an adjoining township to the east. Consequently Messrs. Manchester and Perkins, who established a railroad station at this point, laid out the village of Derby and caused a plat to be made of it, May 1, 1872. The original town plat, which covered something over forty acres of land, was divided into one hundred and ninety-two lots. Within a short time the village began to grow. There was a gradual exodus of people from Freedom, and Derby became quite a trading point. For many years the writer's father conducted a general store in the town; he also operated a grain elevator and shipped large amounts of grain and, to some extent, livestock, to the Chicago markets. Here, also, the writer began the practice of medicine, as did his brothers, Charles and Fred; but time has caused the passing of many things and with it the town of Derby has grown smaller in like proportion to the better traveling facilities of the present age. There is only one physician now residing in the town.

Dr. Samuel H. Stutsman

The first physician to locate in Derby was Dr. Samuel H. Stutsman. He was born in Morgan County, Indiana, in October, 1836, and came to Iowa with the family in 1840. He attended medical lectures in the old University of Iowa, at

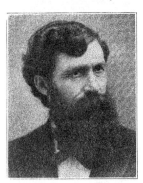

Samuel H. Stutsman, M.D.
1836-1891

Keokuk, Iowa, an institution later known as the College of Physicians and Surgeons, and was graduated from it in the class of 1863. The doctor served as a surgeon in the Civil War. He located in Chariton in 1871, but afterward he moved to Henderson, a spot in the road designated by a postoffice and store building, which was situated some ten miles southwest of the county seat, in Warren township.

Dr. Stutsman was married to Miss Elizabeth Mooney in 1861. They became the parents of

three children, William H.; Lenora; and Carl. The latter afterwards followed in his father's footsteps and became a member of the medical profession. He has resided for many years in Burlington, Iowa.

When the south branch of the Burlington railroad was constructed from Chariton to St. Joseph, Missouri, during the years 1871 and 1872, it passed through the southeastern corner of Union township. When the village of Derby was platted and made a station of the railroad in 1872, the doctor was the first person to purchase a lot from the promoters of the new enterprise. Within a short time he erected a nice home and an office. After four or five years of successful practice, he sold his property and "good will" to Dr. Joseph R. Buffington, and moved to Burlington, Des Moines County, Iowa. He continued to make his home in that city until the time of his death, which occurred in April, 1891. His body was buried in the Burlington Aspen Grove cemetery.

Dr. Alonzo Theophilus West

Dr. Alonzo Theophilus West, born in Knoxville, Marion County, Iowa, April 9, 1854, was a son of Nathan and Marie (Duncan) West. His father was a teacher and taught in the public schools of Knoxville for many years. Alonzo grew up in the town, attended the public schools, and was graduated from the high school. He later began the study of medicine, after which he enrolled in the

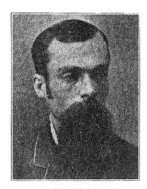

Alonzo T. West, M.D.
1854-1918

Bennett Eclectic Medical College, Chicago, Illinois, and was graduated from that institution in the class of 1874. In the autumn following his graduation, Dr. West came to Lucas County and located in Derby. He was married to Miss Emma

Oehlman, October 12, 1876. She was a daughter of Charles and Dores (Tennis) Oehlman, natives of Hanover, Germany, who came to Lucas County in 1858. After four or five years of practice in and about Derby, the doctor moved to Conway, Taylor County, Iowa. Here he resided until his death, which followed a lingering illness from sarcoma of the shoulder and chest, March 3, 1918. His wife and two daughters survive him.

Dr. Joseph Riley Buffington

Dr. Joseph Riley Buffington was born in Columbus City, Louisa County, Iowa, January 5, 1840. His parents were early pioneers of the west, and located in Iowa Territory in 1838, soon after the close of the Black Hawk War. His father, James Q., was a native of Ohio; his mother, Eliza Ann Sleeth, was a member of one of the old Virginia families. Young Joseph attended the public schools in his home town; later he went to Mount Pleasant for more advanced schooling. He began the study of medicine under the preceptorship of Dr. J. M. Robertson of Columbus City. However, the disturbing influence of the Civil War altered his plans, and in 1862 he enlisted in Company F, 25th Iowa Volunteer Infantry. In time he was made a corporal and later was advanced to sergeant of his company. He served in General Sherman's army, remained with it throughout the war, and received an honorable discharge from the government, June 7, 1865.

On his return to Iowa, following the war, he purchased a farm in Lucas County and was a successful farmer for a number of years. The writer well recalls the farmer-doctor, for he taught three terms of school in the district where Mr. Buffington lived. Not only did three of the Buffington children attend the school at that time, but their father furnished the hickory wood with which to heat the old log schoolhouse, where I had gone to school as a boy and where my father had taught the children of the district years before my time of attendance.

In 1873, Mr. Buffington purchased lots in the new town of Derby. Here he built a nice home for his family and a two-story business building, in which he opened a drug store; but once again the lure of medicine entered his veins, and he became a student of Dr. Samuel H. Stutsman. Following a course of instruction under his new preceptor, he matriculated in the Keokuk Medical College, Keokuk, Iowa, and was graduated from it in the class of 1875. The doctor then returned to Derby where he was associated with Dr. Stutsman until the latter sold out his interest to the

junior member of the firm in 1877, and took his departure for Burlington.

Dr. Buffington continued to practice at Derby until March, 1880, when he moved to Liberty, Gage County, Nebraska. After remaining in that community for ten years, he changed his field of endeavor to Nelson, in Nuckolls County. Here he became associated with a Mr. Knapp in the establishment of a drug store. This partnership continued for ten years. In 1894, the doctor was elected to office in the Nebraska state legislature. This position he filled with dignity and distinction.

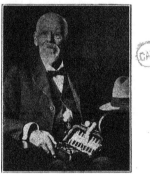

Joseph Riley Buffington, M.D.
1840-1925

Dr. Buffington's first wife was Miss Cyntha Ann Sargent. This union was blessed by three children, Flora E.; William Q.; and George. His second marriage, November 22, 1881, was of considerable interest at the time. The ceremony was performed by means of telephonic communication, as the contracting parties were separated by many miles. The bride was Mrs. Josephine Estella Hickock, of Moline, Illinois. The telephone was somewhat new, and to use the instrument as a means of carrying out a marriage ceremony was a heretofore unheard of procedure in Lucas County and, as such, its use added real zest to the romantic aspect of the marriage institution. Three children were born as a result of this union; Le Roy Alvin; Fred R.; and Nellie. After a life full of activity and service, Dr. Buffington died at his home in Nelson at the ripe age of eighty-five years.

The writer was well acquainted with the parents of Dr. Buffington, for they lived just across the street from him for several years when he was located at Derby. The story of their hardships, endurance and heroism, especially of their surgical experience while pioneering in Iowa, is interesting as related by them many years ago.

The family were moving one day, with a heavily loaded wagon along a sparsely settled trail when David, a babe in arms, fell from the wagon. The mother, hearing his outcry, jumped from the wagon and picked up the child, only to find that a wheel had passed over its thigh. The iron rim of the wheel had torn and lacerated the flesh and crushed the bone to such an extent that the extremity was held by mere strips of skin. There they were, miles from help, with a desperately injured babe; but the parents were equal to the emergency. The mother severed the skin with her scissors and wrapped the stump with a clean cloth. In the hope of finding adequate help, they proceeded on their journey. Some hours later they came to a cabin, where they obtained hot water and received the sympathy of a good woman. The father carefully trimmed away the lacerated muscle tags and loose tendons and, drawing the skin down over the stump, he sewed the flaps together with coarse black thread. The next day the little patient seemed better so they continued their journey. As there was no bleeding from the

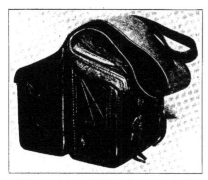

Saddlebags made by David Buffington for the author in 1877

stump and the wound continued to heal, they did not seek further surgical aid. The babe made an uneventful recovery.

When young David grew to manhood he became a harness maker by trade. He made for the writer the first and only pair of saddle-pockets he ever owned. Saddlebags were an essential part of a doctor's equipment in an early day, for they afforded the means by which he could carry medicines and supplies while riding horseback. The

saddlebags made by David Buffington were fashioned after the pair which were owned by my uncle, Dr. William S. Throckmorton, of Nineveh, Pennsylvania. I had carefully taken the measurements of his bags when I was a student in his office. Mr. Buffington was an excellent worker in leather and the saddlebags he made for me were the best and most convenient of any I ever saw. I used them for many years in my practice. They are now in the possession of my son, Dr. Tom.

Another incident which well emphasizes the fortitude with which the father of Dr. Buffington could meet an emergency is illustrated by a story which he told the writer on one occasion. The house in which the family was residing was supported at the corners by stumps of wood set in the ground. For some reason the house had settled in an uneven manner. The elder Buffington, in an endeavor to equalize the supports, took upon himself the task of chopping away the top of one of the stumps. After working an hour or so at the job, with a fair degree of success, he slipped his hand along the top of the stump to clear away the chips. Unfortunately the corner of the house settled just at that moment and his ring finger was caught in such a manner that he could not extricate his hand. Night was rapidly approaching and there were no neighbors for miles around. He finally secured the attention of his wife but she could do nothing to help free her husband. In his desperation he requested his wife to bring a chisel and a mallet. Holding the chisel on the incarcerated finger, he instructed his wife to strike it with the mallet. The amputation of the phalanx was quickly done and the hand was freed from bondage. These stories well reveal the type of parenthood from which Dr. Joseph Buffington sprang.

Dr. Thomas McKaig Wall

Dr. Thomas McKaig Wall was born in Maryland in 1844. He was a graduate of the College of Physicians and Surgeons, Keokuk, Iowa, in the class of 1867. He had served with distinction during the Civil War. He first enlisted in Company K, 14th Iowa Volunteer Infantry and was mustered into service February 20, 1862. Following the battle at Shiloh, Tennessee, the following April, he was reported missing. He was found later and, owing to disability, was discharged July 22. Apparently it was hard to keep down this good and patriotic man, for in March, 1864, he again entered the service of his country; this time with Company K, 2nd Iowa Cavalry. He was wounded at Little Harpeth, Tennessee, December 17, 1864; but he continued to serve throughout the remainder of the war and was discharged from the army at Selma, Alabama, September 19, 1865.

After his graduation in medicine, which followed the Civil War, he practiced for a time at Cincinnati, Appanoose County, Iowa. He then came to Derby in January, 1877, where he remained for about two years. It was during this time that he was married to Mrs. Ellen Scott, a daughter of Isaac Dennis, who was one of the old settlers of the community. The doctor then moved to Smyrna, a little village situated in a good farming community in Clarke County. His stay there was rather short for, with a better opportunity for practice in Wayne County, he located in Humeston. Here the doctor gained a reputation as an ophthalmic surgeon. He successfully operated on an old gentleman, who was practically blind, and removed his crystalline lens. This delicate opera-

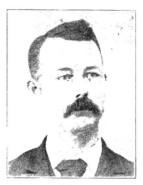

Thomas McK. Wall, M.D.
1844-1917

tion was not being done by country doctors; hence Dr. Wall was entitled to much credit, for his patient received fairly good vision during the remainder of his lifetime. Some years later, the writer was present when the doctor performed a similar operation in the home of a man in Osceola. The patient, who suffered from double cataract, had his vision satisfactorily restored through the doctor's skillful effort. Dr. Wall did not announce himself as a specialist in this line of surgery, but he continued in the field of medicine as a general practitioner.

After practicing a few years in Humeston, the doctor moved to Osceola, Clarke County, Iowa. Here he remained until the time of his death, in November, 1917, an honored and respected gentleman and a true physician. His body was buried in the Osceola cemetery.

Dr. Alburtis P. McCulloch

Dr. Alburtis P. McCulloch, a native of Ohio, came from Brooklyn, Poweshiek County, Iowa, to Derby in 1879. He was a graduate of Rush Medical College, Chicago, in the class of 1868; also of Bellevue Hospital Medical College, New York City, in the class of 1875. The doctor was a well read man in medicine and surgery. Not only had he prepared himself by graduation from two well known medical institutions in America, but he had further pursued his studies abroad by taking a postgraduate course in Edinburgh, Scotland.

During his stay in Derby, which was rather short, Dr. McCulloch was associated with Dr. Joseph R. Buffington. Here he gave evidence of those qualities which marked him as a gentleman and a good surgeon. He left the town to go into partnership with his brother, Dr. George McCulloch, at Humeston, Wayne County, Iowa. After practicing for a time in that community, the doctor returned to his former field of medical activity at Brooklyn, Iowa. We have no further record as to the time, or the place, of the doctor's death.

Dr. William E. Moore

Dr. William E. Moore was born in Ohio in 1852. He came to Iowa in 1882, and located in Derby. He was a graduate of the College of Physicians and Surgeons, Baltimore, Maryland, in the class of 1881. He was married to Miss Agnes Thompson of Derby in 1887. Dr. Moore administered to the sick and afflicted of the town and its surrounding territory for more than twenty-five years. He moved with his family to Lincoln, Nebraska, where he afterwards died.

(To be concluded next month.)

OBITUARIES

ELI GRIMES, M.D.
1867-1934

An Appreciation

In the nineties medical education took a decided step forward. Previous to that time the medical schools, with few exceptions, were rather lax in their requirements. Only a few states had strict medical practice acts. There were many commercial schools turning out doctors who were illy prepared for the care of the sick.

Some far seeing gentlemen, with vast sums of money at their disposal, cast about for some way in which to better their fellow men. They decided to investigate medical education and to exert an influence in supplying the country with better medical care. This brought about a decided advance in the standards of medical teaching. Entrance requirements to medical schools were raised. More intensive teaching of the fundamentals was developed. In the hospitals training at the bedside began.

Eli Grimes was in his early twenties at the time of this medical upheaval. From boyhood on he displayed a very active mind and an intense desire to learn. There was constantly apparent a determination to study consecutively. Everything undertaken was to be followed to a logical conclusion or at least so far as recorded knowledge would go. His father was a minister and, not being endowed with worldly goods, could not give much financial aid; so Eli struggled along. He worked ceaselessly and untiringly to secure the means to advance himself as a student.

After getting what schooling his home town could afford he saved enough money to attend school in Shenandoah, Iowa. This was the beginning. From there he came to Des Moines where he entered Highland Park College, an institution admitting anyone with limited means but with a will to learn and to work. After graduating from this college we learn that, still hungry for knowledge, he entered the State University at Iowa City. There he spent several years in the pursuit of his studies.

He had decided to become a Doctor of Medicine. While carrying out this course he came to realize how helpful a knowledge of chemistry, pathology and botany would be. Not only did he study these subjects, as the medical student of today is required to do, but he went further. As an assistant teacher in these sciences he acquired the information which later gave him a keen insight into disease. His command of this type of knowledge is possessed by few medical men.

After graduating from the State University he located in Des Moines and entered the practice of medicine. He found time to fill a teaching position in Highland Park College and, later on, in the Medical School of Drake University. As a teacher he combined the art of being able to arouse and hold the interest of his pupils with the gift of imparting information.

His study of medicine was pursued with his usual zeal. In his later years unsolved medical problems were of the greatest interest to him. He was constantly surprising his listeners with evidence of his knowledge, its depth and range. He always expressed himself with becoming modesty.

In the sick room Dr. Grimes had full command of his medical equipment. This enabled him to display a diagnostic ability admired by his professional brethren. His presence inspired confidence in his patients and they realized that a master was in attendance. He was always a friend of the younger doctor and enjoyed helping him in times of perplexity.

Cross indexed records covering a period of more than thirty years were of great service to him. He was able, from these records, to gather the histories of patients suffering with any type of disease and to study, individually or collectively, whatever he wished to review.

His reading was extensive and by no means limited to medicine. As a young man he read the Bible through three times. His familiarity with literature, the classics, modern prose, modern poetry and all, was much greater than that of the ordinary professional man. His mind was retentive. That which he studied and that which he read became his own.

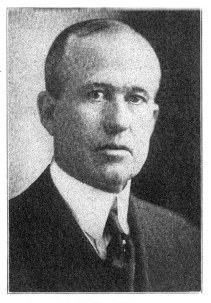

Eli Grimes, M.D.
1867-1934

He was undoubtedly qualified to write in a forceful and convincing manner, and in recent years he derived much pleasure from his writings, both medical and lay. Whether speaking or writing he was capable of maintaining his point. His articles, published in our representative medical journals, are masterpieces both in content and in style.

My acquaintance with Dr. Grimes began about a year after I came to Des Moines. Calling on the late Dr. J. T. Priestley one day, I was introduced to Dr. Grimes who was, at that time, doing Dr. Priestley's office laboratory work. Our professional interests coincided. Many evenings and Sunday afternoons we spent together. During these visits medical subjects were discussed and there never was a time when I did not feel that I had learned something from him. A close friendship was formed, a friendship which was never broken.

Miss Beth Cook, who has been my secretary for more than twenty years, and who has had an opportunity to know Dr. Grimes' worth, wrote the following appreciation. It appealed to me so much that I obtained her consent to add it here.

W. W. Pearson, M.D.

A Tribute

Dr. Grimes is dead. A nobleman of the medical profession has passed on. We shall miss him.

We, who have been wont to depend upon him for comprehensive analysis and keen diagnosis in the solving of obscure medical problems, shall miss him.

We, who have been granted happy, healthful years through his skill and to whom he has been not only a healing physician but an understanding, unselfish and self forgetful friend, shall miss him.

We, with whom he has so generously shared the fruits of his labors that we might be the better equipped for life's struggle, shall miss him.

We, who have loved him and lost him as an intimate personal friend, shall miss him.

The memory of his fine, free thought, his great understanding of humanity, his ready sympathy, his unselfish love for his fellow man, and his unlimited capacity to give always of himself for others, this memory will live on throughout the years.

Dr. Grimes is one of those fortunate few who, all unknowingly, built his own monument, more enduring than granite, which will live ever in the hearts and lives of all those whom his life has touched.

B. C.

HERBERT VICTOR SCARBOROUGH, M.D.
1876-1934

The history of all tuberculosis work in Iowa has not yet been written but when it is, the name of Doctor Herbert Victor Scarborough will appear on nearly every page.

Dr. Scarborough attended Simpson College until he entered the College of Medicine of the State University, from which he was graduated in 1902. The natural step was to enter practice with his father at Grand Junction where he continued until failing health caused him to be admitted to the State Sanatorium in June, 1908. Here he gave his very best efforts until called to a more attractive position in Indiana, July 1, 1930. After two and one-half years as medical director of Sunnyside Sanatorium, he resigned to enter clinical work which he particularly enjoyed. He died suddenly of coronary disease at Norton, Kansas, on New Year's Day. Over a period of more than twenty years I knew him intimately and loved him deeply. His was a noble personality, characterized by kindness, sincerity, goodness and truth. Others will pay a suitable tribute to his life and works. I wish to mention his services in constructive tuberculosis effort.

He was one of the organizers of the Iowa Tuberculosis Association and served continuously on the Board until he left the state. The accomplishments of this outstanding organization is a fitting memorial

to his remarkable genius and constructive foresight. For many years his position as a member of the faculty of the University of Iowa College of Medicine, gave him an unrivaled opportunity to train and stimulate medical students to enter the professional war against tuberculosis. The splendid postgraduate courses given at Oakdale were made possible by his vision and coöperation. His selection for leadership of the Mississippi Valley Sanatorium Association gave testimony of his worth and the appreciation of his fellows. As Superintendent of the State Sanatorium during its developmental years he became a positive force in the organized campaign against tuberculosis; an inspired leader, sympathetic friend, and faithful physician to each and every one of the 7,000 patients who passed through his hands. His wise counsel based upon deep understanding of the human side of tuberculosis and thorough knowledge of its pathology was given freely to the great benefit of the individual patient.

He was courageously assertive in his beliefs, and independent of thought and action; ever devoted to principle; a glorious champion of right and justice for the unfortunate; master of humanitarian attributes; generous and forgiving to a fault—these outstanding qualities must ever distinguish him in the minds of his friends who are left to mourn his untimely death.

John H. Peck, M.D.

HISTORICAL PAPER OF DR. A. G. FIELD
A CORRECTION

In republishing in the January issue, a paper by the late Dr. A. G. Field read before the Polk County Medical Society in May, 1866, several errors were inadvertently overlooked which should be corrected. In 1910 Dr. Field published a collection of papers, including the one under discussion. The collection was titled "Footprints Made in the Dark." It seems likely that when the original paper was republished in 1910, certain philosophic comments were added by Dr. Field in keeping with subsequent knowledge. It is to be regretted that the original paper presented in 1866 is not available.

In the paper mentioned, it is stated "that cholera was due to an animal parasite instead of bacillus or vegetable as later claimed by Dr. Koch." In 1866, Dr. Koch was unknown and had not even graduated in medicine. In another statement, commenting on the great service of Pasteur, reference is made to his work on hydrophobia. The publication of Pasteur on this subject did not appear before 1879. The conjecture that microorganisms were concerned in some way with the causation of disease was no doubt held by medical leaders like Dr. Field in 1866, and at an even earlier date.

W. L. B.

THE JOURNAL BOOK SHELF

BOOKS RECEIVED

ANNUAL REPORT OF THE SURGEON GENERAL OF THE PUBLIC HEALTH SERVICE OF THE UNITED STATES, for the fiscal year 1933. United States Government Printing Office, Washington, D. C. For sale by the Superintendent of Documents, Washington, D. C. Price, seventy-five cents, cloth.

A DIABETIC MANUAL for the mutual use of the doctor and patient, by Elliott P. Joslin, M.D., clinical professor of medicine, Harvard Medical School. Fifth edition, entirely revised. Illustrated. Leo & Febiger, Philadelphia, 1934. Price, $2.00.

MODERN CLINICAL PSYCHIATRY—By Arthur P. Noyes, M.D., Superintendent of State Hospital for Mental Diseases, Howard, Rhode Island. 485 pages. W. B. Saunders Company, Philadelphia and London, 1934. Price, $4.50.

THE 1933 YEAR BOOK OF OBSTETRICS AND GYNECOLOGY. Edited by Joseph B. DeLee, A.M., M.D., professor of

obstetrics, University of Chicago Medical School, and J. P. Greenhill, M.D., associate professor of gynecology, Loyola University Medical School. The Year Book Publishers, Chicago, 1934.

THE SINGLE WOMAN—A medical study in sex education, by Robert Latou Dickinson, M.D., and Lura Beam. The Williams and Wilkins Company, Baltimore, 1934. Price, $5.00.

THE TORCH OF LIFE—By Frederick M. Rossiter, M.D., Licentiate, Royal College of Physicians, London. Eugenics Publishing Co., Inc., New York City. Price, $2.65.

THE YEAR BOOK OF RADIOLOGY—Edited by Charles A. Waters, M.D., associate in roentgenology, Johns Hopkins University, and Ira I. Kaplan, M.D., director, division of cancer, Department of Hospitals, City of New York. The Year Book Publishers, Chicago, Illinois, 1933. Price, $7.00.

BOOK REVIEWS

THE PREGNANT WOMAN

By Porter Brown, M.D., Salina, Kansas. Illustrated, 192 pages. Eugenics Publishing Company, New York City, 1933. Price, $2.00.

This volume has been prepared by a physician of long experience in obstetrics and gynecology. With the avowed purpose "to carry to every woman information about her physical welfare and her function of reproduction," the author begins his discussion by a consideration of some of the common superstitions concerning the menstrual cycle and the pregnant state. This chapter is followed by other sections dealing with sex education of children, childbearing, birth control, the anatomy and physiology of pregnancy, the diagnosis and complications of pregnancy, the care of the mother and newborn infant, and the common infections of tuberculosis, syphilis and gonorrhea.

Upon the findings of the New York Academy of Medicine that 65.8 per cent of maternal deaths were preventable "if the care of the mother had been proper in all respects," the author appropriately concludes his book with a very interesting chapter upon the subject of what the mother should expect of her physician and attendant. This chapter stresses the importance of hospitalization, discusses the various forms of anesthesia, condemns the various injudicious practices of nurse, patient and physician, which may predispose to or cause infection during the lying-in period.

On the whole the book is rather well written and the straightforwardness of the discussion will appeal

to the woman who contemplates pregnancy. The illustrations are all of the line drawing type, and add much to the clearness of the text particularly since the volume is intended for the layman.

THE YEAR BOOK OF GENERAL MEDICINE, 1933

Edited by George F. Dick, M.D., Lawrason Brown, M.D., George R. Minot, M.D., William B. Castle, M.D., William D. Stroud, M.D., and George B. Eusterman, M.D. The Year Book Publishers, Chicago. Price, $3.00.

The Year Book publishers have added two distinguished names to their already prepossessing list of editors for this volume on General Medicine. The newcomers are Dr. George F. Dick, originator of the Dick test, who edits the section on infectious diseases; and George B. Eusterman, gastro-enterologist at the Mayo Clinic, who edits the division of diseases of the digestive system and of metabolism. The co-authorship of this volume by six of America's leading clinicians guarantees its authoritativeness.

To those unfamiliar with the plan of the volume, it may be stated that it is an epitome of modern medical practice as gleaned from a critical survey of the year's literature. Each author, outstanding in his particular field, reviews in abstract the worthwhile literature of the year in his special division. The authors offer generous and critical comments concerning many of the articles abstracted, and this practice adds materially to the usefulness of these abstracts.

One feels somewhat disappointed to find but little mention of the glands of internal secretions. A summary of the year's work concerning the pituitary gland and the adrenal glands would be particularly useful in advancing our knowledge. While much of the literature on these subjects will undoubtedly appear in the volume on therapeutics, it would seem fitting to include some recognition of this work in the volume on general medicine.

However for the physician who is unable to read broadly and critically, this summary of the year's literature will be of untold usefulness. To those having a more generous experience with the literature the volume will serve to crystallize their reading. The volume maintains the high standard set by previous Year Books on general medicine.

———

THE SURGICAL CLINICS OF NORTH AMERICA

Volume xiii, No. 5, Chicago Number, October, 1933. Per clinic year, February, 1933, to December, 1933. Octavo of 254 pages with 93 illustrations. W. B. Saunders Company, Philadelphia and London. Price, paper, $12.00; cloth, $16.00.

This volume presents a number of very interesting clinics, the most noteworthy perhaps being a symposium on important surgical operations in children. This symposium deals with the intracranial tumors of childhood; acute mastoiditis in children; cystic tumors of the neck, especially bronchial and thyroglossal cysts; the surgical treatment of acute empyema and congenital pyloric stenosis; surgery of the urinary tract; and congenital dislocation of the hip.

Of the remaining articles in this number especial mention should be made of the use of x-ray in papillary adenocarcinoma of the ovary; everyday knee injuries; varicose veins and ulcers; and lung abscess. Of the orthopedic subjects presented, that of massive bone graft in the treatment of ununited fractures is particularly interesting.

The volume is very worthwhile but especially outstanding because of the symposium on the surgical operations in children. F. W. F.

VOLUNTARY MOTHERHOOD

A discussion of the various contraceptive methods, with emphasis on generally approved technics. By Antoinette F. Konikow, M.D.. Sold only to physicians for their own use, and for such distribution by them to their patients as may be legally permitted. Buchholz Publishing Company, Boston, 1933. Price, fifty cents.

This small paper bound booklet presents a discussion of the various contraceptive methods with emphasis on generally approved technics. Indicative of the acclaim which has been given this volume since its original publication in 1923 may be cited the fact that it is now in its fourth edition, having been completely rewritten for this printing.

The text of thirty-six pages briefly but critically discusses the means of contraception ordinarily employed, deducing that the safest method and the method of choice is one employing a protective shield in conjunction with a spermicide paste. Full directions are given concerning the use of the methods suggested with a thorough discussion of the precautions necessary to insure its effectiveness.

The book is intended solely for the information and guidance of physicians, and its sale is strictly limited to this group.

———

SURGICAL CLINICS OF NORTH AMERICA

Volume xiii, No. 6. Pacific Coast Surgical Association Number. Per clinic year February, 1933, to December, 1933. Index number, 284 pages with 97 illustrations. W. B. Saunders Company, Philadelphia and London, 1933. Price, paper, $12.00, cloth, $16.00.

This number prepared by the Pacific Coast Surgical Association deals with a wide variety of subjects. Many of the cases discussed are unusual or even rare in surgical experience.

Particularly deserving of citation are the following case discussions: carcinoma of Meckel's diverticulum; rupture of pelvic abscess into the bladder; lacerations of the rectum following contusions of the abdomen; meningopleural fistula following extirpation of the ganglioneuroma of the upper mediastinum; foreign body removed from the abdomen after eighteen years; x-ray burn of leg; value of broth injections (probably foreign protein injections).

It seems particularly fitting that the Surgical Clinics should be chosen for the review and report of these unusual conditions since these clinics are intended primarily to keep the operating surgeon informed concerning progress in this particular field. F. W. F.

INTERNATIONAL CLINICS

Volume IV, Forty-third Series, edited by Louis Hamman, M.D., visiting physician, Johns Hopkins Hospital, Baltimore, Maryland. J. B. Lippincott Company, Philadelphia, Montreal and London, 1933. Price, $3.00.

This number of the International Clinics is one of the most useful which has come to our attention inasmuch as it presents a very practical symposium on the use of endocrine gland products in the treatment of disease. This subject, because of the outstanding achievements reported during the past year, is one which has required rapid and radical revision. For this reason a discussion by some six or seven of the most distinguished workers in this field will be particularly welcome. A discussion of the modern treatment of obesity by Russell M. Wilder, M.D., of Rochester, is particularly useful and timely. The presentation of Paget's Disease of the Nipple by E. M. Eberts, M.D., of Montreal, modernizes our knowledge of this uncommon but interesting condition.

The volume is illustrated.

A TEXTBOOK OF PHYSIOLOGY

By William H. Howell, Ph.D., M.D., Sc.D., LL.D., Emeritus Professor of Physiology in the Johns Hopkins University, Baltimore, Maryland. Twelfth edition, thoroughly revised; 1132 pages with 308 illustrations. W. B. Saunders Company, Philadelphia and London, 1933. Price, $7.00.

It is difficult to review a work of this kind which for a number of decades has continued to be a textbook of unsurpassed excellence in physiology. The only question which naturally arises in the mind of the reviewer is whether the present edition has kept fully abreast of the many rapid advances which have been made in physiology since the last edition, and it is preposterous for a mere clinician to pass judgment on this feature.

The section dealing with the newer physiology of muscle, and that concerned with the recent developments in our knowledge of gonads, was read thoroughly by the reviewer, because of his especial interest in these two subjects. The work in its present form maintains all its former excellence and continues to be the work of choice for medical students as well as for those practitioners of medicine who wish to be informed concerning the newer advances in physiology.   D. J. G.

A MANUAL OF DISEASES OF THE NOSE, THROAT AND EAR

By E. B. Gleason, M.D., LL.D., professor of otology, Medico-Chirurgical College Graduate School of Medicine, University of Pennsylvania, Philadelphia. Seventh edition, revised and entirely reset, 651 pages with 261 illustrations. W. B. Saunders Company, Philadelphia and London. Price, $4.50.

This volume is the seventh edition of an already popular manual for use by students and practitioners in this specialty. In preparing the seventh edition, the sections dealing with the suppuration of the nasal accessory sinuses and the ear have been rewritten to reflect a conservative attitude in the handling of these conditions. The formulary has been amended to include additional therapeutic detail and the pharmacology of some of the more important drugs mentioned in the text.

The original plan of the book has not been altered, since time and experience have proved this plan to be most suitable for teaching purposes. The adequate and enlarged index provides ready reference to the subject matter in the text adding to the usefulness of the volume as a reference guide for the general practitioner.

SURGICAL CLINICS OF NORTH AMERICA

Volume xiii, No. 4, Mayo Clinic Number, August, 1933. Per clinic year, February, 1933, to December, 1933. Octavo of 215 pages with 65 illustrations. W. B. Saunders Company, 1933, price, paper, $12.00, cloth, $16.00.

This number deals largely with rather rare but very interesting pathologic conditions. The following clinics illustrate the type of cases described: hypertrophic stenosis of the pylorus in the adult; chronic duodenal obstruction; retroperitoneal tumors; dermoid cysts of the abdomen; adenocarcinoma of the thyroid, and early renal tuberculosis.

Neurosurgery is given considerable space. The treatment of muscular spasms and painful and trophic lesions of the extremities are described and there is also an interesting article on the experimental production of the syndrome of the spinal cord tumor. Spinal anesthesia is discussed in two articles, one with reference to the use of ephedrine which is advocated, and the other on the use of procaine in spinal anesthesia. The author concludes that spinal anesthesia is practical and safe, and that complications are minor and readily amenable to treatment. A very excellent number.

F. W. F.

IOWA STATE MEDICAL SOCIETY OFFICERS AND COMMITTEES 1933-1934

President..........................Charles B. Taylor, Ottumwa
President Elect................Gordon F. Harkness, Davenport
First Vice President............William E. Ash, Council Bluffs
Second Vice President................Frank H. Conner, Nevada
Secretary..........................Robert L. Parker, Des Moines
Treasurer..........................Harold J. McCoy, Des Moines

COUNCILORS

| | Term Expires |
First District—Felix A. Hennessy, Calmar..................1937
Second District—Lee R. Woodward, Mason City
  (Chairman) 1938
Third District—Frank P. Winkler, Sibley..................1934
Fourth District—James E. Reeder, Sioux City.............1935
Fifth District—William W. Pearson, Des Moines..........1936
Sixth District—Charles W. Ellyson, Waterloo............1937
Seventh District—Arthur W. Erskine, Cedar Rapids......1938
Eighth District—Clyde A Boice, Washington (Secretary)...1934
Ninth District—Harold A Spilman, Ottumwa..............1935
Tenth District—James G. Macrae, Creston...............1936
Eleventh District—M. Charles Hennessy, Council Bluffs....1937

TRUSTEES

Oliver J. Fay, Des Moines.................................1934
John I. Marker, Davenport................................1936
Edward M. Myers, Boone..................................1935

DELEGATES TO A. M. A.

Fred Moore, Des Moines...................................1935
E. D. Plass, Iowa City...................................1934
T. F. Thornton, Waterloo................................1934

ALTERNATE DELEGATES TO A. M. A.

N. G. Alcock, Iowa City..................................1935
W. E. Long, Mason City..................................1934
F. J. Swift, Maquoketa..................................1934

EDITOR OF THE JOURNAL

Ralph R. Simmons................................Des Moines

STANDING COMMITTEES OF THE HOUSE OF DELEGATES

ARRANGEMENTS

Charles B. Taylor, Chairman.........................Ottumwa
Robert L. Parker..................................Des Moines
Harold J. McCoy..................................Des Moines

CONSTITUTION AND BY-LAWS

John H. Peck, Chairman..........................Des Moines
Channing G. Smith....................................Granger
James C. Donahue..................................Centerville

FINANCE

Ernest C. McClure, Chairman..........................Bussey
E. B. Williams.....................................Montezuma
Andrew W. Bennett..................................Iowa City

MEDICO-LEGAL

Frank A. Ely, Des Moines, Chairman....................1935
George C. Albright, Iowa City........................1936
F. Earl Bellinger, Council Bluffs....................1934

PUBLICATION COMMITTEE

Ralph R. Simmons, Editor..........................Des Moines
Robert L. Parker, Secretary.......................Des Moines
Oliver J. Fay, Trustee............................Des Moines
John I. Marker, Trustee..............................Davenport
Edward M. Myers, Trustee................................Boone

PUBLIC POLICY AND LEGISLATION

Thomas A. Burcham, Chairman......................Des Moines
Frank L. Williams.................................Des Moines
Peter A. Bendixen..................................Davenport
Charles B. Taylor....................................Ottumwa
Robert L. Parker..................................Des Moines

SCIENTIFIC WORK

Charles B. Taylor, Chairman.........................Ottumwa
Robert L. Parker..................................Des Moines
Harold J. McCoy..................................Des Moines

SPECIAL COMMITTEES OF THE HOUSE OF DELEGATES

COMMITTEE ON CHILD HEALTH AND PROTECTION

Fred Moore, Chairman.............................Des Moines
E. D. Plass..Iowa City
J. D. Boyd..Iowa City
Lee F. Hill.......................................Des Moines
H. E. Farnsworth...................................Storm Lake

HISTORICAL

Walter L. Bierring, Chairman......................Des Moines
Frank M. Fuller.......................................Keokuk
T. B. Throckmorton...............................Des Moines
Henry B. Young.....................................Burlington
John T. McClintock..................................Iowa City

MEDICAL ECONOMICS

Corwin S. Cornell, Chairman........................Knoxville
James C. Hill..Newton
E. L. Wurtzer.....................................Clear Lake
R. M. Sorenson....................................Cumberland
T. A. Moran,..Melrose

MEDICAL LIBRARY

Felix A Hennessy, Chairman...........................Calmar
C. R. Harken..Osceola
Jeannette Dean-Throckmorton ....Des Moines

MILITARY AFFAIRS

T. F. Suchomel, Chairman........................Cedar Rapids
Mark C. Jones..Boone
Harold A. Spilman...................................Ottumwa

SUPERANNUATED PHYSICIANS

William F. Amdor, Chairman............................Carbon
W. S. Greenleaf.....................................Atlantic
F. G. Murray....................................Cedar Rapids

WOMAN'S AUXILIARY ADVISORY COMMITTEE

Emil C. Junger, Chairman.............................Soldier
O. A. Kabrick.....................................Grandview
James M. Donelan...................................Glenwood
P. B. McLaughlin..................................Sioux City
E. B. Howell..Ottumwa

STANDING COMMITTEE OF THE COUNCIL

SPEAKERS BUREAU COMMITTEE

Daniel J. Glomset, Chairman......................Des Moines
Felix A. Hennessy....................................Calmar
L. C. Kern..Waverly
John C. Parsons.....................................Creston
Dorothy M. Nelson, Secretary.....................Des Moines

SPECIAL COMMITTEES OF THE COUNCIL

MEDICAL EDUCATION AND HOSPITALS

Arthur W. Erskine, Chairman.....................Cedar Rapids
Louis F. Talley.................................Marshalltown
John C. Parsons.....................................Creston

PROFESSIONAL RELATIONS

Prince E. Sawyer, Chairman........................Sioux City
William R. Brock....................................Sheldon
Sydner D. Maiden...............................Council Bluffs

PUBLIC RELATIONS

George B. Crow, Chairman...........................Burlington
Raymond S. Grossman..............................Marshalltown
Harold L. Brereton................................Emmetsburg

The JOURNAL

of the

Iowa State Medical Society

Vol. XXIV   Des Moines, Iowa, March, 1934   No. 3

ERYSIPELOID IN NORTHWESTERN IOWA

Walter F. Harriman, M.D., Sioux City

Erysipeloid, long thought to be an invasion of the skin by a streptothrix, is now known to be a bacterial infection with the bacillus of swine erysipelas. Most of these infections involve the hands or fingers and have frequently been mistaken for a cellulitis of mild but stubborn nature. Incision and drainage, hot packs or ointment dressings have been the usual treatments.

In 1931 Klauder and Harkins reviewed and enriched the literature on erysipeloid. Apparently swine are the favored hosts of this bacillus, but its wide dissemination is extraordinary and the sources of human infection are widespread. It exists as a saprophite or pathogen throughout the animal kingdom. Human infection has been reported from handling fish in fish ponds, game animals, or birds, and from diseased cattle, sheep or hogs.

It would seem that human infection with the bacillus of swine erysipelas is on the increase in this area (region of Sioux City, Iowa), although this increase may be due to the fact that the condition is now more definitely and surely differentiated from other skin and wound infections. Possibly it has existed throughout the United States for many years. Nevertheless it would not seem amiss to suppose that the infection is more prevalent in areas such as this where every farm has its hog-lot with twenty-five to four hundred possible hosts. Fosterman first saw and diagnosed swine erysipelas about 1928 in the neighborhood of Utica, South Dakota, but this was not proved to be true swine erysipelas until the organism was isolated from one of these infected herds in 1930. In the fall months of 1931 Munce and Willey began to isolate the organism from local herds. At the present time (1933) they report widespread infection of swine in this area.

For several years industrial surgeons associated with the meat packing industry in Sioux City have been aware of a peculiar hand or finger infection which occurs regularly among handlers of fresh meat, particularly those handling fresh pork who injure themselves with sharp pork bones. There is a short incubation period in such cases. Within twenty-four hours the skin surrounding the wound assumes a brilliant red color, so characteristic as to have caused the term "red infection" to be applied to it. The color soon darkens to a bluish-red and the patient complains of an aching pain which is augmented by pressure or movement of the infected member. These employees have the best of surgical care. First aid is thorough and the patients are returned to work following the daily dressing of the wound. In these cases the infection is mild and the patient is well in from four to ten days. Yellow oxide of mercury or ammoniated mercury ointment, five per cent mercurochrome and metaphen dressings are efficient. Ultra-violet light is also of value in treatment. However, if the infection is first treated several days after the lesion is well established, the course of the disease is prolonged. The original lesion may heal in a few days only to appear anew on an adjacent finger or area of the hand. Occasionally the infection may pass through several remissions extending over a period of several months. Two such cases (not treated by these industrial surgeons) are known to have resulted in the amputation of a finger. They became secondarily infected following incision in an attempt to establish drainage. Although no separate record of this infection is made, statements of the industrial surgeons in charge of our three packing plants lead me to believe there are about two hundred such infections yearly.

Infection with the bacillus of swine erysipelas is a definite industrial hazard, but it frequently occurs among farmers and in spite of commercial club statements this region is primarily a farming community. My own cases have been farmers or veterinarians; were of two to six weeks' duration when first seen; and had been treated with various local applications without success. The following case is typical.

Mrs. P., a farmer's wife, forty-eight years of age, first noticed a bright red area surrounding a small blister at the base of the right thenar eminence on October 26, 1933. Iodine was applied locally without effect. In a week's time the entire thenar eminence became bluish-red and movement of the thumb was painful. The lesion advanced less rapidly in a proximal direction, but when she consulted a doctor on November 5, 1933, the entire thumb and volar surface of the wrist were involved. Pain was sufficient to interrupt sleep. Her physician incised the thenar eminence over the original lesion. No pus was found. Hot boric packs were applied intermittently for several days and the hand was again incised on November 15. Slight improvement ensued. The hand and forearm were placed in continuous hot packs until November 20, at which time ichthiol ointment was tried. On December 1 a brilliant red area appeared proximal to the old lesion; the patient complained of aching pains in the arm and hand, some soreness in the axilla and her temperature, normal until now, rose to 99.2°.

This patient was first seen by me on December 2, 1933. Her temperature was 99°; pulse, 84. There were no general symptoms other than fever and slight soreness in the axilla. Due to the fact that one of the most characteristic lesions in swine is a vegetative endocarditis her heart was carefully examined. Blood culture was not attempted. The right thumb and anterior surface of the wrist were bluish-red in color, somewhat swollen and movement of the thumb caused pain. The incision wounds on the base of the thenar eminence were fairly well healed. The diagnosis was clear.

Klauder and Harkins reported a few cases which they had treated with an autogenous immune serum with excellent results. No immune serum for human use is made in the United States at the present time. In Germany, where swine erysipelas has been known for many years, an immune serum for human use is available and there are reports of a few cases of human infection which were successfully treated with it. Simple clarified immune serum which is so strikingly successful in the treatment of swine is safe enough to give to humans if one wishes to assume the risk of a possible urticaria or so-called serum sickness.

After the patient had shown no sensitivity to intradermal injections, 20 c.c. of Pitman Moore swine erysipelas antiserum were injected around the lesion in three separate areas. The next day 20 c.c. of the same serum were injected under the loose skin in the lumbar region. In twenty-four hours the patient's temperature was normal, the soreness in the axilla had disappeared and there was visible improvement in the appearance of the lesion. The pain and sensitiveness to pressure was markedly decreased. With no local treatment

other than protective, the patient rapidly improved. She was discharged December 7, 1933.

Two previous cases treated with the same immune serum responded equally well. Three other cases who refused serum treatment returned to their family physician and were finally cured after five, eight and eleven weeks respectively.

It is possible that x-ray therapy may be of value in these cases.

REFERENCES

1 Klauder, J. V., and Harkins, M. J.: Erysipeloid in the United States. Jour. Am. Med. Assn., xcvi:1205-1209.(April 11), 1931.
2. Klauder, J. V., Righter, L. L., and Harkins, M. J.: A distinctive and severe form of erysipeloid among fish handlers. Arch. Dermat. and Syph., xiv:662-678 (December), 1926.
3. Ward, A. R.: The etiology of polyarthritis in swine. Jour. Am. Vet. Med. Assn., lxi:155, 1922.
4. Munce, T. W., and Willey, L. E.: Enzoötic swine erysipelas. North Am. Vet., xiii:No. 3, 1932

DIAGNOSIS OF CEREBRAL VASCULAR ACCIDENTS AND OTHER INTRACRANIAL COMPLICATIONS ARISING FROM TRAUMA*

DORRELL G. DICKERSON, M.D., F.A.C.S.,
Los Angeles

Intracranial vascular accidents resulting from craniocerebral trauma usually determine the immediate seriousness of a head injury. The principal clinical forms of intracranial bleeding are:

1. Hemorrhage from the middle meningeal artery and sphenoparietal sinus
2. Subdural bleeding (acute and chronic) from short communicating cerebral veins
3. Bleeding from larger dural venous sinuses
4. Hemorrhage into cerebral ventricles (from vein of Galen)
5. Subarachnoid hemorrhage.

Other complications arising from trauma to the head usually occur later. Chief among these are:
1. Pneumocephalus, (traumatic äerocele)
2. Traumatic brain abscess
    a. Direct extension from compound fractures
    b. Extension from fracture implicating an air sinus
3. Septic meningitis.

Intracranial bleeding from any source produces symptoms chiefly from pressure. This is usually associated with various degrees of contusion and laceration of brain substance. Localized bleeding within the cranial cavity acts very much the same as a new growth except that the displacement of cerebrospinal fluid and space occupation by the clot is much more rapid. The location, accessibility and the rate of clot formation, to a certain extent, determine the prognosis. Hem-

*Read before the Harbor Branch Los Angeles County Medical Society, Long Beach, California, March 28, 1933.

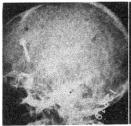

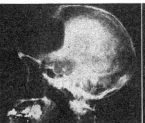

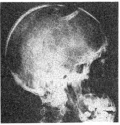

Fig. 1. Metallic drainage tube in abscess of frontal lobe, showing method of treatment in traumatic brain abscess. Recovery.

Fig. 2. Photograph of craniogram showing traumatic pneumocephalus. Duration, five months. Symptoms, headaches, slow pulse rate and maniacal type of psychosis. Air evacuated through frontal osteoplastic flap with suture of dura mater. Recovery.

Fig. 3. Photograph of craniogram showing depressed fracture involving superior longitudinal sinus. Elevation, with recovery.

orrhage into the subarachnoid space, if it becomes stationary before grave pressure symptoms develop, offers a better prognosis than other forms of intracranial hemorrhage. Extradural bleeding, if diagnosed and treated in time offers a fairly good outlook. The prognosis increases in gravity with each succeeding hour after the first two or three. Practically all those patients having suffered from the effects of an extradural hemorrhage for a number of hours with delayed diagnosis, succumb even with operation.

Bleeding from the dural venous sinuses is usually a grave situation. Many die before anything can be done. Hemorrhage into the cerebral ventricles is practically always fatal. On the other hand, delayed clot formation in the subdural space gives the most favorable prognosis if diagnosed and evacuated within a reasonable time after symptoms of increased intracranial pressure have developed.

In those suffering from head trauma, intracranial bleeding may occur from one or a number of points. However, we should be able, clinically, to recognize the principal groups and accordingly classify each case. The failure to recognize hemorrhage from the middle meningeal artery will mean a certain fatality. In a patient who has suffered craniocerebral injury and who subsequently develops signs and symptoms of increased intracranial pressure, the question of bleeding from the middle meningeal artery always arises. This form of hemorrhage offers the most favorable prognosis if diagnosed and corrected early.

The anatomic position of the middle meningeal artery places it in a highly favorable location for injury. It enters the middle cranial fossa through the foramen spinosum and after running a short distance it divides into the anterior and posterior divisions. Anatomic anomalies occur. Its loca-

tion on the outer surface of the dura mater, often lying in a shallow bony groove or bridged over by a thin bony arch, renders it easily susceptible to injury. Usually all extradural hemorrhages are accompanied by fracture and are due to injury of the vessel by a sharp serrated edge of bone. Occasionally a brisk blow on the temporoparietal bones will produce injury by a bending process. Many extradural hemorrhages are due to injury of the sphenoparietal sinus.

During childhood there is little, if any, depth to the bony channel for the middle meningeal artery, but during middle life, and especially in old age, the groove widens and deepens. In early adult life the dura strips with ease from the inner table. In advanced years the dura becomes more adherent and cannot be separated from the inner table without some difficulty. For these reasons epidural hemorrhage is seen more often in young and middle aged adults. Children are rare victims although they are not exempt. The aged are more apt to escape due to adherence of the dura mater to the inner table.

As a rule the clinical picture of epidural hemorrhage is rapid in its development. More than fifty per cent of those suffering from extradural bleeding succumb within the first twenty-four hours. Many are found dead after they have traveled a considerable distance from the scene of the accident. Sometimes they find their way into a police cell and die without recognition of the condition. If there are no superficial signs of external cranial violence it is an easy matter to overlook extradural hemorrhage. There is an unusually high mortality from this form of intracranial bleeding due to poor diagnosis.

Extradural hemorrhage is an old story. It has often been discussed and numerous articles have been written on it, but we should continue to emphasize the necessity for prompt diagnosis.

In the average case of hemorrhage from the middle meningeal artery or the sphenoparietal sinus there is a characteristic picture with the following steps:

1. Loss of consciousness at the time of injury
2. Recovery of consciousness (There are some rare exceptions to this.)
3. Finally, the development of signs of increased intracranial pressure characterized by coma, slowing of the pulse rate and increased blood pressure.

In general, if bleeding is from a torn middle meningeal artery, and it is in most instances, the onset of symptoms is fairly rapid. In some exceptional cases several days may elapse before alarming pressure signs appear. Bleeding from the sphenoparietal sinus is often found in epidural hemorrhage. In fact it accounts for many more hemorrhages of this nature than are usually suspected.

The symptoms of epidural hemorrhage are clear cut. There is the history of a head injury followed by a period of unconsciousness of variable extent; the patient rallies from this and is usually free from symptoms for some time, perhaps a number of hours. During this period the patient usually experiences a dull headache. The masking of the free interval may occur from a prolongation of the period of concussion. As a rule, however, there is complete restoration of brain function following the period of concussion.

The diagnosis is based on the history, roentgenologic examination of the skull showing evidence of a fracture line in the temporoparietal region, progressive slowing of pulse rate, increased blood pressure and perhaps neurologic signs of focal brain irritation; that is, signs involving the motor cortex in the prerolandic face and arm areas. A unilateral pupillary dilatation is of high diagnostic value as indicating the side of injury. Eyeground findings are unreliable as signs of increased intracranial pressure are rarely seen except in the terminal state.

Subdural Hemorrhage. Accompanying many fractures of the base of the skull and, in general, most moderately severe head injuries, subdural accumulations of blood occur. These clots usually gravitate toward the base and, aside from the general symptoms of fracture of the base of the skull, never produce sufficient focal signs to be of practical surgical importance. Injuries to the dural sinuses at the base of the skull account for many of these clots.

There is another form of subdural blood clot commonly referred to as ingravescent subdural bleeding or chronic subdural hematoma. This is invariably due to a previous craniocerebral injury. In many instances a history of trauma may be lacking or else so trivial that it has escaped attention or has been forgotten. These hematomas may be unilateral or bilateral. They are due to a smart blow dislocating the movable cerebrum and thereby tearing one or more of the short cerebral communicating veins entering the superior longitudinal sinus.

These hematomas may also occur from injury to veins elsewhere in the cranial cavity. Usually there will not be any noticeable symptoms for several weeks. During this time the slow accumulation of venous blood becomes encapsulated and forms a virtual tumor mass, mechanically speaking.

Headache is the first symptom. It is dull and aching, very much the same as in tumor of the brain. However, it disappears when the patient is put to bed or is given medication. Emesis and nausea may also occur. As the hematoma compresses the brain, focal as well as general symptoms develop. Mental dullness, retardation of speech and thought and, in many instances, distinct psychotic symptoms develop which may result in the patient being sent to an institution which treats mental disorders.

The eyegrounds may or may not disclose signs of increased intracranial pressure. Likewise, the cerebrospinal fluid offers no positive proof because many show clear fluid and normal pressure. Many will reveal a faint xanthochromic tint with moderate elevation of pressure. Pulse rate may be lowered.

An associated fracture of the skull is rarely found. The neurologic signs are those of an expanding lesion in the cerebral hemisphere. This often accounts for the erroneous diagnosis of tumor. In late cases bilateral neurologic signs develop resulting in bilateral extensor toe signs, abolishment of the deep reflexes of the legs, and the presence of bilateral ankle clonus. In these cases it may become necessary to resort to insufflation of air directly into the cerebral ventricles properly to localize the clot.

Bleeding from Dural Venous Sinuses. Hemorrhage from a dural venous sinus is always a serious situation. If there is no external evidence of fracture, localization of the bleeding point may be impossible and the hemorrhage disclosed only at postmortem. Compound wounds are usually accompanied by terrific hemorrhages.

The lateral and superior longitudinal sinuses are the principal ones exposed to trauma. The superior longitudinal sinus, when torn or occluded, presents a classical neurologic syndrome, which was first described by Sargent and Holmes[1]. Injury to the lateral sinus may provoke symptoms referable to the occipital lobes or the cerebellum. Injury to the superior longitudinal sinus and its lacunae is usually due to a depressed fracture of the vault. Depressed fragments in the middle region of the longitudinal sinus, in addition to injuring the walls of the sinus, occlude the venous system or channels entering the superior longitudinal sinus. This occlusion produces venous stasis which results in symptoms involving the paracentral lobules. There is spasticity of intense degree involving principally the lower extremities, especially the feet and legs. The extremities may be so rigid that extreme extensor adductor spasm may prevent voluntary movement. Involvement of the arms is usually only slight in degree, if at all. Bilateral ankle clonus, Babinski's sign and grossly exaggerated deep reflexes practically always occur. Sensory phenomena of a purely cortical type also occur. As a rule these sensory defects principally affect the lower extremities.

Trauma involving the lateral sinus results principally from direct blows. Velter[2] showed that lateral sinus injuries usually produced fatal results.

Hemorrhage into the Cerebral Ventricles. Hemorrhage into the ventricles from trauma is usually due to injury of the vein of Galen. These form a relatively small group of the clinical subdivisions of head injury patients. Many, when first examined, appear in good condition and present little, if any, evidence of serious intracranial damage. Some of these cases give a history of an occipital blow. The duration of initial unconsciousness may be relatively short or entirely lacking. There is a steady rise in the pulse and respiratory rates and a rapid rise in temperature to a hyperthermic state.

With these symptoms there is headache and vertigo. Later the patients become extremely restless, and stupor finally develops. At first positive neurologic signs are absent but later bilateral extensor toe signs, ankle clonus and spasticity of the lower extremities develop. As the bleeding continues the ventricles fill, cyanosis appears and an extreme state of body rigidity develops. Lumbar puncture yields massive blood stained cerebrospinal fluid under low pressure.

Subarachnoid Hemorrhage. The presence of free blood in the cerebrospinal fluid accompanies many cases of so-called cerebral concussion. The presence of blood in the cerebrospinal fluid gives rise to more or less mild meningeal and cortical irritative symptoms. There are mild rises in temperature, generalized headache, irritability, photo-

phobia and some neck stiffness. Leukocytosis also accompanies the picture. Bagley[3] demonstrated that laked blood injected into the cerebrospinal fluid pathways of dogs produced meningeal irritation. Essick[4] confirmed these observations.

Subarachnoid hemorrhage may vary from a mild, symptomless condition with slight bleeding to profound hemorrhage with early death. A craniocerebral injury with or without skull fracture may cause rupture of the smaller vessels in the pia arachnoid. It is practically always present to some degree in most cerebral traumas and is frequently associated with contusion of the cerebral cortex.

The complications other than vascular, which often confront us in patients suffering from head injuries are about three in number. First in importance are the septic complications. Usually

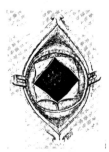

Fig. 4. Drawing of subdural clot exposed through exploratory enlarged burr opening. Symptoms for five months. Localization made by ventriculograms. Bilateral positive Babinski sign and loss of all deep reflexes in legs. Well marked psychosis present. Recovery.

portance are the septic complications. Usually these are traceable to a fracture implicating an air sinus. Septic meningitis is not uncommon in fractures radiating into the mastoid cells. Basal fractures involving the middle ear may be followed especially in children, by septic meningitis. This occurs with relative infrequency but nevertheless is an ever present source of worry even during convalescence.

Infections entering through compound fractures of the vault are common, especially in neglected or improperly treated wounds. It is peculiar that many patients with compound fractures escape septic meningitis. It has been personally observed in some cases of dirty, compound wounds, even with escaping cerebrospinal fluid, that meningitis has only infrequently followed if the wound was given prompt and thorough attention. It is in the least expected case that septic meningitis will make its appearance. The infecting organism is usually the pneumococcus, at times associated with the streptococcus. Purulent leptomeningitis occurring in the wake of a skull fracture practically always can be traced to the pneumococcus. During treatment of a head injury a sudden flare-up of temperature, the development of headache, neck stiffness and hebetude may announce the development of septic meningitis before lumbar puncture clinches the diagnosis. Children under ten years of age are more susceptible to these septic complications than any other group of patients.

There is one point which is of importance from a prognostic standpoint inasmuch as we know that this disease is inevitably fatal; that is, many of these patients will improve after the first two or three lumbar punctures with or without the injection of various forms of sera or antibactericidal preparations. One can avoid an embarrassing situation by withholding a prognosis or else adhering to the original grave outlook since, after a temporary improvement of only a few hours or

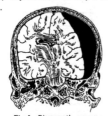

Fig. 5. Diagramatic cross section of head showing large subdural clot extending from vault to base in middle cranial fossa. Duration, symptoms two weeks. Normal eyegrounds. Cerebrospinal fluid pressure ten m.m. (Hg.) Babinski sign was the only positive neurologic finding. Evacuation of clot through burr opening with decompression. Death from hyperthermia and hypostatic pneumonia.

days at the most, these cases settle back and progress to a fatal termination. Very few ever recover.

Brain abscess is practically always chronic. An acute brain abscess following head injury is exceedingly rare. The interval from the date of injury is often from three to six months or more and in some instances, a period of years may elapse before frank symptoms develop. Usually there is a comparatively long drawn out latent interval between the injury and the development of sufficient symptoms to arouse suspicion. These are principally slight rises in temperature occurring periodically with intervals where the temperature may be subnormal. There is also an in-

sidious physical emaciation. The mentality is practically always clear. Focal symptoms may be late in developing or may never appear. One of the most reliable diagnostic signs is a slow pulse rate and subnormal temperature. Headache is dull, deeply seated and paroxysmal. There may be long periods of complete freedom from headache. Localized headache often occurs. Local tenderness and headache is due to congestion and inflammation of the dura mater overlying the abscess. If there is a history of a compound skull fracture or a fissured fracture radiating into an air sinus these symptoms are highly suggestive of an intracranial abscess. The neurologic findings may be exceedingly mild or, as is usually the case, entirely absent. Too much reliance cannot be placed on the absence of eyeground changes.

Traumatic pneumocephalus or äerocele is relatively infrequent. It occurs in injuries implicating the group of frontal and ethmoidal sinuses or the mastoid cells. In frontal fractures a persistent rhinorrhea may be one of the first indications of this condition. Cerebrospinal fluid escaping from the nostrils indicates that there has been a fracture through the frontal sinus or the ethmoidal plate. The accumulation of air over a cerebral hemisphere is a gradual process and the onset of symptoms may extend over a period of several weeks or months after an injury. The patient first complains of headache. Some of them suffer from mental disturbances. Usually the pulse rate is considerably lower than normal and the neurologic signs may be entirely lacking. The diagnosis is made by the craniogram, showing a large pocket of air over the frontal or parietal lobes.

Spontaneous recovery may occur, but very often septic meningitis develops. A considerable number will recover with proper surgical attention. Any condition which increases the intracranial pressure such as laughing, sneezing, straining, or blowing the nose is frequently the beginning of a fatal meningitis.

SUMMARY

The various forms of intracranial hemorrhage together with brain abscess, septic meningitis and traumatic äerocele are considered from the standpoint of complications of head injury. Diagnostic considerations are particularly emphasized.

REFERENCES

1. Sargent, Percy and Holmes, Gordon: Injuries of the superior longitudinal sinus. Brit. Med. Jour., ii:493-498 (January), 1915.
2. Velter, E.: Plaies du crane, Paris, 1917.
3. Bagley, C.: Blood in the cerebrospinal fluid; resultant functional and organic alterations in the central nervous system. Arch. Surg., xvii:18-38 (July), 1928.
4. Essick, C. R.: Formation of macrophages by the cells lining the arachnoid cavity in response to the stimulus of particulate matter. Contributions to Embryology, No. 42, Carnegie Institute of Washington, 272-377, 1920.

3875 Wilshire Boulevard.

INDICATIONS FOR BLOOD TRANSFU-
SION IN PEDIATRICS*

Lee Forrest Hill, M.D., Des Moines

Blood, as a therapeutic agent, offers a most valuable means of treatment, and one that is too often neglected or overlooked. Prior to 1920, transfusions of blood were restricted largely to cases of hemorrhage, and in infants, to hemorrhagic disease of the new born, but since that time the literature contains reference to its use in an ever increasing variety of conditions.

In certain of these conditions blood acts as a specific, comparing in this respect to diphtheria antitoxin, while in many others its good effects can only be attested to by clinical experience. No doubt as time goes on, and the results of transfusion can be analyzed by laboratory exactness as well as by clinical observation, a sharper distinction and more definite classification will be provided to guide the physician in the use of this most important remedy.

When the necessity for a transfusion arises the first step is the selection of a suitable donor. All authorities agree that this must be done with extreme care, in order to avoid serious reactions or possible fatalities. It is desirable that the donor belong to the same group as the patient, but whether groups are determined or not, it is absolutely necessary that cross-matching be done. It is not safe to use group IV, or universal donors, without carrying out this procedure. I should also like to emphasize here that new born infants should not receive blood intravenously until it has been determined by cross-matching that incompatability does not exist, since it has been shown that an appreciable number of infants possess agglutinins in their blood sera at birth. Sidbury[1] believes that hemolysis should be excluded as carefully as agglutination in the proper selection of a donor. It is, of course, assumed that the donor will be a person in good health and free from any contagious disease, particularly lues.

Two methods of giving blood into the vein are in vogue at the present time. Both have their advocates. The direct method, using unmodified blood, requires more technical skill but is said to be freer from reactions. The citrate method is simpler and can be performed by any one accustomed to giving intravenous injections to children. In a recent article Lewishon[2] gives detailed directions for the avoidance of chills following citrate transfusions. The sodium citrate and physiologic salt solution must be prepared with triple distilled water. The utensils used both in collecting and

* Presented before the Eighty-second Annual Session, Iowa State Medical Society, Des Moines, May 10, 11, 12, 1933.

administering the blood must be scrupulously cleaned, boiled in 0.1 per cent sodium hydroxide, rinsed and washed in triple distilled water and carefully autoclaved. When these precautions are taken post-transfusion chills are reduced to as low as one per cent. All transfusions done by us in the series shown have been by the citrate method.

The amount of blood which should be given varies somewhat with the condition for which the transfusion is being performed; 10. c.c. per pound is given by Sidbury as a safe rule to follow. In hemorrhage, and in athrepsia and anhydremia, larger quantities may be desirable; 15 c.c. per pound usually being regarded as safe in such conditions. Generally speaking it may be said that smaller repeated transfusions are safer and more effective than single larger transfusions.

In a strict sense there are few specific indications for the use of blood as a therapeutic measure in children. Among these may be mentioned actual loss of blood as in hemorrhage, hemorrhagic disease of the new born, and severe anemia, either primary or secondary. Experience, however, has shown that in addition to these definite requirements for blood there are numerous other diseases in which transfusion may be of great benefit, and frequently of life saving character. The more familiar one becomes with the use of blood the less frequently is it used as a "last resort" measure.

Unger[3] classifies the indications for transfusion in children under six headings: hemorrhage; diseases of the blood; toxemias; nutritional disturbances; shock and infection.

The necessity for, and the brilliant results obtained by, transfusion in cases of hemorrhage needs no further discussion.

Perhaps the next most important field for the use of transfusions is in the blood dyscrasias. In hemorrhagic disease of the new born, blood transfusion is an absolute specific. Subcutaneous injections of whole blood are sometimes effective but blood transfusion is safer and the earlier it is given the better.

Cases of purpura hemorrhagica are likewise greatly benefited by blood transfusion, either by controlling hemorrhage and restoring lost blood in preparation for splenectomy or, as occasionally happens, as a sole means of treatment. We have had three cases of this disease in the last few years. One of them was so nearly exsanguinated when it first came under observation that the mother readily signed an autopsy permit. Several transfusions, however, so improved the child that splenectomy was successfully performed and in the last four years no further bleeding has occurred. The second was cured by splenectomy alone, and the third was so improved by transfusions that as yet splenectomy has not been performed and no remissions have occurred.

Hemophilia is benefited by transfusion and enables many of these patients to lead a fairly normal life, but the condition is not cured. In congenital or primary anemia of infants, blood transfusion is again a life saving measure.

In the leukemias, transfusions are merely palliative and the same may be said of such conditions as erythroblastic anemia, Banti's disease, Gaucher's disease and Hodgkin's disease, all of which are diseases with a poor outlook under any circumstances. Severe secondary anemia, such as is seen following long drawn out illnesses, is readily relieved by transfusion and results in a quicker establishment of convalescence and a more rapid return to health.

From the literature one gathers that there is not entire agreement as to the value of blood transfusions in acute toxic states such as pneumonia and typhoid fever. Fear of adding to the hyperpyrexia by a reaction following the transfusion, or of overloading the right heart in cases of pneumonia, are the deterring factors in the minds of many clinicians. Offsetting this, however, is always the possibility that the donor's blood may furnish antibodies, increase the oxygen carrying power by added hemoglobin, and improve the blood flow to such an extent that the tide is turned in favor of the patient. We have transfused five children critically ill with pneumonia and have experienced no unfavorable reactions. It is our feeling at present that transfusions should be used more often in

these types of cases. As to the value of blood for its antitoxic properties in such diseases as erysipelas, scarlet fever, and infantile paralysis there can be no question. The protective power of subcutaneous injections of convalescent or parent's serum, or whole blood, in measles is now common knowledge.

Another field in which blood transfusions have proved their worth beyond all question is in the nutritional disturbances of infants and children. The anemia so frequently associated with prematurity is overcome more quickly by small repeated transfusions than by any other method. Likewise in the athreptic infant, with anemia and low food tolerance, transfusions supply the necessary "boost" for a rapid return to a satisfactory nutritional state. Cases of "milk anemia" and Von Jaksch's anemia, respond rapidly to the administration of blood. Perhaps the most spectacular results are achieved in that group of severely ill patients characterized by athrepsia, anhydremia, and acidosis secondary to a parenteral infection. Without blood and glucose the mortality rate is extremely high. Energetic administration of fluid by all possible routes, with the aid of blood transfusions, saves the lives of many of these patients. This same method of treatment is also essential in severe diarrheas and severe cases of dysentery, if the patient is to have every chance for recovery to which he is entitled.

The indication for transfusion in postoperative shock, and in traumatic shock, particularly if accompanied by hemorrhage, is so familiar to every one that no further comment is required. Cases of pyloric stenosis, empyema, and mastoiditis, are frequently benefited by a preoperative transfusion. Less well known and therefore to be especially emphasized is the importance of blood transfusion in combating the shock and toxemia of burns. Many lives would be saved by the instituting of prompt and vigorous intravenous therapy in the severely burned patient.

There remains for consideration a broad group of severely sick patients for whom transfusions are being more and more frequently employed. I refer to cases of so-called septic infections. As examples there might be mentioned mastoiditis, with lateral sinus thrombosis and septicemia, osteomyelitis with septicemia, chronic osteomyelitis, empyema, peritonitis, pyemia, chronic pyelitis, pyelonephritis, septic sore throat, septic scarlet fever, and septic arthritis. In this group of cases, blood may be of value in two ways: first, by overcoming an associated anemia, and second by furnishing antibactericidal or antitoxic properties. Unger has pointed out that the latter may be in-

HEMORRHAGE

	Cases	Deaths
Pneumonia and intestinal hemorrhage	1	0

BLOOD DYSCRASIA

Erythroblastic anemia	1	0
Aplastic anemia	1	1
Hemolytic anemia	1	1
Purpura hemorrhagica	2	0
Unclassified anemia	1	1
Hemorrhagic disease of new born	3	1
Leukemia	1	1

PREMATURITY

Prematurity	2	0

PRE- AND POSTOPERATIVE CONDITIONS

Shock-ruptured spleen	1	0
Pyloric stenosis	1	0
Burns	0	0

INFECTIONS

Pneumonia	5	0
Empyema	2	0
Peritonitis		
Primary	1	0
Secondary to appendicitis	4	1
Septicemia	6	4
Encephalitis	1	0
Congenital lues	1	0
Pyelonephritis	1	0

NUTRITIONAL STATES

Athrepsis with acidosis and anhydremia	3	0
Preceliac with secondary anemia	1	0
Total	41	10

Fig. 1. Illustrative table showing conditions for which blood transfusion has been used by the author.

creased if the donor is first immunized by a vaccine prepared from the organism isolated from the patient's own blood. Unquestionably the outstanding indication for administration of blood in this type of case is anemia. The best results are secured in those cases where the supply of bacteria to the blood stream can be shut off, as in ligation of the jugular vein in lateral sinus thrombosis and mastoiditis. While the results secured by transfusion in such seriously ill patients are bound to be variable, sometimes disappointing, sometimes very gratifying, yet up to the present time it is the best means of treatment available, and until a better one is developed, we should continue to use it.

In conclusion I would emphasize the following points:

1. Transfusion is a valuable therapeutic remedy for many conditions in infants and children.

2. Cross-matching of donor's with patient's blood should be done before every transfusion at all ages.

3. Reactions to transfusions can be largely eliminated if proper precautions are observed.

BIBLIOGRAPHY

1. Sidbury, J. B.: Review of 556 cases of blood transfusion in infants and children. Jour. Am. Med. Assn., lxxxix:855-862 (September 10) 1927.
2. Lewishon, Richard and Rosenthal, Nathan: Prevention of chills following transfusion of citrated blood. Jour. Am. Med. Assn., c:466 (February 18) 1933.
3. Unger, L. J.: Abt's Pediatrics, Vol 4:624.

716 Equitable Building.

INFANT FEEDING*

R. O. HUGHES, M.D., Ottumwa

The only scientific pediatric literature before the beginning of the eighteenth century was handed down by the Greeks. Infanticide was so prevalent elsewhere, that little or no attention was paid to such a thing as infant feeding. With the need for man power, more attention was given to the subject.

There is a note of simplicity in some of the early laws. Soranus (98-117 A. D.) advised against the use of the breast too soon after birth. Breast milk that clung to the finger nail was considered rich in butter fat; if not it was said to be watery. Tobias Katz (1652-1729) advised against too frequent nursing during the day or night. Eberle published a book in 1841, in which he discussed at great length the values of breast milk. The most valuable substitute was cow's milk with water dilutions. The bottle and silver tube was highly recommended in preference to the cup or spoon, because of the dangers of over, as well as

* Presented before the Eighty-second Annual Meeting, Iowa State Medical Society, Des Moines, May 10, 11, 12, 1933.

too rapid feeding. Strong mention is made of the importance of clean bottles, and the discarding of leftover milk. He recognized the deleterious effects, resulting when infants were fed on a stomach not entirely empty, consequently he advocated regulated periods of feeding.

Dewes published a book with views very similar to those expressed in Eberle's work. Both volumes devoted pages to the use of the wet nurse and their necessary qualifications.

An interesting attitude toward artificial feeding taken by a Dr. Clarke seemed very popular, yet possibly was the fundamental basis for many an athreptic. Quoting Dr. Clarke, "It is too presumptuous to assume that the creator of the world acted in error, and that the ignorance of man is capable to correct or make any improvement in his works." Assuming that Dr. Clarke thrived well on breast milk, not all mankind has been so fortunate, and we are still confronted with infant mortality statistics, which should be corrected. Approximately 20 per cent of the deaths of all ages occur during the first year of life; 45 per cent of these deaths are due to disturbances of the gastro-intestinal tract; 80 per cent of the deaths are in the artificially fed babies. This is proof enough that breast feeding, whole or in part, is the best feeding.

In 1898 Heubner, Germany's first pediatrician, proved by the calorimeter that the young infant required one hundred calories per kilogram, or forty-five per pound of body weight. In the breast feeding case then, it is necessary that this equivalent of food be obtained in twenty-four hours. With accurate scales that measure fractions of an ounce, one can readily determine the amount of breast milk obtained by weighing the infant before and after nursing. Care must be taken not to change any article of clothing during the interim. Once the quantity is determined, then calculations can be made as to the number of calories obtained during that particular feeding. This process may be repeated during any number of the twenty-four feedings. If the quantity is insufficient from one breast at any particular feeding, then a shorter period of nursing may be allowed from the other breast. I have made it the practice of interrupting the breast feeding at the end of ten minutes and determining the amount taken in that time. I feel that this procedure gives me some idea as to the most profitable length of nursing period, without lost energy and the swallowing of air on a dry breast. The infant is allowed to nurse the same breast again, to determine its entire contents in the event that insufficient milk was obtained. By this method it is possible to determine the length of nursing time necessary, and whether it becomes necessary to nurse both breasts at each feeding time.

No attention is paid to the quality of the breast milk, as in most instances disturbances are either due to volume underfeeding and its starvation colic, or to overfeeding, associated with swallowed air in the first instance, and gas formation in the latter. For the average baby under two months of age a three hour day schedule and four hour night schedule has been selected as the most adaptable to the mother's routine. If the required number of ounces necessary to fulfill the twenty-four hour caloric requirement is taken, then the condition of the patient is watched. Satisfactory weight gains of the usual five ounces a week or more should be made. Normal secretion and gastrointestinal function depends on regular stimulation. In addition normal growth in the breast feeder, depends upon the gradual increase in the quantity intake, rather than the ever-changing quality, as is true of so many of the artificial feedings. With this view in mind, I began using lactic acid modifications, but found the management difficult, especially in the lower classes, and it became necessary to try some other feeding.

For those babies who are deprived of breast milk, some substitute must be offered that meets certain requirements, i. e., free of injurious bacteria, and containing sufficient protein, carbohydrate, minerals, and vitamins. Cow's milk has been employed for centuries. Any failure to do well was based upon its composition rendering it undigestible. Even with modification, satisfaction was not obtained until the factor of bacterial contamination was considered. Whole citric acid milk with the addition of brown Karo syrup, six to ten per cent, has been employed in every artificial feeding case under my care, for the past two and one-half years. This feeding has been used regardless of the mental ability of the mother, and a personal demonstration is given each mother at the outset either in the home, or at the office. The following day a sample of freshly made feeding is requested as a test of their ability properly to make up the feeding.

The acid is added to the cow's milk in order to alter the size of curd formed in the stomach upon ingestion. The amount of hydrochloric acid in the average baby's stomach, causes whole unacidified cow's milk to form into large curds in contrast to the finer soft curds of breast milk. Milk so altered by citric acid forms a smaller curd, thereby speeding up gastric digestion, and prevents the vomiting of large tough curds so often encountered in non-acidified cow's milk modifications.

The preparation consists in the boiling of the whole cow's milk about three minutes, stirring constantly to prevent scum formation or the sorching of the milk; cool as rapidly as possible, again stirring to prevent scum formation. The milk should be cooled sufficiently to give the sensation of coolness, when dropped on the wrist. At this point the citric acid may be added. I have used the anhydrous form in the proportion of two grams to the pint, or four grams to the quart. As the citric acid is very soluble, four grams is dissolved in one ounce of boiled cooled water and added slowly with a spoon while the milk is being agitated. A fine precipitate will usually form at this point, which necessitates the burning of holes in the nipple, about twice the usual size in order to give freedom of flow.

Whole grade cow's milk or herd Holstein milk is preferred because the fat content more nearly coincides with that of breast milk. I have observed that whole raw milk boiled, makes a much smoother finished product than any of the pasteurized milks.

Whole cow's milk furnishes roughly twenty calories per ounce, and corn syrup one hundred and twenty per ounce. Calculating the caloric intake necessary for twenty-four hours, that amount of milk is usually made up, and divided into equal feedings and kept refrigerated. Ice is not an absolute essential, as a deep well or a cool cellar floor, with an improvised saw dust cooler, will suffice to preserve the acidified boiled milk for twenty-four hours. Each bottle is warmed for feed by setting in warm water; never by heating on the stove.

One should exercise the same care in the preparation of this food, as one would in preparing any other kind of food. Swallowing of air is still possible; over-feeding, gas formation, too frequent or irregular feedings may all occur.

I have observed that at about the fifth or sixth month anorexia develops in many of these babies. When the amount of added acid is gradually lessened, they regain their appetite and continue to digest the milk. I have since used this method of acid decrease, in stimulating the stomach to digest whole unacidified cow's milk. This is done more in the poorer classes, where the cost of the acid is an item of consideration.

Routine examinations are made and as soon as the baby is consuming a quart of milk a day, sieved food feedings are added regardless of the age of the patient. There are certain standards by which babies are judged; often falsely so. If a baby at four months of age attains head and chest measurements the weight and length of a baby, six or seven months of age, should we continue to feed him nothing but milk modifications, merely because of chronologic age? Cereal continues to be a favorite with many of us. However, I feel that those infants who are fed cereal put on weight in excess to length growth, making it very difficult to maintain the proportionate weight and length growth. I feel that vegetables are more valuable, and are the first of the accessory foods injected into the dietary. Spinach is probably the most valuable; however, a wide variety exclusive of potato is soon used. Sieved fruits are also added early, and are well tolerated by infants over five months of age. The accessory foods are given just prior to the milk feeding, either breast or artificial. Orange juice and cod liver oil are given at the end of three weeks or a month, and preferably between morning feedings after bathing. In the event one does not wish to institute accessory foods at such an early age, dried milk preparations may be dissolved into the milk modification, or egg yolks, cooked and stirred into the milk, may be employed to add to its potency.

In conclusion I wish to emphasize a few points. Breast milk has no substitute. When it comes to the use of modifications, it often depends on a "hit and miss" chance, as to what type of feeding is the proper one. Failure does not result so often from the type of feeding, as it does from the regulation of its administration. My experience with citric acid milk modification has proved that this substitute has all the necessary qualifications, because it can be made free of bacteria, concentrated in calories with sufficient protein, carbohydrate, and fat for very satisfactory growth, thus closely simulating breast milk.

LABOR COMPLICATED BY MISPLACED PLACENTA*

JAMES F. TAYLOR, M.D., F.A.C.S., Sioux City

Two years ago I discussed before this society some factors that prolong labor. At the present time I propose to dwell upon the diagnosis and the management of the main factor that prolongs labor—misplaced placenta. In my experience, a misplaced placenta is the main cause of unduly prolonged labor and unless the obstetrician is able to diagnose it in time and is prepared to meet the situation, labor will appear very prolonged and most dangerous for both the mother and the child. In discussing this subject with me, I wish you would remember that we are interested only in practical matters and we do not intend to formulate any rules for the undergraduate medical student.

* Presented before the Eighty-second Annual Session, Iowa State Medical Society, Des Moines, May 10, 11, 12, 1933.

One may distinguish six different positions of the misplaced placenta. The presence of a misplaced placenta influences especially the management of labor in breech presentation and in the posterior occipital position. The misplaced placenta occurs both in the normal pelvis and in the pelvis of the male type. Difficult as it is to manage a case with a misplaced placenta and a normal pelvis, the difficulties are much greater if the misplaced placenta is seen in a patient with a male type pelvis. In the latter case, the ilium is more abrupt and this narrows the transverse diameter, lengthening the anteroposterior diameter. The lumbar curve is deeper in this type of pelvis since there is a slight deformity of the promontory as a result of the fusion of the last lumbar vertebra with the first sacral vertebra.

The main positions of a misplaced placenta are:
1. Left lateral.
2. Right lateral.
3. Low posterior lateral left.
4. Low posterior lateral right.
5. Low posterior.
6. Low anterior.

In normal labor the muscles of the uterus, the abdominal muscles and the normally placed placenta are the main driving forces. The placenta, when misplaced, becomes a retarding factor because of a dissociation of the dynamic function of the uterine muscles. As soon as the membranes are ruptured and the amniotic fluid lost, the abdominal muscles are unable to contribute greatly as a driving force. The child then assumes a position that is compatible with the situation of the misplaced placenta while the head is usually found in the posterior occipital position.

In the presence of a misplaced placenta, I believe that the general idea to allow a woman up to thirty hours to have her baby is erroneous. The longer the delay, the thicker the contraction ring becomes; the baby assumes a more fixed position and the mother becomes exhausted. My experience has shown that waiting twelve hours in such cases is sufficient if no advancement of the head is noticed. I know then that a misplaced placenta is delaying labor and I proceed according to a routine worked out in a long series of cases.

I wrap one or two fingers in gauze and repeatedly wipe out the vagina and the surrounding tissues with liberal amounts of sterile, liquid green soap. Then I change my glove and, using the same soap as a lubricant, I introduce my fingers, one by one, into the vagina until finally my whole hand is in it. Gradually I engage my hand through the cervix up beside the baby's head, where I usually find Bandal's ring around the neck. This ring will vary in thickness according to the length of time of labor. Slowly I work my fingers through the ring and explore the lower segments of the uterus for a misplaced placenta or for a deformity of the pelvis. While in the uterus, my hand is always kept within the ruptured membranes.

LEFT LATERAL POSITION

Let us analyze the management of a case with the placenta placed on the left lateral wall of the uterus. The placenta with its bulging mass of 250 to 300 c.c. of blood pushes the baby over to the right side of the mother's spine; the arms and legs are forced against the right side of the uterine wall with the head in the right oblique lateral posterior occipital position. The delivery may be accomplished by the use of forceps or through version. If one decides to use forceps the head must be pushed back somewhat or rotated sufficiently to place the face in the right oblique. The assistant should be able to feel my hand through the abdominal wall and hold the one blade of the forceps which I have passed alongside my palm and placed on the baby's head; while doing this, I gradually withdraw my hand. The introduction of the second blade is a little more difficult. However, the blades will lock easily, provided the assistant prevents the first blade from slipping. In pulling on the forceps, one must remember the architecture of the pelvis and instead of pulling it straight forward, one must lead the forceps in a curve-like direction downward and then again upward. Such a delivery will cause no harm to the baby and practically none to the mother.

To use forceps in the posterior occipital position is dangerous. Usually the inexperienced obstetrician will place the forceps on the baby's head, will bring the baby out far enough to rotate the head into an anterior position and in such a way will bring the baby on its back on the brim of the pelvis. While doing this the shoulders rotate on the chest-wall with a crushing force. A baby above average weight will always die in such a delivery. In general, these are the cases where I nearly always use internal-external version.

Occasionally, we see that the left lateral placenta brings the baby in the right occipital position with most of the baby's back lying on the iliac fossa. Here, the longer the delay the more oblong the uterus becomes. Out of 1,250 cases I encountered the left lateral misplaced placenta in 20 cases.

RIGHT LATERAL POSITION

The management of these cases is correspondingly the same as in the left lateral group. I have encountered the misplaced placenta in the right lateral position in six cases.

LOW POSTERIOR LATERAL LEFT

When in this position, the placenta is usually situated one-half to one inch from the brim, attached to about the mid-line of the posterior wall, extending up the left side of the uterus. During contraction, the uterus descends sufficiently to bring the placenta down on the brim at the end of the oblique diameter. With an after-coming head, the placenta drags it much farther into the pelvis until the head becomes wedged in, and delivery becomes impossible. To avoid stillbirth in these cases, the only alternative is to rotate the shoulder so that it will throw the face towards the true oblique. One must take care not to bury the face in the placenta. It is evident why it is so important in breech presentation and in delayed labor, to make the examination as early as the cervix will permit. One must remember that all these babies are found in the posterior occipital position except when the child is in the breech position. The low posterior lateral left position, I have encountered in 40 cases.

LOW POSTERIOR LATERAL RIGHT

The same conditions and management prevail here as when found on the opposite side. I have encountered the misplaced placenta in this position in ten cases.

LOW POSTERIOR

When in this position, the placenta is found about one-half to one inch above the promontory and occasionally on the edge of the promontory. This position is easily diagnosed from the constant escape of wine colored blood with each successive contraction. The baby in these cases is found on its back in occiput posterior position. Occasionally, the child's back is in the anterior median line, the head pressing on the pubic bone and the forehead on the placenta. The combined action of the general uterine pressure and fetal axis pressure forces the buttocks towards the mother's abdomen on top of the placenta; while the latter forces the child's knees, arms and cord against the baby's face. Management of this position is the easiest of all since the placenta does not interfere with either oblique diameter. I have seen this position in six cases.

In the majority of the patients, the baby lies on its back while the general uterine pressure and the shortening of the uterus pushes the buttocks forward, pressing the arms, legs and cord under the baby's chin. At the same time, the bulging placenta elevates the shoulders of the baby and holds it in that position. It is obvious that delay here is unavoidable unless the diagnosis of the situation is established early.

In the first position of the lower posterior placenta the application of forceps is dangerous. To apply forceps one would have to shift the baby's head into either oblique, and this carries with it a great danger to the mother's bladder as well as to the baby's neck, since a great deal of force is required to change the position. I have delivered 27 similar cases. A cesarean section may be needed in these cases.

LOW ANTERIOR

Here the placenta is located between the umbilicus and the pubic bones. The majority of the babies are found in occiput posterior position with the back in the median line, with the legs flexed or extended and with the placenta resting on the chest wall. During contractions, the placenta holds the baby in the same position. I have seen this happen in 21 cases of this type. Occasionally, the back is in the anterior median line with the occiput buried in the placenta and the forehead resting on the promontory. Forceps applied in this position are just as dangerous as in the low posterior placenta. In these cases I always do a version. I have seen this position in three cases.

In all the described six positions of the misplaced placenta, we find either the breech or the occiput posterior presentation. I have dwelt more on the latter presentation and it remains to add a few more general words on the breech delivery. One should always make a thorough examination in a primipara as to the outlet and the inlet and this can be easily done when the buttocks are at a transverse diameter. The child can be pushed up, as in the occiput posterior position, and we can ascertain whether or not there is an assimilated pelvis at the inlet or a misplaced placenta. If there is a narrowing of the outlet, it is well to know it before we have to deliver the after-coming head. Through this examination we get the size of the head unless the baby is lying on its back in which case we use Pawlick's grip. If the child is on its back, estimation may be made from the size of its foot since the size of the foot is a fair estimate of the head. According to such an estimate, we decide whether to deliver in the usual way or to resort to a cesarean section.

The morbidity in my cases, notwithstanding the complete examinations, is practically nil; in the whole series I have lost only three babies and no mothers. These three babies I lost in my early years of practice because I did not recognize the misplaced placenta and its effects upon the after-coming head. Since I have learned to appreciate the value of a complete early examination and the influence of a misplaced placenta on the after-coming head, I have lost no babies.

Discussion

Dr. Fred Sternagel, Williamsburg: Dr. Taylor has emphasized that in all his described six positions of misplaced placenta, he finds either breech or occiput posterior presentations. Errors in the diagnosis and treatment of this latter position probably account for more infant deaths and maimed or invalided mothers than any other single obstetrical complication.

At the beginning of labor, 95 per cent of all cases are vertex presentations. In about one-third of this number the occiput is directed posteriorly. Fortunately, in the large proportion of these posterior positions, anterior rotation occurs spontaneously, but not always before the labor has been entirely too prolonged.

DeLee states that not all causes of occiput posterior positions are known or understood. There are many conditions which are believed to influence the baby's head to assume an occiput posterior position. Reason dictates that the misplaced palcenta as a causative factor has not received the consideration it deserves. I cannot understand why this possibility has not been given more thought.

Those of us doing any obstetrics at all, have had several prolonged or persistent occiput posterior positions to conduct through the course of labor. When this problem presents itself, how often we find ourselves confronted with the exasperating experience of trying to deliver that baby. Many times we have felt dissatisfied with our treatment of the case, and too often chagrined at the results.

There are many excellent contributions in the literature on this subject, but unfortunately a large part of them contain no fundamentally new principles. Dr. Taylor has given us a splendid conception of this hitherto neglected factor in prolonged labor. In view of the fact that the treatment especially of persistent occiput posterior positions, is at present by no means satisfactory, his contribution to the management of these cases is both timely and appropriate.

Dr. Emil C. Junger, Soldier: I have known Dr. Taylor for a long time. He is doing excellent obstetrical work in Sioux City. Some of you who have heard me before probably know that my discussions are not always so ultra-scientific.

If I had heard a paper on these various locations of placenta when I was a student, or when I first got out to practice, I probably would have passed up obstetrics or quit studying medicine. Anyway, I would have been scared stiff when I was called to a case of confinement. I think sometimes it is well if we do not know all these obstetric complications.

Dr. Taylor told us of the driving force of the top of the uterus and the placenta as being the main thing for expulsion power. I am located in a small town. All my people are Scandinavians. I have been there thirty-one years. Thirty-one years ago I used to keep some pretty good horses. In those days, in all the obstetric cases, the driving force of the placenta and uterus was so perfect that it was much faster than my driving force, with all the horses I had. I got there late much oftener than on time.

The thing I want to bring out is this: What is the matter now that even in a country town we can hardly ever have a baby without using forceps. No doubt the placentas are up there where they belong, in the fundus of the uterus, but the driving force is lacking. These conditions Dr. Taylor spoke about are scientific, and they are all right, and I appreciate them. I like science. I think any problem that we have is eventually going to be solved by science, but why can't we have babies today as we used to have them? What is the matter with civilization? What is the matter with our women? What is the matter with the way we live? Why isn't the placenta up where it belongs, and why isn't the uterus there and why can't it do its work? I would like to know what has gone wrong with us physically. What has gone wrong with our mode of living that makes obstetrics so difficult now? If this condition had been present thirty-one years ago, I would have quit. I would have left the town if I had had the type of obstetric cases that I have now. Among these young women getting married, there is not one out of ten that can have a baby without lots of help. I can get a whole lot more excited and much more red in the face before I am half through with a confinement, than I am now, and I am plenty excited right now. The only normal case that I have had in years, even among the Norwegians and the Swedes and the Danes was that of a woman last fall. She was out in the field helping with the corn picking, and she really had her baby (the first one) before I arrived. This was the first case of that natural kind in years.

I want to bring out this point: You men and women go home and do some missionary work as to the mode of living of these girls, so that when they get married they can have their babies without killing the doctor.

THE PRESENT STATUS OF MEDICINE*

W. W. BOWEN, M.D., Fort Dodge

Scarcely more than a generation ago there were no laws regulating the practice of medicine. All that was necessary for a young man to practice was for him to read with some doctor for two or three years and then open an office of his own; this without any preliminary education other than the ability to read and write. The American Medical Association studied the matter, and, with the assistance of physicians and others, was instrumental in establishing laws in the various states regulating the practice of medicine. I well remember when there were many doctors who had never been inside a medical school. At first one six months' course of lectures with no clinical or laboratory requirements was sufficient to admit a man to licensure; the minimum was then advanced to two courses and then to three; clinical training and

*Presented before the Eighty-second Annual Session, Iowa State Medical Society, Des Moines, May 10, 11, 12, 1933.

laboratory work were added gradually and the courses lengthened to nine months; and about thirty years ago the present high requirements were made obligatory. The man who wanted to get far in medicine was almost forced by circumstances to complete his studies in Europe.

Up to twenty-five years ago there were many cheap schools, organized usually by a group of doctors without any especial fitness as teachers and with little or no laboratory facilities. They were supported by the fees received from the students. Some of these were conducted at a profit, but their great object was to give the so-called professors a prestige in the community and to provide contacts for their private practice from their graduates. Besides these there were night schools, whereby a truck-driver could attend lectures for a few hours each night and be given a diploma after a time. These were diploma mills, but there were also out and out diploma mills whereby a man could secure a diploma merely by paying a considerable fee without attending the school at all. These were regularly chartered institutions and their diplomas admitted men to practice in some states.

Medical schools were very numerous. There were seven in Iowa; two in Keokuk, two in Iowa City, one in Des Moines, one in Sioux City and one in Council Bluffs. The last two, however, were short-lived. In the main, medical education in the United States was considered a joke in all foreign countries.

After the standards of medical education were raised to their present level, these fake schools rapidly disappeared, and medical education in America is as good and the standards are as high as they are anywhere. The medical profession and teaching institutions cleaned house, and did it well.

Not as many physicians are needed as there were a few years ago because the good roads and rapid transportation allow a doctor to see several times as many patients in rural districts as he formerly could. The same improved facilities for transportation allow patients to be far more readily carried to hospitals and medical centers. Nevertheless, there are more physicians per capita in America than in almost any other nation. The Commission on Medical Education reports that there is in America one physician to every 780 population, while in ten leading European countries there is an average of one to 1,574, with Austria having one to 880, and Sweden having one to 2,890. The Commission also reports that there are in round numbers 156,000 physicians in America and about 121,000 in active practice, and that there are also about 35,000 cultists, many of whom are practicing medicine and all of whom are treating patients. The Commission further finds that there should be one physician to every 1,000 to 1,200 and that there are already about 25,000 doctors (to say nothing of the 35,000 cultists) more than enough to supply the needs of the country.

There are seventy-six medical schools in the United States. Of these there are ten which give only the first two years and therefore graduate none. This leaves sixty-six schools that issue diplomas, and they have graduated an average of 5,224 students a year for the past five years; a few do not enter practice but about 5,000 do. Physicians who have died each year for the past five years number 2,700, and a number have retired so that about 3,000 are eliminated from practice each year, but this still leaves an added surplus of 2,000 doctors a year. In addition to this Canada has nine schools, and from thirty to forty per cent of the Canadian students come here to practice. A considerable number of American students go to European schools for their education and return to the United States to enter practice, so that, all in all, there is a marked increase each year to an already overcrowded profession.

In Iowa there is one doctor to every 928 people. The University of Iowa, College of Medicine has graduated an average of ninety-five students a year for the last five years; an average of seventy-one doctors have died in Iowa each year, so that twenty-one doctors have been added to the profession each year. This is not quite accurate because some doctors have retired and others have moved out of the state, but this variation is compensated for by other doctors moving into the state and by graduates from other schools locating here. However, the fact still remains that our medical school is graduating more than enough to supply the losses by death, retirement and removal.

The population of Iowa remains almost stationary and has done so for some time. Iowa graduates more doctors in proportion than any state in the middle west, and practically every state that has any medical schools, graduates more than the increase in population demands. Besides this Iowa graduates more cultists than regular practitioners.

There are those who contend that the cults do not harm the regular practitioner, but they are certainly mistaken. There have always been cults and quacks. Ordinarily a cult exists from a few years to a generation, but homeopathy lived over a hundred years. Chiropractic is nearing the end. There is now but one school and that one has only a small fraction as many students as it formerly had.

Any cult that begins to imitate the regular school by adding to its curriculum subjects that properly belong to a regular course of study; in other words, any cult that attempts to be scientific, will either go out of existence or eventually fuse with the regulars. This is a logical result because a cult is always based on some theory which has little or no basis, and has not been or cannot be proved by experimentations. For instance, the homeopathic school was based on the theory that a disease can be cured by using a remedy, which when given to a well person, will cause symptoms similar to those of the disease. However, when homeopathic schools introduced pathology and bacteriology into their curriculum it proved that they themselves did not believe in the theory and so homeopathy faded out. Osteopathy is based on the theory that diseases are caused by a partial dislocation of the vertabrae, they call it subluxation. Lately the schools in Kirksville, Missouri, and in Des Moines have added every subject taught in the regular school. True the courses they give are far inferior to similar ones given in the regular colleges, but the fact that they are trying to give them at all, shows that they do not have confidence in their own theory. The people will soon see that. The expense of maintaining such courses, laboratories and so forth are tremendous, and no schools can long stand it without either endowments or state aid. Those schools have little or no endowments, and the likelihood of getting state aid from taxation is very remote, so they appear doomed. At the present time, however, osteopaths constitute a problem to be considered.

An osteopath can by making certain inadequate preparations and passing a board composed of osteopaths be licensed to practice surgery. Sixteen have already been licensed, and eight are now actually practicing surgery in this state. They use any and all drugs. The law states that they shall use no curative drugs internally. They claim that very few drugs are curative, which is correct, and that they have the right to use any other drug they choose, and also have the right to use even curative drugs if they are administered hypodermically or any way other than by mouth, and some of the lower courts have held that their contention is correct. There is, however, no supreme court decision on that point.

The Christian Scientists under the guise of religion are practicing the curative art. They even give "absent treatments." For instance, some of these readers give absent treatments in obstetrics. It is humiliating for a doctor to discover after he has worked twelve or twenty-four hours on a case of labor that some Christian Science reader, giving an absent treatment from sixty miles away has received as much for his services as the physician did. I have actually known this to happen.

This country is over-hospitalized. There are approximately 7,000 recognized hospitals with about 900,000 beds. Besides these there are nearly as many more unrecognized hospitals but they are mostly small hospitals. Hospitals are by their nature semi-charitable institutions and even in good times many of them had a hard time to meet their obligations, so when the depression hit the country the hospitals felt it very early. As conditions became worse the problems of the hospitals became harder and harder until now their condition is deplorable. It was brought out in the meeting of the State Hospital Association in Marshalltown that there are now 4,000 empty hospital beds in Iowa. They have found that as their pay patients became less that the charity patients became more, and that patients who a short while ago would have been pay patients, now do not pay. There are some hospitals, however, that are over filled. They are charity hospitals, state hospitals, and government hospitals.

Our University hospital at Iowa City has a waiting list of over five thousand and it gets larger every month. The primary function of the University Hospital is to provide clinical material for the medical school, but it is getting so far away from its primary function that it is trying to treat all the indigents in the state and is depleting other hospitals everywhere. It is supported by an appropriation and the money is secured by general taxation. The appropriation has been $1,000,000 a year, but the recent legislature decreased it to $900,000 a year. The hospital cost originally $4,500,000, half from the state and half from the Rockefeller Foundation. It would have been better for the state if it had taken the $2,225,000 and built its own hospital. At least the state would have been able to conduct its own hospital and medical school without the influence of the Rockefeller Foundation.

As the Perkins, Haskell-Klaus law now is, the state pays all the expenses of indigent patients at the hospital; their board, room, nursing, drugs, laboratory work, etc., besides transporting them to the hospital and home again together with an attendant when one is necessary, including hotel bills, often a patient is transported back and forth several times.

Too many boards of supervisors and welfare workers are glad to slough off all their indigent patients onto the state because when that can be done, the county is relieved of all expense. It takes considerably more money to send them to Iowa City than to care for them in a local hospital, but the board of supervisors is free of any responsi-

bility. It costs more but the county levy does not need to be so high; yet the same taxpayers pay the bills. The care of the indigent should be a local problem and not a state problem. When it is a local problem the local officers and the local citizens see to it that the county is not looted by the undeserving; when it is a state problem, the local officers and the citizens all tend to push every case onto the state deserving or not.

I do not like the word indigent. These patients should be called paupers, for they are paupers just as much as the inmates of the county home or those on the poor list. People who would never be known as paupers are willing and glad to be taken to the University Hospital as indigents, and abuses of this nature number many hundreds each year.

The conditions arising from the University Hospital are intolerable. They have many times the clinical material they need; they are depleting the hospitals all over the state; they are competing with doctors all over the state; they are making the care of paupers a state function instead of a local function; and they are pauperizing the people over the state by treating people free who are able to pay.

Government hospitals and veterans hospitals are over-filled. The soldier who was wounded or otherwise incapacitated during his service should be cared for, and our government is doing that more lavishly than any government or nation in the history of the world, but the government has been spending hundreds of millions of dollars building hospitals and taking care of veterans who have no service connected disability. This is terribly wrong. There is no reason why these men now in the vigor of manhood should be public charges. President Roosevelt has put a stop to much of it, which a servile Congress never would do. The veterans hospital in Des Moines will soon open. As soon as Congress takes back its authority, now vested in the President, this hospital, and all veterans hospitals will be another menace to other hospitals. If the government elects to take care of all these ex-soldiers it can do so cheaper and better in the hospitals already built and there are ample facilities for doing it in the seven thousand hospitals with their nine hundred thousand beds.

The Committee on the Costs of Medical Care has aroused attention all over the country. The majority report, in brief, is that the doctors, nurses, and dentists be organized around hospitals already existing; they would necessarily be on a salary basis; and that the patients also be organized in groups of 5,000 to 10,000 around the same hospitals; and that they pay for their services in monthly installments by some insurance scheme, or partly by insurance and partly by taxation. Now, part insurance, and part taxation will eventuate in all taxation, and that means that all the curative professions will be on a basis of state medicine. The minority report varies materially from the majority report, and has found favor with the American Medical Association, and with doctors everywhere.

The doctor should meet all these socializing schemes by quiet resistance or non-cooperation, and the means of combating them is the county medical society, which is the unit of all organized medicine, and is most conversant with local affairs. If an attempt is made to socialize medicine in any county, the county medical society need not cooperate. If some of its members incline to favor the proposition, they can be controlled first by moral suasion, and second, by suspension or expulsion from the county society. If the hospital around which the scheme is being organized, is a standardized hospital, a person not a member of the county society cannot be a member of its staff and this action would effectually block it. If the hospital is not standardized it will be more difficult, but any reputable doctor will hesitate for some time before practicing medicine in such a manner that he will be expelled from organized medicine.

Besides this general socialization of all professions connected with health, there are various plans for supporting hospitals by insurance and monthly payments. Some hospitals and some doctors are quite zealous in their favor. There are various plans, the Bailer plan of Dallas, the St. Paul plan, the Milwaukee plan, and numerous others, and they include different amounts of hospital care, some only ward rooms for three weeks, some rooms and laboratory expenses, operating room expenses, anesthetics and everything relating to hositpal expenses, any necessary length of time, and every gradation between these two extremes. Doubtless some of these are workable in some communities. In localities where there are large industries and the patient's assessments can be taken out of the pay checks by the employers and turned over to the hospital without expense of collecting, these plans sound feasible when times are good. However, even in such centers, when times are bad and men are being dropped from the pay rolls rapidly, thus causing lapsed insurance policies, it seems to me that there will be considerable difficulty in making any plan successful. I believe that in Iowa, which is so largely rural, that the expense of organizing and collecting the assessments each month will be so great as to make such a plan unworkable in most communities.

The final answer to all our problems is organized medicine. The state medical society with its con-

stituent county societies is the most important of all organizations to the doctors, whether they realize it or not, and they should pay their annual dues gladly. Our dues are really not high enough to carry on all our functions as they should be, and no one would wish us to discontinue a single function that we now carry on. In these depressed times it is hard for many to pay the dues. I think the so-called Iowa plan for care of the indigent by the county society rather than by individual doctors should be more universally adopted. It is more fair to the doctors and more satisfactory to the board of supervisors as well as to the patients, and it secures a larger membership for each county society. County and state society dues should be removed from the fund received for that work before any other distribution is made. Each man's dues are then paid without any individual effort.

MALIGNANT TUMORS OF THE OVARY, THE SUPRARENAL GLAND AND THE KIDNEY IN CHILDREN*

F. P. McNamara, M.D.

W. A. Henneger, M.D., and C. C. Lytle, M.D.
Dubuque

Because of the rarity of malignant tumors in childhood, physicians often temporize in their treatment, although it is axiomatic that the cure of all malignant tumors demands removal as soon as possible. The following cases are reported not only because of their rarity but to renew interest in them with the hope that tumors of this nature may be more efficiently treated. As two of the cases occurred in a series of twenty-nine necropsies on children, it is not unlikely that they occur more frequently than the reports in the literature would indicate. Probably many cases are undiagnosed or incorrectly diagnosed.

CASE REPORTS

Case 1. The patient, a white girl fourteen years of age, was admitted to The Finley Hospital with a complaint of "colicky pain in the region of the umbilicus and swelling of the abdomen."

Past History: Four months before she had fallen while roller skating and injured her right side. Since that time her menstrual periods which had been regular and not excessive have been associated with considerable pain and caused her to go to bed for two days each month. There was no history of loss of weight.

Present Illness: Four days before entrance she had pain of a mild degree in the region of the

* From the Pathologic and Pediatric Services of The Finley Hospital, Dubuque.

umbilicus. This was followed by nausea and vomiting. During the night she suffered from colicky pain in the region of the umbilicus. The next day she felt better but still had slight pain. She was seen the day before admission when the chief complaint was swelling of the abdomen. At that time she had a temperature of 99.7°.

Physical Examination: The patient was a well developed girl weighing 92 pounds. The general examination was negative. Locally, there was a mass in the abdomen extending from midway between the ensiform cartilage and the umbilicus down into the pelvis. It was approximately 20 cm. in diameter, felt nodular and hard and could be moved slightly from side to-side, athough this caused some pain. On rectal examination the mass

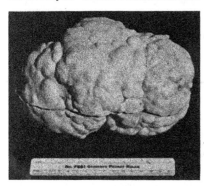

Fig. 1. Ovarian carcinoma; weight, 2,000 grams.

filled the pelvis and was apparently connected with the left ovary. The liver and spleen were negative. A provisional diagnosis of ovarian cyst was made and operation was advised.

At operation a large solid nodular tumor of the left ovary was found (Fig. 1.). The right ovary was cystic and the spleen, pancreas, and the left kidney were enlarged and nodular. Because of the involvement of the other organs only the ovarian mass was removed. The postoperative diagnosis was a malignant tumor of the ovary.

Pathologic Diagnosis: Carcinoma of the ovary.

Subsequent Course: The immediate postoperative course was uneventful and she left the hospital in two weeks. Two years later she returned because of nodular masses throughout the abdomen. She presented cachexia of an extreme degree and she seemed much older than her actual age. X-ray therapy was given and the tumor masses promptly receded. Other treatments were

given as new nodules occurred, and the tumor responded quickly to the x-rays. A few enlarged glands in the groin were more resistant but finally became only the size of peas. The change in the patient was almost dramatic and for a year and a half she seemed like a normal girl of sixteen. The neoplasm then recurred and x-ray therapy had no effect. She failed rapidly and died four years after the onset. A necropsy was refused.

Case 2. The patient, a girl three years and seven months of age, was first seen four months before death because of swelling of the abdomen.

Family History: The patient is a niece of the patient in case one who died from carcinoma of the ovary.

Past History: She was normal at birth and always seemed well.

Present Illness: The only complaint was that the mother had noticed that the patient's abdomen was enlarging. There had been no subjective symptoms and no fever.

Physical Examination: The general examination was negative. The abdomen appeared full in the upper half. There was no tenderness or muscle rigidity. A smooth mass with a definite notch, having the general outline of the liver extended four fingers breadth below the costal border. There were no enlarged lymph nodes and the spleen was not enlarged. The white blood count was 10,600; the red blood count was 4,110,000 and the hemoglobin was 62 per cent. The differential count showed: polymorphonuclears 50, small lymphocytes 30, large lymphocytes 13, eosinophiles 3, basophiles 2, and transitionals 2. A provisional diagnosis of tumor of the liver was made. Subsequently the tumor grew steadily and rapidly. There were no subjective symptoms but the child gradually lost weight. She was able to play until one week before death. The final clinical diagnosis was sarcoma of the liver.

Necropsy Report (No. 119): The positive findings were confined to the abdominal cavity. The peritoneal cavity contained a little blood tinged fluid. A large mass which arose behind the liver filled the upper half of the abdominal cavity. It had pushed the liver downward and to the left. On dissection the tumor was found to be invading the right kidney pelvis but the right adrenal gland could not be found. The liver was adherent to the main mass but had not been invaded. The vena cava contained a tumor mass fused with a postmortem clot of blood. The main mass measured 25x18x10 cms. and was estimated to weigh 3000 grams (Figs. 2 and 3). On section it was soft, very cellular, and in the deeper portions there were numerous small, hemorrhagic areas.

Microscopically the sections showed the neoplasm to be composed of round or polyhedral cells with fairly large nuclei which were rich in chromatin. Mitotic figures were numerous. The stroma was very scant and it was composed of a few connective tissue cells and capillaries. Rarely the tumor cells formed fibrils and very rarely pseudorosettes were seen.

Anatomic Diagnosis: Neurocytoma of the right adrenal gland; invasion of the right kidney and the inferior vena cava.

Case 3. The patient, a white boy fourteen months of age, was admitted to The Finley Hospital with a complaint of pain in the abdomen and loss of appetite.

Past History: He was born after a normal pregnancy and delivery. He always seemed well until about three weeks before admission when his mother noticed that he had become peevish and had lost his appetite. It was thought that his condition was due to teething. He later developed a small abscess of one buttock and he continued to fail.

Physical Examination: The patient was an anemic boy who had evidently lost weight. The skin was loose and the muscles were soft and flabby. There were no enlarged glands in the neck, axillae or groins. On percussion the heart and lungs were normal. On auscultation there were a few bronchial rales in the lower lobe of each lung. The abdomen was flat on the right side but a large, firm mass extended from the splenic region nearly to the brim of the pelvis on the left. The mass did not move with respiration and had the general contour of an enlarged kidney. On admission the patient's temperature was 102° and it fluctuated between 100° and 103° while he was in the hospital. The white blood count was 18,000 and the hemoglobin was 65 per cent. The differential count showed 75 per cent polymorphonuclear cells. An x-ray examination showed infiltrated areas in each lung, which were thought to be evidences of bronchial pneumonia. An exploratory operation was done and the diagnosis of a malignant tumor of the left kidney was made. The patient died ten days after admission.

Necropsy Report (No. 52): The body was that of an emaciated white baby boy. The important findings were those in the lungs, left kidney, liver and lymph nodes. The left kidney was surrounded by a clot of blood of recent origin. The kidney was greatly enlarged and weighed 300 grams. On section the normal architecture was

entirely destroyed by a neoplasm involving all parts of the organ. The growth extended into the pelvis of the kidney and filled the lumen of the ureter. The right kidney was not affected but the retroperitoneal nodes had been invaded by the tumor. Numerous metastases were found beneath the pleura of each lung (Fig. 4). The hilic lymph

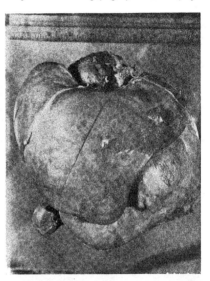

Fig. 2. Neurocytoma; the tumor is seen behind the liver; the tumor weighs 2,800 grams.

nodes showed metastases and a small mass was also found in the liver.

Microscopically the neoplasm was composed of irregularly round, polyhedral cells with large nuclei usually rich in chromatin. They tended to form solid masses and elongated strands which swept through a fairly abundant stroma of connective tissue and numerous small blood vessels.

Anatomic Diagnosis: Composite tumor of the left kidney; metastases to each lung, the liver and to the retroperitoneal and hilic lymph nodes, hemorrhages about the kidney and secondary anemia.

COMMENT

No attempt will be made to make a complete review of the literature on malignant tumors of the ovary, the suprarenal gland and kidney, as such are already available. Only the salient features of each condition will be described. The first case is carcinoma of the ovary. Tumors of the ovary in early childhood are of types similar to those encountered in adults. Cysts (simple, multilocular and dermoid), sarcomas, carcinomas, teratomas, and choriomas have all been reported. Thus, Wiel[1] in 1905, Downes[2] in 1921 and Loeb and Levy[3] in 1931 analyzed the cases reported in the literature for the different periods. Loeb summarized the statistics as follows:

ANALYSIS OF WIEL'S CASES—60 CASES UP TO 1904

Dermoid cysts	21 cases or	35.0 %
Cysts, single or multilocular	19 cases or	31.7 %
Sarcoma	15 cases or	25.0 %
Carcinoma or papilloma	5 cases or	8.3 %

ANALYSIS OF DOWNE'S CASES—26 CASES—1904 to 1921

Carcinoma or sarcoma	16 cases or	61.54%
Dermoid cysts	8 cases or	30.77%
Simple cysts	2 cases or	7.7 %

ANALYSIS OF LOEB'S CASES—35 CASES—1921 TO 1931

OVarian cysts	16 cases or	44.1 %
Teratoid cysts	9 cases or	23.71%
Terato chorio-epithelioma	1 case or	2.9 %
Carcinoma of ovary	5 cases or	14.7 %
Sarcoma	4 cases or	11.76%

Frank[4] in 1932 added two cases of carcinoma and called attention to the accompanying premature sex development. Another indication of the incidence of these tumors is that Lanman[5] found only five cases in 12,260 admissions to the surgical service of the Boston Children's Hospital over a period of ten years.

Tumors of the ovary occur most frequently during active sexual life, but are also encountered at each extreme of life with approximately the same relative frequency. In children the most important clinical sign is an abdominal mass. As in our case the growth sometimes attains considerable size before it is noted by the patient or her family unless some complication arises. Occasionally there are attacks of vague abdominal pain or a slight loss of weight may be noted. Symptoms

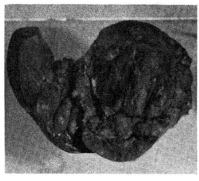

Fig. 3. A section of the tumor from behind; the right kidney is at the lower pole.

due to pressure on the bladder or rectum are seldom present because in children the uterus and adnexa are abdominal rather than pelvic organs. Anemia, constipation or diarrhea and emaciation are late symptoms and usually are due to metastases. At times there is a premature sexual development of a homosexual type (adult distribution of hair, development of breasts and external genitalia, and the initiation of menstruation). The mental age corresponds to that of the child. Other conditions, notably tumors of the pineal body or the suprarenal gland, may result in sexual precocity in children and must be considered in the differential diagnosis. Reuben and Manning[6] have shown that proved cases of pineal gland tumors associated with pubertas praecox have almost always been found in males and therefore they should offer no great difficulty in diagnosis especially if an abdominal tumor is demonstrable. With tumors or hyperplasia of the suprarenal cortex, sexual precocity is of the male type. Thus Hunt and Simon[7] state that if the patient is a male the masculine characteristics are accentuated; if a female the precocity is of a heterosexual type and consists of hypertrichosis, a change in voice and enlargement of the clitoris. Sexual precocity is also encountered in otherwise normal individuals and is thought to be due to hyperfunction of the ovary. Hunt and Simon recommend that such cases should be frequently observed as the precocity may be due to a tumor of the ovary which is not demonstrable at the first examination.

There are no clinical signs which indicate whether an ovarian tumor in a child is benign or malignant. As many of the tumors are malignant, every tumor of the ovary in a child should be assumed to be so until proved otherwise by histologic examination. The tumors metastasize to regional lymph nodes, the peritoneal cavity, the abdominal organs, and the lungs. All authorities agree that a cure demands early extirpation. This should be followed by roentgenotherapy. The neoplastic cells are of an embryonic type and are susceptible to the x-rays. While there is a definite danger of producing eunuchoidism, this should not prevent adequate x-ray therapy after the diagnosis of malignancy has been made. As in all malignant tumors, the prognosis is serious unless the neoplasm is detected early and before metastasis has occurred. There is no reason to defer operation because of the age of the patient.

Case two is an example of another well known but rare tumor of the suprarenal medulla, i. e., neurocytoma or neuroblastoma. Scott[8] in a complete review of the literature found 158 cases reported up to 1933. He added four cases of his own. . In the past these neoplasms have been called sarcoma of the liver or kidney, lymphosarcoma, glioma, malignant hypernephroma, etcetera. In 1910 Wright[9] proved that these tumors were derived from the primitive cell of the sympathetic nervous system and termed them neurocytomas or neuroblastomas. Various other names have been suggested to describe the tumors, but Wright's nomenclature is satisfactory, at least for clinical purposes. Bailey and Cushing[10] prefer the term sympathicoblastoma which indicates that the tumor originates from pluripotential cells of the sympathetic nervous system. Scott suggested a very satisfactory classification based upon the degree of differentiation of the predominating cell in a given tumor. He recognized that many of the tumors showed all degrees of differentiation of the cells. Theoretically these neoplasms might develop in any part of the central nervous system but actually they arise in the sympathetic nerve or its derivatives. The common site is the medulla of the suprarenal gland, but a few tumors have been reported in sympathetic ganglia, the retina and occasionally elsewhere in the body. Usually the tumors are unilateral, but occasionally they are bilateral. The majority are discovered early in life and Hagstrom[11] has reported a case causing fatal fetal dystocia. In Scott's report of 162 cases there were only twelve over the age of ten years. Sex is not a factor in the incidence of the tumors.

There are two clinical forms, known as the Pepper[12] and the Hutchison[13] types. The Pepper type may occur congenitally, but as a rule is discovered before the third year of life. This type tends to remain localized in the abdomen but invades blood vessels and lymphatics, although they do not form distant metastases. They may involve the liver or regional lymphatics and were known as sarcomas of the liver until Wright's studies. The Hutchison type may arise in either suprarenal gland but according to Scott did not arise in both in the cases which he reviewed. He states that the average age when the tumors are discovered is 8.5 years when primary in the left and 3.5 years when primary in the right suprarenal gland. The Hutchison type is characterized by the appearance of metastases in the bones of the skull and especially those about the orbit. As a result unilateral ecchymoses and edema of the eyelids, exophthalmos and frequently swelling in the region of the temporal bone are the first signs noted in the patient. Clinically the picture is similar to that of an injury to the eye, but the x-ray examination demonstrates the true nature of the lesion[14]. The primary tumor may be small and in the past was often overlooked until found at

necropsy. Most cases of each type are diagnosed only in advanced stages and the prognosis is extremely grave. An occasional case has apparently been cured by early removal and therefore the prognosis is not entirely hopeless. X-ray therapy has not been of value in the few cases in which it has been used.

The third case is an example of the most common malignant tumor of childhood, a composite

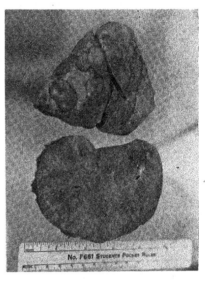

Fig. 4. Composite tumor; a section of the kidney showing replacement by the neoplasm; metastases in the lung (upper).

or mixed cell tumor of the kidney parenchyma. Kretschmer[15] states that Bugbee and Wollstein reported no cases of malignant renal neoplasms in a review of 4,903 necropsies on children; also that Lowsley and Butterfield found no malignant tumors in a series of 100 urologic lesions in infants and children. Kretschmer, however, reported seventeen cases which occurred in the Children's Memorial Hospital and the Presbyterian Hospital of Chicago. Wollstein[16] also reviewed a series of eighteen cases from the Babies' Hospital of New York in children between the ages of three and three-fourths months and six years. Probably many cases have been incorrectly diagnosed in the past. This possibility is evidenced by Kretschmer's review of the cases in the Chicago hospitals. The following histopathologic diagnoses had been previously given: multiple cell type sarcoma, myxomatous tumor, alveolar round cell sarcoma, myxomatous sarcoma and hypernephroma. Birch-Hirschfeld[17] recognized that these neoplasms contained a mixture of epithelial and connective tissue elements which proliferate in an embryonal manner. He believed that they had their origin in remnants of the wolffian body. In 1899 Wilms[18] showed that the tumors were composed of a variety of different tissues; glandular elements, smooth and striated muscles, cartilage, fat, elastic, fibrous and myxomatous tissues were nearly always present. He believed that the tumors arose from cells which had the potential quality to produce all the different types of tissue. The cell tissue was of an embryonal germinal variety still in the first stages of development and he assumed that they were displaced during embryonic life.

Composite or mixed cell malignant tumors of the renal parenchyma are usually unilateral, but are bilateral in rare cases. They retain the outline of the kidney, are encapsulated and are retroperitoneal. As it grows the neoplasm compresses the normal renal parenchyma and ultimately may completely destroy it. Hematogenous metastases are rare unless the original tumor is large and then usually occur in the liver or lungs. The tumor may break through its capsule and the peritoneum and invade the abdominal cavity where it surrounds the viscera, notably the pancreas and the suprarenal glands. The tumor also invades the pelvis of the kidney and blocks the ureter, thus explaining the absence of urinary findings which has been frequently noted.

Clinically the tumors occur before birth or within the first seven years of life. The oldest patients in Kretschmer's and Wollstein's series were six and one-half and six years of age respectively. In the former series there were fourteen boys and three girls; in the latter ten boys and eight girls. Probably sex is not a causative factor in the etiology of these tumors. The predominating sign of the presence of the tumor is a mass in the region of one kidney and rarely in the region of both. Fever and leukocytosis are also present in many cases. Pain in the abdomen, loss of appetite or weight, constipation and vomiting are less frequent symptoms. Urinalysis usually shows an essentially normal urine. In some instances albumin is present and more rarely leukocytes and red cells are found. The diagnosis is made by detecting the mass in the abdomen. Kretschmer states that in his series a palpable mass was present in every case and that in all but one it was the reason for the patient being brought to a physician. Usually the mass was discovered accidentally by the patient's mother or nurse. Kretschmer emphasized that the problems of diagnosis are the same in children as adults and that all cases should be subjected to cystoscopic examination and ureteral catheterization for the purpose of making a pyelogram and in order to determine the function of the opposite kidney. Intravenous pyelograms are also of great value in these young patients. The prognosis is bad but both Kretschmer and Wollstein report one cure each in their series (six per cent).

SUMMARY

Three cases of malignant tumors which occur early in childhood have been described. The true nature of the neoplasms was determined at necropsy in two cases; the other diagnosis was made on the surgical specimen. In the latter the final outcome confirmed the pathologic diagnosis. The patient with the carcinoma of the ovary was the aunt of the patient with neurocytoma of the suprarenal gland. This might indicate a familial tendency toward malignancy. All three tumors are rare but undoubtedly many cases are undiagnosed. As cure depends upon early diagnosis and complete removal, it is very important that every physician should realize the possibility of their occurrence in early childhood. Every abdominal mass in a child should be considered a malignant neoplasm until proved otherwise by microscopic studies.

BIBLIOGRAPHY

1. Wiel, Harry I.: A survey of ovariotomy at extremes of life. Bull. Johns Hopkins Hosp., xvi:102-109 .(March) 1905.
2. Downes, Wm. A.: Tumors of the ovary in children. Jour. Am. Med. Assn., lxxvi:443-445 (February 12) 1921.
3. Loeb, Martin J., and Levy, Walter: Ovarian cysts and tumors in children under ten years of age. Arch. Pediat., xlix:651-666 (October) 1932.
4. Frank, Robert T.: Premature sexual development in children due to malignant ovarian tumors. Am. Jour. Dis. Child., xliii:942-946 (April) 1932.
5. Lanman, Thos. H.: Ovarian tumors in children with a report of five cases. New England Jour. Med., cci:1-6 (September 19) 1929.
6. Reuben, M. S., and Manning, G. P.: Precocious puberty. Arch. Pediat., xxxix:769-785 (October) 1922.
7. Hunt, Verne C., and Simon, H. E.: Carcinoma of the ovary in infancy. Ann. Surg., lxxxvii:84-88 (January) 1928.
8. Scott, Ernest. Oliver, M. G., and Oliver, M. H.: Sympathetic tumors of the adrenal medulla. Am. Jour. Cancer, xvii:396-433 (February) 1933.
9. Wright, J. H.: Neurocytoma or neuroblastoma, a kind of tumor not generally recognized. Jour. Exp. Med., cci:1-6 (July) 1910.
10. Bailey, P., and Cushing, H.: Tumors of the Glioma Group. J. B. Lippincott, Philadelphia, 1926.
11. Hagstrom, H. T.: Foetal dystocia due to metastatic neuroblastoma of the liver. Amer. Jour. Obst. and Gynec., xix:673-676 (May) 1930.
12. Pepper, W.: A study of congenital sarcoma of the liver and suprarenal. Am. Jour. Med. Sci., cxxi:287 (February), 1901.
13. Hutchison, R.: Suprarenal sarcoma in children with metastases in skull. Quart. Jour. Med., i:33-38 (October), 1907.
14. Holmes, G. V., and Dreiser, Richard: Roentgenologic observations in neuroblastoma. Jour. Am. Med. Assn., xci:1246-1248 (October 27) 1928.
15. Kretschmer, Herman L., and Hibbs, W. G.: Mixed tumors of the kidney in infancy and childhood. Surg. Gynec. and Obst., lii:1-24 (January) 1931.
16. Wollstein, Martha: Renal neoplasms in young children. Arch. Path. and Lab. Med., iii:1-13 (January) 1927.
17. Birch-Hirschfeld, F. V.: Sarkomatose Drusengeschwulst der Niere im Kindesalter (Embryonales adenosarkom), Beitr. z. path. Anat. u. z. allg. Pathol., xxiv:343, 1898.
18. Wilms, M.: Die Mischgeschwulste, Leipzig, Arthur Georgi, 1899.

THE FINLEY HOSPITAL CLINICO-PATHOLOGIC CONFERENCE

AMYOTONIA CONGENITA (OPPENHEIM'S DISEASE)

W. A. HENNEBER, M.D., Dubuque

The case to be described presents an interesting diagnostic problem.

CASE REPORT

The patient, a girl 14 months of age, was admitted to The Finley Hospital because of inability to sit up or to hold up her head. She was the first born of young healthy parents. There was no history of a similar condition in children of the relatives. The baby seemed healthy at birth. Later the mother noticed that the baby was weak, and she had to support her head when nursing. It was then noted that she could not sit up. Aside from the weakness she had never been ill.

Physical Examination: The physical examination showed a well developed and nourished but anemic child. The mentality was normal. The general examination was negative except for the condition of the neuromuscular system. The muscles of the arms, legs and thighs, though apparently well developed, felt very flabby. The muscles of the face seemed normal. There was definite weakness of the muscles of the neck, back and extremities, but there was no paralysis. The child was unable to sit up alone and when placed on her back or stomach she was unable to turn over. There was no tenderness of the muscles and joints. The latter were hypermobile. The deep tendon reflexes were absent. The extensor muscles of the forearm were stronger than the flexors and caused a characteristic hypertension of the wrists. There were pad-like swellings about the hands and feet (Fig. 1). The sense of touch and pain seemed normal. The laboratory examination showed a moderate secondary anemia.

Differential Diagnosis: The three diseases that should be considered as possible diagnoses in this case are (1) progressive spinal muscular atrophy (Werdnig-Hoffmann type), (2) myotonia congenita (Thomsen's disease), (3) amyotonia congenita (Oppenheim's disease). There is an hereditary or familial tendency in the first two but not in Oppenheim's disease. The onset of Thomsen's disease is usually in childhood when it is noted that the patient does not play normally. The other two diseases occur during the first year of life. In the Werdnig-Hoffmann type the muscles chiefly affected are those of the pelvic girdle; in Oppenheim's disease the muscles of the extremities and trunk are the ones concerned. The deep tendon reflexes are usually present in the Werdnig-Hoffmann type but are absent in Oppenheim's disease as is true in this case. Mentality and sensations

are normal in all three conditions. In patients with Thomsen's disease, the muscles of the extremities, trunk, face and frequently those of mastication are affected. The muscles feel normal or are hypertrophied, but their contractions are weak. There is also a peculiar stiffness of the muscles when voluntary movements are attempted. In this case the muscles appeared to be of normal size but were very soft, flabby and extremely weak. The tendon reflexes are

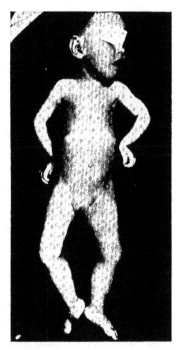

Fig. 1. Photograph of the patient. Note characteristic hyperextension of the wrists and the pads of fat over the insteps. The weakness of the muscles of the trunk, chest and extremities is apparent in the picture.

normal in Thomsen's disease. A sign which was present in our case and which is absent in both the Werdnig-Hoffmann and Thomsen's diseases is hypermobility of the joints. Based on the lack of hereditary or familial influences, the muscles affected, the extreme weakness without paralysis, the hypermobility of the joints and the absence of deep tendon reflexes as well as the age at the time of the onset, a diagnosis of Oppenheim's disease seems to be justified in this case.

Clinical Diagnosis: Amyotonia congenita (Oppenheim's disease).

Subsequent Course: The patient was given a high vitamin diet and ultra-violet ray treatments. Gentle massage was applied to the affected muscles. The child apparently was benefited somewhat and left the hospital for home where treatment was continued. The patient died rather suddenly about six weeks later of what seemed to be respiratory failure.

Necropsy Report: Externally the body appeared as described in the clinical record. There was no rigor mortis after four hours. Grossly the only striking features were the poorly developed, flabby muscles and the anemia. Miscroscopically the cells of the muscles of the extremities and the trunk were atrophic and in some instances had been replaced by connective tissue. Sections of the spinal cord taken at different levels presented similar pictures. The cells of the anterior horns were few in number and in some areas appeared to have undergone lysis. At other times the nuclei appeared pyknotic and occasionally they were surrounded by round cells.

Anatomic Diagnosis: Amyotonia congenita (Oppenheim's disease).

COMMENT

The etiology of amyotonia congenita is unknown. Whether the changes are primary in the muscles or central nervous system is still a matter of controversy. However, the weight of opinion seems to indicate that the muscle changes are secondary to the nerve changes and probably due to trophic changes. The prognosis is always serious though improvement and cure may result in the less advanced cases. Most of the patients succumb to some infection or as the result of respiratory failure. The treatment consists of giving a generous diet rich in vitamins, gentle massage and ultra-violet ray treatment. The child should be encouraged to use all the muscles in the hope of building up their tone.

RESOLUTIONS ADOPTED BY THE CATHOLIC HOSPITAL ASSOCIATION OF THE UNITED STATES AND CANADA

The following item is an excerpt from the resolutions unanimously adopted at the last annual meeting of the Catholic Hospital Association of the United States and Canada:

XXXIX. The Overcrowding of the Nursing Profession and with Relation to the Problem of the Smaller Schools of Nursing.

Whereas, the Council on Nursing Education of the Catholic Hospital Association of the United States and Canada together with its Advisory Committee representing the nursing Sisterhoods, recognizes the present overcrowded condition of the profession of nursing, and

Whereas, from many quarters the suggestion has been made that the number of future graduates in nursing can be effectively reduced by the closing of the smaller schools,

Therefore Be It Resolved as Follows:

First, that while the Council on Nursing Education accepts as a fact the temporary numerical overcrowding of the profession, we must bear in mind the distinction between the overcrowding of the profession and the unemployment in the profession on the one hand and the absolute totals of individuals engaged in the profession and the quality of professional service rendered by those individuals;

Secondly, that it regard this overcrowding as due not so much to the productivity of the smaller schools but rather to other factors among which must be prominently mentioned the relatively excessive enrollment of the larger schools, the concentration of nurses in urban areas, and particularly the nonutilization of the nurse in fields of influence and interest which the nursing profession had a solid right to expect would be open to them in response to the general demand for increased educational facilities already developed or about to be developed through the combined activities of the nursing profession itself and the colleges and universities;

Thirdly, that the Council on Nursing Education and its Advisory Committee regard the general closing of the small school merely because of its size; that is, of any school larger than that of a minimum size even though it is properly equipped as not only inimical to the best interests of nursing and the nursing profession but also as seriously endangering the interest of public health, public welfare, progressive local and national health programs, and as a discouragement to the legitimate ambitions of worthy aspirants in our smaller communities;

Fourthly, that the Council with its Committee favor the immediate creation of new avenues of employment and use of the graduate nurse not only as a measure of remedying the present unemployment situation in the nursing field but also as favoring progressive health and social programs and thereby insuring more effectively the best interests of the public;

Fifthly, that, therefore, this Council and its Advisory Committee view with considerable alarm the policies inaugurated by apparently more than one state for reducing the number of public health nurses in which field there should be rather an enlargement of opportunities for nursing service than a retrenchment if the best interests of the public are to be served;

Sixthly, that an increase of opportunities for service be offered the nurse in school health departments, in industrial health departments, in our hospitals, and in social agencies and in similar organizations and associations;

Seventhly, that, finally, for the better preservation of the small school of nursing, educational facilities be made available by public and private agencies to assist these schools in solving their educational problems and that therefore the Council and this Committee recommend to the Catholic Hospital Association the creation of a special standing committee of the Council to be designated as "The Committee on Small Nursing Schools," which should devote special attention to this problem and should report its findings at frequent intervals in the course of the next year to the Council and formulate a constructive program to be presented to the Council and later to the next annual meeting of this Association.

STATE DEPARTMENT OF HEALTH

THEY ALL BELONG TOGETHER*

"The common interests and the unity of objectives of all groups that are interested and active in public health reminds me of Henry Van Dyke's description of a certain chain of Canadian Lakes. There were many lakes in this chain, each with its own character and its own charm. He describes them. One is 'bright;' another is 'somber;' another is 'transparent;' another is 'severe with fire-scarred mountains and cliffs.' He says, 'there are many more lakes, and all are different. The thread that binds together is the little river flowing from one to another, now with a short leaping passage, now with a longer winding course. You may follow it in your canoe, paddling through the still waters, dropping down the rapids with your setting poles, wading and dragging your boat in the shallows and coming to each lake as a surprise, something distinct and separate and personal. It seems strange that they should be sisters; they are so unlike. But the same stream, rising in unknown springs, and seeking an unknown sea, runs through them all, and makes them all belong together.'

"In public health activities there are four groups of people involved. There are the workers, those who work with the workers, those who are worked upon, and the remainder of the population. I am sure there are no others. Then there are the tools and the materials and the procedures which are used in the process. Finally there are the interrelated effects of the use of materials and tools by the workers and their co-workers upon those worked upon and all the resultant influence upon all the rest of the people. Since no one of these groups can act or change its status without affecting in some measure all the other groups it becomes impossible to establish any method of measurement which will exactly define the effect and influence of any particular activity or group. Nevertheless they influence one another just as truly as do the ripples from four different stones that are cast upon the water within the same sphere of influence. I regard this as one of the fundamental factors in public health. For this reason it becomes extremely important that any contemplated activity be thought through in advance as accurately as possible. It is important to anticipate with all possible accuracy what will be the result of any proposed program upon the several groups of people under the influence of

* Excerpts from an address delivered by Fred Moore, M.D., Des Moines, Iowa, at the Eighth Annual Meeting of the Iowa Public Health Association, Des Moines, November 22, 1933.

that program. Obviously the end results should be of sufficient value to the people at large to make the effort and judgment of conflicting interests worth while.

"The tools of the workers are extremely important. Everything that is done in public health involves the use of something which we might call tools. They are chosen mostly from the fields of science and education and frequently are combinations thereof. It becomes exceedingly important that such tools should stand the tests of scientific accuracy, educational soundness, and the critical review by the most intelligent people of the community in which they are to be used.

"Public health and the practice of medicine are integral parts of medical science. Their development has been interdependent with the other aspects of medical science, no one of which has been retarded or accelerated without having some effect upon all the others. Medical history emphasizes this and reveals how the achievements of the fundamental sciences as applied in the field of medicine have builded the very foundations of public health. Witness the influence of Pasteur and Koch and Virchow and Klebs and Loeffler and Roux and von Behring. Contrast the control of disease of the present day with plagues and pestilence and cholera that devastated Europe in the middle ages; the so-called "ship fever" that made oceanic voyages an extreme health hazard, even within a hundred years, and more recently the ravages of typhoid and malaria and cholera and yellow fever in this country.

"What could have produced so great a change? In summarizing the whole panorama I believe that we will agree that the amazing progress has been due to the discoveries in the fundamental sciences of chemistry, bacteriology and biology and their practical applications by the medical and allied professions. The researches that have led to such marvelous accomplishment have been largely under the inspiration and guidance of men of medicine. The sequence of events, even though the researches were neither concerted nor co-ordinated, reveal how discoveries have emanated from individuals; how they have been applied by the practicing physician to the individual needing treatment; and finally, when measures are sufficiently developed for mass application, how they have become instruments of prevention in the hands of that division of medical science—public health.

"The American Medical Association was organized in New York in 1847 and held its first annual meeting in Baltimore in May of 1848.

"First I want to emphasize that the profession was then determined to improve its status from within. In the second place I want to call attention to the early expression of interest by the profession in public health. At the very first annual meeting in 1848 the constitution was amended to provide for a Standing Committee on Sanitary Improvement. The committee was instructed to present an annual report on the general sanitary condition of the country, compared with that of other localities, embracing as far as practicable the existing arrangements of the Prisons, Hospitals, Educational Institutions, Manufacturing establishments, etc., in their relations to the laws of health and life.

"In my judgment the sole objective in public health is *prevention*. Therefore every activity of public health organizations, be they official or voluntary, should be part of, or allied with, prevention. This viewpoint includes all activities that are related to or productive of prevention.

"At the point where services may be rendered en masse with the same benefit and protection that the individual enjoys when he receives them from his personal physician is where public health begins.

"Men engaged in fundamental fields of science have made great contributions to therapeutics. Public health may render great assistance to the practitioners. The educational profession provides superior technic in health education. The practitioner offers invaluable aid to the educator. Our efforts should not be to kill the isolated opinions and influence of all these different groups nor to control them by censorship. The fundamental thing is to collect and coordinate ideas, develop understanding and appreciation among them and organize their activities for the attainment of a definite objective."

INTEREST NEEDS ONLY PROPER DIRECTION

The officers and the membership of the county medical societies listed below have an opportunity to secure assistance in carrying out diphtheria prevention programs. Since January 1, 1934, inquiries regarding the organization and conduct of such programs have been received by the department from the counties which follow:

County	Community	Inquiry signed by
Appanoose	Exline	Supt. of Schools
Black Hawk	LaPorte	C. W. S. Nurse
Black Hawk	Dunkerton	C. W. S. Nurse
Black Hawk	Hudson	School Supt.
Boone	Boone	School Nurse
Buena Vista	Alta	School Supt.
Cerro Gordo	Clear Lake	M. D.
Cerro Gordo	Plymouth	Mrs. G. Hanson, Box 212
Davis	Pulaski	C. W. S. Nurse
Fremont	Riverton	P. T. A
Guthrie	Panora	M. D.
Guthrie	Guthrie Center	Mrs. J. C. Tallman, R. No. 2
Humboldt	Ottosen	Board of Education
Johnson	Iowa City	Univ. Elem. School Nurse
Kossuth	Swea City	M. D.
Lee	Keokuk	M. D.
Louisa	Wapello	Supt. of School
Lucas	Melrose	M. D.
Lucas	Williamson	Supt. of Schools
Monona	Moorehead	County Nurse
Marshall	LaMoille	P. T. A
Marshall	Clemens	P. T. A
Mitchell	Osage	American Legion
Osceola	Sibley	Co. Supt. of Schools
Osceola	Ashton	Nurse
Page	Clarinda	Seal Sale Com. and Kiwanis
Plymouth	Le Mars	County Nurse
Plymouth	Westfield	School Supt.
Story	Collins	P. T. A.
Scott	(Outside Davenport)	County Nurse
Taylor	Conway	Board of Education
Worth	Manly	American Legion

According to information received at this office, county-wide programs directed by the local county medical society are being organized and conducted in Adams, Cerro Gordo, Clay, Harrison, Jackson, Lucas, Lyon, Osceola, Palo Alto, Scott (rural), Sioux and Union.

PSITTACOSIS

Since the pandemic of psittacosis which caused at least 169 cases and 33 deaths in this country in 1929 and 1930, the disease has been reported in sporadic form in a number of states. During 1933, California reported three cases of this disease. Maryland, Minnesota, South Dakota and Virginia also reported single cases of psittacosis last year. The sudden onset with symptoms of chilliness, fever, severe headache, toxemia and a slight cough with very tenacious sputum, may resemble closely conditions such as influenza, bronchopneumonia and typhoid fever. Of great epidemiologic significance is the history of exposure to parrakeets, love birds or other birds of the parrot family. The incubation period ranges from eight to fifteen days. While birds infected with the virus of psittacosis may show signs of illness, some are known to be "healthy carriers."

FREE MATERIAL OFFER LIBERALIZED

Recently in announcing its policies governing the organization and conduct of county-wide preventive programs the State Department of Health agreed to provide without cost "diphtheria preventive agents in an amount sufficient to treat completely 20 per cent of children availing themselves of this opportunity, . . ." Now the department will provide without cost until July 1, 1934, or such time prior to that date whenever available funds are exhausted, 50 per cent of the toxoid (two dose treatment) and 33⅓ per cent of the alum precipitated toxoid (one dose treatment) required to carry out a county-wide diphtheria preventive program. When a county-wide program of Schick testing is carried out the department will supply all of the ready mixed toxin required without cost. The department hopes by means of this liberal offer of free material to make possible the protection of 45,000 Iowa children, prior to July 1, 1934.

PREVALENCE OF DISEASE

	Jan., '34	Dec., '33	Jan., '33	Most Cases Reported from
Diphtheria	54	56	62	Polk, Woodbury
Scarlet Fever	388	350	142	Polk, Johnson, Davis
Typhoid Fever	5	16	7	Appanoose
Smallpox	25	20	88	Allamakee, Monona
Measles	219	143	10	Fremont, Page
Whooping Cough	148	71	34	Black Hawk, Fayette
Cerebrospinal Meningitis	4	4	19	(For State)
Chickenpox	499	347	204	Black Hawk, Boone
Mumps	208	100	129	Woodbury, Wapello
German Measles	109	1	0	Black Hawk
Poliomyelitis	0	2	0	
Tuberculosis	29	18	26	(For State)
Undulant Fever	7	5	5	(For State)
Syphilis	142	129	158	(For State)
Gonorrhea	192	183	170	(For State)

The JOURNAL of the
Iowa State Medical Society
ISSUED MONTHLY

RALPH R. SIMMONS, Editor.....................Des Moines
PUBLICATION COMMITTEE
RALPH R. SIMMONS, Editor................Des Moines
ROBERT L. PARKER, Secretary................Des Moines
OLIVER J. FAY, Trustee.....................Des Moines
EDWARD M. MYERS, Trustee....................Boone

SUBSCRIPTION $3.00 PER YEAR

Address all communications to the Editor of the Journal,
1122 Bankers Trust Building, Des Moines

OFFICE OF PUBLICATION, DES MOINES, IOWA

Vol. XXIV   MARCH, 1934   No. 3

THE ANNUAL SESSION

Elsewhere in this issue of the JOURNAL will be found an official announcement, over the signature of the president of the Iowa State Medical Society, revealing the plans for the scientific session of the Society to be held in Des Moines, May 9, 10, and 11. It would seem hardly fitting and apparently unnecessary that an invitation be extended to the members of the Society to attend this annual session, since it is your annual session, authorized and conducted by you and designed to be of greatest benefit to the largest number in the Society.

Dr. R. Wesley Scott, professor of clinical medicine, at Western Reserve University School of Medicine, Cleveland, will appear on the program as the guest of the Section on Medicine, and Dr. Verne C. Hunt of Los Angeles, is the guest of the Section on Surgery. The Section on Ophthalmology, Otology, and Rhinolaryngology will follow the same plan of sectional conferences. While these meetings will be separate from those of the general assembly, the guest speaker of the section, Dr. John H. Shea, of Memphis, Tennessee, will address both groups.

Believing that active participation in the program is not only the right but the duty of every member of the Society, and, further, in appreciation of the principle that more speakers permit a more diversified program, the Committee on Arrangements, collaborating with the President, has evolved a scheme of clinics, sectional conferences, and addresses which will generously cover the entire field of medical practice. The guest speakers in surgery and medicine will appear on Thursday and Friday. Their clinics will be limited strictly to cases exemplifying the theme of their addresses. This will permit a more thorough and intensive study of a medical and surgical theme than was possible under the former plan in which

the guest speakers discussed briefly a large variety of conditions.

Each morning session of the meeting will be devoted to the reading of formal papers and the addresses of officers and guests, while the afternoon will be occupied by sectional conferences. Four separate sectional conferences will be held on Wednesday afternoon, the first day of the session, and any member will be permitted to visit the conference of his election. These conferences will discuss cardiovascular diseases and diseases of the chest; pediatrics; abdominal surgery; and urology and gynecology.

On Thursday the five clinical conferences will discuss, respectively, gastro-intestinal diseases and diabetes; neurology and psychiatry; pediatrics and obstetrics; orthopedic surgery; and roentgenology.

While this plan, in many respects, patterns after the plan observed in the meetings of the American Medical Association, the smaller groups attending the several conferences at the annual meeting of our State Society will permit much greater freedom in discussions and give the conference more of a round table character. We feel that the Committee on Arrangements deserves our sincere commendation in the preparation of this program for the annual session, and you will readily agree that the plan not only deserves but demands your support. A hand of hospitality will be extended by Des Moines to the medical profession of the state, and the citizenry of the city unite with the local medical profession in extending to you a most cordial invitation to the Capital City for this annual postgraduate medical feast.

ASPHYXIAL DEATHS

The morning paper proclaims in glaring headlines, "Prominent Business Man Asphyxiated in His Automobile." Public interest is immediately aroused by the calamity. A destitute mother and her three small children are discovered in their shabby kitchen dead from illuminating gas. Society is shocked and promotes an investigation. A new anesthetic fails in the operating room, resulting in death to the patient. Science intervenes and points the way towards safer anesthesia. Within the month, a morning paper proclaims, "Nine Students Killed by Gas in Dartmouth College Frat House." Investigations point to faulty combustion in the coal furnace. In each instance the query naturally arises, "Why should these lives have been lost?"

Statistics reporting the loss of human life through asphyxiation are incomplete and unsatisfactory. Their frequency is not denied, and the figure for the national toll has been placed by some at 50,000 deaths annually, a figure twice that due to automobile accidents. Even if the total loss of human life were only one-half or even one-fourth this figure, we would all be agreed that efforts should be directed towards the conservation of these lives.

Significant of the general interest manifest in the problem of gas poisonings at this time may be cited the organization of a National Society for the Prevention of Asphyxial Deaths,* and the keen interest now shown in the treatment of asphyxiation resulting from the inhalation of carbon monoxide gas by the use of methylene blue. The proposed activities of this national society will undoubtedly extend our knowledge of asphyxial deaths and point the way toward better methods for the prevention and treatment of these conditions. We shall watch their developments with much interest. The introduction of this new therapeutic agent, methylene blue, as a means of treating asphyxial states resulting from carbon monoxide gas has directed attention afresh to this subject and added somewhat to our knowledge concerning this condition. Since any practitioner may be called at any time to attend a case of carbon monoxide poisoning† or to render expert opinion concerning this condition it seems worthwhile to mention briefly some pertinent observations concerning this form of asphyxiation.

Inasmuch as carbon monoxide poisoning, because of its painlessness, and its rapid and comparative sureness, is a favorite mode of suicidal death, and since it is difficult and in many cases impossible to determine the intent behind a monoxide death, damage suits and suits involving accident claims with insurance companies are frequently recorded in court procedures. It becomes immediately apparent from the confusing and often contradictory evidence submitted in medical testimony that our knowledge concerning asphyxiation is incomplete and is but imperfectly understood by the average physician. This fact also stresses the importance of obtaining more accurate and definite information regarding the pharmacology and physiology involved in monoxide poisoning. The medical witness usually recalls the physical characteristics of carbon monoxide; he may remember that the gas is odorless, but he frequently becomes definitely confused by questions

regarding its corrosive, irritative or poisonous qualities and permits inaccuracy to be introduced into his statements. Careful observations indicate that the gas is non-irritative and non-corrosive, and is not itself a poison. The symptoms of carbon monoxide poisoning are those of oxygen starvation of the tissues, or anoxemia, and are the result of changes which disturb the formation of oxyhemoglobin in the blood.

Its symptomatology, its non-cumulative effect and the absence of damage to the organism after recovery, substantiates the thought that carbon monoxide either combines directly with the hemoglobin of the blood, lessening its normal oxygen carrying qualities, or that it paralyzes the catalyst of oxidation (Haldane). Since this combination or compound formed between the blood and the gas is not a stable one as indicated by the relative ease with which it is broken, all authorities agree that the treatment of the condition lies in the replacement of the carbon monoxide in the hemoglobin molecules by oxygen. Rossiter, after observing over two thousand cases of carbon monoxide poisoning, states, "The compound formed between the blood and the gas is not a very stable one and is readily broken up in the presence of oxygen. When the blood is freed of the gas it resumes its normal function again, and the corpuscles are not found to have been destroyed or altered in any way." Because of these facts all treatments heretofore have been directed toward the replacement of carbon monoxide by oxygen by means of respiratory effort. Some have advocated artificial respiration, either manually maintained or by means of a mechanical respirator; others recommend forced respiration with pure oxygen, while still others contend that the best results are obtained with a mixture of oxygen and carbon dioxide in the proportion of 93 per cent oxygen and 7 per cent carbon dioxide.

Benefit from the use of a methylene blue solution injected directly into the venous system was first observed during the treatment of a would-be suicide in which both cyanide and monoxide were considered factors. The favorable results obtained seemed to justify additional observations in cases of uncomplicated monoxide asphyxiation. In the hands of some, good and even brilliant results have been reported in these cases, while others detect no therapeutic benefit or a result not superior in any way to that obtained by former methods. All workers commending the treatment seem agreed that the mechanism by which benefits are derived involve the oxidation-reduction process. How these processes are effected has occasioned debate, and the question is apparently unsettled.

* Incorporated last year in New York and held its first annual meeting in May of 1933. Headquarters: 2 East 103rd Street, New York City. This Society lists in its board and councils medical leaders in private practice, in administrative work, in industries, in the utility and in the insurance field, as well as humanitarians, ministers and officials of the United States Army, the Navy and the public health service.
† "Most of the cases result from illuminating gas, which contains 6 to 10 per cent and is frequently inhaled with suicidal intent; but some come from defective flues of furnaces, coal stoves, charcoal fires, blast furnaces, the running of an automobile engine in a small closed garage and the 'after-damp' of mines and old wells."—Bastedo.

The promise of a new and specific treatment in any field of medical practice immediately spurs clinicians and scientists to redoubled efforts. It is reasonable to predict, therefore, that not only will the truth regarding the usefulness of methylene blue in the treatment of monoxide poisoning be determined and its mode of action revealed with reasonable promptness, but that the sum total of our knowledge regarding asphyxial states will be advanced by these efforts.

THE NORTHWEST MEDICAL CONFERENCE

A meeting of importance to the medical profession of this section of the country was held in St. Paul on Sunday, February 25. The Northwest Medical Conference, of which Iowa has been an integral part for the past four years, is an annual conference of the officers of the state medical associations of the northwest states. The states represented at the 1934 meeting were Illinois, Indiana, Iowa, Minnesota, Montana, Nebraska, North Dakota, South Dakota and Wisconsin.

The value of a discussion of problems which, by geographical proximity and singleness of purpose, are necessarily similar, can scarcely be overestimated. Keynoting and clearly reflected in the St. Paul conference were: first, a growing unrest regarding socialistic trends pointing toward state medicine and second, a renewed emphasis upon the responsibility of the medical profession to maintain its rightful leadership in lay health education.

The past year has brought new problems to the medical profession and for their solution there has been no precedent. The federal government, while offering little interference in the practice of medicine, has, through the Civil Works Administration and the Federal Emergency Relief Act, presented a challenge to the profession which can be met only by the complete cooperation of its individual members. As emphasized in a paper presented to the conference by the chairman of our board of trustees, "The Test of Organized Medicine," the profession in the present crisis is at the mercy of the individual physician. Obvious, then, is the need for a strong and unified organization, as the only possible means of combating the growing forces which would on the one hand disrupt the fundamental precepts of a profession whose ideal has always been service to humanity, and on the other, would place that service in the hands of laymen unqualified to judge its merits. It was apparent in the northwest conference that the officers of the various state organizations are alive to the urgent need for unity of the profession through

its organization. It was equally apparent that organized medicine, having perforce had its attention focused upon economic issues, is actively engaged in a campaign to direct those issues to the best interests of its members.

Dr. C. B. Wright, of Minneapolis, a trustee of the American Medical Association, who has recently spent some time in Washington, brought to the conference an optimistic message regarding the federal administration. It was his encouraging opinion that the administration has no intention of developing any permanent program for the care of the sick; that the present arrangements are only temporary, although tremendous outside pressure is being brought to bear to make the present program permanent.

Iowa is a leader among the states which have organized speakers bureaus offering postgraduate education to the physicians and health education to the laity, the latter by means of radio broadcasts and health talks to lay groups. We have not, however, made use of another medium open to the profession: the newspapers. Our reticence in this respect has been partly due to the meritorious wish of Iowa physicians to avoid any semblance of advertising. Dr. R. G. Leland, Director of the Bureau of Medical Economics of the American Medical Association, warned the conference that commercial interests outside the profession are using more and more space in the newspapers of the country for the publication of material ostensibly for the purpose of providing health education. Some of this is legitimate and of high quality, but much is misleading and pernicious. Dr. Leland urged the increased use of this medium by the organized profession in the interest, not of the physician, but of the public. There can be no question of ethics involved when the material published is purely educational in nature.

Dr. Philip H. Kreuscher, of Chicago, president of the Illinois State Medical Society, was elected president of the conference for the coming year, and Dr. Robert L. Parker, secretary of the Iowa State Medical Society, was elected secretary.

In conjunction with the conference, the annual meeting of the county officers of the Minnesota State Medical Association was held on Saturday, February 24, which guests of the conference were also invited to attend. The officers of the Iowa State Medical Society who were present were impressed with the merit of the informal discussions conducted at the meeting and felt that perhaps the custom of holding such a mid-year conference should be resumed in Iowa. It is possible that the plan may be presented for the approval of the House of Delegates in May.

THE PRESIDENT'S MESSAGE

The program for our state meeting this May will be different. In keeping with the spirit of the times, the Program Committee is offering a new deal. It will be hard for any program to be markedly better than the many good programs that have been planned and presented at our previous meetings. Appreciating this fact, the committee this year decided to present a new type of program which would offer a much greater degree of selection and variety, and it is therefore hoped and believed that it will prove more interesting.

The forenoons of each day will be given over to the regular general session meetings such as we usually have—formal papers and discussions and the medical and surgical clinics. The afternoon meetings present the innovation. They will be devoted to sectional conferences. Conferences on the various phases or fields of medicine, surgery and ophthalmology and otorhinolaryngology will be running simultaneously. In each section there will be given three concise fifteen minute talks each hour, or nine during the afternoon session. With five or six sections being held concurrently in separate rooms, there will be a total of approximately fifty talks each afternoon given by men who are really teachers— one hundred teachers during the two afternoons.

The objects of this new type of program are many: it will make possible more teachers; more practical instruction; a larger number of subjects covered; and an opportunity for a man to select the subjects in which he is most interested. In other words, the program is designed to enhance the scientific value of our state meeting—both to those taking part and to those who come to learn.

Chas B Taylor

President.

SPEAKERS BUREAU ACTIVITIES

POSTGRADUATE WORK

Postgraduate medical education in Iowa still goes on!. The latter part of February and the first of March witnessed the opening of postgraduate courses in three different centers in the state. The tentative outlines of these courses are given below:

I. GENERAL THERAPEUTICS

Creston, Iowa

Wednesday Evenings—7:00 to 9:00 p. m.

Feb. 21 Endocrinology of the Gonads:
Male Gonads—Carl R. Moore, Ph.D., University of Chicago.
Female Gonads—Floyd W. Rice, M.D., Des Moines.

28 Immunology—Paul Cannon, M.D., University of Chicago.

March 7 Cardiac Therapy—Fred M. Smith, M.D., University of Iowa.

14 Diets and Disease—Clifford J. Barborka, M.D., Chicago.

21 Allergy and the General Practitioner— Samuel M. Feinberg, M.D., Northwestern University.

28 Newer Things in Neurology and Psychology—George W. Hall, M.D., Rush Medical College.

April 4 Therapy of Gastro-Intestinal Diseases— George B. Eusterman, M.D., Mayo Clinic.

11 Hypnotics and Sedatives—A. L. Tatum, M.D., University of Wisconsin.

18 General Dermatological Conditions—Oliver S. Ormsby, M.D., Rush Medical College.

25 X-ray Diagnosis—Leo G. Rigler, M.D., University of Minnesota.

II. NEUROLOGY AND PSYCHIATRY

Oskaloosa, Iowa

Thursday Evenings—7:00 to 9:00 p. m.

March 1 Anatomy and Physiology of the Nervous System—T h o m a s B. Throckmorton, M.D., Des Moines.

8 Neurological Diagnosis—Frank A. Ely, M.D., Des Moines.

15 Poliomyelitis — Epidemic Cerebrospinal Meningitis—P. C. Jeans, M.D., University of Iowa.

22 Headaches—C. E. Van Epps, M.D., University of Iowa.

29 Mental Hygiene—A. H. Woods, M.D., University of Iowa.

April 5 Surgical Problems of the Sympathetic Nervous System—A. W. Adson, M.D., Mayo Clinic.

12 Psychoneurosis—A. H. Woods, M.D., University of Iowa.

19 Border Line Cases—William Malamud, M.D., University of Iowa.

26 Insanity—R. A. Stewart, M.D., Independence.

May 3 Tumors of the Central Nervous System— Frank A. Ely, M.D., Des Moines.

III. INFECTIOUS DISEASES

Mount Pleasant, Iowa

Friday Evenings—7:00 to 9:00 p. m.

March 2 Infections—M. E. Barnes, M.D., University of Iowa.

9 Immunity—Julius Weingart, M.D., Des Moines.

16 Some Practical Aspects of Allergy—Fred Gaarde, M.D., Mayo Clinic.

23 The State Department of Health in Relation to Infections—J. H. Kinnaman, M.D., and Carl Jordan, M.D., Des Moines.

The Present-day Management of the Following Diseases:

March 30 Infections of the Lung—John H. Peck, M.D., Des Moines, and H. W. Rathe, M.D., Waverly.

April 6 Infections of the Nervous System—F. H. Lamb, M.D., Davenport.

13 Infections in Childhood—D e n n i s H. Kelly, M.D., Des Moines.

20 Infections of the Gastro-Intestinal Tract —C. W. Baldridge, M.D., University of Iowa.

27 Surgical Treatment of Infections—H. L. Beye, M.D., University of Iowa.

May 4 Treatment of Venereal Diseases—N. G. Alcock, M.D., University of Iowa.
Federal and State Control of Venereal Diseases—F. J. Swift, M.D., Des Moines.

RADIO TALKS

WOI—Fridays, 4:00 p. m.

WSUI—Thursdays, 8:00 p. m.

March 8- 9—Sinus Trouble—J. B. Naftzger, M.D.

15-16—Varicose Veins—A. P. Stoner, M.D.

22-23—The Cause of Eyestrain—H. J. McCoy, M.D.

29-30—Malta Fever—L. R. Woodward, M.D.

April 5-6—Pleurisy—J. C. Painter, M.D.

WOMAN'S AUXILIARY NEWS

Edited by the Press and Publicity Committee

MRS. OLIVER J. FAY, *Chairman*, 10 Thirty-fifth Street, Des Moines

Appanoose County

The Appanoose County Medical Society met Thursday, January 11, with Mrs. W. E. West of Centerville. Officers elected at the business session include: Mrs. C. F. Brummitt, president; Mrs. C. S. Hickman, vice president; Mrs. E. A. Larsen, secretary; Mrs. C. M. Davis, treasurer; and Mrs. J. C. Donahue, chairman of the press and publicity committee. All officers are of Centerville.

Mrs. J. C. Donahue.

Dallas-Guthrie Auxiliary

Thursday, January 18, members of the Dallas-Guthrie Woman's Auxiliary met in conjunction with the Dallas-Guthrie Medical Society, in Adel. While in joint session following the noon dinner, E. J. Butterfield, M.D., of Dallas Center read a carefully prepared paper on Botulism, which could profitably be studied by every housewife. The Auxiliary then adjourned to the home of Mrs. C. E. Mershon where a business meeting was held.

Mrs. E. L. Bower.

Mills County

We hold two regular meetings a year in conjunction with the county medical society, and two for just our own members, that are of a more social nature. We have reviewed many interesting articles from various medical journals and books. We also have had several excellent book reviews, and our association with others of like interests, has developed a splendid feeling of fellowship among the doctors' wives to such an extent that we look forward with pleasure to our meetings, which rate 100 per cent in attendance.

Mrs. D. W. Harman.

Muscatine County Meetings

For the November meeting of the Muscatine Woman's Auxiliary we secured, through the Speakers Bureau of the Iowa State Medical Society, Milford E. Barnes, M.D., of Iowa City, who spoke to us on the Prevention of Diseases in Children. This was a joint meeting with the local Parent Teachers Association.

Mrs. B. E. Eversmeyer was hostess to the Auxiliary for the February meeting of the organization, at which time T. F. Beveridge, M.D., of Muscatine, addressed us on Amebic Dysentery. Two cases had been reported in Muscatine and we were anxious to know more about this disease.

Wednesday, February 14, the Auxiliary was entertained by Mrs. E. L. Emerson at the regular guest day tea. The feature of the afternoon's program was a talk on Holland by Mrs. F. H. Little.

Mrs. A. J. Oliver.

Pottawattamie County

Our year's program has been planned and approved along the regular study lines suggested in the JOURNAL. We have inaugurated a bit of publicity in regard to the two weekly medical broadcasts in the state. We are running the announcements in our Sunday papers on the Woman's Page as auxiliary news, and we feel that this manner of directing attention to the broadcasts will be very valuable. When possible, we will also have short articles from Hygeia published weekly, and hope that they may counteract those written by Drs. Brady, Evans, etc.

Mrs. M. C. Hennessy.

New Auxiliary Organized in Wayne County

Officers of the Woman's Auxiliary to the Wayne County Medical Society, which was organized Thursday, February 15, at a meeting in Seymour, are: Mrs. C. E. Lovett of Lineville, president; Mrs. Arthur E. Davis of Seymour, vice president; and Mrs. J. H. McCall of Allerton, secretary and treasurer.

Woodbury County

The Woman's Auxiliary to the Woodbury County Medical Society entertained the wives of the visiting members of the Sioux Valley Medical Association when that organization met at the Warrior Hotel in Sioux City, January 23 and 24. Mrs. William Jepson was chairman of registration and greeted the guests at the hotel. Auxiliary members were hostesses at a six-thirty dinner Tuesday, at the Warrior Hotel, and presented a program of readings, music and dances. Mrs. R. W. Perkins, president of the Auxiliary, presided over the dinner, which was under the direction of Mrs. P. B. McLaughlin, and Mrs. R. J. Harrington was responsible for a delightful program.

Mrs. R. W. Perkins.

SOCIETY PROCEEDINGS

Calhoun County

Tuesday, February 20, the Calhoun County Medical Society met for the regular monthly meeting at the Court House in Rockwell City. Ten members were present, and the contract with our county supervisors for the care of the indigent sick, and a revision of our county fee schedule was discussed by the various members. Both were accepted unanimously. L. E. Eslick, M.D., of Rockwell City, who was to present a paper on General Medicine, was unable to attend the meeting.

Our next meeting will be held in Rockwell City, Tuesday, March 13, at which time O. R. Prettyman, M.D., of Manson will speak on Urinalysis.

W. W. Stevenson, M.D., Secretary.

Cedar County

Members of the Cedar County Medical Society met in Tipton, Thursday, February 15, to discuss problems arising in the medical care of CWA employees. Arthur W. Erskine, M.D., of Cedar Rapids, councilor of the seventh district, was present to assist in the discussion. E. G. Kieck, M.D., also of Cedar Rapids, read a paper, illustrated with lantern slides showing some of the more common types of skin diseases.

Cerro Gordo County

Leo George Rigler, M.D., associate professor of radiology, University of Minnesota Medical School, Minneapolis, was the guest speaker for the regular meeting of the Cerro Gordo County Medical Society held in Mason City, Tuesday, February 20. His subject was The Early Diagnosis of Cancer in the Stomach.

Chickasaw County

The regular meeting of the Chickasaw County Medical Society was held Friday, February 2, at the Miller Hotel in New Hampton. After a six-thirty dinner, the speaker of the evening, Erwin von Graff, M.D., of Iowa City, presented an illustrated talk on The Dangers of Stump Cancer after Subtotal Hysterectomy.

Paul E. Gardner, M. D., Secretary.

Clinton County

Members of the Clinton County Medical Society met Thursday, February 1, in the Lafayette Hotel in Clinton, for a six-thirty dinner, after which William H. Browne, M.D., of Chicago, spoke on The Management and Treatment of Occipitoposterior Presentations. The speaker stated that he regarded the prognosis in such conditions to be much better than in breech presentations, if the physician used care in making a correct diagnosis. Dr. Browne

explained the proper application of forceps, when indicated, and also the manner of manual rotation.

E. V. Donlan, M.D., Secretary.

Floyd County

Tuesday, January 23, the Floyd County Medical Society met in regular session in Charles City, and the following papers were presented: Obstetrics, M. B. Call, M.D., of Greene; and Tularemia, F. H. Fillenwarth, M.D., of Charles City.

Hardin County

Two Des Moines physicians furnished the scientific program for the Hardin County Medical Society at a meeting held in Iowa Falls, Tuesday, February 20. Ralph H. Parker, M.D., and George A. May, M.D., presented a symposium on The Upper Respiratory Tract.

Johnson County

At the regular monthly meeting of the Johnson County Medical Society held Wednesday, February 7, in Iowa City, Isom A. Rankin, M.D., spoke on Loose Bodies in Joints, and reported a classical case of osteochondromatosis of the shoulder which had been followed for six years. Dr. Rankin's presentation was accorded an enthusiastic reception.

Horace M. Korns, M.D., Secretary.

Linn County Meetings

John H. Musser, M.D., professor of medicine, at Tulane University of Louisiana School of Medicine, New Orleans, is to be the guest of the Linn County Medical Society for its meeting Friday, April 13.

On Thursday, May 3, the program will be furnished by Fred L. Adair, M.D., professor of obstetrics and gynecology, Graduate School of Medicine, Division of the Biological Sciences, University of Chicago.

Louisa County

The Louisa County Medical Society met in Dr. O. A. Kabrick's office in Grandview, Thursday, February 10, for the regular monthly meeting. A departure from the usual scientific program was the presentation of a paper on The Relation of the Patient to the Doctor, by a layman, Mr. A. L. Holiday of Grandview.

Monona County Annual Meeting

Officers elected at the annual meeting of the Monona County Medical Society held in Onawa, Monday, January 29, include: Dr. J. S. Deering of Onawa, president; and Dr. W. H. Fairbanks of Onawa, secretary and treasurer.

Scott County

Paul B. Magnuson, M.D., assistant professor of surgery, Northwestern University Medical School, Chicago, was the speaker at the monthly dinner meeting of the Scott County Medical Society held in Davenport, Tuesday, February 6. His subject was The Type of Arthritis Which is Benefited by Surgery.

Tama County

Two Cedar Rapids physicians were speakers for the Tama County Medical Society when that organization met in Dysart, Friday, February 23. Thomas F. Hersch, M.D., spoke on Common Colds and Their Prevention, and E. G. Kieck, M.D., discussed Common Skin Diseases.

Wapello County Meetings

Tuesday, March 20, members of the Wapello County Medical Society will be addressed by Myron G. Means, M.D., of Ottumwa, on Catarrhal Jaundice; D. T. Rambo, M.D., of Ottumwa will open the discussion. William E. Olson, M.D., of Ottumwa, will furnish the scientific program for the Wapello County meeting Tuesday, April 3, speaking on The Correlation of Simple Laboratory Procedures with Clinical Findings as an Aid to Diagnosis. F. A. Hecker, M.D., also of Ottumwa, is scheduled to lead the discussion on this paper.

Wayne County Meetings

Monday, January 15, Frank A. Ely, M.D., of Des Moines spoke in Corydon before a joint meeting of the Wayne County Medical Society and the Wayne County Parent Teachers Association. His subject was The Value of Social Restraints. This was an easily understood and very educational lecture. Before the regular meeting the physicians and their wives held a covered dish luncheon at the home of Dr. B. S. Walker in Corydon.

Robert O. Hughes, M.D., of Ottumwa was the guest speaker of the Wayne County Society, Thursday, February 15, speaking on The Diagnosis of Acute Diseases of Children. Dr. H. A. Spilman of Ottumwa, councilor of the ninth district, was also present and spoke briefly.

T. D. Englehorn, M.D., Secretary.

Woodbury County

The Woodbury County Medical Society held its regular meeting Thursday, February 15, at the Martin Hotel in Sioux City. Frank Conlin, M.D., of Omaha, Nebraska, addressed the society on the following subject: A Statistical Study of 616 Cases of Diabetes, with Particular Reference to Surgical Complications.

L. E. Pierson, M.D., Secretary.

Wright County

Glen E. Harrison, M.D., of Mason City, spoke before the Wright County Medical Society in Clarion, Monday, February 12, on Infants' and Younger Children's Diseases.

First Councilor District Meeting

Approximately sixty-five physicians from counties in the First Councilor District of the Iowa State Medical Society met in Oelwein, Tuesday, January 30, for an afternoon and evening program. W. Eugene Wolcott, M.D., of Des Moines, spoke in the afternoon on Fractures of the Upper Extremity. Following the six-thirty dinner, Donald C. Conzett, M.D., of Dubuque, gave a lecture on Fractures of the Lower Extremity. Both talks were illustrated by lantern slides.

Sioux Valley Medical Association Elects Officers

Officers of the Sioux Valley Medical Association, elected at the closing session of the recent two-day convention in Sioux City, are: Dr. R. L. Perkins of Sioux Falls, South Dakota, president; Dr. C. C. Telleson of Wynot, Nebraska, first vice president; Dr. Ludwig Sogge of Windom, Minnesota, second vice president; Dr. Roscoe Jepson of Sioux City, secretary; and Dr. W. R. Brock of Sheldon, treasurer.

INTERESTING NEWS
In Brief

Dr. F. G. Banting of Toronto, discoverer of insulin, has been elected to honorary fellowship in the Royal College of Surgeons.

A group of Boston physicians reports favorable results from total thyroidectomy for the relief of congestive heart failure and angina pectoris.

Because of his especial work in furthering the conservation of human eyesight Dr. William H. Luede of St. Louis University School of Medicine, has been awarded the Leslie Dana gold medal.

Adding to our knowledge concerning adrenal physiology, observers at Columbia University state that the cortical substance has an influence on the regulation of salt and water in the body, which is of importance in maintaining the normal volume of the circulating blood.

Observers at the Carnegie Institute of Washington have observed two pituitary hormones affecting the sex glands of young animals. The one causes a premature growth in the sex glands in young animals, while the other has a reverse effect on the ovaries of mature animals.

Discoveries of Chinese life in the medieval period indicate the practice of hygienic methods for the prevention of communicable disease. Careless spitting was taboo; the educated Chinese muffled their mouths and noses when coughing or sneezing; and the individual drinking cup was an order of the Great Khan.

Experiments indicating that the fixed tissues of the body, particularly the skin, are largely concerned in the production of immunity were recently reported by Professor Reuben L. Kahn of the University of Michigan. Up to this time it has generally been accepted that immune substances are the products of blood or blood forming organs.

From observations conducted at the Royal Army Medical College in England a new and somewhat fantastic theory concerning a cause of epilepsy has been evolved. Col. W. P. MacArthur, professor of tropical medicine, believes that the larvae of the cysticercus deposited in the brain is responsible for many cases of epilepsy and may be the etiologic factor in certain cases of mania, melancholia, delusional insanity and dementia.

PERSONAL MENTION

Dr. Walter L. Bierring of Des Moines, gave the first annual address in the Clarence Martin Jackson Lectureship sponsored by the Phi Beta Pi Medical Fraternity, at Minneapolis, Tuesday, February 27. His subject was "Historical Sequence of Medical Events."

Dr. Guy B. Anderson, formerly of Ackley, has located in Ottumwa for the practice of medicine.

Dr. J. H. Sams of Clarion, read a paper on "The History of Medicine and Surgery" before the local Rotary Club, Monday, January 29.

Dr. Jacob Kulowski of Iowa City, is the author of a paper on "Pyogenic Osteomyelitis of the Sacroiliac Joint," appearing in the February, 1934, issue of the *American Journal of Surgery*.

Dr. G. E. Harrison of Mason City, spoke on "Mystery, Magic and Medicine" before the local Lions Club, Wednesday, January 31, and before the Kiwanis Club, Thursday, February 8.

Dr. L. D. Rider has recently located in Estherville for the practice of medicine and surgery. Dr. Rider is a graduate of the University of Nebraska College of Medicine, and has spent four years in general practice in Nebraska. He comes to Estherville direct from Des Moines where he has been associated with the Veterans Bureau since 1930.

Dr. Roland Stahr of Fort Dodge, delivered an illustrated lecture on "Tuberculosis" before the Parent Teachers' Association of Bode, Monday, January 22.

Dr. L. W. Clark, formerly of Chester, has located in Spring Valley, Minnesota.

Dr. C. F. Starr of Mason City, addressed the Tusalata Club of Mason City, Thursday, January 25, on "The Economics of Good Health."

Dr. Eleanor Hutchinson, until recently associated with the State Hospital for Epileptics at Woodward, has moved to Belle Plaine, where she will enter the private practice of medicine.

Dr. M. E. O'Keefe of Council Bluffs, discussed "The Goiter Problem," at a joint meeting of the Lancaster County Medical Society and the Lincoln Medical Society, at Lincoln, Tuesday, February 20.

MARRIAGES

Announcement has been made of the marriage of Miss Grace Edwards of Blairstown, to Dr. L. W. Ward of Fairbank. The ceremony took place October 21, 1933, in Galena, Illinois. Dr. and Mrs. Ward will make their home in Fairbank, where Dr. Ward has been practicing for some time.

The wedding of Miss Lillian Parrott of Chicago, and Dr. Roland B. Morrison of Carroll, took place February 10 in Chicago. Dr. Morrison is a graduate of the University of Iowa College of Medicine, and served his internship at the Washington Boulevard Hospital in Chicago. The young couple will make their home in Carroll, where the groom is associated in the practice of medicine with his father, Dr. O. C. Morrison.

DEATH NOTICES

Hickman, Mack, of Indianola, aged fifty-eight, died January 26, following a long illness. He was graduated in 1906 from the Keokuk Medical College, College of Physicians and Surgeons, and at the time of his death was a member of the Warren County Medical Society.

Hill, Leslie Grant, of Estherville, aged sixty-seven, died February 24, after an extended illness. He was graduated in 1895 from the Hahnemann Medical College and Hospital of Chicago, and at the time of his death was a member of the Emmet County Medical Society.

Wilder, Carleton Victor, of Atlantic, aged eighty-two, died suddenly February 13. He was graduated in 1882 from the Hahnemann Medical College and Hospital of Chicago, and at the time of his death was a member of the Cass County Medical Socoety.

Zinn, George, of Klemme, aged sixty-six, died suddenly January 29. He was graduated in 1897 from the Physio-Medical College of Indiana, Indianapolis, and had long been a member of the Hancock-Winnebago Medical Society.

HISTORY OF MEDICINE IN IOWA

Edited by the Historical Committee

Dr. Henry B. Young, Burlington   Dr. Tom. B. Throckmorton, Des Moines
Dr. Frank M. Fuller, Keokuk   Dr. Walter L. Bierring, Des Moines
Dr. John T. McClintock, Iowa City

The History of Medicine in Lucas County

Tom Morford Throckmorton, A.M., M.D.,
Chariton

Tom Bentley Throckmorton, B.Sc., M.D.,
Des Moines

(Conclusion)

PHYSICIANS WHO HAVE PRACTICED IN DERBY

Dr. Joseph Hagin

Dr. Joseph Hagin came to Lucas County in the early sixties. He located in Warren township, near the village of Freedom, on a farm which consisted of one hundred and twenty acres of land. The doctor was not a graduate in medicine but he soon acquired the confidence and respect of the people who lived in the community. He was a fair country doctor in the 1860's and 1870's. He officiated at the birth of the writer's youngest brother, Dr. R. Fred Throckmorton, April 9, 1869.

Dr. Hagin came to Derby about the year 1884 or 1885, where he remained for two or three years. He then moved with his family to Kansas, where he died soon afterward.

Dr. Charles Michael Throckmorton

Dr. Charles Michael Throckmorton was born, May 3, 1857, in a log house in Warren township within a mile or two of where the town of Derby was afterward located. He was the fourth son of John and Nancy (Lazear) Throckmorton. His early schooling was acquired while attending sub-scription schools and at the Harkness Academy in Garden Grove, Decatur County, Iowa. As a young man Charles taught in the country schools; also, for a few years, he was a clerk in his father's store in Derby. He then went to the Keystone state where he pursued his academic studies in Allegheny College, at Meadville, Pennsylvania. After an absence of two years, he returned home and began the study of medicine under the pre-ceptorship of the writer. This course of instruc-tion was continued for a year and on its com-pletion he matriculated in Rush Medical College, Chicago, Illinois. Here he attended lectures in the summer of 1882 and the winter of 1883; after which time he finished his medical education at

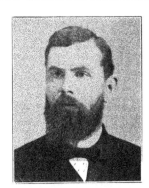

Charles Michael Throckmorton, M.D.
1857—

the Jefferson Medical College, Philadelphia, and was graduated from that institution in the class of, 1885.

He returned home and became associated with the writer in his practice at Derby. This associa-tion was continued for two years; then the doctor moved to Lucas and opened an office for himself. At that time Lucas was a thriving town. The biweekly payroll of the miners employed in that vicinity was the largest of any in the county. Dr. Charles continued to practice in his new location until the autumn of 1891 when he moved to St. Louis, Missouri, where he has since resided.

Dr. Throckmorton was married to Miss Susan McClure, of McClure, Illinois, October 28, 1891. They are the parents of one daughter, Salome; now Mrs. Walter Rohe, of Chicago, Illinois.

Dr. James Calvin Smith

Dr. James Calvin Smith was born in Indiana in 1863. He was a graduate of the Medical Department of the Iowa State University, Iowa City, Iowa, in the class of 1889. The doctor came from Afton, Union County, Iowa, to Derby, in 1889. He remained in the town but a short time. When last heard from in 1925, he was living at Miami, Florida.

Dr. Robert Frederick Throckmorton

Dr. Robert Frederick Throckmorton was born on his father's farm, near the town of Derby, April 9, 1869. He was the seventh son in a family of eleven children. His parents were John

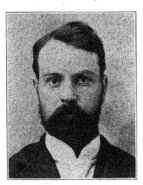

Robert Frederick Throckmorton, M.D.
1869—

and Nancy (Lazear) Throckmorton. As a boy, Fred attended the local schools. When he was sixteen years of age he enrolled in the Northwestern Normal School and Business Institute at Stansbury, Missouri, and continued his studies in that institution for two years. He then returned home and clerked in the general store, owned by his father, at Derby.

In 1889 he matriculated in the College of Physicians and Surgeons, Chicago, Illinois, and received his Doctor of Medicine degree from that institution in the class of 1892. The doctor then served one year as an interne in the United States Marine Hospital Service at Cairo, Illinois; he then returned to Derby and opened an office in the spring of 1893. Realizing the interrelationship of medicine and dentistry, Dr. Throckmorton became a student in the Columbian Dental College, Chicago, Illinois, in 1894, and was graduated from that institution in the class of 1895. He at once resumed his practice at Derby, where he cared for a large and appreciative clientele for over twenty-five years. In 1916 he built the first privately owned hospital in the county.

When the United States entered the World War, the doctor tendered his services to the government and was commissioned First Lieutenant, Medical Section, Officers Reserve Corps, July 6, 1917. He was called to active duty at Camp Dodge, Des Moines, in the following August. Here he served as a surgeon in the Base Hospital for four months; and as attending surgeon for the officers and their families, who were stationed in Des Moines, during the remainder of the war. He was honorably discharged as a Captain in the Medical Corps of the army in February, 1919. He received the commission of Colonel in the Medical Reserve Corps in 1932.

Dr. Throckmorton returned to Derby where he again took up the duties of his practice which had been interrupted because of his army activities; but the lure of the city proved too great for him to remain long in his old locality. He sold his residence and hospital to Dr. George F. Niblock, of Derby, and in the late summer of 1919 he once again became identified with the people of Des Moines.

The doctor was married to Mayme E. Penniwell, at Leon, Iowa, June 30, 1896. She was the daughter of James F. and Barbara (Wadsworth) Penniwell, old time residents of Decatur County. Four children were born to this union: Mrs. Georgia Eaton, James Frederick, Mrs. Barbara Nadine Peterson, and Robert Lazear. One son, James Frederick, followed in his father's footsteps and became identified with the medical profession. He was graduated from the Medical Department of the Iowa State University, Iowa City, in the class of 1925. Both father and son have been associated in the practice of medicine in Des Moines since January, 1932.

Dr. Tom B. Mitchell

Dr. Tom B. Mitchell was born in Monroe County, Iowa, February 27, 1856. He was raised in Lucas County on his father's farm, and received his early education in the public schools; later he attended the Valparaiso Normal School, at Valparaiso, Indiana. He then taught in the Lucas

County schools for several years. Becoming interested in the study of medicine, he became a student in the office of Dr. John W. Culley of Chariton. He later matriculated in the College of Physicians and Surgeons, Chicago, Illinois, and received his Doctor of Medicine degree from that institution in the class of 1884.

Following his graduation, the doctor practiced in Missouri for a year or two; then he moved to Chicago, where he built up a large practice during the twenty years he remained in the city.

When his health began to fail, Dr. Mitchell returned to the scenes of his boyhood days and took up residenceship in Derby. He purchased a farm in the vicinity of the town which afforded him the opportunity of overseeing and managing its care. The doctor died at his home in Derby in 1916.

Dr. George Frederick Niblock

Dr. George Frederick Niblock was born in Wisconsin in 1871. He was graduated from the University of Illinois College of Medicine, March 18, 1900. He came from Marshalltown, Marshall County, Iowa, to Derby, February 14, 1907. In the fall of 1919 he purchased the private hospital and "good will" of Dr. R. Fred Throckmorton, who had practiced in the community for over twenty-five years. With Dr. Throckmorton's removal to Des Moines, Dr. Niblock was left to care for the people in, and about, Derby. He has been the only physician there for the past fourteen years. This situation is in marked contrast to the one which the writer experienced when he was living at Derby, fifty-odd years ago. The community at that time boasted of having at least five doctors, whereas but one is needed today. Good roads, the automobile, the telephone, and who can gainsay but perhaps the airplane, have all aided in bringing about this change. Let us hope it is all for the betterment of mankind.

PHYSICIANS WHO PRACTICED ELSEWHERE
IN THE COUNTY

Lagrange

The town of Lagrange was located in the southeast corner of Cedar township, just west of the Monroe County boundary line. Mr. Samuel Prather, who owned the land, had it surveyed and the town platted in October, 1852. The town, consisting principally of eighty-eight lots, was on one of the main thoroughfares running east and west across the state. The Western Stage Company established a station at that point. Within a short time the inhabitants of the town boasted a post office, two hotels, four drygoods stores, a drug store, two blacksmith shops, a wagon and repair

shop, a cabinet and furniture shop, a shoe shop, and offices occupied by three physicians. For a number of years the town held second position in size in the county. Then came the building of the Burlington and Missouri railroad in 1866, which missed the town by a couple of miles to the south. This unforeseen development sealed the doom of this enterprising and progressive community; and gradually Lagrange passed back into farm land from whence it sprang.

The first physician, who located near the town, was Dr. William Lind. He came from Monroe County to Lucas County in 1856. He remained in the community about twenty-five years.

Dr. Robert Prather was in Lagrange in 1857. Dr. T. B. Brown and Dr. John Hays were residents of the town in an early day. The former died at thirty-two years of age and was buried in the local cemetery; the latter moved to Kansas. Dr. Trobridge was also in practice in the community in 1876. He afterwards moved to Missouri.

There is no record of the qualifications of these pioneer physicians. Much of the information concerning Lagrange and its inhabitants was given the writer by an old time friend, Mr. Charles Noble, who lived in the town from 1855 to 1865.

Freedom

Sometime between 1850 and 1860, a little village sprang into existence in Warren township. It was given the name of Freedom, and was located near the Wayne County boundary line, on Wolf Creek. In an early day it was a thriving inland town and was a trading place for the farmers who lived in that vicinity. It boasted the presence of a sawmill, a gristmill, two or more general merchandising stores, a post office, a school, a church, and a Masonic lodge, Mount Carmel Lodge No. 295. Everything was peaceful and serene with the village inhabitants until the branch line of the Burlington railroad was built from Chariton to St. Joseph, Missouri, in the early seventies. When the town of Derby, some seven miles distant from Freedom, was located on the new railroad, a gradual exodus of the inland town's villagers took place. In time Freedom became but a memory.

Following the close of the Civil War a Dr. Williams came from Missouri and located in the town. There is no record of the medical qualifications of the doctor or the name of the medical school, if any, he had attended. His wife acted in the capacity of a midwife and it was said by some people that her services were superior to those of her husband. Dr. Williams and his wife resided in the town for eight or ten years; after which time they moved to Clarinda, Page County, Iowa, where they eventually died.

Another physician who located in Freedom was a Dr. Wilkinson (or Wilkerson); his exact name is not a matter of record. As far as is known he came from Missouri, but there is no reference as to his qualifications for practicing medicine.

There were other physicians who were located in Freedom at one time or another but no record is available as to who they were, or where they came from, except that a Dr. M. Paul and a Dr. Green practiced in the community for a time.

Last Chance
Dr. Marion Thompson Martin

The first physician to locate in Union township was Dr. Marion Thompson Martin. He was born in Hancock County, Illinois, July 10, 1840. He came with his parents to Iowa the year of his birth, but there is no record of just where the family located their new home. Evidently Marion must have grown to young manhood in the state of Missouri, for we find that he was married to Hannah Josephine Stout, in Sullivan County, Missouri, January 19, 1860. Soon after the outbreak of the Civil War he enlisted in Company A, 23rd

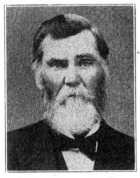

Marion Thompson Martin, M.D.
1840-1925

Missouri Volunteer Infantry, August 17, 1861. He was discharged from the army because of disability at Camp Parole, Alexandria, Missouri, December 7, 1862.

After the close of the Civil War, in 1865, Dr. Martin located at Last Chance, Lucas County, Iowa, a village in Union township which was made up largely of a few houses, a church, a post office, a general store, a blacksmith shop, a sawmill and a "corn-cracker." The latter mechanism was in

common use in an early day as a means whereby the farmers, on bringing their shelled corn to town, could get it ground into coarse meal. It was in this village that the doctor hung out his shingle and, in so doing, he announced to the world that he was ready to care for suffering humanity. He had never attended a course of medical lectures; nor was he the recipient of a medical diploma, as far as records show. Just what qualifications he may have had to warrant his practicing medicine and surgery, other than native ability, must be left to the imagination of the reader. In spite of the apparent lack of medical training, he proved himself to be a successful practitioner and he soon acquired the respect and confidence of the people in the community.

Shortly after Dr. Martin located in Last Chance, the boys in the neighborhood thought that something should be done to announce his arrival. Accordingly, on Hallowe'en, a party of "friends"(?) replaced the good doctor's gig with a pair of timber wheels. The writer recalls the incident quite well for his father brought the unusually large pair of timber wheels, such as were used for heavy logging purposes in Pennsylvania, to Iowa in 1855. The substitution of the timber-logging vehicle for the modest gig, which the doctor owned, produced a very ludicrous effect on the villagers and, with the advertising which followed the oft repeated story of the trade, it gave the newcomer a good start in the community. The doctor took the joke good naturedly, which action increased materially the respect of those individuals who were responsible for the exchange.

The doctor was well liked by the people. He became a member of Chariton Lodge No. 63, A. F. and A. M., at Chariton, in 1867. He officiated at the birth of the writer's younger brother, James Reed Throckmorton, February 24, 1867.

When the town of Woodburn, in Clark County, was laid out as a station point on the main line of what is now the Burlington railroad, Dr. Martin was attracted by the possibilities which the new town offered. Accordingly he left Last Chance and moved to Woodburn, June 19, 1875. Here he stayed during the remainder of his lifetime and died, December 20, 1925, at the ripe age of over fourscore and five years. His body was buried in the Woodburn cemetery.

Oakley

After the Burlington and Missouri railroad had been constructed across Lucas County in the late sixties, the inhabitants of the county were no longer obliged to go long distances for merchandise or food supplies. The railroad facilities removed a heretofore troublesome barrier for the convenient reception of goods. It was but natural that branch roads leading from the main line should, in time, connect this county with other counties on the north and south. In 1877, the construction of the Chariton, Des Moines and Southern Railroad was begun in the endeavor to connect the Capitol of the state with Chariton and the southern counties by way of Indianola. The road passed in a northerly direction through Liberty township. Along its right of way, the Hon. Smith Henderson Mallory, a citizen of Chariton and a promoter of the enterprise, laid out the town of Oakley in 1879. Within a short time its citizens had the convenience of a post office, an express office, a general store, a blacksmith shop, and a shipping point for their grain and stock.

Either the community was slow in growth or else it was cared for sufficiently in a medical way by physicians from Chariton or Lucas, for there is no record to show that any physician located there until 1896. Then came Dr. Ansin Elmer Murphy to care for those needing medical attention. He was a native of Ohio and a graduate of the College of Physicians and Surgeons at St. Louis, Missouri. The doctor practiced in the vicinity for four or five years and proved to be a good, faithful country practitioner. We have no record as to when he left the town or where he may have relocated.

The second physician to locate in Oakley was Dr. William D. Stumbaugh. His parents, the Rev. James and Barbara (Woods) Stumbaugh, came to Lucas County from Ohio in a covered wagon in 1855. They located in Union township where William was born and where he afterward received his early schooling. As a young man he became interested in medicine and began its study under the preceptorship of Dr. William E. Moore of Derby. He later attended a course of lectures in some homeopathic or eclectic school of medicine in Baltimore, Maryland. The certificate or diploma which was issued to him by the Baltimore school was not recognized for a time by the Iowa State Board of Medical Examiners; however, he was permitted later to practice homeopathic medicine by that body, as shown by his certificate which was filed in the county, August 12, 1897. The doctor located at once in Oakley where he continued to practice for a number of years. He then moved to Lacona, Warren County, Iowa. He was married to a Miss Admire, a daughter of Mr. and Mrs. Jacob Admire, who were pioneer settlers in Lucas County. Dr. Stumbaugh died suddenly about 1927.

-Norwood

Otter Creek township is located in the northwest corner of Lucas County. Near its center is a small inland town named Norwood.* The first physician who lived in the township was a Dr. Baker. There is no record of the length of time he remained in the county. Apparently the call of the west proved too alluring to the doctor, for we find that he departed for the far west, presumably to grow up with the country.

A Dr. Molesworth likewise resided in Norwood, or near its vicinity, at one time. There is no record of when the doctor came to, or left, the county.

The writer has no knowledge of any physician being located in Otter Creek township in the last forty years.

Williamson

When the Rock Island railroad extended its line through Lucas County in 1911, the little village of Williamson sprang into existence a few miles northeast of Chariton, and became a station point of the newly built railroad. It was here that Dr. William Clark Fisher located in April, 1927.

Dr. Fisher was born in Salem, Henry County, Iowa, October 22, 1870. His parents were Joseph W. and Lany (Clark) Fisher. Young William attended the public schools in Salem. In 1887 the family moved to Clarinda, where William was graduated from the Clarinda High School in 1890. He received his medical education in the Medical Department of the Iowa State University, Iowa City, Iowa, and was graduated from that institution in the class of 1893. After his graduation, Dr. Fisher began the practice of medicine at Clarinda. Six years later he moved to Rapid City, Pennington County, South Dakota, where he remained until 1907. He then returned to Clarinda, where he continued in the practice of medicine until May, 1917, when he came to Lucas County and located at Tipperary, a small inland mining town. He moved to Williamson in April, 1927 where he has since resided.

Dr. Fisher was married to Miss Lovina S. Osborn, of Clarinda, Iowa, May 10, 1898. Their

*Now that the highway connecting Indianola, Liberty Center and Lucas is completed, we find that Norwood has been left off the main thoroughfare, apparently more isolated from the well beaten path of man than in the days when travel by means of horse and buggy reigned supreme.

family consists of Mrs. Lydia Wilhelmina James, Mrs. Lovina Ellen Enslow, and Merriam Clark. The latter is at present studying dentistry in the Iowa State University.

AFTERWORD

The last chapter of the History of Medicine in Lucas County has been finished. Its pages record a resumé of the settlement of the county since 1848 and the rôle played by those physicians who, at one time or another, have practiced medicine within its borders. Hand in hand with the development of town and farm enterprises, the construction of railroad lines—east and west, north and south—and the establishment of the coal mining industry, there has been found the ever present physician, the harbinger of medical science and skill. The names of one hundred fifty-nine men and women, who have served the people of Lucas County to a greater or lesser extent in the field of medicine during the past eighty-five years, have been recorded. Without doubt, there have been other members of the great profession of medicine who have practiced in the county, but it has been impossible for the authors to obtain any information concerning them. However, no physician, who has ever located in the county, has been overlooked, intentionally. In the compilation of the history, the names of the physicians, with few exceptions, have been arranged in chronologic order as based on the year they began the practice of medicine in the county.

Synchronous with the rôle played by these various physicians there was evolved in the lives of the people that intangible something which became the center around which the history of Lucas County has been built. Of the one hundred fifty-nine physicians whose names are recorded, only fifteen remain to carry on the work so nobly begun by their predecessors. There are ten physicians now living at Chariton; two at Russell; one at Lucas; one at Derby; and one at Williamson. To these individuals, devoted to the great cause of humanity and to the ideals of medicine, the authors would leave this word of admonition. May they never forget the high standard which those physicians, who have preceded them, left as a heritage, nor the subtle influence which their professional acts had on the building of character among the members of the county profession. May they also bear in mind the words of the poet who, in the joy of his heart, exclaimed—

Heights by great men reached and kept
Were not attained by sudden flight;
But they, while their companions slept,
Were toiling upward in the night.

To the individual who, in the dim distant reaches of time, shall take upon himself the task of bringing up to date the History of Medicine in Lucas County, the authors trust that what has been recorded herein may be found of some value to him in carrying on the task which to them has been a "labor of love."

Tom Morford Throckmorton, M.D.
Tom Bentley Throckmorton, M.D.

OBITUARIES

DELBERT WARREN McCRARY
1868-1934

Delbert Warren McCrary, for thirty-three years a practitioner of medicine at Lake City, Calhoun County, died suddenly, January 9, at the age of sixty-six, after a heart attack while on a vacation in Texas.

He was graduated in 1893 from the University of Iowa College of Medicine, and after a brief sojourn at Anthon, Iowa, located in Lake City, where amid the swamps of a prairie country, he endured the hardships of a rural practice which helped to undermine his health. On August 17, 1890, he was married to Miss Anna Encell of Lake City, and to them were born three children, one of whom, Dr. Warren E. McCrary, entered the medical profession. In 1918, Dr. McCrary and his son established the Lake City Hospital. He had been active in the community life, in later years undergoing the trying experiences of a bank president. He was ambitious in his chosen profession, having taken numerous postgraduate courses both in America and Europe.

Dr. McCrary was never one to accept extravagant praise. His keen mind would instantly detect and reject such insincerity. He worked modestly and unassumingly, but hard and long, with eyes ever upon a goal, his Christian faith and practice guiding him away from false paths and questionable practices that would enrich his purse at the expense of his fellow man. Who can doubt that the well equipped, ably manned hospital in Lake City was a dream of his youthful days, that was slowly, even painfully realized through years of toil and sacrifice? To create is the highest aspiration of the human soul. Perhaps his contribution of life blood to the establishment of a hospital in Lake City was at times unappreciated; but insofar as he followed in the path of The Great Physician, his reward is sure.

We mourn the sudden death of Delbert Warren McCrary, our esteemed colleague and friend, and express our condolences to his aged mother, his bereaved widow, and his physician son, who survive him.

P. W. Van Metre, M.D.

THE JOURNAL BOOK SHELF

BOOKS RECEIVED

THE 1933 YEAR BOOK OF THE EYE, EAR, NOSE AND THROAT—The Eye, by E. V. L. Brown, M.D., professor of ophthalmology, University of Chicago; and Louis Bothman, M.D., associate professor; The Ear, Nose and Throat, by George E. Shambaugh, M.D., professor of otology, rhinology and laryngology, Rush Medical College of the University of Chicago; and Elmer W. Hagens, M.D., instructor in otology, rhinology and laryngology, Rush Medical College, University of Chicago. The Year Book Publishers, Chicago, 1933.

THE 1933 YEAR BOOK OF GENERAL SURGERY—Edited by Evarts A. Graham, M.D., professor of surgery, Washington University School of Medicine. The Year Book Publishers, Chicago, 1933.

MODERN CLINICAL PSYCHIATRY—By Arthur P. Noyes, M.D., Superintendent of State Hospital for Mental Diseases, Howard, Rhode Island. 485 pages. W. B. Saunders Company, Philadelphia and London, 1934. Price, $4.50.

ANNUAL REPORT OF THE SURGEON GENERAL OF THE PUBLIC HEALTH SERVICE OF THE UNITED STATES, for the fiscal year 1933. United States Government Printing

Office, Washington, D. C. For sale by the Superintendent of Documents, Washington, D. C. Price, 75 cents, cloth.

A DIABETIC MANUAL for the mutual use of the doctor and patient—By Elliott P. Joslin, M.D., clinical professor of medicine, Harvard Medical School. Fifth edition, entirely revised. Illustrated. Lea & Febiger, Philadelphia, 1934. Price, $2.00.

MEDICAL CLINICS OF NORTH AMERICA, Volume xvii. No. 4. Cleveland Clinic Number, per clinic year, July, 1933, to May, 1934. Octavo of 253 pages with 53 illustrations. W. B. Saunders Company, Philadelphia and London, 1934. Price, paper, $12.00; cloth, $16.00, net.

THE 1933 YEAR BOOK OF UROLOGY. Edited by John H. Cunningham, M.D., associate in genito-urinary surgery, Harvard University Postgraduate School of Medicine. The Year Book Publishers, Chicago, 1934.

TREATMENT IN GENERAL PRACTICE—By Harry Beckman, M.D., professor of pharmacology at Marquette University, School of Medicine, Milwaukee, Wisconsin. Second edition, 889 pages, revised and entirely reset. W. B. Saunders Company, Philadelphia and London, 1934. Price, $10.00.

BOOK REVIEWS

HANDBOOK OF CHEMOTHERAPY

Part One, Metal-Free Organic Compounds. By Dr. Viktor Fischl, departmental director of the Schering-Kahlbaum A.-G., Berlin, and Prof. Dr. Hans Schlossberger, member of the Reich Board of Health, Berlin-Dahlem. H.G. Roebuck & Son, Publishers, Baltimore, 1933. Price, $8.00.

This, the first of three volumes dealing with the very important subject of chemotherapy, discusses the metal-free organic compounds. A second volume will include the metal derivatives, while the third will deal with the theories of chemotherapy.

This volume contains a vast fund of valuable information gleaned from the world's literature on the subject, and evaluated by both a physician and a chemist. It presents discoveries and investigations in this field, which will not become available in textbooks on general therapy for months, or perhaps years to come. While the text is written with due respect to technicalities, chemical formulae and physiologic observations, it is not too specialized to be readily understandable and appreciated by the practicing physician.

Indicative of the general plan of the volume, citations may be made to the chapter dealing with emetin and its derivatives. The authors begin their discussion of this group of drugs by detailing the essentials in its history, occurrence and chemistry. Following this are sections devoted to the pharmacology and

toxicity of the drug, with a generous section devoted to the therapeutic results. The entire discussion, including citation to the literature, covers thirty-six pages of the text.

Being the only authoritative work on this subject available in English, the progressive physician will readily appreciate the significance and worth of this treatise. To the investigator in the field of chemotherapy this volume will be invaluable, and since every physician employs chemotherapy in his daily practice, the work should have a wide appeal.

MEDICAL CLINICS OF NORTH AMERICA

Volume xvii, No. 3, Philadelphia Number, November, 1933. Octavo of 326 pages with 59 illustrations. Per clinic year, July, 1933, to May, 1934. W. B. Saunders Company, Philadelphia and London, 1933. Price, paper, $12.00; cloth, $16.00.

This is the Philadelphia number issued in November, 1933. The opening paper is a report of the encephalitis epidemic which occurred in St. Louis last summer. The subject is considered from the standpoint of the history of preceding epidemics in this country as well as foreign countries which have been visited by this scourge. The St. Louis epidemic was unique in one respect—it was the first time the disease had appeared in epidemic form of large proportion in this country. The writer reports quite fully, going into the symptomatology and type forms of the disease. Other articles of interest are offered on endocrinology and blood and vascular diseases.

F. R. H.

MENTAL HYGIENE IN THE COMMUNITY

By Clara Bassett, consultant in psychiatric social work, division on community clinics, The National Committee for Mental Hygiene, Inc. The Macmillan Company, New York, 1934. Price, $3.50.

In 1931 Ziegler interviewed a "typical" group of physicians to determine the extent of their interest in "nervous" conditions. Over half of those interviewed felt little interest, and about one-quarter more expressed no interest in these conditions. If we can accept as correct the statistics which were collected in New York State in 1927, indicating that of the 11,500,000 population in New York State that year about 500,000 would probably develop serious mental disease requiring hospital treatment, it would seem deplorable indeed that so large a group of physicians should express little or no interest in the problem of neuropsychiatry.

The organized movement for mental hygiene, begun in 1908, with the development of a national committee in 1909, has for its purpose the dissemination of information through many channels concerning mental disease, abnormal mental traits, and remedial conditions which may lead to abnormal mentality. This work has stimulated an outspoken interest in the problems of mental hygiene from educators, social workers, parent teachers associations, club women, and to some extent, the medical profession. That the interest of the medical profession is not greater is to be regretted.

Books such as that written by Clara Bassett are fundamental in character, and if read with due care and thoughtfulness, will go far toward giving a proper insight into the several aspects of the problem of mental hygiene. This comprehensive picture of the relation of mental hygiene to some of the urgent problems of community life presents questions which should be of definite interest to every physician.

Because of these facts we are pleased to recommend the volume to the medical profession.

METABOLIC DISEASES AND THEIR TREATMENT

By Dr. Erich Grafe, professor of medicine and director of the clinic of medicine and neurology at the University of Wurzburg, Germany. Octavo of 551 pages, illustrated with 37 engravings. Lea & Febiger, Washington Square, Philadelphia, 1933. Price, $6.50.

This volume is a translation and revision of a German edition by the same authors a year and a half ago. Since the authors consider that the greatest advances in metabolic diseases during the past few years have occurred in the field of diabetes, they have allotted a large part of their page space to a consideration of this disease.

Part one of the text deals with the consideration of food stuffs and their uses in the body. Part two discusses the nature and treatment of nutritional disorders other than diabetes, while part three continues this discussion with especial references to the condition of obesity and habitual under-nutrition, and introduces the consideration of diabetes mellitus. Part four discusses gout, alcaptonuria, cystinuria and aminuria, while part five is devoted to a consideration of the disturbances of the water and mineral economy in the body.

This delineation of the scope of the text does not give a proper conception of the emphasis which the authors have placed upon the several conditions. To emphasize the important place given the consideration of diabetes mellitus it may be pointed out that of the five hundred and fifty pages of the entire book almost one-half of these pages are devoted to diabetes.

The numerous citations to the literature are about equally divided between the English and German literature.

As a review of the entire field of metabolic diseases, the volume is excellent and will prove a source of handy reference to the practicing physician.

TREATMENT OF THE COMMONER DISEASES MET WITH BY THE GENERAL PRACTITIONER

By Lewellys F. Barker, M.D., professor emeritus, Johns Hopkins University, Baltimore, Maryland. J. B. Lippincott Company, Philadelphia, Montreal and London, 1934. Price, $3.00.

That rare diseases command much of the valuable space in the ordinary text on medical practice has been frequently commented upon, but rarely has an attempt been made to correct this condition. In this book the author has collected a series of lectures prepared and delivered before practicing physicians who desired a review of the treatment of the commoner diseases embodying, insofar as possible, the newer useful and proved observations and technics of the past decade. The name of Barker alone assures the success of such an endeavor.

While the lectures are classified by systems, no attempt has been made by the author to cover completely all phases of any given subject. Illustrative of the formation of this book may be cited his treatment of the common cold. He introduces this discussion by accepting the view of Dochez and others that the common cold is due to an ultra-microscopic (filtrable) virus, and proceeds at once to the preventive and curative treatment of the condition as recognized in modern practice.

The purpose of this volume is obviously to serve the needs of the general practitioner and since it so admirably fulfills its avowed purpose in presenting a modern treatment of the commoner diseases, one predicts a very hearty reception of this volume by practicing physicians everywhere.

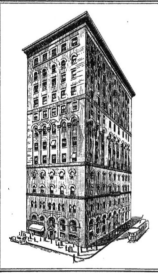

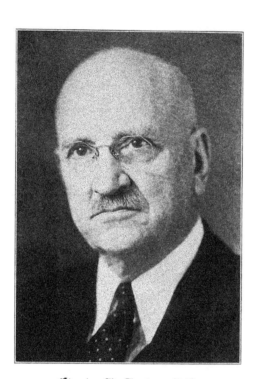

Charles B. Taylor, M.D.
President
Iowa State Medical Society
1933-1934

The JOURNAL

of the

Iowa State Medical Society

VOL. XXIV   DES MOINES, IOWA, APRIL, 1934   No. 4

IOWA STATE MEDICAL SOCIETY
Organized 1850

Eighty-third Annual Session

Des Moines, Iowa, May 9, 10, 11, 1934

Do not fail to Register. Registration Bureau—Hotel Fort Des Moines.

PROGRAM

Wednesday, May 9

8:30 a. m.

West Ballroom

Call to Order—
    CHARLES B. TAYLOR, M.D., President

Invocation—
    REVEREND EUGENE C. BEACH, Ottumwa

Symposium on Arthritis:

  General Considerations—
    JOHN C. PARSONS, M.D., Creston, 8:40-9:00

  Eye, Ear, Nose and Throat Aspect—
    J. K. VON LACKUM, M.D., Cedar Rapids, 9:00-9:20

  Orthopedic Phase—
    ARCH F. O'DONOGHUE, M.D., Sioux City, 9:20-9:40
    Discussion led by M. B. CALL, M.D., Greene, 9:40-10:00

Papillary Cystadenoma of the Ovary—
    C. W. ELLYSON, M.D., Waterloo, 10:00-10:20
    Discussion by J. H. RANDALL, M.D., Iowa City
    W. A. BOICE, M.D., Cedar Falls

Treatment of Pelvic Infections—
    A. C. PAGE, M.D., Des Moines, 10:30-10:50
    Discussion by WM. H. RENDLEMAN, M.D., Davenport
    O. F. PARISH, M.D., Grinnell

Shall Organized Medicine Survive?—
    OLIVER J. FAY, M.D., Des Moines, 11:00-11:20
    Discussion by HAROLD A. SPILMAN, M.D., Ottumwa.
    THOMAS A. BURCHAM, M.D., Des Moines

Presidential Address—
    CHARLES B. TAYLOR, M.D., Ottumwa, 11:30-11:45

Thursday, May 10

8:15 a. m.

West Ballroom

Syphilis as the Cause of Heart Disease and
  Medical Clinic—
    R. WESLEY SCOTT, M.D., Cleveland   8:15-9:15
    Clinical Professor of Medicine, Western Reserve
    College of Medicine, Cleveland.

Surgical Lesions of the Stomach and Duodenum and
  Surgical Clinic—
    VERNE C. HUNT, M.D., Los Angeles, 9:15-10:15

The Significance of Urinary Findings in Nephritis—
    F. P. MCNAMARA, M.D., Dubuque, 10:15-10:35
    Discussion by H. W. RATHE, M.D., Waverly
    JULIUS S. WEINGART, M.D., Des Moines

The Treatment of Gas Bacillus Infection—
    WILLIAM JEPSON, M.D., Sioux City, 10:45-11:05
    Discussion by W. A. ROHLF, M.D., Waverly
    A. B. DEERING, M.D., Boone

The Relationship of Otolaryngology to General
  Medicine—
    JOHN SHEA, M.D., Memphis, 11:15-11:45
    Guest, Eye, Ear, Nose and Throat Section

Sectional Conferences
Wednesday Afternoon, May 9

Time	Cardiovascular and Chest Section (West Ballroom)	Pediatric Section (The Cabin)	Section on Abdominal and Thoracic Surgery (Assembly Room, Third Floor)	Section on Urology and Gynecology (Sample Room "A," Third Floor)	Eye, Ear, Nose and Throat Section (Sample Rooms, "B," "C," "D," "E," Third Floor)
1:30	The Significance of Systolic Apical Murmur— E. L. Wurtzer, M.D., Clear Lake — The Size of the Heart in the Diagnosis of Heart Disease— Elmer E. Kotyke, M.D., Des Moines — The Evaluation of Symptoms in Cardiovascular Disease— Horace M. Korns, M.D., Iowa City	Significance of Pyuria in Children— W. R. Hornaday, M.D., Des Moines — Diaphragmatic Obstetrical Paralysis: Case Presentation— Postinfectious Uremic Convulsions Complicating Hemorrhagic Nephritis with Recovery— Lee F. Hill, M.D., Des Moines — Anemia: Case Report— Dennis H. Kelly, M.D., Des Moines — Hemophilia— — Trichomonas Vaginalis— Diagnosis and Treatment— Helen Johnston, M.D., Des Moines	The Surgical Treatment of Pulmonary Infection— Howard L. Beye, M.D., Iowa City — The Treatment of Empyema— Robert H. Lott, M.D., Carroll — The Relationship of Bronchoscopy to Thoracic Surgery— James A. Downing, M.D., Des Moines	Diagnosis and Treatment of Tuberculous Conditions of the Kidney— L. E. Pierson, M.D., Sioux City — Transurethral Prostatic Resection— N. G. Alcock, M.D., Iowa City	Instructional Conferences — Sample Room "B"—1:30-2:30 — I. Landmarks and Surgical Anatomy of the Neck— E. M. MacEwen, M.D., Iowa City — Sample Room "C"—1:30-2:30 — II. Orbital Tumors— C. S. O'Brien, M.D., Iowa City
2:30	The Diagnosis and Clinical Significance of Auricular Fibrillation— Laurence E. Cooley, M.D., Dubuque — The Relationship Between Coronary Occlusion and Angina Pectoris— B. F. Wolverton, M.D., Cedar Rapids — The Salient Features in the Treatment of Cardiac Failure— H. W. Rathe, M.D., Waverly	Subarachnoid Hemorrhage— Icterus Gravis Neonatorum— James E. Dyson, M.D., Des Moines — Traumatic Rupture of Kidney in a Child of Nine Years— Leonard A. West, M.D., Des Moines — Celiac Disease— Raymond Coppin, M.D., Des Moines — Club Feet— Verl A. Ruth, M.D., Des Moines	Treatment of Burns— N. M. Whitehill, M.D., Boone — Postoperative Accidents and Complications— E. B. Howell, M.D., Ottumwa — The Diagnosis and Surgical Treatment of Pyloric Obstruction in Infants— Howard I. Down, M.D., Sioux City	A Review of Ureteral Surgery— Homer Scott, M.D., Ft. Dodge — Anatomy of the Undescended Testicle— E. M. MacEwen, M.D., Iowa City — The Management of Cases of Apparent Sterility— Ben J. Dimaker, M.D., Fort Madison	Sample Room "D"—1:30-2:30 — III. The Infants' Temporal Bone— Dean M. Lierle, M.D., Iowa City — Sample Room "E"—1:30-2:30 — IV. Discussion of Subjects Suggested by Those in Attendance at the Round Table— W. W. Pearson, M.D., Des Moines
3:30	Non-tuberculous Infections of the Chest— John H. Peck, M.D., Des Moines — The Diagnosis and Treatment of Bronchial Asthma— Julia Cole, M.D., Iowa City	Myer—Torek Operation for Crypto-orchism— Joseph B. Priestley, M.D., Des Moines — Childhood Tuberculosis— Arnold M. Smythe, M.D., Des Moines — Meningitis Secondary to Otitis Media—Possibilities of Operative Procedure— Cecil C. Jones, M.D., Des Moines — Some Unusual Bone Pathology in Children— Harry W. Dahl, M.D., Des Moines	Surgical Procedures for Neoplasms of the Right Half of the Colon— Charles S. Krause, M.D., Cedar Rapids — Acute Intestinal Obstruction— B. Raymond Weston, M.D., Mason City — Tuberculous Lesions of the Gastro-Intestinal Tract— F. R. Petersson, M.D., Iowa City — Management of Appendicitis in the Purulent Stage— Arthur W. Booth, M.D., Elmira, N.Y.	The Newer Treatment of Gonorrhea in Young Girls— Joseph Brown, M.D., Des Moines — Operative Procedures in Malpositions of the Uterus— Donald C. Conzett, M.D., Dubuque — The Proper Treatment for Uterine Malignancies— E. D. Plass, M.D., Iowa City	General Meeting — Sample Room "B"—3:00-5:00 — Presentation of cases with Nose and Throat Pathology by the Broadlawns Staff of the Eye, Ear, Nose and Throat Section of the Polk County Medical Society. — Discussion will be lead by John Shea, M.D., Memphis, Tenn.

Thursday Afternoon, May 10

Time	Gastro-Intestinal and Diabetes Section West Ballroom	Section on Neurology and Psychiatry Sample Room "C," Third Floor	Section on Pediatrics and Obstetrics Sample Room "A," Third Floor	Section on General and Orthopedic Surgery Assembly Room, Third Floor	Section on Roentgenology Sample Room "B," Third Floor
1:30	Diagnosis of Peptic Ulcer— E. G. Senty, M.D., Davenport Diagnosis of Gastric Malignancy— J. T. Straws, M.D., Des Moines Diagnosis of Chronic Gall Bladder Disease and Indications for Surgical Interference— W. A. Rohlf, M.D., Waverly	Headaches— Frank A. Ely, M.D., Des Moines Sciatic Syndrome— John I. Marker, M.D., Davenport The Painful Shoulder Syndrome— Tom B. Throckmorton, M.D., Des Moines	Symposium: Neonatal Deaths and Their Prominent Etiologic Factors; Statistical Data on Neonatal Deaths at the University Hospitals— John H. Randall, M.D., Iowa City Pulmonary Atelectasis— Roy I. Theisen, M.D., Dubuque	Carcinoma of the Breast— J. J. Noonan, M.D., Marshalltown Indications for Thyroid Surgery— T. E. Davinson, M.D., Mason City Spinal Anesthesia— Paul A. White, M.D., Davenport	Irradiation Treatment of Small Fibroids and Menorrhagia— Ben T. Whitaker, M.D., Boone Roentgen Ray Considerations in Injury Cases— W. S. Shegruay, M.D., Atlantic Roentgen Visualization of the Liver and Spleen, with Thorium Dioxide Sol— L. G. Mucksen, M.D., Dubuque
2:30	Roentgenologic Findings in Chronic Gall Bladder Disease— W. H. Gibson, M.D., Iowa City Chronic Appendicitis— Glenn C. Blome, M.D., Ottumwa The Diagnosis and Treatment of Spastic Constipation— C. W. Baldridge, M.D., Iowa City	Clinical Manifestations of Encephalitis— Gregory Barer, M.D., Iowa City The Laboratory Diagnosis of Neurosyphilis— Charles F. Obermann, M.D., Clarinda X-ray in the Diagnosis of Diseases of the Nervous System— A. L. Sahs, M.D., Iowa City	Prematurity— G. A. Hurston, M.D., Des Moines Congenital Heart Disease— Otto N. Glesne, M.D., Fort Dodge Intracranial Hemorrhage— Roy Crowder, M.D., Sioux City	Proper Drainage of Infections of the Hand— McM. Hanchett, M.D., Council Bluffs Wrist Injuries— Douglas N. Gibson, M.D., Des Moines Fractures of the Elbow (Lantern Slides)— Peter A. Bendixen, M.D., Davenport	Tightening the Line of Defense in Making an Accurate Diagnosis— N. L. Hersey, M.D., Independence Fractures of the Wrist in Children— C. L. Gillies, M.D., Cedar Rapids Traumatic Injuries of the Spine— Thomas A. Burcham, M.D., Des Moines
3:30	The Clinical Significance of Hemorrhage from Bowel— William H. Rendleman, M.D., Davenport Treatment of Diabetes: Diet— R. N. Larimer, M.D., Sioux City Insulin— John C. Shrader, M.D., Fort Dodge	Trigeminal Neuralgia and Its Treatment— Walter D. Abbott, M.D., Des Moines The Hematopoietic Diseases and the Nervous System— F. H. Lamb, M.D., Davenport Borderland Psychosis— William Malamud, M.D., Iowa City	Symposium: Infectious Conditions in the Newborn; Sepsis in the Newborn— J. M. Hayes, M.D., Cedar Rapids Skin Infections in the Newborn— James Dunn, M.D., Davenport Conjunctivitis in the Newborn— C. W. Rutherford, M.D., Iowa City Encephalitis and Meningitis in the Newborn— H. E. Farnsworth, M.D., Storm Lake Respiratory Infection in the Newborn— C. A. Waterbury, M.D., Waterloo	Fractures of the Spine— W. Eugene Wolcott, M.D., Des Moines Knee Injuries and Their Treatment— Robert K. Wrenthoff, M.D., Council Bluffs Fractures of the Femur (Moving Picture)— Fred L. Knowles, M.D., Fort Dodge	The Diagnosis and Treatment of Kidney Malignancies— O. V. Butt, M.D., Waterloo Roentgen Ray Diagnosis of Non-opaque Foreign Bodies in the Bronchi— E. L. Rypins, M.D., Iowa City Irradiation Treatment of Superficial Malignancies— H. Dabney Kerr, M.D., Iowa City

Wednesday Evening, May 9

8:00 p. m.

West Ballroom—Hotel Fort Des Moines

Oration in Medicine—
GEORGE B. CROW, M.D., Burlington

Oration in Surgery—
EDWARD M. MYERS, M.D., Boone

Formal Reception in honor of Walter L. Bierring, M.D., President-elect, American Medical Association

Music—Cards—Entertainment

———

Thursday Evening, May 10

ANNUAL BANQUET

West Ballroom—Hotel Fort Des Moines

6:30 p. m.

Toastmaster—
WILLIAM E. ASH, M.D., Council Bluffs

President's Address: Who Are Graduates in Medicine?—
CHARLES B. TAYLOR, M.D., Ottumwa

Address by the President-elect: Why Are We Here, and Where Are We Going?—
GORDON F. HARKNESS, M.D., Davenport

Music—Dancing—Entertainment

———

Friday, May 11

8:30 a. m.

West Ballroom

Surgical Aspects of the Gallbladder and Biliary Tract, and Surgical Clinic—
VERNE C. HUNT, M.D., Los Angeles, 8:30-9:30

Hypertensive Heart Disease and Medical Clinic
R. WESLEY SCOTT, M.D., Cleveland, 9:30-10:30

The Relation of the State Department of Health to the Practice of Medicine—
WALTER L. BIERRING, M.D., 10:30-11:00
Commissioner of Health

Some Causes of Professional Unrest—
R. G. LELAND, M.D., Chicago, 11:00-11:30

Report of House of Delegates

Installation of President

OPHTHALMOLOGY, OTOLOGY AND RHINOLARYNGOLOGY

Wednesday, May 9

1:30 p. m.

Instructional Conferences from 1:30 to 2:30, as listed under the sectional meetings.

3:00 p. m.

Sample Room—Third Floor

Presentation of cases with Nose and Throat Pathology by the Broadlawns Staff of the Eye, Ear, Nose and Throat Section of the Polk County Medical Society.
Discussion led by JOHN SHEA, M.D., Memphis, Tenn.

———

Thursday, May 10

9:30 a. m.

The Cabin—Hotel Fort Des Moines

Chairman's Address: Lacrimal Duct Stenosis—
ROYAL F. FRENCH, M.D., Marshalltown

Cases of Non-Metallic Foreign Bodies in Trachea and Bronchi in Children—
H. E. THOMPSON, M.D., Dubuque
Discussion by SYDNER D. MAIDEN, M.D., Council Bluffs
JAMES A. DOWNING, M.D., Des Moines

Strabismus—General Consideration—
J. B. NAFTZGER, M.D., Sioux City
Discussion by H. B. GRATIOT, M.D., Dubuque
GEORGE A. MAY, M.D., Des Moines

The Relationship of Otolaryngology to General Medicine—Delivered before the General Session—
JOHN SHEA, M.D., Memphis, Tennessee
Guest, Eye, Ear, Nose and Throat Section

———

Luncheon

12:15 p. m.

The Cabin—Hotel Fort Des Moines

Guests of Des Moines Academy of Ophthalmology, Otology and Rhinolaryngology.

———

2:00 p. m.

Two Mastoids—
CARL E. SAMPSON, M.D., Creston
Discussion by DEVOE BOVENMYER, M.D., Ottumwa

The Management of Allergic Manifestation of the Nose and Throat—
JOHN SHEA, M.D., Memphis, Tenn.

Differential Diagnosis of Headaches—
CECIL C. JONES, M.D., Des Moines
Discussion by T. R. GITTINS, M.D., Sioux City

Thrombophlebitis—Secondary to Throat Infections—
SUMNER B. CHASE, M.D., Fort Dodge
Discussion by F. H. REULING, M.D., Waterloo

GUEST SPEAKERS

Eighty-third Annual Session

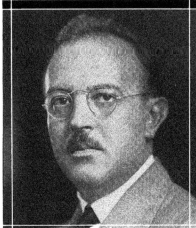

R. WESLEY SCOTT, M.D.
Cleveland, Ohio .

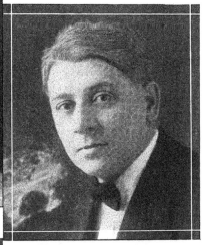

VERNE C. HUNT, M.D.
Los Angeles, California

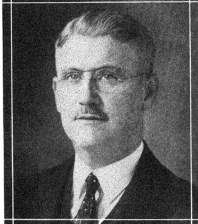

JOHN J. SHEA, M.D.
Memphis, Tennessee

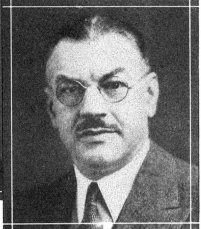

R. G. LELAND, M.D.
Chicago, Illinois

HOUSE OF DELEGATES
American Legion Rooms
Plymouth Building
Wednesday, May 9
4:00 p. m.

Roll Call

Approval of Minutes of Friday Morning Session, 1933

Report of Secretary

Report of Treasurer

Report of Council

Reports of Council Committees

Speakers Bureau Committee—
DANIEL J. GLOMSET, Des Moines, Chairman

Committee on Professional Relations—
PRINCE E. SAWYER, Sioux City, Chairman

Committee on Public Relations—
GEORGE B. CROW, Burlington, Chairman

Cancer Committee—
WILLIAM JEPSON, Sioux City, Chairman

Report of Board of Trustees

Report of the Delegates to the American Medical Association

Reports of Standing Committees of the House of Delegates:

Committee on Constitution and By-Laws—
JOHN H. PECK, Des Moines, Chairman

Committee on Finance—
ERNEST C. McCLURE, Bussey, Chairman

Committee on Publication—
RALPH R. SIMMONS, Des Moines, Editor

Committee on Public Policy and Legislation—
THOMAS A. BURCHAM, Des Moines, Chairman

Medico-legal Committee—
FRANK A. ELY, Des Moines, Chairman

Committee on Necrology—
ARTHUR W. ERSKINE, Cedar Rapids, Secretary

Committee on Medical Education and Hospitals—
ARTHUR W. ERSKINE, Cedar Rapids, Chairman

Reports of Special Committees of the House of Delegates:

Medical Library Committee—
FELIX A. HENNESSY, Calmar, Chairman

Committee on Medical Economics—
CORWIN S. CORNELL, Knoxville, Chairman

Historical Committee—
WALTER L. BIERRING, Des Moines, Chairman

Committee on Military Affairs—
T. F. SUCHOMEL, Cedar Rapids, Chairman

Committee on Child Health and Protection—
FRED MOORE, Des Moines, Chairman

Woman's Auxiliary Advisory Committee—
EMIL C. JUNGER, Soldier, Chairman

Memorials and Communications

New Business

Election of Committee on Nominations

Friday, May 12
8:00 a. m.

Roll Call

Reading of Minutes

Report of Committee on Nominations

Election of Officers

Reports of Committees

Unfinished Business

New Business

Adjournment

ENTERTAINMENT
Wednesday, May 9
8:00 p. m.

Reception in honor of Dr. Walter L. Bierring
West Ballroom—Hotel Fort Des Moines
Physicians and their wives

Thursday, May 10
1:00 p. m.
Auxiliary Luncheon, Younker's Tea Room
All visiting ladies invited
6:30 p. m.
Annual Banquet, Hotel Fort Des Moines
Physicians, their wives and guests

ARRANGEMENTS COMMITTEE

CHARLES B. TAYLOR....................................Ottumwa
ROBERT L. PARKER.................................Des Moines
HAROLD J. McCOY.................................Des Moines
C. B. LUGINBUHL..................................Des Moines
FLOYD B. LANGDON................................Des Moines

LOCAL COMMITTEES

Clinics.......................C. B. LUGINBUHL, M.D., Chairman
Entertainment..............FLOYD B. LANGDON, M.D., Chairman

IOWA STATE MEDICAL SOCIETY OFFICERS AND COMMITTEES 1933-1934

President..........................Charles B. Taylor, Ottumwa
President Elect................Gordon F. Harkness, Davenport
First Vice President............William E. Ash, Council Bluffs
Second Vice President................Frank H. Conner, Nevada
Secretary........................Robert L. Parker, Des Moines
Treasurer........................Harold J. McCoy, Des Moines

COUNCILORS
Term Expires

First District—Felix A. Hennessy, Calmar................1937
Second District—Leo P. Woodward, Mason City.............1935
Third District—Frank P. Winkler, Sibley.................1934
Fourth District—James E. Reeder, Sioux City............1935
Fifth District—William W. Pearson, Des Moines..........1936
Sixth District—Charles W. Ellyson, Waterloo............1937
Seventh District—Arthur W. Erskine, Cedar Rapids
    (Secretary) 1938
Eighth District—Clyde A. Boice, Washington.............1934
Ninth District—Harold A. Spilman, Ottumwa (Chairman)..1935
Tenth District—James G. Macrae, Creston................1936
Eleventh District—M. Charles Hennessy, Council Bluffs..1937

TRUSTEES

Oliver J. Fay, Des Moines...............................1934
John I. Marker, Davenport..............................1936
Edward M. Myers, Boone.................................1935

DELEGATES TO A. M. A.

Fred Moore, Des Moines.................................1935
E. D. Plass, Iowa City.................................1934
T. F. Thornton, Waterloo..............................1934

ALTERNATE DELEGATES TO A. M. A.

N. G. Alcock, Iowa City................................1935
W. E. Long, Mason City................................1934
F. J. Swift, Maquoketa................................1934

EDITOR OF THE JOURNAL

Ralph R. Simmons..............................Des Moines

STANDING COMMITTEES OF THE HOUSE OF DELEGATES
ARRANGEMENTS

Charles B. Taylor, Chairman.......................Ottumwa
Robert L. Parker..............................Des Moines
Harold J. McCoy..............................Des Moines

CONSTITUTION AND BY-LAWS

John H. Peck, Chairman.......................Des Moines
Channing G. Smith...............................Granger
James C. Donahue.............................Centerville

FINANCE

Ernest C. McClure, Chairman.......................Bussey
E. B. Williams................................Montezuma
Andrew W. Bennett.............................Iowa City

MEDICO-LEGAL

Frank A. Ely, Des Moines, Chairman.................1935
George C. Albright, Iowa City......................1936
F. Earl Bellinger, Council Bluffs..................1934

PUBLICATION COMMITTEE

Ralph R. Simmons, Editor......................Des Moines
Robert L. Parker, Secretary...................Des Moines
Oliver J. Fay, Trustee.......................Des Moines
John I. Marker, Trustee........................Davenport
Edward M. Myers, Trustee...........................Boone

PUBLIC POLICY AND LEGISLATION

Thomas A. Burcham, Chairman..................Des Moines
Frank L. Williams............................Des Moines
Harry A. Bailey...............................Davenport
Charles B. Taylor................................Ottumwa
Robert L. Parker.............................Des Moines

SCIENTIFIC WORK

Charles B. Taylor, Chairman......................Ottumwa
Robert L. Parker.............................Des Moines
Harold J. McCoy..............................Des Moines

SPECIAL COMMITTEES OF THE HOUSE OF DELEGATES
COMMITTEE ON CHILD HEALTH AND PROTECTION

Fred Moore, Chairman..........................Des Moines
H. D. Flint...................................Iowa City
J. D. Boyd....................................Iowa City
Lee F. Hill..................................Des Moines
H. E. Farnsworth..............................Storm Lake

HISTORICAL

Walter L. Bierring, Chairman..................Des Moines
Frank M. Fuller..................................Keokuk
T. B. Throckmorton............................Des Moines
Henry B. Young...............................Burlington
John T. McClintock.............................Iowa City

MEDICAL ECONOMICS

Corwin S. Cornell, Chairman.....................Knoxville
James C. Hill....................................Newton
E. L. Wurtzer.................................Clear Lake
R. M. Sorenson...............................Cumberland
T. A. Moran,.....................................Melrose

MEDICAL LIBRARY

Felix A Hennessy, Chairman........................Calmar
C. R. Harken.....................................Osceola
Jeannette Dean-Throckmorton ....Des Moines

MILITARY AFFAIRS

T. F. Suchomel, Chairman....................Cedar Rapids
Mark C. Jones.....................................Boone
Harold A. Spilman................................Ottumwa

SUPERANNUATED PHYSICIANS

William F. Amdor, Chairman........................Carbon
W. S. Greenleaf.................................Atlantic
F. G. Murray................................Cedar Rapids

WOMAN'S AUXILIARY ADVISORY COMMITTEE

Emil C. Junger, Chairman.........................Soldier
O. A. Kabrick.................................Grandview
James M. Donelan...............................Glenwood
P. B. McLaughlin.............................Sioux City
E. B. Howell.....................................Ottumwa

STANDING COMMITTEES OF THE COUNCIL
SPEAKERS BUREAU COMMITTEE

Daniel J. Glomset, Chairman...................Des Moines
Felix A. Hennessy................................Calmar
L. C. Kern......................................Waverly
John C. Parsons..................................Creston
Dorothy M. Nelson, Secretary..................Des Moines

SPECIAL COMMITTEES OF THE COUNCIL
MEDICAL EDUCATION AND HOSPITALS

Arthur W. Erskine, Chairman..................Cedar Rapids
Louis F. Talley.............................Marshalltown
John C. Parsons..................................Creston

PROFESSIONAL RELATIONS

Prince E. Sawyer, Chairman...................Sioux City
William R. Brock................................Sheldon
Sydner D. Maiden...........................Council Bluffs

PUBLIC RELATIONS

George D. Crow, Chairman.....................Burlington
Raymond S. Grossman........................Marshalltown
Harold L. Brereton...........................Emmetsburg

HEADQUARTERS

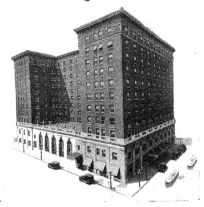

HOTEL FORT DES MOINES

MEETING PLACES

Headquarters—Hotel Fort Des Moines

General Meeting—West Ballroom, Hotel Fort Des Moines

Sectional Meetings—West Ballroom, The Cabin, The Assembly Room, Sample Rooms, Hotel Fort Des Moines

House of Delegates—American Legion Rooms, Plymouth Building

Eye, Ear, Nose and Throat Section—Sample Rooms, Third Floor, Wednesday; The Cabin, Thursday; Hotel Fort Des Moines

Registration and Commercial Exhibits—Mezzanine Floor, Hotel Fort Des Moines

Scientific Exhibits—Green Room, Hotel Fort Des Moines

Headquarters for Woman's Auxiliary—Hotel Fort Des Moines

———

SPECIAL MEETINGS

County Secretaries Conference Luncheon
Wednesday, May 9
Des Moines Club, 12:15 p. m.

———

Military Surgeon's Dinner
Wednesday, May 9
Des Moines Club, 6:30 p. .m.

———

Eye, Ear, Nose and Throat Section
Thursday, May 10
The Cabin—Hotel Fort Des Moines
12:15 p. m.

———

Iowa Pediatric Club
Friday, May 12
Place to be announced, 12:15 p. m.

Section Chairmen and Reporters

Section on Medicine—
Chairman, FRED M. SMITH, M.D., Iowa City

Section on Surgery—
Chairman, LESTER D. POWELL, M.D., Des Moines

Section on Ophthalmology, Otology and Rhinolaryngology—
Chairman, ROYAL F. FRENCH, M.D., Marshalltown

Reporter, General Sessions—
MASTER REPORTING COMPANY, Chicago

Reporter, Eye, Ear, Nose and Throat Section—
MASTER REPORTING COMPANY, Chicago

Reporter, House of Delegates—
MASTER REPORTING COMPANY, Chicago

OUR GUESTS

R. WESLEY SCOTT, M.D., Cleveland, Ohio
VERNE C. HUNT, M.D., Los Angeles, California
JOHN J. SHEA, M.D., Memphis, Tennessee
R. G. LELAND, M.D., Chicago, Illinois

Rules for Papers and Discussions

With the exception of the papers or talks given by the guest speakers, no paper on the general sessions program shall occupy more than twenty minutes in its delivery; discussions of papers are limited to five minutes and no member shall speak more than once on any subject.

Each paper shall be typewritten, and deposited with the Secretary after the paper or talk has been given; if this is not done, it will not be published.

On rising to discuss a paper, the speaker will please come forward and announce his name and address plainly.

———

REGISTRATION

Do not fail to register.

Please bring your membership card for presentation at the registration desk.

6:30 p. m.
Banquet, Hotel Fort Des Moines
Physicians, wives and guests

Friday, May 11
10:00 a. m.
Business Meeting, Woman's Auxiliary ·
Assembly Room, Hotel Fort Des Moines

Election of Officers—

Installation of Officers—

Postconvention Meeting held upon adjournment of
this meeting—

This program, social and business, is for all visiting women. All eligible women are urged to become members.

State Society
of
Iowa Medical Women

Thirty-seventh Annual Meeting, Des Moines

Tuesday, May 8, 1934

Grace Ransom's Tea Room

Greetings—
LEONE M. SCRUBY, M.D., Des Moines

Dinner
6:30 p. m.

Call to Order—
ELEANOR M. HUTCHINSON, M.D., President, Belle Plaine

Business Meeting

Reading of the Constitution—
JEANNETTE DEAN-THROCKMORTON, M.D., Des Moines

Program

What Can Be Done for Race Betterment—
ELEANOR M. HUTCHINSON, M.D., Belle Plaine

Child Nature and the Child's Emotional Needs—
MARTHA LINK, M.D., Dubuque

Superstitions of Pregnancy—
ALICE H. HATCH, M.D., Des Moines

Peptic Ulcer in Children: Case Report—
PAULINE MOORE, M.D., Solon

OFFICERS

President....Eleanor M. Hutchinson, M.D., Belle Plaine
Vice President...................Pauline Moore, M.D., Solon
Secretary   Julia Ford Hill, M.D., Des Moines
Treasurer—
Jeannette Dean-Throckmorton, M.D., Des Moines

A Convention Preview

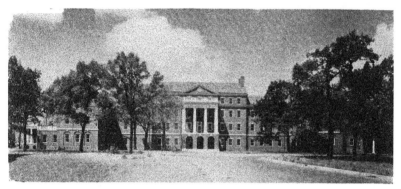

UNITED STATES VETERANS' HOSPITAL, DES MOINES

The Eighty-third Annual Session of the Iowa State Medical Society to be held in Des Moines, May 9, 10 and 11, 1934, marks a new epoch in the development of the program for the state meeting. The sectional type of program, which has been used extensively for national meetings, is this year being initiated in Iowa. The morning sessions are to be conducted on the same plan as in the past years but the sectional conferences, which feature the afternoon meetings, are a decided departure from previous programs.

Des Moines is expecting and preparing for an unusually large attendance at the State Medical Society meeting for several reasons. First, there is a great increase in the number of people taking part in the program; second, the selection of talks afforded by the sectional meetings should interest a larger number of doctors; and last, but not least, during the past few months there have been a few rifts in the dark clouds of depression which will be reflected in the attendance at the annual session.

There are to be other innovations in the program this year which will add to the interest of the meeting for both the doctors and their wives. The Iowa State Medical Society has the distinction this year of having, for the first time in its history, one of its members assuming the office of president of the American Medical Association. On Wednesday evening, it has been arranged to hold a formal reception in honor of Dr. Walter L. Bierring, so that the doctors and their wives throughout the state who have not yet met him

may do so, and so that his many friends may congratulate him on having earned the highest recognition which the medical profession can bestow on one of its members. Just before the reception and in keeping with the dignity of the occasion, the old custom of having a surgical and a medical oration is being re-established.

The program itself is of a very high order. Every paper is one of great interest. The guest speakers, Drs. John Shea, R. Wesley Scott and Verne Hunt are highly qualified in their respective fields and Dr. Hunt is a former Iowan. We are fortunate in having with us Dr. Leland of the Bureau of Medical Economics of the American Medical Association to discuss medical economic problems. Another distinguished guest on the program is Dr. Arthur Booth of Elmira, New York, who is one of the trustees of the American Medical Association. He is to be in the state visiting friends at the time of the state meeting and has very kindly consented to contribute to one of the sectional programs.

The Woman's Auxiliary Program Committee is planning a most interesting and entertaining program for the doctors' wives. With the increasing activities of this group, their program has lengthened until they now have a short session each afternoon and evening during the meeting.

The State Society of Iowa Medical Women is to have a short dinner meeting the evening of Tuesday, May 8, in order that they will be free to attend the general meetings on the 9th, 10th and 11th.

With all of these meetings being held in the short space of two and one-half days, even the Hotel Fort Des Moines, which is the headquarters for the meeting, is pushed to capacity for meeting space. The general morning meetings will be held in the large ballroom; the afternoon meetings will be held there and also in the Cabin on the eleventh floor, in the Assembly Room on the third floor and in the several large sample rooms on the third floor. The House of Delegates will meet in the American Legion Rooms in the Plymouth Building, which is located diagonally across the street from the Fort Des Moines Hotel. The registration desk and information bureau will be located in their usual place on the mezzanine floor.

The women attending the meeting will find many interesting activities when their meetings are not in session. When the scientific and business sessions of the doctors are not being held, they will find the commercial and scientific exhibits, located on the mezzanine floor, of great value. Another feature, new in Des Moines, which should prove very interesting to all physicians is the Veterans Hospital, which has just been opened. A visit to the hospital will reveal many beautiful buildings, and the hospital is reputed to be one of the most modern and best equipped institutions of its kind in the United States. A trip to the hospital would be both interesting and worthwhile.

The program for the annual meeting of the State Medical Society has been planned for the individual member—the Program Committee has tried to keep in mind his interests and likes. The success of the meeting is dependent upon the support of the members. An innovation such as the sectional meetings involve many detailed arrangements and the cooperation of the doctors is essential to their running along smoothly and according to schedule. The members are urged not to overcrowd any one section but to visit as many of those in which they are interested as possible. The meeting rooms will be spread over three floors, but will be centered mainly on the mezzanine and the third floor. A huge chart, outlining all of the sectional meetings and indicating exactly where and when each will be held, will be placed near the registration desk. There will be several people on hand to direct the doctors to the various meeting places. Much confusion in the meetings can be avoided if no one enters or leaves a room during a talk but does so during the short interval between talks.

If this new type of program is well liked by the members of the Iowa State Medical Society, it will be continued and probably amplified next year. If it is not popular, the old type of program will undoubtedly be resumed. Give the program a fair trial; make concessions for its youth and inexperience, but be sure and express your opinion for the guidance of those who plan next year's meeting.

The meeting in May, 1934, has the opportunity of making medical history in Iowa. Every member of the Society should have some part in it.

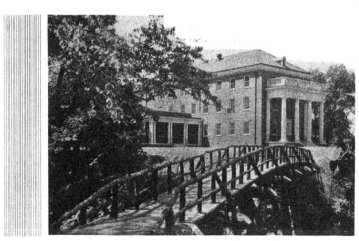

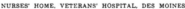

NURSES' HOME, VETERANS' HOSPITAL, DES MOINES

INTRATHORACIC TUMORS

A REPORT OF FIVE CASES AND REVIEW OF
THE LITERATURE*

W. D. RUNYON, M.D.
M. C. WHEELOCK, M.D.
Sioux City

In the brief space of four months, five different intrathoracic new growths were seen in our office. They were classified as follows: mediastinal Hodgkin's disease, a mediastinal lymphosarcoma, an endothelioma of the pleura, an hemangio-endothelioma of the lung, and a metastatic adenocarcinoma of the lung. The histories of these cases are briefly reviewed.

K. H., a nurse, thirty-eight years of age, a single woman was seen because of an eruption of two years' duration which started first on the thighs, the buttocks, and the back, and then spread to the ankles and legs. The maculae which first appeared were followed by small hard papules and ended as nodules with white centers. There was marked pigmentation and excoriation. The skin over the thorax had a vitiliginous appearance. The itching was intense; it even interfered with sleep and was only partially relieved by the usual procedures. She had lost fifteen pounds. Her menstrual periods had increased in frequency and amount of flow. Examination showed a tall, asthenic middle-aged woman. There was no adenopathy. The lungs were found clear and the heart normal. A small fibroid was found in the uterus and the right kidney was felt low down. There was a secondary anemia; 3,820,000 erthrocytes with a hemoglobin of 73 per cent; leukocytes numbered 14,600 with a normal differential count; urine, blood chemistry and basal metabolic rate were normal. Several Wassermann reactions were negative. There were no symptoms pointing to a mediastinal involvement. Diagnosis was made of scabies, secondary anemia, ptosis of the right kidney and fibroid. Treatment did not affect the skin lesions or the intense pruritus. A dermatologist diagnosed the condition as lichen planus hypertrophicus. Three months later she mentioned that an aggravating cough was causing her difficulty. Suspicions were aroused and an x-ray picture showed a widening of the mediastinum with several large irregular nodes projecting into the shadows on both sides of the hilus. The radiologist diagnosed the condition as mediastinal Hodgkin's disease.

The intense unrelieved itching should have suggested the solution. At the same time we know that enlarged mediastinal glands do not cause

*A complete bibliography of pertinent literature will be found in the authors' reprints.

symptoms unless they exert pressure on important structures. Lemon and Doyle[31] feel that a diagnosis of Hodgkin's disease should not be made without microscopic study. Because there were no enlarged glands this procedure was not feasible. On the other hand Wessler and Greene[53] Symmers[44] and Cooper[7] state that involvement of the superficial glands is not always present. Hence the diagnosis depended entirely on the roentgenogram. The patient obtained relief by x-ray treatments and then left for another city. We learned later that she committed suicide. A postmortem examination was not performed.

W. W., a farmer, thirty-three years of age, married, was seen because of a twenty-five pound weight loss, weakness, and afternoon rise in temperature (as high as 99° to 101°), and a severe unproductive cough of three months' duration. Later there was difficulty in breathing. Examination showed a definitely ill young man, somewhat cachectic in appearance. There was no adenopathy. The chest was symmetrically expansive, resonant throughout except for slight dulness posteriorly over the paravertebral area. The breath sounds were asthmatic in character over the entire chest posteriorly. The cough was obstructive in type. What little sputum was expectorated showed no tubercle bacilli. The only laboratory finding was a leukocytosis of 23,600 with 89 per cent neutrophils, which resulted from an infected finger. Diagnosis was made of an obstructive lesion. An x-ray picture showed an infiltrating type of pathology radiating from the left hilus into the lower half of the chest and several large mediastinal nodes. The roentgenologist specified that it was a mediastinal lymphosarcoma. Relatives were advised that the outlook was poor, but radiotherapy was suggested to alleviate symptoms. Temporary relief was obtained but death occurred about six months later. There was no autopsy.

D. G., a salesman, fifty years of age, was first seen because of weakness and a "run down" condition following an attack of influenza about three weeks before examination. He had not been well since the preceding summer when he suffered from ease of fatigability and breathlessness. This symptom had grown progressively worse. He was unable to lie on the left side because of dyspnea. His appetite also had failed. Examination showed a rather well nourished male adult, nicely developed and not acutely ill. The lower teeth were in poor condition. The chest showed a wide costal arch; on the right side, bulging of the interspaces in the base, limited expansion, flatness from below the scapula down the axilla and obliquely forward to the fifth rib. The breath sounds were distant and tubular in the upper chest. No râles were heard.

The heart was in normal limits, but displaced to the left. The lower border of the liver was felt pushed downward. Both epididymi were swollen and tender. Fluoroscopy showed the left lung clear, the diaphragmatic excursion free, the entire right chest up to the level of the third rib posteriorly densely cloudy and a haziness along the third rib. The flat plate showed a fluid level up to the sixth rib, anteriorly, cloudiness with soft infiltration of the lung and below this the entire lung filled with fluid; the esophagus was pushed forward and the mediastinal space displaced to the opposite sides with a mottling of the left chest. On thoracentesis, 1,530 cubic centimeters of a hemorrhagic fluid were aspirated. Staining of the sediment showed an enormous number of large non-nucleated cells measuring from fourteen to twenty-five micra in diameter with a densely staining blue nucleus in a lighter blue solid cytoplasm; many underwent mitotic division. The x-ray picture at this time showed a suspicious area along the pleura on the right, suggestive of a neoplasm. Two days later 1,400 cubic centimeters of fluid were aspirated and 400 cubic centimeters of air injected. A stereoscopic study showed an infiltrative type of pathology in the right lung confined chiefly to the lower two-thirds, a definite fluid level in the lower half of the chest and several areas which appeared to be on the pleural surface. On the basis of the x-rays this was an endothelioma of the pleura with fluid in the pleural cavity. Stained sediment of the second fluid showed the same type of cells as in the first. The pathologist, after a study of the cells, concurred with the radiologist. Roentgen ray therapy delayed the process but death resulted eight months later. Necropsy was refused. A diagnosis of tuberculosis with effusion had been previously made in this case.

A. B., a child, two years of age, was brought in because of difficulty in breathing, and in crying, of two days' duration. The left chest was flat to percussion over the upper part, the heart was displaced nearly into the right chest and breath sounds were heard only over the right chest. An x-ray picture showed the heart to be displaced toward the right by a large amount of fluid in the left pleural cavity, and a clear right lung. Thoracentesis resulted in a bloody fluid containing many white specks, with lymphocytes predominating up to 90 per cent. On the succeeding day 60 cubic centimeters of what was apparently pure blood was drawn off and in the last portion many white flakes resembling tissue were seen. An x-ray picture made following this aspiration showed a mass in the left side of the chest, apparently arising from the mediastinum. Microscopic examination of the white material showed an hemangio-endothelioma of the lung.

Radiotherapy was advised and used with little success. She was seen in another city and an adenocarcinoma was diagnosed. Accordingly slides were sent elsewhere. Two pathologists substantiated the hemangio-endothelioma and one the adenocarcinoma. The child died three months later and a postmortem examination showed the presence of an hemangio-endothelioma in the lung.

S. M., a housewife, seventy-three years of age, came in complaining of an aggravating cough, breathlessness, pain in the chest under the sternum and in front of the spine, orthopnea of necessity, loss of weight of about twenty-five pounds and loss of strength for a period extending over a year. Examination showed innumerable enlarged glands behind the sternomastoid and along the anterior border which were discrete, freely movable and very hard. There was limited expansion on the right side, flatness over the right chest anteriorly from the level of the third rib up and posteriorly over the same area. Over the left apex there was relative dulness. Over the whole area on the right side there were harsh breath sounds occurring through the whole inspiratory and expiratory phase. There were no râles and no cavities. Biopsy, made from one of the cervical nodes, revealed an adenocarcinoma. An x-ray picture showed an irregular nodular mass extending out from the right hilum into the upper and the middle right lobes which had all the appearance of malignancy. In both lung fields numerous small lesions were present which had the appearance of a blood-borne metastasis, and the pleura at the right base was adherent to the diaphragm. This was diagnosed as a metastatic adenocarcinoma involving both lungs. Because of her poor general condition further examinations were deferred. The primary site was considered to be in the stomach. Radiotherapy was not successful and she died four months later at her home. Necropsy was not permitted.

It was unfortunate that autopsies could not have been obtained since much information could have been secured from this source. Little is known concerning the etiology of Hodgkin's disease and lymphosarcoma. They are considered by Mac-Carty, quoted by Lemon, to be different manifestations of a similar process. Lemon feels that Hodgkin's disease and tuberculosis are unrelated. True carcinoma of the lung is on the increase according to Brunn[5], Greenberg [20], Arkin[1] and Mc-Crae, Funk and Jackson. Grove and Kramer[21] report an incidence of 0.15 per cent or more of all autopsies; about one per cent of all carcinoma and two per cent of all deaths from pulmonary diseases. Various factors such as repeated attacks of influenza, cigarette smoking, gas from tar products and inhalation of various gases are considered as causes. Fortune feels that there is no relation between tuberculosis and cancer of the lung. Wells and Cannon report a case of carcinoma of the lung following trauma. Fried[18] lays stress on chronic inflammation of the lung and an hereditary tendency. At present the last word has not been written concerning pneumonoconiosis and its relation to primary carcinoma of the lung. It is still a disputed question. Further, it must be realized that the increase in the number of postmortem examinations is demonstrating more pathologic findings in the lung. The x-ray has also proved to be a valuable aid in diagnosis.

Rose[42] in an admirable study has outlined the location of the more frequent mediastinal new growths and the results of pressure which they exert on the various structures. This should be reviewed by all who intend to increase their ability to determine the presence of tumors in this region. Since nearly every type of tissue is found here, nearly every kind of tumor is possible of development. Hodgkin's disease and lymphosarcoma are fairly frequent. The latter was found by Symmers to develop in the thymic remains; hence in the anterior mediastinum. The former develop in the tracheobronchial nodes; hence anywhere. Leukemia may also develop in these nodes. Thymomata are found in the superior mediastinum; less commonly lesions of a substernal thyroid may be found here. Chondromata and chondromyxomata, fibromata and fibromyxomata, are found in the anterior and the posterior mediastinum. Teratoma and ciliated epithelial cysts are found in the anterior mediastinum; ganglioneuromata in the posterior, and lipomata, xanthomata and carcinomata anywhere. Arkin[1] classifies carcinoma of the lung thus: endobronchial, hilar, mediastinal, central, lobar, pleural and rheumatoid. Histologically, cancer of the lung, according to Ewing as quoted by Greenberg[20], arises from the mucous membrane of the bronchi, from the mucous glands of the bronchi, or from the alveolar epithelium. Blumgarten prefers the simple arrangement of hilar and pleural carcinoma. Some writers question the possibility of a definite neoplasm arising from the alveolar cells. Concerning the pleura proper, Aschoff as quoted by Heur[25] differentiates between an hemangio-endothelioma, a lymphangoendothelioma and a peri-endothelioma. Various tumors have been reported; Lemon[32], an hygroma, a fibroma, a lipoma, a myxoma, a neurofibroma, an osteochondroma and a chondroma; Wollstein, a multiple hemangioma of the lung; MacMahon and Mallory, a fibrosarcoma of the pleura; Smith and Stone, a mesothelioma and a teratoma; Catron, a leiomyosarcoma of the pleura; Klemperer and

Coleman[29], a mesothelioma; and Yater and Lyddane, a lipoma of the mediastinum.

The outstanding symptoms are varied. There may be none in some cases, the lesion being discovered as the result of a routine x-ray examination or fluoroscopy; because of a sudden hemiplegia, or persistent joint pains, the result of brain and bone metastasis, respectively. If the new growth is located in the mediastinum it is more likely to be discovered provided pressure is exerted on definite structures. Dyspnea occurs in about 93 per cent of the cases. It is more marked if an anterior mediastinal tumor is present and very severe if the lesion is a hilar carcinoma. It may pass on to an orthopnea. It is usually of long duration, without cardiorenal complications or other causes. Cough occurs in 90 per cent and is most marked if an anterior mediastinal tumor or a hilar pulmonary cancer is present; is unproductive if pleural in nature, but produces thick profuse sputum if hilar in nature. It may be so violent as to cause pain and vomiting, and often produces paroxysms. Early in the process it is difficult to explain. The so-called "prune juice" sputum is rare. The resemblance is more that of currant jelly. It occurs in about 60 per cent, although it is usually late. Thin mucosanguineous sputum over a period of weeks or months with little fever and no chills or night sweats, should suggest a bronchial ulceration from a new growth. Pain is very common, is more severe if the lesion is malignant even though very small, becomes progressively worse, is unrelieved by opiates, and is usually intercostal, substernal, clavicular or limited to the affected area. Cyanosis is supposed to occur fairly early and is present in 50 per cent of all cases. It is due to venous compression. Osteo-arthropathy takes place in 25 per cent, so that clubbing of the fingers in a person of cancer age should excite suspicion. Hoarseness is more common in mediastinal Hodgkin's disease and the lymphosarcoma due to pressure on the recurrent laryngeal nerve. In this pleural type there are the symptoms of an idiopathic pleurisy, with or without effusion, in 50 per cent. In primary lung tumors cachexia is late; in the metastatic variety it is early. Mix[37] feels that in the presence of an operative scar and any pneumonic symptom, a metastatic pulmonary lesion should be suspected. Horner's syndrome is not nearly so frequent as formerly supposed. Vascular disturbances are uncommon.

The physical findings are not always conducive to an easy diagnosis. In the hilar involvement there are diminished breath sounds and dulness to percussion. In the pleural type there is dulness and absent breath sounds. In some cases a small area of consolidation may be outlined. Behier quoted by Barron[2], speaks of a peculiar tubular breathing due to a narrowing of the bronchus from compression which he calls "cornage." This is very significant if a bloody sputum accompanies it. Hoffman, Aufrecht and Rosenbach describe an asymmetry of the two halves, a degree of curvature, ironing out of the interspaces, retraction of the ribs and overlying dulness. Rogers[41] states that 7.5 to 10 per cent show evidence of a palsy of the phrenic nerve (more often on the left side) with paralysis of the corresponding side and an accompanying paradoxical respiration; a tracheal deviation toward the affected side, hyper-resonance in the remaining lung tissue, lesser respiratory excursion on the affected side, and every possible type of breathing or râle. In considering the metastatic aspect Craver[9] suggests a complete examination of the lungs for all patients with a carcinoma of the breast or an osteogenic sarcoma, to save any unnecessary operations.

Fishberg[13] places the most faith on the history and the physical findings. Often the physical findings are not suggestive. The x-ray picture is most important and views should be made from various angles. Fluoroscopy will aid in ruling out a pulsating mass. If a hemorrhagic pleural effusion recurs frequently, the sediment should be stained and studied thoroughly. Fishberg[13] found cancer cells in 70 per cent of the hemorrhagic fluids from patients with neoplasm. The sputum should be examined, because in 60 per cent the tumor cells may be found. Fishberg recommends diagnostic pneumothorax in certain questionable cases. If any enlarged glands are present one should be removed for biopsy. Bronchoscopy in the hands of competent men is of inestimable value in diagnosing carcinoma of the bronchus. Vinson[46] has shown how absolutely essential it is, although he calls attention to the possibility of fatal hemorrhage following it. Weller[51] has three requisites for the diagnosis of carcinoma of the lung, which are difficult to satisfy; necropsy, the nature of the lesion verified by the microscope and the establishment of the fact that the lesion is not secondary. Ford points out that carcinoma of the cervix will metastasize to the lung. Phillips[40] depends entirely on inspection and palpation. Farrel[12] has outlined briefly and concisely the manner in which the roentgenogram will aid in the diagnosis. Summarizing the above opinions, it is apparent that as many of these signs as can be obtained should be secured and analyzed. The intrathoracic lesion should be definitely stated as to degree of malignancy, type of growth, location, and accessibility to surgery.

Metastases from primary carcinoma of the lung pass to the nearby lymph nodes, the opposite lung, the liver, the pleura, the kidney, the brain, the bones, the adrenal gland, and the heart. If the lesion is a metastatic involvement of the lung the growth usually continues there profusely, although regional glands may be involved. Hodgkin's disease and lymphosarcoma will usually involve other nodes in the body if death does not occur too quickly. However, Dunlap states that malignant tumors situated in the lung or kidney are especially prone to run an asymptomatic course.

Complications are infrequent. From carcinoma of the bronchus, a severe hemorrhage may occur; from compression of the bronchus due to exogenous or endogenous new growth, there may be an atelectasis followed by bronchiectasis; and a pleural effusion, usually hemorrhagic, follows a malignant involvement of the pleura.

The outlook is poor in the malignant type; but favorable in the benign type if removal is possible. The outlook in Hodgkin's disease according to Symmers[44] is hopeless death occurring in six years on an average. Jacobs[28] reports that at least ten per cent of teratomata undergo sarcomatous or carcinomatous transformation. Baron[2] sees a hopeless outlook in carcinoma of the lung with an average of one and one-half years of life. Lymphosarcoma and metastatic carcinoma are definitely incurable.

The treatment of malignant intrathoracic tumors is based on radium and x-ray with a very small percentage amenable to surgery. Desjardins[10] says that radiotherapy provokes the quickest response in the lymphocytic mediastinal structures; hence the Hodgkin's disease and the lymphosarcoma; it is not nearly so satisfactory for epithelial tissue. Heur[25] reports eight patients operated upon for intrathoracic tumors, of which six recovered from the operation and two died, one from a ruptured aneurism and the other from coronary embolism. Of the six who recovered, one died four months later, and one, ten months postoperatively, from extension; two are alive and well five years later, and two alive and well two years, postoperatively. Harrington[24] reports thirty-eight patients, from whom intrathoracic new growths were removed surgically. Three deaths resulted; one a neurofibromata, on the fourth day due to pneumonia and bloody effusion, the second, also a neurofibromata on the sixth day because of bronchopneumonia and hemorrhage into the spinal cord, and the third, a dermoid cyst undergoing malignant changes, because of cerebral embolism. Sixteen are living and have been completely relieved of symptoms for three months to six years. Neuhof reports six patients who were operated upon, of which one lived. Vinson and Leddy[40] diagnosed seventy-one cases of bronchogenic carcinoma by biopsy. Twenty-nine of the patients received no treatment and died, an average of five plus months after the condition was discovered. Forty-two had radium or x-ray treatments or both, and of these thirty-two lived an average of eight months; while the ten patients who received x-ray therapy alone are living from fifteen months to four years with an average of twenty-three months. Wharton reported a case of generalized edema following x-ray therapy of a lymphosarcoma. It is not necessary to state that the control of the x-ray and radium therapy should be in capable hands. There is no treatment for the metastatic variety other than to alleviate symptoms as well as possible.

In conclusion we feel that all should be more cognizant of the fact that intrathoracic new growths are fairly frequent, that the benign type in a fair percentage will become malignant, that surgery has more to offer than before and that radiotherapy even though it will not cure, will prolong life; hence early diagnosis is the essential factor. In none of the five cases outlined could resection have been carried out. Nevertheless, lesions will be seen subsequently which can be treated thus.

BIBLIOGRAPHY

1. Arkin, Aaron: Bronchus Carcinoma. Medical Clinics of North America, W. B. Saunders and Company, p. 1255, (March) 1930.

2. Barron, Moses: Carcinoma of the lung. Arch. Surg., iv: 624 (May) 1922.

3. Blumgarten, A. S.: Diagnosis of primary lung tumors. Am. Jour. Med. Sc., clxii:376 (September) 1921.

5. Brunn, Harold: Primary carcinoma of the lung. Arch. Surg., xii:406 (January) 1926.

7. Cooper, DaVid A.: Hodgkin's Diseases of the Mediastinum. Medical Clinics of North America, W. B. Saunders and Company, p. 993. (January) 1931.

9. Craver, Lloyd F.: Simulation of acute respiratory diseases by secondary lung tumors. Am. Jour. Med. Sc., clxix:792 (May) 1925.

10. Desjardins, Arthur U.: Values of radiotherapy in mediastinal tumors, California and West. Med., xxxii:377 (June) 1930.

12. Farrel, John T., Jr.: Roentgen diagnosis of intrathoracic neoplasms. Radiology, xiii:1 (July) 1929.

13. Fishberg, Maurice: Discernment of intrathoracic neoplasms by aid of diagnostic pneumothorax. Jour. Am. Med. Assn., lxxvi:581 (February 26) 1921.

18. Fried, B. M.: Primary carcinoma of the lungs. Arch. Path., viii:46 (July) 1929.

20. Greenberg, David: Pulmonary neoplasm. Am. Jour. Med. Sc., clxix:648 (May) 1925.

21. Grove, J. S., and S. E. Kramer: Primary carcinoma of the lung. Am. Jour. Med. Sc., clxxi:250 (February) 1926.

22. Harrington, S. W.: Intrathoracic new growths results of surgical treatment. Surg. Gynec. and Obst., li:647 (November) 1930.

24. Harrington, S. W.: Surgical treatment of mediastinal tumors. Ann. Surg., xcvi:843 (November) 1932.

25. Heur, George J.: Intrathoracic tumors. Ann. Surg., lxxix: 670 (May) 1924.

26. Hoffman, F. L.: Cancer of the lungs. Am. Rev. Tuberc., xix:392 (April) 1929.

28. Jacobs, William F.: Malignant mediastinal teratoma. Am. Jour. Path., v:275 (May) 1929.

29. Klemperer, P. and C. B. Robin: Primary neoplasms of pleura. Arch. Path., x:385 (March) 1931.

31. Lemon, W. S. and J. B. Doyle: Clinical observation of Hodgkin's disease with special reference to mediastinal involvement. Am. Jour. Med. Sc., clxii:516 (October) 1921.

32. Lemon, W. S.: Rare Intrathoracic Tumors. Medical Clinics of North America, W. B. Saunders and Company, p. 17, (July) 1931.

33. Lemon, W. S., P. P. Vinson and H. J. Moersch: Primary carcinoma of the bronchus. Southwestern Med., xvi:485 (December) 1932.

36. MacRae, Thomas, E. H. Funk and Chevalier Jackson: Primary carcinoma of the bronchi. Jour. Am. Med. Assn., lxxxix: 1140 (October) 1927.

37. Mix, C. L.: Metastatic Carcinoma of the Lung. Medical Clinics of North America, W. B. Saunders and Company, p. 1681, (May) 1922.

40. Phillips, John: Differential diagnosis of diseases of the mediastinum. Jour. Am. Med. Assn., lxxviii:1355 (April 6) 1922.

41. Rogers, W. L.: Primary cancer of the lung. Arch. Int. Med., cxxx:1058 (January) 1932.

42. Rose, E.: The Effects of Pressure within the Mediastinum. Medical Clinics of North America, W. B. Saunders and Company, p. 999. (January) 1931.

44. Symmers, Douglas: Clinical significance of pathological changes in Hodgkin's disease. Am. Jour. Med. Sc., clxvii:313 (March) 1924.

46. Vinson, P. P.: Differentiation of Primary Carcinoma of the Bronchus and Unusual Types of Pulmonary Tuberculosis. Medical Clinics of North America, W. B. Saunders and Company, p. 1501 (May) 1929.

49. Vinson, P. P., and E. T. Leddy: The roentgen treatment of primary malignant disease of the tracheobronchial tree. Ann. Otol. Rhinol., and Laryngol., xli:1259 (December) 1932.

50. Weiss, Edward: Differential diagnosis of primary and secondary carcinoma of the bronchi. Am. Jour. Med. Sc., clxxvii: 487 (April) 1929.

51. Weller, C. V.: Pathology of primary carcinoma of the lung. Arch. Path., vii:478 (March) 1929.

53. Wessler, H., and C. M. Greene: Intrathoracic Hodgkin's disease: its roentgen diagnosis. Jour. Am. Med. Assn., lxxiv: 445 (February 14) 1920.

THYMIC DISTURBANCES IN CHILDREN*†

G. E. Harrison, M.D., Mason City

The Index Medicus for the past seven years contains 457 references to articles concerning the thymus gland. There are articles on the anatomy; articles on the pathology; articles on the experimental physiology; in fact, articles covering every conceivable phase of the subject. The majority of these papers advance theories and describe symptom complexes and syndromes arising from thymic disturbances. There are a few, however, that refute these theories and deny the very existence of such symptoms or syndromes. While it is dangerous to be dogmatic about anything in the realm of scientific medicine and while no doubt there is much to be said in favor of each side of the controversy, I believe that we will soon see the day when we will accept with more reluctance, and make with more caution, diagnoses of thymic dysfunction.

It is not necessary, perhaps, to remind you that the thymus gland is triangular in shape and occupies the superior anterior portion of the mediastinum; that its base is in close relationship to the base of the heart; that its relationship to the great vessels, major nerves, and trachea is necessarily most intimate and that like most parenchymatous organs, is capable of great variation in size, shape and weight. In 80 per cent of the cases, according to Noback[30], the apex becomes cervical in relationship, extending through the so-called critical space of Grawitz from the thoracic cavity. This space, bounded by the unyielding sternum and

*Presented before the Eighty-second Annual Session, Iowa State Medical Society, Des Moines, May 10, 11, 12, 1933.
†A complete bibliography of pertinent literature will be found in the author's reprint.

vertebrae, is quite small, averaging some 2.9 cm. in diameter in the newly born infant. It is conceivable without a great stretch of the imagination, that a hyperplastic gland might become wedged in this space, thus compressing the aforementioned structures and producing obstructive symptoms. However, it is conceded that this action occurs only occasionally.

For many years the thymus gland was considered necessary for growth, sexual maturity, nutrition and what not. Many laboratory animals were sacrificed in extirpation experiments. Park and McClure[32] in 1918, by a monumental piece of work, concluded that this gland was not necessary for life; that its removal altered in no way the development of hair, teeth, body contour, muscle and osseous systems. It is significant, I believe, that later investigators found their work so complete that extirpation experiments have almost totally disappeared from the literature.

The secretions of the thymus gland have had their part in the controversy. Their possible presence and their probable action are still matters of hypotheses. The brevity of this paper does not permit a review of the work on experimental physiology. It may be said, however, that there seems to be some inter-relationship between the thymus gland and the glands of internal secretion, notably the suprarenal gland. Suprarenalectomy in the rabbit produces a syndrome comparable to that of status thymicolymphaticus in children; but even so, what of it? Cannot the symptoms of hypotonicity, susceptibility to infection, and vagotonic manifestations usually ascribed to this syndrome be explained on the basis of deficient adrenal secretion, the consequence of which we know a little, rather than on the hypersecretion of the thymus gland of which we know less? It is obvious in the final analysis, that whatever the thymic secretion is, no one fully understands it, and it only follows, therefore, that it is difficult to determine when there is too little or too much.

Symptoms for which the thymus gland is reputedly responsible are: flabbiness of muscle, lack of resistance to infection, convulsions, eczema, mental retardation, to say nothing of pylorospasm, colic, constipation, apnea, cyanosis, laryngeal spasm, stridor and many others too numerous to mention. It is comforting for us physicians to have a convenient doorstep at which to lay obscure, confusing symptoms. It is equally comforting, perhaps more so, to apply a convenient dose of x-ray therapy to the thymic region as a cure for these perplexing symptoms; then because many cases improve, as they no doubt would anyway, our scientific consciences are appeased, we become enthusiastic and are convinced of the relationship of the thymus gland to these symptoms. The doctrine of *Post Hoc, ergo propter hoc* is a dangerous one and has lead many a practitioner into disastrous pitfalls. True, remarkable improvement sometimes appears to follow such treatment. The hypothesis has been advanced that protein end products of the tissue destruction are responsible in some way for this improvement. The important point is that as good results can be obtained by irradiation over any parenchymatous organ, the spleen or the pylorus of the stomach. This fact alone should be a strong argument against too hasty diagnosis of thymic dysfunction or too hasty attribution of symptoms to a supposedly enlarged thymus gland. Unfortunately, thymic enlargement is associated with sudden death in the minds of the laity as well as in those of many medical men. Have we not all seen nervous mothers made miserable by the knowledge that their child has an enlarged thymus? They are unable to sleep; they get up at night to see if their child is still alive. If we are convinced in our own minds that irradiation of the thymic area is of benefit in certain conditions, is it not better to use the treatment purely empirically than to chance parenteral misery and our own scientific prostitution?

There is a great need for the revision of our ideas concerning a normal thymus gland. Kinney and Taylor[28], after a study of 150 infants in their first twenty-four hours of life, came to the conclusion that there are no normal constants as to size, shape or density. In general, it can be said that the thymus gland varies with the nutrition of the patient. The definite relationship of the size of the thymus gland to disease has been pointed out by Edith Boyd[3] who has collected data on 1,891 thymus glands. She states that whatever the cause of death, the weight of the gland decreases with the length of illness and this decrease is well under way by the end of the first week. She feels that the large glands, heretofore associated with status thymicolymphaticus, are really normal, and that x-ray pictures of such glands should be considered evidence of good health and nutrition. If such a premise can be accepted, and I believe it can, it explains the frequency in which apparent enlargement is found. Peterson and Miller[37] found 57 per cent of their newly born children with shadows considered larger than normal. Liss, Wasson and Shannon[39] have shown that wide thymic shadows, considered evidence of thymic syndromes, are common in healthy and symptom free children. In Cooperstock's[7] series, there was even compression of the trachea in 50 per cent of the infants who presented no symptoms at all. In our clinic, over a period of twenty-two months,

297 babies were delivered. Of these, 200 were delivered by members of the staff and x-ray pictures were taken on the fourth day in a search for enlargement of the thymus gland. Of this number, 76 infants, or 38 per cent, apparently had enlarged glands. By the greatest stretch of the imagination, ten of these 76 had one or more symptoms ascribed to thymic dysfunction. While my series with its 38 per cent fails to equal Miller's 57 per cent and Cooperstock's 50 per cent, it is still difficult to see how even 38 per cent of our babies are born with a pathologic state.

That the practice of x-raying all children at birth is worthless is made apparent, further, by the unique piece of work by Hasley and De Tomasi[42]. These workers, with a Cin-ex camera which takes exposures on a roll of film at the rate of four per second have demonstrated by their serial roentgenograms that the size of the thymus gland varies with the respiratory phase, the position of the diaphragm, systole and diastole of the heart, engorgement of the pulmonary artery, aorta and the vena cava. A picture plucked at random from any series may well be taken by the ordinary standards to show an enlarged gland; another from the same series, but in a different cardiac and respiratory phase, will appear, by the same tokens, perfectly normal. Thus it is apparent that much of the statistical data of the past on the x-ray incidence of enlarged thymus glands must be revised. It is equally evident that pictures showing the apparent shrinkage of the gland after exposure to x-rays are worth but little, because, if the identical cardiac and respiratory phases are not represented, the comparisons are not significant.

The question might well be asked, if not the thymus gland, then what?

Certainly the upper respiratory passages should be searched for adenoids, abscesses, adenitis, and congenital anomalies of the larynx in cases of stridor. Pancost has demonstrated by the fluoroscope and carefully timed lateral roentgenograms that there is a great collapse of the trachea and pharynx at the end of expiration and the beginning of inspiration. It is quite probable that this abnormal laxness of soft tissue may be responsible for many stridors. Cyanosis and apnea should demand an investigation of the circulatory and central nervous systems; colic and constipation, require regulation of diet, and so we could go through the entire list of symptoms. Something can usually be found to explain all symptoms if we search for it and are not obsessed with the probability of thymic pathology.

In conclusion, it may be said that first, there is a great variation in the size and weight of the thymus gland according to the state of health and nutrition of the patient; second, that there is possibly some inter-relationship between the thymus gland and the glands of internal secretion; third, that there is a dire need of a revision of our ideas of what constitutes an enlarged thymus gland and the symptoms arising thereof; and finally that there is no definite evidence of a thymic secretion and that symptoms ascribed to its excess or absence can often be explained on some other basis.

May we bear these facts in mind and make the diagnosis of thymic enlargement or dysfunction with more caution and more care, so that this "fetish" of "enlarged thymus gland" will soon be cast into oblivion where it rightfully belongs.

BIBLIOGRAPHY

3. Boyd, Edith: The weight of the thymus gland in health and disease. Amer. Jour. Dis. Child., xliii: 1162-1214 (May) 1932.

7. Cooperstock, M.: Present concepts of enlarged thymus and status thymicolymphaticus. Jour. Mich. State Med. Soc., xxix:21-24 (January) 1930.

23. Kinney, Mila J. and Raymond G. Taylor: Observations on eight years' experience in the treatment of the thymus gland in infants and young children. Am. Jour. Roentgenol., xxi: 263-270 (March) 1929.

30. Noback, Gustave J.: A contribution to the topographic anatomy of the thymus gland, with particular reference to its changes at birth and in the period of the new-born. Am. Jour. Dis. Child., xxii:120-144 (August) 1921.

32. Park, E. A., and R. D. McClure: The results of thymus extirpation in the dog. Am. Jour. Dis. Child., xviii:317 (November) 1919.

37. Peterson, Reuben and Norman F. Miller: Thymus of the new-born and its significance to the obstetrician. Jour. Am. Med. Assn., lxxxiii:234-238 (July 26) 1924.

39. Shannon, E. H.: Some observations on thymus in early infancy. Can. Med. Assn. Jour., xxii, 775-785 (June) 1930.

42. Symposium on the Thymus. (a) Review of literature relative to animal experimentation regarding thymic disturbance, Clement A. Smith. (b) Clinical aspects of diseases of thymus gland in childhood. W. C. C. Cole. (c) Present concepts of enlarged thymus and status thymicolymphaticus, M. Cooperstock. (d) Cin-ex camera studies of thymus in infants and children, C. K. Halsey and R. Q. DeTomasi. (e) The use of x-ray in the treatment and diagnosis of enlarged thymus, S. W. Donaldson and J. M. Barnes. Jour. Mich. State Med. Soc., xxix:11-36 (January) 1930.

FUNCTIONAL DISTURBANCES ASSOCIATED WITH THE MENOPAUSE*

DELLA G. DRIPS, M.D., Division of Medicine
The Mayo Clinic, Rochester, Minnesota

In our conception of the menopause certain clinical manifestations are associated: first, irregularity and finally cessation of menstruation; second, vasomotor disturbances, and third, atrophy of the genitalia and tissues of the breasts. We have assumed that these manifestations were evidences of cessation of ovarian activity. However, when substitution treatment has been given by means of ovarian extract in an attempt to control the severity of the menopausal symptoms, particularly vasomotor disturbances, contradictory and confusing results have been obtained.

In recent years, treatment has been gradually

*Presented before the Thirty-sixth Annual Meeting, State Society of Iowa Medical Women, Des Moines, May 10, 1933.

placed on a more logical basis. Studies of the blood and urine of women during the menopause to determine the amounts of ovarian estrogenic and pituitary anterior lobe hormone present, have done more than anything else to explain the physiologic phenomena, and thus throw light as to when substitution treatment is of value. Zondek, as a result of such determinations, has divided the climacteric into three periods.

Period 1. In this period an excess of the ovarian estrogenic hormone is found in the urine. It is assumed that the ovary during this period can no longer respond to the stimulus to luteinization from the anterior pituitary lobe and so fails to produce sufficient luteal hormone to balance the estrogenic hormone produced. This is, then, secreted in excess. During this period, menstruation is often more profuse or more prolonged, and the bleeding is irregular. The uterus, in such cases, is often larger and softer than normal, and curettage reveals hyperplasia of the endometrium. After such a diagnostic curettage has been made and the diagnosis of menorrhagia of the menopause established, it may be possible to control the bleeding with some preparation of ovarian luteal hormone. The only active preparation on the market at present is sistomensin. The action of sistomensin seems to be increased by the addition of calcium. If this medication does not take care of the bleeding, a menopausal dose of radium within the uterus or roentgen rays over the ovaries will be effective.

Period 2. In this second period the secretion of ovarian estrogenic hormone begins to fail also; only a small amount or none is found in the blood and urine. The menses become farther apart and scantier, finally ceasing entirely. The vasomotor disturbances reach their height during this period, and it is in this period that preparations of the ovarian estrogenic hormone should produce good therapeutic effects. Aschheim[1] feels that the pure estrogenic hormone which is made in Germany from the urine of pregnant mares, has given especially good results in the treatment of the vasomotor disturbances of this period. He gives it orally in divided daily doses up to 1000 or 1500 mouse units daily until an effect is produced. At times, only small amounts are required.

Kurzrok[4] has reported a group to 100 women suffering from the vasomotor disturbances of the menopause, and found that only those without ovarian estrogenic hormone in the urine were benefited by ovarian medication. This consisted of 2 c.c. of sistomensin containing ten rat units of estrogenic hormone, once a week, intramuscularly (sistomensin contains a standardized amount of the estrogenic hormone, together with a nonstandardized amount of the ovarian luteal hormone).

This is a very small dose of estrogenic hormone. As yet, little is known concerning the sensitivity of the vasomotor center. It is possible that it may require more ovarian estrogenic hormone to inhibit the vasomotor impulses at the beginning of this period than at the end, when hormone is not present in the urine. I have found that individuals vary greatly as to the dosage necessary to control the vasomotor disturbances. The best results are attained if patients are treated within the first year after the cessation of the menses; the earlier the treatment, the better the result. The hot flashes which recur at intervals for several years after cessation of the menses may probably be continued because the vasomotor center has acquired a bad habit; they are best controlled with sedatives such as phenobarbital or bromides.

Period 3. The urine in this period contains an excess of the follicle-ripening hormone of the anterior pituitary lobe. The presence of this hormone in excess in the urine is significant of complete ovarian failure; it may be present for several months. The hot flashes usually subside during this period and the atrophic changes in the genitalia due to the continued lack of ovarian estrogenic hormone, may become pronounced. Symptoms such as pruritis vulvae, which may be associated with this atrophic change, are sometimes relieved by preparations of ovarian estrogenic hormone.

The headaches of the menopause may be the result of neurasthenia or they may be an aggravated migraine type, but there is, without doubt, a headache like that which occurs with the menses, that is, glandular. The administration of various preparations of ovarian estrogenic hormone and the combination of estrogenic hormone with luteal or preparations of whole ovary, have not seemed to be of benefit.

The increase of weight after the menopause has not been explained. It, likewise, has not been influenced by substitution treatment by means of ovarian extract. Kaufmann[3] has isolated a hormone from the liquor folliculi which apparently influences fat metabolism. There may be another ovarian hormone, as yet not isolated, which has to do with metabolism. The tendency has been to consider the thyroid gland responsible for this obesity. Because the gland enlarges with puberty and pregnancy, it has been linked with ovarian function and there has been a tendency to believe that it became hypo-active after ovarian function ceased. This hypothesis has not been substantiated. The relationship between the ovaries and the thyroid gland as far as fat metabolism is concerned is not yet known. The suprarenal glands, and pituitary glands no doubt are likewise concerned.

Study of the basal metabolism should be continued during the menopause. I have found that some women after artificial or spontaneous menopause have low basal metabolic rates. This may be due to an extreme state of fatigue, the result of continued vasomotor disturbances. The fatigue and low rate may have been preëxistent, only aggravated by the menopause. Such women often feel much better when their basal metabolic rate is raised and held at a normal level. They feel less tired. The nervous system apparently becomes more stable and as a consequence, the hot flashes subside. Apparently, a vicious circle has been broken.

It has seemed to me that the neurosis of the menopause is built up on some sensation associated with the vasomotor disturbances called "hot flashes." Zondek[5] describes the "klimakterische Wallungen" which apparently correspond to what we call "hot flashes," but "waves" is a better term as it implies more than a sensation of heat. The sensation begins in the epigastrium and passes to all parts of the body, ending with a feeling of heat followed by perspiration; a sense of oppression, faintness, air-hunger, palpitation and finally heat and perspiration; one or all may be experienced in the minor waves. With more intense stimulations, there may be associated alterations of the psyche, depression, increased irritability, restlessness, impairment of memory, inability to concentrate, easy mental fatigue and other mental symptoms. The phenomenon has been explained as originating in the vasomotor center. A stimulus is transmitted along the splanchnic nerves. The entire vascular system of the abdomen is contracted and a large amount of blood is suddenly forced into the peripheral vessels. Active vasodilatation of the peripheral vessels seems to occur at the same time. As a result of the sudden displacement of such a large volume of blood from the center of the body to the periphery the symptoms of faintness, oppression and air-hunger, anxiety, palpitation, heat and perspiration have a true physiologic explanation. It is not surprising that a woman experiencing one of these vasomotor waves for the first time should become frightened. Her fear becomes directed to one of the organs of the body, depending on which sensation makes the most impression. Often, it is the heart, because of the palpitation. This makes her heart-conscious for the first time. The idea that she has heart trouble becomes fixed in her mind. She visits a physician and complains of rapid and irregular beating of the heart; a sensation of the heart "turning over," and "stopping,"

sufficient to keep her awake at night, and shortness of breath with any exertion, so that she is unable to do her work. She may not mention the hot flashes or other disturbances, her mind being fixed on her heart. The hot flashes may even have subsided and left only the neurosis of the menopause; this neurosis will require the same treatment as any other. After every examination possible is made to rule out organic heart trouble, a great deal of time must be taken to explain to the patient the origin of the "heart trouble," assuring her in a kindly but impressive way that it is not organic. If any medication is given, which would be only a sedative, she must be assured that it is not for heart trouble but to help her to get some rest so that she can better forget her heart. It would be useless and unscientific to use the ovarian extract in the treatment of such neurotic residual manifestation.

Women who have previously been unstable nervously and mentally, or women who are in a state of chronic fatigue when the menopause overtakes them, may have exaggerated nervous and mental manifestations. It is always wise in such cases to examine carefully the previous history, as these women may need some special guidance to carry them through the menopause without a complete nervous breakdown.

All sorts of queer notions and fears exist in the minds of the laity and even among certain physicians concerning the menopause. It is called the "second great crisis" in a woman's life. One hears expressions such as the "storm of the menopause," or "calm after the menopause." Gertrude Atherton has recently revived the impression that women go through some degenerating process of mind and body during the menopause and must be "reactivated" following it in order to live a worthwhile life after the age of fifty. If a woman is in good nervous and physical health, the approaching menopause need not be given a thought. Her disability may be so mild that she will be scarcely aware of it. If it becomes somewhat troublesome in the way of unusual bleeding, or flashes, a sensible physician can give her the needed help to make her quite as normal as before. Many women express themselves as feeling better after the change than they ever did before and are able to accomplish much more. One is reminded of the oft quoted words of Currier[2]: "All that tends to develop and strengthen the physical part of woman, to render her insensitive to the ordinary ills of life, to make her forgetful of self, is favorable to a normal menopause."

BIBLIOGRAPHY

1. Aschheim, S.: Personal communication to the author.
2. Currier, A. F.: The Menopause, a consideration of the

phenomena which occur to women at the close of the childbearing period, with incidental allusions to their relationship to menstruation. D. Appleton and Co., New York, 1897. p. 325.
    3. Kaufmann, C.: Weibliche Keimdrüsen und Fettstoffwech-
sel. Arch. f. Gynaek., cxliv:285-291, 1930-1931.
    4. Kurzrok, R.: Follicular hormone in the urine as index of
therapy in the menstrual dysfunction. Endocrinology. xvi:361-
365 (July-August) 1932.
    5. Zondek, Bernhard: Die Hormone des Ovariums und des
Hypophysenvorderlappens. Julius Springer, Berlin, 1931, p. 343.

THE DIAGNOSIS AND TREATMENT OF TRIGEMINAL NEURALGIA*

WALTER D. ABBOTT, M.D., F.A.C.S., Des Moines

There is no clinical entity which is more distressing to the patient than the painful affliction
of trigeminal neuralgia. This symptom complex
is characterized by stabbing, throbbing and lancinating pain of the face, and although most common after the fourth decade, it has been known to
occur in as young an individual as nine and as old
a one as ninety years of age. In spite of the fact
that this condition can readily be relieved with
a minimal risk, there is still much confusion relative to the diagnosis, and it is the purpose of this
paper to present the salient features of this clinical entity with the hope that it will lead to earlier
recognition and relief of suffering.

HISTORY

Avicenna, about 1000 A. D., is credited with the
original description of this disease when he called
it *tortura facies*, and in 1773, Fothergill described
a "painful affection of the face." Many other
authors reported this condition, but little was
added to the original contributions. Until Bell,
in 1883, outlined his experiments, proving that
the trigeminal nerve supplied sensation to the
face, this disease was considered the result of a
disorder of the facial nerve. Mears was the first
to suggest radical treatment for trigeminal neuralgia in an operation consisting of an intracranial
approach through the foramen ovale with partial
avulsion of the Gasserian ganglion. Rose, in 1892,
approached the ganglion through the floor of the
middle fossa of the skull, but both of these procedures were attended with considerable hemorrhage and mortality. In 1891, Horsley attempted
an avulsion of the sensory root; however, because
of the death of the patient, little recognition followed his effort. Hartley, in 1892, performed a
section of the second and third branches of the
nerve peripheral to the ganglion but this was not
a permanent result. Krause advocated extradural
exposure of the ganglion, avulsion and division of
the peripheral branches. All of these formidable
procedures were of little value until, in 1898,
Spiller and Keen proposed section of the posterior
sensory root. Then, Frazier and Spiller in 1900,

* Presented before the Eighty-second Annual Session, Iowa
State Medical Society, Des Moines, May 10, 11, 12, 1933.

and von Gehucten in 1903, demonstrated that
division of the posterior sensory root would result in permanent anesthesia of the face and that
regeneration of the fibers did not occur.

Since that time, the radical operation has
changed from ganglionectomy of the Krause-
Cushing type to simple division of the posterior
root chiefly through refinements in the technic by
Frazier, Adson and Peet with a reduction in mortality to less than one per cent. More recently,
Dandy has advocated an approach through the
posterior fossa with a partial division of the sensory root near the pons in an effort to preserve
the tactile sensation. However, this type of operation carries a greater hazard and there have
not been sufficient reports to justify a change from
the accepted temporal route.

For a number of years prior to the development of a satisfactory radical operation, palliative peripheral neurectomy was practiced. However, Schlosser, in 1903, demonstrated that alcoholic injection of the nerve roots was of greater
advantage and did not produce mutilating scars.
In 1914, Hartel described a technic for alcoholic
injection of the ganglion and there are still some
advocates of his method despite the dangers
fraught by the possibility of a keratitis or paralysis of other cranial nerves.

The most satisfactory palliative method was
evolved by Levy and Boudouin in 1906, when they
described their technic of injection of the peripheral branches of the nerve at the foramina.
This was later modified by Patrick.

ETIOLOGY

The cause of trigeminal neuralgia is not known.
Horsley believed that this disease was the result
of an ascending neuritis following infection of the
teeth, but this theory cannot be accepted because of
the occurrence of this condition in the absence of
dental caries and its persistence after the radical
extraction of teeth. Frazier considered this condition as a sequel of sclerosis of the ganglion, and
Dana thought it was a result of degenerative
changes in the ganglion. However, the experiences of the pathologists do not conform with this
hypothesis. Adson has suggested that arteriosclerosis might be a causative factor as this disease occurs in the later decades of life. The fact
that trigeminal neuralgia does occur in young people, though rarely, would preclude this theory.
In a previous paper, I have advanced an additional theory, that based upon the presence of
sympathetic fibers in the trigeminal nerve, might
cause an imbalance of the blood supply causing
these painful spasms.

DIAGNOSIS

Trigeminal neuralgia is characterized by shooting, stabbing, lightning-like pains radiating along the distribution of one or more branches of the fifth cranial nerve. These pains occur in paroxysms lasting from a few seconds to one or two minutes. The attacks of pain may be so frequent that they seem almost constant, but there is always a brief interval between the paroxysms in true trigeminal neuralgia.

The attacks may be provoked by talking, chewing of food, washing the face or teeth, touching the face, or even a draft of cold air. It is not uncommon to see a patient, who is usually meticulous about appearance, with the face unwashed or unshaven because of the dread fear of producing this painful spasm. During the attack, the patient will either sit immobile and tense, or suddenly clasp the hand to the face. Some patients have even rubbed the skin from the affected side of the face in an effort to alleviate their suffering. Often there is a particularly sensitive area on the face or gums, known as a "trigger zone," and touching this region will initiate an attack. These people learn to shun all types of stimuli and become veritable recluses in their attempt to ward off this agonizing pain. Unfortunately, radical extraction of teeth or sinus operations will not relieve this pain, and careful and painstaking examination is necessary to distinguish this condition from other types of facial or head pain.

One of the most confusing types of head or facial pain is migraine which produces pain through the eyeball or cheek. However, trigeminal neuralgia is not associated with headache, and a careful history in conjunction with a more constant pain will suffice to distinguish a bizarre type of migraine from true neuralgia. Pain from an infected sinus or tooth is more constant and a diligent search will reveal the underlying pathologic process. Glossopharyngeal neuralgia is similar to trigeminal neuralgia in the fact that both conditions are intermittent. However, the pain of glossopharyngeal neuralgia is provoked by yawning, swallowing, or talking, and the radiation is into the ear drums instead of in the branches of the fifth nerve. Cocainization of the tonsillar fossa, which is the trigger zone of glossopharyngeal neuralgia will serve as a ready and simple means of differentiation. Trigeminal neuralgia is unaffected by cocainization of the throat while glossopharyngeal neuralgia is immediately relieved.

The "lower half headache," sphenopalatine neuralgia, as described by Sluder is a different type of head pain, characterized by a more constant pain in the malar bone, radiating to the sphenoid region and down the neck. Cocainization of the sphenopalatine ganglion will afford temporary relief in this condition and alcohol injection produces favorable results. Undoubtedly the sympathetic fibers carry pain impulses from the face as shown by Mixter and White, Flothow and Abbott. There may be some relation between these atypical facial neuralgias and trigeminal neuralgia and, when there is extreme doubt, alcohol injection of the peripheral branches of the fifth nerve will conclusively establish a ready means of diagnosis.

TREATMENT

Palliative Treatment. There is no form of medication which will give prolonged relief in trigeminal neuralgia. Inhalation of trichlorethylene will give temporary relief in a small number of cases. Opiates may minimize the paroxysms of pain but they should not be administered continuously, because even massive doses will not afford comfort as the pain progresses in frequency and intensity. The most satisfactory method of palliative treatment is alcoholic injection of the nerve branches. Superficial injection does not afford relief as long as the deep injection of the nerves. In the deep injection, relief is obtained for a period of nine to twelve months, and with each injection the duration of relief is shorter. However, at least one injection should be performed prior to operation, because it allows the patient to become accustomed to the anesthesia which follows section of the posterior root. It is unwise to repeat the deep alcoholic injection indefinitely unless there is a distinct contraindication to surgery, because a certain amount of scar tissue forms around the nerve and sooner or later complete failure will result.

Technic of Injection. The prevailing custom is to place the patient under partial anesthesia because severe pain results when the nerve is approached. The mandibular branch is injected at its exit from the foramen ovale by inserting the needle under the zygoma at a point two and one-half centimeters in front of the external auditory meatus. The needle is directed up and back along the floor of the skull until the foramen is encountered at a depth of four centimeters. The point of entry for injection of the maxillary branch is 0.5 cm. anterior to the site of injection for the mandibular division. The needle is directed vertically to the anteroposterior axis of the skull and slightly upward to a depth of five centimeters where the foramen rotundum is reached. Two cubic centimeters of 95 per cent alcohol are injected into each nerve and it is then my custom to inject two cubic centimeters of air to prevent dripping the alcohol along the course of the needle as it is removed. The ophthalmic division should be injected superficially in the supra-orbital foramen because it is not safe to inject large amounts of alcohol around the orbit. A satisfactory injection will result in anesthesia in the distribution of the branch or branches injected.

Radical Treatment. Prior to operation, it is often necessary to place the patient in the hospital for several days in an effort to combat the previous period of starvation or dehydration so common in patients with this condition, since many will not eat for fear of provoking a paroxysm of pain. The operation consists of division of the posterior sensory root. Since the original operation, there have been numerous refinements such as preservation of the motor root by Frazier, Cushing and Adson. In 1922, Kanavel and Davis discussed the anatomy of the trigeminal nerve with reference to preserving the motor root and injury to the superficial petrosal nerve and geniculate ganglion of the facial nerve by traction on the Gasserian ganglion. Adson, in the same year, published a method of preserving the motor root and a means of avoiding trauma to the superficial petrosal nerve by incising the arachnoid sheath above the ganglion. Frazier has advocated subtotal division of the sensory root when the ophthalmic branch has not been involved and has thus prevented complications which occasionally arise when the cornea is insensitive. Some authors prefer local anesthesia in this operation, but it is my impression that avertin is more satisfactory because it reduces operating time and lessens the psychic shock in a patient who is pain-racked and apprehensive.

The patient is placed on the operating table, on his back, with the head in a ganglion headrest. The table is elevated until the zygoma is parallel with the floor. This position will enable the surgeon to be oriented at all times and will obviate difficulties encountered in an abnormal floor of the middle fossa. An incision is made from a point five centimeters above the helix of the ear down to a point one centimeter anterior to the tragus. The temporal fascia and muscle are incised and the skull is trephined. The opening is enlarged to a diameter of four centimeters in a downward direction so that the approach may be made along the floor of the middle fossa. The dura is elevated gently with dry dental rolls and retracted upward. The middle meningeal artery is encountered at the foramen spinosum. This artery should be ligated or the foramen plugged with stiff bone wax previously heated in hot saline so that it can be moulded into the foramen and allowed to harden. Immediately beyond the fora-

men spinosum, the third branch of the trigeminal nerve is exposed. The dissection is carried upward and posteriorly until the lower edge of the ganglion is observed. At this point, the dura is incised along the anterior surface of the petrous bone. When pulsations are encountered, the arachnoid is incised and the posterior sensory root is exposed. Retraction of the sensory root with a right angle hook will disclose the motor root mesially and in an oblique direction. The sensory root is then divided and iodoform strips are inserted to prevent venous oozing. The wound is closed with interrupted silk sutures. If a total division of the sensory root is performed, then it will be necessary to apply an eye shield to prevent corneal ulceration. The eye is washed with boric acid twice daily and on leaving the hospital the patient is fitted with a corneal shield devised by Adson and Schroeder.

CASE REPORTS

The following two typical case reports illustrate the danger of alcoholic injection of the Gasserian ganglion and the satisfactory result after section of the posterior sensory root.

Case 1. A white woman, seventy-eight years of age, complained of sharp, lancinating pain in the second and third branches of the right trigeminal nerve, of fourteen years' duration, attacks of pain occurring on eating, washing the face or talking. Trigger soreness was in the right upper lip. She had tried trichlorethylene with no results, and submitted to ten superficial alcohol injections with average relief of pain for nine months. The first deep alcohol injection was in April, 1931, with subsequent anesthesia in the second and third branches, and relief from pain for nine months. The second injection was in February, 1932, because of recurrence of pain, with relief until September, 1932. At this time, the pain also involved the ophthalmic branch of the right trigeminal nerve, and an alcohol injection of the Gasserian ganglion was performed. Following the injection, there was complete anesthesia in all three branches. However, the patient developed corneal ulcer, and paralysis of the right sixth, seventh and eighth nerves. Function in the right sixth and seventh nerves has gradually returned so that at present there is only a residual weakness of the right face. There has been no return of pain.

Because this woman was in very poor general condition, an alcoholic injection of the Gasserian ganglion was performed, but the sequela of the injection seemed far worse than the risk of operation.

Case 2. A male, farmer, forty-six years of age, complained of sharp, shooting pains in the second and third divisions of the right trigeminal nerve of four years' duration, pains provoked by talking, eating, washing the face or laughing. A deep alcohol injection in November, 1929, afforded relief for one year. On July 28, 1931, section of the posterior sensory root was performed under ether anesthesia with preservation of the motor root. There was complete anesthesia in all three branches of the right trigeminal nerve, and there has been no return of pain since the operation.

This is the typical result of the radical surgical procedure, and there is no group of patients more grateful than those individuals who have obtained permanent relief from such pain.

SUMMARY

Trigeminal neuralgia is a classic entity characterized by paroxysms of stabbing, shooting or darting pains in one or more branches of the nerve. The treatment consists of two measures: alcoholic injection of the nerve as a palliative means and preliminary to operation, and section of the posterior sensory root which affords permanent relief with a surgical mortality of less than one per cent.

Discussion

Dr. Harry M. Ivins, Cedar Rapids: The case which I am reporting caused me to go into the literature rather extensively, and put me in a position to appreciate how thoroughly Dr. Abbott has presented the subject. I have only praise for his paper and the work done on it. I would like to bring out the point that I do not think trifacial neuralgia is so easily diagnosed as the text might lead one to believe. Eventually, it seems to me, the diagnosis must be made, but there seem to be no symptoms that must definitely run their course before the diagnosis can be made.

It is very easy to say that trifacial neuralgic pains are stabbing, throbbing, piercing, staccato-in-kind, and if they are not, it is not trifacial neuralgia; but trifacial neuralgia is a distinctly subjective disorder, and being such the patient may not understand what the doctor means when he speaks of paroxysms, or the doctor may not understand just what the patient means, and it has been my experience that when these patients are going through these seizures their minds are not so keen on interpretation, and what is a staccato pain to the inquisitive doctor is a continuous pain to the patient. Then again I find that authorities differ. For instance, as to the duration of the paroxysms; our texts state that the paroxysms last one-fourth to one-half minute, yet Patrick says he has had patients in which the pain lasted for fifteen minutes, and Jelliffe reports them as lasting for a day, or even for a few days. These are discrepancies either in symptoms or in interpretation, and being a subjective disorder it may be that the patient is at fault. To such a patient I am of the opinion that the rapid paroxysms, with no let-up, seem after a while like a constant pain, and he might so report it.

The patient came to my office February 20, 1933, holding his jaw and complaining of paroxysmal pain on left side of face, covering the branches of the fifth nerve. His own statement follows: Very sharp-shooting pains on the left side of the face that came suddenly and left suddenly with very tender spot in front of external canal, which he would not let me touch. The pain extended up over the temple and above the eye, directly forward under the eye and over the upper lip, down the inferior jaw, and back behind the ear and down the neck.

This man's trouble seemed to begin the first of January when he was ill with influenza for a week to ten days. Following this he had seizures of pain which came suddenly and ceased suddenly, but were not particularly severe, and in the beginning seemed to be worse in the temporal region than in the lower jaw. However, as time advanced, (you will note it covered about a month), these paroxysmal seizures became more severe and more frequent with a tendency to pass from one seizure to the next, and he spoke of it as "lasting most of the time," rather than in a staccato manner, which, according to the hard and fast rule, would seem to argue against trifacial neuralgia.

On February 19, 1933, the paroxysms were so constant as to keep him in pain most of the day and night, so that when he came into my office on February 20 he was a sad-looking sight with swelling in front of his ear which he would not permit me to touch, and although he was quite free from pain when he came in, manipulation of his mouth started up the pain again, and he was sorry he came in. This condition was characteristic as any manipulation in the mouth seemed to revive the pain. I gave him trichlorethylene which relieved him for the time being. Manipulation of the mouth may irritate any one or all three of the branches of the third division, the dental, buccal or lingual. However, there was no apparent pathology in the mouth and throat except, perhaps, his tonsils. These were submerged with red anterior pillars, no pus or food deposits. His teeth had just been cleaned and x-rayed, and one tooth had been filled by a dentist of excellent reputation. I wish you to note that examination of his teeth did not help us to find any focal infection.

When the pain first developed in January, he thought perhaps his trouble was caused by his teeth as the pain at times seemed to be more in the lower jaw. However, the teeth were negative to all tests; that is, they were not sensitive and the x-ray pictures were negative. He had a lower molar in which there was an old silver filling, and this filling was removed and a gold one put in. When he came into my office, knowing the dentist and his good reputation, we were perhaps misled. At any rate, another x-ray picture was taken of this tooth although it was not tender and did not bother him with heat and cold, and we found no shadow. Yet during the period in which I had him under observation, manipulations in his mouth caused the paroxysmal seizures to start.

He had a fair night on February 21, and on February 22 he did not have much pain, but on February 23 he again came to my office and reported that the pain had been practically constant during the previous night and that his lower jaw was very sore. The lower molar referred to was removed at once, and the pain disappeared like magic. On the apex of one of the roots a slightly roughened area was discovered which cast no shadow but which was the beginning of an abscess. The tooth was split and the nerve was in a degenerated condition, and away went my trifacial neuralgia.

It is one of the simplest things in the world to say that a neuralgic pain is one that is stabbing, hits like a shot and goes away quickly, and unless the pain conforms to this stereotyped rule it is not trifacial neuralgia; but I am sure that this case showed every symptom of trifacial neuralgia until the last day when the tooth became the prominent factor.

Dr. Gordon F. Harkness, Davenport: Dr. Abbott in this admirable presentation has answered part of my questions. Davis and Pollock in their experimental work where analgesia did not persist after section of the posterior root and was only accomplished by an accompanying cervical sympathectomy, concluded that the sympathetic system did not contain antidromic fibers. Nelson and Frazier, however, noting an increase of deep pressure sense after posterior root section, felt that antidromic fibers do exist. I wonder what Dr. Abbott proposes to do when section of the posterior root does not give complete relief. Will you then attack the superior ganglion?

Dr. Walter D. Abbott (closing) : I have enjoyed Dr. Ivins' case report. I think it leads us into rather dangerous territory. Some cases of true tic douloureux will disappear like magic when nothing has been done, and the short period of time elapsing since the tooth has been removed would make me want to keep this patient under observation for a year or two lest the pain return. It is probably true that the tooth was the offending factor.

When we are confronted with an atypical pain like that, we have one means of diagnosis, and that is alcoholic injection of the nerve. If it is not true trigeminal neuralgia the patient must still have pain. If it is true trigeminal neuralgia the pain will be relieved.

We also enter into a dangerous territory when we consider these atypical neuralgias, and I only mention them briefly, and that is our sympathetic nerve pain which Temple Fay, McClintock, Frazier and Peet have described. Various procedures on the sympathetic system have been advocated and carried out, such as stripping of the carotid artery, alcoholic injection of the adventitia of the carotid artery, removal of the sympathetic ganglia. As yet the reports are so conflicting that I do not believe we can lay down any definite rule.

In regard to Dr. Harkness' remarks, there is a great deal of contention over that. Frazier and Adson feel that the seventh nerve does carry some deep pressure sensation. I have in mind a case reported by Temple Fay two or three years ago which will probably answer your question. The patient had what appeared to be typical trigeminal neuralgia, and the fifth nerve root was cut with complete anesthesia. The patient still had pain. The seventh nerve was cut and the patient still had pain. The tenth nerve was cut and the patient still had pain. Then Temple Fay, under local anesthesia, exposed the carotid artery at the bifurcation with the stripping of the adventitia into the external and internal carotid. In stripping the adventitia the pain was relieved. On the other hand, Frazier reported twenty-eight cases of atypical facial neuralgia in which he removed the superior cervical ganglion or the middle or the inferior, and found that in all twenty-eight cases the results were unsatisfactory. Peet, Adson and Flothow contend that if Frazier had explored the sympathetic system from the posterior approach rather than going through the inferior cervical triangle he might have achieved a complete severance of all the sympathetic fibers.

Flothow has reported one case of pain like this which responded to removal of the stellate ganglion consisting of the inferior cervical and first thoracic sympathetic ganglia. I have had a similar case in which alcoholic injection of the stellate ganglion relieved the pain, and in the December, 1932, issue of the *Annals of Otology, Rhinology and Laryngology*, Temple Fay has a splendid article in which he reviews this whole subject and advocates exposure of the carotid artery at the bifurcation, with the stripping of the adventitia and also removal of the inferior cervical and first thoracic ganglia.

A SIMPLE METHOD FOR APOTHECARY-METRIC TRANSCRIPTION

Milton A. Bridges, B.S., M.D., F.A.C.P.
New York

In the course of graduate teaching, the question often arises as to the facility with which the older practitioner can learn to write prescriptions in the metric system. Due to the frequency of this question, as well as the evident unwillingness on the part of the practitioner to study properly the metric system, as is required in the medical schools today, it is my desire to refurnish with amplification the so-called "Standard Prescription" as noted in Eggleston's "Essentials of Prescription Writing."

It is well recognized that the older practitioner thinks exclusively in the apothecary system. The exemplified "Standard Prescription" as hereafter detailed will serve the purpose of providing a ready means of immediate and accurate apothecary-metric transcription.

Several fundamentals must be firmly and irrevocably borne in mind, as follows:

EQUIVALENTS

Household	Apothecary	Metric
One teaspoon	One dram (60 m.)	4.0 c.c.
One dessertspoon	Two drams (120 m.)	8.0 c.c.
One tablespoon	One-half ounce	15.0 c.c.
Two tablespoons	One ounce	30.0 c.c.
One wineglass	Two ounces	60.0 c.c.
One wineglass	Four ounces	120.0 c.c.
One wineglass	Six ounces	180.0 c.c.
One wineglass	Eight ounces	240.0 c.c.
One wineglass	Fifteen grains	1.0 Gm.
"Fifteen drops"	Fifteen minims	1.0 c.c.

(It is universally acknowledged that drops, due to varying specific gravities, are subject to marked differences.)

THE PRESCRIPTION OF SOLIDS OR LIQUIDS

The following axiom is the sole basis of the transposing from the apothecary to the metric system in prescription writing:

"When fifteen doses of a solid or liquid are prescribed, the individual dose, in the apothecary system (in grains or minims), is equivalent numerically to the number of total metric doses (in grams or c.c.)"

When thirty doses are prescribed, the total metric dose is equivalent to double the individual apothecary dose. When forty-five doses are prescribed, the total metric dose is equivalent to triple the individual apothecary dose. In prescribing less than fifteen doses; i. e., three, five, ten, and so forth, the total metric dose is equivalent to the ratio of the number of doses prescribed over fifteen; i. e., ten doses equal 10/15 ($\frac{2}{3}$) of the single apothecary dose. This axiom is applicable equally to solids and liquids.

Solids

If it is desired to prescribe fifteen capsules each of which is to contain three grains of acetphenetidin, it should be written as follows:

	Single Apoth. Dose	Metric
	m.	c.c.
	gr.	Gm.
R Acetphenetidini	gr. III	3.0

Misce et pone in capsulas No. 15.
Sig: One capsule as directed.
(The apothecary dose is duplicated.)

If the dose is to be thirty capsules (articles), it should be written as follows:

	Single Apoth. Dose	Metric
	m.	c.c.
	gr.	Gm.
R Acetphenetidini	gr. III	6.0

Misce et pone in capsulas No. 30.
Sig: One capsule as directed.
(The apothecary dose is doubled.)

If the dose is to be forty-five capsules (articles), it should be written as follows:

	Single Apoth. Dose	Metric
	m.	c.c.
	gr.	Gm.
R Acetphenetidini	gr. III	9.0

Misce et pone in capsulas No. 45.
Sig: One capsule as directed.
(The apothecary dose is tripled.)

If the dose is to be ten capsules (articles), it should be written as follows:

	Single Apoth. Dose	Metric
	m.	c.c.
	gr.	Gm.
R Acetphenetidini	gr. III	2.0

Misce et pone in capsulas No. 10.
Sig: One capsule as directed.
(The apothecary dose is multiplied by two-thirds.)

When a q.s. menstruum is employed, no additional change is indicated; for example, for fifteen doses it should be written as follows:

	Single Apoth. Dose	Metric
	m.	c.c.
	gr.	Gm.
R Pulvis Opii	gr. I	1.0
Oleum Theo.	q.s.	q.s.

Misce et Fac. Suppositoria No. 15.
Sig: As directed.
(The apothecary dose is duplicated.)

For five doses it should be written as follows:

	Single Apoth. Dose	Metric
	m.	c.c.
	gr.	Gm.
R Pulvis Opii	gr. I	0.33
Oleum Theo.	q.s.	

Misce et Fac. Suppositoria No. 5.
Sig: One suppository as directed.
(The apothecary dose is multiplied by one-third.)

For thirty doses it should be written as follows:

	Single Apoth. Dose	Metric
	m.	c.c.
	gr.	Gm.
R Pulvis Opii	gr. I	2.0
Oleum Theo.	q.s.	

Misce et Fac. Suppositoria No. 30.
Sig: One suppository as directed.
(The apothecary dose is doubled.)

When prescribing thirty powders or other articles where a q.s. is not employed, the following is self-evident:

	Single Apoth. Dose	Metric
	m.	c.c.
	gr.	Gm.
R Mag. Oxidi	gr. V	10.0
Calcii Carbonatis	gr. III	6.0
Natrii Bicarbonatis	gr. XV	30.0

Misce et pone in chartalas No. 30.
Sig: One powder as directed.
(The apothecary dose is doubled.)

Liquids

As previously mentioned, the same axiom applies to liquid prescriptions.

The number of doses prescribed is readily determined by the division of the total volume of the prescription by the amount prescribed at each dose; for example: in a four ounce mixture (which is equivalent to 120 c.c.) when a teaspoon dose (4.0 c.c.) is prescribed, the total doses are thirty. [In reality an error creeps in when a teaspoon dose is ordered, owing to the fact that the average teaspoon holds closer to 5 c.c. than 4 c.c. (1 dram). This inconsistency in the metric system is equally applicable to the apothecary system.] As a teaspoon is considered 4.0 c.c., then its multiple in 120.0 c.c. is thirty.

EXAMPLES

For thirty doses the prescription should be written as follows:

	Single Apoth. Dose	Metric
	m.	c.c.
	gr.	Gm.
R Drug No. 1	gr. I	2.0
Drug No. 2	mns. V	10.0
Drug No. 3	gr. IV	8.0
Drug No. 4 q.s.	drms. I (M60)	120.0

Misce et Sig: One tsp. (4 c.c.) P.R.N.
(The apothecary dose is doubled.)

For fifteen doses the prescription should be written as follows:

	Single Apoth. Dose	Metric
	m.	c.c.
	gr.	Gm.
R Drug No. 1	gr. I	1.0
Drug No. 2	mns. V	5.0
Drug No. 3	gr. IV	4.0
Drug No. 4	drms. I (M60)	60.0

Misce et Sig: One tsp. (4 c.c.) P.R.N.
(The apothecary dose is duplicated.)

For forty-five doses the prescription should be written as follows:

		Single Apoth. Dose	Metric
		m.	c.c.
		gr.	Gm.
·B	Drug No. 1	gr. I	3.0
	Drug No. 2	mns. V	15.0
	Drug No. 3	gr. IV	12.0
	Drug No. 4	drms. I (M60)	180.0

Misce et Sig: One tsp. (4 c.c.) P.R.N.
(The apothecary dose is tripled.)

In the preceding prescriptions, it is to be noted that the total volumes are 120 c.c., 60 c.c., and 180 c.c. One dram (4 c.c.) is given at each dose. This makes the various volumes yield thirty, fifteen and forty-five doses, respectively. The axiom notes that the total metric dose is numerically equivalent to the individual apothecary dose, when fifteen doses are prescribed. Hence the individual apothecary dosage is doubled, duplicated or tripled.

Infrequently, it is necessary to give more than one dram at a dose. This is customary when using rhubarb and soda, or cod liver oil as a vehicle. The following prescriptions exemplify dessertspoon [drams 2 (8.0 c.c.)] doses:

EXAMPLES

For fifteen doses the prescription should be written as follows:

		Single Apoth. Dose	Metric
		m.	c.c.
		gr.	Gm.
B	Tinct. Nux. Vomicae	mns. V	5.0
	Misturae Rhei et Sodii	drms. II (M120)	120.0

Misce et Sig: One dessertspoon (2 drams—8.0 c.c.) p.c. (15 doses).
(The apothecary dose is duplicated.)

Naturally, economically, it is considered poor policy to prescribe such a small total volume with an increased dosage. For thirty doses the prescription should be written as follows:

		Single Apoth. Dose	Metric
		m.	c.c.
		gr.	Gm.
B	Tinct. Nux. Vomicae	mns. V	10.0
	Misturae Rhei et Sodii q.s.	drms. II (M120)	240.0

Misce et Sig: One dessertspoon (2 drams—8.0 c.c.) p.c. 30 doses.
(The apothecary dose is doubled.)

For forty-five doses the prescription should be written as follows:

		Single Apoth. Dose	Metric
		m.	c.c.
		gr.	Gm.
B	Tinct. Nux. Vomicae	mns. V	15.0
	Misturae Rhei et Sodii q.s.	drms. II (M120)	360.0

Misce et Sig: One dessertspoon (2 drams—8.0 c.c.) p.c. (45 doses).
(The apothecary dose is tripled.)

In the event that a tablespoon (½ oz.—150.0 c.c.) dose is indicated, the following example shows the method of procedure:

		Single Apoth. Dose	Metric
		m.	c.c.
		gr.	Gm.
B	Pot. Chlor.	gr. III	3.0
	Tinct. Ferric Chlor.	gr. IV	4.0
	Glycerini	drms. II (M120)	120.0
	Aqua Dest. q.s.	drms. IV (M240)	240.0

Misce et Sig: One tbsp. [(½ oz.)—16 c.c.] in water every 4 hours. (15 doses.)
(The apothecary dose is duplicated.)

It is to be observed that in the previous examples fractional doses have been entirely omitted.

It has been found that the simplest way in which to handle fractional doses is to have the prescribing physician visualize the fraction utilized in the terms of dollars and cents. For example, if it is desired to prescribe in each dose a gr. ss. of codeine sulphate, this individual dosage should be visualized as one-half a dollar—fifty cents; i. e., 0.50. In this way immediate transposition with the greatest ease can be accomplished. For fifteen doses the prescription should be written as follows:

		Single Apoth. Dose	Metric
		m.	c.c.
		gr.	Gm.
B	Drug No. 1	gr. ss	0.50
-	Drug No. 2	gr. 1/10	0.10
	Drug No. 3	gr. 1/50	0.02
	Drug No. 4	gr. 1/200	0.005
	Drug No. 5	gr. 1/3	0.33

Misce et pone in capsulas No. 15.
(The apothecary dose is duplicated.)

For thirty doses the prescription should be written as follows:

		Single Apoth. Dose	Metric
		m.	c.c.
		gr.	Gm.
B	Drug No. 1	gr. 1/20	.10
	Drug No. 2	gr. 1/50	.04
	Drug No. 3	gr. 1/3	.66
	Drug No. 4	mns. II	4.0
	Drug No. 5	gr. VI	12.0
	Drug No. 6 q.s.	drm. I (M60)	120.0

Misce et Sig: One tsp. (4.0 c.c.) as ordered. (30 doses.)
(The apothecary dose is doubled.)

The preceding prescription consists in a mixture of fractions and whole numbers. The total doses are thirty. The total metric quantity required, according to the axiom, is numerically twice the individual apothecary dose.

THE METRIC EQUIVALENT IN PERCENTAGE SOLUTIONS

The prescription writing of percentage solutions in the metric system is exceedingly simple. The following examples should fully clarify and demonstrate the facility with which this may be accomplished.

A one ounce (30 c.c.) solution of varying desired strengths is to be written as follows:

		Percentage Desired	Metric
			c.c.
			Gm.
B	Drug	20%	6.0
	Drug	10%	3.0
	Drug	5%	1.5
	Drug	2%	0.6
	Drug	1%	0.3
	Drug	1/2%	0.15
	Drug	1/10%	0.03
	Aqua Dest. q.s.	oz. 1	30.0

A four ounce solution of varying desired strengths is written as follows:

		Percentage Desired	Metric
			c.c.
			Gm.
B	Drug	20%	24.0
	Drug	10%	12.0
	Drug	5%	6.0
	Drug	2%	2.4
	Drug	1%	1.2
	Drug	1/2%	0.6
	Drug	1/10%	0.12
	Aqua Dest. q.s.	oz. IV	120.0

As can be seen, the procedure consists in simply altering the decimal point, and multiplying or dividing by cardinal numbers.

A MEANS OF TRANSPOSING TOTAL METRIC INTO INDIVIDUAL APOTHECARY DOSAGE

Frequently, a physician is presented with a prescription written in the metric system, and is desirous of being able to determine readily the individual dose of each of the prescribed drugs in the apothecary system. When this occasion arises, the reverse of the foregoing procedure is observed; for example:

		Single Apoth. Dose m. gr.	Metric c.c. Gm.
℞	Drug No. 1	?	1.0
	Drug No. 2	?	0.5
	Drug No. 3	?	9.0
	Drug No. 4	?	60.0
	Drug No. 5 q.s.	?	120.0

Misce et Sig: One tsp. (4 c.c.) P.R.N.

It is evident that the preceding prescription contains thirty doses. Therefore, in its formation it was necessary to double the individual apothecary dose in order to form the total metric quantity. (Refer to axiom.) Hence the individual apothecary dosage for the preceding prescription is numerically one-half of the total metric dosage as follows:

		Single Apoth. Dose m. gr.	Metric c.c. Gm.
℞	Drug No. 1	gr. ss	1.0
	Drug No. 2	gr. 1/4	0.5
	Drug No. 3	gr. IV ss	9.0
	Drug No. 4	drm. ss (M30)	60.0
	Drug No. 5 q.s.	drm. I (M60)	120.0

The following prescription presents a mixture of most all practical variations in dosage. It is a combination of both liquids and solids with fractional and whole grain doses together with a vehicle.

		Single Apoth. Dose m. gr.	Metric c.c. Gm.
℞	Drug No. 1	?	0.02
	Drug No. 2	?	0.10
	Drug No. 3	?	0.01
	Drug No. 4	?	10.0
	Drug No. 5	?	20.0
	Drug No. 6	?	0.66
	Drug No. 7	?	14.0
	Drug No. 8	?	30.0
	Drug No. 9	?	60.0
	Drug No. 10 q.s.	? q.s.	120.0

Misce et Sig: One tsp. (4.0 c.c.) as directed.

This prescription also contains thirty doses. Therefore, in order to have obtained the noted metric dosage the individual apothecary dose must have been doubled. The following shows the steps by which reduction to the individual apothecary dose is obtained:

		Metric c.c. Gm.	Multiple	Cents	Dollars	Single Apoth. Dose m. gr.
℞	Drug No. 1	0.02	.01	1	1/100	1/100
	Drug No. 2	0.10	0.05	5	1/20	1/20
	Drug No. 3	0.01	0.005	1/2	1/200	1/200
	Drug No. 4	10.0	5.0	500	5	5
	Drug No. 5	20.0	10.0	1000	10	10
	Drug No. 6	0.66	0.33	33	1/3	1/3
	Drug No. 7	14.0	7.0	700	7	7
	Drug No. 8	30.0	15.0	1500	15	15
	Drug No. 9	60.0	30.0	3000	30	30 (drm. ss.)
	Drug No. 10	120.0	60.0	6000	60	60 (drm. 1)

		Single Apoth. Dose m. gr.	Metric c.c. Gm.
℞	Drug No. 1	1/100	0.02
	Drug No. 2	1/20	0.10
	Drug No. 3	1/200	0.01
	Drug No. 4	V	10.0
	Drug No. 5	X	20.0
	Drug No. 6	1/3	0.66
	Drug No. 7	VII	14.0
	Drug No. 8	XV	30.0
	Drug No. 9	LX (zss)	60.0
	Drug No. 10 q.s.	XXX (zss)	120.0

Misce et Sig: One tsp. (4.0 c.c.) as directed.

Whereas the preceding appears complicated in explanation, in reality the entire procedure is purely mental and astoundingly simple in practice.

580 Park Avenue.

TUBERCULOSIS IN INFANCY*

ARNOLD M. SMYTHE, M.D., Des Moines

Tuberculosis, primarily a lymphatic disease, is also an infectious and communicable disease which is transmitted from person to person by direct contact. This direct contact is particularly important with infants who are fondled and kissed repeatedly by their admirers, the latter little suspecting that the infants are receiving infective doses of tubercle bacilli until it is too late. The reaction of a host to a primary infection, and reinfection with tubercle bacilli, is the same whether it occurs in infants, children or adults.

In order to have a clear understanding as to how the primary tuberculous infection reacts in the host, a brief review of the important anatomic relations of the lymphatic system in the lungs and the formation of the tubercle will be discussed. Miller's classical study of the structure of the lungs demonstrates that the walls of the peripheral air sacs, the atria, the sacculi alveolares, and the alveoli pulmonis, do not contain lymphatic vessels. The distal portion of the lymphatic system in the lungs begins as a small collection of lymphoid cells located at the distal end of the ductulus alveolares. On the floor of the peripheral air sacs are found large mononuclear cells called alveolar phagocytes, histiocytes or clasmatocytes, whose function is to ingest and remove foreign bodies from the air spaces. These cells appear in the air sacs a few hours after birth.

*Presented before the Eighty-second Annual Session, Iowa State Medical Society, Des Moines, May 10, 11, 12, 1933.

Tubercle bacilli lodged in the air sacs of the lungs are immediately attacked by the alveolar phagocytes and engulfed. Attempted destruction of the tubercle bacillus begins at once. These alveolar phagocytes, with their engulfed tubercle bacilli, start migrating to the distal portion of the ductulus alveolares and lodge in the microscopic mass of lymphoid tissue at this anatomic location. Once lodged in this mass of lymphoid tissue, primary tuberculosis begins at once, that is, the formation of the tubercle of Küss or Ghon. According to Fried's experimental work the first stage of the primary tubercle is formed within five minutes. The formation of the primary tubercle is briefly characterized by a dense wall of epitheloid cells thrown around the infecting agent. Around the epitheloid cells, fibroblastic tissue forms, which becomes infiltrated with lymphocytes. There is no direct circulatory connection with the central portion of the tubercle. Some of the central cells degenerate or necrose with the formation of giant cells. The formation of a tubercle requires from eight to fifteen days. The primary tubercle may be summarized as a proliferating reaction of the host to the infective organism. This type of a reaction does not, to our knowledge, produce symptoms of clinical tuberculosis. In this respect it is directly contrary to reinfection as we will shortly see.

During the formation of the primary tubercle, a changed condition of the body cells results and to this characteristic reaction, Pirquet applied the term "allergy," which means "changed condition or different action." This hypersensitiveness is produced by the formation of a primary tubercle within the body. At the time the sensitiveness develops, a specific immunity against the tubercle bacilli is acquired. Natural and passive immunity are never present. Therefore, the formation of the primary tubercle creates a state of allergy, produces specific immunity which enables the host to resist infection.

What resistance has an infant against the tubercle bacillus? He has the native, or natural, reaction of tissues to any foreign body in host; a mechanical resistance which depends upon the strength possessed by the walls of the tubercle in keeping the tubercle bacilli localized; and specific or acquired immunity which is formed as the result of the body becoming sensitized to the tubercle bacilli.

Krause has shown that primary infection may result from a dozen or more tubercle bacilli, whereas it takes many thousands of tubercle bacilli to reinfect the host. What, then, is the nature of the reaction of the sensitized host to reinfection by tubercle bacilli? Wherever the reinfecting tubercle bacilli are lodged, they are immediately met by a marked inflammatory reaction which tends to stop the progress of the tubercle bacilli. Small reinfections are apparently overcome, while in massive doses, some of the tubercle bacilli survive to produce secondary types of tuberculosis. The marked inflammatory process, caused by reinfection, is equally as dangerous to the host as to the infecting agent. Clinical symptoms, chills, fever, malaise, anorexia, loss of weight, etc., develop. Therefore reinfection by the tubercle bacilli is characterized particularly by a severe tissue inflammation producing toxic manifestations.

The mortality of tuberculous infants according to textbooks and hospital records, is very high. By using the tuberculin test, x-rays, etc., it has been demonstrated that tuberculosis in infancy is far from always being fatal. Statistics are now accumulating in our juvenile tuberculosis clinics over the country, showing that large numbers of the infants infected with the tubercle bacillus regain perfect health under proper hygienic measures. Infants developing tuberculous bronchopneumonia, tuberculous meningitis and miliary tuberculosis, usually die. These types of tuberculosis are due to a caseous gland rupturing into the blood stream or bronchi, followed by a marked inflammatory reaction, characteristic of reinfection.

It is evident that we have two types of tuberculous infection in infants; the primary infection which produces no symptoms and is characterized pathologically by proliferation with tumor formation; and the reinfection or super-infection type which produces clinical symptoms and is characterized pathologically by severe inflammatory reaction of the tissue against the reinfecting tubercle bacilli. The latter type of infection produces the mortality.

Much emphasis should be placed upon an early diagnosis of tuberculosis in infants and children so that proper hygienic measures may be instituted immediately. The tuberculin test, particularly the Mantoux or intradermal test, should always be used in making the diagnosis of primary tuberculosis because clinical symptoms do not occur in this type of infection. This test is a harmless procedure. A positive tuberculin test proves that the host has been infected with tubercle bacilli. The next most valuable aid in making a diagnosis is the x-ray. Frequently it is negative in the primary infection because Ghon's nodule is too small to cast a shadow and calcification is seldom present. History and laboratory findings are important. Since the primary nodule produces no symptoms, and the x-ray is frequently negative and the history and laboratory findings are secondary adjuncts, it is evident that the tuberculin test is of primary importance in making an early diagnosis of tuberculosis.

911 Bankers Trust Building.

HERNIA OF THE JEJUNUM THROUGH AN APERTURE IN THE MESENTERY OF THE SMALL INTESTINE

·S. W. BARNETT, M.D., Cedar Falls

Since strangulation of the small intestine through an opening in the mesentery of the small intestine is an uncommon occurrence, and having noted the report of one case in the August issue of the JOURNAL OF THE IOWA STATE MEDICAL SOCIETY, I am reporting one additional case at this time.

Present Complaint: The patient, a white man, twenty-six years of age, had been out on a "beer party" on the night of April 23, 1933, drinking new, green beer. Both he and his fellow companions became ill at the stomach, with nausea and vomiting. He called at a physician's home on the evening of April 24, complaining that he had been vomiting all day and had cramps in his stomach. He also had many loose bowel movements. He was sent home, advised not to eat anything, to take an enema, and report to the office in the morning if he was not better. The afternoon of April 25, the physician was called tò the patient's home because of severe vomiting and pain in the abdomen. There had been no bowel movements, even though a number of soap-suds enemata had been given. A diagnosis of intestinal obstruction was made and he was transported to the hospital. Shortly after entering the hospital he had projectile vomiting of dark, foul-smelling, intestinal contents, and some bright red blood.

Past History: The past history was essentially negative. The patient had had no illness since childhood; no operations, and no stomach distress of any type.

Family History: No relevant facts were obtained under this classification.

Physical Examination: April 24, he walked to the physician's home and seemed at ease except as he stated, that he was nauseated all the time. He was not carefully examined at this time. When seen at his home at 3:00 p. m., April 25, the patient had a continuous desire to vomit. His temperature was 99°; pulse 80; respiration 18; heart and lungs negative for pathologic findings; abdomen, scaphoid; some voluntary rigidity; rectal examination: negative. At the hospital the patient

did not act ill ·but looked haggard. Findings at this time were temperature 99°; pulse 72; respiration 18; blood pressure 108/62; head and neck, negative for pathology; heart, not enlarged, no murmur, rate regular; lungs, normal for breath sounds and percussion note, expansion, good and equal; abdomen: scaphoid, firm, tenderness in epigastrium, but not extreme tenderness, no tumors or masses felt, liver, spleen and kidneys not felt, no tenderness in hypogastrium or lower abdomen, area of tenderness not definitely localized but in the region of the umbilicus or slightly lower; rectal findings, negative; neurologic examination, negative; pupils reacting normally, reflexes and sensations responding normally; urine: specific gravity, 1030, albumin, a trace, sugar, negative, casts, a few hyaline and few epithelial cells; blood findings: red blood count, 4,480,000; white blood count, 16,000, definite shift to the left.

Diagnosis: Intestinal obstruction, cause unknown.

An operation was performed and on opening the abdomen, a collapsed small intestine appeared, as well as a distended small intestine. The obstruction was found in the lower portion of the jejunum, approximately three inches being strangulated in an opening in the mesentery of the small intestine. The aperture easily admitted the index finger. The intestine was hyperemic in this area, but not gangrenous, and normal circulation returned after a few minutes of warm wet toweling.

The postoperative convalescence was uneventful and he was discharged from the hospital on the tenth postoperative day, in good condition.

THE FINLEY HOSPITAL CLINICO-PATHOLOGIC CONFERENCE

TUBERCULOSIS OF THE KNEE JOINT

DONALD C. CONZETT, M.D., Dubuque

This case was previously presented at an earlier conference, and was reported as Case No. 3 in the September issue of THE JOURNAL OF THE IOWA STATE MEDICAL SOCIETY.

CASE REPORT

A man, twenty-one years of age, complaining of pain and moderate swelling of the knee of five weeks' duration, was first seen eight months ago. There was no history of injury or infection. The family history showed that one sister had had pulmonary tuberculosis but was considered cured. An x-ray examination of the patient revealed a cystic area at the upper end of the tibia with otherwise normal joint spaces and smooth cartilaginous surfaces. After the knee was immobilized in a plaster cast for six weeks, the roentgenologist reported that the

defect had filled in but that he was unable to determine the nature of the process. Clinically the patient
had recovered. At that time our conclusions were:
"It is our opinion that this was a low grade Brodie's
abscess which absorbed and was replaced by bone
following treatment of rest, immobilization and constitutional support."

Subsequently the patient returned to his work as
a drug clerk and continued for four months without
complaint. Three and a half months later he was
seen because of a fall on a slippery sidewalk which
had occurred two weeks before. As the result of
the injury there had been immediate pain and swelling in the knee. Liniments and massage had only
aggravated the condition while the swelling had
further increased. Examination of the knee revealed
a diffuse and uniform swelling of the entire joint.
Exquisite pain was elicited over the area of the anterior attachment of the internal meniscus. The remainder of the knee was not tender. Flexion was limited

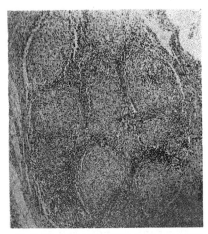

Fig. 1: Low power microphotograph of synovial membrane
showing proliferative tubercles.

to 90° and extension to 170°. There were no constitutional symptoms and no temperature elevation. The
boy had gained weight since his first examination.
Because of the definite history of trauma and the
distinct localization of tenderness, it seemed likely
that he had suffered an injury to the cartilage, although the swelling seemed disproportionate to the
other symptoms. Operative treatment was advised
but the patient insisted on conservative management.
The limb was therefore immobilized in extension for
two weeks. At the end of that time no change was
noted; the swelling and localized tenderness persisted.
X-ray examination was made of both knees and also
a visualization of the chest because of the family
history of tuberculosis. The roentgenologist reported

as follows: "X-ray examination of both knees shows
the right to be entirely normal. The left, however,
shows a marked narrowing of the articular space,
especially on the lateral side. In addition, there is a
haziness about the joint and marked soft tissue
swelling. There is an area of destruction which is
very small on the upper anterior lip of the tibia.
Although the narrowing of the articular process suggests a displaced semilunar cartilage, I am very
suspicious of an early tuberculosis of the synovial
or peri-articular type because of the swelling, destruction and haziness present. The x-ray examination of the chest shows an old pleurisy at the left
base and thickening of both hilus regions suggestive
of an old, healed, childhood tuberculosis. There is
no evidence of active tuberculosis. Conclusions: 1.
Probable early tuberculosis of the left knee. 2. Possible displaced semilunar cartilage. 3. Thickened
pleura at the left base. 4. Healed, childhood tuberculosis."

The following day under ethylene anesthesia, the
knee was opened. A Fischer incision was used curv-
ing medially toward the internal margin of the
patellar tendon. This allowed a view of the meniscus
and permitted visualization of the joint cavity. On
incising the capsule, a large amount of dark red,
polypoid material, which appeared to be hypertrophied
synovia, presented itself. The internal semilunar
cartilage showed no irregularities and its anterior
attachment was firm. A considerable amount of this
synovia was removed and the knee closed in layers
using a fine 00 plain catgut for the capsule. The
limb was then dressed in extension with a posterior
splint in place. A diagnosis of tuberculosis of the
joint was made and the tissue sent to the laboratory
for histologic examination and guinea-pig inoculation. The pathologic report was as follows: "Grossly:
the specimen consists of several pieces of synovial
membrane that are dark red. No tubercles can be
seen, but the membrane appears thickened. Microscopically: sections from the several pieces were
taken and they show all parts involved by a chronic
inflammatory exudate. In two of the sections there
are numerous typical early tubercles (Figs. 1 and 2).
Anatomic Diagnosis: tuberculosis of synovial membrane."

COMMENT

This case is a good illustration of the problem
presented by tuberculosis of bones and joints. While
tuberculosis was suspected when the patient was first
seen, the fact that the bony changes disappeared as
judged by symptoms and x-ray examination led us
to believe that possibly we were in error. Seven
months later after a fall, the patient returned with
a swollen, painful knee. The physical examination
was indefinite; the roentgenologist's conclusion after
the examination was that the condition was very
suspicious of an early tuberculosis. The family history indicated the possible source of infection. At
operation the changes in the synovia while suggestive of tuberculosis were indefinite. A positive diag-

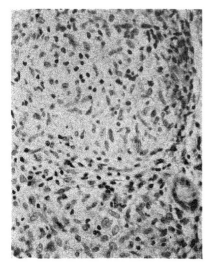

Fig. 2: Higher power microphotograph showing epitheloid cells, wandering cells and a single giant cell.

nosis was made only after the histologic study. This difficulty in reaching a diagnosis is quite characteristic of tuberculosis of bones and joints especially in the early stages. While the disease has been known for centuries up until recent times the diagnosis was largely made on clinical signs and macroscopic examination of tissue. Since the beginning of the present century the x-ray examination became an important diagnostic accessory. In recent years the accuracy of the diagnosis of tuberculosis of joints has been questioned by several workers. Thus Sundt[1] states that diagnosis of primary, chronic monarticular lesions of joints is one of the most difficult diagnostic problems. Milgram[2] in a review of 142 cases of proved tuberculosis found only 87 (60 per cent) diagnosed clinically. In 42 cases with a sudden onset 60 per cent were incorrectly diagnosed. Evidently cases with the sudden onset of pain offer the greatest difficulties in diagnosis. X-ray examination is an important aid in reaching a diagnosis but in the early stages of the disease it may be misleading. However, it is very necessary in ruling out other conditions which might be responsible for the symptoms. An important diagnostic aid, but one which has been greatly neglected, is the tuberculin test. It should be utilized in all indefinite bone and joint conditions. Most authorities agree that biopsy should be done in all doubtful cases in adults. Many other investigators also believe that biopsy should be done in children. Unfortunately the microscopic studies are not definite in all cases.

Very frequently only chronic inflammatory tissue is seen. Therefore some method of demonstrating the tubercle bacilli should be utilized. Guinea pig inoculations and cultures of the material removed should be used. If the possibility of any acute or chronic pathology of bones or joints being tuberculous is kept in mind, and if the various diagnostic procedures are fully utilized, an accurate diagnosis should be made in practically all cases. The treatment is either conservative or surgical. Most American authorities reserve conservative treatment for children. The trend, however, is to include children in cases selected for surgical treatment. Operative treatment is generally considered most suitable, largely for economic reasons. The end results of months or years of conservative treatment of bones or joints are usually the same as those after a few weeks of surgical treatment. Therefore arthrodesis of the joints or fusion operations for tuberculosis of the spine in patients without other active tuberculous lesions have shown good results. Rarely amputation may be required because of extreme pain, hopeless loss of function, and persistent draining sinuses about a joint. Obviously the results of treatment will be better if an early and accurate diagnosis is made.

REFERENCES

1. Sundt, H.: The diagnosis and frequency of tuberculous disease of the knee. Jour. Bone and Joint Surg. xiii:740-757, (October) 1931.

2. Milgram, J. E.: Diagnostic inaccuracy in tuberculosis of bone, joint and bursa. Jour. Am. Med. Assn., xcvii:232-235, (July 25) 1931.

AMERICAN ASSOCIATION ON MENTAL DEFICIENCY

The annual meeting of the American Association on Mental Deficiency will be held at the Hotel Waldorf Astoria, New York, May 26, 27, 28 and 29, 1934. The Saturday session, May 26, will be given over to the sociologic, psychologic and the special educational aspects of the problem in order that local social workers and school teachers may have an opportunity to attend without interfering with their regular duties. The Tuesday afternoon session will be a conjoint meeting with the American Psychiatric Association. Data as to the program may be obtained from the Secretary, Dr. Groves B. Smith, Godfrey, Illinois.

ANNUAL MEETING OF THE IOWA HOSPITAL ASSOCIATION

The annual joint convention of the Iowa Hospital Association, the Iowa Dietetics Association, the Iowa Record Librarians, and the Iowa League of Nursing Education, will be held in Council Bluffs, April 30 and May 1. Visitors of national prominence in all fields will attend, and Mr. Robert Jolly of Houston, Texas, president-elect of the American Hospital Association, will be the guest speaker.

SPECIAL ARTICLE

THE TEST OF ORGANIZED MEDICINE*

Oliver J. Fay, M.D., Des Moines

Within the next fortnight we shall round out the first year of what is popularly termed "the new deal." Whether you and I approve of that deal, whether it represents evolution or revolution is rather beside the point, since accept it we must. Perhaps the changes are evolutionary in that the foundations for them were undoubtedly laid in an indefinite past, over an incalculable period of time; certainly they are revolutionary in that they affect profoundly the very fiber of our social structure, in that they encompass every business, every profession, every individual in every walk in life. We of the medical profession have been inclined to feel a false sense of independence, a spurious security because under the provisions of the NRA and of the CWA, our profession has been specifically exempted from regulation. In reality, I believe that we are merely on probation, that we are standing at the cross roads and that now, today, we are facing a crisis that must profoundly affect the entire future of our profession, that will either open to it wider fields of service, or will make of it a mere trade. If we would choose wisely, or if we would be permitted even a voice in determining our professional future, we must seek a clear understanding of the pending issues, must face them squarely, and must meet them in the strength of solidarity.

During the past few years, the medical profession has been under a continuous fire of criticism. There is nothing new in that, for we may safely assume that there were those in the tribe who essayed to tell the first medicine man how he should have conducted his medicine making; but in these later years we have been subjected to something more than casual sniping. There has been a continuous gruelling cross fire, indulged in not only by disgruntled individuals and intolerant sects, but by a wide and fairly representative cross section of the periodical and daily press. Moreover, this muck-raking campaign has too often had the support of a minority section of our profession, for the most part that section which is devoted to the academic rather than to the clinical practice of medicine. Some idea of the extent and effect of that campaign may be had from a study of the Report of the Committee on the Investigation of the Costs of Medical Care, a report that did not confine itself to the subject ostensibly under discussion but developed into propaganda for state

*Presented before the Northwest Medical Conference, Saint Paul, Minnesota, February 25, 1934.

medicine. The report, like the press attacks which preceded and followed it, was unfortunate and destructive in that it tended to undermine the confidence of the public in the medical profession, a confidence which is vital to the welfare, not alone nor chiefly of the physician, but to an even greater extent to the welfare of the public. It was fortunate and constructive in that it roused the medical profession, always lethargic in matters not intimately concerned with the care of the sick, too often myopic in viewing even those public policies which affect their professional interests, to a realization of the danger which threatens it and, through it the best interests of the people. For the first time, the average physician saw state medicine not as the chimerical bogy he had long considered it, the butt of his jokes or, depending on his mood, the peg upon which he might hang his oratory, but as the menacing bureaucratic octopus it has become; not as something which might be of possible interest in the remote future, but as something with which he stands face to face, with which he must come to grips now. For him it has ceased to be a visionary scheme for supplying ideal medical care to an indifferent populace at some indefinite future time, and has become an immediate threat to that intimate relationship that exists, that always has existed, between physician and patient, which it would replace by a mechanized, centralized bureau—call it a community clinic, if you will. The physician may have dreamed of a day when medical research could be carried on unhampered by lack of private funds, when the man who had a vision, who had something vital to contribute to medical research, might carry on his work without seeing his family suffer privation; certainly, he had not envisioned a future in which the scientist would become a mere automaton under bureaucratic control.

The effect of the loss of confidence in the physician for which the much publicised report of the so-called Committee on the Costs of Medical Care was responsible is something which we have no method of evaluating. The effect of the report on the medical profession itself is more apparent to the thoughtful observer. At once there sprang up a mushroom growth of so-called clinics in various parts of the country, the personnel of which was not for the most part in the best of professional standing, but which purported to give the public much for little. Various hospitals and laymen at once organized plans for the care of the sick on some group insurance basis. These schemes varied widely in details and scope, but they inevitably had one basic principle in common—the exploitation of the physician for the profit of the layman or of the hospital. To thoughtful physicians with a deep and humanitarian interest in their profession, however, the report came as a call to arms; it gave them that feeling of professional solidarity which has unfortunately been lacking among the members of our profession. I believe the reaction to that report which, by the way, carefully avoided discrimination between the physician and practitioners of our so-called left handed schools of healing, has been manifest in a better morale among the rank and file of the medical profession. It has given them a keener appreciation of their community of interests, of their responsibility to the public, of the urgent need of themselves establishing a sounder basis for medical practice. The medical profession should have a unique power, a unique opportunity of influencing legislation and public policy where the health of our people is concerned, for there are few men in public life who do not repose particular confidence in some one physician, who are not approachable by him. The very fact that we as a profession keep free from political entanglement should but add force to our word when we speak on some medical issue, but we have been lamentably slow to speak that word when it has been needed. Even in the face of some crisis it has seemed impossible to arouse general professional interest, to obtain any unanimity of opinion, any concerted action from our profession. If the Report of the Committee on the Costs of Medical Care has actually succeeded in awakening and unifying a large part of our profession, it has accomplished something of real value.

The past months which have brought basic changes and government control to so many fields of endeavor have, on the contrary, brought apparent endorsement to the medical profession. In the bulletin issued by the Federal Civil Works Administration, entitled "Rules and Regulations, No. 5," it is specifically stated under the head of Medical Treatment that: "In locations where neither public nor designated medical facilities exist, or where the number of such facilities is inadequate to furnish the service required, local Civil Works Administrators are authorized to arrange for medical care by reputable private physicians. This does not include the use of osteopaths or chiropractors unless treatment by such practitioners is recommended by the government or by designated private physicians." The recognition of the essential difference between medicine and the left-handed schools of so-called healing, a vital difference predicated not upon prejudices and antiquated taboos

but upon recognized scientific criteria and long years of prescribed training, is something which we have failed to attain in our own state, and which many other states have failed to establish. To me at least it is most gratifying that at this time such recognition should have come to us from the Federal Government.

In still another matter, in its handling of the medical phases of the CWA work, the government has given the medical profession a gratifying vote of confidence. While its regulations provide fixed fees to be paid for hospital care, for laboratory work, for x-ray examination, they do not fix a medical fee schedule beyond providing that: "The fees charged shall not be in excess of those charged patients in the same income class as the injured person." It is as though the government recognized that in its Hippocratic code the medical profession already possessed all needed regulations, that this great professional code of necessity transcends any lesser regulations that might be provided by the NRA, the CWA, the PWA, or what not.

We of the medical profession dare not, however, assume that this method of caring for the injured is a closed issue. There is nothing permanent, nothing unchangeable about the present regulations. If tomorrow the government should find that certain physicians are failing to live up to the spirit of the Hippocratic code, it can provide new regulations. It can take over the entire medical work of the various units under its control, and by arranging to have their work done by salaried government employees, it can go far towards establishing state medicine on a permanent basis. At the risk of appearing old-fashioned I must confess that I can see little to be gained and much to be lost by the extension of communism to the scientific fields, in other words, by turning the practice of medicine over to the state. Yet a relatively small number of physicians who, through petty greed fail to play fair in their handling of federal cases, may precipitate the issue of state medicine. In brief, you and I, the members of the medical profession as a whole, are at the mercy of the individual physician. The question of whether you and I are to be permitted to continue as free members of a great profession, or are to become mere cogs in the machinery of state medicine depends upon whether each and every member of our profession is willing to play the game. Unless we are mere visionaries, we must admit that there is no large group of humans, in or out of the medical profession, that is 100 per cent perfect. We must face the fact that there are always those who are willing to seek personal profit at the cost of group welfare, who are tempted to betray their profession for a mere handful of silver. We, as individuals, are powerless in the face of such betrayal. In childhood's fairy tales, right always triumphs, but in a world of cold realities, we often see its colors dragged in the dust because those who should champion its cause sit idly by in supine anticipation of some eleventh hour miracle. The problem can be coped with only through organization, through strong group control. There is nothing new or revolutionary about the idea of group activities and control. Industry has long recognized the value of the principle, and under the new regime it is assuming even larger proportions. Only we of the medical profession have desperately tried to hold onto our haloes, to convince those about us by assuring ourselves that there is something other-worldly about the physician and his profession, that for him alone natural laws are abrogated, that his profession alone is not subject to the fundamental laws, such as that of supply and demand, which govern all other human activities. In the past twenty-five years we have taken one step in the right direction. More stringent regulations governing the equipment and conduct of medical schools and the licensing of their graduates have resulted in the closing of the doors of most of those medical schools with inadequate equipment organized by avaricious medical staffs for the revenue from their diploma mills. The number of medical colleges in this country has been reduced from 162 in 1906 to 76 in 1932, and the number of those graduating from medical colleges decreased from 5,364 in 1906 to 4,735 in 1931, but in these years the total number of physicians in the United States increased from 121,484 to 156,440, an increase of some 35,000. It is true that in approximately the same period of time, the population of the United States increased from 84,154,000 to 122,275,000, so that the ratio of physicians to the population decreased from one to every 692 inhabitants in 1906, to one to every 786 in 1931. In reality, however, the individual physician's field has been narrowed, and not widened during this quarter century. The control of many contagious diseases has not only greatly decreased the morbidity among the population, but the building of better roads, the remarkable development of automotive transportation, the concentration of our population in towns and cities, and the enormous increase in the hospitalization of the sick has made it possible for one physician to serve a much larger number of people. He must have this increased professional field if he is to have an income which will make it possible for him to meet the higher standards of training, procure equipment demanded in modern practice and continue postgraduate study. It cannot be denied that adequate medical care is lacking in many sections of our country, but this is not due to any shortage of physicians, rather it is due to the fact that these territories offer too little inducement to the physician. If starve he must, the physician usually prefers to starve in some medical center rather than out in the wide open spaces, perhaps on the old theory that misery loves company. The fact remains that the country as a whole has more physicians than it needs or can adequately support. The effect of overcrowding is to be deplored from the standpoint of the profession and public alike. Having invested one's youth and patrimony in a medical education, the physician must perforce seek to wrest a living from his profession, and if that living cannot be legitimately gained, it is inevitable that an attempt should be made to gain it by sharp practices. Overcrowding in the profession breeds the advertising quack, the contract surgeon, and the fee splitter. I resent the statement that half of the appendectomies performed in this country are performed needlessly, and I can find no justification for that statement when it comes from someone outside the clinical practice of medicine who can offer no statistical proof of his libelous statement. However, if unnecessary operations are performed, if vicious practices creep into our profession, if financial considerations instead of high principles have a voice in too many professional decisions, I believe that those responsible for the conduct of our medical colleges are not equally but more responsible for this regrettable condition than is the medical profession itself. It is not enough that we have reduced the number of our medical colleges by more than half, if those remaining are engaged in a competitive campaign of expansion, requiring more money to build greater clinics to accommodate more students that still greater clinics may be built to provide for an even larger number of students, so that these students must enter an increasingly overcrowded professional field. It is not enough to provide better training for our medical graduates if when these medical graduates enter the field of practice they must choose between starvation and sordid compromises. It is not enough that our medical schools prate of high ideals, of cooperation and of fair play if these same schools, with clinics subsidized by endowment or by the taxpayers' money, enter into the field of private practice as competitors of their own graduates.

I believe that our medical schools have three legitimate functions and only three: first, the training of the needed number of medical students; second, the advancement of medical research; and third, the cooperation with the practicing physicians in the territory the school serves in the solving of problems beyond his scope. The training of a greater number of medical students than the number needed to supply the medical needs of our populace may increase the prestige of the school, may satisfy the ambitions of its dean and faculty, but it undermines the foundations of sound medical practice and it violates every economic law. Medical research is a legitimate function of the medical school, and one which should have the whole-hearted support of the profession and the general public. We should and must look to our medical schools as centers of scientific advancement. The clinical training of our students is important, and it follows that our medical schools must be supplied with adequate clinical material for such training. This must not be construed, however, to mean that the medical school should function as a private clinic; it does not justify the competitive practice of medicine by the school, nor should such practice be condoned under whatever guise it may appear. Only a few days ago, an attempt was made to defend such clinics on the ground that they were not money making, that they did not in fact pay their way. I am at a loss to know which condition is the more pernicious— a center of medical training that profits by competing with its graduates in private practice, or one which undermines the profession by providing medical service at less than the cost of such services, meeting its deficit from private endowment and from the taxpayers' pockets. In every field of endeavor, whether it be agriculture, merchandising, or caring for the sick, it is unsound to countenance underselling or selling at less than cost. The poor we have always with us, and today as always in the past, they must be cared for; but the man who is self-respecting and self-supporting should not be educated away from, but educated towards paying an honest fee for services honestly rendered. He should consider it as wounding to his pride to be a patient in a free clinic as to stand in the bread line. Indigent patients, and only indigent patients, should be cared for by the clinics of a medical school.

In admitting some of the shortcomings of the medical profession, in calling attention to some of the unfortunate conditions which help to foster those shortcomings, I have no desire to align myself with the carping snipers on the side lines. We have had too much of criticism. I believe that we as a profession are aware of and ready to admit our shortcomings, but this is not enough. We must set our own house in order, or we must face the probability of devastating regulation from without, regulation by those who have little conception of, or feeling for the intangible values that go to make up the spirit of medical practice. We must raise the standards of medical practice, but we can raise them only by raising the standards of living, by insuring a decent living to the physician who plays the game. This is possible only through providing that graduates be scaled down to the needs of our population and not up to the ambitions of our medical colleges. This is a problem of the immediate future but we must keep down sharp practices within our ranks, not when these other desiderata have been attained, but now, today, or we must face the probability that the federal government will rescind its tacit endorsement of a free medical profession, and will federalize its medical work.

If you ask me how we are to obtain these vital objectives I have but one answer—through organization. God knows we do not lack medical organizations, but we do lack organization. We have countless medical and pseudo-medical societies, but for the most part we have failed to grasp the significance and power of group action. The very nature of our work has made us individualists. It has made us too prone to feel that in our profession it must be every man for himself; but the day of the individualist has passed. We have need, a vital need, for organization, for strong organization in medicine if we as a profession would survive. As individuals, we can do nothing to stem the tide if it turns to state medicine, although we may have a firm conviction that state medicine would mean the decadence of the art if not the science of medicine. As members of a great national organization, the American Medical Association, we can do much. That association has unique strength, unique power, but we dare not forget that it is strong, that it is powerful only as the individual state societies of which it is composed are strong and powerful. These state societies in turn are strong or weak, powerful or pusillanimous as the county medical societies which make up their membership are strong or weak, powerful or pusillanimous. And the strength or weakness of these county societies, their loyalty or indifference, rests with each individual member, is dependent upon you and me. It is for you and me to decide whether at this critical time, the component county societies are to show their strength and loyalty, are to hold their membership to the spirit of the Hippocratic code. If we fail today as members of a great professional organization, how shall we tomorrow escape membership in a mere trade union under federal control, call it state medicine if you will?

STATE DEPARTMENT OF HEALTH

Expected Morbidity from Communicable Diseases in Iowa During 1934

M. E. BARNES, M.D.

Professor of Hygiene and Preventive Medicine, State University of Iowa and Director of State Hygienic Laboratories

It is obvious that the measurement of progress in the control of communicable disease requires an historical record as to their actual incidence. The conclusions which are warranted from such data are dependent upon the accuracy of the diagnosis and the completeness with which the various diseases are reported.

In addition to the historical value of such records, they may have a prophetic value for the reason that certain diseases have a definite rhythmical or cyclical trend. In such cases we can anticipate, on the basis of past experience, that they will show a rising or declining trend in certain years. Thus, a rough forecast may be made as to the years when measles or scarlet fever may be expected to rise above their basic levels. What are the basic levels of the various diseases? To arrive at this, some method must be found to avoid the distortion caused by epidemic prevalence.

A commonly used measure, known as the tricentral mean, may best be illustrated by an example. In Iowa during the nine years from 1925 to 1933, inclusive, the reported cases of diphtheria in January were 91, 86, 139, 85, 47, 55, 46, 92, 62. Rearranged in order of magnitude these figures are: 139, 92, 91, 86, 85, 62, 55, 47, 46. The average of the tricentral group (86, 85, 62) is 74. Thus should 74 cases of diphtheria occur in January, 1934, it would be in keeping with past experience as representing years

in which exceptionally high and exceptionally low prevalence were excluded. This same procedure is applied to each month, and for each disease for which we desire to determine a basic level.

The results of such computations are set forth in the table below. Assuming that the diseases are being adequately reported, by comparing the reported incidence with the "excepted" incidence one can determine at a glance whether the disease in question is prevailing at a rate above or below its basic level. In proportion as it exceeds this level, the disease shows epidemic incidence.

Comparison of the observed and expected incidence for January and February indicates the following:

1. Diseases showing a markedly excessive incidence above their basic levels: chickenpox, measles, mumps and whooping cough.

2. Diseases showing a markedly decreased incidence; diphtheria and smallpox.

3. Diseases prevailing at close to basic levels: scarlet fever, cerebrospinal meningitis, poliomyelitis, and typhoid.

There are decided limitations to the value of such comparisons, but by giving us a rough measure of what to expect in a "normal" year as based on the preceding nine years, they give us an additional means of appraising the significance of current morbidity reports.

EXPECTED AND OBSERVED MORBIDITY IN IOWA, 1934 (9-YEAR TRICENTRAL MEAN)

	Diphtheria		Scarlet Fever		Chicken Pox		Smallpox		Cerebro-spinal Meningitis		Measles		Polio-myelitis		Mumps		Typhoid		Whooping Cough	
	Exp.	Obs.	Exp.	Obs.	Exp.	Obs.	Exp.	Obs.	Exp.	Obs.	Exp.	Obs.	Exp.	Obs.	Exp.	Obs.	Exp.	Obs.	Exp.	Obs.
January...	74	54	324	388	232	498	174	25	8	4	113	219	1	0	102	208	5	5	69	148
February...	54	32	335	299	197	337	185	22	6	4	85	481	1	2	146	228	3	5	60	116
March......	46		328		169		164		7		141		0		184		5		88	
April......	34		247		164		182		3		196		1		187		4		65	
May........	35		175		154		145		3		303		0		136		2		68	
June........	26		121		89		98		2		184		0		80		8		64	
July........	20		59		31		70		2		46		1		28		9		72	
August....	24		43		10		20		3		6		8		12		21		55	
September..	38		77		14		16		2		9		21		10		24		34	
October	77		171		109		29		3		10		19		33		19		40	
November ..	78		220		232		104		3		12		8		48		13		58	
December ..	77		298		348		145		3		48		4		94		8		62	
Total.....	583		2398		1749		1332		45		1153		64		1060		121		735	

SCARLET FEVER EPIDEMIC TRANSMITTED BY RAW MILK

An outbreak of scarlet fever occurred at Hampton, Franklin County, Iowa, shortly after the middle of March. The first cases to be reported took sick on March 17. At least thirteen patients developed illness on March 18 and 19. A total number of 34 cases had been reported by March 27. The main symptoms were headache, sore throat, nausea and vomiting, followed by a rash and nearly all cases showed the typical appearance of scarlet fever. Infection was of moderately severe grade.

The explosive character of the epidemic and occurrence of illness in preschool children and adults, convinced attending physicians that contact was not responsible for the spread of infection. It was learned that all patients had used raw milk from the same dairy. Moreover, illness was reported among members of the dairyman's family. W. K. Long, M.D., Health Officer of Hampton, ordered that the milk supply concerned be shut off, and reported the situation to the State Department of Health.

Investigation was made on March 20 and March 21, in cooperation with the local health officer and attending physicians. A visit to the dairy farm revealed an active case of scarlet fever as well as a number of convalescent cases. No physician had been called to the home and as a consequence, quarantine had not been established. Throat cultures were taken from twenty patients and forwarded to the state laboratories. Hemolytic streptococci were reported as being present in almost pure culture in thirteen instances, and in large numbers in four additional cases. Twelve of the patients were under nine years of age, the smallest being a child of nine months.

The milk supply in question represented about twenty per cent of the total amount distributed in the city. Equipment for pasteurization was being ordered. People were warned in the meantime to boil all raw milk before use.

This outbreak of milk-borne infection indicates unmistakably that a raw milk supply, even though of superior quality, represents a hazard to community health. Careful pasteurization of all dairy products is essential as a final safeguard against disease transmission.

Carl F. Jordan, M.D., Epidemiologist.

DIPHTHERIA LITERATURE

The diphtheria literature which the department provides without cost has been approved by the Committee on Child Health and Protection of the Iowa State Medical Society. The material available includes: the consent slips, certificates of immunity, a pamphlet entitled "Protect All Children Against Diphtheria," and two leaflets entitled "Toxoid Preferred to Toxin-Antitoxin" and "Suggested Technique for the Administration of Preventive Agents."

The leaflets are available only to physicians. Consent slips and certificates of immunity are supplied by the department only after the county medical society has approved a plan for a diphtheria prevention program. The pamphlet, giving general information about diphtheria and its prevention, is available upon request.

PREVALENCE OF DISEASE

	Feb. '34	Jan. '34	Feb. '33	Most Cases Reported From
Diphtheria	32	54	45	Polk, Shelby
Scarlet Fever	299	388	175	Polk, Johnson
Typhoid Fever	5	5	2	Appanoose
Smallpox	22	25	160	Winneshiek
Measles	481	219	20	Pottawattamie, Page
Whooping Cough	116	148	42	Black Hawk, Dubuque
Cerebrospinal Meningitis	4	4	6	(For State)
Chickenpox	337	498	161	Black Hawk, Boone
Mumps	228	208	190	Woodbury, Wapello
German Measles	637	109	0	Black Hawk, Hardin
Poliomyelitis	2	0	0	Calhoun, Webster
Tuberculosis	28	29	26	(For State)
Undulant Fever	5	7	6	(For State)
Syphilis	132	142	165	(For State)
Gonorrhea	145	192	142	(For State)

VENEREAL DISEASE INFORMATION

For a number of years the United States Public Health Service has been publishing, for the information of physicians, health officers, and others, a monthly abstract journal known as "Venereal Disease Information." This publication usually contains one original article on a subject of general interest in connection with venereal diseases and numerous abstracts from the current literature pertaining to these diseases. In the preparation of this abstract journal more than three hundred and fifty of the leading medical journals of the world are reviewed and abstracts made of the articles on this subject.

The cost of "Venereal Disease Information" is only fifty cents a year, payable in advance to the Superintendent of Documents, Government Printing Office, Washington, D. C. It is desired to remind the reader that this nominal charge represents only a very small portion of the total expense of preparation, the journal being a contribution of the Public Health Service in its program with state and local health departments directed against the venereal diseases.

ANNUAL SECRETARIES' CONFERENCE

The annual conference of county society secretaries will be held on Wednesday, May 10, in conjunction with the annual session of the Society. All county society secretaries will be the guests of the Society at a 12:15 luncheon at the Des Moines Club on that day. Following the luncheon a program of discussions concerning state and county society activities and problems will be directed by Dr. Robert L. Parker. The conference is planned to be of mutual interest and benefit to all participating secretaries, and of assistance to them in performing their official duties. It is hoped that every county society secretary in the state will be present.

The JOURNAL of the
Iowa State Medical Society
ISSUED MONTHLY

Ralph R. Simmons, Editor....................Des Moines

PUBLICATION COMMITTEE

Ralph R. Simmons, Editor....................Des Moines
Robert L. Parker, Secretary..................Des Moines
Oliver J. Fay, Trustee.......................Des Moines
John I. Marker, Trustee......................Davenport
Edward M. Myers, Trustee.........................Boone

SUBSCRIPTION $3.00 PER YEAR

Address all communications to the Editor of the Journal,
1122 Bankers Trust Building, Des Moines

Office of Publication, Des Moines, Iowa

Vol. XXIV   APRIL, 1934   No. 4

IT IS YOUR PARTY

If you had prepared a sumptuous banquet, had completed all details with your butcher, your caterer, and your baker, and had fully instructed your servants concerning the time and place, would you then attend and enjoy the repast? Would you require a special invitation? Your plans executed by competent and trusted servants would assure epicurean delights too pleasant to miss. Only the most severe dyspeptic could be induced to forego that dinner.

Just as surely, the educational banquet spread for the members of the Iowa State Medical Society at the Eighty-third Annual Session, planned by the entire Society and executed by a competent group of trusted servants, assures intellectual and fraternal delight too pleasant to miss. It is·your party and my party. It is just as much your party as it is the program committee's party, or the officiaries' party, or the party of the speakers appearing on the program.

These facts cannot be gainsaid. Need we, then, issue you a formal invitation to attend? Elsewhere in this issue of the Journal we publish the detailed program announcing subjects and speakers and indicating, so far as an announcement can, the scope and excellence ·of the meeting. Think of it! Over one hundred teachers, covering not only the fields of general medicine and surgery, but also the various specialties. It is a sumptuous banquet indeed.

Will you attend your party?

CHANGES IN THE PERKINS, HASKELL-KLAUS LAWS

In the January issue, the Journal published the majority and minority reports and recommendations of the committee appointed under House Joint Resolution No. 7 of the Forty-fifth General Assembly, for the investigation of the indigent patient problem in Iowa. The extra session of the legislature has now adjourned and has left in its wake the enactment into law of several· of the recommendations made by that committee. The physicians of the state will want to familiarize themselves with the enacted amendments as they affect the commitment of indigent patients to the University Hospitals and the care in their local communities of those who are not committed.

The county part-payment plan, endorsed by the Iowa State Medical Society at the 1933 annual session, and included in the recommendations of the majority report, was rejected by the legislature. The quota system of distribution of hospital service among the several counties, according to population, was legalized by the insertion of Section 4018-f1 in Chapter 199 of the Code. This amendment permits each county to commit an additional 10 per cent of patients beyond its allotted quota and provides for commitments in excess of that number at the expense of the county. Obstetric and orthopedic cases are excluded from this and other requirements of the law as amended.

Responsibility for the determination of indigency is now placed upon the county board of supervisors.

A thirty-day threshold for admissions is allowed in all but emergency cases. This provision does not apply to obstetric and orthopedic cases. If a patient cannot be admitted to the University Hospitals within a period of thirty days after application, or if in an emergency case, he cannot be admitted immediately, responsibility for medical or hospital care locally is now placed by law upon the county authorities.

Other minor changes have been made in the Perkins, Haskell-Klaus laws, such as the reduction of the physician's examining fee from five to three dollars; the reduction of escorts' wages from three to two dollars per day; and provision for the collection of debts due the county for hospitalization of indigent patients if and when they become collectible.

The complete text of the law as amended will be included in the annual report of the Committee on Public Policy and Legislation.

FEDERAL EMERGENCY MEDICAL RELIEF IN IOWA

Des Moines, Iowa, March 13th, 1934.

To Whom It May Concern:

In connection with Federal funds being used for medical aid for indigent and destitute families in the State of Iowa, we have taken the attitude that it was preferable and advisable for the local county or other local political subdivisions to carry this load rather than to make it a federal matter. Our reason for this is that we believe the supervision of medical attention near at home has a tendency for better results. Federal treatment, in our opinion, becomes more or less complicated. The principal reason, however, for my attitude in this case is that all of our federal funds are allocated to us on a matching basis, and up to this time we have never had sufficient funds for the payment of state and federal medical care in addition to other requirements.

To illustrate my point in this connection, our legislature has just passed a bill appropriating $3,000,000 for emergency relief of unemployed persons in the state of Iowa. This is the maximum amount that will be raised between now and the next session of the Iowa legislature for this purpose. If we are fortunate enough to receive from the federal government an additional $3,000,000, which is the maximum which can be hoped for, in our opinion this $6,000,000 will not be sufficient to take care of the food, fuel and clothing requirements of the unemployed and destitute people of the state between now and the next session of Congress and our legislature.

I base my opinion for this matter very largely on present conditions, which, of course, may and we hope will change for the better. However, with the betterment of conditions generally, the need for medical relief would also lessen, and the necessity for federal aid along this line would therefore not be so great.

As to some states receiving federal medical aid, namely the Dakotas, their situation is not at all similar to ours. Practically all of the Dakota territory is drought stricken and without any available funds for commodities or assistance to the poor in any way. Iowa is in a much better condition, and it is my contention that we should continue to do as much for ourselves as we possibly can.

Yours very truly,

E. H. Mulock, Chairman, ISERC and
State Administrator, CWA.

The above communication is an open letter from E. H. Mulock, chairman of the Iowa State Emergency Relief Commission and State Administrator of the CWA, in regard to the supplying of medical care, along with food, fuel and clothing, as a measure of federal relief. Mr. Mulock's opinion, voiced in answer to inquiries from doctors in many sections of Iowa, that medical attention can best be supplied by the county or other local authorities, may come as a disappointment to many physicians who have honestly felt that medical attention, since it is one of the necessities of life, should be supplied as are food, fuel and clothing. On more deliberate study of the principles involved, it appears that his arguments in regard to the difficulties of administration and the limitation of funds are not only well founded, but that there are other less obvious, but perhaps even more vital objections from the standpoint of the medical profession itself.

There can be no question but that the doctor has been forced to assume an undue share of the burden in caring for the sick poor. It has too often been taken for granted that while the provision of food, fuel and clothing for the indigent is a duty to be shared by all taxpayers, among which the physician is, of course, included, the medical care of the sick poor is a burden to be borne by the physician alone. This belief is so patently unjust and fallacious, that it is mentioned here only to point out its obvious faults. The provision of medical care is clearly to be ranked with the provision of other necessities of life, as a common duty to be shared by all. While this is a general truth, it applies not only to the present emergency but to that post-depression period to which we all look forward so hopefully. If the federal government were to assume the duty of supplying medical care as an emergency measure, such relief would obviously be hedged around with many safeguards and arbitrary rulings including the establishment of a fee schedule, and a very modest one. Assuming that in the press of times like these many physicians would consider this preferable to no fees at all, it cannot be gainsaid that the establishment of such a fee schedule, or arbitrary federal regulation of medical practice would constitute a formidable menace to the future development of medicine as a free profession. State medicine in any form must inevitably handicap scientific advance, the further development of an honored profession. In this present emergency, as in the future, it would seem that the profession should be united in securing contracts with the proper county authorities providing for the care of indigents who are charges upon the county by the members of the county society on a basis which is not only fair to the taxpayers but to the profession as well.

PHYSICIANS' FEES AND THE RETAIL SALES TAX

The following legal opinion regarding the Retail Sales Tax Act, and its effect upon physicians who are dispensing medicines, has been obtained by the Society in response to the many inquiries received at the central office. This opinion has been concurred in by the State Board of Assessment and Review and can therefore be considered by the physicians of Iowa as authoritative.

Des Moines, Iowa, March 7, 1934.

Dr. Robert L. Parker,
Secretary, Iowa State Medical Society,
Bankers Trust Building, Des Moines, Iowa.

Dear Sir:

Where a physician carrying a stock of medicines and drugs prescribes a certain agent as a remedy after diagnosing a patient's ailment, and adds to his regular fee, the price of the medicine or drug, is he required to make a report and pay a tax under the provisions of the Retail Sales Tax Act recently passed by the Forty-fifth Extra General Assembly?

In answering the question submitted, I desire to quote from the Act as follows:

"Sale" means any transfer, exchange, or barter, conditional or otherwise, in any manner or by any means whatsoever, for a consideration.

"Retail Sale" or "Sale at Retail" means the sale to a consumer or to any person for any purpose, other than for processing or for resale, of tangible personal property and the sale of gas, electricity, water, and communication service to retail consumers or users.

"Business" includes any activity engaged in by any person or caused to be engaged in by him with the object of gain, benefit, or advantage, either direct or indirect.

"Retailer" includes every person engaged in the business of selling tangible goods, wares, or merchandise at retail, or the furnishing of gas, electricity, water and communication service, and tickets or admissions to places of amusement and athletic events as provided in this division.

"Section 38. Tax imposed. There is hereby imposed, beginning the first day of April, 1934, and ending April 1, 1937, a tax of two per cent (2%), upon the gross receipts from all sales of tangible personal property, consisting of goods, wares, or merchandise, except as otherwise provided in this division, sold at retail in the State of Iowa, to consumers or users . . ."

Section 2538, Code of 1931, sets out the "prescribing or prescribing and furnishing medicine for human ailments constitutes the practice of medicine" and in addition thereto, the courts of this country have uniformly held that the practice of medicine included the following:

1. Judging the nature, character and symptoms of the disease.

2. Determining the proper remedy for the disease.

3. Giving or prescribing the application of the remedy to the disease.

So that if the physician diagnosing a case also gives or furnishes medicine to a patient without making a separate charge for the same, each of his acts constitutes a part of the practice of medicine which is rendering a service and could not be construed as a retail sale for the reason that he receives his compensation for services rendered and not through the sale of tangible goods, wares or merchandise, and therefore no tax would be collectible on any part of the service rendered by a physician while actually and in good faith practicing his profession.

However, where medicine is sold by a physician to an individual as a separate and distinct act, not a part of the practice of medicine, then the sale would be taxable to the same extent as those sales of drugs or medicines made by a registered pharmacist, as this would constitute a sale of tangible personal property.

The distinguishing features governing the interpretation of this act in so far as you are interested would be whether the physician included in his charge the cost of the medicine or material furnished, or whether he made a separate charge for the medicine or material; in the first instance no tax would be collectible, but in the second, a record should be kept and a tax paid the state upon the sale. In other words, no additional charge for material furnished should be made by the physician, but he should make his original fee cover his total service, including any material or medicine necessary to combat successfully the abnormal condition existing with his patient.

A physician is in the position of independent contractor, and he either may charge a flat fee for the entire service rendered the patient or charge a flat fee for each office or house call, and if in either of these cases he furnishes as part of his services certain medicines or materials essential to such service, it would not constitute a sale under this act any more than would those materials furnished by dentists, or papers and files furnished by an attorney, or by a building contractor who furnishes both material and labor on a construction project under contract for a certain specified amount.

The State of Michigan has had in operation for some time a sales tax law comparable to the new Iowa law and the following is taken from the Supplementary Rulings and Decisions of the State Tax Board of Michigan, and which bears out the thought hereinbefore expressed as far as the same pertains to certain professions.

"Persons engaged in the professions of and known as opticians and optometrists, physicians, dentists, architects, artists and veterinarians are deemed to be rendering a service and not selling at retail. They are considered to render and receive compensation primarily for services the receipts of which are not taxable.

The sale to such persons of such tangible personal

property as they may use or consume incidental to the rendering of such services, are "sales at retail," the gross receipts from which are taxable.

Where members of the professions enumerated above sell tangible personal property to consumers for use apart and distinct from the rendering of a service they are liable for tax on gross receipts from such sales."

So that I am of the opinion that in answer to your question herein submitted, there would be no tax upon any drug or medicine sold a patient as a remedy for a disease where the same was incidental and a part of the service rendered by the physician after diagnosing the patient's condition, and that a physician would only be liable for the tax where drugs and medicines were sold separate and apart from his services.

Yours truly,
Gerald O. Blake, Attorney at Law.

E. D. C.

This title has for the past six years designated the Early Diagnosis Campaign which means the organized effort to promote the early recognition of tuberculosis. The Iowa Tuberculosis Association has joined with similar groups all over the country to create interest in and stimulate investigation for the detection of this common and dangerous disease. The campaign has been largely educational through the laity by means of speakers and newspaper publicity, posters, films, slides and various forms of literature.

The medical profession has a responsible and highly important place in the project. We must be prepared to demonstrate our clinical ability to make an exact and definite early diagnosis when the opportunity is presented; to that end the modern physician appreciates that whenever a case of tuberculosis is discovered every contact should be examined. To support the profession in this practice, tuberculosis associations throughout the country are striving to focus public attention, through the medium of this educational campaign, upon the communicability of tuberculosis. Last year's slogan was, "Tuberculosis—From whom did he get it—To whom has he given it—Examine and protect every contact." This was a variation, with modification of the previous year's slogan— "Tuberculosis causes tuberculosis—every case comes from another." The recognition of this fact has done more to change conditions with respect to the incidence of tuberculosis than all of the steps that have been taken toward the control of the disease. The unfortunate fact remains that, although we have known that the disease was highly communicable, we have not always used this knowledge wisely in the expenditure of funds and in the dissemination of publicity intended for tuberculosis control.

The Iowa Tuberculosis Association has this year developed and promulgated an intensive medical program aimed at the "earlier discovery" of tuberculosis through following every case of tuberculosis back to its source. We have found that tuberculosis is a group disease rather than an individual problem; thus where tuberculosis exists in a family, thorough investigation of every member of the family group is essential if we are to discover the source of the disaster.

With the best of contact examination work, many cases of tuberculosis elude the vigilance of the physician and the health department. The most helpful supplementary device for finding cases is that of examining school children routinely with diagnostic tuberculin, followed by an x-ray film of all reactors. By this means early cases of tuberculosis are found among apparently healthy school children; and, as a result of examination of contacts in the home, previously unknown active cases are discovered.

Tuberculin testing of school children by the Mantou method is now in progress in many communities in Iowa. For obvious reasons only the pupils in the grades from seven to twelve have generally so far been contacted. Instead of the long recognized dictum that practically all children of high school age have been infected by the tubercle baccillus, we find that less than ten per cent react to the highly specific tuberculin. The vast majority of these reactors show calcification of the primary nodules and the lymph nodes of the hilus, but only rarely is parenchymal disease demonstrated on the x-ray film. Unfortunately the necessity of obtaining parental consent before giving the tests, has interfered with the general application of this harmless procedure.

A valuable by-product of mass tuberculin testing of school children has been the almost universal acceptance of the test by the teachers. A striking illustration of the danger of association with open tuberculosis in the schoolroom was found recently in routine testing of junior high pupils in an Iowa county seat. A tuberculous teacher, who had continued her work as long as she was able, had infected nearly 50 per cent of her pupils. Many workers in this field believe that the reactors among children furnish the major percentage of tuberculous disease in adult life; hence every effort should be made to find primary tuberculosis so that appropriate preventive measures may be instituted to prevent the development of clinical disease. John H. Peck, M.D.

THE PRESIDENT'S MESSAGE

The program is now a very complicated affair, covering many more subjects, and more phases of some subjects than ever before.

It will be impossible for any member to attend all the sections. Study the program as published in this issue. You will find exactly what you want to hear discussed. Please mark those conferences which most interest you. Even pencil your second and third choices, and bring this marked program with you. This will enable you to go quickly to the rooms where your subject or subjects of choice are being discussed. Assistants from the office force will direct you and give you all possible aid.

Your Program Committee has worked unceasingly to give you the latest and best in all phases of medicine and surgery. Vast advances have been made in the treatment of arthritis and we are attempting to present the practical advances so that every practitioner who must deal with arthritis may profit. Beginning with the first forenoon in the general session, when the subject of arthritis is treated as a symposium, until the last paper on the Friday morning session, when present-day medical economic problems are discussed, the entire program is one of value and interest.

The committee has had perfect cooperation from the men in the field from every quarter of the state. It now comes up to the final stage. If the committee can get the teachers and those to be taught together without friction, it feels that there will be no need for apologies as to the results.

Bring your wives and attend the reception given to Dr. Walter L. Bierring, president elect of the American Medical Association. The banquet will be different, and the committee believes you will want to attend.

This has been a glorious year for your president. He has been shown courtesies and accorded a reception far beyond his deserts. For all this he is thankful and prays that the work accomplished will justify this fine reception.

Chas B Taylor

President.

SPEAKERS BUREAU ACTIVITIES

POSTGRADUATE COURSE NOTES

Enthusiastic reports are being heard from the members of the Iowa State Medical Society who are taking the three postgraduate courses being offered by the Speakers Bureau this spring. The doctors enrolled in these courses are learning the most recent facts about old and new subjects and are having new methods of treatment of diseases excellently demonstrated.

The group taking the course at Creston was privileged to learn the results of several years experiments in diet and disease made by Dr. Clifford J. Barborka of the Northwestern University Medical School—facts which are just now in the process of being printed but which these doctors heard first hand before the book comes off the press.

At Mt. Pleasant Dr. Rathe of Waverly had a tank of commercial oxygen to illustrate his lecture on the newer treatment of pneumonia to the members taking the postgraduate course on Infectious Diseases.

The lectures of the postgraduate group at Creston are scheduled to be held from 7:00 until 9:00 p. m. on Wednesday nights. This makes it possible for the lecturers from out of the state who come by train to leave on the 9:30 p. m. train, following the meeting. However, the lectures have been so excellent and the doctors were so interested that in two instances the lecturers were forced to cancel their reservations for the 9:30 train and take one leaving two hours later.

All of the doctors who are lecturing on these courses, whether they are from Iowa or from other states, have commented on the splendid attitude of the men taking the courses; have noted their sincerity, interest and eagerness in keeping abreast of the latest advances and knowledge in their profession.

The doctors taking the course on Neurology and Psychiatry at Oskaloosa are going to "quiz" themselves to see if they are getting the most out of the lectures. One week they had a lecture on the subject of "Headaches"; the following week they had prepared some case reports—giving only the history and laboratory findings, and withholding the diagnosis. Each doctor was given a copy of these case reports at the next meeting. The cases were discussed and the doctors tried to diagnose them from the facts presented. This served as an excellent means of reviewing the lecture of the previous week.

These reports indicate the value of postgraduate courses and show what a vital part they are playing in the medical postgraduate work in Iowa. Requests are already beginning to come in for fall courses; if the doctors in your locality are interested in having a course near you, it would be wise for the secretary of your society to get in touch with the Speakers Bureau at the earliest possible moment.

1934 PROGRAM

The Speakers Bureau wishes to take this opportunity to congratulate the Program Committee on the excellent program they have arranged for the annual meeting this year. The Bureau feels that the best program is one which provides for the development of the greatest number of men and one which gives the most in value and interesting facts to those who are listening. The program this year most admirably combines these two features. The program this year is decidely not a one-man's program—it is everyone's. If you are not contributing to it in any other way, you can support it by your presence at the state meeting. You will be well repaid.

DISTRICT MEETINGS

Eight district meetings and one district meeting of deputy councilors have been held already this year. Three of the districts in the state hold regular quarterly district meetings and are enthusiastic about the plan. Such meetings are undoubtedly a potent force for good in our medical organization. They do much to promote unity among wider and wider groups of members of the medical profession. Doctors' from all sections of the district meet together, eat together, talk together; frequent meetings develop a tolerance for the other fellow's viewpoint, develop friendships and build for much better feeling within the profession.

Furthermore, district meetings provide an excellent opportunity for the scientific advancement of the doctors in that district. It is a distinct honor to be asked to give a talk before such a large group of one's fellow practitioners and those preparing talks are inspired to do the best they can, which makes the program of double value—to those speaking and those listening.

Finally, these district meetings serve as an excellent clearing house for matters affecting the profession as a whole. Many important matters of policy and business, economic and ethical problems arise from time to time which involve every member of the State Medical Society. The discussions and opinions of those attending these district meetings do much to settle these problems.

RADIO TALKS

WOI, Ames—Fridays, 6:45 p. m.
WSUI, Iowa City—Thursdays, 8:00 p. m.

April 5- 6 Pleurisy—J. C. Painter, M.D.
      12-13 Health and Happiness—Frank M. Fuller, M.D.
      19-20 Winning Health Essay.
      26-27 Nephritis—W. M. Fowler, M.D.
May 3- 4 Sleeping Sickness—Jesse L. Sauer, M.D.
      10-11 Mother's Day—Joseph H. Kinnaman, M.D.

WOMAN'S AUXILIARY NEWS

Edited by the Press and Publicity Committee

MRS. OLIVER J. FAY, *Chairman*, 10 Thirty-fifth Street, Des Moines

HEALTH ESSAY CONTEST

The Health Essay Contest in the public high schools in Iowa, which was sponsored by the Woman's Auxiliary and the Speakers Bureau, came to a close Thursday, March 15. One hundred ninety-five essays were submitted from all parts of the state and from all high school grades. These essays represent only a small fraction of the actual number of students who participated in the contest. The rules of the contest allowed only three papers from any one school to be submitted. For this reason, the greatest elimination took place in local schools. All the essays which had been written in any one school were examined and evaluated, and only the three best were sent to represent that school in the state contest. In one small town one hundred students wrote essays and from this group only three were selected to be sent in.

Of these one hundred ninety-five girls and boys, twenty-three will win prizes: first prize, $15.00; second prize, $10.00; third prize, $5.00, and twenty prizes of $1.00 each. These are the prizes to be awarded by the Woman's Auxiliary. The Speakers Bureau is making an additional award to the first prize winner of a trip to either Ames or Iowa City to read the winning essay over the radio during regular broadcasting periods of the Iowa State Medical Society.

The preliminary checking and judging of these essays by the members of the Woman's Auxiliary has already been done. The final judging will be done by the following committee: A member of the State Department of Health, a member of the State Department of Public Instruction, a member of the Iowa Parent-Teacher Association, a member of the Iowa State Medical Society and a member of the Woman's Auxiliary. The final judging is to take place in the near future and the prize winners' names will appear in the Des Moines *Register and Tribune*. The winning essay will be broadcast from station WOI, Ames, on Friday, April 20, at 6:45 p. m., and from WSUI, Iowa City, on Thursday, April 19, at 8:00 p. m.

The Woman's Auxiliary is especially pleased with the whole-hearted interest manifested in such a worthwhile educational project. Health is undoubtedly the greatest asset man can possess. Only by beginning to build for health in our youth can we expect to retain it in our later life. Youth tends to take health for granted. If by this contest these girls and boys who have written essays have been inspired to reflect more seriously on the value of health and the methods by which one can attain this quality, the contest has been a great success.

This contest was made possible through the co-operation of the Speakers Bureau, the State Department of Public Instruction, the State Department of Health and particularly of the individual instructors, educators, principals and superintendents of the various local schools. It was because of their approval, endorsement and organization of the contest in their own schools that we were able to conduct this state-wide project. To them goes the sincere appreciation of those who sponsored the Health Essay Contest.

Cerro Gordo County

The Woman's Auxiliary to the Cerro Gordo County Medical Society has been organized for two years. We hold our meetings regularly, with talks and book reviews. At our last meeting, which was held at the home of Mrs. L. R. Woodward, with thirty-two present, we elected the following officers for the coming year: Mrs. T. E. Davidson of Mason City, president; Mrs. C. M. Franchere of Mason City, vice president; Mrs. Draper Long of Mason City, secretary; and Mrs. E. L. Wurtzer of Clear Lake, treasurer. Plans are being made for a summer picnic.

Mrs. T. E. Davidson

Howard County

Officers elected at the meeting of the Woman's Auxiliary to the Howard County Medical Society, held Saturday, March 10, are: Mrs. C. F. Snopek of Cresco, president; Mrs. W. A. Bockoven of Cresco, vice president; and Mrs. L. W. Clark of Chester, secretary and treasurer.

Muscatine County

Mrs. E. L. Emerson was named president of the Woman's Auxiliary to the Muscatine County Medical Society at a meeting held Monday, March 19. Other officers are: Mrs. A. L. Bryan, president-elect; Mrs. W. W. Daut, secretary; Mrs. R. M. Arey, treasurer.

Pottawattamie County

The Woman's Auxiliary to the Pottawattamie County Medical Society met in Council Bluffs, Tuesday, March 20, and the following program was presented: The Organization of the Iowa State Board of Health, Mrs. F. Earl Bellinger; The New Drug and Cosmetic Bill, Mrs. Grant Augustine; What Shall I Believe in Regard to Advertisements of Patent Medicines, Mrs. Joseph B. Thornell; and Radio Advertisements of Medicines and Cosmetics, Mrs. C. V. Edwards.

Webster County

Monday, March 5, members of the Woman's Auxiliary to the Webster County Medical Society met for their regular annual meeting, and elected the following officers: Mrs. E. D. Morrison, president; Mrs. E. N. Zinn, vice president; Mrs. F. L. Knowles, secretary; and Mrs. O. N. Glesne, treasurer. Dr. L. L. Leighton, president of the Webster County Medical Society, addressed the group on the Copeland-Tugwell pure food, drug and cosmetic act, which is now being presented to Congress.

SOCIETY PROCEEDINGS

Black Hawk County

Tuesday, March 20, the Black Hawk County Medical Society met in Waterloo, with the following program: A Consideration of Renal Malignancies with Special Reference to Their Treatment, N. G. Alcock, M.D., Iowa City; discussion by A. G. Fleischman, M.D., Des Moines; Arthur W. Erskine, M.D., Cedar Rapids; and Otis W. Britt, M.D., Waterloo.

Boone-Story Society

Members of the combined Boone and Story County Medical Societies met in Nevada, Tuesday, March 20, for the regular dinner meeting. H. P. Elmquist, M.D., of Cambridge, presented a paper on Diseases of the Blood, and George J. Severson, M.D., of Slater, spoke on Purpura Hemorrhagica.

Calhoun County

The Calhoun County Medical Society held its monthly meeting at the Court House in Rockwell City, Tuesday, March 13. The scientific program was as follows: Urinalysis, O. R. Prettyman, M.D., of Manson, and General Practice, L. E. Eslick, M.D., of Rockwell City. These papers were both interesting and practical and were freely discussed by the nine members who were present at the meeting. The next meeting will be held at the McVay Hospital in Lake City.

W. W. Stevenson, M.D., Secretary

Cerro Gordo County

S. Marx White, M.D., professor of internal medicine at the University of Minnesota School of Medicine, Minneapolis, was the guest speaker for the Cerro Gordo County Medical Society at its meeting held in Mason City, Tuesday, March 20. Dr. White spoke on Heart Disease Among Elderly People. The next meeting will be held Tuesday, April 17, with W. A. Fansler, M.D., assistant professor of surgery at the University of Minnesota School of Medicine, as guest speaker.

Clinton County

Clifford J. Barborka, M.D., of Chicago, was the speaker of the evening Thursday, March 1, when the Clinton County Medical Society met in Clinton. His talk followed a six-thirty dinner. Dr. Barborka, formerly of the Mayo Foundation, Rochester, and now associate professor of medicine, Northwestern University Medical School, Chicago, is a specialist on diet and nutrition. He presented an illustrated address on The Present Conception of the Relation of Diet to Health and Disease, which was exceedingly interesting and instructive.

E. V. Donlan, M.D., Secretary

Davis County

When the Davis County Medical Society met in Bloomfield, Friday, March 9, F. L. Nelson, M.D., of Ottumwa, furnished the scientific program, speaking on The Diagnosis of Surgical Urology.

Decatur County

The Decatur County Medical Society was host to Dr. Charles B. Taylor, of Ottumwa, president of the state society, at a dinner meeting held Wednesday, February 7. The scientific paper of the evening was presented by Edward B. Hoeven, M.D., of Ottumwa, who spoke on The Modern Treatment of Eclampsia. Dr. H. A. Spilman, also of Ottumwa, and Dr. J. C. Donahue, of Centerville, spoke briefly to the group.

The Decatur County Medical Society is cooperating with the Red Cross and the CWA in presenting a series of classes in first aid.

J. E. McFarland, M.D., Secretary

Floyd County

The regular meeting of the Floyd County Medical Society was held at the Hotel Hildreth in Charles City, Tuesday, February 27. Two papers were presented; one on Cancer of the Breast by Norman C. Flater, M.D., of Floyd, and one on X-ray Studies by Vernon Moore, M.D., of Charles City.

J. B. Miner, Jr., M.D., Secretary

Fremont County Meetings

On Friday, January 19, the Fremont County Medical Society met in the offices of Drs. Wanamaker and Wanamaker in Hamburg. Each one of the twelve doctors present reviewed one or more interestin cases that had come under his observation in recen practice. The following officers were elected for 1934: Dr. H. P. Cole, of Thurman, president; Dr G. L. Roark, of Tabor, vice president; and Dr. A. E Wanamaker, of Hamburg, secretary and treasurer

A very satisfactory meeting of the Fremont County Medical Society was held at the home of Dr. and Mrs H. P. Cole in Thurman, Thursday, March 22. Th occasion was Dr. Cole's birthday. After a very fin dinner, the wives adjourned for a social meeting, whil the physicians held their scientific session. Verno: L. Treynor, M.D., of Council Bluffs, gave an excellen talk on Diabetes, and M. C. Hennessy, M.D., of Coun cil Bluffs, councilor for this district, spoke at lengt on the problems connected with the CWA. At th close of the dinner Dr. Cole was presented with token of respect and esteem in the form of a beauti ful fountain pen desk set.

A. E. Wanamaker, M.D., Secretary

Johnson County

The Johnson County Medical Society met at th Jefferson Hotel in Iowa City, Wednesday, March with the following program: Peptic Ulcer in Children, Pauline V. Moore, M.D., of Solon; discussion opened by Mark L. Floyd, M.D., of Iowa City; Immunity in Scarlet Fever, Philip C. Jeans, M.D., of Iowa City; and What the Practitioner Should Know About Quarantine Laws, Milford E. Barnes, M.D., of Iowa City.

___

Lee County

Thursday, March 15, members of the Lee County Medical Society met in Keokuk, with an afternoon session at the Graham Hospital, and an evening meeting at the St. Joseph's Hospital. Paul G. Dick, M.D., of Chicago, was guest speaker for the society, taking as his subject, Examination of the Stomach by X-Ray. Other papers on the program were: Cesarean Section, John T. Hanna, M.D., of Burlington; So-called Enlargement of the Thymus Gland in Infants, Francis E. Sultzman, M.D., of Hannibal, Missouri; and The Leukocyte Blood Picture in Acute Infections, Marcus P. Neal, M.D., professor of pathology, University of Missouri School of Medicine.

Linn County Meetings

John H. Musser, M.D., professor of medicine at Tulane University of Louisiana School of Medicine, New Orleans, is to be the guest of the Linn County Medical Society for its meeting Friday, April 13. He will speak on The Treatment of the Various Kinds of Anemia.

On Thursday, May 3, the program will be furnished by Fred L. Adair, M.D., professor of obstetrics and gynecology, Graduate School of Medicine, Division of the Biological Sciences, University of Chicago.

Marshall County

Howard L. Beye, M.D., of Iowa City, addressed the monthly meeting of the Marshall County Medical Society, held in Marshalltown, Tuesday, March 6, on Acute Empyema.

Page County Annual Meeting

Dr. R. D. Smith, of Clarinda, and Dr. F. H. Clark, also of Clarinda, were named president and secretary, respectively, at the annual meeting of the Page County Medical Society held in Clarinda, Monday, March 5.

___

Pottawattamie County

Tuesday, March 20, members of the Pottawattamie County Medical Society met at the Mercy Hospital in Council Bluffs for their regular dinner meeting. The following program was presented by Council Bluffs physicians: Management of Prostatic Obstruction, Gerald V. Caughlan, M.D.; Head Injuries, Joseph Stech, M.D.; discussion opened by William E. Ash, M.D.; and Some of the Present Phases of Infant Feeding, Isaac Sternhill, M.D.

Arnold L. Jensen, M.D., Secretary

Polk County

The regular monthly meeting of the Des Moines Academy of Medicine and Polk County Medical Society was held at the Hotel Fort Des Moines, Tuesday evening, March 27. Joseph C. Ohlmacher, M.D., professor of bacteriology and pathology and administrative head of the University of South Dakota, was the guest speaker. He gave an illustrated lecture on The Functional Basis of Certain Kidney Disorders with a Brief Consideration of the More Important Kidney Lesions. Preceding the scientific lecture a number of the local physicians met in the Tap Room for a dinner in honor of Dr. Ohlmacher. Approximately 150 members and guests were in attendance at the meeting. The usual social hour was enjoyed by a number of the members following the meeting.

___

Sac County

With guests from Sioux City, Glidden, Lake City and other towns, the Sac County Medical Society held a most successful meeting at the Park Hotel, Tuesday, March 20. The speaker of the evening was Fred Knowles, M.D., of Fort Dodge, who discussed Care and Fracture of the Neck of the Femur, and showed moving pictures of his technic and cases. Thirty doctors were present and listened with great interest, several of them participating in the discussion, which was led by James W. Graham, M.D., of Sioux City.

At the business session, a contract with the Board of Supervisors for the care of the poor was approved. Dr. J. R. Dewey of Schaller was elected delegate, and Dr. J. J. McCarl of Sac City, and George W. Anderson of Early, were named alternate delegates.

J. R. Dewey, M.D., Secretary

Scott County

Carl A. Hedblom, M.D., professor of surgery at Northwestern University School of Medicine, Chicago, was the speaker at the monthly meeting of the Scott County Medical Society held in Davenport, Tuesday, March 6. His subject was The Treatment of Pulmonary Abscess and Empyema.

___

Wapello County Meetings

On Tuesday, April 17, Ralph Selman, M.D., of Blakesburg, will speak before the Wapello County Medical Society on Early Frontier Medical Experiences. Discussion of the address will be opened by Murdoch Bannister, M.D., of Ottumwa.

W. E. Anthony, M.D., of Ottumwa, will furnish the scientific program for the Wapello County Medical Society, when that organization meets Tuesday, May 8. He will speak on Dyspnea as a Diagnostic Symptom, and the discussion will be led by R. O. Hughes, M.D., also of Ottumwa.

Evon Walker, M.D., Secretary

Washington County

The Washington County Medical Society held its monthly meeting, Tuesday, March 6, at which time H. Dabney Kerr, M.D., of Iowa City, gave an address on X-Ray Treatment of Skin Malignancies. A review of the x-ray pictures of other conditions, and general discussion followed. A business meeting and oyster supper closed the session.

W. S. Kyle, M.D., Secretary

First Councilor District Meeting

A meeting of the First Councilor District was held in Charles City, Tuesday, April 3, at the Hotel Hildreth, with the following program: Correlation of Child Health and the State Department of Health, Fred Moore, M.D., Des Moines; and The Treatment of Infectious Diseases in Children, Dennis Kelly, M.D., also of Des Moines. Dr. F. A. Hennessy of Calmar is councilor for the district.

Second Councilor District Meeting

A joint meeting of the Wright County Medical Society and the Second Councilor District was held at Clarion, Tuesday, March 27. The success of this type of program is becoming more pronounced with each repetition. The three papers presented at this meeting were extremely well prepared on pertinent subjects, and were well discussed. The program consisted of: Case History of Cerebral Thrombosis, B. L. Basinger, M.D., of Goldfield; Bandl's Contraction Ring, with case report, Nelle Thomas Schultz, M.D., of Humboldt; and Colitis, M. G. Bourne, M.D., of Algona. Dr. Charles B. Taylor president of the state society, Dr. Robert L. Parker, secretary of the state society, and Dr. H. A. Spilman, chairman of the council, were present as guests, and spoke briefly to the group.

L. R. Woodward, M.D., Councilor

Sixth Councilor District Meeting

Tuesday, March 13, a joint meeting of the Poweshiek County Medical Society, and other members of the Sixth Councilor District, was held in Grinnell at the Hotel Monroe-Gifford. P. E. Somers, M.D., of Grinnell, read a paper entitled, The Light Under the Bushel, which was discussed by T. U. McManus, M.D., of Waterloo, and Aaron C. Conaway, M.D., of Marshalltown. Oliver J. Fay, M.D., of Des Moines, presented an address on The Test of Organized Medicine, which was followed by a general discussion. Announcements were made by Dr. C. W. Ellyson, councilor of the sixth district.

Eleventh Councilor District Meeting

A. G. Pohlman, M.D., head of the department of anatomy, Creighton University School of Medicine, Omaha, was guest speaker at the meeting of the Eleventh Councilor District held in Shenandoah at the Hotel Delmonico, Wednesday, March 21. Dr. Pohlman spoke on The Adaptation of the Circulatory System. A. A. Johnson, M.D., of Council Bluffs, read a paper on Amebic Dysentery and Its Complications; and W. H. Maloy, M.D., of Shenandoah, talked on Nephritic Retinitis. Dr. M. C. Hennessy of Council Bluffs is councilor for the district.

INTERESTING NEWS
In Brief

The vasodilator substance of the blood and body tissues has been subjected to critical chemical study at Harvard Medical School and is now identified as adenosine triphosphate.

A statistical study completed by the Travelers Insurance Company indicates that about 13,500 persons were killed last year in collisions between automobiles and pedestrians.

Said to be the oldest known prescription for remedial drugs, a stone tablet has been found dating to 3700 B. C. which bears directions for making an inhalant for the treatment of head colds.

Because of his thoroughness and the far-reaching quality of his observations in genetics, Dr. Thomas Hunt Morgan of the California Institute of Technology was awarded the 1933 Nobel Prize in Medicine.

Studies at the Rockefeller Institute for Medical Research in New York City indicate that the olfactory nerves are the chief paths for the transmission of the virus of poliomyelitis from the nasal cavity to the brain.

The American College of Surgeons, long interested in the statistical study of cancer, has collected the records of over 12,000 cancer patients who have remained alive over a five year period following surgical treatment.

A statistical analysis made by the Metropolitan Life Insurance Company indicates that the mortality from diabetes is increasing throughout the world, and that this increase in practically all instances is limited to women during and after the menopausal ages.

PERSONAL MENTION

Dr. J. W. Myers, who has been practicing medicine in Sheldon for nineteen years, moved his practice and family to Postville.

Dr. Ludwig Gitler, of Fairfield, spoke before the Fairfield Forum Club, Wednesday, February 28, on "Psychopathic Cases and Their Treatment."

Dr. H. S. Miner, after eight years of practice in Green Mountain, is moving to Beaman.

Dr. Ralph L. Irwin, formerly of Sioux City, has located in Paullina for the practice of medicine. Dr. Irwin was graduated from the State University of Iowa College of Medicine in 1925, and has spent four years in Boston, where he was engaged in hospital work.

Dr. Raymond Rice, city health officer of Council Bluffs, spoke before the Kiwanis Club, Tuesday, March 20, on the history and development of immunization methods for diphtheria by scientists since the early part of the seventeenth century.

Dr. James W. Wetzel has come to Sac City from Chicago, to be associated with Dr. L. B. Amick at the Sac City Hospital. Dr. Wetzel was graduated in 1929 from the University of Illinois College of Medicine, and has practiced medicine in Lorain, Ohio, for three years.

Dr. and Mrs. R. R. Hansen, of Marshalltown; Dr. Otis R. Wolfe, of Marshalltown, and Dr. J. E. O'Keefe and, family, of Waterloo, are among those sailing on the S. S. Pennsylvania for a Carriban cruise. Brief stops will be made in Cuba, Jamaica, Panama, Colombia, Venezuela and Puerto Rico.

MARRIAGES

The marriage of Miss Marian Knapp, of Detroit, Michigan, to Dr. R. Lawrence Knipfer, of Brandon, Iowa, took place Tuesday, March 13, at the home of the bride's aunt, in Detroit. Mrs. Knipfer will complete her nursing course at the Herman Keifer Hospital in June, at which time she will join Dr. Knipfer in Brandon, where he has been practicing for several months.

DEATH NOTICES

Frear, Edwin D., of Danbury, aged seventy-nine, died March 19, after an illness of six years' duration. He was graduated in 1882 from the State University of Iowa, and was for several years a member of the Woodbury County Medical Society.

George, Abel Benson, of Burlington, aged fifty-five, died December 29. He was graduated in 1900 from the University of Illinois College of Medicine, and at the time of his death was a life member of the Des Moines County and Iowa State Medical Societies.

Juen, Joseph A., of Ossian, aged fifty-nine, died March 11, from a cerebral hemorrhage following a short illness. He was graduated in 1904 from the College of Physicians and Surgeons, St. Louis, and at the time of his death was a member of the Winneshiek County Medical Society.

Pond, Issi Otto, of Perry, aged sixty, died suddenly March 15. He was graduated in 1901 from the State University of Iowa College of Homeopathic Medicine, and at the time of his death was a member of the Dallas-Guthrie Medical Society.

Reynolds, John William, of Creston, aged fifty-nine, died suddenly March 14. He was graduated in

1898 from the Kansas City Medical College, and had long been a member of the Union County Medical Society.

Thomas, Samuel W., of Melcher, aged eighty-five, died March 6, after a lingering illness of a year's duration. He was graduated in 1880 from the Kentucky School of Medicine, Louisville, and at the time of his death was a life member of the Marion County and Iowa State Medical Societies.

Valenta, Joseph A., of Cedar Rapids, aged sixty-two, died March 17, after a short illness. He was graduated in 1896 from the State University of Iowa College of Medicine and at the time of his death was a member of the Linn County Medical Society.

Wiley, Edward B., of Grinnell, aged seventy-five, died March 5, following a long illness. He was graduated in 1882 from Hahnemann Medical College and Hospital of Philadelphia, and at the time of his death was a member of the Poweshiek County Medical Society.

CANCER ROUND TABLE CLINICAL AND PATHOLOGIC CONFERENCE

Broadlawns General Hospital

Tuesdays—7:30-9:00 P. M.

April 10	The Historic Background of the Cancer Problem
17	Cancer of the Breast
24	Cancer of the Stomach
May 1	Cancer of the Intestines
8	Cancer of the Uterus

All physicians, nurses and health agencies are urged to participate. The period will consist of a brief introductory lecture followed by clinical round table discussion.

WARNING

Two men have recently called on railway surgeons and attorneys in Knoxville purporting to represent the Rock Island Railway. These men attempted to collect donations from railway physicians and attorneys to be used for the benefit of the unemployed. The only identification which they presented was a railroad time book. The Iowa officials of the Rock Island Railway have stated that they have no knowledge of these two men and that their credentials are not adequate. Dr. Samuel Plummer, Chief Surgeon of the Rock Island, has given the JOURNAL permission to issue this warning to the physicians of Iowa, in case they extend their operations to other parts of the state, and has assured us that legitimate representatives of the railway are furnished obviously authentic credentials. It is suggested that if any physician is solicited by these men, he immediately notify the local Rock Island office.

HISTORY OF MEDICINE IN IOWA

Edited by the Historical Committee

DR. HENRY B. YOUNG, Burlington   DR. TOM. B. THROCKMORTON, Des Moines
DR. FRANK M. FULLER, Keokuk   DR. WALTER L. BIERRING, Des Moines
DR. JOHN T. McCLINTOCK, Iowa City

Diphtheria in Iowa in 1881

The following letter to the first State Board of Health of Iowa, bearing the date of October 24, 1881, should be of particular interest at this time in view of the increased activities and interest in diphtheria immunization in Iowa. At the time this was written the organism causing diphtheria had not been discovered. The keen observation and careful analysis, at a time when the aid of a laboratory was not available to the men in the field, is indeed interesting. Dr. Ward Woodbridge, the author of the letter, is now retired and resides at Central City, Iowa.

"Diphtheria In Waubeek, Linn County, and Vicinity—Reported by Ward Woodbridge, M.D., Health Physician of Waubeek

"Diphtheria is prevailing in the village of Waubeek and vicinity, now, for the fourth time in two years and three months. In August, 1879, it made its first appearance in twenty years, and at that time the first case appeared in a family out of town. There was no school, and as far as could be told the case was one of spontaneous development. It proved fatal, and all the other members of the family, including the mother, the father being at that time in the Black Hills, were attacked with it, but all recovering. At the same time, a serious epidemic was prevailing in Cedar Rapids, and the next two cases were undoubtedly imported from there, both proving fatal. There were a few light cases following, and it declined. The people knew nothing at all of it, and sympathizing with their neighbors visited them, and public funerals were held. Proper cautions were not taken in cleansing, etc., and in December following, another and more severe epidemic broke out, resulting in fourteen deaths. Two physicians, Drs. Crawford and Gremm were here at the time and battled manfully with the disease, Crawford being an able young man, Gremm an 'irregular.' At the time this epidemic prevailed, I was away at school and

no record was kept of it. So my facts have to be gathered from any and every source available; but there was no importation in the beginning of the second epidemic. There were a few unimportant cases following in the fall and winter of 1880 and 1881. In April, 1881, I settled in Waubeek, in Dr. Crawford's place, Dr. Gremm having previously moved away. June 14, on returning home from the meeting of the Iowa Union Medical Society I was summoned to see a child fourteen years of age and found him suffering from a very severe attack of diphtheria. This case occurred at school, as did also the first case of the second epidemic referred to above. My first case was in the family of a merchant of the town, and both he and his wife came down into the store from the sick room (living over the store); and I am told that the mother of the next case was in the store with her two children, aged two and one-half years, and eight months, respectively; and that the lady took the children in her arms. This she denies to me, so I give it for what it is worth, which is not much, as we shall see presently. The first case made a good recovery, but the next two were fatal, one dying of diphtheritic laryngitis. From this, the disease spread, and seven cases proved fatal in the village and five around it. Some rather remarkable evidence of its contagiousness may as well be spoken of here. A little girl, aged about ten years, had some relatives living in town, and she came to stay all night with them. In the night one of the children was taken sick with diphtheria. She returned home, went to school, and in five days took sick at school. Six days following, two cases occurred in two separate families, and soon two more, all proving fatal. The little girl first taken made a slow tedious recovery. A baby in the same family died with it. There were forty one cases in all. The disease gradually declined and in six weeks had entirely disappeared. During its prevalence, I tried to impress on the people the necessity of using great caution. No publi funerals were allowed, and everything used about the sick burned or thoroughly smoked with sulphur fumes and then washed. October 8 I was again called to see a case, which took sick at school. On returning home, I sent my own children at once to their grandparents to isolate them from it if possible, but on the evening of the 7th my girl, aged eight, was taken sick with it and died the morning of the 10th, and tonight as I pen these lines, I am watching over another one of my children lying very sick with it. There have been, so far, thirteen cases, with three deaths, and it is still ranging. This makes fifty-four cases which have been in my hands since the 14th of June, with fifteen deaths. Now this epidemic has not by any means been confined to Waubeek and vicinity, but has been all around us, both in towns and country.

"The village of Waubeek is situated on the southwest bank of the Wapsipinicon River, Maine township, Linn county, Iowa, and contains about three hundred inhabitants. The ground is lower than it is west and northwest, but on a level south and southeast. It is located on a ledge of rocks, which in places crop out, and there are several fine rock quarries in and around it. There is a fine farming country all around the village, except to the east, and a community of good, intelligent farmers. There is a good water privilege and a mill; a creamery in

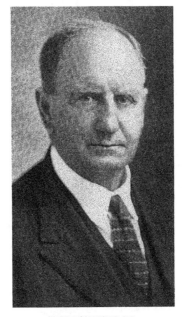

WARD WOODBRIDGE, M.D.
(Rush Medical College, 1881)

almost the center of the town, to which I shall have occasion to refer again. It is not, strictly speaking, a thrifty village. While there are a great many industrious people, there are, also, a great many who seem to live from hand to mouth; and some rather untidy housekeepers which, of course, is very inviting to contagious and infectious diseases. Malaria enters largely into all forms of sickness throughout the community, either primarily or as a complication. In

very many of the cases of diphtheria I have noted the intermittent character of the fever, and often more than the initial chill, with gastric irritation, showing distinction, it seems to me that the malaria is adding to the severity of the disease. The health of the community in general this year, has been at a very low standard—or, in other words, 'below par.' Neuralgia, rheumatism, gastric catarrh, malarial and typhus malarial fevers. Erysipelas sores not healing kindly, but persistent and stubborn, have been prevailing to a much more than usual extent for the past six months. Scarlet fever has also prevailed about eight miles south of us, to some extent.

"We refer to the well-known physical law, 'That no effect can be the result of a single cause,' and so I fully believe in regard to diphtheria— that no single cause for it will ever be demonstrated; but, rather, that a multiplicity of causes will always be found operating for its production. I do not refer to the specific character of the disease; for that, of course, is well defined, but to the causes operating to bring on an epidemic. I see the United States Board of Health agree that it is at first a strictly local disease. With the greatest respect for the opinions of those very able gentlemen I am not prepared to agree with them. On the other hand, there are very able and experienced investigators who maintain that it is always primarily a constitutional disease, with a local manifestation. This I also deny. I think the 'golden mean' is to be found between the two extreme opinions; viz., that a great number of cases are primarily constitutional, and the throat symptoms secondary. Others again, manifest very mild throat symptoms, with little or no constitutional disturbances; intense fevers, reaching 105° F., pulse 140, or even higher, with great prostration, aching head, back and limbs, and profound disturbance of the nervous system, with the throat symptoms entirely in abeyance for twenty-four or thirty-six hours, and the cases proceed rapidly to a fatal termination. This, it seems to me, could be accounted for in no other way than that the diphtheritic virus had invaded the whole economy, and that the onset of the disease was so violent as to be incompatible with life. I remember one case very distinctly, of this kind, in which the membrane on the tonsils never exceeded the size of the thumb nail, yet it was fatal. Perhaps it is unwise to occupy space in arguing this point further, and it is of no use for me to attempt to speak of the specific character of the virus—to tell what it is, or what it is not. Volumes have already been written upon it. The question is: Why does it prevail so often, persistently and fatally about Waubeek? First, the influence of contagion must be admitted. We cannot, of course, tell the manner of its operation. Can we even say that it is capable of being widely diffused? It seems to hang around certain places and things, in a manner perfectly surprising. I have said that it was not confined to Waubeek and its vicinity. It is prevailing now in and about Anamosa, twelve miles distant; in and about Springville, eight miles distant; and in the country eight miles distant both west and northwest; also, to some extent in Marion and Cedar Rapids before it appeared in Waubeek. There are no swamps near our village; no new land being broken up; but all under a high state of cultivation. The creamery spoken of above, was not kept in the best possible condition. There was a cistern to receive the sour milk, which was allowed to go foul. The owners were requested to clean it out, and wash it with copperas water once a week, which they very kindly did. The mill-dam was injured during the high water in the spring, and a new water-course cut its way through and left the old bed lying next the town, with some stagnant water in it. The mill company repaired it, and it is now full of water, removing that possible source of infection. Nearly all the drinking water is from wells drilled from forty to sixty feet in the solid rock. Indeed, I cannot see that there is anything in the village, or its surroundings, that especially invites the contagious germ of diphtheria, that they do not have in all the towns and villages about us, and so they have diphtheria too. It certainly was not carried from Waubeek to them. So, there must be a multiplicity of causes, with health generally at a low ebb.

"The prevalance of disease of all kinds, and especially of an infectious character—for even typhoid fever has been prevailing southwest of us to an alarming extent—will show the causes can hardly be atmospheric, as it will break out, and run four or six weeks, then decline, and nothing more be heard of it for a longer or shorter interval, when it will break out again. Moreover an epidemic will be declining in one place, at its height in another, and commencing in another. So, it would seem that whatever the circumstances are that so favor its development and progress, they could not bring it about without the presence of its own peculiar contagious germ. (Some gentlemen may object to the term, germ; they may call it something else). So epidemic and contagion could hardly be separated. There are isolated cases occurring all the time. Sporadically—sometimes one; sometimes a few in a place. Only last week a girl fifteen years old died with it, and no case had been within five miles of the locality for three months, they living in the country, several miles from all towns. Thus, after all, we are obliged to say that the diphtheritic germ is present with us, and that occasionally an assemblage of circumstances favor its development, and that the nature of both are unknown to us. In its nature it is worse than scarlet fever, for it is sporadic, epidemic, and contagious; and there seems no possible escape from it. I am often asked, as I presume all physicians are: 'Is there no preventive?' My invariable reply is: only, to get the general health up to as high a standard as possible, so that in case an attack should come, perhaps it may lighten it. It is a terrible scourge, snatching away the youth, beauty and promise of our land, and the disease is assuming alarming magnitude, not only with us here in this vicinity, but all over the country, and in fact the world. There have been, in the two years and three months, twenty-nine deaths in and around Waubeek, and doubtless as many more in a radius of ten miles. It will be a happy time for the human family when the profession finds some plan of treatment that will more nearly control it than any now known; but at present there is a large class of cases, and doubtless always will be, that the medical arm is too short to reach; for when we reach the point when science is equal to disease, death will be banished from the land—a point inconsistent with nature, and never designed by 'Him who doeth all things well.'

"Respectfully and fraternally yours,
"WARD WOODBRIDGE, M.D.
"Waubeek, Linn County, October 24, 1881."

THE JOURNAL BOOK SHELF

BOOKS RECEIVED

ALLERGY IN GENERAL PRACTICE—By Samuel M. Feinberg. M.D., F.A.C.P., assistant professor of medicine, Northwestern University Medical School, Chicago. Illustrated with 23 engravings and a colored plate. Lea & Febiger, Philadelphia, 1934. Price $4.50.

ANNUAL REPORT OF THE SURGEON GENERAL OF THE PUBLIC HEALTH SERVICE OF THE UNITED STATES, for the fiscal year 1933. United States Government Printing Office, Washington, D. C. For sale by the Superintendent of Documents, Washington, D. C. Price, seventy-five cents, cloth.

EXTERNAL DISEASES OF THE EYE, by Donald T. Atkinson, M.D., consulting ophthalmologist to the Santa Rosa Infirmary and the Nix Hospital, San Antonio, Texas. Octavo of 704 pages, illustrated with 479 engravings. Lea & Febiger, Philadelphia, 1934. Price, $7.50.

LOVE—A TREATISE ON THE SCIENCE OF SEX ATTRACTION—By Bernard S. Talmey, M.D. Fifth edition, newly revised and enlarged, with 52 illustrations. Eugenics Publishing Company, New York, 1933.

MEDICAL CLINICS OF NORTH AMERICA—Volume xvii, No. 1. Cleveland Clinic Number, per clinic year, July, 1933, to May, 1934. Octavo of 253 pages with 53 illustrations. W. B. Saunders Company, Philadelphia and London. Price, paper, $12.00; cloth, $16.00, net.

MODERN CLINICAL PSYCHIATRY—By Arthur P. Noyes, M.D., Superintendent of State Hospital for Mental Diseases, Howard, Rhode Island. 485 pages. W. B. Saunders Company, Philadelphia and London, 1934. Price, $4.50.

MEDICO-MILITARY SYMPOSIUM, 1934—Conducted under the auspices of the Kansas City Southwest Clinical Society and the Medical Department, Seventh Corps Area, United States Army, at the General Hospital, Kansas City, Missouri, March 12-17, 1934. Brown-White, Publishers, Kansas City, 1934.

THE 1933 YEAR BOOK OF GENERAL THERAPEUTICS—Edited by Bernard Fantus, M.S., M.D., professor of therapeutics, University of Illinois College of Medicine. The Year Book Publishers, Chicago, 1934. Price, $2.25.

THE 1933 YEAR BOOK OF NEUROLOGY AND PSYCHIATRY Edited by Peter Bassoe, M.D., clinical professor of neurology, Rush Medical College; and Franklin G. Ebaugh, M.D., professor of psychiatry, University of Colorado School of Medicine. The Year Book Publishers, Chicago, 1934.

THE 1933 YEAR BOOK OF UROLOGY—Edited by John H. Cunningham, M.D., associate in genito-urinary surgery, Harvard University Postgraduate School of Medicine. The Year Book Publishers, Chicago, 1934.

OUR MYSTERIOUS LIFE GLANDS AND HOW THEY AFFECT US—By William J. Robinson, M.D., consultant to the department of genito-urinary diseases and dermatology, Bronx Hospital, New York. Eugenics Publishing Company, New York, 1934. Price, $2.50.

SURGICAL CLINICS OF NORTH AMERICA, Volume xiv, No. 1, Philadelphia Number, February, 1934. Per clinic year, February, 1934, to December, 1934. 225 pages with 62 illustrations. W. B. Saunders Company, Philadelphia and London, 1934. Price, paper $12.00; cloth, $16.00.

BOOK REVIEWS

A DIABETIC MANUAL

For the mutual use of the doctor and patient, by Elliott P. Joslin, M.D., clinical professor of medicine, Harvard Medical School. Fifth edition, entirely revised. Illustrated. Lea and Febiger, Philadelphia, 1934. Price, $2.00.

In the light of our present knowledge regarding the treatment of diabetes, the instruction of the patient and his education concerning his own disease and its management are of paramount importance. For this reason, the medical profession enthusiastically welcomed the first edition of Dr. Joslin's Diabetic Manual.

This manual, now in its fifth edition, has been thoroughly revised and rendered more useful to both the patient and his physician. Following a general consideration of diabetes and the discovery of insulin, the author presents diabetic arithmetic and the methods of figuring suitable diets for the diabetic patient. Later chapters discuss acidosis and diabetic coma, the hygiene of the diabetic with a very happy outlook on prognosis which will go far towards encouraging the faithful adherence to the diabetic program. The two final chapters of the text deal with foods and their composition, and selected laboratory tests useful in diabetic treatment.

The author has at no time sacrificed accuracy for the sake of brevity or simplicity. He has, on the other hand, presented the subject in a very comprehensive fashion and omitted technicalities and theories. Dr. Joslin's Diabetic Manual will continue to be one of the most outstanding and the most useful reference book for the diabetic patient.

INTERNATIONAL CLINICS

Volume I, Forty-fourth Series. Edited by Louis Hamman, M.D., visiting physician, Johns Hopkins Hospital, Baltimore, Maryland. J. B. Lippincott Company, Philadelphia, Montreal and London, 1934. Price, $3.00.

These International Clinics have been so conspicuously helpful in bringing postgraduate medicine to the physician's desk that they are generally accepted as outstanding in their particular field.

With the latest number of this clinic a new and valuable feature has been announced, patterned in a fashion after the famous Cabot Case Reports. The editors of the International Clinics, in collaboration with the Pittsburgh Diagnostic Clinic, furnish with every volume a supplement reporting two full case histories. Additional data and an analysis of the case, as made by the staff of the Pittsburgh Diagnostic Clinic, are furnished upon request. This new feature, in furtherance of the Clinic's plan, promises to be valuable indeed.

Especially interesting in this volume are several clinical papers upon cardiac diseases. Particularly worthwhile is the clinic on functional heart disease by William S. Love, Jr. The section on pediatrics is devoted to a symposium on lead poisoning. The Address in Medicine, by A. Cantarow of Philadelphia, and the Address in Surgery by Donald C. Balfour of Rochester, will be of general interest, since each in a way summarizes the advances in medicine during the past year.

TREATMENT IN GENERAL PRACTICE

By Harry Beckman, M.D., professor of pharmacology at Marquette University, School of Medicine, Milwaukee, Wisconsin. Second edition, 889 pages, revised and entirely reset. W. B. Saunders Company, Philadelphia and London, 1934. Price, $10.00.

Reprinted on five different occasions, the first edition of this volume "broke all records for sales of a book of this kind," and made it desirable that a new revision be prepared. This new edition has been completely rewritten and brought entirely up-to-date. It contains hundreds of new and approved treatments, many of which are not found in other books.

The general plan of the book has remained unchanged. Following the usual grouping of diseases the authors have presented the indications for treatment and the various therapeutic drugs and remedies employed for both prophylaxis and cure.

Its broad scope and encyclopedic character places the volume more in the category of reference works, rather than that of the textbook, but inasmuch as its avowed and accomplished purpose is to place the essentials of therapeutics in its modern form on an equal footing with the other fundamentals of medicine, the volume should meet the needs of the student and practitioner alike.

The carefully prepared cross-reference index adds materially to the usefulness of the volume.

THE 1933 YEAR BOOK OF GENERAL SURGERY

Edited by Evarts A. Graham, M.D., professor of surgery, Washington University School of Medicine. The Year Book Publishers, Chicago, 1933.

This is a review of the progress and development in surgery in the past year and consists of a discussion on methods, technics and results.

The field of general surgery is thoroughly covered. Many chapters could be selected for comment but this is scarcely possible under the circumstances. The chapter on pancreatitis offers much that is encouraging in the operative handling of these cases which not long ago were in a hopeless

surgical category. The surgery of hyperinsulinism and hypoglycemia is also discussed. Malignancy comes in for an extensive consideration but little in the way of new information is brought out.

The book is useful not as a textbook but rather as a handy reference book for latest methods and their results.   F. R. H.

THE 1933 YEAR BOOK OF OBSTETRICS AND GYNECOLOGY

Edited by Joseph B. DeLee, A.M., M.D., professor of obstetrics, University of Chicago Medical School, and J. P. Greenhill, M.D., associate professor of gynecology, Loyola University Medical School. The Year Book Publishers, Chicago, 1934.

Like all other volumes in this series this Year Book of Obstetrics and Gynecology presents a review of the worthwhile literature written on these subjects during the year 1933, together with the name of the author and the journal in which the article was originally published.

The value of the book is greatly enhanced by the terse comments of the editors. These editorial notes are prompted both by a generous clinical experience and a long observance of the general literature in this field, and for these reasons are frequently as helpful or even more helpful than the epitome of the original article.

This volume is a great timesaver when a short review of any article on the subject is needed, yet the original article may be read if desired. It is one of the handiest and most valuable books available on the subject.

F. W. R.

THE SINGLE WOMAN

A medical study in sex education by Robert Latou Dickinson, M.D., and Lura Beam. The Williams & Wilkins Company, Baltimore, 1934. Price, $5.00.

This volume is presented by the National Committee on Maternal Health as one of its publications "on certain medical aspects of human fertility." Inasmuch as this study deals with such fundamentals as physiology and anatomy this is a medical study; yet it is more comprehensive than the adjective medical implies. It deals with the whole patient as a human being. There is psychology, where environment, where emotional life, where conflict cause refugees from that conflict. The approach to this problem is based for the most part on 1,078 case records drawn from a practice extending over fifty years.

Part One deals with health. Case histories are here analyzed insofar as they bear upon the sex life of the patient, since in many cases the abnormal sex adjustment was due all or in part to local pelvic disturbances.

Part Two deals with sexual experiences of various kinds, as revealed by these extensive records and as they throw light upon normal and abnormal sex development.

Part Three deals with those creative problems of family, religion, art, and work, insofar as they reflect an outlet for biologic, sexual deprivation.

Part Four presents an interpretation of the various groups studied and attempts to establish a definite pattern of sexual experience.

Since the material embodied in this volume has been collected and reviewed with unmistakable care and insight, and since no comparable study of the single woman and her sex problem has heretofore appeared, this work immediately commands the attention of the physician and the sociologist. It follows and supplements the study of sex adjustment begun by the same authors in "A Thousand Marriages" (reviewed in this section of the Journal, June, 1932).

_____

THE 1933 YEAR BOOK OF THE EYE, EAR, NOSE AND THROAT

The Eye, by E. V. L. Brown, M.D., professor of ophthalmology, University of Chicago; and Louis Bothman, M.D., associate professor; *The Ear, Nose and Throat*, by George E. Shambaugh, M.D., professor of otology, rhinology and laryngology, Rush Medical College, University of Chicago; and Elmer W. Hagens, M.D., instructor in otology, rhinology and laryngology, Rush Medical College, University of Chicago. The Year Book Publishers, Chicago, 1933.

This volume contains 466 headings under which are briefly discussed important questions about the eye, including the effect of drugs, experimental studies of physiology, pathology and pharmocology, and various common and some very uncommon diseases of the eye. Bacteriology of the conjunctiva and a citation of a micro-organism found for the first time is mentioned. Tumors, benign and malignant, are reported, as well as many types of therapy for given diseases and derangements of the eye.

The ear has 96 headings with brief descriptions of new therapeutic measures for ear diseases and new observations in otology. The nose and throat have 96 headings with somewhat longer descriptions of various diseases. Vitamin calcium therapy used for increasing the resistance of respiratory mucosa to infection is mentioned.

There is a report of the committe on eye, ear, nose and throat tumors. Allergy has its fair share of consideration in this 1933 issue, a subject about which much is written and little known.

The larnyx has 43 headings under which is emphasized the direct laryngoscopic examination of laryngeal disorders as well as bronchoscopic studies of chronic bronchial disease. Esophagoscopy is recommended for the study of strictures, tumors and other diseases of the esophagus.

A physician should be well grounded in fundamentals of medical practice before taking too seriously all that is said in this book.

H. J. McC.

_____

THE 1933 YEAR BOOK OF PEDIATRICS

Edited by Isaac A. Abt, M.D., professor of pediatrics, Northwestern University Medical School. The Year Book Publishers, Chicago, 1934.

We quote from the introduction to this volume: "Medical literature has attained such dimensions that it is no longer possible for an individual to master it as a whole. Even the literature of a special branch, such as pediatrics, is so voluminous that no physician can be expected to know all of it." Upon such a concept the Year Book Publishers, through the medium of carefully selected editors, have from year to year offered the practicing physician collected and condensed articles of merit from the world literature.

With the rapid growth of any particular phase of medical practice the problem of editing the particular volume covering this subject is multiplied many times. In this volume on pediatrics, great discrimination is required to include all of the worthwhile citations to the literature, and at the same time weed out the scores of articles which have only a limited value or interest.

Maintaining the high standard of efficiency shown in former issues of this Year Book, the authors have produced a resumé of the literature of 1933 which is to be commended. The busy practitioner, as well as the specialist in pediatrics, will be agreeably surprised by the wealth of information contained in this volume.

_____

THE 1933 YEAR BOOK OF DERMATOLOGY AND SYPHILOLOGY

Edited by Fred Wise, M.D., professor of dermatology and syphilology, New York Postgraduate Medical School and Hospital of Columbia University; and Marion B. Sulzberger, M.D., associate in dermatology and syphilology. The Year Book Publishers, Chicago, 1934. Price, $2.25.

Incorporated in this volume are two innovations, besides the usual abstracts and editorials. The first is a brief article presented by the editors, sketching the practical aspect of modern therapeutic procedures in the management of a common disease of the skin. In this particular issue, this editorial summary covers the treatment of acne vulgaris.

The second change embodied in this issue, the mention of the volume and page number of almost all articles abstracted. This makes it possible to refer directly from the review without looking up the original article. While this will serve as a short-cut to the occasional author, the reviewer feels that the writer in failing to read the original article himself may lose more than can possibly be gained by this short-cut.

The bibliography in this volume does not appear in page footnotes as heretofore, but is grouped together at the end of the volume.

Since this number of the Year Book reviews the literature on allergy and immunology, the volume will have an increased value to every physician.

THE TORCH OF LIFE

By Frederick M. Rossiter, M.D., Licentiate,

Royal College of Physicians, London. Eugenics Publishing Co., Inc., New York City. Price, $2.65.

On the basis of a "lamentable lack of knowledge that largely prevails among the medical profession of the ars amandi," and upon the belief that "a frank and honest presentation of the facts relative to the art of love must be a contributing factor in safeguarding, the morals of the young generation," this author presents an intimate discussion of the psychology and physiology of the sex act.

The discussion begins by a discourse on the need of definite sex knowledge by married persons, particularly young married persons. Succeeding chapters discuss the physiology and anatomy of the sex organs, furnishing a foundation for chapters designated, "The Love Drama," and "The First Night."

The book is quite readable, and where it seems desirable to recommend such a book the physician may cite this one along with the several others which have recently been published covering this same field. We believe the physician should carefully read the volume before recommending it to a patient, since in some instances the injudicious distribution of such a book may do much harm.

TRANSACTIONS OF THE COLLEGE OF PHYSICIANS OF PHILADELPHIA

Fourth series, fifty-fifth volume. Containing the papers read before the College from January, 1933, to December, 1933, inclusive. Edited by Walter G. Elmer, M.D. Published for the College in Philadelphia, 1933.

This is number one of the fourth volume, fourth series and contains the necrology list with memoirs for the preceding year as well as the roster of the membership of the society. The only article appearing in full is that by Hans Zinsser of the Harvard Medical School on "Recent Advances in the Study of Typhus Fever," although a number of other articles appear in abstracted form. The general tone and level of the contents are up to the standard which is characteristic of the papers presented before this society.   F. R. H.

·MERCK ANNOUNCES APPOINTMENT OF DR. EUGENE MAIER

The Merck Institute of Therapeutic Research, Rahway, New Jersey, announces the appointment of Dr. Eugene Maier as Chief Bacteriologist. Dr. Maier is a graduate of the University of Tuebingen, Wuertemberg, Germany, and completed his studies at the University of Erlangen, Germany. He was associated with the Rockefeller Institute of New York as Research Assistant from 1926 to 1930. Since 1931 Dr. Maier has been at Bellevue Hospital, New York, in the department of pathology, as bacteriologist for the Tuberculosis Division of Columbia University.

LEADER IN PHARMACEUTICAL FIELD DIES

Word has just been received in the State Society office, of the death of Mr. E. Mead Johnson, on Tuesday, March 20. Mr. Johnson, as president of the Mead Johnson and Company, was a pioneer in the field of pharmacy. His death will be a distinct loss to the pharmaceutical and medical professions.

SEMICENTENNIAL OF THE ARCHIVES OF PEDIATRICS

The Archives of Pediatrics, a monthly publication devoted to the diseases of infants and children, is this year observing a "Semicentennial"—the first issue of this journal bore the date January 15, 1884, and the publication of the journal has continued without interruption to date. These facts have been considered of sufficient importance to warrant the dedication of the February issue of this journal to the pediatric pioneers of 1884. Reproduced in this issue are a number of original communications, clinical lectures and clinical memoranda from such pioneers as William T. Plant, A. Jacobi, F. Forchheimer and L. Emmett Holt. Students of medical history and pediatrics will find this unique number of especial interest.

Editor, Iowa State Medical Journal:

I am making a survey on the incidence of cretinism in the United States, and would greatly appreciate it if you would insert a notice in your JOURNAL to this effect and ask any of your readers who might have records of such cases to communicate with me.

No one has ever attempted to make a survey of this kind and it will only be through the cooperation of the medical journals and the profession that it will be possible to make such a survey. I will be especially interested to receive any photographs of these cases. I am asking that the names and addresses be given in order to eliminate the duplication of cases. When this data is compiled, I expect to turn it over to the American Medical Association, where it may be filed for further reference and study.   Arnold Jackson, M.D.
        Madison, Wis.

The JOURNAL

of the

Iowa State Medical Society

VOL. XXIV   DES MOINES, IOWA, MAY, 1934   No. 5

AN OVERLOOKED FACTOR IN SUSCEPTIBILITY TO THE COMMON COLD

ARTHUR E. EWENS, B.S., M.D.,

Atlantic City, New Jersey.

There is probably no more formidable enemy to human health and comfort than the common cold, the widespread incidence of which continues to defy both etiologic explanation and prophylactic control. This ubiquitous malady not only inflicts upon this country a direct economic loss of four hundred and fifty million dollars annually,* but paves the way to a host of refractory catarrhal difficulties that impose a further sacrifice of occupational efficiency and an ever increasing need for the largest group of specialists in the entire field of medical practice.

Recent efforts to curb the ravages of this universal plague have been focused upon the possible identification of a specific causative agency, the assumption being that prospective laboratory findings offer about the only hope of success. There has been no definite proof, however, that a distinct bacterial cause exists, and even if one were ultimately isolated it is questionable whether the perplexities of the problem would be materially lessened. It is rather difficult to visualize serologic protection against a disease which itself tends to augment, rather than diminish, subsequent susceptibility. More readily conceivable are the altruistic possibilities that might accrue from the detection of an eliminable anatomic factor in man's vulnerability to catarrhal infections. Theoretically, a structural abnormality could induce lowered resistance to organisms normally present in the nose and throat and, if common to a great many individuals, might more logically explain the prevalence of "colds" than the supposed aggressiveness and specificity of an undiscovered bacterium or virus. Such an hypothesis is quite

*Based upon statistics of the United States Public Health Service.

consistent with the negative results of bacteriologic investigation, and is by no means a vain conjecture. It is actually true that clinical research has overlooked one correctable somatic impairment whose predisposing influence is empirically and convincingly demonstrable, and whose delayed recognition seems measurably responsible for the erstwhile futility of the fight against the common cold.

This overlooked factor is none other than that apparently innocuous structure, the uvula, so often carelessly designated as "the palate" by both the laity and the profession. This devitalized and physiologically superfluous appendage has never received any critical consideration beyond that accorded it by Hippocrates, who recognized its frequent elongation as a mechanical cause of paroxysmal coughs and advocated staphylotomy as a corrective measure. Unfortunately, Hippocrates' suggestion has never attained great popularity. Had its practical utility in dealing with innumerable cases of convulsive coughing and incessant clearing of the throat been properly appreciated, a vastly more important potentiality of this procedure would inevitably have come to light long before the twentieth century. The main impediment to this revelation has been, and still is, a superstitious and erroneous conception of the functional importance of the uvula, in consequence of which staphylotomy has been inadequately performed even when "cautiously" resorted to.

A customary degree of hesitancy and conservatism dominated the writer's early employment of staphylotomy but it soon became apparent that a bolder procedure involved none of the dreaded risks and was much more efficacious and dependable. Gradually this was found to be true to the point of removing the uvula in its entirety, an operation which has since been performed many hundreds of times, and with results as unprecedented as the operation itself. Routine use of *staphylectomy* for the relief of habitual clearing of the throat and an amenable type of paroxysmal cough eventually revealed the rather amazing fact that it also exercised a remedial influence upon catarrhal conditions of the entire upper respiratory tract. Primarily, this was not an objective disclosure, nor was it even a suspected possibility. It was purely accidental. The original observation must be accredited to patients themselves, who, repeatedly called attention to various unanticipated benefits conferred by staphylectomy, notably a relative freedom from "colds"—but whose alleged experiences were at first regarded as sheer products of the imagination. Except for the repetition and enthusiasm of these incredible contentions they might not have aroused the slightest interest, for there seemed to be, at that time, no logical reason to suppose that the mere removal of a small piece of redundant tissue from the faucial arch could produce the remote and phenomenal effects which these patients were wont to ascribe to it. About twenty years have now elapsed since a skeptical investigation of this apparent myth was thus inaugurated, and the unique experience to which it led has afforded incontestable proof of the provocative rôle of the uvula in uncontrollable recurrences of the common cold and in the intractability of other catarrhal difficulties involving both the nose and throat.

By painstaking follow-up methods and the helpful cooperation of interested patients it has been determined that staphylectomy checks susceptibility to "colds" in excess of fifty per cent. In occasional instances a complete absence of recurrence has been reported for periods of several years, and rarely have indifferent results been observed. Exact percentages of efficiency cannot be tabulated, the controls in this investigation having necessarily been in each case the past experiences of the subject himself. Patients are seldom able to state accurately the number of attacks a year they have previously encountered, but they can make postoperative comparisons that are sufficiently definite for practical purposes; and the contrast is usually so sharp that a precise ratio becomes relatively unimportant. What applies to the comparative frequency of "colds" before and after staphylectomy is equally true concerning the abated intensity and duration of infections that may develop after the uvula has been removed. A peculiar phase of the latter observation is the mildness or entire absence of sinusitis in cases where this had invariably been a troublesome accompaniment or sequel of rhinitis prior to operation.

The effectiveness of complete removal of the uvula has been substantiated not merely through subjective information, but by significant and unmistakable changes in both pharyngeal and nasal structures. The most conspicuous of these visible effects are so prompt and decided in some instances as literally to defy belief. Chronic postnasal engorgement is reduced to a degree that definitely facilitates nasal breathing, and the characteristic signs and symptoms of pharyngeal and nasopharyngeal catarrh are rendered *permanently* less pronounced. These clearly discernible effects are more than suggestive of a contributory culpability of the uvula in marked catarrhal tendencies; in fact they have been so constantly observed as to admit of no other interpretation.

The part played by the uvula in predisposition to the common cold and kindred affections may not appear so strange and inexplicable if we take into consideration the extremely poor vascularity of this structure and its other correspondingly sparse histologic components, which would unavoidably render it less resistant than the substantial and well vascularized portions of the pharynx. Furthermore, its anatomic location is especially favorable to the accumulation of ceaseless installments of bacteria,—dangling directly in the pathway of both respiration and deglutition. It is thereby subjected also to more or less mechanical abuse, particularly in the act of snoring. These combined characteristics make the uvula an ideal bacterial nidus upon which micro-organisms gain a flourishing surface foothold, subsequently invading in overpowering numbers the posterior nares and other contiguous areas that might otherwise be capable of maintaining a relatively healthy status. (In striking conformity with these practical considerations is the well known fact that the earliest symptom of an incipient coryza is not referable to the nose, but is almost invariably a sensation of dryness and pruritic discomfort in the vicinity of the soft palate, nasal involvement being a somewhat delayed development.)

This line of reasoning may appear fundamentally defective in that it wholly ignores the supposed functional requisites of the uvula; but does the uvula really serve any distinct or valuable purpose in the human being, or is it a superfluous and rudimentary structure? In lower animals it is essential as a reflex expulsive mechanism of vital importance. During the act of panting it thus affords protection against the hazardous ingress of flying insects and other foreign material, but aside from its participation in this highly necessary defense of the larynx and pulmonary tract it serves no other purpose for which the major portion of the normal velum palatinum does not alone suffice. The life and habits of primi

There is no preoperative means of gauging the pathogenic culpability of the uvula in cases of marked susceptibility to the common cold. Neither its size nor any other observable characteristic affords a dependable index to the advisability of excision, for it has been found that an exceptionally small uvula may be a source of pronounced disturbance and that it is not the elongated type only that definitely contributes to lowered nose and throat resistance. Staphylectomy may therefore be considered a justifiable and advantageous procedure in practically all cases exhibiting aggravated catarrhal tendencies, its efficacy being determined by the thoroughness of the operation and not by the dimensions nor the consistency of the tissue removed.

Denunciation of this radical proposal may be dictated by popular prejudice, but a practical and reliable estimate of its alleged rationality and merits is readily available to every member of the profession. The means is extremely simple and clinical material everywhere abundant.

Staphylectomy is such a minor procedure that it hardly admits of a technical description. It exacts no unusual skill of the operator nor does it demand special facilities. The topical employment of cocaine, or larocaine (Roche), in sufficiently generous amounts renders the operation practically painless. The use of both hands being essential, it becomes necessary for the patient to manipulate the tongue-depressor, which he or she can be instructed to do even more expeditiously than a trained assistant. Active hemostatic measures have never been required, although the possibility of their need has at times been anticipated. Ordinarily, only a trivial amount of bleeding is witnessed and spontaneous arrest usually takes place in one to five minutes. In many instances there is practically no hemorrhage at all. Postoperative care is a negligible consideration, but patients have, when practicable, been kept under daily observation until the wound was fully healed. The importance of removing the uvula in toto cannot be too strongly emphasized, as no compromise between staphylotomy and *staphylectomy* will yield results clearly confirmatory of the original findings reported.

Superstitious aversion to complete removal of the uvula has for ages obscured the possibility of an epochal rhinolaryngologic achievement, for only through the experimental employment of staphylectomy will it be possible to glean the facts that are indispensable to success in the long attempted conquest of "colds" and related nose and throat disturbances. This obstructive prejudice, although universal, is entirely unwarrantable.

Over two thousand stahpylectomies have revealed not the slightest justification for it. In the hands of the writer the procedure in question long ago passed from the stage of experimentation to that of established clinical utility, the enormous scope of which will prove no less astounding to future investigators than it has in the course of this anomalous experience.

3600 Pacific Avenue.

THE DIAGNOSTIC SIGNIFICANCE OF CEREBROSPINAL FLUID EXAMINATION*†

WILLIAM MALAMUD, M.D., Iowa City

The use of the cerebrospinal fluid for diagnostic and research purposes has a comparatively short history. Although its existence has been known for centuries, it was only through the introduction of the *lumbar puncture* in 1891 by Quiricke that this relatively simple and safe method of obtaining the fluid opened up the possibility of investigating the conditions of the spinal fluid in the living human being. The knowledge which has been gained since then, however, has proved to be of such importance in clinical work that at present no final diagnosis of a mental or nervous disease, or a differential diagnosis between them and diseases of other systems, is justified without an investigation of the cerebrospinal fluid. Of the different aspects of this work the most successful research has been done on the composition of the fluid and the variations that it may undergo in different types of diseases. For the purpose of ascertaining this composition a number of tests have been devised, some of which are simple enough so that they lend themselves even to general office work, while others are more complicated and require a more elaborately equipped laboratory. The evaluation of the results of most of these tests simply as diagnostic criteria has been rendered comparatively easy by the empirical standardization on the basis of a large number of cases. The understanding of these tests and their significance in relation to the function of the cerebrospinal fluid, however, requires an appreciation of the anatomic and physiologic factors concerned in this function, and for that purpose it is probably best to begin with a few brief statements concerning these. It must be emphasized that, because of the relatively short period of time since these studies have been started, very few of the theories concerning the anatomy and, especially

*From the Psycopathic Hospital, State University of Iowa.
†Presented before the Johnson County Medical Society, January 3, 1934.

the physiology of the cerebrospinal fluid system, have been universally accepted. In this brief discussion we shall present only those facts that are most widely accepted without attempting to go into a discussion of the disputes that have arisen in each case.

Anatomic considerations: The most important structures concerned in the production, absorption, and circulation of the cerebrospinal fluid are the meninges, the ventricular system, the choroid plexuses, and the lymph and perivascular spaces. The meninges consist of three membranes. (See Fig. 1.) The dura or hard membrane encloses the whole cerebrospinal axis and lies next to the bony structures. It stretches over the brain and cord, bridging over most of the separations between their subdivisions and sending only four processes into the underlying structures: the falx cerebri between the two cerebral hemispheres, the falx

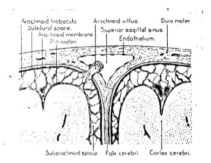

Figure 1. Diagram of a coronal section of the meninges and the cerebral cortex, showing the relation of an arachnoid villus (pacchionian body) to the venous sinus (Weed).

cerebelli between the two cerebellar hemispheres, the tentorium cerebelli, and the diaphragma sellae. The arachnoid, or spider-web membrane, encloses the cerebrospinal axis next to the dura and is separated from it by the narrow subdural space. It is in closer contact with the brain structures, but it, too, bridges over most of the fissures and irregularities of the central nervous system structures. The third membrane, the pia, lies next to the central nervous system tissue, following all its irregularities and fissures so that the area between the arachnoid and pia, the so-called subarchnoid space, thus gains a large number of exaggerations in capacity where the arachnoid passes over two more or less widely separated parts of the nervous system. The largest of these spaces are known as cisternae and are designated according to thei anatomic positions. The most important of these are the cisterna chiasmatica, the cerebello-medullaris, and the interpeduncular. The subarachnoid space with all its cisternae forms a containing vessel for the so-called external spinal fluid. The internal spinal fluid is contained in the ventricular system, consisting of the four ventricles of the brain and the central canal of the spinal cord. (See Fig. 2.) These two (i. e. the external and internal compartments) are connected by three foramina: the foramen of Magendie and the two foramina of Luschka. The external space, furthermore, communicates with the venous sinuses, especially the superior sagittal by the so-called pacchionian bodies. (See Fig. 1.) These are formed by arachnoid processes which protrude into the sinuses, pushing the dura ahead of them, and the communication is, therefore, not a free one but through the double membrane consisting of arachnoid and dura.

The plexuses consist of highly convoluted vascular bodies which dip into the ventricles from the blood vessels supplying the brain. Of these we have the plexus of the fourth ventricle which gains entrance into it by forcing the roof of the hind brain ahead of it, the plexus of the third ventricle which gains a similar entrance through the roof of the midbrain, and the two plexuses of the lateral ventricles which gain entrance through the medial walls of the cerebral hemispheres. In addition to these we have the perivascular and lymph spaces throughout the central nervous system tissue.

Physiologic considerations: The cerebrospinal fluid is not a rigidly fixed substance but is continually produced, circulated, and absorbed. The rate of production and absorption may be increased, depending upon certain physiologic or pathologic conditions such as, for instance, the removal or loss of spinal fluid or the occurrence of inflammatory and other diseases of the central nervous system. Both the production and the absorption of the spinal fluid are matters of discussion, but the following theories are the most widely accepted ones.

The main source of the spinal fluid is formed by the four plexuses of the ventricular system. The fluid is produced by them and discharged into the ventricular system. From there it gains access to the subarachnoid space, and thence it reaches the venous sinuses through the pacchionian bodies. This, however, does not altogether exhaust all the possibilities. In addition to its producing function, the plexus may also absorb some of the spinal fluid, and some investigators feel that its main function is that of absorption. Furthermore, the pacchionian bodies in addition to their

function of absorption may also have some producing functions. Finally, the meninges throughout the central nervous system, the lymph spaces, the perivascular spaces, and the brain tissue itself most probably play some rôle, both in the production and absorption of the spinal fluid, and some authors have considered each one of these as the main source or exit of the spinal fluid.

The circulation of the spinal fluid has also been a subject of dispute. Since this fluid it produced and absorbed at a certain rate, we can easily see that a certain amount of circulation must be postulated coming from the source and leading toward the point of absorption. In addition to this, the movements of the brain tissue associated with the heart-beats, respiration, movements of the head and body, and so on, contribute certain mechanical impulses for such circulation. Whether this motion takes place only within the external and internal spaces coming from the ventricles through

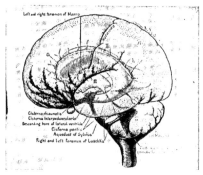

Figure 2. Diagram of ventricles of the brain and subarachnoid cisternae (Dandy).

the foramina into the subarachnoid space, or whether, in addition to this, there is also a certain amount of circulation through the brain tissue itself, as for instance von Monakoff suggests, at present remains questionable.

The main function of the cerebrospinal fluid is to serve as a water cushion for the tissues of the central nervous system. These tissues are, so to speak, suspended in the fluid which helps to safeguard them from jolts against the hard cranial and spinal cavities. In addition to this, it helps in regulating the variations in pressure within this system. Whenever the contents of these cavities are increased, as for instance by an increased flow of blood into them or the development of a new growth, or when they are decreased by loss of fluid or tissue, the cerebrospinal fluid compensates for these variations either by a decrease or increase in its amount. It is needless to say, of course, that this ability to compensate is only within certain limits, and, furthermore, that the fluid itself, if blocked in some manner, may cause an increase in intracranial pressure. It has been suggested that in addition to these functions the fluid also serves the purpose of nutrition. This has especially been stressed by the school that considers the possibility of circulation through all the tissues of the central nervous system. No incontrovertible proof has been advanced that such a function exists, although it is a possible one.

Opinions differ as to the nature of the development of the cerebrospinal fluid. Some observers consider the spinal fluid as being produced in a purely physicochemical manner by an interchange of substances between the blood and the spinal fluid spaces through the producing membranes, the amount and consistency of the fluid being regulated by the laws of osmotic pressure. The most widely accepted theory is that advanced by Mestrezzat who considers the spinal fluid as a dialysate, although some others consider it as a filtrate, a transudate, and so on. Others are of the opinion that the fluid is produced mainly by a process of secretion. Weighty proof and argument have been brought both in support of and against these theories. At present it is probably best to consider the production of the spinal fluid as being governed primarily by the laws of dialysis, but that some physiologic activity must be present to explain certain of the characteristics of this process.

The manner of obtaining the cerebrospinal fluid is rendered possible by the fact that at certain points in the central nervous system comparatively large spaces are formed that are filled with spinal fluid and where the introduction of a needle can be effected without serious injury to the nervous tissues. Of these the most important are the following three spaces:

1. The lateral ventricles—A needle can be introduced through a trephine in the skull, through the cerebral cortex into the large lateral ventricles.

2. The cisterna cerebello-medullaris—A needle can be introduced here between the lower border of the foramen magnum and the upper border of the first vertebra into the cerebello-medullary cistern.

3. The lumbar route—Since the spinal cord ends about the level of the first lumbar vertebra and the sack containing cerebrospinal fluid proceeds further down, a needle can be safely introduced through the spaces between the second and third and third and fourth lumbar vertebrae without any danger of injuring the cord and yet reaching the cerebrospinal fluid.

The latter is the safest and easiest method of obtaining the fluid, although the former two are sometimes used, especially when there is reason to believe that the upper fluid differs in consistency from the lower, or where there is a block between them. These points are also utilized when medication is to be introduced into the cerebrospinal system.

Under normal conditions the spinal fluid is colorless, of a specific weight, and viscosity only slightly different than water. It comes out under a pressure of up to 200 mm. of water when the patient is in a horizontal position. The reaction is weakly alkaline, and it contains a number of organic and inorganic substances. The most important of these for test purposes are: the cells (lymphocytes) none to five; protein, 13 to 30 mg. per 100 cc.; chlorides, about 730 mg., and sugar, about 60 mg.

METHODS OF INVESTIGATION IN CLINICAL WORK

The above enumerated physical and chemical characteristics of the spinal fluid vary a great deal in different cases of nervous and mental diseases. The tests that have been devised for the examination of the fluid depend primarily upon these variations and can best be interpreted in terms of deviations from the normal. The most frequent of these are as follows:

1. *The pressure.* Physiologically the pressure will vary with the position of the patient, his activities such as struggling, disturbances in breathing, resistiveness, and so on. When these are eliminated, disturbances in pressure indicate the presence of organic diseases of the central nervous system. An increase of pressure above 200 mm. should be considered as pathologic if no physiologic reason can be discovered for it. It occurs most frequently in cases of neoplasms, but may also be found in inflammatory diseases where a block is produced by the inflammatory proliferation, or where there is an increased production of cerebrospinal fluid. Decreases in pressure may occur in cases of new growths, especially, of the spinal cord where the fluid from above the growth is blocked and cannot enter the lower portion of the cerebrospinal axis.

2. *The color.* The normal fluid is colorless, and the occurrences of any degree of tinging should be considered as pathologic. One must be careful to exclude the possibility of injuring a blood vessel while doing the puncture. In such cases, of course, the spinal fluid will be tinged with blood, but this will be readily separable from the fluid when it is allowed to stand, and, fur-

thermore, as the fluid is allowed to run in the needle the color decreases in intensity. Where hemorrhages into the spaces containing the fluid have taken place there may be various discolorations, depending upon the period of time that has elapsed between the hemorrhage and lumbar puncture. In old hemorrhages there is a slightly yellowish tinging of the fluid which is known as xanthochromia. This color does not disappear upon allowing the fluid to stand, and microscopically one cannot find blood cells in it. In addition to hemorrhages it may also be found in new growths. In some cases xanthochromic fluid when allowed to stand may coagulate to a greater or lesser degree of intensity, and this is known as the Froin syndrome. It is found in cases of occlusions of the subarachnoid space caused by spinal tumors, compressing vertebral diseases, and meningitic adhesions. One usually finds a more or less normal fluid above the block and the Froin syndrome in the fluid below it.

3. *The cell count.* This is determined by mixing the fluid in a white blood counting pipette with a special stain (crystal violet, glacial acetic acid, five per cent phenol. and aq. dist.). A drop of the mixture is placed in a Fuchs-Rosenthal chamber, the cells in the entire ruled area are counted, and the total divided by three. As was stated above, the normal fluid should contain anywhere from none to five small lymphocytes. An increased cell count is known as pleocytosis, and it is usually considered that anything above ten cells is pathologic, although some observers (Nonne) consider anything above five as abnormal. In cases of pleocytosis it is important for diagnostic purposes to ascertain not only the number of cells but also the type. In inflammatory diseases without pus formation and in meningitic irritations one usually finds a relatively smaller number of cells and they do not contain any leukocytes. The most important diseases where such increases occur are the syphilitic affections of the central nervous system. In these, outside of the acute syphilitic meningitis, one may find anywhere from 20 to 100 cells, most of them being small lymphocytes and some plasma cells. In tubercular meningitis larger amounts of cells are found (300 to 400 or more), but they are also mainly lymphocytes. In the purulent meningitides one finds very large amounts of cells, 2,000 and 3,000, a considerable number of which are leukocytes. In tumor formations one may find tumor cells in the spinal fluid.

4. *Protein content.* Within recent years a great deal of attention has been paid to the investigation of the protein content in the cerebrospinal fluid. The most frequently used method consists

in mixing one cc. of a 60 per cent spinal fluid solution in distilled water with one cc. of a five per cent sulphosalicylic acid. This precipitates the proteins, and the intensity of the cloudiness is then read in the colorimeter against a standard suspension containing a known amount of protein. The total protein should range from 13 to 30 mg. per 100 cc. in the normal individual. Anything above 30 is suspicious, and quantities over 40 are indicative of some disease of the central nervous system. Increased protein content is found, of course, in a great many different types of organic diseases, inflammatory as well as degenerative. Any process that is accompanied by the destruction of tissues within the central nervous system, or vascular lesions that permit the passage of proteins from the blood stream may give rise to an increased protein content. It was found that in

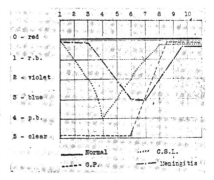

Figure 3. Chart representing four typical gold sol curves. The figures 1 to 10 on the upper margin refer to the tubes containing the various concentrations. The figures 0 to 5 at the left hand margin refer to the different degrees of discoloration of the solution.

a large number of cases where no other pathologic signs could be discovered, where the cell count and color were normal, and even the pressure was not increased, there might be a definite increase of the protein content. It is also important in the determination of proteins to investigate the relative proportions of the different types of proteins present. The most important special protein constituent to be determined is globulin. It is usually demonstrated by placing one cc. of cerebrospinal fluid in a test tube and adding a layer of saturated ammonium sulphate on top of that. A white ring at the junction of the two fluids is a positive reaction and should always be considered as pathologic. In some cases, as for instance in general paralysis, the globulin is markedly increased out of proportion with the rest of the proteins. In purely destructive processes very little globulin may be found but there is a large increase in the total protein.

5. *The colloid reactions.* The most important of these is the gold sol reaction. In this test a specially prepared colloidal gold sol containing gold chloride, potassium carbonate, oxalic acid and formaldehyde in distilled water, is used as the reagent. Five cc. of this reagent are added to each of ten tubes containing solutions of spinal fluid in 0.4 per cent NaCl solutions. The spinal fluid concentration in these tubes starts out with a 1:10 ratio in the first, half of this in the second, and so on up to the tenth tube in which the concentration is 1:5,120. This test depends upon the fact that normal spinal fluid does not affect the gold sol, no matter what the concentration may be. In a large number of the organic diseases of the central nervous system, however, the gold sol is affected, and its color changes from the original red through a series of reddish blue, violet, blue, light blue, and colorless, depending upon the concentration and upon the type of disease. With the use of the above technic special forms of reaction can be found to be characteristic of certain diseases. Figure 3 shows the gold sol curves characteristic for the three most commonly occurring syndromes (general paralysis, meningitis, and cerebrospinal lues) as well as the curve for the normal spinal fluid. The preparation of the reagent requires very careful technic and chemically pure ingredients and is, therefore, best carried out by specially trained technicians. At present the chemistry of this and other colloid tests is not well understood, but it is most probably dependent upon the pathology of the protein components of the fluid. Of the less frequently used colloid reactions the normomastic and the benzoin tests are the most important.

6. *Chloride content.* The determination is made by the Van Slyke method by the use of nitric acid and silver nitrate. The normal fluid contains about 720 to 740 mg. per 100 cc. In certain diseases such as tubercular meningitis, we find a decrease of the chloride content, and in others, such as cardiorenal disease, an increase of the chlorides may be found.

7. *Sugar.* The method is the same as is used in the blood sugar determination. Normally the spinal fluid sugar is of a concentration slightly over one-half of that in the blood. In some cases of meningitis we may find a decrease of the sugar in the spinal fluid. In other cases such as encephalitis or diabetes an increase of the sugar content is found.

8. *The blood cerebrospinal fluid barrier.* As was mentioned above the cerebrospinal fluid is sep-

arated from the blood by a series of membranes, but as it ultimately comes from the blood most of the substances that are found in it must come from the blood. This passage of substances from the blood into cerebrospinal fluid is regulated in such a way that some enter freely, others not at all, and still others enter in smaller proportions than they are found in the blood. This presupposes the existence of a barrier between the two, and in some diseases of the central nervous system a disturbance of this barrier may take place, with a

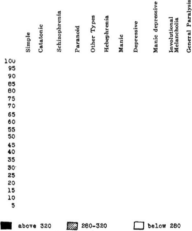

Figure 4. Graphic presentation of the changes in the blood cerebrospinal fluid barriers in the more common mental diseases. Each column represents a special syndrome. The figures on the left hand margin refer to the proportions of cases in terms of percentage. The first six columns represent 303 cases of schizophrenia, with its five subdivisions. In all of these there is a large proportion of decreased permeability (those above 320 and very few cases of increased permeability (those below 280). The seventh, eighth and ninth columns represent 231 cases of manic depressive psychosis, and here the bulk of the cases show a normal permeability (between 280 and 320). The tenth column is that of involutional melancholia, and the eleventh represents 53 cases of general paralysis, most of which show an increased permeability (those below 280).

resulting increase or decrease of the passage of substances. One of the most successful attempts of determining the function of this barrier has been devised by Walter and is known as the Walter bromide test. Bromides are introduced into the system by oral administration, and when they enter the blood will then find their way into the spinal fluid. Normally only one-third of the concentration of bromides in the blood should be found in the spinal fluid. When the barrier disturbed in such a way that the passage of substances is increased, then more bromides are found in the spinal fluid, and vice versa. It has been determined that the amount of bromides found

upper abdomen, and it is common knowledge that these patients are occasionally operated upon for some intra-abdominal lesion. Another early sign is the increase in respiration. Temperature rises rapidly during the chill, going as high as 104 degrees or even 105 degrees within the first twelve hours. During the first few days the temperature may not vary more than one or two degrees, or a distinct remittent temperature may be present from the beginning. Dyspnea accompanies the hurried respiration in nearly all cases. A short, unproductive and painful cough accompanies the early signs. In a day or two it usually becomes productive, and the mucus becomes blood-streaked, with a characteristic reddish brown or rusty sputum. The pulse ranges up to 100 or 120. If it is persistently over 120 the outlook is serious.

During the early stages of the disease the pathologic picture in the lungs is one of congestion, with loss of elasticity of the alveolar walls and consequent dilitation of the alveoli which may contain serum and blood cells. During this stage there may be some impairment of motion on the affected side. The percussion note at this time is hyper-resonant and even tympanic, due to the "resonance chamber" effect of the stretched alveolar sacs. Dulness does not develop until true consolidation becomes definite.

In the early stage the chief physical sign is the crepitant râle which is heard on deep inspiration. It is only of significance, of course, when it is associated with a chill, fever, cough and other early symptoms of pneumonia. After consolidation takes place the typical bronchial breathing begins. A diagnosis of lobar pneumonia, therefore, may be made shortly after the onset, upon the history of a sudden chill, a high temperature, a dry cough, pain in the chest and prostration, and upon finding an acutely ill patient, with some dyspnea and a rapid respiratory rate, slight impairment of motion on one side of the chest, a slight or moderate hyperresonance on percussion, distant breath sounds, fine crepitant râles and perhaps a friction rub. So much for the diagnosis of lobar pneumonia.

The mode of onset in bronchopneumonia is essentially different from that of lobar pneumonia, the one developing insidiously in the course of, or at the conclusion of another disease, the other setting in abruptly in an individual in good health. Lobar pneumonia is usually unilateral, while bronchopneumonia is bilateral.

In the early diagnosis of bronchopneumonia we have a very different picture to deal with. Since the disease frequently develops as a sequel to acute bronchitis it is usually more prevalent during the winter and early spring months. At this time, respiratory infections are more common than at other seasons of the year and in this respect bronchopneumonia is no exception. Inasmuch as bronchopneumonia is usually an incident in or occurs at the conclusion of a preceding disease process, the symptomatology is complex. For example, the physician must carefully distinguish between uncomplicated measles, influenza, and bronchitis, and the cases in which a secondary infection has involved the actual lung parenchyma.

The primary form occurs almost exclusively in children. In the secondary form, at the onset usually there has been present an acute bronchitis either alone or as a complication of one of the acute infections, particularly measles and whooping cough. During the winter and spring months when pulmonary diseases are most common, even trivial respiratory symptoms are to be viewed with suspicion. The transition from the minor to the more serious affection is gradual and the first thing to arouse suspicion as to the presence of bronchopneumonia may be the increase in respiratory rate and the increase in temperature. *The patient with acute bronchitis who continues to have a temperature·for more than forty-eight hours, must be seriously considered as a bronchopneumonic subject.* The next most common symptoms are dyspnea and cough. Physical examination may show the presence of a diffuse bronchitis with or without patches of consolidation. In many instances there is a complete absence of physical signs or they may be so indefinite as to escape notice entirely. The diagnosis is made from the symptoms and general condition rather than to confuse it with some other disease. The disease is nearly always bilateral. The consolidation hardly ever involves an entire lobe even when large areas are present. It tends to involve lower lobes and the degree of consolidation varies from day to day.

In a patient convalescing from an acute infectious disease, particularly acute bronchitis and influenza, the occurrence of fever, cough, rise in respiratory rate, cyanosis, toxemia and physical signs marked in the lower lobes, especially the presence of fine, crackling râles, even without evidence of consolidation, are sufficient to warrant a diagnosis of bronchopneumonia. In a typical case of secondary bronchopneumonia we have a picture which as a rule is fairly clean cut. An individual previously in good health is taken ill with an acute upper respiratory disease. After a few days the patient becomes definitely conscious of a lack of well being, chilly sensations, prostration, generalized aching and fever. After several more days localizing symptoms begin to develop, namely: cough, dyspnea, perhaps pain in the chest and

expectoration. If an examination is made in the first twenty-four hours following the onset of these symptoms there is usually little to be found physically, except the general evidence of an acute febrile disease, prostration, fever and rapid pulse. The examiner is often in doubt, but his attention is called to the lungs by the appearance of cyanosis, increased respiration and a few fine râles over one or more areas especially in the lower lobes. During the succeeding few days it becomes evident that there is trouble in the lungs. The cough increases at this time and the mucous has a characteristic greenish mucopurulent appearance in contradistinction to the tenacious rusty discharge of the lobar type. Following this, the evolution of the physical signs in the lungs is gradual. Without any sudden or extensive percussion changes, showers of fine râles appear. The signs may never progress beyond this point, or the breathing may become definitely tubular, indicating large areas of solidification. Bronchitis alone is not serious; the temperature is normal, or just slightly raised, there is no dyspnea, no cyanosis, and only coarse râles are present, whereas the presence of fine crackling râles, especially in the lower lobes with a continued temperature for several days, always suggests pneumonia. In other words *a severe bronchitis with marked general features is usually a bronchopneumonia.* In a protracted case, the occurrence of apical involvemen must always place one on the look out for tuberculosis. A bronchopneumonia due to the hemolytic streptococcus (influenza) is characterized b marked toxemia, dyspnea, cyanosis, bloody sputur and a high respiratory rate, a rapid onset and general picture of a severe septic infection.

Pain is rarely a marked feature in this form o pneumonia and in many cases it is entirely absen It usually occurs in the form of a dull aching sei sation over the site of the pulmonary lesion. Tl temperature is usually moderately high and ma be remittent in type. It may be of a short dur tion, a week for example, but it generally las considerably longer, ending not by crisis as lobar pneumonia but by lysis. The pyrexia m last for two, three or more weeks and there m be relapses.

It is always difficult and at times impossible determine the exact time at which acute bronchi merges into bronchopneumonia. The heighten temperature, increased respiratory rate, dyspn and prostration are the symptoms of greatest valt If, coupled with these, one finds localized resona râles at the base of the lungs, one is justified making a diagnosis of pneumonia. In short the the patient with simple bronchitis looks much le ill than one with bronchopneumonia, the temper

under all conditions, whether it is mild or severe, must be considered as a heavy drain on the patient's general health. Months are required to build up the resistance torn down during the week or two the disease goes through its various stages. One thought which I wish to emphasize is that severe bronchitis can become bronchopneumonia without any great, sudden changes and when it does, it should be treated strictly as a case of severe pneumonia, rather than as one of acute bronchitis.

ACUTE GONORRHEA IN THE MALE*

GEORGE DEWAYNE JENKINS, M.D., Burlington

Gonorrhea is one of the oldest and yet one of the most common diseases that comes to the attention of all physicians; not only to the general practitioner, but to the men in the various special branches of medicine. However, since it is one of the oldest diseases it is still looked upon with disgrace in most circles. In this day and age of more liberal thinking, moving pictures on sex, broadminded discussions of sex delinquencies, and contraceptive literature, gonorrhea is still referred to as the "social disease."

One of the main reasons for its prevalence is the ignorance on the part of the boy and girl, man and woman, as to its significance, the method of transmission, and the dire results that may ensue from such an infection. It is commonly thought that gonorrhea is a disease of filth and that the better classes are immune to such an infection. All of us have had the experience of an individual saying that he could not possibly have been infected by so and so because she was clean and a high type of individual. It therefore rests with the medical profession to see that such information is given the public in such a manner that it will be properly and scientifically understood. If we can impress upon the individuals that come under our care the necessity of treatment until the disease is irradicated in order to minimize sterile marriages, the infection of the innocent wife, and the broken morale we will have accomplished a great deal in the suppression of the disease.

In order that we may understand the course of the disease we must understand the anatomy of the genito-urinary tract in the male. It is the lower genito-urinary tract in which we are especially interested, although the upper urinary tract occasionally becomes infected secondarily. The upper portion of the lower genito-urinary tract is the bladder. From the bladder the prostatic ure-

*Presented before the Tri-County Medical Society, Fairfield, November 16, 1933.

thra empties into the bulbous urethra. Emptying into the prostatic urethra are the prostatic ducts and the ejaculatory duct. From the bulbous urethra the penile urethra opens into the fossa navicularis.

The fossa navicularis is usually lined with stratified squamous epithelium for a distance of about one centimeter. The anterior urethra to and including the bulbous urethra is of columnar type of epithelium. The membraneous urethra, prostatic urethra and bladder are lined with transitional epithelium. The urethra, as far as the bulbous portion, is lined with many glands of Littre and it is these small indentations that often harbor the infection and prolong the course of the disease.

The gonococcus has several special characteristics and because of these its identification can be made in most instances without much difficulty. It is a gram negative diplococcus and is intracellular. Of the other organisms that simulate it in morphologic appearance, the meningococcus and the micrococcus catarrhalis are notable. The meningococcus is not found in the urethra without the presence of meningitis. The micrococcus catarrhalis is occasionally found in the female genital tract, but is said to be extracellular. However, its occurrence is very rare in the male, and the only positive means of identification is by culture. It is possible to identify all positively with means of culture. In the case of the male, for all practical purposes, the gram stain will suffice, and with the clinical picture of gonorrhea and history of exposure, the ordinary methylene blue stain will give a working diagnosis.

The incubation period of the disease again depends upon the characteristics of the gonococcus. Since the gonococcus produces only an endotoxin the organism must go through the entire life cycle before the symptoms begin. It is usually thought that the incubation period allows only for the penetration of the organisms into the tissues; however, there is one further step that must take place and that is the destruction of the gonococcus in order that the endotoxin may be liberated. After the liberation of the endotoxin the tissue makes an effort to respond to this toxin. In order for the entire life cycle to take place a period of from forty-eight to seventy-two hours must elapse. Therefore, any case which has an incubation period of less than forty-eight hours cannot be a new infection. The average incubation period is from three to seven days, although it may be a period of one or two days, or in rare instances, three weeks. In the later instance the rule is that the symptoms were of such a mild nature that the individual was not cognizant of the disease and it

took an alcoholic debauch or sexual excess to brin the infection to his attention. It is this endotoxir liberated from the gonococcus, that is responsibl for the symptoms, through tissue response to th toxin, much in the same manner as is the respons to any toxin through the formation of pus, swel ing and inflammation.

Prophylaxis plays a very important part in th treatment of gonorrhea. If all the individual who were exposed to gonorrhea would take prope prophylactic treatment there would be very littl gonorrhea for us to treat. The efficacy of th prophylaxis varies directly as to the time tha elapses between the time of exposure and the tak ing of the treatment. The optimum time fo prophylaxis is immediately following exposure For this purpose urethral instillations of ten pe cent argyrol, two per cent protargol, two per cer mercurochrome, or five per cent silver nucleinat are all of about equal value. Each should be hel in the urethra for a period of time, not less tha five minutes. In addition to this the externa genitalia should be cleansed and anointed wit thirty per cent calomel ointment, which should b allowed to remain in place for several hours, as prophylaxis against syphilis.

The symptoms of the disease are as variable a is the course of the disease. Typically three t seven days following exposure the patient wi experience a burning or itching of the externa meatus and upon examination of the meatus wi note that the lips of the meatus are swollen an reddened. This will last for one or two day after which a urethral discharge is first notice At times there may be a general reaction in th form of malaise or a slight rise in temperatur With the onset of the urethral discharge the may be burning and smarting on urination. Ho ever, these symptoms are variable and many p tients will have absolutely no symptoms except t urethral discharge.

The urethral discharge is also variable. Oft one hears the expression that there is a macr scopic characteristic to the gonorrheal discharg This statement is not correct, since the dischar from a nonspecific urethritis may be yellow, crea and profuse, or it may be scant and only serous nature. The only positive means of identifyi the etiologic agent is by making a stained sme and examining it microscopically.

The psychologic control of the patient is a ve important factor. Fright characterizes the fi stage of the disease; an inferiority complex ma the second stage, and this is finally followed the "I don't care" attitude. It rests with the phy cian to talk the entire situation over with the

urethra, since we must be very careful that none of the solution goes beyond the bulbous urethra. In addition to this the urethra must not be distended, allowing the fluid to flow in easily and flow out freely. After irrigations the irrigating fluid is drained out of the urethra and an antiseptic solution instilled into it. For this instillation I have had the best results from neutral acriflavine 1.100 in ten per cent gelatin. It is allowed to remain in the urethra for five minutes. Other drugs that may be used are protargol, one-half of one per cent; neosilvol, ten per cent; argyrol, ten per cent; and silver nucleinate, five per cent. In instilling the drug into the urethra only a small amount should be used; not more than enough to fill the anterior urethra, but *not distend it.* Since our treatment is local to the anterior urethra, we should not get too enthusiastic and push the infection back into the posterior urethra. This treatment should be continued daily for a period of ten to fourteen days. In addition to this if the patient is intelligent and can be taught the proper way to instill the urethra I have the patient administer protargol, one-half of one per cent, three times a day.

During the time that the patient is on active treatment he should wear a good fitting scrotal supporter. This is one of the best means to prevent epididymitis. He should also refrain from active exercise such as golf, horseback riding, or long walks. Of course, the best results will be obtained if the patient can be hospitalized, because absolute control of the patient can be obtained.

There is not much that needs to be eliminated from the diet of the patient, except alcohol in any form. It is also a good plan to eliminate spicy foods. The fluid intake should be increased until the patient is getting as much liquid as he can take comfortably. Sexual excitement and coitus, aside from transmitting the disease, are among the things that the patient should abstain from absolutely. One of the surest ways to produce complications is for the patient to indulge in an alcoholic debauch or to have sexual excitement of any nature. The patient should be informed of the dangers of gonorrheal ophthalmia and instructed to wash his hands thoroughly with soap and water after each urination or handling of the genitalia. He should be cautioned as to the dangers of infecting others by leaving his secretions on towels, toilets and bath tubs. If such a plan of treatment is followed diligently by the patient, the infection should be cleared up in a period of two to four weeks.

After the subsidence of the urethral discharge

the patient should be allowed a one week rest without medication, and then a small sound should be passed into the urethra just to the bulbous urethra. If there is no recurrence of the urethral discharge after a week's time has elapsed, he should return and another sound should be passed into the urethra and the urethra gently massaged over it. If there is no recurrence of the discharge following this examination, it is a good plan to massage the prostate once a week for a period of two to three weeks, in order to preclude the possibility of a latent infection. The patient should finally be instructed not to have coitus without using a condom for a period of three months.

If the foregoing principles are carried out I believe that we will be able to reduce the complications of acute gonorrhea in the male from about 90 per cent to approximately 15 or 20 per cent.

FRACTURE OF THE SPINOUS PROCESS OF THE SIXTH CERVICAL VERTEBRA

CASE REPORT

A. A. EGGLESTON, M.D., F.A.C.S.
J. C. McKITTERICK, M.D., F.A.A.Ped.

Burlington

The small spinous processes of the cervical vertebra, supported as they are by the ligamentum nuchae, and interspinous ligaments, and the trapezius, longissimus cervicis, spinalis and semispinalis muscles, are not subject to injury except from trauma exerted at an unusual angle.

The literature has little to say about such fractures.

REPORT OF CASE

L. A. G., a white male, forty-two years of age, while driving July 6, 1933, was severely thrown about within his car when it left the road and turned over. Although shaken and bruised he was apparently not badly hurt and was able to drive his car over fifty miles to the office of a physician, where careful examination disclosed numerous bruises and sore spots, a bump on the top of his head, and a tender area just above the vertebra prominens. Pressure upon this area was painful and gave him the sensation of his eyes "bulging out." There was no restriction of motion, no abnormal reflexes and no other pathologic findings, and he was told to report the next day. In describing the accident he mentioned that a stout wooden bow in the top of the car just above his head was broken, apparently by force from within.

On reporting again he complained of pain and a "catch" in the back of his neck. An x-ray picture (Fig. 1) disclosed a fracture of the spinous

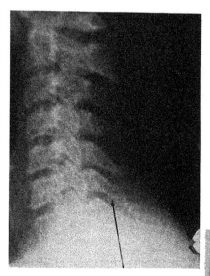

Figure 1. Roentgen ray picture, July 8, 1933, showing fracture and partial separation of fragment.

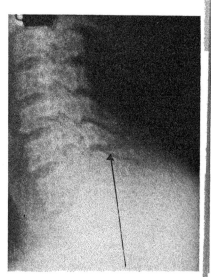

Figure 2. Roentgen ray picture, July 22, 1933, showing complete separation of fragment.

process of the sixth cervical vertebra. A cast was immediately applied.

For the next few days there was no great improvement; restless sleeping, irritability, and on the thirteenth day following, the circular cast was removed and the neck again examined by x-ray. This time the fragment was entirely separated from the stump (Fig. 2). The patient was adrised to have it removad; and a supparting sast was temporarily applied. This gave very little relief, and on August 3, under local·anesthesia, the fragment was removed.

Convalescence was uneventful after the subsidence of the initial soreness. The "catch," painful motion, local tenderness and sleep disturbance disappeared by the twelfth day; the wound healed without trouble, and the patient was discharged as cured on August 25, 1933.

The case is presented because of the following unusual factors it shows:

1. Trauma from above resulting in a fracture of the sixth cervical spine, a rare injury.

. 2. The gradual increase of symptoms, local and general, accompanied by loss of sleep and definite nerve shock, relieved rapidly and entirely by the removal of the fragment.

Iowa State Bank Building.

CALCIUM THERAPY IN PRE-ECLAMPTIC TOXEMIA*

ERWIN C. SAGE, M.D., Eagle Grove

Eclampsia has long been known as a disease of theories.[18] Students of this interesting symptom complex have attempted to place the blame for its development on foci of infection, chemical poisons or toxins formed by the metabolic activity of fetus, placenta, mammae, liver, kidneys, or uterus. Others have ascribed it to anaphylactic shock, thyroid deficiency, and so on. Practically every organ in the body has passed through the gamut of investigation, and nothing has been proved except that this syndrome does affect all bodily tissue. In 1910 Mitchell[13] suggested that eclampsia was caused by a lack of calcium. In other words, eclampsia is a deficiency disease in the pregnant woman due to a shortage of systemic calcium.

McLester[12] tells us, "The mineral diet of the American people is more likely to be deficient in respect to calcium than any·other element." The minimum requirement to preserve a safe balance is .45 grams a day and .75 grams should be taken each day. We do not know the fetal requirements

*Presented before the Second Councilor District Medical Society, Hampton, October 26, 1933.

but a growing child requires four times as much calcium as an adult. We can safely say that one to one and one-half grams should be ingested each day by the expectant mother to meet her needs and·those of the growing fetus. In terms of milk this would be equal to about one and one-half liters.

Several factors have induced us to believe that a calcium deficiency may be responsible for at least a large percentage of pre-eclamptic and eclamptic manifestations. The symptoms appear most frequently in the third trimester of pregnancy when the calcium demands of the fetus are greatest. The incidence is greater in multiple than in single pregnancies, one observer reporting as many as one-fourth of them being pre-eclamptic and one-ninth of all multiple pregnancies progressing to the convulsive state. A survey of my own cases has further shown that all pre-eclamptics disliked and did not drink milk, our chief source of calcium, and many .avoided the vegetables richest in that mineral.

Many reports in the literature discuss the effect of calcium therapy in symptoms analogous to those of eclampsia but occurring in other diseases. We must go to these reports to acquire our knowledge of the clinical and experimental effects of calcium since little study has been made on this subject from an obstetric standpoint.

Let us first consider hypertension. The exact cause of hypertension is obscure; however, the explanation of Evans[3] will serve us. "It is probable," he says, "that high blood pressure is first due to a widely distributed spasm of the arterioles caused by chemical stimulation of the pressor nerve supply to these vessels." May we apply this to pre-eclampsia? The sedative action of calcium is well understood. In this respect it acts as an antagonist to the irritant action of sodium. When the systemic calcium is reduced the. sodium preponderance stimulates the·pressor nerves to the arterioles and in turn produces a spasm of the arterioles with the resultant hypertension. Clinically, Davis[7] reported a group of cases of essential hypertension in which calcium therapy alone caused a drop in blood pressure to a normal level.

Andrews[3] produced in experimental animals a syndrome similar to eclampsia, with hypertension, edema, and finally convulsions, by injecting hypertonic sodium chloride into the vascular system of dogs. These symptoms could be relieved at will by washing the sodium chloride from the blood and adding calcium salts. He concluded that the symptoms produced were due to a disturbance of the calcium sodium balance. While his experiments were done in connection with study on uremia, the findings apply equally as well in eclampsia where the terminal symptoms are the same. Minot[17] produced a symptom complex similar to eclampsia by giving carbon tetrachloride to dogs fed on lean meat. With the intravenous administration of calcium chloride the dogs recovered in thirty minutes. In contradistinction to this, Harding and Van Wyck[11] administered hypertonic sodium chloride intravenously to three eclamptic patients with disastrous results.

Bennett[3] reports a case of uremia in which a low blood calcium persisted. He suggested the relationship between the twitchings and convulsions of uremia with tetany. About twenty-five years ago, McCallum[13] proved that tetany was due to a systemic poverty of calcium. Many of the symptoms of pre-eclampsia are so similar that one authority[2] states, "Tetany plus convulsions equal eclampsia."

The blood findings in the pre-eclamptic syndrome are of little value to us. The calcium content of the fetal blood is higher than it is in the maternal blood. The maternal blood calcium varies only slightly from the normal in severe eclamptic patients. This does not mean that the intercellular calcium balance is not disturbed. The entire content of blood calcium is only five-tenths of a gram[14] and during pregnancy the blood stream simply acts as a conveyor from the tissues to the fetus. The fetus is a calcium parasite and its demands must be met even though the host perish.

Edema is a second cardinal symptom of pre-eclampsia. The cause of edema is not definitely established although recent studies on cell permeability throw much light on the subject. Internists have long felt that a sodium chloride free diet favored the early relief of edema. O'Donnell and Levin[15] reported a series of cases in which edema and ascites in children were promptly relieved by the injection of calcium gluconate. Albuminuria, the third cardinal symptom, is undoubtedly the result of edema of the kidney stroma and when the edema disappears the urine will become clear unless the condition persists long enough to cause permanent kidney damage. The eye symptoms, epigastric pains, and cerebral manifestations are likewise due to an edema of the affected part and occur at times in all diseases of which edema is a symptom.

Before discussing the use of calcium in pre-eclampsia, I would like to survey the commonest forms of treatment now in use. The Straganoff treatment is the choice of some. This is the outgrowth of the old chloroform treatment. It consists in paralyzing the patient with subtoxic doses of morphine. Naturally this treatment is often

fatal to the fetus and sometimes to the mother. Sodium amytal and magnesium sulphate are similarly used in an effort to narcotize the mother to the point where she can no longer have a convulsion. Sedation is a temporary measure, aimed at giving the mother an opportunity to go into labor or if that does not occur, to allow time for an induction of labor. Recently, Arnold and Fay[1] have advocated the use of a dry diet in these cases together with free purgations. The results have been very satisfactory. They have managed to reduce the edema and hypertension in many cases. In contrast to this is the old standard milk diet treatment, which has been successfully used by many. Of course, here we have a paradox; a fluid free diet and a high fluid diet producing identical results in the same disease. It is apparent that some element must produce the desired effect other than the fluidity or non-fluidity of the diet. Glucose and gum acacia used intravenously increase the viscosity of the blood and act as a dehydrating agent to the edematous tissues. Blood letting, a treatment of long standing in eclampsia, mechanically relieves hypertension by reducing the total blood volume.

In view of the fact that there is no appreciable relationship between blood calcium and eclampsia, how and where does the disturbance of the calcium balance occur? Cantrow, Montgomery, and Bolton[5] express the opinion that although the total calcium remains the same, there is a decrease in the ratio of the diffusible to the non-diffusible cal cium, and this in turn affects the cell permeability There is little doubt that in eclampsia the cel permeability is changed. However, it seems mor reasonable to suppose that the fluid bathing the cel becomes dominated by the sodium ion, as sodiun chloride. This, following the laws of osmoti pressure, increases the amount of fluid within th cell and often distends the cell beyond its norma limit of elasticity. As a result the cell wall lose its tonus and its permeability is increased. Whei the proper calcium balance is maintained, experi mental evidence indicates that cell distension doe not occur.

Cameron[4] feels that the blood calcium is low especially during the eclamptic state. He believe that with an increased calcium excretion there i an excessive acid production. In connection wit Alexander Daly, he has adopted a routine treat ment for pre-eclamptic patients in which he give calcium lactate, sodium bicarbonate, and potassiu citrate to all mild cases. In the severe cases, ca cium acetate or gluconate is given intravenousl, The effect is dramatic. Blood pressure falls, an the edema and albuminuria disappear as if b magic. Daly[6] reported 18 cases with 161 in his control series. Most cases responded to oral medication, and labor was induced in those cases in which treatment was not effective. The patients were kept on a normal diet. Only two per cent required induction of labor as compared with 66 per cent in the control series. Eleven per cent of the births were premature as compared with 63 per cent in the control series. We feel that his results were due entirely to the amount of calcium ingested. Dieckmann[8] in his recent report states that he can find no change in the acid base equilibrium in pre-eclamptic patients unless there is an actual nephritis present and other observers have felt that calcium is absorbed more rapidly when the contents of the small bowel are kept acid.

Recent studies concerning calcium metabolism demonstrate the fact that calcium deficiency is not always due to a shortage of calcium in the diet but is at times due to a failure to utilize the calcium that is available. For this reason, in my cases, my patients have received viosterol in connection with calcium lactate. Enough calcium lactate is given to make certain that the patient will receive more than the minimum daily requirement for herself and the growing fetus—about one and one-half grams. With this treatment they are kept on a normal diet. I would like to report five cases. Cases one and two are mild pre-eclamptic patients; three, four and five are severe cases. We were taught that patients who had two or three cardinal symptoms were pre-eclamptic, that is a blood pressure of 140 or more, edema, and albuminuria. I now treat as pre-eclamptic those patients who show a rather slight increase of pressure and a rather slight edema. We know that the normal tendency of blood pressure is to drop during pregnancy. A rise of ten or fifteen mm. in the presence of edema now indicates to me that the ionic balance is being disturbed and I feel that the sooner prophylactic measures are begun, the better.

Case 1: The patient was a primipara, twenty years of age. The general physical examination and history were negative. She was first seen on November 16, 1931, and her estimated date was May 27, 1932. On April 29 her pressure was 128/80 and she was edematous. On May 19 her pressure was 150/100. She was given 15 minims of viosterol daily and 60 grains of calcium lactate. She was also instructed to go to bed and to remain there until given permission to be up. She did not stay in bed, however, but her pressure dropped to 120/80. Her edema disappeared overnight and did not recur.

Case 2: The patient was a primipara, twenty-one years of age. The history and physical examination were negative. She was first seen on June 10, 1932, and her date was estimated for September 2, 1932. Her pressure was normal until August 21, when it

had risen to 140/80. Marked edema was present and the urine contained one plus of albumin. She stated that her weight had increased twenty pounds in two weeks. She was given calcium lactate and viosterol on which she lost twelve pounds in forty-eight hours; her albumin became negative, and her blood pressure was normal until her delivery occurred on August 30.

Case 3: The patient was a multipara, thirty-six years of age, this pregnancy being her sixth. Physical examination was negative except for a slight edema and a blood pressure of 135/90. When she first consulted me on July 21, 1931, she was estimated to be due on November 12. This patient had a very dramatic obstetric history. With her first pregnancy she had three convulsions but delivered a full term baby who died at the age of two years of convulsions. Her second pregnancy resulted in a miscarriage at six and one-half months. With her third pregnancy she delivered a full term baby but was in bed for two months on a milk diet. With her fourth pregnancy she was again on a milk diet and her edema was very severe. She had a fall in the middle of the seventh month, and two weeks later delivered a macerated dead fetus. Her fifth pregnancy resulted in a full term baby but again she was very edematous. Her blood pressure was 170 and she was on a milk diet for two months. Returning to her present pregnancy, on August 19, 1931, her pressure was 142/95 and she became very edematous. She was put to bed on a milk diet; her pressure dropped to 128/85 in two days. On September 3, however, it went to 150/90. She was again put to bed on a milk diet with no improvement. On October 1, she was given 20 minims of viosterol daily and 60 grains of calcium lactate daily. Her blood pressure dropped to 120/80; her edema disappeared and she felt so good that she quit taking the medicine after about a week. On October 18, her pressure again went up to 160/100. As this was the first patient on whom I had used this type of therapy, and knowing that the baby was viable, I induced labor with a Vorhees' bag.

Case 4: The patient was a primipara, twenty years of age. History and physical examination were negative. She was first seen on June 1, 1932, and her estimated date of labor was November 18. Her blood pressure on examination was 110/70. It was normal until October 18 when it rose to 130/90 and she became very edematous and had a trace of albumin in her urine. She was given calcium lactate and viosterol in the usual dose. Her pressure became normal in forty-eight hours and the edema and albumin disappeared. On November 1, she exhausted her supply of medicine. The edema gradually recurred and she called me. Her blood pressure was then 170/100. The edema was very severe and her albumin two plus. She was put to bed and an attempt was made to load her with calcium by mouth. As she was very nauseated, she did not retain this well. She went into labor on November 7; when her pressure had dropped to 150/100.

Case 5: The patient was a primipara, twenty-six

years of age. The history and physical examination were negative. She first consulted me on September 3. On December 2, she began to show signs of toxemia, with a blood pressure of 150/100. With calcium therapy her pressure dropped to 140/90 on December 8. Two days later it went up to 170/110 for no apparent reason. She had no edema or albuminuria at this time, but did have a slight cold. On December 14, her pressure was 130/90 but it began to rise gradually. As the calcium therapy did not seem to help her, she was put on Arnold and Fay's dry diet, also without improvement. She never developed an appreciable edema but by January 7 the urine was loaded with albumin. She developed an anuresis, terrific epigastric pains and labor was induced by the Vorhees' bag. Why we failed in this case, we do not know. Could the slight cold which the patient developed have produced a pure nephritis on an already injured kidney? Her albuminuria persisted for three months after delivery and she was the only patient in this series in whom symptoms were present postpartum. This patient had also a bicornate uterus and the placenta was full of enfarcts. This, of course, brings to mind recent studies on the relationship between placental enfarction and eclampsia.[2]

In conclusion, certain facts indicate that eclampsia may be a calcium deficiency disease. I feel that with the cooperation of the patient and proper prenatal care, for which there is no substitute, eclampsia is a disease which should never occur. When the available therapeutic measures do not avail in the treatment by pre-eclamptic patients, labor should be induced. Calcium therapy is, I believe, if not a specific, at least a distinct, aid in the treatment of pre-eclamptic toxemia.

BIBLIOGRAPHY

1. Arnold, J. O., and Fay, Temple: Eclampsia; its prevention and control by means of fluid limitation and dehydration. Surg. Gynec., and Obet., lv:129 (August) 1932.
2. Bartholomew, R. A., and Kracke, R. R.: The relation of placental infarcts to eclamptic toxemia. Am. Jour. Obst. and Gynec., xxiv:797 (December) 1932.
3. Bennett, T. I.: Nephritis; its problems and treatment. The Oxford Press, London, 1929.
4. Cameron, Samuel J.: An aid in the treatment of toxemia of pregnancy. Lancet (London), ii:731 (October) 1932.
5. Cantarow, A., Montgomery, T. L., and Bolton, W. W.: Calcium partition in pregnancy, parturition and toxemias. Surg., Gynec., and Obst., li:469 (October) 1930.
6. Daly, Alexander: An aid in the treatment of toxemia of pregnancy. Jour. Obst. and Gynec. of British Empire, xl:209 (April) 1933.
7. Davis, N. S. III: Hypertension: the value of calcium salts plus diet in its management: a possible classification and an historical perspective. Jour. Am. Med. Assn., xcvii:543 (October) 1931.
8. Dieckmann, William J.: Comparative studies of the blood in the nonconvulsive toxemias of pregnancy. Am. Jour. Obst. and Gynec., xxvi:543 (October) 1933.
9. Drennan, Jennie. G.: If the abstraction of calcium salts from the mother's blood by the fetus is the cause of pueperal eclampsia in the former, then the eclamptic mother should not nurse her infant. Am. Jour. Obst., lxiv:259 (August) 1911.
10. Feinberg, Samuel M., and Lash, Abraham F.: The blood calcium in eclampsia. Surg., Gynec., and Obst., xlii:255 (February) 1926.
11. Harding, J., and Van Wyck, H. B.: Canadian Med. Assn. Jour. (May) 1931. Reviewed by De Lee and Greenhill in Practical Medicine Series, Obstetrics and Gynecology, pp. 104-106, The Year Book Publishers, Chicago, 1931.
12. McLester, J. S.: Nutrition and Diet in Health and Disease, p. 94. W. B. Saunders Company, Philadelphia, 1928.
13. Mitchell, James R.: A new theory of eclampsia. Med. Rec., lxxviii:906 (November 19) 1910.
14. Nixon, W. C. W.: Calcium therapy and the toxemias of pregnancy. Lancet (London), ii:291 (August 8) 1931.
15. O'Donnell, William S., and Levin, Samuel J.: The treatment of edema: effect of calcium gluconate on edema in children. Jour. Am. Med. Assn., xcvi:837 (March 14) 1931.
16. Talbot, John E.: A theory on the etiology of the toxemia of pregnancy with or without convulsions. Surg., Gynec. and Obst., xxviii:165 (February) 1919.
17. Theobald, G. W.: The causation of eclampsia. Lancet (London), i:1115 (May 24) 1930.
18. Williams, J. W.: Textbook of Obstetrics, D. Appleton and Company, New York, 1930.

AUTOTRANSFUSION FOLLOWING RUPTURE OF THE SPLEEN

CASE REPORT

WENDELL DOWNING, M.D.,

WILLIAM LARSEN, M.D.,

Le Mars

Autotransfusion or reinfusion of a patient with his own blood which has accumulated in the serous cavities from an internal hemorrhage was first suggested by Theis, a German, in 1914. Extensive literature has been developed on this subject in Germany, but few articles have appeared in American periodicals. It has long been known that blood which has accumulated in the peritoneal or pleural cavities does not clot readily even after several hours. This fact makes it possible to retransfuse the patient who has had a serious internal hemorrhage by filtering the blood and introducing it into his veins. With such a procedure there is no question of an unsuitable blood grouping and there is no delay and no expense for a donor.

From a review of the literature, we find that autotransfusion has been used chiefly in cases of ruptured ectopic pregnancy, rupture of the spleen or liver and less frequently in hemothorax. Reactions after transfusions have been slight and the procedure is entirely safe. Contaminated blood should not be used. Amounts varying from a few to two thousand cubic centimeters of blood have been reinfused. The effused blood may be given by the direct method or it may be mixed with sodium citrate in the usual way. The blood is always carefully filtered through layers of gauze before retransfusing and it is then introduced into the median basilic vein as in other transfusions.

The following case report of traumatic rupture of the spleen with a severe internal hemorrhage illustrates the value of autotransfusion. A boy fourteen years of age at 9:00 p. m., while swinging on a trapeze fell several feet striking the front of his left chest against the rim of a steel barrel.

He was unable to get up and showed immediate shock. He was carried to his home where he was seen by his physician. He complained of pain in his left chest which was increased by deep breathing and he was pale and restless. His temperature was 98° and pulse 68. He drank large quantities of water which he promptly vomited. His pallor and restlessness gradually increased. When seen by one of us at 12:30 a. m. his pulse was 90 and blood pressure 90/60. There was slight tenderness over his left chest and in his left upper abdominal quadrant. There was dulness in the flanks but no fluid wave was elicited. Pallor was marked. He was given morphine sulphate Gr. 1/6 and was taken to the hospital at once.

On arrival his pulse was 120 and of poor quality, respirations were 30, temperature 97°, and his blood pressure had fallen to 60/40. A fluid wave was easily made out and the abdomen was dull except for a small area in the epigastrium. Blood count revealed hemoglobin 60 per cent, red cells 2,000,000, and white cells 19,000. A group four donor was secured in case of need. Under nitrous oxide and ether anesthesia the peritoneal cavity was opened through a long left rectus incision and it was found filled with blood. The wound margins were retracted upwards and about fifteen hundred cubic centimeters of blood were dipped out with a cup into a basin containing sodium citrate solution. The spleen was then found to be displaced downwards and showed multiple tears in the parenchyma and capsule, one tear almost bisecting the organ. The pedicle was exposed and clamped and the spleen removed. Approximately three thousand cubic centimeters of blood were present in the peritoneal cavity. As soon as the bleeding was controlled reinfusion was begun. The blood which contained very few clots was filtered twice through eight layers of gauze, and one thousand cubic centimeters of blood and two hundred cubic centimeters of saline were introduced into the median basilic vein by gravity method.

By the time the patient's wound was closed his color was much improved. His pulse was 110 and of good quality, and his blood pressure was 100/60. He had no post-transfusion reaction, his highest fever was 101° and was normal after the fifth day. His convalescence was uneventful and he made a complete recovery.

THE FINLEY HOSPITAL CLINICO-PATHOLOGIC CONFERENCE

CARCINOMA OF THE OVARY

H. M. PAHLAS, M.D., Dubuque

The case to be presented is that of a rapidly developing ascites in a woman thirty-four years of age.

CASE REPORT

The patient, a white woman, was admitted to The Finley Hospital, March 9, 1934, with a complaint of "fluid in the abdomen."

Family History: The patient's husband and one child of six are living and well. Her father died of a ruptured appendix. Three sisters, two brothers, and her mother are living and well.

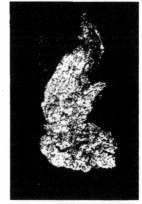

Figure 1. Photograph of a portion of the omentum, showing replacement by large numbers of carcinoma implantations.

Past History: The patient has always had good health except for an occasional cold in the winter time. Her child was born after a normal pregnancy and there have been no miscarriages. Her menstrual cycle has varied between twenty-four and twenty-eight days and has lasted about six days. The flow has been moderately profuse but there never has been a frank hemorrhage.

Present Illness: About six weeks ago while telephoning, the patient had a sudden sharp pain across the lower abdomen. She thought it was due to gas and took hot peppermint water which gave her some relief. That night she took magnesium citrate solution and during the next two days she had numerous liquid stools. An examination at that time showed her abdomen to be tympanitic, but there were no points of tenderness. The liver was not enlarged. She was given a prescription for the diarrhea with considerable benefit, but she still complained of gas and distention. On examination the next day, the abdomen was dull and evidently contained considerable fluid. A vaginal examination was unsatisfactory because of the fluid in the abdomen. The body of the uterus and the uterine cervix seemed normal but the ovaries could not be felt. She was advised to enter the hospital but refused, and she was then given ammonium chloride and salyrgan in an attempt to decrease the fluid in the abdomen. The ascites diminished considerably for two weeks and then began to increase. She finally entered the hospital for an abdominal paracentesis and further study.

Physical Examination: The patient is a very thin woman who does not appear to be suffering. Her eyes react to light and accommodation. There are no enlarged glands in the neck and the thyroid gland is of normal size. The lungs are clear and resonant throughout. The heart is not enlarged; the sounds are clear, regular and there are no murmurs. The abdomen is markedly distended; shows a definite fluid wave and on percussion there is dulness throughout, except in the upper portion. The extremities are negative. The systolic blood pressure is 120 and the diastolic is 70 mm. of mercury. The temperature is 99.4°, the pulse is 100, and the respirations 20. The

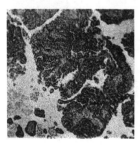

Figure 2. Low power microphotograph showing the papillary formation of the neoplasm.

white blood count is 11,000 with 74 per cent polymorphonuclear leukocytes. The red blood count is 4,600,-000; hemoglobin, 78 per cent; color index 0.84; the urine is negative.

Course in Hospital: The day after admission, 10,-000 cc. of faintly blood tinged, amber fluid was obtained by an abdominal paracentesis. The laboratory examination of the fluid showed it to be sterile and to contain a moderate number of red cells but did not clot. A differential cell count showed 70 erythrocytes, 21 lymphocytes, and nine polymorphonuclear leukocytes. Large amounts of fluid were centrifuged and the sediments studied for malignant cells. A moderate number of cells with large vesicular nuclei were seen, but since there were no mitotic fig-

ures they were thought to be desquamated peritoneal cells.

After removal of the fluid a vaginal examination showed the uterus and adnexa to be fused and fixed in the pelvis. It was thought that the left ovary was considerably enlarged. An x-ray examination of the lungs showed no evidence of metastases. An exploratory operation was advised.

Preoperative Diagnosis: Carcinoma of the ovary with peritoneal metastases or tuberculous peritonitis.

Operative Notes: There was a large cyst of the left ovary with solid papillary-like masses growing over the surface. The cyst was bound to the uterus and to the intestines by adhesions. The entire peritoneum was studded with small neoplastic masses which tended to fuse. The omentum had been almost entirely replaced by the neoplasm (Fig. 1). The omentum was removed and the abdomen closed.

Pathologic Report: The sections of the omentum show the neoplasm to have a papillary formation. There is a central core composed of connective tissue and blood vessels which is surrounded by heaped up epithelial cells, rich in chromatin and showing numerous mitotic figures. Occasionally the epithelium tend to form small glands and in some instances they tend to form solid masses. (Figs. 2 and 3.)

Anatomic Diagnosis: Peritoneal implantations (ovarian carcinoma).

COMMENT

This is a case of rapidly developing ascites in a young woman who had previously been well. With the absence of evidences of heart disease, nephritis, pregnancy and enlargement of the liver, the first diagnosis which should be considered is that of malignant disease of the peritoneum. The second possibility is tuberculous peritonitis. The several other possible causes of ascites are easily ruled out and the exploratory operation especially in view of the blood tinged fluid was obviously the procedure of choice.

Carcinomas of the ovary may occur at any age but are encountered most frequently during active sexual life. It is often stated that they occur in the greatest number between forty and fifty years of age. Actually they develop at all ages and the safest rule is to consider all ovarian tumors malignant until they are proved otherwise by histologic examination. Approximately 20 per cent of all ovarian tumors are carcinomas. The incidence of carcinoma according to cyst type is variable, but of the pseudo-mucinous cysts, about 15 per cent are carcinomas; of the serous cysts 35 per cent, and of the papillary cysts 40 per cent. In addition to the carcinomas arising in cysts there are solid neoplasms which usually form small masses not unlike brain substance in their general appearance. In addition the ovary is frequently the site of metastatic carcinoma. All the primary neoplasms whether arising in cysts or as solid tumors tend to break through the wall of the cyst or the capsule of the ovary. The chance of cure is obviously better when they are removed while still encapsulated. When the neoplasm breaks through the capsule the cells are disseminated through the abdominal cavity and become implanted on the peritoneum

Implants on the peritoneum may be benign or malignant. When actually invasive death occurs in a short time. In cases with benign implants twenty-five years may intervene before a "recurrence" takes place. In such cases symptoms are present only when secretion is faster than absorption. Malignant transformation may occur later or the implants may be killed by overgrowth of fibrous tissue. Fifty-eight cases of the latter have

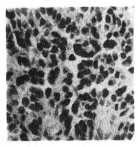

Figure 3. High power microphotograph showing type cells of the neoplasm.

been recorded. As a rule, however, the peritoneal implantations are malignant and during removal of any cyst or tumor of the ovary, it is imperative to prevent contamination of the peritoneum by the contents of the cyst or the cells of a solid tumor. The treatment of all carcinomas is removal of both the ovaries and a supravaginal hysterectomy (Graves). The presence of peritoneal inplantations does not contraindicate the removal of the original ovarian tumor, for the implantations even when malignant sometimes regress and disappear after the removal of the primary gowth.

CONCLUSION

A case of ovarian carcinoma with peritoneal implantations has been described. The importance of ascites as the first symptom of the condition has been emphasized. The treatment of these neoplasms depends upon early diagnosis and complete removal.

REPORT OF CASES FROM THE
BROADLAWNS GENERAL
HOSPITAL, DES MOINES

JULIUS S. WEINGART, M.D., JOSEPH BROWN, M.D., FRANK W. FORDYCE, M.D., Hospital Staff Committee

Authors' Note.—It is the purpose of the staff of Broadlawns General Hospital in the following reports and those which will appear from time to time in the JOURNAL to present some of the most interesting, puzzling, and unusual cases which we have been called upon to treat at this hospital. Like the stories in the Sunday School books, these tales have a moral, as will be evident to those who will take the time to study them. We have not tried to disguise our mistakes, or to claim credit for diagnoses not made before autopsy, nor has any attempt at overelaboration been made. Only the essential part of the history is given, and a pedantic review of the literature has been studiously avoided.

REPORT OF CASE NO. 30185

This patient, a white man, wrapper in a bakery, thirty-one years of age, was admitted to Broadlawns Hospital on September 7, 1933, about 10:00 a. m., in a restless and irrational state. He died about one hour and fifteen minutes later. The chief entrance complaint when seen in the out patient department was "just sick" for two weeks. No history was obtained from the patient because of his mental and physical state, but the following facts were obtained from the wife and other relatives.

On August 24, 1933, the patient had an intestinal upset with diarrhea and vomiting which lasted for only one day. This followed, supposedly, the eating of a green apple. The vomitus was composed of apple and some bile stained fluid. The next day, August 25, he felt fairly well, and worked at his job all day. On August 26, he had another intestinal upset similar to the first. Constipation followed, associated with weakness, but no pain. His appetite was poor. He would take orange juice and water, but no solid food. The above condition continued for ten days. On September 6, the hands and feet became numb and tingling. At no time did the patient complain of pain or any distress. There was an infection in the eyes for the last three days, but no photophobia.

Past medical history: Essentially negative.

Social and family history: Negative

Physical examination: Examination revealed a

well developed but poorly nourished white male who was very restless and tossed about in bed. He did not seem to be oriented, and although very thirsty, only took a swallow each time he was given water. He appeared ill. The eyes were sunken, the pupils were partially dilated, and they reacted only sluggishly to light. A purulent discharge from both eyes was present, and the conjunctival vessels were congested. There was no photophobia; and pathology in the ears, nose, and pharynx was absent. The mucous membrane of the mouth was cyanotic. The chest was clear. X-ray films showed the lower border of the heart to be at the midclavicular line, but we were unable to hear heart sounds in any position. We were also unable to read the blood pressure or to get the count or contour of the pulse. The abdomen was negative. All reflexes were absent, delayed or impaired, and there was a sensation of pain over the legs. The white blood count was 16,000; the Kahn test was negative; and the Widal test was negative.

Course while in hospital: The patient was put to bed immediately. He was extremely restless, and his temperature was 99.8°, taken rectally. As mentioned before, no information could be obtained from the patient. His condition remained about the same for an hour, after which he became quiet, and it was apparent that he was dying. In fifteen minutes he was pronounced dead.

Clinical diagnosis: Undetermined. Acetanilid poison and typhoid were considered possibilities.

Autopsy findings: The autopsy was performed one hour after death. The body was as described in the physical examination. There was rigor mortis, one plus, and postmortem lividity, two plus; no edema was present, and the external marks were as previously described. The peritoneal, pericordial, and pleural cavities showed no adhesions; there was a small amount of straw colored fluid present; and the linings were smooth and shiny. The heart was normal in size, musculature, color and consistency. The lungs were crepitant throughout. The gastro-intestinal system was normal, and no injection or distension of the intestines or stomach was noted. The mucous membrane of the stomach showed no injection or ulceration. The liver was a purplish-blue color, but of normal consistency. On cut section, much thick cyanotic blood poured out. The kidneys were normal, capsule strips easily leaving a smooth surface. Both the adrenal glands were enlarged to three times their normal size, firm in consistency with the medulla destroyed. On cut section, the gland was found to be infiltrated with a gray, granular, homogeneous material, but no gross necrotic areas were seen. At no place could any

medullary tissue be seen grossly. A microscopic examination showed the major portion of the tissue to be composed of caseous material with no definite structure. There was an infiltration of monocytic cells. Typical tubercle formations could be seen at places, and normal adrenal gland tissue was only seen occasionally.

Microscopic diagnosis: Tuberculosis of the adrenal glands.

This case was most unusual in that the clinical history was so short. This patient died of Addison's disease, and had worked within ten days of his death, the first symptoms appearing sixteen days before death occurred. There was little, if any, bronzing of the skin. It is very doubtful if a diagnosis could have been made without an autopsy. Even at autopsy, the diagnosis might have been missed if the adrenal glands had not been examined, but the history of weakness and gastro-intestinal disturbances, especially directed attention to these organs. These glands contained the only definite tuberculous lesions in the body. A small amount of fairly normal tissue was found in one of the adrenal glands, and the patient had probably lived for some time only on this small margin.

REPORT OF CASE NO. 66699.

This patient was a man, fifty-three years of age, who entered the hospital, complaining of a dull pain in the epigastrium of six years' duration. The pain had been periodic, and had been absent at times for a year. During the last few months, he had been bothered more with nausea, vomiting and tarry stools. Belching, as well as food and alkali, gave him relief. Three months before admission, the patient experienced a period of three weeks during which he vomited after practically every meal. A physician prescribed powders, pills, and milk between meals. This treatment gave him relief until two days before admission, at which time the pain recurred and the patient vomited once. He had never vomited blood. The patient said his skin had become yellowish during the last three months.

Nothing in the past history gave a clue as to the cause of his illness. He had some tingling of the hands and feet with cramping of the leg muscles for three months. There was no fever, and aside from his paleness, the physical examination was essentially negative. A laboratory examination showed the presence of a severe anemia; red blood count, 2,150,000; white blood count, 5,000, with 88 per cent polymorphonuclears; 12 lymphocytes; hemoglobin, 50 per cent; urine, a specific gravity of 1.010, with a slight trace of albumin; sediment was negative.

This patient was at first regarded as anemic due to a bleeding gastric ulcer, but no blood was found in his stools. His history as given would lend credence to this diagnosis if we did not remember that every now and then a history hinders more than it helps us. We then considered the possibility of pernicious anemia, and he was given a course of liver extract, which produced no essential improvement in his blood count, or even a rise of his reticulocytes. It was then that Dr. Peisen, who had been studying him with us, noticed that the single specimen of urine had been found to have a specific gravity of 1.010, and suggested the possibility of nephritis. A Mosenthal test showed a fixed specific gravity for the twenty-four hours, an average of 1.010. The seven specimens in the twenty-four hours ranged from 1.009 to 1.012. The urea nitrogen in the blood was 45 mg. per cent, and the phenol red test showed a total return of only ten per cent in two hours.

This patient evidently had marked secondary anemia due to renal insufficiency. The diagnosis was delayed for some time because there was little in his history to suggest it. His blood pressure was only 145/75 and we had not paid attention to the rather low specific gravity of his urine. It is possible that his gastric symptoms were really due to his uremia. It has been noted before by many observers that an abnormal concentration of urea in the blood may sometimes act as a depressant to the blood forming tissues. The above case was a good illustration of this. He was discharged from the hospital about one month after admission with a diagnosis of chronic nephritis complicated by secondary anemia. He died two months after his discharge.

J. S. W.

ANNUAL MEETING OF THE AMERICAN ASSOCIATION FOR THE STUDY OF GOITER

The Annual Meeting of the American Association for the Study of Goiter will be held in Cleveland, June 7, 8, and 9, 1934. Headquarters are at the Wade Park Manor, and scientific sessions are open to any members of the medical profession in good standing. A registration fee of $2.00 will be charged. A special program of entertainment is being arranged for visiting ladies.

Mornings are to be devoted to clinics in the Cleveland hospitals, the University hospitals, and The Cleveland Clinic. Dr. R. M. Howard of Oklahoma City, will deliver his presidential address, Thursday, June 7. Friday afternoon, the Van Meter prize essay award will be issued for the best essay based upon original research work on any phase of goiter. This year marks the fifth anniversary of this essay contest, and it is hoped that the contest will stimulate

valuable research work, especially in regard to the basic cause of goiter.

A feature of the annual dinner, held at the Wade Park Manor, Friday evening, June 8, will be an illustrated lecture by Professor Francis H. Herrick of Cleveland, on "The Life History of the American Eagle."

Officers of the society are: Dr. R. M. Howard of Oklahoma City, president; Dr. Allen Graham of Cleveland, president elect; Dr. Thomas M. Joyce of Portland, Oregon, vice president; Dr. J. R. Yung of Terre Haute, Indiana, corresponding secretary; Dr. F. B. Dorsey, Jr., of Keokuk, Iowa, recording secretary, and Dr. W. B. Mosser of Kane, Pennsylvania, treasurer.

IOWA CONFERENCE ON CHILD DEVELOPMENT AND PARENT EDUCATION

The Eighth Iowa Conference on Child Development and Parent Education will be held in Iowa City, June 19, 20, and 21, 1934. The conference is sponsored by the Iowa State Council for Child Study and Parent Education with the cooperation of the Iowa Child Welfare Research Station and Extension Divisions of the State University of Iowa, Iowa State Teachers College, and Iowa State College of Agriculture and Mechanic Arts. The program will present some of the issues of the new educational deal. It is open to all persons interested in studying children. No admission fee will be charged for any of the conference sessions.

Conference speakers will include the following: Dr. William E. Blatz, Director, St. George's School of Child Study, Toronto, Canada; Dr. Paul H. Douglas, Professor of Economics, University of Chicago, Chicago; Miss Agnes Samuelson, State Superintendent of Public Instruction, Des Moines, Iowa; Dr. David M. Trout, Dean of Men, Hillsdale College, Hillsdale, Michigan; Dr. Edna N. White, Director, Merrill-Palmer School, Detroit, Michigan; Dr. George F. Zook, United States Commissioner of Education, Washington, D. C., and Professor Frances Zuill, Head of the Department of Home Economics, State University of Iowa, Iowa City, Iowa.

For further information address the Iowa Child Welfare Research Station, State University of Iowa, Iowa City.

A.M.A. GOLFERS PLAY JUNE 11TH

The American Medical Golfing Association will hold its twentieth annual tournament at the Mayfield Country Club in Cleveland on Monday, June 11, 1934.

All male Fellows of the American Medical Association are eligible and cordially invited to become members of the A.M.G.A. Write the Executive Secretary, Bill Burns, 4421 Woodward Avenue, Detroit, for an application blank and full details of the 1934 tournament.

The twentieth tournament of the American Medical Golfing Association promises to be a happy affair, attended by some two hundred medical golfers from all parts of the United States.

STATE DEPARTMENT OF HEALTH

The State Department of Health at the Annual Meeting of the Iowa State Medical Society

Exhibit

At the coming meeting of the Iowa State Medical Society the State Department of Health will exhibit five block models which show interesting facts about some of the principal causes of death in Iowa. The mortality from diseases of the heart, cancer, accidents (all forms) and tuberculosis by years for the period from 1923 to 1933, inclusive, and by age groups will be pictured by this method. In addition, the mortality for cancer by sex for the years 1932 and 1933 will be shown. A master model giving facts about the deaths of infants under one year of age during 1933 has been made. Neonatal mortality by age groups, by sex, and by principal causes of death form a part of this large model. The influence of the period of pregnancy at which the mother first consulted the doctor, the effect of the type and place of delivery, and classification of the medical attendant on infant mortality will be shown.

This will be the first time that such models have been shown to the membership of the Iowa State Medical Society. Original and unique methods of displaying these three dimensional models and of producing lighting effects have been devised by Mr. McAllister of the Division of Public Health Engineering. This exhibit by the department will be instructive and attractive as well. Those interested in the subject "neonatal deaths and their prominent etiologic factors" will want to study the feature model on infant mortality before attending the symposium on that subject.

Information Desk

In connection with its exhibit the department will maintain an information desk. Here medical practitioners may secure information about the rules and regulations of the State Board of Health, the duties of local health officers, the literature available without cost and other subjects. Request for supplies (free silver nitrate ampules, literature request cards, death and birth records, etc.) are solicited.

Representatives of Department Participating in and Attending the Meeting

Representatives of the department will appear on the formal program. Walter L. Bierring, M.D., Commissioner of Public Health, will give an address Friday, May 11, at 10:30 a. m. on "The Relation of the State Department of Health to the Practice of Medicine." Jos. H. Kinnaman, M.D., will speak briefly to the pediatric section on "The State Department of Health and Preventive Programs." F. J. Swift, M.D., Deputy Commissioner of Health; Carl F. Jordan, M.D., Director, Division of Communicable Diseases and Epidemiologist; M. E. Barnes, M.D., Iowa City, Iowa, Director, Hygienic Laboratories, and other representatives of the department, will attend the meeting. The members of the department invite the membership of the society to discuss informally public health problems with them at that time. The department has just completed a special study and analysis of the infant mortality for Iowa during 1933. Data available from this study will be referred to by speakers included in the symposium on "Neonatal Deaths and Their Prominent Etiologic Factors."

Open House at the Offices of the Department

Why not visit the offices of the State Department of Health at 1027 Des Moines Street (one block north of the State Capitol Building), while you are in Des Moines?

TRACING THE SOURCE OF TYPHOID INFECTION

In typhoid fever, regardless of whether it be a single case, several cases or an epidemic, there is a definite source of infection. The source, if discovered, is usually found to be a typhoid carrier. With the help of attending physicians, the State Department of Health obtains information relative to reported cases of typhoid fever, in the effort to establish the source of infection. The following account is of interest as it illustrates the cause and effect relationship so often observed, between typhoid carriers and cases.

A two-year-old boy took sick with fever on March 13, 1934. He was seen by Dr. D. S. Burbank of Pleasantville and later admitted to a Des Moines hospital, where Dr. Lee F. Hill was the attending physician. The child was suffering from typhoid fever. Through the kindness of Dr. Hill, the patient was seen in the hospital on March 26. Information relative to the probable source of infection was obtained from the child's mother.

The patient's family includes himself, a sister seven years of age, the father and the mother. Neither of the parents, nor the other child, have had typhoid fever in the past. The patient's maternal grandmother had this disease about eighteen years ago, in 1916. Her son and daughter suffered an attack before her recovery. The other daughter (mother of the two-year-old patient), was away at the time, attending school in another city. The following year, 1917, a second son developed typhoid fever and died. The grandmother of the child now sick in the hospital, visited in the child's home several weeks prior to the onset of the illness and helped with the housework and care of her grandchildren.

It was suspected that the patient's grandmother might prove to be a typhoid carrier. A letter was directed to Dr. Burbank, requesting that he arrange for the procuring of specimens of feces and urine from this woman. A supply of stool containers, with postage attached, was forwarded by the State Department of Health. The desired specimens were sent to the State Laboratory at Iowa City. On April 6, 1934, a report was received from the laboratory, stating that B. typhosus had been isolated from a fecal specimen. Laboratory tests demonstrated that this woman is a typhoid carrier, and established with a high degree of certainty, the source of infection in the grandchild of two years with typhoid fever.

TYPHOID FEVER IN NEWARK TOWNSHIP, WEBSTER COUNTY, IOWA

Dr. J. P. Sharon, of Fort Dodge, recently completed a typhoid survey of Newark township in the northeast corner of Webster county. With the aid of Dr. Carroll Parsons, of Vincent, by a study of records and through inquiry in the community, Dr. Sharon ascertained how many typhoid fever cases and deaths have occurred in the township from 1905 to 1933, inclusive. There were five deaths from the disease during this period. The number of cases and years of occurrence are indicated in the following table:

Year	Typhoid Cases	Year	Typhoid Cases
			Carried forward..13
1905	2	1920	1
1914	1	1921	4
1915	1	1925	1
1916	3	1926	2
1917	4	1927	3
1919	2	1933	5
	13	Total	29

In addition to the total number of 29 cases, 3 other patients in the township suffered illness in past years resembling typhoid fever.

A number of persons, former typhoid patients, provided specimens, which were forwarded by Dr. Sharon to the State Laboratory. Typhoid bacilli were reported as being present in a fecal specimen from a woman 65 years of age, who together with her husband, acquired typhoid fever in Oklahoma in 1901.

It was possible in all but one of the 29 cases to trace the probable source of infection to this woman, who was discovered to be a carrier. Six cases occurred among her relatives and four among farm hands who were employed at different times on her husband's farm. Two cases of typhoid fever occurred among persons who were near neighbors and four more among men who became ill several weeks after threshing on this farm. Six people developed typhoid fever following church or school picnics, at which this woman helped with the preparation and serving of food. In addition, six patients represented secondary cases occurring in various homes, making the total number, twenty-eight.

In 1927 it was suspected that this woman was a carrier, but laboratory specimens failed to demonstrate the fact. The recent survey in Newark township was of particular significance, in that a definite source of typhoid infection, known to give rise to many cases of the disease over a period of years, was discovered. Continued supervision of the known source is also a matter of importance, so that the occurrence of future cases may be prevented.

PREVALENCE OF DISEASE

	Mar., '34	Feb., '34	Mar., '33	Most Cases Reported from
Diphtheria	27	32	41	Woodbury, Linn
Scarlet Fever	352	299	186	Polk, Franklin
Typhoid Fever	3	5	1	Des Moines, Keokuk, Marion
Smallpox	37	22	174	Palo Alto, Winneshiek
Measles	884	481	42	Plymouth, Pottawatamie
Whooping Cough	222	116	65	Black Hawk, Plymouth
Cerebrospinal Meningitis	10	4	10	Dickinson, Polk, Woodbury
Chickenpox	307	337	204	Woodbury, Montgomery
Mumps	367	228	292	Woodbury, Hamilton
Poliomyelitis	1	2	1	Mitchell
Tuberculosis	32	28	38	(For State)
Undulant Fever	22	5	8	Linn, Cerro Gordo
Syphilis	131	132	213	(For State)
Gonorrhea	160	145	187	(For State)

The JOURNAL of the
Iowa State Medical Society

ISSUED MONTHLY

RALPH R. SIMMONS, Editor.....................Des Moines

PUBLICATION COMMITTEE

RALPH R. SIMMONS, Editor.....................Des Moines
ROBERT L. PARKER, Secretary..................Des Moines
OLIVER J. FAY, Trustee.......................Des Moines
JOHN I. MARKER, Trustee......................Davenport
EDWARD M. MYERS, Trustee.....................Boone

SUBSCRIPTION $3.00 PER YEAR

*Address all communications to the Editor of the Journal,
1122 Bankers Trust Building, Des Moines*

OFFICE OF PUBLICATION, DES MOINES, IOWA

Vol. XXIV   MAY, 1934   No. 5

AN IMPROVED INFANT MORTALITY RATE

During the past half century, statisticians figure that the average span of human life has been extended ten years. This does not mean that the expectancy among adults has been extended ten years. In fact, statistics indicate that adult expectancy has changed but slightly during this period. The conservation of life predicating this statement of life extension is based entirely, or nearly so, upon the marked saving in infant and juvenile lives.

Statistics of a reliable character upon this problem have been available for only a relatively short time. For this reason a recent study of a prehistoric village located in New Mexico is particularly interesting and significant. Under the direction of the School of American Research at the University of New Mexico, excavations have been conducted since 1926 in the Jamez Canyon at Rockpoint and Indian Village, the site of prehistoric settlements inhabited for not more than four generations. Observers agree from their intensive study of these sites that thirty-six per cent of the village inhabitants died in infancy. Differently stated, this indicates that at this early time, out of every three babies born, one would die in infancy.

Observations such as these emphasize the strides in progress made by civilization and modern science. It would be an interesting study to follow the trends in infant mortality by successive steps, from this early time with its appalling infant death rate down to the modern time. Unfortunately, the evidence is missing to link these data with those collected under our modern registration system. A justifiable pride may be had in the fact that "infant mortality has been decreasing since comparable annual statistics have been collected in the United States. As recently as 1915, one infant of every ten born in the registration area died before reaching its first birthday; in 1920, one out of twelve died; in 1925, one out of fourteen; in 1930, one out of fifteen; in 1931, one out of sixteen; while in 1932 only one out of every seventeen babies died before the expiration of its first year."

ADDING INSULT TO INJURY

Newspaper comment would permit the conclusion that Norman Baker, formerly of Muscatine, Iowa, not only profited materially by his alleged cancer cure, but also from various commercial enterprises sponsored by him. To secure a mouthpiece for his blatant tirade against the "medical trust" and to further publicity regarding his alleged cancer cure, Baker sought the ownership of a newspaper. Unsuccessful in his attempt to purchase an established paper in Muscatine, Baker launched the Muscatine *Free Press*, permitting former patients and other gullible investors to share his success in the Progressive Publishing Company. When the mills of the law had ceased their grinding Baker was so shorn of authority and his ballyhoo style was so cramped that he decided to retire across the border into Mexico, where he hoped to find people more appreciative of his outstanding discoveries and his philanthropic proclivity. To collect a sum aggregating over $80,000 Baker, through the Norman Baker Investment Company, a corporation organized for the purpose of consolidating his many holdings, petitioned foreclosure of the Progressive Publishing Company to satisfy his claim. His friends and former patients, so graciously allowed to invest with him in this project, will now be permitted to sacrifice their investments in his favor, if his petition is sustained. Were it not for the serious and even tragic aspect of this matter, one might be tempted to dismiss the entire subject with a shrug of the shoulders, but the wastage of human life and the blasting of an innocent hope must prompt serious reflection. Baker, safely across the Mexican border, has eluded federal officers patiently awaiting his attempt to return to the United States, but he continues to suck a hearty nourishment from the veins of Iowa citizens.

A public consciousness sufficiently aroused could prevent the repetition of such a calamity.

MEDICINAL WHISKY

The repeal of the Eighteenth Amendment introduced the problem of meeting the demand for properly aged whisky without the benefit of the years required for the natural aging of this product. The available supply of good whisky in American warehouses was limited and entirely insufficient to meet the new demand. To supplement our meager supply by permitting the importation of aged whisky from abroad, at a price which would be a challenge to bootleg whisky, would waive tariff provisions and jeopardize home industry.

The obvious solution to the problem was to permit the sale of several different grades of whisky for beverage purposes, each a product safe in its chemical constituents but varying in fineness and the process of manufacture. This would permit the sale not only of the fully aged, fine whiskys of domestic and foreign makes, but also of various blended whiskys and whiskys artificially aged or synthetically prepared. In creating these several products a satisfactory price range could be established and the demand immediately met. Such a plan was recently authorized by the Federal Alcohol Control Administration and became effective at once.

This liberalization in the requirements of whisky for beverage purposes as outlined by the Federal Alcohol Control Administration would apparently contradict the provisions of the Food and Drug Act in their definition of whisky, and destroy the effectiveness of this law. To explain the apparent conflict in the rulings of these two agencies the Food and Drug Administration has just issued a statement (February 6, 1934) intended to clarify the specific requirements of the Federal Food and Drug Act as they apply to medicinal whisky. It shows that whisky sold for drug purposes is subject to requirements which do not apply to an article intended exclusively for beverage use.

The Food and Drug Administration emphasizes that the requirements it enforces in regard to medicinal whisky are not administrative rulings, but are set forth in the Food and Drugs Act which requires that drugs listed in United States Pharmacopoeia shall conform to the definition in that authority. The definition for whisky in the United States Pharmacopoeia is more rigid than the definition for "straight whisky" which the Federal Alcohol Control Administration issued (February 6, 1934) in that whisky defined in the pharmacopoeia must be aged four years in charred wood containers, and its alcoholic content must be not less than 16 per cent and not more than 57 per cent by volume of absolute alcohol. Medicinal whisky which does not conform to the pharmacopoeial standard must be labeled to differentiate it clearly from the official product.

The text of the ruling follows: A drug sold within the jurisdiction of the Federal Food and Drugs Act as "Whisky," "Spiritus Frumenti," or "Sp. Frum." must comply exactly with the definition for "Whisky" in the United States Pharmacopoeia and otherwise satisfy the provisions of that authority for "Whisky." It must be labeled with a statement of the quantity of alcohol in terms of the percentage by volume of absolute alcohol.

A drug varying from the pharmacopoeial specifications for "Whisky" in strength, quality or purity (but not in the identity of its constituents or of the materials from which it is made) may be sold as "Whisky not U.S.P." if the label carries a declaration of its own standard of strength, quality and purity. It may be first, an article conforming to the definition in the United States Pharmacopoeia except with respect to time of aging, percentage of alcohol and content of acids and esters, or second, a mixture of the above with grain alcohol or grain alcohol and water, or third, a mixture of U.S.P. whisky with grain alcohol and water. It may not contain alcohol from non-grain sources nor may it contain any substance not present in U.S.P. whisky. Such a drug may be labeled as in the following three examples, assuming it to be of the indicated composition in each case:

WHISKY—NOT U.S.P.

Aged............years. Alcohol by Volume, ...%

WHISKY—NOT U.S.P.

........% straight whisky aged............years,
........% neutral spirits from grain
TOTAL ALCOHOL BY VOLUME, ...%

WHISKY—NOT U.S.P.

....% U.S.P. Whisky, ...% neutral spirits from grain
TOTAL ALCOHOL BY VOLUME, ...%

Diluted alcohol (from whatever source) with or without artificial flavor and color, is not entitled to the name "Whisky," however qualified, if sold as a drug; but may be sold as a drug under any other name which is not false or misleading in any particular.

A pharmacist filling a prescription for "Whisky," "Spiritus Frumenti" or "Sp. Frum." must fill it only with whisky conforming to the requirements of the United States Pharmacopoeia. If a physician prescribes "Whisky not U.S.P." and specifies the standard of strength, quality or purity desired, the prescription must be filled with a product conforming to such specifications.

CARBON MONOXIDE AND "MYSTERY" ACCIDENTS

In the March JOURNAL, editorial comment was made of carbon monoxide in asphyxial accidents. The accidents dealt with in that article were those of a serious and often fatal character —the immediate or direct result of massive doses of this gas. Reasoning that perhaps lesser degrees of asphyxiation might occur if this dangerous gas were present in automobiles, several agencies have studied the rôle which carbon monoxide may play in the production of unexplained or "mystery" accidents with automobiles. In 1933, there were 58,900 unexplained automobile accidents in which cars driven off the highway, for no apparent reason, killed 3,260 persons and injured 53,240 others.

A critical investigation made by the Motor Vehicle Department at Hartford, Connecticut, showed that fully seven per cent of the motor vehicles designated as "the run of the road," contain, while in operation, enough carbon monoxide to cause symptoms of asphyxiation in the driver.

There appears to be a grave probability of serious accidents if the drivers in these cars are exposed to the dangerous atmosphere for several hours at a time. The present frequent use of the automobile for long pleasure trips and the use of trucks for distant hauling make the hazards of long exposure particularly significant. At least eighty per cent of the automobiles tested in Hartford contained measurable quantities of carbon monoxide gas when the car was in operation. While difficult of proof, their observations no doubt explain why so many drivers lose control of their cars with resulting accidents.

Inasmuch as the poisoning from carbon monoxide is an insidious one and is accompanied by a marked slowing down of mental processes, headache, and faulty vision, it does not seem at all far fetched to offer the presence of carbon monoxide poison as an explanation of these "mystery" accidents with automobiles.

These observations made at Hartford have been confirmed and substantiated by researches conducted by the Travelers Insurance Company and the Cities Service Oil Company. They further demonstrated that dangerous concentrations of carbon monoxide may quickly accumulate within a car which is following another at usual trailing distance and that the gas may enter the trailing car whether its windows are open or shut. An appreciation by the physician of these hazards of carbon monoxide asphyxiation of milder degrees, which may result indirectly in serious or even fatal accidents, and the proper dissemination of this knowledge to the laity may go far towards lessening this large number of "mystery" accidents over which we may be justly concerned.

Like many another blessing to humanity, unless intelligently operated and properly safeguarded, the automobile may become an instrument of death and destruction.

THE ETIOLOGY OF RICKETS

Prior to the studies of Mellanby in 1919, rickets and its handmaiden, malnutrition, were considered as inter-reciprocal parts of the same disease mechanism. As elements in a vicious cycle, rickets was considered the result of malnutrition, and in turn an ever-increasing malnutrition was the constant sequel to rickets. During the three or four years immediately following Mellanby's observations a large volume of confirmatory evidence was accumulated in many clinics and laboratories, so that by 1922, Vitamin D had been separated from Vitamin A and its anti-rachitic properties were well understood. During the past ten years these results have won for Vitamin D a place among the truly specific therapeutic agents and the deficiency of this vitamin has been thoroughly established as the principal factor in the production of rickets.

Lending additional evidence to the fact that rickets is not the result of under-nourishment or malnutrition may be cited a recent study made by the United States Childrens' Bureau of the children in Puerto Rico. The Bureau reports an observation of 584 children over a period of three years in Puerto Rico, where the majority of children are greatly under-nourished, some even to the point of starvation. Of this group only five were found during this period to have definite rickets. They conclude that the absence of rickets in these children, in spite of their poor state of nourishment, is due to the fact that they spend most of their time in the tropical sunshine. It is further suggested from this observation that tropical sunshine offers greater protection against rickets than the conventional amounts of cod liver oil or other Vitamin D derivatives.

This latter statement is supported by observation made in the United States where children who received generous amounts of cod liver oil were found suffering from slight rickets. The Childrens' Bureau proposes a complete study of the factors operating in this latter group, but believes that malnutrition plays no essential part. These American children are, for the most part, of normal or very slightly subnormal weight. Apparently the last word has not been said concerning either the etiology or prevention of rickets, and the researches of the Childrens' Bureau are to be commended.

SPEAKERS BUREAU ACTIVITIES

ROLL OF HONOR

For some time, it has been the feeling of the members of the Speakers Bureau Committee that some recognition should be given the doctors who are supporting the postgraduate courses sponsored by the Bureau. These physicians are devoting their time and money in the interests of scientific medicine to the end that they may become better doctors. Many of them drive long distances in all kinds of weather to attend these courses once a week, when given in their locality.

The three postgraduate courses which the Speakers Bureau offered this spring have just been completed. In recognition of their interest in keeping abreast of medical progress, the Speakers Bureau is publishing a list or an honor roll of the doctors who took these courses.

Doctors Taking the Complete Course at Creston

C. A. Ayres, Lorimor	J. G. Macrae, Creston
C. L. Bain, Corning	J. E. McFarland, Leon
A. S. Beatty, Creston	R. S. McKean, Murray
Howard Beatty, Creston	John C. Parsons, Creston
F. Binder, Corning	V. Powell, Red Oak
A. S. Bowers, Orient	D. L. Raffington, Creston
A. W. Brunk, Prescott	C. C. Rambo, Creston
W. H. Cash, Lenox	W. S. Reiley, Red Oak
H. A. Child), Creston	E. O. Reynolds, Greenfield
C. A. Conklin, Garden Grove	C. B. Roe, Afton
G. A. Cooper, Red Oak	C. E. Sampson, Creston
J. C. Cooper, Villisca	H. E. Story, Osceola
J. W. Fry, Creston	F. W. Sells, Osceola
J. H. Gasson, Red Oak	E. K. Sexsmith, Greenfield
H. V. Golden, Clarinda	C. E. Sixbury, Lamoni
Martin Sukov, Clarinda	H. M. Smith, Clarinda
C. F. Obermann, Clarinda	J. T. Stanton, Mt. Ayr
C. R. Harken, Osceola	J. B. Stoll, Creston
J. N. Goodman, Osceola	T. F. Thomsen, Red Oak
J. A. Harper, Greenfield	E. Tinsman, Orient
O. B. Hawley, Corning	J. H. Wallahan, Corning
J. W. Hill, Mt. Ayr	E. J. Watson, Diagonal
K. R. Huff, Lenox	A. F. Watts, Creston
C. N. Hyatt, Humeston	Adam Weaver, Cumberland
M. E. Johnson, Corning	R. E. Wiley, Fontanelle
W. K. Keith, Creston	

The Following Doctors Attended One or Two of the Lectures

W. F. Amdor, Carbon	J. S. Coontz, Leon
I. Taylor, Earlham	C. B. Hickenlooper, Winterset
F. K. Burnett, Clarinda	J. D. Shively, Osceola
F. H. Clark, Clarinda	O. L. Fullerton, Redding
B. S. Walker, Corydon	F. A. Bowman, Leon
F. S. Bowen, Woodburn	M. W. Rogers, Leon
J. F. Aldrich, Shenandoah	J. F. Veltman, Winterset
E. E. Shaw, Indianola	G. J. Anderson, Winterset
Max Witte, Bangor, Maine	

Doctors Taking the Entire Course at Oskaloosa

C. N. Bos, Oskaloosa	Lyle Venable, New Sharon
Walter Campbell, Oskaloosa	W. N. Wright, Rose Hill
L. F. Catterson, Oskaloosa	D. S. Burbank, Pleasantville

M. Childress, Oskaloosa	P. E. Newport, CCC Camp
G. H. Clark, Oskaloosa	D. L. Grothaus, Delta
P. M. Day, Oskaloosa	J. C. Kepler, Kirksville
F. A. Gillett, Oskaloosa	John Maxwell, What Cheer
M. R. Greenlee, Oskaloosa	J. A. Dulin, Sigourney
F. J. Jarvis, Oskaloosa	T. G. Dulin, Sigourney
B. O. Jerrel, Oskaloosa	A. P. Johnson, Sigourney
K. L. Johnston, Oskaloosa	F. B. Ralston, Knoxville
C. H. Merrill, Oskaloosa	F. M. Wright, Knoxville
L. A. Rodgers, Oskaloosa	Harry P. Engle, Newton
E. B. Wilcox, Oskaloosa	J. A. W. Johnson, Newton
E. M. Williams, Oskaloosa	J. E. Traister, Eddyville
B. G. Williams, Oskaloosa	E. S. Macrae, Eddyville
Manley Forsyth, Fremont	L. A. Prewitt, Ottumwa
G. E. Bartlett, New Sharon	J. J. Sybenga, Pella

Those Taking One or Two of the Lectures

C. L. Heald, Sigourney	C. I. Fox, Pella
J. C. Hill, Newton	Ralph McLaughlin, Monroe
H. C. Payne, Pella	F. D. Walk, South English
C. Aschenbrenner, Pella	F. L. Nelson, Ottumwa
E. C. McClure, Bussey	

Doctors Taking the Complete Course at Mt. Pleasant

O. A. Geeseka, Mt. Pleasant	F. R. North, Winfield
S. W. Huston, Mt. Pleasant	J. S. Gaumer, Fairfield
J. W. Laird, Mt. Pleasant	K. G. Cook, Fairfield
C. W. Gardner, Mt. Pleasant	L. D. James, Fairfield
F. M. Edwards, D.D.S., Mt. Pleasant	R. G. Swinney, Richland
	I. F. Thompson, Donnellson
F. V. Coles, Mt. Pleasant	J. L. Saar, Donnellson
J. R. McKirahan, Wayland	E. J. Lessenger, New London
E. C. Allen, Wayland	J. M. Howe, Hillsboro
F. C. Harrison, Winfield	D. H. King, Batavia

Those Attending One or Two of the Lectures

F. H. Mehler, New London	G. H. Gilfillan, Cantril
W. S. Lessenger, Mt. Pleasant	Geo. B. Crow, Burlington
W. A. Sternberg, Mt. Pleasant	J. N. Patterson, Burlington

Especial recognition should be accorded Drs. John C. Parsons, Creston; L. A. Rodgers, Oskaloosa; L. F. Catterson, Oskaloosa, and J. W. Laird, Mt. Pleasant, who have had charge of the local arrangements for these postgraduate courses and whose splendid cooperation greatly contributed to the success of the work.

RADIO TALKS

WOI—Fridays, 6:45 p. m.

WSUI—Thursdays, 8:00 p. m.

May 3- 4—Sleeping Sickness, Jesse L. Saar, M.D.

10-11—Mother's Day—J. H. Kinnaman, M.D.

17-18—Posture—Malcolm Royal, M.D.

24-25—Our Glands and Ourselves—J. W. Billingsley, M.D.

WOMAN'S AUXILIARY NEWS

Edited by the Press and Publicity Committee

MRS. OLIVER J. FAY, *Chairman*, 405 Thirty-seventh Street, Des Moines

CONTEST WINNERS

The final judging of the essays submitted in the Health Essay Contest, recently sponsored by the Woman's Auxiliary and the Speakers Bureau, was completed just as last month's JOURNAL was being printed. Auxiliary members are undoubtedly anxious to know which ones of the two hundred contestants were judged the prize winners.

Miss Eleanora Liljegren, senior, of Harcourt, was awarded first place and a prize of fifteen dollars. Second place and ten dollars went to Mildred Mauer, of Minden, and Paul McGiveren, of Alburnett, won third place and five dollars.

In addition to these three main prizes, a prize of one dollar was awarded to each of the students writing the twenty next best essays. Those achieving this honorable mention are:

Wilma N. Axel, Muscatine
Cella Conklin, Avoca
LaNora Dippel, Marion
Jeneva Flayharty, Mt. Union
Helen Mary Hinsch, McGregor
Gertrude Kuhn, Ft. Atkinson
Dorothea League, Perry
Ruth McCullough, Wapello
Otto Matthias, Anamosa
Maxine Merkel, Ankeny
Harriett Miller, Quimby
Madonna Miller, Lawler
Helen Ann Morrison, Dubuque
Phyllis Nelle, Le Mars
John Ott, Sanborn
Francis Otto, Preston
Jack Peterson, Truesdale
Charlotte St. Onge, Sioux City
Margaret Seddon, Melcher
Jane Veitch, Schaller

The essay winning first place was broadcast over both radio stations WOI and WSUI. Through the courtesy of the Speakers Bureau, Miss Liljegren was sent to Ames personally to present her essay over WOI on the regular broadcasting period of the Iowa State Medical Society on April 20, at 6:45 p. m. Mrs.

W. A. Seidler, President of the Woman's Auxiliary, introduced Miss Liljegren and gave a brief account of the contest before the essay was read. Miss Liljegren wrote a letter thanking the Auxiliary and the Speakers Bureau for the money sent her and in the letter remarked that "The privilege of broadcasting was a pleasant experience which I shall long remember."

It is hoped that the interest which has been shown in this contest will carry over until next year and that the Health Essay Contest may become an annual event.

MEDICAL EXHIBIT

Through the efforts of the Woman's Auxiliary, the American Medical Association is to have an exhibit at the annual meeting of the National Congress of Parents and Teachers which is to be held in Des Moines immediately following the annual meeting of the Iowa State Medical Society. In addition to the exhibit, free copies of *Hygeia* will be distributed to all those registering at the meeting.

THE CLEVELAND MEETING

The Woman's Auxiliary to the American Medical Association will hold its annual meeting in conjunction with that scientific body, in Cleveland, Ohio, June 11-15, 1934. It is hoped that many members of the Woman's Auxiliary to the Iowa State Medical Society will be able to attend and profit from the many interesting sessions which have been arranged. Auxiliary headquarters will be at the Carter Hotel, and all members are requested to register there immediately upon their arrival.

NEW AUXILIARY IN MARION COUNTY

Officers of the newly organized Woman's Auxiliary to the Marion County Medical Society are: Mrs. H. C. Payne of Pella, president; Mrs. E. C. McClure of Bussey, secretary; and Mrs. D. S. Burbank of Pleasantville, treasurer.

SOCIETY PROCEEDINGS

Boone-Story Society

A meeting of the Boone and Story County Medical Societies was held Tuesday, April 17, at the Holst Hotel in Boone. Following the seven o'clock dinner, James F. Edwards, M.D., of the Iowa State College at Ames, reported on Student Health Activities, and John F. Morse, M.D., of Nevada, spoke on Fractures.

Buchanan County

The regular meeting of the Buchanan County Medical Society was held in Independence, Thursday, April 5. Dinner was served at six-thirty, after which F. P. McNamara, M.D., of Dubuque, gave an illustrated talk on Observations of Interesting Cases that come to Necropsy. The paper was discussed by John L. Kestel, M.D., of Waterloo, and F. R. Mulsow, M.D., of Cedar Rapids.

M. C. Melrose, M.D., Secretary.

Calhoun County

The Calhoun County Medical Society held its monthly meeting at the McVay Hospital in Lake City, Tuesday, April 17. Preceding the scientific program a dinner was served at one of the local restaurants. Warren McCrary, M.D., of Lake City, presented a very interesting paper on Gallbladder Disease, which was freely discussed by the members present. Since the state meeting in May, and the Twin Lakes District meeting in June conflict with future meetings, it was decided to have our next meeting in July, at which time arrangements will be made for a picnic preceding a scientific program.

W. W. Stevenson, M.D., Secretary.

Cerro Gordo County

Thirty-eight members of the Cerro Gordo County Medical Society met at the Hotel Hanford, Tuesday, April 17, for the regular monthly meeting. Walter A. Fansler, M.D., assistant professor of surgery at the University of Minnesota School of Medicine, presented the scientific program, speaking on Cancer of the Rectum. The address was illustrated with lantern slides.

The next meeting will be held Monday, May 14, with Verne C. Hunt, M.D., of Los Angeles, California, as guest speaker. His subject will be Cancer of the Breast.

Clinton County

The members of the Clinton County Medical Society held their monthly meeting at the Lafayette Hotel in Clinton, Thursday, April 5. After a dinner in the main dining room, we enjoyed a talk given by G. K. Fenn, M.D., of the Northwestern University School of Medicine, Chicago, on Some Experimental and Clinical Considerations of the Coronary Circulation. Dr. Fenn illustrated his lecture by the use of lantern slides. L. O. Riggert, M.D., Coroner of Clinton County, also spoke briefly on his experiences with coronary disease as a coroner. A short business session was held and the Iowa sales tax insofar as it applies to physicians was discussed.

Eugene V. Donlan, M.D., Secretary.

Dallas-Guthrie Society

Thursday, April 19, the Dallas-Guthrie Medical Society met in Panora, and the following program was presented: Fractures of the Bones of the Arm, W. Eugene Wolcott, M.D., of Des Moines; and Neurological Examination Methods, Frank A. Ely, M.D., also of Des Moines.

Fayette County

D. W. Ward, M.D., of Oelwein, was the speaker of the evening when the Fayette County Medical Society met in West Union, Tuesday, March 27. The subject of his talk was Abnormalities of the Abdomen.

Floyd County Meetings

The regular scientific meeting of the Floyd County Medical Society was held at the Hotel Hildreth, Tuesday, March 27, and the following two papers were presented: Kerosene Poison, C. H. Cords, M.D., of Rudd, and The Surgical Importance of Pockets, Julius Niemack, M.D., of Charles City.

Tuesday, April 24, the Floyd County Medical Society met at the Y. M. C. A. at 8:00 p. m. The meeting was preceded by a six-thirty dinner at the Garden Cafe. Ray A. Fox, M.D., of Charles City, gave a paper on Biliary Diseases with Special Reference to Complications. The following case reports were presented by Charles City physicians; Culdesac Hernia and Garrulity, A. F. Kober, M.D.; Frontal Sinus Complicated by Nonspecific Meningitis, F. H. Fillenwarth, M.D.; Epidemic Meningitis, C. W. McQuillen, M.D., and Surgery of Pulmonary Tuberculosis, H. A. Tolliver, M.D.

James B. Miner, Jr., M.D., Secretary.

Jasper County

J. W. Young, M.D., of Newton, read a paper on Socialized Medicine, at a meeting of the Jasper County Medical Society held in Newton, Tuesday, April 3.

Jefferson County

Robert O. Hughes, M.D., of Ottumwa, furnished the scientific program for the Jefferson County Medical Society, when that organization met in Fairfield,

Wednesday, April 18. He spoke on Methods of Diagnosis of Diseases of Children.

Johnson County

Harry L. Alexander, M.D., associate professor of medicine, at Washington University School of Medicine, St. Louis, and editor of the *Journal of Allergy*, addressed the Johnson County Medical Society, Wednesday, April 4, on the subject of Allergy from the Standpoint of the General Practitioner. Dr. Alexander's refreshingly sane attitude and thorough grasp of his subjct, together with his pleasing delivery, made a deep impression on his audience.

Horace M. Korns. M.D., Secretary.

Keokuk County

Members of the Keokuk County Medical Society, and the Keokuk County Dental Association met in joint session, Monday, April 16, at the Sigourney Hotel in Sigourney. The meeting was held in honor of Dr. Charles B. Taylor, president of the Iowa State Medical Society, who was formerly a resident of Keokuk County and practiced at What Cheer. The guest speaker was R. A. Fenton, D.D.S., of Iowa City, who spoke on Focal Infections.

Linn County

William J. Mayo, M.D., of Rochester, Minnesota, will be the guest speaker of the Linn County Medical Society at its meeting to be held in Cedar Rapids, Thursday, June 7.

Louisa County

The Louisa County Medical Society met Thursday, April 12, at Letts. After the six-thirty dinner, Mrs. Charles Herrick read a paper on The Relation of the Nurse to the Doctor, and Roy E. Tandy, M.D., of Oakville, spoke on The Relation of the Doctor to the Nurse.

Madison County

The Madison County Medical Society, on the date of its regular monthly meeting, Monday, April 9, honored Dr. W. H. Thompson of Winterset at a dinner given in the local Rotary Club rooms, in observance of his fifty years of service in the practice of medicine. The meeting was called to order by the president, Dr. Arnold L. Nelson, who on behalf of the society presented the honored guest with a basket of flowers. In recognition of his long and faithful service, Dr. Thompson was voted an honorary membership in the Madison County Medical Society, and our delegate to the annual session was instructed to make application for a life membership for Dr. Thompson in the Iowa State Medical Society. The meeting was then turned over to Dr. Channing G. Smith of Granger who presided as toastmaster over a program consisting of short congratulatory talks interspersed with musical numbers, and an address by Dr. Thompson, reminiscent of the past fifty years.

C. B. Hickenlooper, M.D., Secretary.

Marshall County

Albert M. Snell, M.D., of Rochester, Minnesota, presented Early and Late Sequelae of Operation on the Gallbladder, before the Marshall County Medical Society, Friday evening, April 6.

Polk County

The regular monthly scientific meeting of the Des Moines Academy of Medicine and Polk County Medical Society was held at Hotel Fort Des Moines, Tuesday evening, April 24.

The meeting was opened with the presentation of clinical cases. Lester D. Powell, M.D., presented three cases of perforated duodenal ulcer; Daniel J. Glomset, M.D., discussed a case of auricular flutter; and Lawrence D. Smith, M.D., reported a case of abruptio placentae.

William E. Sanders, M.D., called attention to a Round Table Cancer Conference being held at Broadlawns General Hospital and urged members of the society to attend. The scientific program was opened with a paper on Trichomonas Vaginalis Vaginitis by Helen Johnston, M.D. Discussion was opened by Floyd W. Rice, M.D., and continued by Drs. Joseph Brown, Lawrence D. Smith and Henry E. Kleinberg.

Edward J. Harnagel, M.D., lectured on Jaundice. Discussion was opened by Julius S. Weingart, M.D., and Arnold M. Gordon, M.D., made some additional comments regarding the disease.

Approximately 125 members were in attendance at the meeting, and a large number of them remained for the usual social hour.

Pottawattamie County

Members of the Pottawattamie County Medical Society met at the Chieftain Hotel in Council Bluffs, Thursday, April 26, at which time the following program was presented by Council Bluffs physicians: Indications for Tracheotomy, Jack V. Treynor, M.D.; The Estimation of Disability in Injured Workmen, Karl Werndorff, M.D.; and Report of the Chicago Meeting of the American College of Physicians, A. A. Johnson, M.D.

Arnold L. Jensen, M.D., Secretary.

Scott County

David S. Hillis, M.D., assistant professor of obstetrics, Northwestern University Medical School, Chicago, was the speaker at the monthly meeting of the Scott County Medical Society held in Davenport, Tuesday, April 3. Dr. Hillis spoke on Obstetrics and the General Practitioner.

Washington County

The Washington County Medical Society held its regular monthly meeting, Tuesday, April 3, in the court house at Washington. Erwin von Graff, M.D., of Iowa City, spoke on Ectopic Pregnancy, and exhibited specimens. It was very interesting and instructive. At the close of the meeting, Miss Marian

Baker, social welfare worker of the county, held a conference with the doctors on the relief work which is being accomplished.

W. S. Kyle, M.D., Secretary.

Woodbury County Meetings

The Woodbury County Medical Society held its regular monthly meeting, Thursday, March 29 at the West Hotel in Sioux City. J. W. Graham, M.D., of Sioux City, discussed a paper on Fractures of the Radius and Ulna.

Thursday, April 19, members of the society met at the West Hotel in Sioux City, at which time the scientific program was presented by members of the Pottawattamie County Medical Society. In exchange for this interesting program, members of the Woodbury County Medical Society will present a program before the Pottawattamie County Medical Society next month at Council Bluffs. The program was as follows: The Traumatic Abdomen, Arnold L. Jensen, M.D.; Transurethral Prostatic Resection, Gerald V. Caughlan, M.D.; and The Education of the Diabetic Patient, Raymond Rice, M.D. This program was very much appreciated by all those present and it is earnestly hoped that these exchange meetings may become an annual custom.

Lawrence E. Pierson, M.D., Secretary.

INTERESTING NEWS
In Brief

Recently published figures indicate an increase of over $18,000 in Linn County's medical relief costs for 1933 over that of 1932.

A donation of $300,000 has been received by the University of Wisconsin Medical School to finance an elaborate laboratory for the study of cancer.

A report of the state auditor indicates a saving of over $20,000 in the operating costs of the State Hospital at Cherokee for the year 1933 over that of 1932.

Research on filterable virus diseases of the eye will be carried on at the University of Iowa under terms of a $300 grant from the American Medical Association.

More than 15,000 visits were made by physicians connected with the Woodbury County Medical Clinic during a eight and one-half months' period ending January 1, 1934.

The Division of Vital Statistics of the Iowa State Health Department reveal a decrease in both the death and birth rates in Iowa in 1933, with 38,000 births and 25,000 deaths.

Studies directed toward the physiologic activity of schizophrenic patients indicate that the metabolic rate varies markedly without apparent cause, and that the blood pressure, pulse rate and red blood count are consistently lower than in the normal individual.

Dr. William H. Park, veteran director of the New York City Department of Health, has been given the Public Welfare Medal of the National Academy of Sciences in recognition of his work in research and disease prevention.

Of 1,453 students tested with tuberculin by the Von Pirquet skin test at Iowa State College, 90 per cent of the men and 83 per cent of the women gave negative reactions. Of the 179 who gave a positive reaction, 70 per cent were essentially negative by x-ray examination.

Terminating a service established in 1924, the Washington County supervisors recently voted to discontinue the health unit in Washington County. Because of the opposition among the taxpayers it is expected that this action may be reconsidered by the county supervisors.

A new and as yet unnamed anesthetic has been demonstrated at Sinai hospital, Baltimore, by Dr. A. E. Goldstein. A satisfactorily narcotizing sleep is produced in twenty minutes after intravenous injection of this anesthetic substance. Recovery is said to be prompt and without nausea or other undesirable after-effects.

Doctors William J. and Charles Mayo, surgeons of Rochester, Minnesota, recently announced a donation of $500,000 to the University of Minnesota to be used in the furtherance of medical science. In confirming the donation the Doctors Mayo stated that inasmuch as the money came from the sick "we believe it should return to the sick."

Rivaling the late plant wizard, Burbank, but in an entirely different fashion, two Canadian scientists have recently produced a potato containing little or no starch. This result has been accomplished by the introduction of proper enzymes into the stalk of the growing potato plant. What use there may be for the starchless potato remains to be determined.

Charging conspiracy, a Wisconsin physician and his wife have sued the Hotel Congress and Dr. Herman Bundeson, Chicago Health Commissioner. Each of the plaintiffs suffered attacks of dysentery said to have been contracted while they were guests at the hotel. Dr. Bundeson was accused of negligence and conspiracy in failing to announce the dysentery outbreak at an earlier date.

Johns Hopkins' well known professor of biology, Dr. Raymond Pearl, recently attracted newspaper attention by a report which showed that "under present-day conditions of life the average birth rate is lowered 73 per cent below its natural level." Explaining this statement he indicated that in his study of 5,000 married women, 48 per cent practiced birth control and "produced only planned and wanted babies exactly when they wished to have them."

Have you missed the oily voice of John R. (Goat Gland) Brinkley over your radio?' His high-power station located in Villa Acuna, Mexico, just across the Rio Grande from Del Rio has been silenced by the Mexican government, who charge Brinkley with the illegal practice of medicine without permit. It would appear that Brinkley must pack his radio station on to a flat boat and tow it out into the Atlantic Ocean beyond the twelve-mile limit, if he wishes to continue restoring pristine vigor to decrepit old men by way of his gland transplantations.

PERSONAL MENTION

Dr. Otis Wolfe of Marshalltown, while on the lecture cruise of the Pan-American Medical Association to Caribbean and South American countries, gave an illustrated lecture on "A Journey to Spain" before the General Assembly, and a paper on "The Modified Barraquer Cataract Technic" before the Section on Ophthalmology.

Dr. A. B. Phillips 'was recently elected mayor of Clear Lake.

Dr. Joyce G. Schmidt of Postville, who for the past four years has been associated in the practice of medicine with her father, the late Dr. A. A. Schmidt, has retired from active practice, and is leaving for Galva, Iowa, to join her husband and establish a home at that place.

Dr. R. Parker Noble, who has practiced medicine at Norway, Iowa, for the past two years, will enter general practice at Cherokee, devoting special attention to children's diseases.

Dr. Eugene Smith of Waterloo, spoke on "Mental Hygiene" at the meeting of the Registered Nurses Society of Black Hawk County, Wednesday, April 18.

Dr. Jacob Breid, head of the Indian sanatorium and superintendent of the Sac and Fox agency in Marshalltown for the past fourteen years, has resigned his position, and is leaving for Trenton County, Missouri, where he will spend the summer. He plans to spend next winter in California. He will be succeeded by Dr. Ira D. Nelson, who for the past four years has been physician and superintendent at the Indian hospital in Claremore, Oklahoma.

Dr. Stella Mason of Mason City, sailed from Seattle on April 28 on the President Jackson for Yokahama, Japan. After a short visit there, she will sail for Vladivostok to begin a long inland journey across Siberia to Russia, after which she will go to Warsaw and Berlin. Dr. Mason plans to be away six months.

Dr. A. V. Hardy of Iowa City, connected with the hygiene and preventive medicine department of the State University of Iowa College of Medicine, has left for Chicago, at the request of the United States

Public Health Service, where he will spend the next three months studying the outbreak of amebic dysentery, which centered about Chicago last fall.

Dr. F. W. Mulsow of Cedar Rapids, was the guest speaker at the Cedar Rapids Lions Club, Tuesday, April 10. His subject was "Microbes."

Dr. Laydon Wentworth has located in Marble Rock, where he has purchased the equipment and practice of Dr. E. E. Lashbrook, who has moved to Estherville. Dr. Wentworth is a graduate of the State University of Iowa College of Medicine, and has just completed a three years' internship at the Henry Ford Hospital in Detroit.

Dr. Philip C. Jeans of Iowa City, discussed "New Knowledge in the Physical Care of the Child" at the regular monthly meeting of the Child Study Club, Saturday, April 7.

Dr. John Walter Martin, formerly of Des Moines, is returning to that city from Baltimore, Maryland, where he has resided for the past five years, and where he was engaged as surgical director and vice president of the United States Fidelity and Guaranty Insurance Company. He will resume private practice upon his arrival in Des Moines.

Dr. John G. Goggin of Cedar Rapids, has located in Ossian, where he has purchased the office equipment and practice of the late Dr. J. A. Juen.

Dr. C. H. Graening of Waverly, spoke at Janesville, Wednesday, April 18, for a community meeting arranged by the American Legion Auxiliary. His subject was "Prevention of Contagious Disease and Child Care and Development".

Dr. E. D. Plass of Iowa City addressed the Tri-City Alumnae of the Normal College of Physical Education, at Indianapolis, Saturday, April 21. His lecture was on "Physical Education and Its Relation to the Biological Functions of Women".

MARRIAGES

Miss Elizabeth Jane Lutz of Des Moines and Dr. Joseph B. Priestley of Des Moines were married at the home of the bride's mother, Mrs. Walter Blackburn Lutz, Saturday, April 14. Dr. and Mrs. Priestley left immediately after the ceremony for a two weeks' trip after which they will be at home in Des Moines, where the groom has been engaged in the practice of medicine for the past two years.

DEATH NOTICES

Huntoon, DeWitt Clinton, of Waterloo, aged sixty-one, died April 17, as the result of a stroke. He was graduated in 1903 from Rush Medical College, Chicago, and at the time of his death was a member of the Black Hawk County Medical Society.

King, Thomas Wayne, of Lamoni, aged fifty-three, died March 28, as a result of a skull fracture incurred in a fall some time ago. He was graduated in 1905 from Ensworth Medical College, St. Joseph, Missouri, and had been a member of the Decatur County Medical Society.

McCreight, Arthur Henry, of Fort Dodge, aged sixty-eight, died March 28, after a several weeks' illness of pneumonia. He was graduated in 1897 from Rush Medical College, Chicago, and at the time of his death was a member of the Webster County Medical Society.

Sanders, Charles Willard, of Northwood, aged seventy-four, died March 27, following a stroke of apoplexy. He was graduated in 1884 from Rush Medical College, Chicago, and recently completed fifty years of practice in Worth County. At the time of his death he was a member of the Worth County Medical Society.

Shultz, Charles S., of Spirit Lake, aged seventy-one, died April 12, after a short illness of pneumonia. He was graduated in 1891 from the State University of Iowa, College of Medicine, Iowa City, and at the time of his death was a member of the Dickinson County Medical Society.

OBITUARIES

ISSI OTTO POND, M.D.
1873-1934

Dr. I. O. Pond, for thirty-three years a surgeon and general practitioner of medicine, first at Sioux Rapids, Iowa, and later at Perry, Iowa, died suddenly from an acute heart attack at his home at Perry, Thursday, March 15, 1934.

He was graduated in 1901 from the State University of Iowa College of Medicine, and then went to Sioux Rapids, Iowa, where he opened a private hospital. In 1905 he attended the Chicago Polyclinic School of Surgery.

Dr. Pond moved to Perry in 1914 where he was Surgeon in Chief of the King's Daughters' Hospital for many years. He was also the Dallas county surgeon from 1920 to 1934, and surgeon for the Chicago, Milwaukee and St. Paul Railway. He was affiliated with many professional and social organizations. It was through Dr. Pond's untiring efforts and efficient management that the Perry hospital was brought from a weak institution to one of strength.

During his lifetime he had ministered to thousands and until his health was partially broken some months ago, responded to all demands for his knowledge and service without thought of the cost. He was a true friend, and many in poverty can testify to his deeds of kindness and healing ministry. Dr. Pond had en-

deared himself to members of his profession in Perry and Dallas county. He was often called in consultation, since diagnosis was his speciality. Dr. A. J. Ross, Perry, one of his closest associates, says that he was a surgeon of considerable note and had unusual ability and perception enabling him to perform operations of a delicate nature, successfully. Dr. Pond was a man of versatile mind. His interests included philosophy, modern problems of economics and studies suited to the scholar. All these things made him a doctor admired for his skill, a citizen with an interesting personality, and a man of the highest moral and spiritual order.

He is survived by his wife, a son, Waldo, who is a student of Drake law school, a daughter, Almeda Florence, and a daughter, Helen M.

S. J. Brown, M.D.

ARTHUR HENRY McCREIGHT, M.D.
1866-1934

At a meeting of Webster County Medical Society held April 19, the following resolution was passed in regard to the death of Dr. A. H. McCreight of Fort Dodge, and it was recommended that a copy be forwarded to the Iowa State Medical Society for publication in the JOURNAL.

"In memory of one who has finished his work, fought the good fight and gained the victory over death, we offer the following resolution:

"*Whereas,* Dr. Arthur H. McCreight has passed on to a more perfect existence, and has left hearts that are lonely and a place that cannot be filled,

"*Be It Resolved,* That we, the Medical Society of Webster County, express our sense of loss and loving sympathy to the family and friends who will miss his companionship and sympathetic understanding."

John C. Shrader, M.D.

WARNING!

A Delaware County physician has recently advised us of the activities of one W. J. Canning, giving an Iowa address at Davenport and purporting to represent the Alicante Vineyards Company, 20 West Jackson Blvd., Chicago. Our informant reports that this agent is visiting doctors, selling wine flavors in small keg lots. He collects a deposit at the time the order is taken and the purchaser agrees to pay the remaining sum on delivery from Chicago. It appears that Solicitor Canning is acting without authority since our informant received no merchandise and his letters to both the solicitor and the Chicago company are unanswered.

The central office of the Iowa State Medical Society would be glad to receive information concerning the operations of this solicitor.

HISTORY OF MEDICINE IN IOWA

Edited by the Historical Committee

DR. HENRY B. YOUNG, Burlington   DR. TOM. B. THROCKMORTON, Des Moines
DR. FRANK M. FULLER, Keokuk   DR. WALTER L. BIERRING, Des Moines
                    DR. JOHN T. MCCLINTOCK, Iowa City

History of the Iowa State Board of Health

FREDERICK J. SWIFT, M.D.,
Deputy Commissioner—State Department of Health
Des Moines, Iowa

The first meeting of the newly created Iowa State Board of Health was held at the State House in Des Moines on May 5, 1880.

For several legislative sessions state societies representing the regular, homeopathic and eclectic schools of medical practice had been active in sponsoring a State Board of Health bill in connection with a Medical Practice Act, but without success.

On January 29, 1880, in the 18th General Assembly, Mr. Palmer of Guthrie County introduced House File 258 and Senator Ham of Dubuque introduced Senate File 98 entitled "An Act to establish a State Board of Health in the State of Iowa, to provide for collecting vital statistics and to assign certain duties to local boards of health, and to punish neglect of duties." This bill was referred to the Senate Committee on Medicine and Surgery and reported out for passage; but, on motion of Senator Larrabee it was re-referred to the Committee and a substitute bill was prepared. This substitute bill passed the Senate on February 27, 1880, the House on March 25, 1880 and was signed by Governor John H. Gear on March 26, 1880.

The Act provided that the Board should consist of nine persons one of whom should be the Attorney General (by virtue of his office), one a civil engineer and seven physicians. The term of the office was fixed as seven years, and in the case of physician members, the term of one should expire each year.

The following appointments were made: William S. Robertson, M.D., Muscatine; Phillip W. Llewellyn, M.D., Clarinda; Wilmot H. Dickinson, M.D., Des Moines; Henry H. Clark, M.D., McGregor; Justin M. Hull, M.D., Lake Mills; Ephraim M. Reynolds, M. D., Centerville; George

F. Roberts, M.D., Waterloo; James F. Loring, civil engineer, Dallas Center; John F. McJunkin, attorney general, Washington. At the first meeting a permanent organization was perfected, and

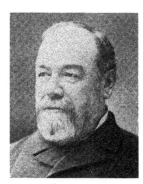

DR. W. S. ROBERTSON
President State Board of Health
1880-1887

Dr. W. S. Robertson was elected president and Mr. L. F. Andrews as secretary.

Dr. Robertson was a graduate of Jefferson Medical College, Philadelphia, a Civil War veteran and Professor of Theory and Practice of Medicine of the Medical Department, State University of Iowa. He had been a member of its faculty since 1869, and had taken an active part in its organization.

On taking the chair as president he addressed the Board as follows:

"Gentlemen: We have come together at the call of the Governor for the purpose of organiz-

The annual appropriation for the first State Board of Health was $5,000.00 with the provision that the secretary's salary should not exceed $1,200.00 per year. The following year the law was changed requiring the secretary to be a physician. Mr. Andrews was elected assistant secretary and served as such for eighteen years. While with the State Board Mr. Andrews prepared and ᴀᴀᴛᴜʀᴇᴅ ᴛʜᴇ ᴘᴀᴀᴀᴀɢᴇ ᴀf ᴛʜᴇ ʟᴀᴡ ʀᴇɢᴜʟᴀᴛɪɴɢ ᴛʜᴇ ᴀᴀʟᴇ and use of oils for illuminating purposes and the making and sale of linseed oil.

Dr. R. J. Farquharson, of Davenport, Iowa, was, on May 5, 1881, elected the first medical secretary of the State Board. Dr. Farquharson was well qualified for this important position and served with honor and distinction. It was a fortunate choice because he brought to the new department the advantage of a cultural education and extensive experience in the practice of medicine. At his untimely death three years later Dr. William D. Middleton of Davenport, Iowa, wrote a tribute which is published in this issue and indicates the high character of the first secretary.

(To be continued)

BIOGRAPHICAL SKETCH

of

ROBERT JAMES FARQUHARSON, M.D.

By W. D. MIDDLETON, M.D.

(Reprinted from the Proceedings of the Davenport Academy of Natural Sciences, Vol IV.)

Dr. Robert James Farquharson was born in Nashville, Tennessee, on the 15th of July, 1824. His father, one of the early settlers of the State, was a Scotchman and his mother a native of Kentucky.

He was an exceedingly apt scholar as a boy, which was shown in his entering the University of Nashville at the early age of fourteen and graduating from that institution in 1841, or when only seventeen years of age. In that period he found time to take an extra course in higher mathematics at the earnest desire of the professor of that branch of instruction, the president speaking of him as "always first in his class" and another from Prof. Troast which testifies to his "application" and his "love for the Natural Sciences." Dr. Farquharson read medicine in the office of Dr. Jennings of his native place, repairing to Philadelphia, then the center of medical education in this country to attend lectures and graduating from the medical department of the University of Pennsylvania in the spring of 1844.

At twenty Dr. Farquharson entered Blackley Hospital to serve for a year, meeting nearly all great lights in medicine of that time on an intimate footing. He graduated from the hospital service with honor and had found time, also to obtain the diploma of the Obstetric Institute, a hospital institution for practical instruction in that branch of science. Paul Goddard and Robert Morris, great physicians of that day, testify to his "high professional qualifications as well as his uniformly amiable and gentlemanly deportment." George B. Wood, M. Clymer, Richard Ashhurst, W. E. Homer, Samuel Jackson, and N. Chapman speak in affectionate terms of his professional attainments and scholarship.

In 1845 he was moved to New Orleans and did regular work in his profession both in private practice and hospital service. In 1847 he entered the U. S. Navy as assistant surgeon. Letters to his father still exist, showing his extensive travel in many parts of the world. While on duty on the Schooner Yancy on the coast of Africa, Dr. Farquharson contracted the deafness, which was, in his own estimation, a great affliction and which caused him to shrink from embracing so many opportunities because of a hypersensitive idea he felt that communication with him was laborious and annoying. Letters from superiors in service during this period speak highly of him.

In 1855 Dr. Farquharson resigned from the navy to marry Mary Lydia Smith of Nashville; after a happy married life of nearly thirty years' duration, she with four children still survive him. After marriage Dr. Farquharson settled in Nashville to practice his profession till the outbreak of the Civil War. He often spoke of the impossibility of conveying how one who had served his country as an officer and taken the oath required prior to such service could ever turn against that flag. This made his life in the south among his old associates unpleasant to him. He was a confidential friend of Andrew Jackson and after occupation of Nashville by the Federals, was employed in military hospitals, having been appointed by Johnson surgeon of his own regiment, 4th Tennessee Infantry; but his deafness caused his resignation very shortly. In 1863 and 1864 Dr. Farquharson was in charge of an extensive hospital at Nashville Military Railroad System, which closed in January, 1865.

After rebellion, he found the largest part of a fair fortune swept away; he moved to Arkansas, doing active and laborious county practice until 1868, when he moved to Davenport. Joining the Academy of Sciences in its first year of existence he took active part until his removal to Des Moines

in 1880. Dr. Farquharson was president of the Academy of Sciences in 1878, a librarian three years, a member of its Library and Publishing Commission six years and of the Commission on Museum three years. He represented it at its meeting in Detroit in 1875, at the American Association for the Advancement of Science, of which he was a permanent member and left in its published proceedings the following papers: Vol. I, "Do Rifle-balls Burn When Striking the Animal Body?", "A Study of Skulls and Long Bones from Mounds Near Albany, Illinois," "Recent Archaeological Discoveries at Davenport, Iowa," Vol. II, "The Inscribed Tablets found by Rev. J. Gass," "Post Mortem Examination of a Boa-Constrictor," "Formation of Ground Ice on the Rapids of the Mississippi," Vol. III, "Annual address, as President, in January 1879."

Dr. Farquharson presented a series of the reports of the French Academy in the original. In 1880 he was appointed by the French Societie Ethnographique—its member for Iowa, with power to recommend any further additions to its membership; this he always considered one of the highest honors ever paid him. His retiring disposition and the singular sensitiveness he displayed in regard to his deafness rendered his strictly professional work somewhat meager and unproductive. The bulk of this was done as a consulting physician. From 1870 he remained a member of the visiting staff of Mercy Hospital until his removal to Des Moines where he was transferred to the consulting staff. Dr. Farquharson planned and supervised construction of the outlying ward for contagious diseases known as St. John's. Plans for this building have since been published and commended by all sanitary authorities of the country and in several places adopted. For years he had thrown the best energies of his active mind into the prevention of disease.

In 1881 Dr. Farquharson was elected Secretary of the State Board of Health and removed to Des Moines. He was also a member of the Sanitary Council of the Mississippi Valley and the American Public Health Association. His worth as a leader in sanitary methods was fully confessed; and as a member of the Iowa State Medical Society, he left his impress on its proceedings in several important papers, an account of original observations on "Leprosy in the State of Iowa" attracting much attention. Dr. Farquharson died in Des Moines, Iowa, September 6, 1884, of dysentery; he was buried in Nashville, Tennessee at Mount Olivette Cemetery.

THE JOURNAL BOOK SHELF

BOOKS RECEIVED

THE BASIS OF PASSIONAL PSYCHOLOGY—By Dr. Jacobus X. French Army Surgeon. Privately printed, American Anthropological Society, 70 Fifth Avenue, New York City, 1934. Price, $4.00.

EXTERNAL DISEASES OF THE EYE, by Donald T. Atkinson, M.D., consulting ophthalmologist to the Santa Rosa Infirmary and the Nix Hospital, San Antonio, Texas. Octavo of 704 pages, illustrated with 479 engravings. Lea & Febiger, Philadelphia, 1934. Price, $7.50.

I KNOW JUST THE THING FOR THAT!—By J. F. Montague, M.D., medical director, New York Intestinal Sanitarium, The John Day Company, New York, 1934. Price, $2.00.

LOVE—A TREATISE ON THE SCIENCE OF SEX ATTRACTION—By Bernard S. Talmey, M.D. Fifth edition, newly revised and enlarged, with 52 illustrations. Eugenics Publishing Company, New York, 1933.

MEDICAL CLINICS OF NORTH AMERICA—Volume xvii, No. 4. Cleveland Clinic Number, per clinic year, July, 1933, to May, 1934. Octavo of 253 pages with 53 illustrations. W. B. Saunders Company, Philadelphia and London. Price, paper, $12.00; cloth, $16.00, net.

MEDICAL CLINICS OF NORTH AMERICA, Volume xvii, No. 5, New York Number, March, 1934. Per clinic year, July, 1933, to May, 1934. Octavo of 324 pages with 32 illustrations. W. B. Saunders Company, Philadelphia and London, 1934. Price, paper, $12.00; cloth, $16.00.

MEDICO-MILITARY SYMPOSIUM, 1934—Conducted under the auspices of the Kansas City Southwest Clinical Society and the Medical Department, Seventh Corps Area, United States Army, at the General Hospital, Kansas City, Missouri, March 12-17, 1934. Brown-White, Publishers, Kansas City, 1934.

THE 1933 YEAR BOOK OF GENERAL THERAPEUTICS—Edited by Bernard Fantus, M.S., M.D., professor of therapeutics, University of Illinois College of Medicine. The Year Book Publishers, Chicago, 1934. Price, $2.25.

THE 1933 YEAR BOOK OF NEUROLOGY AND PSYCHIATRY—Edited by Peter Bassoe, M.D., clinical professor of neurology, Rush Medical College; and Franklin G. Ebaugh, M.D., professor of psychiatry, University of Colorado School of Medicine. The Year Book Publishers, Chicago, 1934.

THE 1933 YEAR BOOK OF UROLOGY—Edited by John H. Cunningham, M.D., associate in genito-urinary surgery, Harvard University Postgraduate School of Medicine. The Year Book Publishers, Chicago, 1934.

SURGICAL CLINICS OF NORTH AMERICA, Volume xiv, No. 1, Philadelphia Number, February, 1934. Per clinic year, February, 1934, to December, 1934. 225 pages with 62 illustrations. W. B. Saunders Company, Philadelphia and London, 1934. Price, paper, $12.00; cloth, $16.00.

SURGICAL CLINICS OF NORTH AMERICA, Volume xiv, No. 2, New York Number, April, 1934. Per clinic year, February, 1934, to December, 1934, 293 pages with 71 illustrations. W. B. Saunders Company, Philadelphia and London, 1934. Price, paper, $12.00; cloth, $16.00.

BOOK REVIEWS

ALLERGY IN GENERAL PRACTICE

By Samuel M. Feinberg, M.D., F.A.C.P., assistant professor of medicine, Northwestern University Medical School, Chicago. Illustrated with 23 engravings and a colored plate. Lea & Febiger, Philadelphia, 1934. Price, $4.50.

There is perhaps no field in the practice of medicine or surgery where the physician does not daily encounter some of the manifestations of the allergic phenomena. It is indeed timely, then, that the subject of allergy should be presented in a readily understandable fashion for the guidance of the practitioner who does not devote special time or consideration to allergy.

The author of this book had in mind just such a class and has successfully discussed the manifestations and problems of allergy with brevity and clearness, so much desired for the rapid understanding of this subject. One feature of the volume which will be found helpful in understanding the protean character of this group of conditions, is the extensive section of the book devoted to the presentation and discussion of case histories. The review of these cases from the author's experience serves to crystallize and make more readily useful the discussion contained in the earlier chapters of the book.

While by no means the most complete or extensive

of the several volumes which have recently appeared on this subject, none of a more practical or helpful character than this one has come to the reviewer's attention. For its qualities of terseness, clearness and thoroughness, this book is recommended to those physicians who would know practical allergy.

ANNUAL REPORT OF THE SURGEON GENERAL OF THE PUBLIC HEALTH SERVICE OF THE UNITED STATES

For the fiscal year 1933. United States Government Printing Office, Washington, D. C. Price, seventy-five cents, cloth.

This report covers the work done in the eight divisions of the public health service. The report of the division on scientific research and that of the division on venereal diseases are perhaps of greatest interest to the general practitioner. Under the former heading is reported the original investigation of the service into such diseases as cancer, leprosy, malaria, heart and nutritional diseases, with reports from the National Institute of Health.

The report of the division on veneral diseases contains a study of untreated syphilis in the negro. This study indicates that syphilis of the cardiovascular system, the central nervous system and the nervous system are common manifestations.

The factual accuracy of the report, together with

its broad scope, makes it particularly valuable to physicians.

――――

MODERN CLINICAL PSYCHIATRY

By Arthur P. Noyes, M.D., Superintendent of State Hospital for Mental Diseases, Howard, Rhode Island. 485 pages. W. B. Saunders Company, Philadelphia and London, 1934. Price, $4.50.

Fully appreciating the needs of the advanced medical student in the field of psychiatry, the author has presented in this volume a highly practical and easily understood discussion of the fundamental principles in this specialty.

His classification of mental abnormalities and psychopathic states appears to be an entirely rational one, and this subject loses much of its traditional abstractness when it is supported by his clear and forceful description of the characteristic symptomatology of each condition.

After a terse description of the physical and psychic elements which enter into the production of a given abnormal mental state, the author reviews its symptomatology and differential diagnosis. In each instance a section suggesting appropriate treatment concludes his discussion. Each chapter carries its separate bibliography.

While this volume might appeal to the well trained psychiatrist as being of an elementary character, it will undeniably appeal to those having a lesser interest in the subject because of its simple, straightforward approach, its clearness of description and its complete lack of tedious discussion or debate concerning either the etiology or the treatment of the several conditions discussed.

――――

OUR MYSTERIOUS LIFE GLANDS AND HOW THEY AFFECT US

By William J. Robinson, M.D., consultant to the department of genito-urinary diseases and dermatology, Bronx Hospital, New York. Eugenics Publishing Company, New York, 1934. Price, $2.50.

Written primarily for the layman, this popular treatise on the glands of internal secretion, their functions and abnormalities, presents a very vivid and readily understandable discussion of this subject. For the most part the author has adhered very strictly to demonstrated facts concerning the physiology and pathology of the several glands. Well aware of the fickleness of human attention and interest, the author has in a few instances digressed somewhat into the theoretical and, in order, no doubt, to maintain the reader's interest, has dwelt at more length than appears justifiable on the ground of frequency, in the discussion of some abnormalities resulting from glandular deficiencies. It is particularly true in the chapter entitled "Homosexuality."

The chapter discussing the present status of rejuvenation is particularly well written and timely

because of many false conceptions accepted by the laity, the result of over-enthusiastic but ill-advised newspaper publicity concerning this subject. An extensive glossary defining technical terms common to this discussion permits the author to maintain a more scientific and more accurate viewpoint in his writing.

Five full chapters are devoted to a discussion of the vitamins, which, while not anticipated in the title of this volume, pleasingly round out his discussion of the "mysterious" secretions of the body now commanding a prominent position in popular fancy. The book is illustrated.

――――

PSYCHOANALYSIS AND MEDICINE

A Study of the Wish to Fall Ill. By Karin Stephen. The MacMillan Company, New York, 1933. Price $2.50.

This book deals with subjects that are given little or no time in the curriculum of the American medical school. Dr. Stephen developed her book from a series of lectures, which was presented to Cambridge students, stressing the medical aspects of psychoanalysis. With commendable lucidity she discusses psychoanalysis as a discipline for investigating unconscious mental processes as well as an instrument for treating certain forms of mental illness. The various basic psychoanalytic concepts such as primitive sexuality, the oedipus complex and defense mechanisms are taken up in detail.

With the uninitiated reader constantly in mind, the author explains questions that arise frequently in regard to this much disputed subject matter. She rightly insists upon a differentiation between psychoanalytic theory, which is subject to modification, and the sound empirical facts. On the therapeutic side, the prolonged nature of the treatment as well as its applicability only to selected cases is emphasized. This is the best general work on psychoanalysis that the reviewer has seen.

M. S.

――――

PSYCHOLOGY OF SEX

A Manual for Students. By Havelock Ellis. Long and Smith, Inc., New York, 1933. Price $3.00.

This volume deals with the psychology of the normal and abnormal sexual impulses. Among the problems discussed are the biology of sex, homosexuality, and marriage. The book is intended for students and general medical men, and gives a list of publications in English at the end of each chapter for further reading. Himself a pioneer and arduous investigator of sexual phenomena, Havelock Ellis has also incorporated the more advanced work of other writers in this field, giving full cognizance to Freud and the psychoanalytic school.

In these days of strong eugenic movements it is worth pointing out that Ellis considers homosexuality to have a well marked hereditary basis.

M. S.

The JOURNAL

of the

Iowa State Medical Society

| Vol. XXIV | Des Moines, Iowa, June, 1934 | No. 6 |

THE PRESIDENT'S ADDRESS—WHO ARE GRADUATES IN MEDICINE?*

Charles B. Taylor, M.D., Ottumwa

"The man who sees keenly, hears clearly, and whose senses, powerful at the start, are sharpened and refined by constant exercise"—Gomprez—if this man be a medical man, he is in a way to become a graduate.

Graduation time, whether in the arts, sciences, law or medicine, has always demanded a vast amount of explanation. The candidate has been inclined to consider himself a finished product. He wonders that the crowd does not say: "Behold the Man."

This is all perfectly natural. For years he has striven to master the sciences included in the curriculum, and has fought the nightmare of being conditioned. He has won, and against great odds. He is told by his college that he is a graduate of medicine. He is recognized by his state as being a graduate. He is registered as a graduate. The convocation orator, alone, tells him he has not graduated; that he has only reached the first mile post; that he has been given the first lecture in his initiation into the medical order; that the mysteries of the cult will only be revealed to him as he is able to understand them—and the convocation orator is the only one who is right.

Is he a graduate, then "Generosity he has, such as is possible to those who practice an art, never to those who drive a trade; discretion tested by a hundred secrets; tact tried in a thousand embarrassments"—Stevenson. This is impossible of accomplishment for one who has just been handed his diploma.

To me it has become increasingly evident that graduate study has been too expensive; too difficult of accomplishment; too much time loss; too much lost motion; that only the very aggressive would get far in graduate study. I can see a phy-

*Presented before the Eighty-third Annual Session, Iowa State Medical Society, Des Moines, May 9, 10, 11, 1934.

sician—and his name might be legion—whose practice is not extremely lucrative; whose families might easily gravitate to his competitor; I can see such a physician easily convincing himself that he can in no wise afford a week, a month, or three months' study in some medical center with all its attendant expense. Facilities have not been provided in college and hospital centers that might meet any large demand in an orderly way.

Who of us has not gone to a city, taken subways and elevated trains to distant hospital centers, and seen only some indifferent work by an interne or resident physician, carrying with it no instruction? Yet this has been about our best way to contact clinical instruction—unless we go to the far distant institutions and register for a lengthy and expensive course costing more than the above designated physician can net in years of practice. But who needs instruction more than he? How can he deliver what he does not have? Perhaps he is a reader. If so he can go far, but few continue with consecutive reading without the stimulus of authoritative contact. Once convinced that he cannot afford graduate study, and unless he is a consistent reader, he becomes complacent, content, egoistic, *in status quo*. The mind that was once fertile is now becoming sterile. Mentally he has become "sickly, stale and unprofitable." Wit he may have but wisdom none. His mind has died by asphyxiation. He has taken his mental life by a lethal dose of non-cerebration, or perhaps like Lazarus, "he is not dead but sleepeth."

It is in the hope that he only sleepeth or in the hope that such sleep can in the future be prevented, that I would gladly welcome some scheme by which every physician can voluntarily inoculate himself with the hormone of knowledge or, if he fails in this, that he be inoculated by state authority. Castor oil may be just as effective when forced as otherwise.

I want it definitely understood that I am describing those physicians who refuse knowledge when it is within their reach.

"Under the old conditions the isolation of the practitioner in many districts, the necessity of dealing with every situation single handed or with the minimum of help of neighboring colleagues, created a type of man, self reliant, skillful, observant, who must surely be ranked among the best that the profession of medicine has produced. They have lived and worked and died, unhonored save in the lasting esteem and memory of the community which they served so faithfully."—Le Flemming.

In Iowa there is no such isolation any more. Yet facilities for training are inadequate. The Commission on Medical Education says, "Keeping physicians aware of and competent to use new knowledge and methods is one of the most important factors in a complete and satisfactory medical service for the community. And the responsibility of providing opportunities for the continuing education of physicians must be shared by the medical profession and the medical schools if they are to work out this essential feature." An extensive survey in Michigan showed that fifty per cent of physicians had had no postgraduate work. No such survey has been made elsewhere, but percentages probably differ little in other states.

A number of states, through the medical societies, are carrying on graduate education similar to the work done by our Speaker's Bureau. Seventy per cent of physicians in the New York State Society have been reached by 116 courses with 632 lectures. Our bureau has been a practically self sustaining institution. The chairman, and others interested, besides those teachers who have made these courses a possibility, have given their time more freely than they should. I am convinced that some plan should be evolved by which extension work might be furnished to all medical men in the state. This should be so arranged that no unreasonable burden would be loaded on any one man or any set of men. The business of instructing *under-graduates* still rests with those professors who are now aiding in this graduate teaching under this bureau. The University Medical Department is not sufficiently manned for both these services. It is manifestly unfair to ask these men to "double time" to the point of exhaustion.

In my opinion, however, this two fold function, to train new physicians, and to continue the training of the practicing physicians, is a duty of a state owned and state operated medical school. I do not believe that it should be done without expense to the receiving physicians, and fair minded and intelligent physicians would not object to paying a reasonable fee for such instruction. But the instruction should be placed within the reach of

every physician, and I believe that some stimulus, bordering closely on compulsion, should be exerted so that physicians might avail themselves of the teaching. No argument is necessary to convince intelligent men that both life and health would be conserved by this plan. The beneficiaries are the people themselves who are treated more intelligently and whose lives and health are saved by better treatment.

There are well trained men in practice in every section of the state, who might be tied in with the extension department of the University. All expenses should be paid and perhaps a reasonable remuneration for time should be allowed. Such teaching practitioners would profit by such a plan. They would themselves become more learned and they would increase their consultation practice— both legitimate considerations. A faculty of twenty-five men outside the state school, and yet representing it; and a definite extension department within the school, coordinating their work and giving credits where earned, would raise the standard of medical practice immeasurably.

The specialist is more inclined to keep abreast of the times than is the general practitioner. The specialist hangs out a sign which verily howls that he knows his field, so that he is stimulated to live up to his advertising. The "Physician and Surgeon" sign covers the human race—some field! The psychology of this sign is: 'it can't be done'; therefore the owner often ceases to try. Yet it is conceded that the general practitioner is, and, by necessity must be, not only the backbone, but the entire skeletal structure of medicine. If scientific medicine stands the stress and exigencies of Time's fast driving, it will be because the general practitioners are structurally sound.

The physician must function in almost every exigency of life; the accident; the fever; the complications of birth; the manifold dysfunctions of the various working parts; and if the physician fails to function, disaster is the result. We have no powers to compute the damage—only the Infinite Mathematician can do that, but a serious and an alert mind that does function, as a mind in such responsibility should, has no need for worry. However, a strange anamoly, those least competent often assume the most responsibility and when the inevitable breakdown occurs, are the least disturbed. In such situation there is no wind tempered to the shorn lamb.

We have, unfortunately, a small class of physicians who will not be benefited by education. Education makes them more adept in unworthy practices. They are a part of "that unfortunate bi product of the creator's early work." They ar the offal. They smell to heaven. They lead o

are members of the "gang." They do not have machine guns, but patients are hijacked just as surely. Their motto is: "Get his money; save him if you can; but do not fail to get his money." The fact that the patient has confidence makes the game safe. Duke University is making an attempt to eliminate those students without character. There are vast difficulties inherent in such a plan. Those born without moral sense and without the sense of obligation may be very intelligent and capable of concealing their defects, but the University has made a start in the right direction. There was Brutus, there was Iago, there was Judas, but is it not comforting that there was also Caesar, Othello and Jesus.

In religion, science, art, medicine and literature everywhere there are these conflicting forces; but thanks be—the dominant forces are for honesty and decency and this holds true very positively in medicine. The infinite possibilities for trouble in the human body and mind make the physician's lot more difficult than any other.

Every individual reacts differently from every other; and each, in turn, reacts differently at different times. Multiply these by each functioning cell in the body and by every mental and emotional process and one wonders that the best physician accomplishes so much. Medicine deals with processes which may be seen or elicited or may be hidden in the innermost recesses of the body or mind. The responsibility for this body and mind to continue in their functioning is the physician's. If this be his responsibility then who is the graduate in medicine except him who has in labors abundant and in the travail of new thought, brought forth a constantly renewing life.

THE PRESIDENT ELECT'S ADDRESS
WHY ARE WE HERE AND WHERE ARE WE GOING?*

GORDON F. HARKNESS, M.D., Davenport

Was it prophetic wisdom on the part of those who formulated our constitution, that Article 2 gives as some of the purposes of our organization, the extension and advancement of medical knowledge and science, the enactment and enforcement of just medical laws, the promotion of friendly intercourse between ourselves, the guarding and fostering of our material interests, the enlightenment and direction of public opinion, and increasing our usefulness to the public in the prevention and care of disease and the prolonging and adding comfort to human life? So regardless of where we go we can remain strict constitutionalists, in

*Presented before the Eighty-third Annual Session, Iowa State Medical Society, Des Moines, May 9, 10, 11, 1934.

spite of the fact that there seems to exist a modern tendency to discard constitutions.

What brings most of us here? To learn and to participate in the extension of medical knowledge and the desire to meet together as friends. There is nothing controversial about such a purpose nor does it offer future problems, and may our scientific programs continue to merit the approval of our members. There are some who would contend that this suffices, and that with this we justify our past, present, and future existence as an organization. Such individuals have failed to discern that there has been developing a social attitude toward medical service and the traditions of our profession that assumes the proportions of a fundamental conflict. Society no longer regards the work of the physician from a purely individual viewpoint. Years ago Disraeli stated that "the public health is the foundation upon which rests the happiness of the people and the welfare of the State." Blackstone renders the legalistic interpretation as follows: "The right to the enjoyment of health is a subdivision of the right of personal liberty, one of the absolute rights of persons." With modern trends there are many who would consider adequate health and medical service not a social necessity but a social right of the individual to be furnished by his government, analogous to education and police protection.

If we are to be heard and our opinions are to carry weight regarding medical matters of public concern, if society is to accept the guiding hand of the medical profession as to the health of its members, then we must act as never before in a collective way through our medical organizations. We must learn to view dispassionately the changing order as we encounter the socializing factors that are rapidly entering our entire governmental fabric, with the fear in many minds that State Medicine is just around the corner. Here we must consider the changes that scientific medical advancement has brought in what constitutes present day medical practice. Here we encounter the changes that modern methods of transportation have made in the practice of medicine. Here we encounter the present day cost of medical care, hospitalization, nursing, et cetera, as contrasted with the past few decades. Here we encounter the increasing ratio of medical practitioners to our population. Again a formidable array of problems that we can discuss under our constitutional authority. We must be constructive in our attitude, for many do not seem to realize that our future position in society will not be determined by ourselves but by the society we are serving. We must be able to convince society that our ideas offer a better health program than any other.

Intense individualists we may be, but only through organized medicine can we accomplish our purposes.

The medical profession is the only guild that has survived the centuries from medieval times. A guild, you know, was an organization, the members of which were pledged to improve their craftsmanship, to furnish their products in a sufficient amount to supply the needs of the community, and each member of the guild, if he developed an improvement in his craftsmanship, was pledged to give it freely to his fellow guild members. Furthermore, the guild protected its members by not admitting to membership more than were necessary to supply the needs of the community. We, as a guild, have been negligent in supplying sufficient opportunities for our members to improve themselves and have done nothing as to the limitation of members. The voluntary raising of the qualifications for membership has not served to limit the number of applicants to our guild.

The pioneer physician, who constituted a local board of health, though not so named; who was a self-constituted medical charity organization, but without a press agent; who battled epidemics of diphtheria and typhoid and so forth, has gone to his reward. The medical profession was the first to realize that certain phases of public health were better handled by governmental agencies. Our profession early recognized the need for and gave unselfish support in organizing certain social service agencies and has continued to give as has no other group gratuitously of our time and skill to help the unfortunate. There is not a physician here who is not still serving gratuitously those in his private practice who are unable to pay for services.

We must not permit professional isolation to blind us as to what constitutes the public welfare. As citizens of the commonwealth we constitute the only group that is doubly taxed, first our normal taxes, and secondly our free services to charity patients. Even those who differ with us admit that large numbers of medical practitioners are inadequately remunerated. Governments, while theoretically accepting the responsibility of medical care as one of the essentials of life, have largely left the cost of this burden to the medical profession. There is evidence that the public is beginning to appreciate this and has expressed a certain willingness to accept part of this burden.

As an organization we feel that the physicians should be the arbiters as to their services and not under the orders of some salaried layman, social worker, or organization. We feel that the physician best serves his calling primarily as an individualist and best serves his patients as individual

human beings and not as numbered cases in an institution. We feel the incentive to personal ambition remains in the physician's individuality as expressed to his clientele. We feel that governmental institutions supported by taxpayers, to which group the physician belongs, may properly have the cooperation of the medical profession, but have no place as active competitors in the private practice of medicine. We feel that indigency is a local responsibility, although in these days of financial depression, this responsibility has passed even state boundaries to the national government. May God forbid that it is anything but an emergency change. We feel that the physician, individually competitive, is entitled to remuneration according to his ability and should not be prevented from making a decent living through socialistic paternalism.

We appreciate as no other group the scientific advances in medicine, and we know the art of the practice of medicine as no layman can know it. We feel that no other group can as well distinguish between scientific medicine and the frills of medical care. We deplore the establishment of great governmental bureaucracies since governmental institutions are notorious for their economic inefficiencies. Consider our postal service deficit as an example. The quality of any service depends on the integrity and ability of its personnel. Governmental bureaucracies, dominated perhaps by politicians, fill us with misgivings.

As a nation we are not a homogeneous group. We are an Iowa organization. Our problems are primarily Iowa problems, not national problems, and in this day when paternalism in government seems to have such a vogue, can it be that we have been sapped of that rugged individualism of our forbears that made this state what it is today? Not that we do not seek information, not that we would not adopt willingly that which is good from without if applicable to Iowa; but has Iowa's intelligence so fallen, even though our literacy is the highest in the nation, that we cannot solve our own problems? Are we to be standardized? Are New York's problems our problems? They are not. Do we have to sit supinely by and have salaried employees from a foreign environment, whose very jobs depend on the changes they can suggest, come to us, tell us just what we should do, and should we blindly accept their decisions as gospel truth? Do we need a survey by so-called experts who are not living Iowa's problems to tell us when to get up, sit down, and roll over? A member of the faculty of our University, not of the College of Medicine, recently gave me a definition of an expert. He said, "An expert is a man a long way from home." No, as Iowans, let u face our problems and if we disagree let us settle our disagreements and work together. We have educational and economic problems that are peculiarly Iowa problems. Your organization is the only one in Iowa that can officially act for you as a group.

As to the enactment and enforcement of just medical laws, we have been working on this problem for a long time and as yet do not have a satisfactory medical practice act. Organized medicince does not ask a monopoly. It does ask that those who practice any form of healing art should meet certain preliminary educational qualifications. Our profession has of its own accord increased the qualifications required of its own members. It does, asking only simple justice, demand that those who have not met these qualifications, be not permitted while practicing under this or that sectarianism to invade the practice of medicine. What is the reason for our failure to obtain simple justice? We have had committees and members who individually have labored faithfully, but the real blame has been elsewhere. Turn to an organization, more or less in disrepute, which has been rebuffed not because of its organization but rather because of the greed associated within its administration, Tammany Hall. Tammany Hall has suffered rebuffs before and has come back, and it will come back again because the real strength of its organization is not in its official heads but in its precinct captains. The real fault of failure of our medical practice act legislation has been because each individual member of our organization has not been made to realize that he is a precinct captain. I doubt that there is a doctor in Iowa who if he would acquaint himself with the proposed medical practice act legislation could not go to three or four laymen of influence in his community, show them the justice and the public welfare that such legislation embodies, and gain their active support. With it there would come success. Let no member who does not realize his individual responsibility offer criticism of the representatives of our organization if they fail.

The raising of the standards of undergraduate medical education has had the endorsement of organized medicine in Iowa, but the actual development and working out of this problem we have left to the small group of medical educators. Organized medicine does, however, feel that medical education only begins with the conferring of the title of Doctor of Medicine. Stagnation and deterioration comes to him who does not realize this. The rapid advances in scientific medicine made during the past two generations, greater than in several of the preceding centuries, makes the need of some form of postgraduate study not a luxury

but a necessity for the individual physician in order that he may render an adequate health service to his patients. Some may be able to keep abreast of the times by individual reading, but far more need the incentive and encouragement offered by organized methods of instruction. Quoting C. C. Bass, Dean of the College of Medicine of Tulane University, "At the present time only an insignificant proportion of physicians take postgraduate courses every year." However, the physician is not entirely to blame, for continuing the quotation, "Unfortunately, the facilities and qualified personnel for good postgraduate instruction are entirely inadequate for more than a small fraction of the physicians who should have it." Wasting time attending major operations or listening to lectures by specialists, promoting, innocently perhaps, their own field, does not constitute good postgraduate instruction. Where is the physician desirous of receiving a short, intensive course in good postgraduate instruction, given for a modest fee, going to turn?

Your organization has instituted as an aid to the physician who is desirous of improving his education, postgraduate courses provided on little more than a cost basis. May I pause to pay tribute to one of our members whom many of you do not realize has given unstintedly of his time and efforts with an ever bubbling enthusiasm to promote these courses. It is little that I can do when I call to your attention the services that Dr. Daniel Glomset has rendered your organization in this particular field of activity. Your organization has made use of the services of teachers in our College of Medicine. This has been made available through the individual efforts of faculty members and administrative authorities. For this our organization should be and is truly grateful. There is, however, a limit to the type of postgraduate instruction that your organization can institute. It must be practically a didactic course. Clinical postgraduate instruction is what is lacking. We have but to turn to our State Agricultural College to have demonstrated the practicability of short courses of instruction. There are two factors necessary to the success of such a program. The first is a realization that medical education and medical practice in Iowa should go hand in hand, that their interests are mutual, and secondly, that the administrators of medical education themselves realize and believe in this enlarged scope of usefulness of a tax supported state institution. It of necessity demands full cooperation between organized medicine and medical education, it means the respect of one for the other, recognition of the problems of each group, and a willingness to work together to solve these problems.

What has all this to do with Iowa's problems? What Iowa needs is greater opportunities for Iowa physicians to improve themselves through increased facilities as to good clinical postgraduate instruction. A medical teacher said to me, "There never were too many good doctors and there are too many poor doctors." Granting some truth to the statement, my reply is that most of the blame can be laid at the doorstep of medical educators, that medical educators have failed in a proper perspective. They have concentrated on the undergraduate but have woefully neglected the postgraduate student.

We have in Iowa one medical school, a state institution, tax supported, and the recipient of philanthropy from without the state. It received its philanthropy because through the enactment of certain state legislation, it was carrying on the interesting experiment of conducting a good medical school in a small center of population. Clinical material essential to the very life of the College was possible only through such legislation. Some have questioned the wisdom of such an experiment. It seems to me that raising such a question now is comparable to a man debating with himself after twenty-five years of married life as to whether he should have married the girl he did. He's married and what is he going to do about it? Just make the best of his bargain.

Iowa has certain responsibilities in our sisterhood of states. Medical education is particularly expensive in Iowa, yet it is one of Iowa's responsibilities. We should not ask other states to educate the doctors of Iowa up to a number required to maintain a ratio such as Iowa needs for proper medical service. As Iowans we should have a justifiable pride in maintaining an excellent College of Medicine. No one should expect a teaching hospital to be able to compete economically with an ordinary hospital. The teaching hospital may bring its per diem charge per patient down to a comparable figure but the extra hospital days that are given in a teaching hospital increase the total cost. Endowed medical schools and hospitals in large centers of population relieve local governments of indigency responsibilities and costs. The taxes we pay in Iowa are the only means by which we can have medical education in Iowa, and forced as we are to draw the necessary teaching material from a wide area, medical education must of necessity be an expensive proposition.

The relationships between the College of Medicine and the medical profession have not attained that unity of action which should be of great mutual advantage. Having expressed myself that differences of opinion should be settled in conference rather than before legislative committees, and that such a course would be of lasting benefit to all, I was invited to meet with the Executive Committee of the Faculty for an interchange of views. It is only fair that the medical profession should be acquainted with the attitude of medical educators in Iowa. Proposals have come to the University administrative authorities from official committees of our organization and from official committees without our organization. Some of these proposals, which I feel were offered in good faith as constructive measures for the future welfare of the University, the medical profession, and for the public good, were accepted and some were rejected. The present law places no restrictions on the admittance of patients to the University Hospital, except the limitations of state appropriated funds. There are no legal restrictions as to cost or private patients.

The University administrative authorities, realizing that absolute dependence on adequate clinical material comes through the operation of the Perkins, Haskell-Klaus laws, which operated entirely by means of state levies, have been reluctant to have changes made that would place part of the cost of indigent patients back to the counties from which the patient came. The law operated inefficiently as demonstrated by the development of a waiting list of approximately 5,000. This was due to county governments, who do not worry about state levies, being willing to neglect their indigents, in the hope that eventually the cost would be paid by state taxation. Some counties discovered, however, that their share of the state tax was more than they were getting from the University in the way of indigency care. When this became known to the taxpayers the University administrative authorities became alarmed as to consequences and instituted the quota plan. The quota plan attempts to equalize the cost between the counties. In doing this it attempts to eliminate the unfair distribution of the state tax. The exempting of certain departments interferes with fair distribution. It fails, however, to recognize the local responsibility of indigency, insofar as the citizens of county governments being made tax conscious of their indigent costs.

There is one outstanding reason for the University authorities maintaining this position, and that is because, through no fault of theirs, the supplying of clinical material is necessarily an expensive proposition for the taxpayers of Iowa. Even though the contention may be made otherwise before legislative committees, the facts controvert such an assertion. The total costs are known but comparative costs are not known to the taxpayer.

Let me give you the comparative costs of patients whom we hospitalized in Scott county and those we sent to the University Hospital.

	Scott County 1933	University July 1, 1932 July 1, 1933
Number hospitalized	406	385
Total hospital days.....................	2,678	8,150
Average hospital days per patient	6.6	21.1
Total cost (without fees, transportation)	$9,015.01	$29,942.85
Transportation, fees, etc.		4,204.51
Total cost	9,015.01	34,147.36
Average per diem cost (excluding transportation)	3.37	3.68
Average patient cost.....................	22.20	77.77
Obstetric cases		140
Obstetric cases, hospital days...........		3,510
Obstetric cases, days average per mother		25
Babies		142
Babies, average hospital stay...........		11
Cost of mothers' care (excluding transportation)		$11,732.16
Average cost of mothers' care...........		83.80
Average cost of babies' care...........		16.25
Total average cost (excluding transportation, average mother and baby)........		100.05
Cost of babies..........................		2,317.50
Total cost mothers and babies (excluding transportation)		14,049.66
University figure, 406 patients, estimated	Same ratio	31,564.62
Transportation, fees		4,433.52
Total		36,998.14
Total surgical hospitalized, Scott County..	156	Estimated Same ratio
Selected group similar to University cases	191	191
Hospital days	1,798	4,640
Cost	$5,859.28	$14,477.80
Average cost	30.67	75.80
Average cost per day.................	3.22	3.68
Average stay in days.................	9.4	20.6
Transportation and fees, $10.90 per patient		$ 2,081.90
Total cost with transportation........		$16,559.70

As to total number of cases, the ratio of costs were over four times our local cost. This, however, would not be fair because of some differences in types of cases, but taking 191 cases which were comparable, the ratio was nearly triple local costs, and if one considered comparable cases and obstetric cases, the ratio of cost under state care would be between three and four times our local care costs. This, the difference in local and state costs, I believe, is the reason that the University administrative officials rejected a county part payment plan.

There is nothing in these comparative figures that should be taken as an inference that there is any criticism offered to the cost of caring for patients at the University. It is expensive, but within limitations, it is worth it. It does emphasize that indigency should be a local responsibility and that the supply of clinical material for the College of Medicine should be limited to the educational and teaching needs of the College, and that the University Hospital has no economic reason for serving our indigents beyond the numbers needed for clinical instruction.

County governments do not worry themselves about state levies, but we pay them. Yet county responsibility owes something to the state. It owes something to state educational institutions and in the case of the University Hospital should be willing to grant it enough of an advantage in the division of hospital expenses so that no county government, in order to save some dollars, would refuse to contribute to the teaching needs of the College of Medicine.

The administrators of medical education in Iowa, where medical education through no fault of theirs must necessarily be expensive, should, if given assurance of sufficient clinical teaching material in the way of Iowa's indigents, be glad to give real assurances that there will be no attempt to exceed in hospital services those beyond the teaching needs of the College. By that I mean that the hospital should be established definitely as an educational institution and not a state institution for indigency. It seems inconsistent that an institution should exist for the purpose of training physicians for Iowa and then enter into active competition with these graduates in the practice of medicine. I am not inferring that there has been any marked abuse along these lines, but in these days lay influences from various sources are advocating the socializing of medicine, and when, as occurred this last winter, a so-called foreign expert employed by the state of Iowa publicly advocated throwing open the University Hospital to private practice; it then behooves Iowa's medical administrative authorities to give to the medical profession some assurance that they do not favor such a program.

It is unfair to the taxpayers of Iowa to be asked to support an expensive type of medical school and educate more than the number of students required to maintain in Iowa a proper ratio of physicians to our population. It is unfair to the graduates of the institution, but more important it is economic extravagance. Apropos of this particular phase of the subject, I quote C. R. Bardeen, Dean of the University of Wisconsin Medical School, speaking of state supported medical schools, "In the long run they are not likely to receive requisite state support if they seek to educate a much larger number of physicians than are necessary to meet state needs. The problem of an adequate supply and proper distribution of physicians, therefore, is a vital concern of those in charge of such schools." State university medical schools serve a most important part in equalizing the opportunities for medical education, since the fees required from residents is materially less than that of endowed schools. Paradoxical as it may seem, in 1932 and 1933 the number of graduates from the twenty-two state universities giving complete medical courses was 1,524, which was less than one-third of the total number of university graduates (4,895). In creating this oversupply we must realize that the state universities play a relatively minor part. The limiting of medical graduates to the needs of the community is not as simple as one might think, and time does not permit a further discussion of the difficulties that present themselves; but certainly the first requisite is to subscribe to the principle that a state supported institution should not expect or ask its taxpayers to pay for the educating of more physicians than are necessary to supply the needs of the state. This we have a right to expect. It is useless to strive to improve the ethics of a profession if you so overcrowd the group that many are denied a decent living. Starving physicians and high ethics will never go hand in hand.

To this principle the Executive Committee of the Faculty could not subscribe; and to be fair, let me state that the limitation of medical students is a controversial subject. There are those who sincerely do not subscribe to any artificial limitation. The contention of the Executive Committee was that as medical educators the only limitation they could be expected to maintain was one of high scholastic requirements; that anything beyond that was without the province of the medical educator; and that the expense of medical education in Iowa was in no way a determining factor. They contended it was rather the province of the state government to limit the number that should be licensed to practice each year and then they would bring the number of graduates within those limits; and further, that with a limited faculty that medical education. in Iowa could be improved with a smaller number of students.

The University Hospital on March 27 had a total of 721 patients, classified as follows: 614 indigent patients, fifty-seven cost patients, forty-one private patients, and five staff patients. The hospital is built to accommodate about 200 more patients. The Association of Medical Schools places five.to six beds per clinical student as a requirement. There are at present 141 students in clinical years; so the present number of beds are sufficient for the present number of clinical students. The same association prescribes fifteen obstetric cases for each senior student. Last year the obstetric department had 874 deliveries, which did not quite meet the qualifications. Senior students make up this deficiency elsewhere. This obstetric educational cost if the Scott county ratio is maintained, totals over $97,000.00 for obstetric clinical material alone. If the hospital were operated to capacity as some have advocated, the per diem charge could be reduced, but the total cost to the state would be increased. More logical would be limiting the number of beds to the requirements of clinical students and utilizing the unoccupied part of the hospital for some other purpose.

The Executive Committee expressed the opinion that there was no desire to increase the bed capacity beyond the required needs for clinical students, and that the present hospital occupancy was all sufficient for the present number of students. In other words, the state and private philanthropy have built a larger hospital than we need for medical education in Iowa.

The cost patient in a state supported institution offers the opportunity for abuse by the individual and by the institution. The referring physician is often to blame, or he may be the victim of circumstances when he hesitates to refuse a request for such an application. The University desires to adhere to the rule that no cost patients will be received without a request for the same from a local physician; and they further expressed themselves as favorable to the patient being required (as in Wisconsin) to sign a financial statement, preferably at his home.

As to the private beds, the Executive Committee gave an assurance that, as long as there was sufficient clinical material, they were going to adhere to the rule of limiting private beds (including gratuitous cases) to five per cent of the hospital's beds. They felt that this was sufficient assurance that there was no attempt being made to capitalize the institution or teaching positions to build up private practices, which could be considered as competing with the medical practitioners in Iowa.

Does the taxpayer have the right as a private patient to demand the services of the University Hospital? As an educational institution, the writer would say, he does not. Yet the equipment and personnel of the institution may be able to offer something as to treatment or opinion that should not be denied the patient. The Executive Committee of the Faculty expressed the opinion that they preferred to receive private patients through the reference of the patient's physician, but that they did not feel they were warranted in refusing private patients who came individually. To illustrate, cases were cited where patients had consulted two physicians, receiving advice from one that did not coincide with that given by the other, and that members of the faculty were called upon to render a sort of referee's decision. Certainly official connection with the University does not bestow any official prerogatives as refereeing between the practitioners of Iowa. While acting in this capacity is doing no more than is done every day in the practice of medicine, yet medical educators are in a position to be *ultra ethical*, if you please. The highest type of professional courtesy asks assurance of a patient that he has released himself of all obligations from his previous physician. Surely we can ask that courtesy of Iowa's medical educators; and even more if they are cognizant of what good will and friendship of the medical profession means to the University's future. I believe they could do much to cement that friendship by limiting the private patients to those referred by practitioners in the field.

Earlier reference was made to the lack of facilities for postgraduate instruction. The present faculty has made a few attempts in the way of postgraduate instruction. The present personnel is inadequate to carry on such work regularly. With proper personnel added it would have the cooperation of the present faculty. It offers the opportunity to enhance the educational value of the College of Medicine to the state, and through it the development of a 100 per cent cooperative spirit between the medical profession and the College of Medicine. The impetus for the establishing of short postgraduate courses should come from the medical profession showing an interest in and a desire for the same.

In conclusion, I would emphasize that we in Iowa should look at our medical problems primarily as Iowa problems, not national problems. Medical education and the practice of medicine have so much in common, can be so mutually helpful, that a division of the two means that each will be the loser. Medical education in Iowa is particularly expensive. The administrators of medical education are conscious of this fact and are most sensitive to the reaction of the same upon the taxpaying public. Our medical administrators and educators are fine, earnest men, placed in the peculiar position of maintaining a school in a small center of population absolutely dependent upon clinical material through the operation of certain statutory laws. The fact that the operation of these laws necessitates an expensive type of indigency care is beyond their control. Since the very existence of the College is dependent on some kind of a state indigency law, our medical educators have been too fearful of suggested changes. This fear has demanded a free hand, it has opposed the local community becoming tax conscious of their indigency care. In reality, they have been living in fear of the taxpayer, and minimizing the benefits to be derived from the enthusiastic friendship of the medical profession. It has been suspicious of organized medicine as something destructive. As long as there is adequate clinical material, the attitude of Iowa's medical educators is to work with the profession, and avoid abuses as to cost and private patients. Adequate clinical material is, however, their primary concern to which all else would be sacrificed.

It is our job to dispel this fear that something, that even the medical profession, wants to interfere with the flow of their very life blood. We have a pride in medical education; as a profession we should enlist and strive to perpetuate the high standard of Iowa's contribution to medical education. As taxpayers we are ready to contribute to its necessary high cost in Iowa. Through our professional positions we are the first group of taxpayers to recognize the costs. An aroused taxpayer often becomes a destructionist. The permanency of medical education in Iowa, I believe, will depend on serving the needs of Iowa, and only Iowa.

The medical profession in Iowa stands today, as it has in the past, a true friend of medical education. It does not consider educational institutions as primarily institutions for the care of indigency, because when so used in Iowa they become economic extravagances. It is the hope and the prayer of some of us that the medical profession and medical education can be made to realize their interdependence, so that in the future our differences will be as small family differences and to the commonwealth we can appear as one.

PANCREATIC LITHIASIS

REPORT OF A CASE

HARRY A. COLLINS, M.D., F.A.C.P., Des Moines

Pancreatic lithiasis is a rare condition. It has been indirectly responsible for one of the epoch-making discoveries in medicine. The diagnosis is difficult. A review of the eighth case of pancreatic lithiasis which was diagnosed preoperatively may enable a diagnosis to be made more often in the many patients who harbor this trouble in the pancreas. Pancreatic stones, resulting in obstruction of the pancreatic ducts, lead to atrophy of the pancreas, but the islands of Langerhans remain intact even when the acini disappear completely, and as a rule, glycosuria does not develop unless an interstitial pancreatitis is superimposed. This interesting finding led Banting to the discovery of insulin.

Pancreatic calculi are not common, only 107 cases being reported in the literature up to 1932. Of these 107 cases, only six cases were diagnosed clinically before surgery or autopsy.

As early as 1815, Christopher R. Pemberton wrote that he had been favored with a pancreatic calculus which in its component parts differed from that of the ox, as it consisted entirely of calcium carbonate. The first case reported was by Graff in 1667. Osler was able to collect seventy cases in 1900. Kennicutt and Killoch each reported one case in 1902, and Phillips reported one case in 1904. Mueller reported a case in 1903, Atkinson and Hirsch reported one case in 1910, Pforringer, Bissell and Barron each reported a

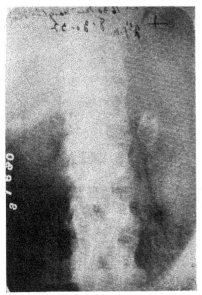

Fig. 1. Note shadow to the left of the spine.

case respectively in 1912, 1913 and 1920, and Seeger reported two cases in 1925. F. B. Ackman collected seven more cases in 1932, which included four cases reported by Hartman in 1925, one case by Charvat and Felkova in 1926, one case by Lindsay in 1929, and one case by Ackman and Ross in 1932. Opie's report on 1,500 autopsies in 1910 revealed only two cases.

It is generally agreed that pancreatic stone is the result of stasis, infection, altered secretion of the pancreas, or obstruction of the pancreatic ducts. The composition of the stones is usually calcium carbonate, which is not a normal secretion of the pancreas.

Pende, in 1907, ligated the pancreatic ducts in a series of rabbits, and he found stones in a large percentage of the rabbits whose ducts were dilated. The usual time for formation of the stones was twenty-eight days. Man and Giordano, in a clas-

sical experiment on animals, showed that a reflex of bile into the pancreatic ducts did not cause pancreatitis. Double ligation of pancreatic ducts in animals did not result in formation of stone.

Pancreatic stones are more common in females than in males, and the average age at the appearance is about forty-three years. The stones are usually multiple, and as a rule are found where the ducts enter the duodenum. In a few instances, the entire gland has been found to contain stones. Gaillard reported a stone in the tail which ulcerated into the stomach. Clayton reported a stone which had ulcerated into the peritoneal cavity, and Molierre and Nichols reported a case with hemorrhage from the duodenum due to ulceration as a result of a pancreatic abscess which was secondary to pancreatic stone. These stones vary in size from that of fine sand to two and one-half inches in diameter. They are usually white or a yellowish gray, irregular in shape, and very similar to sali-

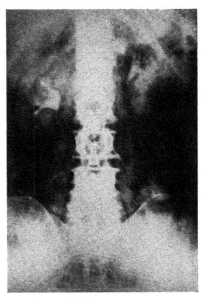

Fig. 2. Showing the stone outside of the left kidney.

vary calculus. The pancreas at first shows very marked interlobular inflammatory changes with round cell infiltration which is followed later by fibrosis. The islands of Langerhans are the last to be involved. The most common complications in reported cases were abscess of the pancreas, pancreatic cysts, carcinoma, cholelithiasis, appendicitis and duodenal ulcer. The pancreas may be enlarged or atrophied, and fat necrosis was reported in only one case.

The clinical diagnosis is most difficult; in fact, Moynihan writing on pancreatic calculi in 1902 said it was impossible to give an accurate portrayal of symptoms as so few cases had been recorded. Pain is an important symptom, but is variable in severity and duration. It may be acute, paroxysmal, dull or constant. Pancreatic pain,

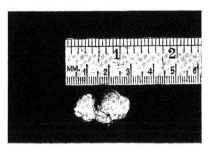

Fig. 3.

however, does have one rather common characteristic, and that is that it radiates to the left. Glycosuria is more constant in advanced cases. In Osler's series of seventy cases, twenty-two presented glycosuria, and Lazarus reported thirty-six cases showing glycosuria out of eighty cases reviewed. The stool changes are noted, but not constant. Kennicutt and others have made a diagnosis by finding stones in the feces. Fatty stools were present in three patients who were operated upon and reported by Seeger. Weight loss was noted in nine out of twenty-two cases reviewed by Seeger, and jaundice was not common. Mueller was of the opinion, after a very extensive investigation, that the absence of fat splitting in the stool without cachexia was very suggestive of pancreatic calculi. Mayo Robson suggested the use of the x-ray in diagnosis of pancreatic stone because of the large amount of calcium. Hartig reported a case in which the x-ray examination was negative and yet a stone was found at operation. Lindsay reported a case with a stone shadow outside of the stomach. Postoperative x-ray pictures for Lacoutie and Charbonel's patient, and one reported by Hartman, showed overlooked pancreatic stones. Kuhler in 1928 reported only two cases of lithiasis of the pancreas in which there was roentgenologic evidence of the condition. Sennett in 1929 made a diagnosis of pancreatic

stone by x-ray, but the case was not verified at operation or autopsy. Graham, in 1932, reported a case diagnosed as pancreatic calculi by x-ray and confirmed at operation. In the case which I am reporting, a diagnosis of pancreatic calculi was made. We had some difficulty confirming this diagnosis even after the abdomen was open. Dr. L. D. Powell was of the opinion that it was a gland. Sistrunk, Danzig, Ackman, Ross, Seeger and others all report cases in which one or more operations were performed. Laparotomies were performed, and in each instance the stone was overlooked and found at necropsy. It is evident, therefore, that even after laparotomy, palpation is uncertain. Seeger reviewed twenty-two cases in which stones were removed from the pancreas. There were two deaths in this series, or a mortality of 8.5 per cent.

May I repeat that pancreatic lithiasis is a very rare condition. A review of the literature shows that this case report is the 108th reported pancreatic stone, and the eighth case in which a clinical diagnosis was made before operation and confirmed at operation.

Mrs. M. E. B., seventy-three years of age, presented herself for examination on August 30, 1932, at which time she was complaining of attacks of severe upper abdominal pain. Her family history was essentially negative. She had been married thirty years and had six children. She had had no operations, no serious illness, and went through the menopause at forty-five years of age.

She stated that for many years "off and on" she had attacks of severe upper abdominal pain. The pain would frequently radiate through to the back, and not infrequently, she said the pain would radiate to the left of the midline of the abdomen. The pain was so severe that those who saw her during these attacks stated that the patient would turn blue at that time. Morphine was required for relief on several occasions. There was no history of chills or fever. She had much bloating and belching, and a certain amount of food idiosyncrasy. There was no history of jaundice, and there was no evidence of fat in the stool or undigested food. For the two years prior to the time I saw her, the patient had complained of having severe attacks of weakness occurring before meals. At times, it was difficult for her to get to the table, but as soon as she was able to get a little food in her stomach, this weakness and trembling would subside. There was no evidence of any urinary disturbance, and her weight was lowered about ten pounds within the year.

On physical examination, this patient seemed somewhat obese, and her color was rather poor. Examination of the heart and lungs showed nothing significant, her blood pressure was 140/80, pulse 88, and temperature 99.4°. Examination of the abdomen revealed very definite tenderness in the epigastrium, especially to the left of the midline, but there were no palpable masses. Examination of the pelvis and rectum was negative, and her reflexes showed nothing abnormal. Urinalysis showed a specific gravity of 1.005, acid reaction, a trace of albumin, negative for sugar, and negative microscopically. Her blood count showed hemoglobin to be 80 per cent, red blood cells 4,150,000, and leukocytes 6,000. The blood sugar taken at 11 a. m., the patient having had breakfast, was 148 mg. per 100 c.c.

The x-ray examination of the chest showed no evidence of disease, the x-ray examination of the stomach was negative, and the x-ray examination of the gallbladder showed a pathologic gallbladder, but no stones. It was noted on the gallbladder plates that there was a definite shadow to the left of the spine (see Figure 1) at about the location of

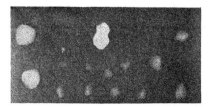

Fig. 4.

the second and third lumbar vertebrae. The question immediately arose as to whether or not this was a kidney stone or a pancreatic stone. With this in mind, an intravenous pylogram was done and x-rays taken which showed very conclusively that the stone shadow was outside of the left kidney (see Figure 2).

I, therefore, made a diagnosis of pancreatic lithiasis and chronic cholecystitis, stones questionable. The patient was referred to surgery, and after the usual preoperative preparation, was operated upon by Dr. L. D. Powell. When the pancreas was palpated, the surgeon was of the opinion that he felt a hard gland in the body of the pancreas, but it was only after an incision was made through the capsule that the stone shown in Figure 3 was delivered from the tail of the pancreas. The gallbladder contained multiple stones. Figure 4 is a picture of the stones, taken postoperatively, showing the marked difference in density between the pancreatic and the biliary stones.

The patient did not do well after operation, and

died of postoperative shock and liver insufficiency on the third postoperative day.

820 Equitable Building.

BIBLIOGRAPHY

1. Hodgson, H. K. Graham: X-ray diagnosis in a case of pancreatic calculus. Brit. Jour. Radiol., v:783 (October) 1932.
2. Kennicutt, F. P.: Pancreatic lithiasis, with report of a case. Am. Jour. Med. Sc., cxxiv:948 (July-December) 1902.
3. Moynihan, B. G. A.: On pancreatic calculus. Lancet (London), ii:355, 1902.
4. Opie, E. L.: Disease of Pancreas. Pemberton's Treatise, 1815, p. 68.
5. Seeger, S. J.: Pancreatic Lithiasis. Radiology, x:126 (February) 1928.
6. Seeger, S. J: Pancreatic Lithiasis. Surg. Gynec., and Obst., xl:841 (June) 1925.
7. Sistrunk, W. E.: The surgical removal of pancreatic stones. Ann. Surg., lxxiv:380 (September) 1921.

THE PHYSICIAN'S RESPONSIBILITY IN RECTAL CARCINOMA*

WALTER A. FANSLER, M.D., F.A.C.S.

Minneapolis

The responsibility of a physician lies not only in making a correct diagnosis in cases of carcinoma of the rectum and colon, but also in seeing that the patient secures proper treatment at the earliest possible moment. Only too often have I had patients consult me after the loss of much valuable time spent with some charlatan or quack, although the diagnosis had been made months before by some reputable physician. This is very often due to the fact that the first physician had not taken the necessary time, or used the tact and patience necessary to explain carefully the situation to the patient. The fact that certain methods of treatment were necessary and that any delay greatly increased the danger were not brought home to him. The patient is always looking for an easy way out and it is hard for him to accept the fact that there is no easy way in rectal carcinoma.

Upon discovering a cancer, the first question arising in the physician's mind is how and to whom the information should be given. My opinion is that in most cases, the patient himself should be told although it may be desirable to lead up to the question gradually and to discuss it first with his family. After all, the patient is the one most concerned and sooner or later he must know the truth. I think in most cases where the family keeps this information from the patient, they are only deceiving themselves, and the sufferer simply plays the game with them. If the patient is the head of the family there is little choice, for it is usually important that business affairs be rearranged and provisions made for the family in case of untoward results. The patient is facing a serious ordeal and the final decision as to the course to follow is his. To make this decision he should be in possession

* Presented before the Linn County Medical Society, Gedai Rapids, January 11, 1934.

of the facts at least before operative procedures are actually instituted.

Upon being told that a cancer exists, the first thought in the mind of the patient is whether or not there is hope of cure. Unless the case is obviously hopeless the physician should be as cheerful and reassuring as possible. The patient's courage is already at a low ebb and it is necessary to give him renewed hope and spirit. In cases of this kind nothing can possibly be gained by pessimism. Except when it is obvious that a generalized carcinomatosis exists, we cannot be even reasonably sure as to whether the disease has spread until the abdomen is explored. On the other hand we do know that 55 per cent of all rectal carcinomas are suitable for operation, and of this group, 70 per cent may expect a five year cure or better. Thus considering the condition with which we are dealing we have every reason to be encouraging. Even in those cases which are so far advanced, or for other reasons are not suitable for radical operation, the outlook is not hopeless. A colostomy followed by x-ray or radium therapy will often improve the patient's health and give him months and even years of comfort. I recall one patient who for physical reasons, could have only a colostomy done, yet he lived for five years with no other therapy and enjoyed good health until a few months before his death. Periods of two and three years of life following simple colostomy are not at all unusual. We have definite figures available as to percentage of cures, longevity, etc., but in dealing with an individual case it is a different matter. There are so many variations from the expected that the more carcinomas I see the more hesitant I become to make a very definite prognosis in a given case. After grading the tumor, following microscopic examination of the tissue, we may prophesy more accurately, but even then there is ample room for error. Since the prognosis is uncertain, it would seem then that the physician is fully justified in giving the patient every encouragement as to the possibility of an actual cure, or at least prolonged existence.

The next problem is the operative procedure necessary to secure the best results. It is here that the firmness, patience and tact of the physician may be tried to the utmost. Unless he is firm and patient and tactful, the patient is quite likely to go to someone who will make impossible promises of an easy method of cure. The only result will be a loss of valuable time and further progress of the disease, perhaps to the point of inoperability. The physician should tell the patient that he is confronting an extremely serious problem and that to solve it successfully he must submit to two operative procedures, which are not without

danger and which involve an appreciable stay in the hospital. He should be told that one of these operations will likely involve the formation of a permanent colostomy. In my experience the colostomy is the hardest thing for the patient to accept and it is usually upon this issue that he leaves the reputable physician and seeks the quack. He must be made to realize that a colostomy is the price he must pay to enable the surgeon to perform an adequate removal of the growth and the adjacent glands. It must be explained that the omission of this operation greatly decreases his chance of a permanent cure. As a matter of fact, the patient's feeling against a colostomy is largely mental and based on lack of knowledge. Almost without exception, patients soon become accustomed to a colostomy and really have very little inconvenience from it. Most animals have a bowel movement after eating and with the loss of our sphincter muscle whose chief function is to enable us to live up to the dictates of polite society, or perhaps finish a rubber of bridge before attending to a duty which should have immediate attention, our colon goes back to its normal animalistic routine. By changing the colostomy dressings two or three times a day there is little inconvenience. A simple elastic belt without any bag or other fancy gadget is usually the most satisfactory contrivance for caring for a colostomy. As a rule, diet will take care of gas, which at most is little worse than the normal rumbling of our intestine, and except in cases of diarrhea, our patient has little complaint. If the reasons for a colostomy and what may be expected after it is performed are carefully explained, the patient usually accepts it. The patient sometimes objects to the time needed for his case, but with the colostomy settled this is usually not difficult to arrange. The knowledge that failure to allow sufficient time greatly increases the operative risk and may be the determining factor in success or failure of the surgeon's efforts, will usually suffice. Eight to ten weeks is probably the average hospitalization period for two stage procedures, and five weeks for the one stage abdominoperineal operation. The one stage operation must be limited to the exceptionally good risks, but I am convinced that with improved operative technic and preoperative care, this group can be increased in number. It is, of course, the ideal procedure where operative mortality can be kept within reason. Whether the operative mortality, which varies from five to fourteen per cent in two stage procedures, should be discussed with the patient is open to question. He knows it is a serious operation and unless the question is asked directly, I see no use in mentioning it, although it should be explained to some other member of the family. Almost invariably the patient brings up the question of the possibility of being cured by radium or x-ray therapy. It is possible to eradicate locally a not too extensive rectal cancer by use of radium. However, we can never be certain that metastases are not present even where the local lesion is small. Thus we are taking chances in the use of radium in those very cases where it would seem most likely to produce a cure. For that reason, except in the most minute lesions, I do not advise its use, other than for palliation. In large rectal lesions it is impossible to apply radium with sufficient accuracy to destroy all the tumor mass even if metastases do not exist. Where large doses are used in growths of this type the mortality rate is almost as high as from surgical procedures.

It should also be remembered that in many cases severe pain often results from the extensive use of radium. This frequently lasts for months and is far more prolonged and severe than that resulting from operation. X-ray is excellent for palliation and as an adjunct to surgery. It is valuable between the first and second stages, postoperatively or following colostomies in inoperable cases. Frequently a large fixed tumor will markedly decrease in size and become movable. If these facts are carefully explained the patient is usually willing to dispense with radium and x-ray, except where the surgeon thinks advisable, and will submit to the necessary surgical maneuvers.

Assuming that the necessary operations have been successfully completed the duty of the physician is still not discharged. As long as the patient lives, he always has the thought of the possibility of recurrence. This is made worse because he hears from time to time of persons dying with cancer. It is necessary to his peace of mind that he have periodic examinations and reassurance. In those unfortunate cases where recurrence does occur some therapy is necessary. I have seen many patients made happier by small doses of x-ray or some form of hypodermic medication even though the physician and family knew it had no actual effect on the course of the disease. To the average patient the abandonment of treatment means the abandonment of hope. Eventually these patients may have pain, and if so, morphine should be used in sufficient doses to secure relief. No matter how large or how frequent the dose, the relief of pain should be secured.

In conclusion then let me repeat the opening paragraph of this paper. It is the duty of the physician not only to diagnose the presence of rectal cancer, but to see that the patient secures proper and adequate treatment. If he does not see a case through to this conclusion, regardless of the time, patience and tact necessary, he has not fulfilled his entire obligation to that patient.

RECTAL CONSTIPATION

Charles J. Drueck, M.D., Chicago

When hunger is satisfied digestion begins. The delicate mechanism which governs the change from food to flesh and blood is still somewhat a mystery. Even more obscure are the factors which separate the useable from the refuse and the discharge of the waste. If these factors fail to operate harmoniously, and it becomes necessary to invoke the aid of outside help the method of choice will always be the one that reproduces normal evacuation as closely as possible. To attain this object, drugs, physical therapy or surgery may be necessary to build up the vital functions and to refresh and invigorate our patient. It is alleged that more than twenty-five per cent of all cases of chronic constipation are caused or aggravated by mechanical obstructions in or about the intestinal tract.

While serious obstructions do occur at any and all parts of the digestive tract, by far the larger number occur in the rectum and anus; yet this terminal bowel is about the last place we look for such interference. Perhaps this is because we are looking for big causes instead of little ones; for major instead of minor lesions.

We have groped about in the abdomen for Jackson's membranes, Lane's kinks, mobile cecums, visceroptosis and adhesions, as mechanical obstructions to fecal transit, when the real cause was usually to be found within a finger's length of the anal outlet. Even when such obstructions to the lumen of the abdominal bowel are present, they are much less productive of constipation than are similar conditions in the pelvic portion of the intestine. The increasing consistency of the feces as they near the outlet makes obstructions in the rectum and anal canal much more troublesome than when they occur higher up.

Pelvirectal fecal stasis was first described by Barnes[1] in 1878 who coined the word dyschesia from the Greek words "difficult" and "to go to stool." Later Hertz[2] revived the term. The condition is recognized clinically by finding the rectum filled with feces and also roentgenologically by the barium meal being emptied from the upper portions of the colon in the proper time but retained in the sigmoid flexure and rectum for perhaps days. (See Fig. 1)

Rectal constipation is a condition that may be encountered at any time of life, due to a congenital malformation at birth, a kink in childhood, a diffuse inflammation in adult life or a neoplasm in the bowel in advanced age, and at all ages is influenced by diet. It frequently accompanies or follows disturbances of the stomach or upper digestive tract as expressed by the atony, spasticity or mechanical abnormalities found roentgenologically, but rectal disease frequently precedes upper digestive disturbances and in many instances the

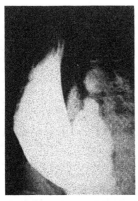

Fig. 1. The stomach is prolapsed into the pelvis.

constrictions, ulcerations, distentions and catarrhal inflammation of the colon, small intestine or stomach are but late manifestations of rectal obstruction.

Obstruction is, of course, always a relative matter; a disproportion between the power of expelling the feces from the pelvic colon and rectum, and the resistance to that force. So many causative factors enter into the production of obstruction of the bowels, and the domination of the clinical picture by one symptom varies so much according to the personality of the afflicted individual, and to the region of bowel involved, that volumes have been written on this subject.

Various predisposing causes lead to irregular bowel evacuations, such as improper food and drink, the upright posture of man and his mobile, elongated sigmoid flexure, habitual neglect of the natural stimulus to bowel movement, lowered vitality, nervous disease, lack of sufficient exercise, and in women the effect of childbirth stretching the abdominal muscles and weakening the pelvic floor. Such factors are present in many individuals having normal evacuations, and in the absence of additional exciting factors, constipation will often disappear following hygienic and dietetic care. It cannot therefore be classed as habitual constipation.

Rectal constipation frequently has a definite date of onset, months or years previous, and a history of rectal pain and bleeding, attacks of diarrhea, anal or rectal inflammation and loss of muscular tone in the affected area, which weaken the bowel and blunt the rectal reflex thus rendering rectal evacuation incomplete and eventually leading to severe constipation, straining at the stool, small poorly formed evacuations, with "piles" which protrude and obstruct the bowel outlet when the rectal contents pass, together with rectal pain and backache, while the habitual taking of cathartics, especially salts, produces soft irritating evacuations which damage both the intestinal tract and the general nutrition.

Secondary results of rectal constipation are direct and reflex. Back pressure upon the bowel causes dilatation of the sigmoid, colon and cecum, and weakens their musculature. This is followed by stagnation of the bowel contents and inflammation of the colon and appendix. The ileocecal valve is often insufficient and the colonic contents pass back into the small intestine, causing increased nutritional and toxic symptoms. (See Fig 2) Reflexly the stomach is irritated, hyperacidity and prolonged closure of the pyloric outlet occur, and pain and discomfort after eating lead to a mistaken diagnosis of stomach ulcer, gallbladder disease, or appendicitis. In advanced cases, the pig-

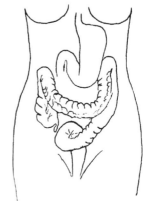

Fig. 2. Ptosed stomach and transverse colon.

mented skin, cold hands and feet, traces of albumin and an excess of indican in the urine, poor physical condition, and nervousness, indicate intestinal catarrh and toxin absorption.

INEFFICIENT POWERS OF DEFECATION

Weak Abdominal or Pelvic Muscles: Inefficient powers of defecation are to be suspected when constipation dates from pregnancy, or is associated with ascites, large abdominal tumors or obesity. It is often easy to ascertain the condition of the abdominal muscles by simple palpation in the horizontal position; and during the examination the discovery of a movable kidney, a prolapsed stomach (See Fig. 3) or a dropped liver

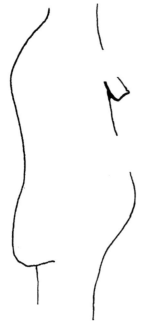

Fig. 3. Body contour of enteroptosis.

would suggest that the abdominal muscles are weak. The patient should next be told to raise her head from the couch; the recti muscles contract and their strength can be ascertained, and any separation between them recognized. Finally, the patient should be examined standing up; when bulging of the abdomen below the umbilicus shows that visceroptosis is present and that the abdominal muscles are weak. The patient often complains of abdominal discomfort which is relieved by lying down or by pressing the lower abdomen upwards.

In all cases in which a woman whose bowels have previously been regular, becomes constipated after the birth of a child, the condition of the

pelvic floor should be investigated, as well as tha of the abdominal wall. The anus is normall slightly retracted; the retraction being increase and the anus drawn slightly forward when th levator ani muscles are contracted by making th movement required in the attempt to begin defeca tion. If these muscles are weak the retractio from the condition of rest is absent or diminished On straining the whole perineum projects furthe than it should, and in severe cases the uterus ma be more or less prolapsed; in such cases no furthe evidence is necessary to show that dyschesia i partly due to weakness of the levator ani muscle:

Painful Abdominal or Pelvic Diseases: In ou consideration of rectal constipation numerous in stances will be found associated with painful con ditions of the abdomen or pelvis; such as an in flamed prostate or uterine disease. These induce reflex inhibition of the intestine and seriously in terfere with normal peristalsis.

Weak Diaphragm: When constipation is pres ent in asthmatic or very emphysematous peopl it is partly due to the fact that the great rise i intra-abdominal pressure required for defecatio cannot be produced by contracting the diaphragn as the latter is already as low as it can go.

ABNORMAL RESISTANCES TO DEFECATION

Abnormal resistances to defecation are of tw types; functional obstruction and organic obstru tion. The latter strictures are of two types, b nign and cancerous. Many of the benign lesio frequently produce no other symptom than that constipation and the presence of the underlyi condition is quite likely to be overlooked if think of every case of constipation as a habit r sulting from sedentary life, errors of diet or ne lect of the natural calls. Of extreme importan is the frequency with which cancer reaches an a vanced stage without manifesting any sympto other than constipation. In every case of cons pation that does not promptly yield to ordina measures a digital examination of the rectu should be made, and in cases of doubtful origin t rectum and pelvic colon should be examined wi a proctoscope and sigmoidoscope.

Stricture of the rectum affects females mo frequently than males; Wallis[3] says five or times as frequently. Poelken, who collected 2 cases, reported that 25 were men and 190, or per cent, were women. Hartmann[4] reporting cases of a general surgery practice, noted that were women. Rosser[5] found the so-called beni strictures to be ten times that of the malign strictures among those that might offer a diagn tic problem because of their annular nature a similar location.

In form these stenoses may be:

1. Annular, like a ring. They involve only a short length of the longitudinal axis of the bowel, but they completely surround it.

2. Tubular, sometimes called cannular. This involves upwards of three inches of the rectum in its entire circumference and in all of its coats.

3. Linear. This is a cicatricial or fibrous deposit and invades but part of the circumference. It constricts the lumen by the size of the deposit, or through contraction of the walls.

4. Spastic. This is due to spastic contraction of the sphincter muscle because of painful lesions in the anal canal.

5. Valvular. This may be a congenital deformity by a fold of mucous membrane or a fibrous band extending across the lumen of the rectum, or hypertrophy of Houston's valve.

Any of these may produce large or small calibered stenoses, even to actual obstruction of the rectum. Constrictions which allow but a small channel past them produce well known and easily diagnosed symptoms, but minor obstructions which cause but a moderate degree of stenosis are constant sources of neuralgic and reflex symptoms which may be difficult to relieve. Small cicatricial or connective tissue deposits in the walls of the rectum are constant sources of irritation because of the friction produced by the passage of fecal matter over them. It is not necessary that the caliber of the canal shall be so constricted as to form an obstruction in order to produce irritating symptoms.

Etiologically strictures may be classified as follows:

1. Congenital
2. Spastic
3. Traumatic
4. Chemical
5. Inflammatory
   a. Amebic
   b. Chronic Ulcerative Colitis
   c. Lymphogranuloma Inguinale (Proctitis obliterans)
   d. Tubercular
   e. Venereal
6. Malignancies

The pathologic changes in the benign strictures are inflammatory and ulcerative in character with leukocytic and lymphocytic infiltration. They are very similar in type regardless of the etiology and the specimen is therefore not differentially diagnostic.

The influence of venereal disease is a much disputed question. Syphilis is considered a major factor by Asman[6], Gant[7], Cripps[8], Ball[9], and Hartmann[10] and as emphatically denied by Lockhart-Mummery[11]. Gonorrhea, however, may be a frequent cause. Hayes[12] made smears in 78 of his cases of rectal stricture and found 54 of them (69.23 per cent) positive for gonorrhea. He found 83.18 per cent of his rectal strictures in women. Tuttle[13] also reported a large preponderance of strictures in women; 216 women in 313 cases. Women suffering with gonorrhea have a vaginal discharge which escapes out over the perineum. As the sphincters relax for defecation the anus is patulous and the mucosa everts. The squatting posture and the contractures of the pelvic muscles at stool force materials from the vagina, and the cleansing efforts after defecation wipes material on the skin about the perineum and anus into the anal canal. It is thus very evident how vaginal discharges may be wiped into the anus.

Trauma, a sequence of previous rectal treatments or operations is a very frequent cause of stricture. Of 258 cases studied by Buie[14] 148 patients gave histories of having had operations upon the rectum and 63 of them had been treated or operated upon for hemorrhoids. Buie emphasizes that strictures do not develop so much because of the amount of tissue which is sacrificed at hemorrhoidectomy, as because of sloughing when the wound is not cared for properly. This same statement applies to other rectal operations such as fistulas especially when involving the vagina or urethra. Inflammatory disease of the pelvic fascias, also prolonged labor, radium applications and scalding rectal drips must be remembered.

While simple diarrhea probably never leads to permanent deformity of the bowel, chronic ulcerative colitis frequently is associated with stricture, and many authorities regard bacillary and endamebic infections as the early stages of chronic ulcerative colitis.

REFERENCES

1. Barnes, Robert: Clinical History of the Medical and Surgical Diseases of Women. London, 1878, p. 145.
2. Hertz, A. F.: Constipation and Allied Intestinal Disorders, London, 1909.
3. Wallis, Fred C.: Surgery of the Rectum. Wm. Wood and Company, New York, 1907, p. 85.
4. Hartmann, Henri: Inflammatory strictures of the rectum. Lancet, (London), i:307 (February 18) 1932.
5. Rosser, Curtis: Benign stricture of the rectum. Texas State Jour. Med., xxvii:777 (March) 1932.
6. Asman, Bernard: Syphilitic stricture of the rectum. International Clinics, iii:1357 (October 20) 1923.
7. Gant, S. G.: Diagnosis and Treatment of Diseases of the Rectum, Anus and Contiguous Textures. F. A. Davis Company, Philadelphia, 1895, p. 399.
8. Cripps, W. H.: On diseases of the Rectum and Anus. J. and A. Churchill, London, 1913, p. 588.
9. Ball, C. B.: The Rectum. H. Frowde and Hodder and Stoughton, London, 1908, p. 332.
10. Hartmann, Henri: Inflammatory stricture of the rectum. Lancet, (London) i:307 (February 18) 1932.
11. Lockhart-Mummery, P.: Diseases of the Rectum and Colon. Wm. Wood and Company, New York, 1923, p. 381.
12. Hayes, H. T.: Stricture of the rectum. Tr. Am. Proct. Soc., xxxii:173, 1931.
13. Tuttle, James: Diseases of the Anus, Rectum and Pelvic Colon. D. Appleton and Company, New York, 1903, p. 455.
14. Rankin, Bargen, Buie: The Colon, Rectum and Anus. W. B. Saunders Company, Philadelphia, 1932, p. 372.

VAGINAL HEMORRHAGE IN THE NEWBORN*

HENRY E. KLEINBERG, M. D., Des Moines

There are many deviations from normal physiology that do occur and that are often passed by unnoticed. One of these variations is the vaginal hemorrhage of the newborn, and particularly that more frequent group which might be termed functional or endocrinologic. The amount of hemorrhage varies from a mere spotting of serum to the severe bleedings that terminate fatally.

Vaginal hemorrhages may be classified as follows:

1. Traumatic.
2. Hemorrhagic disease.
3. Sepsis neonatorum.
4. Syphilis congenitalis.
5. Congenital anomalies of the circulation and viscera.
6. Precocious menstruation.
7. Premature menstrual bleeding.

The *traumatic factor* has a bearing in some of these cases. Forceps, pituitrin, difficult labors, contracted pelves, cord compression, atelectasis, and asphyxia, all play a part in its causation. Breech presentations have a double liability here as the literature shows that physicians do at times lacerate the vaginal opening, mistaking it for the mouth in a vertex; and in other deliveries due to the very rapid moulding, plus fast forcible extraction often aided by forceps, cause intracranial injury at the brain base, near the pituitary body. Peculiarly, in China, midwives frequently force open the vagina of the newborn with their fingers, and cause bleeding.

Hemorrhagic disease, such as hemophilia and leukemia, is noted in about one case in two hundred. It is found equally in the sexes, and frequently begins during the first week. It is progressive without treatment, though at times treatment is of no value. Whereas the normal coagulation time of a newborn infant is five to ten minutes, in these hemorrhagic diatheses it is prolonged to thirty to ninety or more minutes. The blood platelet count is decreased.

Sepsis neonatorum at times produces and is associated with vaginal bleeding. In institutions it may become epidemic in proportions. These cases are marked by fever, leukocytosis, and the offending organism may be isolated from the blood stream. It usually occurs in the second week.

Congenital syphilis is associated at times with vaginal bleeding, due to an increased coagulation time, blood platelet decrease, circulatory disturb-

* Presented before the Osler Club, Des Moines, April 26, 1933.

ances, and visceral pathology. Prenatal routine blood examinations should eliminate this cause.

As to the *congenital anomalies of the circulation and viscera,* Pearce says[1] that it is possible that any condition which would materially interrupt the normal flow of the blood stream in the newborn during or immediately after birth, or any condition which would interfere with an interchange of the chemical elements of the blood would be conducive to bleeding. In this category would be included the cardiac defects, aneurisms and varices, and pelvic maladjustments encouraging venous stasis.

Precocious menstruation, per se, should be considered as the rarest of all the causes of vaginal bleeding. Kerley[2] says that a child may menstruate even at birth and be more or less regular. He mentions 150 cases of Lenz, and 36 cases of Morse in which regular menstruation began between birth and the second year. The children are usually large, and tend to have large breasts, axillary and pubic hair, and prominent mons veneri. Ovulation is associated with these menstruations. Though the etiology is not known, some disturbance of the pituitary gland seems likely to exist.

Premature menstrual bleeding is the most common vaginal hemorrhage of the newborn. Although it does occur in general practice, it is usually noted only in hospital practice where closer observation of infants is kept, and even there vaginal spotting may be disregarded as of no moment. DeLee[3] says: "We have, certainly once every month, a little baby that menstruates for a few days." Lippman[4] has observed its incidence as one in three hundred, in children that are quite healthy. From local sources, the frequency is variously estimated from five per cent to one in two hundred. It begins about the third to fifth day after birth, and lasts for one to five days, ceases and does not recur. It is not a precocious menstruation, but may be considered as a pseudomenstruation. Possibly this bleeding may be the defervescence of a lone or sporadic precocious ovulation, although the menstruation is most likely independent of it. Halban[5] and Zappert[6] theorize that the bleeding is an analogy to the mammary and pelvic changes that take place in the mother, and have shown the same histologic processes of uterine menstruation in its various stages. At birth the child's uterus is hypertrophied, involution taking place within three weeks. It appears that hormones in the placenta and maternal blood, which are physiologic to the mother, are powerful enough to evoke menstruation in the newborn. This hormone acts like the follicular hormone of the anterior pituitary gland, and fits in with the researches of Wirz[7] who recently found that the pituitary glands of the newborn contain the follicular pituitary hormone, but not the luteal hormone. A surplus of this hormone when present at birth causes the menstruation, and is then eliminated through the kidneys. Subsequent menstruation then develops at puberty when the anterior pituitary hormones plus the ovarian hormones become more powerfully developed

CASE REPORT

In seventeen years, I have observed five cases of menstrual bleedings of this type. Four of them were mild, but the last one was quite severe. This led me to review the literature which was surprisingly scarce. On February 28, 1933, I was called in consultation to deliver a gravida two, who had been in labor for forty-eight hours presenting a left occipitoposterior position. Midforceps extraction was reasonably accomplished and a nine and a half pound baby delivered without noticeable damage. On the third day this baby began to menstruate, passing a moderate typical menstrual blood. This increased until the sixth day so abundantly that the baby became pale and began to lose weight. Being Sunday, the blood tests were omitted, and 43 cc. of paternal blood was injected into the baby's hips. Within twenty-four hours the flow was stopped. The amount lost was about 200 to 250 cc. It has not recurred to date. Convalescence was normal and the baby was sent home on the tenth day. There was no sepsis, no hemophilia, and no syphilis.

The prenatal care of the mother and its relation to the fetus is important. The correction of maternal defects, and correction of any pathology is paramount. The maintenance of a sufficient calcium and Vitamin D intake is necessary. Active treatment in these premature menstrual bleedings, should be whole blood transfusions, possibly the use of ergot and pituitrin, and finally and most logically the exhibition of the luteinizing pituitary hormone as is to be had in Antuitrin "S" or follutein.

CONCLUSION

These cases of vaginal bleeding of the newborn are not uncommon. The premenstrual bleeding type is probably due to a "hormonal spillover" from the mother. It is rarely fatal. Closer observation will show a greater incidence than was formerly believed.

1118 Equitable Building.

REFERENCES

1. Pearce, N. O.: Pediatrics, Isaac A. Abt. Vol. II, Chap. xix, 1923.
2. Kerley, C. G.: Practice of Pediatrics, Third edition, p. 516.
3. Personal communication to the author; April 20, 1933.

4. Lippman, G.: W. Bull., St. Louis Med. Soc., v:307 (September) 1911.
5. Halban: Zentralbl. f. Gynak., No. 43, (October) 1904.
6. Zappert: Wien Med. Wehnschr., p. 1478, 1903.
7. Wirz, P.: Zeitschr. f. Geburtsh. u Gynak., No. 104, p. 293 (January) 1933.

GYNECOLOGIC UROLOGY*

ERWIN VON GRAFF, M.D.

Department Obstetrics and Gynecology,
Iowa City, Iowa

The close topographic relation between the female genital and urinary tracts has compelled the obstetrician and gynecologist, more than any other specialist, to devote his attention to the physiology and pathology of the function of bladder and kidneys. This interdependence was manifested at a time when urology was only at the beginning of its amazing development.

Forty years ago, G. Kolischer, in Vienna, first recognized the significance of cystoscopy for the gynecologist. In cooperation with Latzko, he discovered and correctly interpreted the condition since known as "bullous edema." Later, W. Stoeckel, acknowledged as the founder of gynecological urology, and H. A. Kelly in this country, developed this subject into an uncontested border territory between gynecology and urology. Much pioneer work in the development of modern urology has been carried forward by gynecologists and obstetricians, and we do not feel ourselves intruders in this field. In using urologic diagnostic methods and executing conservative or operative treatment, we are, in a sense, harvesting, for the benefit of our patients, the fruit of a soil tilled by one of our own kin.

An enumeration of the most important and frequent female diseases affecting the urinary tract will best explain the significance and necessity for gynecologic urology.

Urinary incontinence, so frequently encountered, is due in a large number of cases, to congenital malformations, such as epispadias (i. e., incomplete closure of the anterior wall of the urethra), abnormal width of the urethra in cases of atresia, or partial or complete aplasia of the vagina. This latter condition often leads to the use of the urethra for sexual intercourse, and it is astonishing how long this abuse may occasionally continue without the knowledge of the participants, and especially without immediate incontinence. Sooner or later, however, incontinence leads to the discovery of the abnormality. These cases demonstrate best, that the complicated mechanism of the closure of the urethra is not effected by an ordinary circular sphincter muscle, but by the cooper-

* Presented before the American Clinical Society of Genitourinary Surgeons, Iowa City, November 17, 1933.

ation of two groups of muscles, situated anteriorly and posteriorly to the urethra, which compress its walls in the fronto-occipital direction.

In other instances, incontinence (many cases of nocturia) is caused by a congenital weakness of the entire muscular apparatus, together with laxity of the connective tissue and fascial fixation (Bonney) of the urethra. The most effective treatment, advised by Goebell-Stoeckel, is the suspension of the urethra by two fascia-muscle strips containing the pyramidalis muscles.

The same type of incontinence may develop as the result of injuries to the muscle fascia system during childbirth, and, in this connection, it must be pointed out that the laxity of the urethra, not the degree of prolapse, is the essential factor.

Frequent micturition during the climacterium is often due to a nervous irritability of the bladder, and has nothing to do with prolapse frequently present at this time. In the postmenopausal period, eversion of the urethral mucosa (urethra caruncle) may cause burning, smarting, and other urinary disturbances.

Pregnancy and childbirth are often accompanied or followed by urologic complications. The pyelitis of pregnancy, characterized by an initial dilatation of the ureters and the kidney pelves, and followed by infection with B. coli by way of the bloodstream or lymphatics, is still a problem not definitely solved. Various peculiarities of pregnancy seem to contribute to the condition, especially the purely mechanical compression by the uterus, together with hypertrophy and relaxation of the ureters, and an increased tendency to dilate, as well as a reduction in the frequency and intensity of their peristalsis.

During delivery the bladder may be injured in the course of instrumental delivery, or be subjected to prolonged compression resulting in puerperal vesicovaginal fistula.

In gynecology, parametrial abscesses perforating into the bladder frequently require cystoscopy to establish the diagnosis and prognosis. In cancer of the cervix cystoscopy with catheterization of the ureters is indispensable in order to avoid errors as to the extent of the lesion and the prognosis, and to determine the choice of treatment. The very first sign that the tumor has involved, if only very superficially, the wall of the bladder, is the bullous edema of the mucosa.

Finally, injuries of the ureter must be mentioned in connection with operations, especially abdominal total hysterectomy. If a ureter has been cut not too far from the bladder, implantation into the bladder usually proves successful. However, if the injury has been overlooked, or implantation is impossible, the best one can hope

for is the development of a ureterovaginal fistula, which almost always requires the extirpation of the kidney, since the results of a secondary implantation into the bladder are very poor. The same holds true for ureteral fistulas which develop during the second week following operations as a result of blunt injury during operation, or from slow abrasion by a suture leading to a decubitus in the wall of the ureter. In all such cases, secondary implantation of the ureter is extremely difficult because of peritoneal adhesions and scarred tissue. Moreover, hydro-ureter, and hydronephrosis, if not pyonephrosis, may render the implantation inadvisable. Experience has shown that a secondary ureteral fistula may close after "autonephrectomy" or after spontaneous healing of the fistula as long as three months after operation, and that any sort of interference must be postponed for at least that long.

This short review shows that gynecologic urology is a field deserving recognition. Its peculiarities and limitations are best designated when one considers that, given a gynecologic or obstetric condition, the urologic examination is required to complete the diagnosis. As only the gynecologist is in a position to draw the proper conclusions from added urologic findings, it is reasonable for him to be familiar with the modern diagnostic possibilities of urology and be able to use them himself. Needless to say, the greatest benefit for the patient will result from the willing cooperation of both specialties.

INTERSTITIAL PREGNANCY

M. L. McCREEDY, M.D., Brighton, and
R. J. SWINNEY, M.D., Richland

Definition. When the impregnated ovum lodges and develops within that portion of the fallopian tube which lies within the wall of the uterus, it is called interstitial pregnancy. This portion of the tube is approximately one and one-half centimeter in length and is the smallest in diameter. It has been further subdivided by Schauman into three parts; the inner, outer and middle one-thirds. The type of pregnancy resulting, according to this classification, depends upon the location of the implantation. The inner third is called uterointerstitial; the outer third, tubo-interstitial; and the middle third interstitial. To me this additional subdivision seems more academic than practical, due to the shortness of this portion of the tube and to the fact that the pregnancy will migrate along the line of least resistance.

History. Cases of interstitial pregnancy are not found in the early literature because postmortem examinations were prohibited.

The earliest described case is an autopsy report written by Pierre Dionis[11] in 1718. It is doubtful if the author fully understood the true condition which led to the patient's death from intra-abdominal hemorrhage. About a hundred years later Breschet [10] saw a patient at autopsy and read of a similar case in the German literature which he reported with wood cuts to the Royal Society in 1825. Mojon[3] in the same year collected four known cases and wrote a thesis on the subject. The first case reported in America was by Fitz[2] in 1875 before the Boston Medical Society. This was followed by several more in the next twenty years. Prior to 1890 the literature contained only twenty authentic cases and they were all discovered at autopsy. In 1882 Doran[1] could find only six specimens in the six leading museums of England. On October 15, 1893, Traub performed the first surgical operation for the treatment of a ruptured interstitial pregnancy, and a few days later Lawson Tait,[8] independently, performed the second such operation. Since the introduction of surgery into the field a few cases have been reported each year. In 1922 Moore[4] compiled 79 cases which had been treated by surgery. Of this group, twenty patients had been operated upon before rupture took place.

Etiology. Interstitial pregnancy is the rarest type of ectopic pregnancy, with the possible exception of ovarian pregnancy. In a series of 1,547 cases of ectopic pregnancies Wynne[9] found only 1.16 per cent of the interstitial type. So rarely is it found that many men go through a lifetime practicing without seeing a single case. It is said that Lawson Tait, a man who made ectopic pregnancy famous, saw only one case of interstitial pregnancy. The white race furnishes 90 per cent and the colored races 10 per cent of the reported cases. The age limits are 18 and 44 years, with the most of the cases falling between 25 and 35 years. Multipara are more susceptible than are primipara. Previous pregnancies or abortions predispose to the condition. Infections of the genital tract, especially endometritis and endosalpingitis with the destruction of the cilia, are predisposing agents. Mechanical obstructions such as adenoma in the lumen or near it may cause obstruction to the passage of the ovum. Plugs of mucus in the lumen or diverticulae may also interrupt the progress toward the uterine cavity. The ovum itself may be over developed when it passes into the interstitial portion, or the ovum may be normal and the tube be of the infantile type. Richardson[7] reported a case where the ovum lodged in the stump of a tube that had been removed five years previously and he is the authority for the state-

ment that at least three similar cases had been reported.

Course and Termination. The course and termination of an interstitial pregnancy depends upon the site of implantation and the line of least resistance to its growth. If it develops toward the tubal end its course will be very similar to that of a tubal pregnancy, except that it will go a longer period of time before rupture. The average length of time before rupture is a month longer in an interstitial pregnancy than in a tubal pregnancy. If the ovum attaches in the middle third and does not migrate, it usually develops a sac of its own in the muscle fibers and may go to term, or it may rupture into the uterine cavity or into the abdominal cavity late. If the attachment is in the inner third or the resistance is less toward the uterine cavity, the mass will develop in that direction and the termination may be an abortion into the uterine cavity. This may be further passed from the uterus and, not knowing the origin, we speak of it as an abortion. On the other hand it may only be partially aborted into the cavity and develop as a normal intra-uterine pregnancy. In spite of the scarcity of these cases in the literature I feel that there must be at least as many of this type as there are ruptures into the abdominal cavity. It seems only probable that a goodly proportion of them would migrate toward the uterus, dilating the tubal orifice. The reason we do not find them is that we are unable to examine the uterine cavity after an abortion. Occasionally we find a case that goes to term with the child in the cavity and the placenta either wholly or partially within the tube. Gilbert[3] and Munde[5] have reported such cases and I shall report my findings a little later in the article. In addition to the three locations in which the ovum may develop there is always the possibility of the ovum dying at any point in the developmental process and decomposing. The death of the ovum may be brought about by hemorrhage or pressure or some other factor. If this death occurs early it may form a mole or a hematoma, while if it occurs later the ovum may decompose and the remains, that is the fetus, may remain in the sac for some time. Such remains have been removed many months after the normal period of pregnancy is past.

Symptoms and Findings. The symptoms are not unlike those of any tubal pregnancy except that they are later in manifesting themselves. The most constant symptom is pain in the pelvis, especially in the affected side. At times this is severe while at other times it is simply a discomfort. Irregular bleeding which is often mistaken for menstruation may be a symptom. After rupture the symptoms are those of intra-abdominal hemorrhage and shock. The findings are almost entirely reached by bimanual examination. There will be tenderness in the pelvis especially on the affected side and there is usually an asymmetrical enlargement of the uterus.

Diagnosis. The most important point in the diagnosis of interstitial pregnancy is to bear in mind its possibility in all cases with abnormal menstruation. At times, it is impossible to diagnose the condition before laparotomy. The most important thing is repeated examination if one is not sure of a diagnosis. The condition can easily be confused with appendicitis if the pregnancy is on the right side. In fact, cases have been found in which the patient was operated upon for an acute appendix, but this embarrassing situation can often be prevented if a bimanual examination is done. A fibroid tumor in one cornua of the uterus will often mislead one in the examintion. However, the history will explain the situation and repeated examinations will soon rule out other possibilities. If a diagnosis cannot be made and the patient seems to be suffering, an exploratory laparotomy is indicated. After rupture, the diagnosis is made easily from the picture of pain, the shock, and the finding of a baggy, bulging culdesac.

Treatment. The treatment for interstitial pregnancy is immediate surgical interference. If the condition has developed very far the operation of choice is a supravaginal hysterectomy, while if it is found earlier a resection may be possible. If the pregnancy goes beyond the sixth month without rupture, the chances are that it will be delivered through the natural route, or a section may be done at term. Hodge[6] reported a case in which he dilated the cervix, ruptured the dividing membrane between the sac and the uterine cavity, and delivered the child with recovery of the mother. In case the child has migrated into the uterine cavity the delivery will be normal, except possibly during the third stage, as in my case.

Prognosis. Before 1893 when surgery was introduced into the treatment of the condition the prognosis was exceedingly grave. The mortality was from 95 to 100 per cent as far as recorded cases were concerned. There may have been cases that aborted but all ruptured cases were fatal. Occasionally a case is found before 1893 where Faradic currents were used with recovery but this is questionable.

Since the introduction of surgery, the mortality has fallen to around ten per cent for all cases, and those patients operated upon before rupture took place have no higher a death rate than those on whom an exploratory laparotomy is performed.

If a positive diagnosis could be made at an early date, there would be very few deaths from this condition.

CASE REPORT

The patient was a normal, well developed primipara. She was twenty-six years of age, white, and denied any venereal history or any previous obstetric episodes. The pregnancy was normal throughout, except for a great deal of pain in the right side. At times it was severe while at other times it was only a discomfort. It seemed to ascend as the pregnancy progressed and at term the pain was at the right costal margin. Early, she had some irregular bleeding but thought nothing of it. When confined she delivered a normal baby weighing seven pounds without any complications other than that the cord was very short and broke in two when the baby was born, with the free end retracting into the vagina.

After delivery the uterus seemed to contract to about the normal size, yet the placenta did not present itself. Since the cord was retracted there was no way to determine the progress of the third stage. There was little hemorrhage and it was decided to wait, in the hope that the placenta would pass spontaneously. After waiting some two hours the patient was anesthetized with chloroform and the vagina was entered. We expected to pick up the free end of the cord, but this was not found, so the cavity of the uterus was explored. It was found to be empty and was symmetrical as far as the origin of the tubes was concerned. The left orifice was not large enough to admit the tip of the small finger, while the right one was large enough to admit the index finger. Coming through this opening was the cord. There were about two inches of cord free in the cavity, but there was an attachment outside the uterine cavity.

Palpating through the abdominal wall, which was relaxed and thin, a mass about as large as the uterus itself could be felt to the right and attached to the uterus. Holding this mass with the free hand the opening of the right tube was dilated and there was found to be a diaphragm of tissue separating two cavities. The placental tissue was separated by blunt dissection with the finger, and removed piecemeal. There was some bleeding but not as much as would be expected. The cavity was explored following the removal of the placenta and seemed well cleaned out. Much to our surprise her postpartum course was normal. She developed very little rise of temperature, there was but little bleeding, and she was able to be up and around in the usual length of time.

CONCLUSION

I feel that this is a case where the migration was toward the uterine cavity; one in which the child developed in the cavity while the placenta developed in the interstitial portion of the tube. It does not seem illogical to imagine that there may be cases where the migration is a little more complete, and with the placenta developing partly within the cavity and partly within the tube, being expelled normally by the contraction of the uterus.

I am indeed grateful to Dr. R. G. Swinney, of Richland, Iowa, for his assistance in this case, and to Dr. Jeanette Dean-Throckmorton for looking up the literature and shipping me some 125 books and magazines.

BIBLIOGRAPHY

1. Doran, Alban: Tran. Obst. Soc. London, xxxvii:228-239, 1882.
2. Fitz, R. H.: Amer. Jour. Med. Sc., lxix:95-103, 1875.
3. Gilbert, T. C.: Texas State Jour. Med., xviii:546-547 (March) 1923.
4. Moore, G. A.: Boston Med. and Surg. Jour., clxxxvii:284-288 (August 24) 1922.
5. Munde, P. F.: Am. Jour. Obst., xii:330-333, 1878.
6. Parre, I. S.: Extra Uterine Pregnancy, H. C. Lea Publishing Co., pp. 266.
7. Richardson, I. A.: Lancet (London), ii:296-297 (August 9) 1930.
8. Tait, Lawson: The Lancet (London), i:89 (January 13) 1894.
9. Wynne, H. M. V.: Bull. Johns Hopkins Hosp., xxix:29-35 (February) 1918.
10. Breschet, Gilbert: Mémoire sur une nouvelle espèce de grossesse extrautérine, pp. 27, E. Duverger, Paris, 1826.
11. Dionis, Pierre: Cited by Wynne. Traité général des accouchemens, qui instruit de tout ce qu'il faut faire pour être habile accoucheur, pp. 488, C. M. d'Houry, Paris, 1718.
12. Mayer: Beschreibung einer Graviditas interstitialis uteri, nebst Beobachtungen über die merkwürdigen. Veränderungen welche die weiblichen, Genitalien und namentlich der uterus in hohen Alter erleiden, Bonn, 1825.

Case Report

UNILATERAL FUSED KIDNEY

OTTO N. GLESNE, M.D., Fort Dodge

Unilateral fused kidney is one of the rare types of congenital malformation. A review of the literature with a collection of all cases reported was made by L. E. Pierson in 1932 and 103 cases were reported by him, including 58 reported by Kretschmer in 1925. Stewart and Lodge found one example in their series of 6,500 autopsies. Henry Morris, et al., have reported finding one in 15,908 autopsies.

M. S., born May 2, 1933, at 7:02 A. M., died at 10:30 A. M. the same date, weight 2 pounds, 12 ounces. After delivery it was noted that the child was very cyanotic and respirations were difficult. Carbon dioxide and oxygen were administered frequently with no change in the condition. Alpha-lobeline was administered, but the cyanosis continued. Respirations gradually became less and death occurred at 10:30 A. M., three and one-half hours after birth.

Examination of the child at birth revealed that heart tones were best heard to the right of the sternum. Breath sounds were absent over the entire left chest, and were very faint on the right side:

Examination at autopsy revealed the body of a female infant of very small stature, having a normally shaped trunk and head, with normal genitalia and anus. Meconium was noted appearing at the anus.

Upper Extremities: On the right hand there was an extra thumb protruding proximal to the normal thumb. This thumb was the same length as the normal thumb and had much the same ap-

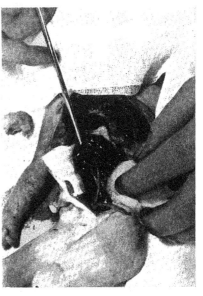

pearance. On the right hand there was a deformity present between the index finger and the ring finger, causing an angulation of about 45 degrees when in the resting position.

Lower Extremities: Difficulty was experienced in getting the left lower extremity to assume the natural position of the right, probably because of a congenital dislocation of the left hip joint. The feet were abnormal, in a position known as talipes valgus, more pronounced on the left foot than on the right.

The liver was abnormally large and practically filled the whole of the upper abdominal cavity. On removal of the anterior chest wall, examination of the diaphragm revealed a diaphragmatic hernia on the left side with the greater portion of the transverse colon, two-thirds of the ileum, and the spleen, in the pleural cavity. A very small portion of the lung was aërated. The heart and other contents of the mediastinum were pushed to the right, accounting for the impression of a dextrocardia. The right lung was expanded, although not as much as it should have been. Further examination of the heart revealed the aorta and the pulmonary artery to be in normal position. However, the intraventricular septum was patent as well as the foramen ovale. After removal of the liver a mass was noted in the right lumbar region which upon dissection proved to be a kidney with two pelvises and two ureters leading from it, the one ureter from the lower pole going underneath the ureter from above, crossing the vertebral column, going posteriorly to the rectum and entering the bladder in a normal manner on the left side. The ureter from the upper pole of this kidney descended in the normal manner and entered the bladder normally on the right. The anterior surface of this fused mass was very much lobulated. (The photograph shows the kidney in the position found with ureters dissected free). Examination for a kidney on the left side showed an absence of kidney in this position. However, a gland about the size of a half dollar, which was thought to be a suprarenal gland, was noted; this assumption was later proved, on microscopic section. No suprarenal gland was found on the right side above the kidney.

THE FINLEY HOSPITAL CLINICO-PATHOLOGIC CONFERENCES

TRAUMATIC RUPTURE OF THE INTESTINES

NECROPSY FINDINGS IN TWO CASES

F. P. McNAMARA, M.D., Dubuque

The cases to be described are examples of lesions that may result from external trauma to the abdomen. Of late years this type of injury has become of increasing importance because of their frequency due to automobile accidents. These injuries often present puzzling clinical problems and the surgeon frequently hesitates to perform a laparotomy because of the vagueness of the symptoms or because of the degree of shock. As early operation is the only treatment for a ruptured intestine, the necropsy findings in these two cases are described in the hope that they may aid in the better care of similar cases in the future.

CASE 1

Chief Complaint: The patient, a white boy nineteen years of age, was admitted to The Finle Hospital, September 18, 1931, with a complain of "severe abdominal pain as the result of a fille milk can falling on his abdomen."

Family history and past history: Irrelevan

Present illness: The patient was lifting a fille milk can from a wagon when he slipped and fe on his back. The milk can weighing approx mately 100 pounds, struck directly on the boy abdomen. When seen shortly afterwards he wa in a state of severe shock and was sent to th hospital at once.

Physical examination: The general examina tion was negative except for evidence of shoc There was no sign of external injury to the ak dominal wall. There was moderate rigidity ove the left central and upper abdomen, but it was n board-like. There was moderate tenderness i the upper abdomen and about the umbilicus.

Course in hospital: The patient continued t complain of severe pain in the abdomen. Th pulse which was very weak and thready varie between 120 and 140 per minute. The temper; ture was 97 degrees F. and the respirations wer 28 per minute. The white blood count was 7,00 Shortly after admission he had an emesis of brigl red blood. He then complained of considerab thirst and nausea. The surgical shock was com bated by supportive measures, heat and elevati of the foot of the bed. The patient did not 1 spond, failed rapidly, and died twelve hours aft admission.

Clinical diagnosis: Trauma of the abdom with gastric hemorrhage; possible rupture of abdominal viscera.

NECROPSY (No. 128)

At necropsy the abdominal cavity was found contain fecal material and a little acute inflamn tory exudate over the coils of the intestine of 1 upper abdomen. A ragged tear extending arou three-fourths of the jejunum was found five cer meters below the duodenum. It was surrounc by clotted and fluid blood. A small perforati was also found on the greater curvature of stomach which contained considerable chan; blood. Otherwise the necropsy was unremarka

Anatomic diagnosis: Traumatic rupture of jejunum and stomach; gastric hemorrhage acute peritonitis.

CASE 2

Chief complaint: The patient, a boy seven ye of age, was admitted to The Finley Hospi January 31, 1933, with a complaint of hav been struck in the abdomen by a fender of an automobile twenty-four hours previously.

Family history and past history: Irrelevant.

Present illness: Twenty-four hours ago while crossing a street he was struck in the abdomen by a fender of an automobile. When seen by a physician he complained of pain in his lower abdomen. He was nauseated and vomited small amounts of watery fluid. He was sent home and kept quiet and only allowed to take small sips of water. Six hours before admission to the hospital he was transported fifty miles, but since he felt well he was left at the home of relatives. There his symptoms became worse and he was advised to enter the hospital.

Physical examination: The patient was in moderately severe shock. The pulse was 140 and the respirations were 42 per minute. The temperature was 105 degrees F. The general examination was negative. The abdomen was slightly distended and tympanitic. There were no points of tenderness or dulness.

Course in hospital: The patient remained in shock in spite of treatment. His temperature fell to 101 degrees within twelve hours, but then rose to 104 degrees. The pulse became more and more thready. The distention of the abdomen decreased. He had an emesis of 500 c.c. of fresh and changed blood. He became very restless and later delirious. He failed progressively and died fifteen hours after admission.

Clinical diagnosis: Probable ruptured abdominal organ with peritonitis.

NECROPSY NO. 163

The general examination was negative. On opening the peritoneum a very small amount of blood tinged fluid was found between the coils of intestine. There was no evidence of peritonitis. A laceration involving two-thirds of the circumference of the descending portion of the duodenum was found. The impression was obtained that the duodenum had been pinched between the automobile fender and the vertebral column. Extending downward from this area a fibrino-purulent exudate could be traced retroperitoneally toward the right kidney. On dissection the latter was found to be practically surrounded by purulent exudate although the kidney substance was not involved.

Anatomic diagnosis: Traumatic rupture of the descending portion of the duodenum; retroperitoneal cellulitis with perinephritic abscess.

COMMENT

In each case there was a history of injury to the abdomen which was followed by pain, shock, nausea, and vomiting of blood. The pulse also

became progressively more rapid and thready in each instance. In the first the temperature was subnormal; in the second the temperature was high, indicating infection. As suspected the most likely site of the infection would be the peritoneal cavity, but there were no definite clinical signs of peritonitis in either case. In the second case the absence of peritonitis was explained by the site of the rupture of the duodenum which was retroperitoneal. Evidently the infection had spread with great rapidity down, toward, and around the right kidney. In neither case was surgery considered advisable because of the vagueness of the clinical signs, and especially because of the degree of shock.

GENERAL DISCUSSION

Rupture of the stomach may occur from within due to excessive distention, or from without due to external violence. If the stomach is filled with food, violent pressure from the outside may result in rupture. Rupture of the intestine is usually due to crushing or tearing because of injury. Rarely there may be injury of the mesenteric blood vessels with secondary gangrene and perforation of the intestine. In 1932 Cooke* collected from the literature about 700 cases of traumatic rupture of the intestines not due to automobile accidents. He reported twelve cases due to automobile injuries which came to necropsy in a ten year period. They constituted more than five per cent of the 210 fatal automobile accidents. Undoubtedly many cases have been undiagnosed, sometimes because of the vagueness of the signs and symptoms and sometimes because of a failure to consider rupture of the intestines as a possibility, since there was no external injury to the abdomen. As successful treatment demands prompt surgical intervention it is important to make a diagnosis as quickly as possible no matter how slight the injury appears to be. Cooke quotes Lund as stating that "a surgeon is justified in doing an exploratory laparotomy in all cases of suspected traumatic rupture of the intestine without waiting for a definite diagnosis."

Diagnosis: The diagnosis depends upon the history of an injury to the abdomen. Often the patient belittles the injury, but a perusal of the literature will indicate how frequently a comparatively slight trauma to the abdominal wall may result in rupture of the intestine. The skin over the abdomen often shows no evidence of injury, probably because of the protection of clothing. At times there may be abrasions, lacerations, or a hematoma of the abdominal wall. Cooke states that the early

* Cooke, H. Hamilton: Traumatic rupture of the intestines caused by automobile accidents. Ann. Surg., xcvi:321-329 (September) 1932.

signs and symptoms may be due to shock, rupture of the intestine or intraperitoneal hemorrhage. In early cases, especially those with small perforations of the intestines, serious symptoms may be lacking. In the two cases presented the outstanding symptoms were shock, pain in the abdomen, emesis of blood and a rising pulse. An x-ray examination using a flat plate is exceedingly important and should be made in every case. It will serve to demonstrate free air in the peritoneal cavity which, of course, comes from the intestine. The air will move depending upon whether the patient is standing or lying down.

Treatment: Without early surgical treatment death is inevitable, and is due to hemorrhage, peritonitis, or shock. Therefore, the preoperative treatment should be directed to combat shock and hemorrhage. The patient should be kept warm, moved as little as possible and be given a blood transfusion. The peritonitis is controlled by early laparotomy, the location and repair of the rupture or ruptures, ligature of all bleeding points, careful cleansing of the peritoneum, and closure with provision for drainage. When all bleeding points have been tied off, physiologic salt solution or whole blood may be given freely. The prognosis is very serious, depending upon the extent of the injury to the intestine, the amount of hemorrhage, and how widespread the peritonitis is, as well as the amount of shock. Except for the latter it is obvious that the earlier a case is operated upon the better will be the control of the first three factors. Even with operation the prognosis is very serious.

Note: I wish to express my appreciation to Doctors R. R. Harris and H. M. Pahlas of The Finley Hospital Medical Staff for the use of their histories.

REPORT OF CASES FROM THE BROADLAWNS GENERAL HOSPITAL, DES MOINES

JULIUS S. WEINGART, M.D., JOSEPH BROWN, M.D., FRANK W. FORDYCE, M.D., Hospital Staff Committee

REPORT OF CASE NO. 65700

This patient was admitted to Broadlawns Hospital on October 5, 1932. The history gave no clue to the cause of his illness. It was essentially as follows. He had not felt well since about three years ago, when he had begun to have epigastric pain. It occurred as soon as he started to eat, and was relieved by belching or by taking soda and vinegar. It was present every day, being more severe at times, and occasionally keeping him awake at night. Nausea was now and then present, but he never vomited. Gradually he became weaker, and

had night sweats. Three days before admission he took to his bed.

There was fever on admission, and during the first week of hospitalization.

Physical examination showed only that he looked ill, had evidently lost weight, and that the spleen edge was palpable. He had a leukocyte count of 5,000 with 94 per cent polynuclears and six per cent lymphocytes; and a slight anemia, with a red blood count of 3,150,000, and 60 per cent hemoglobin. All other laboratory tests were negative. The blood smear seemed normal, and the stomach contents showed no free hydrochloric acid. Blood culture and agglutination tests for undulant fever were negative. Various diagnoses were made by the staff but none was corroborated. After a week of normal temperature he was sent home.

He returned to the hospital on November 27, 1932. He said that he had become weaker, and his appearance was that of a very ill man. He complained of some pain in the hips, and in the chest, and of some coughing. He said he had coughed up some blood. He had had one profuse night sweat and one attack of diarrhea. His temperature curve at this time is shown above. He seemed, even after the cessation of fever, to be losing ground. At this time the possibility of Hodgkin's disease with Pel-Ebstein fever was considered. There were no palpable superficial lymph nodes, and further studies, including an x-ray examination of the thorax, stomach and duodenum gave no help in diagnosis.

He was sent to the University Hospital at Iowa City. The medical staff reported that his temperature was normal on admission, that all examinations by physical and laboratory means were negative, and that he seemed to improve for a while. On December 26, however, he had a drenching night sweat, and began to run a fever which varied from 98 to 103 degrees. The pulse and respiration became rapid. The spleen again became palpable, and a few superficial lymph nodes could be felt. One of these was removed, for they, too, suspected Hodgkin's disease. Sections of this were reported as normal, except for some chronic inflammation. The patient died on February 24, 1933. Autopsy revealed malignant lymphoma of the Hodgkin type, bronchopneumonia and arteriosclerosis.

REPORT OF CASE NO. 69968

This patient was a man, fifty-four years of age, who entered the hospital complaining of cough for the past four months. Recently he had had some pain in the chest also. With the cough he had raised a considerable amount of non-odorous sputum, as much as two cupfuls at a time. He was blind and therefore unable to describe it. He had lost about twenty pounds in weight, and had become somewhat weaker.

The past history is of no interest except that he had smallpox three years before the

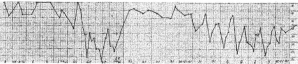

Fig. 1.   Case No. 65700

present illness which produced opacities of both corneas, leaving only light perception in each eye. Physical examination showed an enlarged and rather hard lymph node in the inner angle of the right supraclavicular space. A few scattered coarse râles were heard in both lungs. Examination of the heart showed nothing definite. It was thought that the edge of the spleen could be felt. The above chart shows the course of his temperature.

The white blood cells ranged from 10,000 to 20,000. Other laboratory tests, including agglutination tests for undulant fever, were negative. Several x-ray pictures were taken of the thorax. The first one showed the lung hilus shadows large and dense, with some fibrosis, and cloudiness at both bases. One taken three weeks later showed

a similar mass of enlarged lymph nodes along the upper border of the pancreas. The mesenteric nodes, and the retroperitoneal nodes, especially those along the lower part of the aorta were similar. The liver also showed a few nodules. The spleen was enlarged to about three times its normal size, and contained nodules like those in the lungs and liver.

Even at autopsy the diagnosis from the gross findings was not certain. Not until microscopic sections were examined were we rather surprised to find that we had been dealing with a case of Hodgkin's disease. Sections from various nodes, and from the nodules in lungs, liver and spleen, all showed the typical histologic picture of this disorder.

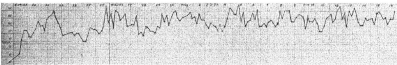

Fig. 2.   Case No. 69968

a considerable increase in the shadow at the right hilus. Another taken three weeks later showed still further increase in these shadows, and mottled densities throughout both lungs. Because of the progression the pulmonary lesions, carcinoma of the lung was strongly suspected. Biopsy of the node in the neck was suggested, but in a few days this had receded, and the matter was dropped. He died with no member of the staff suspecting cause.

At autopsy there were numerous enlarged lymph nodes about the hilus of each lung and in the superior mediastinum. These varied in size from a pea to a walnut. On section they seemed partly replaced by fibrous tissue and partly necrotic. The lungs contained numerous nodules averaging one centimeter in diameter. Many of these contained yellowish granular centers. There was

COMMENT

The above cases illustrate the great difficulty of making a positive diagnosis in certain cases of Hodgkin's disease. Indeed it must sometimes be a mere suspicion, when a continuous or intermittent fever is explainable by nothing else. In any case, biopsy of a lymph node is the only certain method; but in the first case no superficial enlargements were present, and in the second only one was found. The change in this after diagnostic x-ray, as viewed now in retrospect, was significant. It was disregarded at the time, for the lung lesions, the great quantity of sputum, and the fever, due, as we thought, to bronchial obstruction, seemed to warrant the presumption of pulmonary cancer.

Experiences like the foregoing emphasize the fact that the diseases of the lymphatic system are so protean in the pathologic distribution, and so variable in their symptomatology that their recognition ante mortem may be difficult or impossible.   J. S. W.

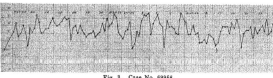

Fig. 3.   Case No. 69968.

STATE DEPARTMENT OF HEALTH

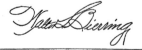

Infantile Paralysis*

It is likely that no other infectious disease has aroused greater interest in the past few years than poliomyelitis, commonly known as infantile paralysis. This is no doubt due largely to the fact that President Roosevelt himself suffered an attack of this disease a number of years ago. An article in a recent issue of the *Literary Digest* mentions that funds totaling over a million dollars were raised on the occasion of the President's last birthday, January 30, 1934. This entire amount will be devoted to the care of patients and to further the continued study of infantile paralysis. These funds will provide better equipment and facilities for the enlargement of the work now being done for crippled children in the hospital at Warm Springs, Georgia. A fund of $100,000 will be used to stimulate further research work and investigation of this disease. Poliomyelitis, although it most often affects little children, also attacks older persons. The disease is no respecter of persons and in a sense this is fortunate. The deep interest which the President takes in this cause must be based to no small degree on his own personal experience. Because he suffered, he is able to do much for others who are affected with this disease.

How long has medical science known about infantile paralysis?

As long ago as the Revolutionary War, in 1776, a physician in his writings referred to a paralysis of children. Sir Walter Scott is thought to have had infantile paralysis. Nearly a century ago, in 1840, a physician named Von Heine described the injurious effects of this malady on certain nerve cells of the spinal cord.

How prevalent is this disease?

Fortunately, actual cases of infantile paralysis are extremely rare, even in the presence of a severe outbreak. In 1905, an epidemic of 1,000 cases occurred in Sweden and Norway. Iowa and

Minnesota experienced a severe epidemic in 1910, and New York in 1916. Several years ago, the disease was prevalent to an unusual degree in Iowa, 222 cases being reported in 1930 and 167 cases in 1931. In 1932 and 1933 reports of 51 and 45 cases respectively, reached the State Department of Health. The number of cases as compared with the total population, is therefore very small. It is unusual for the condition to affect more than one member of a household.

What causes infantile paralysis?

The disease is due to a very minute, living agent, called a virus, so small that it cannot be seen with a microscope of the highest magnification. In respect to its minuteness and nature, this virus resembles that of smallpox, chickenpox, measles and influenza, all of which are regarded as virus diseases.

What are some of the symptoms of this disease which serve to warn parents of the possible nature of a child's illness?

Headache is a common symptom and a chief complaint in a child old enough to tell parents how he feels. Constipation is the rule although intestinal trouble such as diarrhea may affect children when infantile paralysis is prevalent in a community. Pain, soreness of muscles and tenderness of the skin may be present. Stiffness of the neck serves as a warning sign. The child is usually restless, irritable and feverish. There may be muscle twitching and, in the case of a baby, convulsions. In a condition of this kind, it is essential that medical advice be sought as soon as possible. The physician may be able to assure parents that sickness is due to some other cause. A thorough examination must be made and it may be advisable to draw a small amount of fluid from the spinal column. The spinal fluid in infantile paralysis contains white blood cells which help to establish an early diagnosis. It is a fortunate thing that among children who suffer an attack of this disease, only a small percentage develop signs of paralysis. This thought should be reassuring to

* Radio talk, Station KSO, Monday, May 28, 1934, given by Carl F. Jordan, M.D., Director of Division of Communicable Diseases, State Department of Health, Des Moines, Iowa, under the auspices of the Des Moines Academy of Medicine and Polk County Medical Society.

parents. If the disease should be prevalent, with one or several known cases in the community, people will accomplish more by trying to be calm and retain presence of mind rather than to give way to feelings of fear and panic.

How does infantile paralysis spread from person to person?

This disease, like typhoid fever and diarrhea of infants, is more prevalent during the summer. Although cases may occur in any season of the year, over half of the total number of patients take sick in August, September and October. Investigators have for years thought of the possibility of insects playing a part in the spread of infantile paralysis. It was but natural to think of flies and mosquitoes because these are abundant at the same time that the disease is most prevalent. Experiments have been carried out with mosquitoes, the house fly, stable fly and other insects, in the attempt to transmit the disease to monkeys. There is however, no convincing evidence pointing to insects as playing a rôle in the spread of this infection.

The possibility of this sickness being transmitted from animals to human beings, has also been considered. Paralysis has at different times been reported as affecting domestic animals, such as horses, cows or chickens, along with a case of infantile paralysis in a farm home. Here again, there is no satisfactory evidence associating paralysis of animals with the human type of this disease.

Physicians and investigators who have had years of experience in observing and studying epidemics of infantile paralysis, agree that close association or contact is the chief factor in the spread of infection. The germ or virus is present in secretions of the nose and throat of infected people, and it is thought to be transferred from one person to another through speech, cough or sneeze. The condition in its manner of spread, therefore resembles diphtheria, the common cold, and many other of the so-called respiratory diseases.

What about immunity to this disease?

Immunity is regarded as playing a very important part in a community whenever infantile paralysis is prevalent. The patient who suffers an attack of the disease acquires a permanent immunity. This is likewise true of the mild cases in which children have the beginning symptoms, but escape paralysis. In addition and strangely enough, many children and older persons who have been exposed to this infection, not only escape illness but develop a life-long protection. This widespread form of immunity which nature confers upon people in the midst of an outbreak, is little short of astonishing.

What can be done to control infantile paralysis?

Control measures, as exercised by city and local health departments are largely confined to the patient himself and to members of the family or others known to have been exposed. The period of isolation for the patient is twenty-one days. Children who have been exposed and removed from the quarantine area, are kept under observation for ten days before being allowed to mingle with the public. In addition to patients and known contacts, other people may be healthy carriers of the virus or germ. The problem of discovering these carriers is a very difficult one. For this reason, control measures are at present limited in their accomplishment.

What means of prevention are used in infantile paralysis?

The need for prompt medical care during the pre-paralytic stage has already been stressed. Early diagnosis with administration of preventive measures may help to prevent the onset of paralysis. The value of convalescent serum in the prevention of paralysis has not been conclusively demonstrated, but results in many instances have been gratifying. Health departments and laboratories serve a useful function in the preparation and distribution of this serum.

Should weakness of certain muscles develop, careful medical and nursing care are indicated. In some cases, paralysis is temporary and may be followed by complete recovery. Massage treatments should be given only on advice of the attending physician. If weakness or paralysis persists in the muscles of an arm, leg or other part of the body, other measures need to be instituted. Remarkable results are often obtained through orthopedic appliances, operative procedures, such as muscle transplantation and other efforts to restore or rehabilitate muscle and nerve function. An encouraging thing is that disability in infantile paralysis is only physical and that mental powers following such an affliction are likely to be augmented.

Suffering and disappointment may enter some of our homes. Should this happen, it may be that the patients, inspired by the example of our President, will overcome a great handicap and finally emerge triumphant. May we not hope that funds expended for the purpose, and the continued efforts of devoted workers and of those highly trained in this field of medical science, will lead to additional means of preventing this malady.

From the standpoint of the community, it may be mentioned in summary that the reporting of cases of infantile paralysis and observance of quarantine regulations are of importance. From

(Continued on page 306)

The JOURNAL of the
Iowa State Medical Society

ISSUED MONTHLY

RALPH R. SIMMONS, Editor.....................Des Moines

PUBLICATION COMMITTEE

RALPH R. SIMMONS, Editor.....................Des Moines
ROBERT L. PARKER, Secretary..................Des Moines
OLIVER J. FAY, Trustee.......................Des Moines
JOHN I. MARKER, Trustee......................Davenport
EDWARD M. MYERS, Trustee.......................Boone

SUBSCRIPTION $3.00 PER YEAR

*Address all communications to the Editor of the Journal,
1122 Bankers Trust Building, Des Moines*

OFFICE OF PUBLICATION, DES MOINES, IOWA

Vol. XXIV   JUNE, 1934   No. 6

MEDICAL UNITY A REQUISITE FOR
PUBLIC SERVICE

*"The public health is the foundation upon which
rests the happiness of the people and the welfare
of the state."*—DISRAELI.

During the past year much publicity, chiefly of
an unfortunate character, has been given to differences of opinion which have arisen between the
general practitioners of medicine scattered
throughout the state and the authorities of the
College of Medicine at the State University. The
newspapers would lead one to believe that the
differences were unsurmountable. I repeat that
this appears decidedly unfortunate since the ultimate purposes of the two groups are identical and
the much heralded differences are not so grievous
but what an intelligent conference between representatives of the two groups would iron out the
several problems satisfactorily.

Why should there be any differences between
these two groups? The College of Medicine is
commissioned to qualify students in the art and
science of medicine so that they may take their
places in the ranks of general practitioners as the
need arises. In furthering this commission, the
College of Medicine has acted with diligence and
effectiveness, as is attested by the high standing
of the College and the success achieved by its graduates. Can it be, then, that the school is ignorant
or unmindful of the problems of the general practitioner?

It would appear that fundamentally three activities of the College have aroused criticism:

First, it is contended that the College of Medicine is not serving in a full measure when its edu-

present personnel is inadequate to carry on such work regularly." "The impetus for the establishment of short postgraduate courses should come from the medical profession, showing an interest in and a desire for the same."

Indicative of this impelling demand, Dr. Harkness cites the enthusiastic reception accorded the graduate courses furnished to the Iowa profession by the Speakers Bureau of the Iowa State Medical Society. Certainly President Harkness believes that the time is ripe for the College of Medicine to declare actively and positively in favor of "postgraduate courses provided on little more than a cost basis."

As a background for a clear understanding of medical costs affecting undergraduate education, President Harkness introduced a survey of treatment costs, which clearly indicates that in the care of comparable cases the costs in the State Hospital are between three and four times the cost of caring for the same patient locally. "This, the difference in local and state costs," he states, "is the reason that the University administrative officials reject a county part-payment plan." He further points out, "that no county government, in order to save some dollars, would refuse to contribute to the teaching needs of the College of Medicine." He concludes, "The hospital should be established definitely as an educational institution and not as a state institution for indigency." It is evident to the student of this problem that, "the state and private philanthropy have built a larger hospital than we need for medical education in Iowa," but this fact does not warrant the University in asking taxpayers to pay for the education of physicians in excess of Iowa's needs, nor in using the excessive number of beds for the care of the indigent sick in excess of the teaching needs.

Discussing the matter of private practice in the University Hospital he states, "It seems inconsistent that an institution should exist for the purpose of training physicians for Iowa and then enter into active competition with these graduates in the practice of medicine."

That a lack of unity of opinion should exist between the medical profession and the College of Medicine is to be deplored. A mutual understanding of the problems of each, weighed without prejudice and inter-related thoughtfully, will not only present a solidarity of purpose to the lay public, so necessary in engendering confidence, but will also guarantee that unity of action indispensable to the welfare of each group. He states, "Medical education and the practice of medicine have so much in common, can be so mutually helpful, that a division of the two means that each will be the loser."

LIQUOR PERMITS FOR PHYSICIANS

With the repeal of the eighteenth amendment provision is made for the sale and use of alcoholic beverages subject to the laws established in the several states. At the last session of the Iowa legislature, laws were enacted regulating the distribution and use of alcoholic beverages in Iowa. These laws are referred to as the Iowa Liquor Control Act, and their execution has been placed under the administration of the Iowa Liquor Control Commission.

Inasmuch as the Iowa Liquor Control Act recognizes the special needs of the physician in the use of alcoholic beverages, it appeared particularly timely that an interpretation of this enabling act be obtained for the information of the physicians of the state. In the following letter, Attorney Gerald O. Blake, formerly of the attorney general's staff, outlined those features of the Liquor Control Act especially affecting physicians and hospitals:

May 10, 1934

Committee on Public Policy and Legislation.

Gentlemen:

You request an opinion relative to the purpose and privileges authorized under the special permit feature to physicians, pharmacists, etc., provided under the Iowa Liquor Control Act and which is called to your attention by letter from the Iowa Liquor Control Commission under date of May 8, 1934.

In reply I might say that under the Iowa Liquor Control Act, two permits are provided for; one is called the individual permit, and the other a special permit for physicians, pharmacists, dentists, veterinarians and manufacturers using alcoholic liquors, and as far as these pertain to the physician, he will, if he desires to secure any liquor for his individual use, be required to secure an individual permit. As to the special permit provided for, it can only be used to purchase liquors for compounding purposes. The special permit does not authorize a physician to resell any liquor to his patients, unless the same is compounded medicinally and in such a form that it cannot be used as a beverage.

Liquor purchased under an individual permit cannot be used professionally, but I might add that it is not necessary for a physician to have either an individual or a special permit to prescribe liquor for his patients who may, when liquor is prescribed, purchase the same from the State Liquor Store under their (the patient's) own individual permits.

Neither does the special permit authorize the purchase of liquor from any other source than from the state liquor store by the holder thereof.

Under the special permit there is no limit to the amount a physician can purchase, and in the event there is no liquor store available, he can make his purchase from the Central Liquor Store in Des Moines, Iowa, and the liquor will be shipped to him. Under the present statute, it is not necessary for any permit holder, individual or special, to report the amount of liquor used, or how the same was disposed of.

There are very stringent penalties for the resale of liquor, regardless of whether the party selling the same holds an individual or special permit.

In fact, the only advantage of a special permit to a physician is that he may purchase liquor from the State Liquor Control Commission for compounding purposes only, as under the law he cannot use the liquor he purchases under his individual permit for any other purposes than his own consumption, and as a permit is not necessary in order to authorize him to prescribe liquor, he would only need a special permit in the event he was compounding his own medicines and dispensing them to his patients.

Trusting this answers your request, I am,

(Signed) Gerald O. Blake.

The foregoing letter did not treat upon the interpretation of the Iowa Liquor Control Act insofar as the use of alcohol by hospitals or physicians is concerned. Supplementing the letter reproduced above, Attorney Blake, under date of May 18, 1934, supplemented his interpretation with the following statement:

"Due to the many requests relative to the purchase of alcohol by hospitals, I feel I should make an additional opinion to the one recently written to you regarding the purchase of liquor by physicians.

"I might say upon investigation, I find that hospitals desiring to purchase alcohol will have to order the same from the Iowa Liquor Commission. The Commission will then forward their order to the distillery which in turn will ship to the hospital the amount of alcohol ordered. The Liquor Commission will then bill the hospital for the alcohol, but has made arrangements with the federal government whereby no federal tax will be paid by the hospital on alcohol purchased.

"Alcohol purchased by physicians may be bought from any of the state liquor stores but it will be necessary for the physician to pay in addition to the price of the alcohol, the federal tax.

"Alcohol in small quantities will be kept on hand by the liquor commission for sale to physicians and dentists."

In the meantime, the foster mother rabbit was prepared for the reception of the fertilized ovum by mating with a sterile male. The fertilized ovum from the glass vessel was then transferred to her uterus where it became implanted and developed exactly as though it had been produced and fertilized within her body. To preclude the possibility of error in technic and the misinterpretation of observation, the true mother and true father used in the experiment were of one breed, whereas the foster mother and the sterile male rabbits used in the experiment were of an entirely different breed. In each instance the litter of young rabbits was of the same breed as the true mother and father.

The experiments are not only of the most interesting character, but open up an avenue of observation which will undeniably be of great value in furthering the sum total of our knowledge concerning genetics and inheritance. However, one is not justified in the assumption that this work will be productive in opening the way for ectogenetic reproduction in the human being despite the apparently increasing demand upon the part of many potential mothers to be relieved of the burden of child-bearing. Haldane's dream of ectogenetic babies is still far from being realized.

LEGISLATIVE AID SOUGHT IN PREVENTING BLINDNESS

It is estimated that there are more than 100,000 blind persons in the United States. Of this number an increasingly large per cent of blindness has been found to result from trauma to the eye from flying particles of glass in automobile accidents. Realizing the importance of this hazard, five states, New York, Pennsylvania, Michigan, Nebraska and Massachusetts, have made it mandatory for automobiles to be provided with non-shatterable glass as a means of safety. The National Society for the Prevention of Blindness has been active in sponsoring bills in several states, notably, Iowa, urging similar action. There appears to be little doubt that such legislation would not only reduce the number of cases of accidental blindness, but would also go far toward reducing the number of fatal or mutilating accidents. During the past year this organization, in advancing eye hygiene as a part of the general health program, sent representatives into Iowa, Nebraska, South Dakota, Wyoming, Nevada, California, Mississippi and North Carolina. In Iowa, the Society has furthered the training of teachers, particularly at the teachers colleges and normal schools, so that they may provide an adequate course on eye care and hygiene in the health department of the existing curricula.

THE SAMUEL D. GROSS PRIZE

The Philadelphia Academy of Surgery has announced that essays in competition for the Samuel D. Gross Prize of fifteen hundred dollars will be received until January 1, 1935. The conditions annexed by the testator are that the prize "shall be awarded every five years to the writer of the best original essay, not exceeding one hundred and fifty printed pages, octavo in length, illustrative of some subject in surgical pathology or surgical practice founded upon original investigations, the candidates for the prize to be American citizens.

It is expressly stipulated that the competitor who receives the prize shall publish his essay in book form, and that he shall deposit one copy of the work in the Samuel D. Gross Library of the Philadelphia Academy of Surgery, and that on the title page it shall be stated that to the essay was awarded the Samuel D. Gross Prize of the Philadelphia Academy of Surgery.

The essays, which must be written by a single author in the English language, should be sent to the "Trustees of the Samuel D. Gross Prize of the Philadelphia Academy of Surgery, care of the College of Physicians, 19 S. Twenty-second Street, Philadelphia," on or before January 1, 1935. Each essay must be typewritten, distinguished by a motto, and accompanied by a sealed envelope bearing the same motto, containing the name and address of the writer. No envelope will be opened except that which accompanies the successful essay. The Committee will return the unsuccessful essays if reclaimed by their respective writers, or their agents, within one year. The Committee reserves the right to make no award if the essays submitted are not worthy of the prize. Trustees of the Academy are Drs. William J. Taylor, Edward B. Hodge, and John H. Gibbon.

NEW OFFICERS FOR IOWA MEDICAL WOMEN

Dr. Edna K. Sexsmith of Greenfield, was elected president of the State Society of Iowa Medical Women, at the thirty-seventh annual meeting held in Des Moines, Tuesday, May 8. Other officers are: Dr. Rose Butterfield of Indianola, vice president; Dr. Cora W. Choate of Marshalltown, secretary, and Dr. Jeannette Dean-Throckmorton of Des Moines, treasurer.

INSTITUTE OF REGISTERED NURSES

Sixty nurses attended the first institute of district number nine, Iowa Association of Registered Nurses, held in Council Bluffs, Wednesday, May 2. The institute was arranged to give the nurses newer aspects of medical knowledge and nursing technic. The following program was presented: Newer Aspects of Neurology, Gerald V. Caughlan, M.D., of Council Bluffs; Education of the Diabetic Patient, Raymond Rice, M.D., of Council Bluffs; and Hourly Nursing, M. A. Tinley, M.D., and Isaac Sternhill, M.D., both of Council Bluffs.

SPEAKERS BUREAU ACTIVITIES

LABORATORY COURSE

Because of numerous requests for a laboratory course, the Speakers Bureau is contemplating offering one. The proposed course will last two weeks and will consist of mornings devoted to instruction in laboratory technic and afternoons devoted to lectures on the clinical evaluation of laboratory tests.

The schedule for the first week of the course will include the routine as well as the newer procedures in clinical hematology, urinary examinations, renal tests, technic of clinical bacteriology, and stool examinations with particular reference to parasitology. During the second week, the mornings will be given over to laboratory demonstrations and instructions in electrocardiography, basal metabolism and roentgenology, and the afternoons to the discussion of the clinical evaluation of these procedures.

The clinical lectures will be given by various Iowa clinical pathologists, such as: F. H. Lamb, Davenport; F. P. McNamara, Dubuque; Julius Weingart, Des Moines; H. W. Rathe, Waverly; and A. C. Starry, Sioux City. The subject of roentgenology will be handled by Thomas A. Burcham, Des Moines; Harold A. Spilman, Ottumwa; and H. Dabney Kerr of Iowa City.

The expense of this course has not been definitely determined yet, but the object is to give it, like the usual Bureau courses, on a cost basis. If fifty enroll for the course, the fees should be about twenty dollars. If any member wishes to have his technician take this course, arrangements can be made accordingly.

This course will be given only if a sufficient number of doctors indicate their interest in taking the work. The Bureau must know at once if enough are interested so that arrangements may be completed.

All physicians interested in such a course are urged to write the Speakers Bureau, 1122 Bankers Trust Building, Des Moines, immediately for further and more complete information. If the course is desired it will be given during the second and third weeks of July.

CONGRATULATIONS!

In a recent issue of the Decorah *Public Opinion* appeared a column entitled "Our Health," which discussed the problems of posture. At the head of the column was a paragraph stating that this health column would appear from week to week in an attempt to give authoritative information regarding health and the progress made in recent years in the prevention of disease.

These articles are supplied to the Decorah paper by the Winneshiek County Medical Society, and as far as we know, it is the only society in Iowa which is sponsoring such a program of health education. The Winneshiek County Medical Society also conducts a weekly radio program of health broadcasts over station KGCA at Decorah.

Both the editor of the Decorah *Public Opinion* and the members of the Winneshiek County Medical Society are to be congratulated on the service they are rendering the public in making available this valuable health information.

MEETINGS OF MERIT

The Louisa County Medical Society has held two very interesting and worthwhile meetings in the past few months. At their meeting at Grandview on February 10, a layman discussed the subject of "The Relation of the Patient to the Doctor," and at their meeting at Letts on April 12, one of their local nurses talked on "The Relation of the Nurse to the Doctor," and in reply Dr. Roy E. Tandy of Oakville, spoke on "The Relation of the Doctor to the Nurse." It is always well for these three factions of the public health circle to work in harmony and a clear understanding of their proper relation to each other is particularly important in these days of a changing social and economic order. Those who plan the programs for the Louisa County Medical Society are to be congratulated upon selecting such subjects for discussion before and by members of their society.

RADIO TALKS

WSUI—Iowa City, Thursdays, 8:00 P. M.
WOI—Ames, Fridays, 6:45 P. M.

May 31-June 1—Care of the Feet,
Arthur Steindler, M.D.

June 7-June 8—Pale People,
C. W. Baldridge, M.D.

June 14-June 15—Amebic Dysentery,
C. B. Hickenlooper, M.D.

June 21-June 22—Mental Hygiene,
R. A. Stewart, M.D.

June 28-June 29—A Safe and Sane Fourth,
Donald C. Conzett, M.D.

WOMAN'S AUXILIARY NEWS

Edited by the Press and Publicity Committee

MRS. OLIVER J. FAY, *Chairman*, 405 Thirty-seventh Street, Des Moines

The Fifth Annual Meeting of the Woman's Auxiliary to the Iowa State Medical Society, held in Des Moines, May 9, 10, and 11, proved to be a most worthwhile and successful meeting from every standpoint. Approximately two hundred members and guests registered during the three-day convention, over which our president, Mrs. William A. Seidler of Jamaica, presided in her usual efficient manner.

Business sessions were held Wednesday morning and afternoon, Thursday morning and Friday morning. Wednesday evening, the members of the Auxiliary joined their husbands in the reception honoring Dr. and Mrs. Walter L. Bierring. The annual banquet for physicians, wives and guests was attended Thursday evening, after which dancing was provided for those present. The luncheon meeting held at Younkers, Thursday afternoon, was well attended. Music was furnished by the Polk County Woman's Auxiliary, and Miss Agnes Samuelson, superintendent of the State Department of Public Instruction, delivered the address of the afternoon.

The outstanding feature of the business session was the presidential report given by Mrs. Seidler, which included a resumé of the work which was accomplished during the year, and the progress which had been made in the various lines of endeavor. It was increasingly evident that not a little of the success and progress of the past year has been due to the ability and enthusiasm of our president, who entered so wholeheartedly into her work.

An innovation was made in the governing policy of the organization, when a motion was passed including county society presidents as members of the executive board. Because of the cordial reception of the health essay contest, which was inaugurated during the past year, it was unanimously decided to make this contest an annual affair, and a new committee was created to take charge of this activity. Mrs. Seidler was named chairman of this new group, called the Essay Contest Committee. Several changes were made in the constitution and by-laws. These will be recorded in this section at some future date.

Mrs. James A. Downing of Des Moines, who was named president-elect at last year's meeting, was installed as President of the Woman's Auxiliary to the Iowa State Medical Society, Friday morning, at the general business meeting. Other officers who were elected at that time are:

President Elect
    Mrs. Charles B. Taylor, Ottumwa

First Vice President
    Mrs. M. C. Hennessy, Council Bluffs

Second Vice President
    Mrs. T. I. Wigim, Muscatine

Third Vice President
    Mrs. E. D. Morrison, Fort Dodge

Fourth Vice President
    Mrs. L. R. Woodward, Mason City

Secretary
    Mrs. A. C. Starry Sioux City

Treasurer
    Mrs. Russell Doolittle, Des Moines

Director
    Mrs. J. C. Donahue, Centerville

Delegates to the National Auxiliary Meeting
    Mrs. Thomas A. Burcham, Des Moines
    Mrs. W. A. Seidler, Jamaica
    Mrs. H. A. Spilman, Ottumwa

Alternates to the National Auxiliary Meeting
    Mrs. E. L. Bower, Guthrie Center
    Mrs. William S. Carpenter, Altoona
    Mrs. D. H. Hopkins, Glidden

SOCIETY PROCEEDINGS

Black Hawk County

Verne C. Hunt, M.D., of Los Angeles, California, was the guest speaker for the Black Hawk County Medical Society when that organization met in Waterloo, Tuesday, May 15. His subject was Surgical Lesions of the Colon and Rectum.

Boone-Story Societies

Members of the Boone and Story County Medical Societies enjoyed a picnic, Friday, June 1, at the Y. M. C. A. Camp, north of Boone. The afternoon scientific program was presented by A. W. Adson, M. D., of Rochester, Minnesota, who spoke on Acute Injuries of the Head and Spine, and Clifford G. Grulee, M.D., of Chicago, whose subject was Intracranial Hemorrhage and Other Conditions of the Newborn.

Cerro Gordo County

More than fifty members and guests of the Cerro Gordo County Medical Society met in Mason City, Monday, May 14, at which time Verne C. Hunt, M.D., of Los Angeles, addressed the group on Cancer of the Breast. The next meeting of the society will be held Thursday, June 21, with Donald P. Abbott, M. D., of Chicago, as guest speaker.

Clinton County

Thursday, May 3, members of the Clinton County Medical Society met at the Lafayette Hotel for a six-thirty dinner, after which we enjoyed a talk on the subject of Endometriosis, given by George H. Gardner, M.D., of the Northwestern University Medical School, Chicago. Dr. Gardner stressed the importance of proper diagnosis and treatment of this new disease entity. A short business meeting followed the speech, and plans for our meeting on Thursday, June 7, were discussed. Howard Hartman, M. D., of the Mayo Clinic, Rochester, will be the principal speaker. E. V. Donlan, M.D., Secretary.

Hardin County

Dennis H. Kelly, M.D., of Des Moines, furnished the scientific program for the Hardin County Medical Society, Tuesday, May 1, at Iowa Falls, speaking on Infectious Diseases. W. E. Marsh, M.D., Secretary.

Linn County

The regular meeting of the Linn County Medical Society was held at the Hotel Montrose in Cedar Rapids, Thursday, June 7, with the following program: Some of the Physical Properties of Water, William J. Mayo, M.D., of Rochester; Current Conception of Nephrolithiosis, James T. Priestley, M.D., of Rochester; and Ambulatory Treatment of Hernia by the Injection Method, Thomas F. Suchomel, M.D., Cedar Rapids. The first meeting of the society after the summer recess will be held Wednesday, September 12, with Dean D. Lewis, M.D., of Baltimore, president of the American Medical Association, as the guest speaker.

Louisa County

Carl J. Lohmann, M.D., of Burlington, spoke before the Louisa County Medical Society, Thursday, May 17, in Oakville, on the subject, Electrical Surgery.

Marion County

The medical staff of the Veterans Administration Hospital at Knoxville, entertained the Marion County Medical Society, Tuesday, April 24. The following program was presented: The Psychoses of Shakespeare's Characters, C. L. Whitmire, M.D., The Blood Sedimentation Test, H. N. King, M.D.; Localization of Brain and Cord Tumors, M. H. Goldman, M.D.; and Gallbladder Diseases, C. M. Schiek, M.D.

O'Brien County

The O'Brien County Medical Society held a special meeting at Primghar, Thursday, May 17. A motion was unanimously carried endorsing the proposed basic science law, recently approved by the House of Delegates at the annual session.

Pottawattamie County

Sioux City physicians furnished the scientific program when a joint meeting of the Pottawattamie County and Woodbury County Medical Societies was held at the Jennie Edmundson Hospital in Council Bluffs, Tuesday, May 29. The program was as follows: Duodenal Stasis, George W. Koch, M.D.; Tubal Pregnancy, Charles P. McHugh, M.D.; Our Responsibility to a Cross-eyed Child, J. E. Dvorak, M.D.

Arnold L. Jensen, M.D., Secretary.

Scott County

Mark Jampolis, M.D., of Northwestern University School of Medicine, was the speaker for the Scott County Medical Society at its meeting held in Davenport, Tuesday, May 1, taking for his subject, Preventive Measures in Pediatric Practice.

Henry A. Meyers, M.D., Secretary.

Wayne County

Members of the Wayne County Medical Society met in the office of Dr. C. N. Hyatt in Humeston, Tuesday, April 24, and listened to and discussed the following papers: Undulant Fever, C. E. Lovett, M.D., of Lineville; and Intestinal Obstruction, B. B. Parker, M.D., of Allerton.

Woodbury County

The regular monthly meeting of the Woodbury County Medical Society was held Thursday, May 17, at the West Hotel in Sioux City. Dinner was served at six-thirty with approximately sixty members present. William E. Cody, M.D., of Sioux City, presented a paper on Spinal Anesthesia, which was discussed by many members of the society.

L. E. Pierson, M.D., Secretary.

Fort Madison Medical Society

Dr. I. W. Traverse was elected president of the Fort Madison Medical Society, Thursday, May 24. Other officers elected are: Dr. F. W. Noble, vice president, and Dr. H. C. Cleary, secretary.

Four County Medical Society

The Four County Medical Society, composed of physicians in Buena Vista, Cherokee, Ida and Plymouth counties, met for the annual meeting in Cherokee, Tuesday, May 22. The program was as follows: Present Day Knowledge of Strabismus and Its Treatment, J. E. Dvorak, M.D., of Sioux City; Treatment of Acute Middle Ear Disease, M. J. Joynt, M.D., of LeMars; Ante Partum Hemorrhage, T. R. Campbell, M. D., of Sioux Rapids; and Toxemia in Pregnancy, R. B. Armstrong, M.D., of Ida Grove. The present officers of the society were elected to serve another year, and are: Dr. M. J. Joynt of LeMars, president; Dr. H. E. Farnsworth of Storm Lake, vice president; and Dr. J. H. Wise of Cherokee, secretary and treasurer.

Northwest Iowa Medical Society

The spring meeting of the Northwest Iowa Medical Society was held in Sheldon, Tuesday, April 24. After a six-thirty dinner, the following program was presented: Medical and Surgical Problems in Proctology for the Practitioner, Louis A. Buie, M.D., of Rochester; and Cardiac Insufficiency in Obese Individuals, Harry L. Smith, M.D., of Rochester. The open forum was led by Dr. Robert L. Parker of Des Moines, secretary of the Iowa State Medical Society.

Tri-County Medical Society

The Tri-County Medical Society, composed of physicians in Henry, Jefferson and Washington counties, held its May meeting in Washington, Tuesday, May 1. Following a six-thirty dinner, a skin clinic was conducted by J. F. Auner, M.D., of Des Moines. Several patients were presented by attending physicians. The program was interesting and practical, and was enjoyed by all present.

W. S. Kyle, M.D., Secretary,
Washington County Medical Society.

INTERESTING NEWS
In Brief

The Baltimore College of Dental Surgery is the proud possessor of a set of artificial teeth worn by George Washington.

The adolescent acceleration of growth begins, apparently independent of age, when girls and boys reach an average height of 50 and 53 inches, respectively.

Recent investigations indicate that the injection of the drug acetylcholine prevents the fatal toxic effect in benzene poison observed particularly among dry cleaners.

For the discovery of heavy hydrogen, Professor Harold C. Urey of Columbia University, forty-one years of age, will be decorated with one of the highest honor of science, the Willard Gibbs Medal.

To provide an adequate supply of pure oxygen for the treatment of pneumonia in the Wisconsin State General Hospital, pipes leading from a central supply depot will carry this gas direct to the rooms of the institution.

All of the vitamin health-giving properties of fresh cod liver is said to be retained in a chocolate bar which has recently been manufactured in Canada under the direction of the Canadian Department of Fisheries.

Observations conducted at the University of Toronto School of Hygiene direct attention to the economical source of scurvy-preventing Vitamin C in turnip juice. In Toronto one cent will buy 1,100 Vitamin C units in this form.

A trust fund of approximately $200,000 has been created by anonymous donors to be used over a period of ten years for the establishment and maintenance of a department of cancer research at the Hebrew University in Jerusalem.

With the recognition of triple weight hydrogen, the discovery of Lord Rutherford in England, it becomes possible, at least theoretically, to form eighteen kinds of water by various inter-relationship of the molecules of hydrogen and oxygen.

A recent survey conducted by the United States Bureau of Narcotics indicates that about 1,700 handlers of narcotic drugs, mostly physicians, violated the Harrison Narcotic Law by using the narcotics themselves or supplying the drug to addicts.

Researches at the University of Pennsylvania would indicate that "One out of three persons of a typical college group has within his body an ameba parasite similar to the sort that caused the amebic dysentery epidemic in Chicago last summer."

Observing identical twins in the same home environment, the one with a birth injury and the second without physical handicap, Dr. Richard L. Jenkins of Chicago, records mental dulness in the one, which he believes definitely assignable to the birth injury.

PERSONAL MENTION

Dr. W. M. Fowler of Iowa City, attended the twenty-sixth annual meeting of the American Association for Clinical Investigation, held recently in Atlantic City, New Jersey, and presented a paper on "The Effect of Theophyllin Ethylenediamine in Experimentally Induced Infarction in the Dog." Assisting Dr. Fowler in the preparation of this paper were Drs. Fred M. Smith and H. M. Hurevitz, both of Iowa City.

Dr. L. B. Bacon, who for forty-five years has been the only physician in Pacific Junction, has retired from active practice because of ill health. He has gone to Westboro, Massachusetts.

Dr. J. Sam Newton, who was graduated in 1931 from the State University College of Medicine, has located in Keota for the practice of medicine. Dr. Newton served his internship at the City Hospital, Cleveland, Ohio; was later resident physician in the Peoples Hospital, Detroit, Michigan; and is now completing a term as assistant surgeon at the Ohio Soldiers and Sailors Hospital, Sandusky, Ohio.

Dr. James P. Sharon of Fort Dodge, spoke at a local Parent-Teacher Association meeting on "Communicable Diseases."

Dr. A. B. Kuhl, Jr., for the past two years director of public health in Davenport, is in New York taking special work in operative surgery at the New York Polyclinic Hospital. He expects to be in the east several months.

Dr. Philip C. Jeans of Iowa City, spoke before the forty-sixth annual meeting of the American Pediatric Society, held in Asheville, North Carolina, May 3 to 5, on the subject, "The Prevalence of Vitamin A Among Iowa Children."

Dr. C. J. Snitkay and **Dr. Don H. Newland**, both of Belle Plaine, have announced their removal into new offices situated in the old Corn Belt Trust Savings Bank.

Dr. William J. Connell of Dubuque, addressed the Dubuque Lions Club Wednesday, May 2, on "The Increased Span of Life."

Dr. Andrew H. Woods and **Dr. Erich Lindemann**, both of Iowa City, presented papers before the American Psychiatric Association at the annual meeting of that society held in New York City, May 27 and 28. Dr. Woods spoke on "Mental Diseases in Shakespeare's Plays," and Dr. Lindemann discussed "Effects of the Drug Adrenalin in Mental Diseases."

DEATH NOTICES

Fauth, Karl John, of Wellsburg, aged thirty-six, died May 17, as the result of double pneumonia complications. He was graduated in 1925 from the State University of Iowa College of Medicine, and had been a member of the Grundy County Medical Society.

Franchere, Frederick Erasmus, of Sioux City, aged sixty-seven, died April 28, after an illness of several weeks' duration. He was graduated in 1890 from the University of Minnesota Medical School, and at the time of his death was a life member of the Woodbury County and Iowa State Medical Societies.

Prescott, Lee Washbon, of Sloan, aged fifty-two, died May 5, after a week's illness of pneumonia. He was graduated in 1905 from the State University of Iowa College of Medicine, and at the time of his death was a member of the Woodbury County Medical Society.

INFANTILE PARALYSIS

(Continued from page 297)

the viewpoint of the patient, early and adequate medical and nursing care are of great significance, especially in the pre-paralytic stage. If paralysis occurs, adequate and proper medical care are likewise indicated, followed by supervised rehabilitation.

For all of us, an attitude of hopefulness will go far toward assuring progress in the struggle of mankind against infantile paralysis.

TRICHINOSIS

Three cases of trichinosis were recently reported to the State Department of Health, by Dr. E. Pfeiffer, of Hartley, Iowa. The patients were adults, all of whom recovered. Infection was acquired from pork sausage, which on examination in the laboratory, showed large numbers of the encysted forms of Trichina spiralis. Butchering was done at home. Cases and outbreaks of trichinosis occur in Iowa from time to time. It is hoped that reporting of cases of this disease may be more complete.

PREVALENCE OF DISEASE

	April, '34	Mar. '34	Apr. '33	Most Cases Reported From
Diphtheria	39	27	43	Polk
Scarlet Fever	243	352	140	Polk, Lee
Typhoid Fever	0	3	1	
Smallpox	26	37	70	Humboldt
Measles	976	884	115	Pottawattamie, Cass
Whooping Cough	267	222	53	Black Hawk, Plymouth
Cerebrospinal Meningitis	9	10	10	Polk, Cass
Chickenpox	245	307	179	Montgomery, Dubuque
Mumps	313	367	391	Woodbury, Hamilton
Poliomyelitis	0	1	0	
Tuberculosis	24	32	34	(For State)
Undulant Fever	8	22	23	Cedar
Syphilis	117	131	198	(For State)
Gonorrhea	131	160	150	(For State)

HISTORY OF MEDICINE IN IOWA

Edited by the Historical Committee

Dr. Henry B. Young, Burlington   Dr. Tom. B. Throckmorton, Des Moines
Dr. Frank M. Fuller, Keokuk   Dr. Walter L. Bierring, Des Moines
                    Dr. John T. McClintock, Iowa City

History of the Iowa State Board of Health

Frederick J. Swift, M.D.,
Deputy Commissioner—State Department of Health
Des Moines, Iowa

(Continued from last month)

Following the death of Robert J. Farquharson on September 6, 1884, Josiah Forrest Kennedy, A.M., M.D., was elected Secretary of the Board on May 14, 1885. Dr. Kennedy was born near Landsburg, Pennsylvania, on January 31, 1834. He was educated at Williamsburg Academy and Dickinson College, and was graduated from the Medical Department of the University of New York City in 1858. That same year he settled at

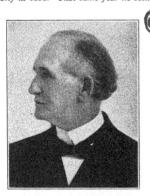

DR. JOSIAH FOREST KENNEDY
Secretary State Board of Health
1885-1907

Tipton, Iowa, and engaged in the general practice of medicine. In 1861 he was made an Assistant Surgeon in the Army, being stationed at Georgetown, S. C., and for two weeks was in charge of the wounded from Antietam. He resigned from the Army in 1862 and returned to Tipton, Iowa. In 1869 he was elected professor of obstetrics in

the Medical Department of the State University of Iowa.

For many years he was an active member of the Polk County and the Iowa State Medical Societies and held various important offices in the American Public Health Association. It was said of him that "his courteous manner and conscientious devotion to duty endeared him to his many associates and colleagues as well as to his professional ministration." During his tenure of office there were many developments in scientific medicine and public health administration. Dr. Kennedy served as Secretary of the Iowa State Board of Health and State Board of Medical Examiners from May 5, 1885 to January 31, 1907, a period of twenty-two years.

With the adoption of a medical practice act, the State Board of Medical Examiners was created and began operation on July first of that year. The law provided that the physicians of the State Board of Health together with the Secretary should be the State Board of Medical Examiners. Later the law was changed so that the Secretary ceased to be a member of this Board, but by virtue of his connection with the State Board of Health, he became Secretary of the Board of Medical Examiners.

FIRST MEDICAL PRACTICE ACT

Prior to 1886 there was no law regulating the practice of medicine in Iowa. However, an act to regulate the practice of pharmacy and the sale of medicine and poisons was passed in 1880, and an act to regulate the practice of dentistry was enacted in 1882.

The medical practice act authorized the State Board of Medical Examiners to grant three forms of certificates:

1. To those who were graduates of medical colleges recognized by the Board as of good standing;

2. To those who had, at the time of the passing of the act, been not less than five years in continuous practice in the state, three years of such practice having been in one locality; and

3. To those who, not having these qualifications passed a satisfactory examination before the Board.

This act was amended in 1897 requiring that after January 1, 1899, all persons beginning the practice of medicine in Iowa must submit to an examination and all persons receiving their diploma subsequent to January 1, 1899, must present evidence of having attended four full courses of study of not less than twenty-six weeks each, no two of which to have been given in any one year.

New duties were from time to time imposed upon the State Board of Health and the reports show that they gave much time and attention to the enforcement of quarantine, and to the investigation and study of typhoid fever, tuberculosis, malaria, the adulteration of food and drugs, pollution of water, and general sanitary conditions throughout the state.

In 1904 the Thirty-second General Assembly amended a previous act passed by the Thirtieth

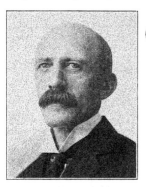

DR. LOUIS A. THOMAS
Secretary State Board of Health
1907-1910

General Assembly which provided that the Bacteriological Laboratory of the Medical Department of the State University should, in addition to its regular work, perform all scientific analyses and tests, etc., which might be required by the State Board of Health. Dr. Henry Albert was appointed Director of the Laboratory.

On Dr. Kennedy's resignation as Secretary on January 31, 1907, Dr. Louis A. Thomas of Red Oak, Iowa, was appointed Secretary of the State Board of Health. Dr. Thomas was born in Dunkirk, France, in 1862, of English parents and came to the United States in 1882. He served as Second Lieutenant in the British Navy for four years and was stationed in Calcutta, India, for a time. He received his medical training at the College of Comparative Medicine, Chicago, and at St. Bartholomew's Hospital at London. During his term

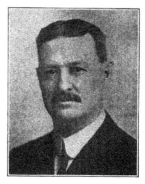

DR. GUILFORD H. SUMNER
Secretary State Board of Health
1910-1913

as Secretary of the Board he took an active part in sponsoring medical legislation.

An act to provide for the examination and regulation of graduate nurses and to regulate the practice of nursing was passed by the Thirty-second General Assembly and became a law in July, 1907. The Thirty-third General Assembly enacted a law regulating the practice of optometry which went into effect July 4, 1909. On January 1, 1910, Dr. Thomas tendered his resignation as Secretary and Dr. Guilford H. Sumner was appointed as his successor.

Dr. Sumner was born at Marengo, Illinois, in 1856. He came to Iowa in the early seventies and taught school in Delaware County at Manchester, Iowa, for a number of years. He was graduated from Valparaiso College where he received a B.S. degree and from the Medical College at the University of Iowa in 1896. After graduation he began the practice of medicine in Waterloo, Iowa, where he served as health officer for many years.

The Thirty-fifth General Assembly in 1913 provided many changes in the membership of the State Board of Health to go into effect July 1, 1913. It was enacted that the Board should consist of the Governor, Treasurer of State, Secretary of State, Auditor of State and the Secretary, Executive Officer of the State Board of Health as ex-officio members. The active members were to consist of four physicians and one sanitary engineer, the term of office to be five years, one member appointed each year. The Secretary of the Board was given the title of Commissioner during the interim of the Board meetings.

Members of the State Board in 1913 were: Dr. Walter L. Bierring, president, Des Moines; Dr. George F. Severs, vice president, Centerville; Dr. John L. Tamisiea, Missouri Valley; Dr. Henry A. Dittmer, Manchester, and Lafayette Higgins, C.E., Sanitary Engineer, Des Moines.

(To be continued)

WILLIAM HENRY WELCH, M.D.
1850-1934

On April 30, 1934, Dr. William Henry Welch died in the Johns Hopkins Hospital, Baltimore, bringing to a close a half-century of leadership in American medicine.

Four years ago the medical profession throughout the world, by special meetings, by ceremonies at Washington, D. C., and through the medical press, paid respect to Dr. Welch on his eightieth birthday. Heralded as the "Dean of American Medicine," Dr. Welch was acclaimed as the greatest single factor in the modernization of American medicine.

Dr. Welch was born in Norfolk, Connecticut, April 8, 1850, and was early inspired to a career in medicine by a father and four uncles who had successfully practiced this profession. He was graduated in 1870 from Yale University with the degree of Bachelor of Arts, at the age of twenty years. He was graduated from the College of Physicians and Surgeons in 1874 and the same year entered Bellevue Hospital for internship. During the succeeding years he studied abroad and began a teaching career which carried him into the faculty life of several of America's leading medical colleges. After his affiliation with Johns Hopkins University in 1916, he occupied successively several teaching chairs in this institution, climaxing his career in the foundation of the Institute of the History of Medicine in Johns Hopkins University School of Medicine as one of his last acts before his retirement in 1931, when he became emeritus professor in this institution.

The hundreds of students scattered throughout America who have felt the vital influence of this master as teacher, the thousands of physicians who have been inspired by the personality of this leader, and the hosts who have come to know Dr. Welch through his able and significant writings, join in one accord in paying tribute to the "Dean of American Medicine." A noble and useful life is ended, but the spirit of this great physician will, through his achievements, continue to encourage and inspire future students in the medical profession.

INVESTIGATION OF CONGENITAL MALFORMATIONS

It is common for mothers of congenitally malformed infants to ask: "If I should give birth again, what is the chance that my next child will also be defective?" The Gynecean Hospital Institute has undertaken a study of families possessing congenitally malformed children in an attempt to answer this question. Important objects of this investigation of malformations are: (a) To determine their frequency of recurrence in the same family. (b) To study the nature of the defects. (c) To throw light upon their etiology.

Families in Pennsylvania possessing one congenitally malformed child have been located through medium of death certificates. Data from this source are being augmented by those from their hospital records, their family physicians, and from home visits. Undoubtedly, some of these families will exhibit recurrences of malformations, but the number of the latter families probably will be small. In order to locate as many additional families as possible, which possess two or more defective offspring, it seems necessary to broadcast the fact that the study is being made.

Physicians who have knowledge of any such families are urged to communicate with: Dr. Douglas P. Murphy, Gynecean Hospital Institute, University of Pennsylvania, Philadelphia, Pennsylvania.

THE SEVENTH ANNUAL GRADUATE FORT-NIGHT OF THE NEW YORK ACADEMY OF MEDICINE

The Seventh Annual Graduate Fortnight of the New York Academy of Medicine which will be held October 22 to November 2, will be devoted to a consideration of gastro-intestinal diseases. Sixteen important hospitals of the city will present coordinated afternoon clinics and clinical demonstrations. At the evening meetings prominent clinicians from various parts of the country will discuss the various aspects of the general subject. A complete program and registration blank may be secured by addressing Dr. Frederick P. Reynolds, 2 East 103 Street, New York.

REUNION OF KEOKUK GRADUATES

Monday, June 18, has been selected as the date for the reunion of all graduates of medicine, dentistry, pharmacy, and nursing of the old College of Physicians and Surgeons, Keokuk Medical College, and those combined institutions which in 1908 were consolidated with Drake University, and later with the State University of Iowa. This reunion will be the fourth to be held in Keokuk; the first being in 1927, the second in 1928, and the third in 1930, at which time twenty per cent of all living graduates were in attendance. It is the sincere wish of the committee in charge of arrangements, that each graduate will endeavor to be present, to contribute to the success of the meeting. Additional details may be secured through Dr. William Rankin of Keokuk, chairman of the publicity committee.

THE JOURNAL BOOK SHELF

BOOKS RECEIVED

THE BASIS OF PASSIONAL PSYCHOLOGY—By Dr. Jacobus X. French Army Surgeon. Privately printed, American Anthropological Society, 70 Fifth Avenue, New York City, 1934. Price, $4.00.

EXTERNAL DISEASES OF THE EYE, by Donald T. Atkinson, M.D., consulting ophthalmologist to the Santa Rosa Infirmary and the Nix Hospital, San Antonio, Texas. Octavo of 704 pages, illustrated with 479 engravings. Lea & Febiger, Philadelphia, 1934. Price, $7.50.

I KNOW JUST THE THING FOR THAT!—By J. F. Montague, M.D., medical director, New York Intestinal Sanitarium, The John Day Company, New York, 1934. Price, $2.00.

LOVE—A TREATISE ON THE SCIENCE OF SEX ATTRACTION—By Bernard S. Talmey, M.D. Fifth edition, newly revised and enlarged, with 52 illustrations. Eugenics Publishing Company, New York, 1933.

MEDICAL CLINICS OF NORTH AMERICA—Volume xvii, No. 4. Cleveland Clinic Number, per clinic year, July, 1933, to May, 1934. Octavo of 253 pages with 53 illustrations. W. B. Saunders Company, Philadelphia and London. Price, paper, $12.00; cloth, $16.00, net.

MEDICAL CLINICS OF NORTH AMERICA, Volume xvii, No. 5, New York Number, March, 1934. Per clinic year, July, 1933, to May, 1934. Octavo of 324 pages with 32 illustrations. W. B. Saunders Company, Philadelphia and London, 1934. Price, paper, $12.00; cloth, $16.00.

MEDICO-MILITARY SYMPOSIUM, 1934—Conducted under the auspices of the Kansas City Southwest Clinical Society and the Medical Department, Seventh Corps Area, United States Army, at the General Hospital, Kansas City, Missouri, March 12-17, 1934. Brown-White, Publishers, Kansas City, 1934.

THE 1933 YEAR BOOK OF GENERAL THERAPEUTICS—Edited by Bernard Pantus, M.S., M.D., professor of therapeutics, University of Illinois College of Medicine. The Year Book Publishers, Chicago, 1934. Price, $2.25.

THE 1933 YEAR BOOK OF NEUROLOGY AND PSYCHIATRY—Edited by Peter Bassoe, M.D., clinical professor of neurology, Rush Medical College; and Franklin G. Ebaugh, M.D., professor of psychiatry, University of Colorado School of Medicine. The Year Book Publishers, Chicago, 1934.

THE 1933 YEAR BOOK OF UROLOGY—Edited by John H. Cunningham, M.D., associate in genito-urinary surgery, Harvard University Postgraduate School of Medicine. The Year Book Publishers, Chicago, 1934.

SURGICAL CLINICS OF NORTH AMERICA, Volume xiv, No. 1, Philadelphia Number, February, 1934. Per clinic year, February, 1934, to December, 1934. 225 pages with 62 illustrations. W. B. Saunders Company, Philadelphia and London, 1934. Price, paper, $12.00; cloth, $16.00.

SURGICAL CLINICS OF NORTH AMERICA, Volume xiv, No. 2, New York Number, April, 1934. Per clinic year, February, 1934, to December, 1934, 293 pages with 71 illustrations. W. B. Saunders Company, Philadelphia and London, 1934. Price, paper, $12.00; cloth, $16.00.

BOOK REVIEWS

OBSTETRIC MEDICINE

The Diagnosis and Management of the Commoner Diseases in Relation to Pregnancy. Edited by Fred L. Adair, M.D., professor of obstetrics and gynecology, University of Chicago; and Edward J. Stieglitz, M.D., assistant clinical professor of medicine, Rush Medical College of the University of Chicago. Illustrated, Lea & Febiger, Philadelphia, 1934. Price, $8.00.

This book is what its name implies, a treatise on obstetric medicine. In it are discussed diseases which accompany pregnancy, but are not attributable to pregnancy. In this way it differs materially from discussions that appear in texts on obstetrics.

These conditions which accompany pregnancy are divided into two parts; first those diseases which antedate pregnancy and are aggravated by it, and second, those diseases which arise during pregnancy as accompanying conditions. Those in the latter class are modified by pregnancy, but are not peculiar to it. In such a manner this book fills the gap between obstetrics and medicine.

The book is divided into twelve sections of several chapters, and each chapter is written by an authority on his subject. The sections are divided as follows: general considerations; specific infections; nonspecific infections; disorders of the nervous system; disorders of the respiratory system; disorders of the circulatory system; disorders of the alimentary system; disorders of the urinary system; disorders of

endocrine balance; disorders of the blood; disorders of body mechanics, and disorders of the skin.

Illustrations are few since the clearness of the text seems to make them unnecessary.

For the use of any practicing physician whose work includes obstetrics, this book should prove exceedingly valuable because it discusses in a clear and concise fashion, the problems so commonly slighted in textbooks on obstetrics.   F. W. R.

LOVE—A TREATISE ON THE SCIENCE OF SEX ATTRACTION

By Bernard S. Talmey, M.D., Fifth edition, newly revised and enlarged, with 52 illustrations. Eugenics Publishing Company, New York, 1933.

This volume is the outgrowth of study made by the author in the field of normal and abnormal sex impulses and sex practices. The author presents several aspects of normal sex activity, discussing at length both psychic and physical aspects of the sex act. Much space is devoted to the presentation of various pathologic sex impulses and sexual practices, and the treatise is concluded by a discussion of education in sex hygiene.

The subject matter is clearly presented and will readily be understood by the average intelligent adult reader. The physician desiring an elementary insight into the study of sex and sex relations may profitably read this volume, although it is obviously intended for the lay student.

tions. Again the author exercises good judgment in reserving final appraisal as to the usefulness of these therapeutic aids. This book is particularly valuable as a reference aid and a very important addition to a complete library. W. R. H.

TRANSACTIONS OF THE COLLEGE OF PHYSICIANS OF PHILADELPHIA

Fourth Series, Volume Two, Number One. The Medical Profession and the Public. Joint Meeting of the College of Physicians and the American Academy of Political and Social Science, February 7, 1934. Philadelphia, Printed for the College, 1934. Price, $1.00.

This volume of the transactions is a most important and timely one inasmuch as the ten addresses reproduced are focused about the subject of socialized medical practice. Representatives of the Milbank Memorial Fund and the Julius Rosenwald Fund present the viewpoints of these philanthropic bodies, advocating the adoption of a socialized scheme of medical practice.

Presenting the view of organized medicine, Dr. Morris Fishbein speaks under the caption, "The Doctor and The State." Reflecting the experiences of other countries in a program of socialized practice, Dr. Henry E. Sigerist of Johns Hopkins University and Dr. Grant Fleming of McGill University, speaks from a background of extensive study and research.

The address of Dr. Roger I. Lee of Boston, entitled "The General Practitioner—His Place in the Medical Profession," is of such a fundamental character in a consideration of this problem that it should be read by every physician.

MEDICO-MILITARY SYMPOSIUM, 1934

Conducted under the auspices of the Kansas City Southwest Clinical Society and the Medical Department, Seventh Corps Area, United States Army, at the General Hospital, Kansas City, Missouri, March 12-17, 1934. Brown-White, Publishers, Kansas City, 1934.

For the past twelve years the Kansas City Southwest Clinical Society has been devoting its efforts to educating the physician. In combination with the military training course of the Seventh Corps Area the Society has given its spring clinical symposium, resulting in postgraduate education of an outstanding order.

This volume presents fifty short abstracts of the papers presented in the spring of 1934. A survey of this small volume of abstracts convinces the reviewer that the Kansas City Southwest Clinical Society has been signally successful in its avowed purpose "of continuing education of the physician."

COUNTY MEDICAL SOCIETY OFFICERS

COUNTY	PRESIDENT	SECRETARY	DEPUTY COUNCILORS
Adair	L. H. Ahrens, Fontanelle	A. S. Bowers, Orient	A. S. Bowers, Orient
Adams	O. B. Hawley, Corning	J. H. Wallahan, Corning	W. F. Amdor, Carbon
Allamakee	J. W. Thornton, Lansing	M. E. Kallman, Postville	J. W. Thornton, Lansing
Appanoose	W. L. Downing, Moulton	C. S. Hickman, Centerville	C. S. Hickman, Centerville
Audubon	R. H. Payne, Exira	P. E. James, Elk Horn	W. H. Halloran, Audubon
Benton		G. R. Woodhouse, Vinton	G. R. Woodhouse, Vinton
Black Hawk	J. R. Thompson, Waterloo	F. Harold Entz, Waterloo	A. J. Joynt, Waterloo
Boone	Mark C. Jones, Boone	B. T. Whitaker, Boone	Mark C. Jones, Boone
Bremer	F. J. Epeneter, Denver	J. E. Whitmire, Sumner	F. R. Sparks, Waverly
Buchanan	W. M. Barrett, Independence	M. C. Melrose, Independence	C. W. Tidball, Independence
Buena Vista	M. A. Armstrong, Newell	J. H. O'Donoghue, Storm Lake	H. E. Farnsworth, Storm Lake
Butler	E. A. Kepler, Allison	H. G. MacLeod, Greene	M. B. Call, Greene
Calhoun	F. W. Hobart, Lake City	W. W. Stevenson, Rockwell City	P. W. Van Metre, Rockwell City
Carroll	D. H. Hopkins, Glidden	Walter A. Anneberg, Carroll	W. L. McConkie, Carroll
Cass	Harry H. Penguite, Massena	R. L. Barnett, Atlantic	R. L. Barnett, Atlantic
Cedar	W. H. Jenks, Tipton	E. J. Van Metre, Tipton	E. J. Van Metre, Tipton
Cerro Gordo	T. E. Davidson, Mason City	William C. Egloff, Mason City	S. A. O'Brien, Mason City
Cherokee	John M. Pope, Cherokee	G. Dean Tipton, Cherokee	Paul Allen, Cherokee
Chickasaw	P. E. Stuart, Nashua	P. E. Gardner, New Hampton	Paul E. Gardner, New Hampton
Clarke	J. D. Shively, Osceola	J. N. Goodman, Osceola	
Clay	G. W. Adams, Royal	Charles C. Collester, Spencer	E. E. Munger, Spencer
Clayton	A. E. Beyer, Guttenberg	J. W. Hudek, Garnavillo	W. H. Hudek, Garnavillo
Clinton	Ralph F. Luse, Clinton	Eugene V. Donlan, Clinton	R. T. Lenaghan, Clinton
Crawford	W. A. Garner, Kiron	J. James Duffy, Denison	C. L. Sievers, Denison
Dallas-Guthrie	George McMahon, Waukee	Samuel J. Brown, Panora	S. J. Butterfield, Dallas Center
			S. J. Brown, Panora
Davis	C. D. Fenton, Bloomfield	H. C. Young, Bloomfield	H. C. Young, Bloomfield
Decatur	J. W. Wailes, Davis City	J. E. McFarland, Leon	J. E. McFarland, Leon
Delaware	J. I. Jones, Manchester	C. A. Carroll, Manchester	
Des Moines	C. J. Lohmann, Burlington	F. H. Aid, Burlington	John T. Hanna, Burlington
Dickinson	Don E. Rodewig, Spirit Lake	Ruth F. Wolcott, Spirit Lake	W. E. Bullock, Lake Park
Dubuque	L. H. Fritz, Dubuque	D. F. Ward, Dubuque	P. P. McNamara, Dubuque
Emmet	W. E. Bradley, Estherville	Smith C. Kirkegaard, Ringsted	M. T. Morton, Estherville
Fayette	James Parker, Fayette	C. C. Hall, Maynard	C. C. Hall, Maynard
Floyd	A. F. Kober, Charles City	J. B. Miner, Jr., Charles City	Ray Fox, Charles City
Franklin	W. R. Arthur, Hampton	J. M. Burger, Hampton	W. E. Long, Hampton
Fremont	H. P. Cole, Thurman	A. S. Wanamaker, Hamburg	A. S. Wanamaker, Hamburg
Greene	B. C. Hamilton, Jr., Jefferson	John R. Black, Jefferson	B. C. Hamilton, Jr., Jefferson
Grundy	M. H. Thielen, Grundy Center	R. T. Spain, Conrad	M. H. Thielen, Grundy Center
Hamilton	W. B. Lewis, Webster City	M. B. Galloway, Webster City	M. B. Galloway, Webster City
Hancock			Thomas McMahon, Garner
Winnebago	A. J. Peterson, Forest City	W. F. Missman, Klemme	A. J. Irish, Forest City
Hardin	E. C. Fraser, Iowa Falls	W. E. Marsh, Eldora	J. C. Koeneman, Eldora
Harrison	A. C. Bergstrom, Missouri Valley	F. E. Hanson, Magnolia	Elmer J. Cole, Woodbine
Henry	F. C. Allen, Wayland	W. A. Laird, Mount Pleasant	W. A. Sternberg, Mount Pleasant
Howard	J. W. Clark, Chester	W. A. Bockoven, Cresco	Wm. A. Bockoven, Cresco
Humboldt	Ivan T. Schultz, Humboldt	Arthur D. Jensen, Humboldt	A. J. Coddington, Humboldt
Ida	E. S. Heilman, Ida Grove	W. P. Crane, Holstein	E. S. Parker, Ida Grove
Iowa	C. H. Hermann, Amana	J. F. Sinn, Williamsburg	J. J. Sinn, Williamsburg
Jackson	John W. Jordan, Maquoketa	William Lawder, Maquoketa	F. J. Swift, Maquoketa
Jasper	E. A. McMurray, Newton	S. E. Hinshaw, Newton	H. F. Engle, Newton
Jefferson	S. S. Gauner, Fairfield	F. G. Cook, Fairfield	I. N. Crow, Fairfield
Johnson	Matt Ware, West Branch	Horace M. Korns, Iowa City	George C. Albright, Iowa City
Jones	C. R. Smith, Onslow	W. F. Dolan, Anamosa	T. W. Redmond, Monticello
Keokuk	H. L. Grothaus, Delta	W. P. Stirlen, Delta	W. P. Stirlen, Delta
Kossuth	Robt. L. Williams, Lakota	Pierre Sartor, Titonka	W. T. Peters, Burt
Lee	Frank R. Richmond, Fort Madison	F. B. Dorsey, Jr., Keokuk	F. M. Fuller, Keokuk
			Robert L. Feightner, Fort Madison
Linn	H. J. Jones, Cedar Rapids	T. F. Hersch, Cedar Rapids	M. M. Downing, Cedar Rapids
Louisa	L. E. Weber, Wapello	H. J. Chittum, Wapello	J. H. Chittum, Wapello
Lucas	J. A. Hills, Russell	H. H. Jarvis, Chariton	R. C. Gutch, Chariton
Lyon	L. L. Corcoran, Rock Rapids	A. P. Stewart, Inwood	L. L. Corcoran, Rock Rapids
Madison	Arnold L. Nelson, Winterset	C. B. Hickenlooper, Winterset	C. B. Hickenlooper, Winterset
Mahaska	E. M. Williams, Oskaloosa	G. S. Catterson, Oskaloosa	F. Catterson, Oskaloosa
Marion	E. P. Bell, Pleasantville	G. S. Cornell, Knoxville	G. S. Cornell, Knoxville
Marshall	A. R. Lynn, Marshalltown	G. Meyer, Marshalltown	R. S. Grossman, Marshalltown
Mills	R. B. Dye, Glenwood	M. M. Donelan, Glenwood	B. Lacey, Glenwood
Mitchell	John O. Eiel, Osage	G. G. Walker, Riceville	E. S. Walker, Riceville
Monona	J. S. Deering, Onawa	W. H. Fairbanks, Onawa	E. C. Junger, Soldier
Monroe	W. Gray, Albia	F. Moran, Melrose	A. Moran, Melrose
Montgomery	B. F. Gillmor, Red Oak	R. E. Thomsen, Red Oak	L. J. Cooper, Villisca
Muscatine	B. E. Eversmeyer, Muscatine	R. R. Goad, Muscatine	T. F. Beveridge, Muscatine
O'Brien	W. R. Brock, Sheldon	H. Brackney, Sheldon	W. R. Brock, Sheldon
Osceola	E. F. Farnum, Sibley	H. B. Paulsen, Harris	L. H. Heetland, Sibley
Page	C. D. Smith, Clarinda	F. H. Clark, Clarinda	J. F. Aldrich, Shenandoah
Palo Alto	W. J. Brereton, Emmetsburg	J. H. Powers, Emmetsburg	Harold L. Brereton, Emmetsburg
Plymouth	W. W. Shepard, LeMars	L. C. O'Toole, Le Mars	W. W. Larsen, Le Mars
Pocahontas	A. W. Patterson, Fonda	J. C. Riordan, Pocahontas	J. H. Hovendon, Laurens
Polk	Fred Moore, Des Moines	Leonard A. West, Des Moines	Ralph H. Parker, Des Moines
Pottawattamie	C. F. Baumeister, Avoca	Arnold D. Jensen, Council Bluffs	J. J. Treynor, Council Bluffs
Poweshiek	E. J. Reagan, Brooklyn	J. F. Lawton, Grinnell	C. Y. Lawton, Grinnell
Ringgold	A. J. Watson, Diagonal	J. W. Hill, Mount Ayr	J. Watson, Diagonal
Sac	Henry Fobes, Auburn	R. Dewey, Schaller	L. H. Jones, Wall Lake
Scott	H. Lamb, Davenport	Henry A. Meyers, Davenport	A. P. Donohoe, Davenport
Shelby	Helge Borre, Shelby	A. L. Nielson, Harlan	A. L. Nielson, Harlan
Sioux	John DeBey, Orange City	B. Bendixen, Ireton	D. J. Gleysteen, Alton
Story	H. W. Bowers, Nevada	W. B. Sperow, Nevada	E. B. Bush, Ames
Tama	C. S. Stoakes, Dysart	P. W. Gessner, Dysart	A. Pace, Toledo
Taylor	T. Maloy, Bedford	G. W. Rimel, Bedford	G. W. Rimel, Bedford
Union	Howard Beatty, Creston	H. A. Childs, Creston	John C. Parsons, Creston
Van Buren	Coffin, Farmington	J. N. Stephenson, Milton	C. R. Russell, Keosauqua
Wapello	A. Kepler, Kirkville	Evon Walker, Ottumwa	Evon Walker, Ottumwa
Warren	C. H. Mitchell, Indianola	W. E. Shaw, Indianola	J. E. Loosbrock, Lacona
Washington	M. Braden, Wellman	W. S. Washington	R. E. Stuteman, Washington
Wayne	N. Hyatt, Humeston	J. D. Englehorn, Lineville	T. D. Englehorn, Lineville
Webster	L. L. Leighton, Fort Dodge	John C. Shrader, Fort Dodge	Roland Stahr, Fort Dodge
Winneshiek	A. F. Barfoot, Decorah	Edward F. Ragan, Decorah	A. F. Fritchen, Decorah
Woodbury	L. H. Tripp, Sioux City	Lawrence E. Pierson, Sioux City	
Worth	G. S. Westly, Manly	R. L. Olsen, Northwood	S. S. Westly, Manly
Wright	B. L. Basinger, Goldfield	J. R. Christensen, Eagle Grove	G. E. Schnug, Dows

6-10-34

The JOURNAL
of the
Iowa State Medical Society

Vol. XXIV   Des Moines, Iowa, July, 1934   No. 7

ORATION IN SURGERY

Animating Factors in Surgical History*

E. M. Myers, M.D., Boone

The past is the depository of all that has been. It may seem only a sepulchre full of dead men's bones, yet it holds the achievements of the great workers of all time. It furnishes the steps on which we rise to new discoveries. Although slow and conservative, it struggles on to power under every disadvantage.

The great past comes to us rich with experiments, wise with experience, full of victories and heroism. Not the least of our obligations is the veneration of its greatness. Our wealth consists in the toil of its workers, the thought of the thinkers, and the creations of the gifted ones who have wrought themselves into human history. Thus, we turn to it for a lamp to guide our steps and we sit at its feet as at the feet of a great teacher.

No more fascinating and inspiring story has ever been told than the one which describes the conditions, delineates the characters and portrays the ambitions and the antagonisms in the creative centuries of surgical history. We have spread before us at this session, a great feast of clinics, scientific papers and discussions reflecting the results of proved theories in research and experiment as well as the practice and experience in medicine, surgery and the specialties. What have been the forces at work in the past, to bring these things to pass? They are many and diverse, and standing out against the background of history, more availing than others perhaps, we see the ethical document of Hippocrates, the progressive qualities of the great leaders, their rugged individualism, the advancement of the science, the perfection of the art of surgery, the passion for research, the quest for truth and not least of all, love for the humanities—all, the gradual unfolding

*Presented before the Eighty-third Annual Session, Iowa State Medical Society, Des Moines, May 9, 10, 11, 1934.

of thought and action, an evolution, as it were; having the initial impulse to aid humanity up the ascending scale of life.

Turning for a moment to the times when our profession had few of the characteristics of a science; when it merely observed and guessed; when professional influence was invested in charm and incantations; when medical men relied on nature and sought arbitrary remedies, let us consider briefly some of the influences that vitalized and illumined the profession of surgery until it has become one of the most progressive and beneficent forces of civilization. In so doing, we may have an appreciation of the emotions of the immortal Goethe, which prompted him to say, "The best we derive from history is the enthusiasm it excites in us."

The dead monotony of animal history is written in the meadows or the mountain side, in the hieroglyphics of nature, but great scientific truths come to us incarnated, in living, earnest-seeking, couragous men. Indeed, any truth to forge its way to the front, must sparkle in the brain and burn in the heart of some great man. It must have a human heart to pulsate in union with other hearts, and tender hands to lay hold of other hands.

Hippocrates, whose power of observation and depth of conviction gave him intellectual authority surpassing any other man of his time, saw the vision and felt the need of his beneficence, and from this necessity was formulated "the most memorable of human documents," the Hippocrates Oath. Entering, as it did, the field of moral purpose and personal sacrifice, it became a creed—an ethical guide and an inspiration throughout the ages, as effectual and indispensable today as it was twenty centuries ago.

I know that these are the days when it is popular to say that creeds are nothing; that men have outgrown them; that our profession is a life, not some printed words on parchment; but we surely have not grown to such liberty and looseness. We need a creed as much as we need a skeleton, with a strong spinal column, well covered with muscle and sinew and cuticle, molded into a symmetric creation—an embodiment of beauty and strength and central to some great dominating conviction. Whether or not the Hippocrates Oath was the product of one man's brain is not so vital as the truth that it came into being in response to great human need, and by its very nature is adaptable to the varying changes of society through the centuries.

History was once the mere narrative of insignificant events in the lives of royalty who had neither learning, courage or achievement, but there came a time when it had to do with the elements of civilization, the principles that govern them; the motives that inspire them, with the forces they have subjugated, the sciences they have mastered, the institutions they have established and the liberties they have maintained. These are the events that make great men a necessity. There are many characters in surgical history immortal for the structure of their minds and the sweep of their work.

It takes a strong character to impress the world. Only a few men in a century are big enough to make a bend in the stream of human history. To see men so filling the field of vision that thinkers will soberly discuss the question of them being recognized forces in shaping the ambitions and destinies of the human race is to determine their phenomenal greatness. They must be great enough to be epoch makers, and such were the leaders in medical thought in the bloody travail of fifteen centuries.

The difficulties and antagonisms that hedged their way were only the superstructure used in building their characters and strengthening their purposes. Where is the scaffolding used in piling the Pyramids? Gone, forty centuries ago, but the Pyramids tower over the sands of Egypt as grim and grand as when they received the first royal mummy. So are the creatures and the circumstances that assailed these heroic leaders, gone and forgotten, leaving only a perspective of magnificent achievements.

Measured by the difficulties they surmounted, the plans they executed, the criticisms they received, these worthies are preëminent in surgical history. Their lives seem to be the embodiment of the thought of that great statesman who said, "I would rather have the inspiration of a great idea than to wear any worldly crown for a thousand years." Such inspirations are resistless, and it matters not in what field of human want, they are sure to leave enduring monuments of their greatness. If it is government, they leave constitutions; if it is holy heroism, they leave crusades;

if it is worship, they leave temples and cathedrals; if it is the most gratifying of all impulses, philanthropy, they leave schools, hospitals, sacrificial service and organized benevolences in every field of human need.

Hippocrates, teaching his inductive method, and Galen, the exponent of the deductive method, were supreme in their time, but their rule was tyrannical because it denied the minds of men freedom of expression. "To deny authority or dissent from their teaching was not only heterodox, it was heresy punishable by death." As a result, surgery for more than a thousand years was almost barren of notable achievement. So oppressive and far-reaching was this autocratic rule that it called for rare courage for Mandville, in a frenzy of disapproval, to exclaim, "Surely God did not exhaust all his wisdom in the creation of Galen."[1]

Nor can we forget that as late as the sixteenth century, Servatus, the discoverer of pulmonary circulation, was burned at the stake in Geneva, as a heretic. Vesalius was attacked because he taught a new anatomy; Paré was criticized bitterly for his simplified treatment of wounds; The entire French Academy derided Harvey for his theory of the circulation of blood and Pott inveighed against Hunter's operation for hernia. Frequently ostracism, always ridicule and contempt greeted the doctrines, practices and virtues of the surgical teachers who were at variance with these despots.

How shall we speak of such heroism? Their suffering moves our pity; their courage inspires our purpose and challenges our admiration, and we reverently exclaim, "Oh, that heroes' work should be so dear and the trials of these valiants so abundant!"

What an inspiration it is to contemplate these worthies! They meant conquest and expected victory because they worked from an inner impulse and so rose superior to every disadvantage and found their fields of labor everywhere. Through these turbulent centuries, their individualism was not to be denied—first a conviction, then a purpose, then a revolution, and then a new epoch. Truly, we have a great ancestry—we are born of heroes!

Notwithstanding the fortitude which these leaders exhibited in this long period of intellectual darkness, it is not difficult to understand why the discovery by Harvey, for example, which gave physiology a new birth and which firmly laid the scientific foundation of surgery, had eluded his predecessors. Many before him had stood on the very brink of this discovery, but they were devoid of any spark of investigation, they preserved old

ether, were guided by the experience of previous trials, half success and half failure.

In the pre-anesthetic days, the surgeon had to move with celerity, undeterred by struggles or hemorrhage. There is no need for such qualities now—the spectacular in surgery has gone with the men who fostered it. Surgical success is no longer measured by the number of minutes required for operating, but by the condition of the patient many days after. The triumph of the old surgeon was immediate, and scarcely reached beyond the amphitheater; the triumph of the modern operator is deferred, and is found in the wards and convalescent homes. Truly, the changes that this discovery has wrought in the method, the confidence, and the gentleness of the modern operator, are as wonderful as the discovery itself.

The patient labors of Lister, under the inspiration of Darwin's theory, brought him imperishable honors, yet none was more ready than he to acknowledge how much the antiseptic methods of wound treatment owed to the researches and discoveries of Pasteur.

To the fortunate, life in the eighteenth century meant easy going enjoyment in the broad sunshine of life, in the midst of delightful paintings of Gainsborough and Mozart's symphonies. But the eighteenth century was also the age of successful quacks, high infantile and adult mortality rates, devastating epidemics, and the worst hospital management on record. Even under the brilliant teachings of men like John Hunter, there had been few advances in surgery because "beliefs were formed more on authority than on facts."[2]

It is sad to think that before the era of antisepsis there stood behind the earnest surgeon, a shadow which rendered hopeless, his kindliest effort. The possibility of a revolution in scientific knowledge was unthought of, and to many indeed, inconceivable.

Such were the conditions when Lister did his work, and became an apostle of a new doctrine and a defender of a new faith. It is hardly possible to speak of the results of his amazing work, in measured terms. Operations which Lister neither contemplated nor dared to perform are now done every day—operations which now permit us to study at leisure the morbid processes during the lifetime of the patient. A "pathology of the living" has been created; a close correlation has been established between visible structural changes and the symptoms to which they give rise. "Surgery has indeed become the strong arm of research."

Probably the most notable change in surgery which has come as a result of Lister's work has been the creation of new knowledge of visceral disorders, and practically all was gained by experimental science of which the actual material was the human patient. Yet the contributions of the laboratory in these conditions were almost negligible, a fact which prompted Sir Thomas Lewis to remark, "physiology is lagging too far behind, too much concerned with the laboratory, too little with hospital wards and men."

Profiting by such experience we are learning to concern ourselves with early recognition of disease. We have been too much engaged in terminal events; our hospital wards have been filled with examples of advanced disease. Research work and clinical inquiry lie too much apart; surgical advance depends not on the clinician alone nor on laboratory workers alone, but on their union in decisive activity.

However, as close as this relationship may be, we must not fail to realize that it is chiefly clinical judgment that must govern our decisions and that laboratory research is chiefly ancillary rather than a controlling influence. It is a very grave error to allow the clear evidence of clinical experience to become subservient to the disclosures of the laboratory. Let us not forget that we practice an art, and never allow theories however ingenious, or statistics however conclusive, or authority however venerable, to take the place of experience.

From time to time, some of the greatest surgeons have expressed a belief that surgery had reached the limit of efficiency as a method of treating disease, but that is not new. Erickson made such a prediction when Listerism first became established. Twenty-five years ago, Sir F. Treves, still in his fifties announced his retirement thus, "Surgery has become stale, flat and unprofitable—only minor technical advances are possible." Yet, Horsely had just removed the first spinal cord tumor; the thorax was still unopened and mutilating operations were being done on the mouth, tongue and jaw, a field now almost entirely surrendered to radio therapy and cautery.

There can be no limit to surgery; if it would live, it must advance. It is not unlikely that much of this progress will lie in the direction of intelligent cooperation between physician and surgeon. Indeed, it would almost seem that the object of the surgeon of the future will be the abolition of surgery. It is too visionary to say a medical cure may be found for exophthalmic goiter, which is a toxic process, or that gastric and duodenal ulcers should be cured without operation? We have only to look beyond the boundaries of speculation, however, to find many tangible evidences of surgical progress.

There has been real advance in the systematized treatment of fractures and the period of incapacity has been definitely reduced. Rapidly alternating diathermy current now renders possible the ablation of brain tumors, formerly considered inoperable. The delicate technic of the abdominal surgeon is immeasurably superior to that of his predecessor 25 years ago, because he realizes that it is vital to conserve every drop of blood, to prevent undue exposure of viscera, to diminish afferent nerve stimuli, and to avoid sacrificing efficiency for speed. The cooperation of internist and surgeon in preoperative preparation and postoperative care is another noteworthy advance.

New conceptions arising from this knowledge will naturally restrict operations, but the field of surgery will enlarge to include what are now regarded as medical diseases. Witness the progress in cranial surgery, through the work of Horsely, Kocher, Cushing and others, in revealing the peculiarities of the cerebral circulation, and clarifying cerebral lesions. Until recently, the chest was considered out of bounds to the surgeon, but the development of radiology, the use of lipiodol, artificial pneumothorax and new knowledge of respiration and gas exchange has widened the field of thoracic surgery, so that removal of tumors of the lung, pleura and mediastinum, draining deep seated abscesses and even lobectomy is now being accomplished. The brilliant work now being done on the sympathetic nervous system, on arthritis and osteomyelitis, in plastic surgery, on the endocrine glands, the renal system, on nerves and blood vessels, in industrial surgery not to mention surgery in special fields, gives us only a gleam of infinitely greater achievements. The fact that we have no definite knowledge of the future, no clear vision of the direction in which surgery may advance, does not justify the prediction that no improvement can or will take place.

It is the conviction of many that the advancement of the art of surgery will not come with the invasion of new anatomic fields nor with furthe perfection of technic, but will come with increase knowledge of the cause and prevention of disease with improvement in diagnostic methods, the exer cise of better surgical judgment and broade knowledge of medicine. At least, these source from which advancement might come, are th fields in which we especially need to work.

The fear of sepsis will no longer command th thoughts of the surgeon; they will be directed t his studies in lives, splenic and pancreatic func tion, of sugar, of nonprotein content, of hormone. or of metabolic rates, for these are the factor which enable us to understand the patient's pecu liarities, his perverse symptoms, his unfavorabl reactions, and his resistance, so that we may prepare him for or deny him an operation and guide him to a successful convalescence.

If surgery is to be something more than a craft; if it is to continue to be a means of research, those who practice it should not be rendered impotent by provincialism. The great moving force of our profession through all the centuries has been individualism. Nothing so easily destroys a man's capacity for thought and action as the restriction of his mental efforts. There are today groups who would socialize us and divest us of our individualism, and make our profession machine powered, under bureaucratic control. We are confronted with a new and serious problem, and it must be met and answered.

This transformation of attitude toward our profession on the part of bureaucracy is bound to come; it lies with us to say by which way it will come. If we, as a profession do not display adequate sensitiveness to social values and adequate statesmanship in meeting these social issues and ourselves lead and administer this evolution, we may be sure that we in turn will inevitably be led and governed.[3]

Standing boldly against the forces of bureaucracy which are moving upon us from all quarters, threatening the foundations of our profession, is the report of the Commission of Medical Education, of which our distinguished and honored Dr. Bierring is a member. A worthy document: "It represents professional idealism, it extols individualism, and is rich in constructive thought toward overcoming the faults of the proposed system" of the Committee on the Costs of Medical Care.[4] In these ominous times, we must not fail to perpetuate the spirit of our ancestors and match their victories, for we have mightier agencies within our reach, stronger weapons and wider fields if we will but use them, and our responsibilities are measured by our opportunities. The threatened danger of destroying the very element which can assure close and enduring personal relation between surgeon and patient, and substituting for it fallacious methods by which other public services are being purged, ought to arouse us to renewed courage and united activity.

Manifestly, there are doubts, even thoughts of despair, but is man, profession, or nation to be judged by unusual behavior in this period of unrest? We should find encouragement in this seething restlessness and criticism of social forms, for they constitute evidence of growth rather than decay, but they must be wisely administered and firmly controlled.

Let us not be disheartened; the direction of our vision is everything. In our progress toward idealism, we may overcome every stronghold of bureaucracy; destroy every temple of cultism and quackery; burn every altar of hypocrisy and commercialism; purge our ranks of every corruption. We may advance our science, encourage research, beautify our art, establish our individualism, and we will have yet done nothing if we are indifferent to the humanities, those instrumentalities that not only afford culture and lend dignity to the profession, but also those impulses which inspire benevolence.

There occur here and there throughout history, outstanding sentences which seem to epitomize the dominant thought as motives of life. There is a sentence in the writings of Hippocrates, over which many commentators have lingered: "the love of humanity associated with love of his craft; the joy of working joined to a true love of his brother." That is the animating spirit of surgery—the endowment of its ascendency.

To stand, as it was once my cherished privilege, by the side of a master surgeon and look upon the warping spine of an only infant son, twisted by disease into a helpless disfigurement; then to behold this surgeon, with despairing and almost rebellious hand, lift that frail body, with every drop of his blood boiling into one purpose; and every fiber of his being, tense in one everlasting determination, at all costs, to place that child above want and certain of social recognition; to have such experiences and relationships with great leaders in our profession, is to catch that spirit and to have a new conception of the worth and duty of our profession, when Nature's defeated harmonies need restoring.

"Surgery is more than science—more than art. In dealing with menacing realities, the surgeon must possess courage and humility and work with an exactitude that approaches piety. We, who seek to alleviate pain, restore health and turn the hand of death aside, have a sacred trust."[5]

Let us rise to the worth of our heritage and be true to our trust; to foster science, to perfect the art; to respect our ethics; to venerate the humanities, to seek the truth, to labor always for progress and elevate our calling in the eyes of men, so that, in the repose from our labors, in the cool and shade of the evening of our professional life, when the memories of those animosities and scorns which exhaust and defeat, bear upon us, and we feel we have not come near enough to our professional reward to hear the music and enjoy the feast, we may yet have the unspeakable satisfaction of having had as the guiding principle in our life and work, this comforting sentiment, "The spark of life we tend is a part of the divine—and immortal."

SHALL ORGANIZED MEDICINE SURVIVE?*

Oliver J. Fay, M.D., Des Moines

The assembly of a medical society, be it local, statewide, or national in scope, has always seemed to me particularly inspiring. It signifies organized medicine, and organized medicine has always stood for science and progress, efficiency and human service. It is true that medicine had its birth in the fears and superstitions of primitive man, and it continued to be nine-tenths cant and credulity, and one-tenth philters and folklore so long as the practice of medicine continued to be dominated by religion and philosophy. Though the painted mask and the tom-tom gradually gave way to the impressive costume by day and the mystic voice in the temple by night, though the propitiatory offering changed from skins and provender to votary tablets and coin of the realm, there was little essential progress until the physician had freed himself from religious and philosophic control. Not until then did he establish for himself ideals of truth and service and through those ideals awaken to consciousness of medical fraternity and solidarity.

In those first centuries of progress the disciples of a great physician and teacher honored him as founder of a school and thus became a group united by common interests and a common cause. The medical guilds followed the social pattern of a later age, and if they sometimes overstressed ethics they yet perpetuated the idea of fellowship. State and national medical societies, formed for the express purpose of furthering scientific advancement, stressing community of interests, and emphasizing internationalism in medicine, were a development of the nineteenth century, and it is only within our own times that these societies have a measure of the support they deserve, have begun to realize the dreams of their founders in their support of scientific progress, a broadening field of service, and a deepening fellowship. Perhaps in no field of human endeavor have there been so many and such signal achievements to record; yet today organized medicine is once more in peril of philosophic control. In spite of their proud record, mere men of science are, the public is assured by the ballyhoo of the subsidized sociologists, incapable of carrying on except under the direction and control of our doctors of philosophy —those men who have nothing in common with the medical profession save the title of "doctor," and who with their large salaries are as alien to

* Presented before the Eighty-third, Annual Session, Iowa State Medical Society, Des Moines, May 9, 10, 11, 1934.

the under privileged upon whom they base their case.

For the past several years, the medical profession has been a favorite target. If now and then a faint voice has been raised in sentimental praise of the achievements of medical science and the selfless devotion of its disciples, that voice has been drowned out by the thundering chorus of criticism and condemnation. The infant and maternal mortality rate is too high, and the medical profession has lamentably failed to lower it; more, it is by its own confession in part responsible for that mortality rate. The physicians of our country are unevenly distributed throughout the land; a century ago, the doctor was content to spend his days and a large part of his nights traveling rough trails on horseback, but his modern prototype prefers the comforts and contacts of the city, so that while our urban districts are oversupplied, many sparsely settled districts are in desperate need of physicians. One day it is suggested that this rural shortage be overcome by permitting men with a shortened period of training to enter upon the practice of medicine there. The next, there are loud lamentations because too many people are cared for by poorly qualified physicians. Again it is proclaimed that a large part of our populace is too poor to pay for needed medical care; or that while the very poor are well provided for in free clinics and endowed hospitals, our great middle class is unable to obtain adequate medical care at a price it can afford to pay. Even the rich are not forgotten. Now and again a voice is raised condemning physicians for having a graduated fee schedule; it is unfair that the man of wealth should be asked to pay more than his poor neighbor; service is service, it is proclaimed, and is worth only so much regardless of the social and financial position of the person to whom it is rendered. After undertaking an arduous survey—amply financed by various funds and foundations—our doctors of philosophy have even discovered what any mere doctor of medicine could have told them off-hand, namely, that the income of the average physician is insufficient to provide an adequate return on and eventually amortize his investment in education and training, to meet necessary expenses, and allow for the further study that will keep him in touch with medical advances, to say nothing of permitting him to accumulate a competency for his old age.

It avails little to point out the fallacies in this arraignment. That a group of physicians has made a careful study of the problem of maternal mortality and its causes, and has had the courage to make public its conclusion that the medical pro

costs of medical and hospital care because such expenses are unpredictable; one family may be entirely free from any such expenses in any given year, or even for many years, while another family may be called upon to meet an emergency that would seriously cut or even wipe out its income for the year. It must be admitted that the sun riseth on the evil and on the good, and that the rain falleth alike on the just and the unjust, but under our present social order what other assurances of absolute equality do we have? Which of our sociologists feels it incumbent upon himself to reduce his income to the level of the rag-picker's; or believes that if the latter's income were raised to the level of his own, the rag-picker would so administer his affairs as to train his children to useful citizenship and lay aside a competence for his old age; or would in his years of good health and good fortune provide for medical care if and when good health fails him? But this, your sociologist will argue, is the most convincing argument in favor of the state's administration of medical affairs; adequate medical care, in health and in disease, is one of the basic needs of a people and as such, should be provided by the state. Sanitary lodging, proper food, adequate clothing must outrank medical care as basic needs. Is the state to provide all these, not only in an emergency such as the one we are facing, but as a permanent institution? If your sociologist answers "No," then we have a right to question the singling out of medical care as a basic need when the very essentials of life itself are not provided by the state; and if he answers "yes," then we have indeed reached the ideal of the communist, and it may well be asked whether even the sociologist is ready to accept a social state in which even he would lose his exalted position and be reduced to the rank and file. The provision of medical care by the state under sociologic direction and control, of course, would be a horse of a different and far more acceptable color, elevating the sociologist to that overlordship in the practice of medicine for which, having made a cursory survey of the field, he modestly feels himself far better fitted than the medical man who has merely made it his life's work.

Dr. James H. S. Bossard, a Ph.D., and a sociologist, of course, points out that the large amount of free medical care given to children in the schools, the soldiers in the World War, and workers in industrial plants, and the increasing participation of the government in medical practice have caused the public to look on medical service as they do on education and police protection, and that in considering the public demand for socialized health service, we must consider the weight of numbers—only 150,000 doctors as compared with 122,000,000 patients. We admit the weight of this latter argument for the physician has long been schooled in the precept that his own welfare is always secondary to the welfare of the group; but we do question Dr. Bossard's right to state that *"over against* this newer public demand for a socialized health service . . . stands a very old profession dominated by individualistic conceptions." We have as yet no reason for subscribing to his inference that the best interests of the public and of the profession are in reality antagonistic unless we are willing to accept the sociologists' mere assumptions as gospel. We are willing to plead guilty to the charge, if charge it be, that we are individualists, but who among you, with first hand knowledge of the sick has found a patient other than an individualist? Once he has an injured eye, or an aching stomach, it becomes distinctly *his* eye, or *his* stomach; he is not content with treatment of *an* eye injury, or *a* gastric ulcer; *his* injury, *his* hunger pains are things apart, and he is not only himself acutely conscious of this distinction; he must feel that his medical attendant is also aware of the unique nature of his suffering. He may not be averse to having the state pay his bills, but he is far from desiring a mechanized medical service. And who, having had experience with the bureaucratic brand of service that we have come to associate with state control, can question that socialized medical service would be mechanized service?

In the numerous sociologic surveys, two fundamental issues seem to have been lost in the fog of miasmal radicalism. One fundamental which has been ignored is an economic principle of which we have heard much in other fields; the control of surpluses. We have learned, and it has been a painful lesson, that the havoc which ensues when we continually produce more foodstuffs than we can consume or export, affects not alone the farmer but everyone. It has apparently occurred only to the thoughtful few that the overproduction of physicians, which we are permitting our medical schools, often at the taxpayers' expense, not only works a hardship upon the physicians themselves but is also responsible for many of the unfortunate phases of medical practice directly affecting the public. I believe that a majority of men entering the practice of medicine have the scientist's love for truth seeking, are honestly activated by the desire to serve their fellowmen, but they would be more than human if they could retain these bright ideals untarnished through the years when their work fails to bring them a live-

lihood, to care for their children, to provide a competence for their old age. Let our sociologists who would appoint themselves our overlords turn their attention to putting a brake upon the competitive ambitions of our medical schools, and insist upon restricting the number of their graduates to the small additional number needed to care for the nominal increase in our population. Recognizing that the poor we have always with us, and that they must continue to have what they have always had since medicine became an organized profession, free care, let our sociologists devote their talents to placing the burden of such care where it belongs, upon the community as a whole. Thus will they contribute something tangible to the solution of the cost of medical care. It is axiomatic that man attaches small value to that which is his without effort and without price. Except among the very poor, who are acknowledgedly already receiving free medical care, we cannot hope to raise our health standards by offering the public free health service. The public which, our sociologists would have us believe, demands free medical service as its right, is so little interested in health problems that free lectures on health topics are notoriously little attended. Let our sociologists devote the resources of their great funds and foundations to an educational campaign directed towards making the general public health-conscious, towards arousing in them a sense of their own responsibility for their physical well-being. Neither the primitive attitude of placing the entire responsibility with the gods, nor the sociologic one of thrusting such responsibility upon the state is calculated to insure the cooperation of the individual, and his cooperation we must have if we are to accomplish anything tangible.

A second fundamental which has been ignored, perhaps because it does not accord well with the contemplated sociologic overlordship, is a recognition of the local character of many of these problems. Thus in sparsely populated regions, medical attendance can be provided only if the physician is assured a livelihood. His income from private practice must be supplemented by certain grants or subsidies from the state, or some political subdivision. This, and calling a halt on the continued annual over-production of physicians, will tend to alleviate some of our urban problems also. In many cities the outpatient departments of our hospitals, dispensaries and clinics, maintained always with the best of intentions but too often with an entire lack of sociologic discrimination, create special problems and seriously interfere with the establishment and maintenance of high ethical and professional standards. It is not only the soldier who must fight on his belly—anatomically men are built much on the same pattern, whatever their trade or profession. During those halycon days before the Great Depression, optimism and over-expansion were not limited to individuals and industry; many of our hospitals also sought to materialize their castles in Spain and as a result have found themselves confronted by a financial crisis. They have found comfort and moral support in some of the schemes fathered by our sociologists; the idea of building insurance or community clinics about our hospitals naturally appeals to hospital boards and superintendents, and they, along with the sociologists, are inclined to lose sight of an important and basic consideration; that the physician is after all an essential part, more, he is *the* essential part of any scheme for medical care.

The sociologist himself could not be considered a menace to medical progress. His voice, whether raised in peans of praise or in vituperation would not be heard outside the circle of his own kind, for the public finds sociology in the abstract of even less interest than it finds medicine. The campaign of the sociologists is a danger, and a very real one, only because it is backed by the almost limitless resources of such foundations as the Twentieth Century, the Milbank, and the Rosenwald Funds. They have attacked and have the avowed intention of undermining organized medicine. Through publicity and the press, they seek to arouse public opinion in support of their program of so-called socialized medicine. Through specious presentations of the professional aspects of state medicine, they seek recruits among those who are striving desperately to establish themselves in practice. By insidious propaganda through men who, although ostensibly physicians, having found easy chairs at a safe distance from the firing line, they strive to give the impression of a grave schism within the ranks of the medical profession. It is amusing but perhaps not relevant to recall that the fortunes which made possible these sociologic foundations were not made by applying their socialistic principles to industry. What we dare not forget is that as *individuals* we are helpless, we may be forced to dance to the tune the sociologist would pipe, but as a *profession* we cannot be forced into any scheme which would exploit the physician, which would make him the puppet under brain trust control. Under the systematic campaign of disruption, can organized medicine survive? There can be but one answer: in the interests of enduring fellowship, of humane service, of scientific progress, organized medicine must survive.

THE LEUKOCYTE BLOOD PICTURES IN ACUTE INFECTIONS*

M. Pinson Neal, M.D.†
Columbia, Missouri

The differential blood count combined with and in its relation to the total white cell count is a valuable diagnostic and prognostic aid in both acute medical and surgical diseases. From experience under properly controlled conditions we know this fact to be true, yet one frequently finds articles condemning the leukocyte count as being of little or no value, or of being misleading. The common error is for an author to criticize the leukocyte count as a guide to infection on the basis of his using the total cell enumeration for that interpretation. Another error, which is even more serious, is for the differential cell percentages to be estimated on the basis of counts of 25, 50, or even 100 cells. We frequently find supposedly well trained men counting 25 white blood cells and multiplying the individual numbers by four, and recording this as the percentage of cells. This is like walking across a corner of a forest, seeing three elms, one oak, and two sycamore trees, and then saying that the forest is made up of only these types of trees and in such proportion.

In the performance of blood counts, meticulous care in every detail must be insisted upon. Adherence to standard technic, counting 100 squares for total cell values, and obtaining the differential percentages from at least a 300 cell count, is our routine procedure.

We are convinced that properly interpreted, such leukocyte counts constitute a means to the saving of lives, shortening of hospital periods, diminishing needless suffering, and preventing unnecessary operations. The findings and conclusions herein are based upon gross and histopathology of the lesions where surgical conditions are concerned, since this is the only exact method of diagnosis. Conclusions drawn from leukocyte counts not so controlled cannot be accurate. Blood counts and other morphologic blood studies are identical with the histologic studies of fixed tissues, and are therefore, not for the untrained and inexperienced to make final interpretations upon. To carry the comparison further, the cells characteristically seen in the local reaction in disease, as in pyogenic infections, syphilis, typhoid fever and the leukemias, are the cells causing the modification in the blood picture in such diseases.

The following methods of choice and corresponding interpretations will be found helpful:

* Presented before the Lee County Medical Society, Keokuk, March 15, 1934.
† Professor of Pathology, University of Missouri, Columbia.

1. Total white cell count; an index to resistance.

2. Differential cell enumeration; a neutrophilia indicates pyogenic infection, with the degree, dose and virulence of infection being shown by a rise in the percentage of neutrophils.

3. The septic factor (neutrophil-eosinophil ratio); a supplementary index to the presence of pyogenic infection.

4. The estimation of young and immature neutrophils; a guide to pyogenic infection, and when increased in numbers, indicates hyperplasia of bone marrow meeting the call for these cells.

5. Graphic method of recording total count and neutrophil percentage; demonstrating by a curve the degree of resistance as weighed against the infection.

The Total Count Variations and Indications. The total count is normal or below in uncomplicated tuberculosis, typhoid fever, malaria, measles, influenza and agranulocytosis, diseases from which acute pyogenic lesions often are largely differentiated by the blood findings. A hyperleukocytosis occurs after hemorrhage, after injections of bacterial vaccines, during the late stages of pregnancy, in the puerperium and in the leukemias, which are not conditions of pyogenic character.

Normal or subnormal total counts are often seen in highly virulent, massive, or very severe cases of infection, as peritonitis, pneumonia and septicemia, and in gangrenous or perforating lesions, as appendicitis. The total cell count is often little or not at all increased in cases of acute infection where there is little or no resistance on the part of the patient, and in those with slight infections.

These facts reveal the fallacy of relying upon total leukocyte counts in the diagnosis of infection and as a guide to operation. Yet it is still used with little, and in many cases, no reference to the differential percentage. It is not uncommon to find hospitals with standing staff orders that the differential cell count need not be done when the total count is 10,000 or less. We have seen patients held under observation because of total counts of 10,000 and less, and when an operation was finally performed there was found a ruptured or gangrenous lesion like an appendix, a peritonitis, or a spreading infection. Total counts depended upon to indicate infection are dangerous. They should be given no value except when considered with the differential count, and the two then weighed in conjunction with clinical findings.

The total leukocyte count is a guide to the resistance of the patient against infection in medical and surgical conditions.[1] With a good resistance the total count is high, and as long as the infection

trophils and the total count run parallel. The increase in neutrophils indicates the presence of infection and a corresponding increase in total count shows a favorable reaction to the infection.

Eosinophils (polymorphonuclear eosinophils). An absence of eosinophils or a decrease in their percentage, associated with a rise in neutrophils, termed by Simon,[3] the septic factor, is a definite aid in deciding upon the presence or absence of pyogenic infection. The presence of the normal or of an increased percentage of eosinophils is a favorable sign that no acute infection is present. The falling eosinophil values in acute infection are often sharp from existing high percentages seen in bronchial asthma, and parasitic or skin diseases. An increase or the reappearance of eosinophils after a previous drop, or their disappearance, indicates the "dawn of convalescence" and is often the first evidence of improvement. The post-infective eosinophilia is of great importance in prognosis. Their return in numbers above normal is a sure indication that the infection has been overcome or completely removed.

Variation in Lymphocyte Percentages. In interpreting lymphocytic percentages, one must remember that their values are above normal in childhood, in the lymphatic leukemias, and the diseases associated with toxic manifestations such as syphilis, tuberculosis, toxic goiters, measles, whooping cough and typhoid fever. Lymphocytes are not phagocytic or protective in acute pyogenic infections. In fact, as the neutrophil percentage increases in streptococcic, pneumococcic, staphylococcic and meningococcic infections the lymphocytes decrease, resulting in a lymphopenia. This has been used as the neutrophilic-lymphocytic index. As the acute process is removed or overcome, the neutrophils decrease and the lymphocytes increase to normal or above. This ratio or index is not as dependable as is the neutrophil-eosinophil index.

The Estimation and Recording of Young and Immature Cells. Arneth made the first effort to interpret young forms and place a clinical interpretation upon their significance. Von Schilling modified the Arneth index. Technical methods of both are unwieldy for practical purposes, often cause delay where intervention is needed, and are subject to wide discrepancies through factors of personal interpretation. Long before the Schilling count was introduced, I used a more general method of determining young cells. Since blood cell studies correspond to the histologic study of fixed tissues, the measurements of immaturity have been the same as in tissue pathology, particularly in tumor diagnosis. We take into considera-

tion the size of the cell and the nucleus, their ratio, the staining reaction of each, and whether the nucleus is non-lobated as in myelocytes, merely indented, or definitely lobated. Recently the terms "segmented," or "nonsegmented" and "filamented" or "nonfilamented" are accepted as descriptive of adult and mature cells, or young and immature cells. In general, the interpretation of young cells versus adult cells has been limited to the polymorphonuclear neutrophils, where 90 to 95 per cent of the adult forms show two or more lobations. Myelocytes and myeloblasts must be recorded as such, for when present, they indicate an added degree of gravity to the case of infection, or otherwise establish a diagnosis of leukemia.

Under normal conditions the proportion between young and mature forms is one to ten, with the maximum limit being one to five, which value is also considered normal for young children. A ratio of one to three, or one to one, indicates the presence of pyogenic infection, and the greater the number of the young forms, the more severe the condition. A proportion of one immature to one or less mature cells indicates marked severity.

In the very early stage of acute infection, mature neutrophils are drawn from the storage center in the bone marrow and may give in the transport system, that is, the blood, a neutrophil percentage of 85 or more, with a possible total cell count of 20,000, and yet maintain a low ratio of the young or immature forms. This interpretation is often missed because by the time a blood count is made, the young forms have increased and the ratio may definitely point to an infection. While the estimation of the young and immature forms has rarely been found necessary where early and repeated counts are obtained, it has been of much value in their absence, and in cases of questionable findings.

The Erythrocyte Sedimentation Rate. The erythrocyte sedimentation rate has been used by some gynecologists, phthisiologists and others as a guide to infection and to determine the degree of activity of the disease if and when present, and as an aid in determining the proper time for operation. The test has its values, particularly in gynecology and in tuberculosis. It does, however, fall short of permitting certain interpretations from the differential and total leukocyte count, and in its use there are other limitations. It cannot replace the methods advocated for the diagnosis and prognosis of acute infections and of the leukemias.

Repeated Counts. Repetition of counts is a necessity in watching the doubtful case (compare counts 1 and 2 in Chart 1). They show in acute pyogenic infections the rising neutrophilia, the falling eosinophil values and the waning of a lymphocytosis that may have been present. Not uncommonly we see a blood count with a neutrophil percentage of 45 to 50, and three hours later a count of 60, or even 70. The second count showing the rise in neutrophil values of 50 or more per cent is a very emphatic indication, yet the values of the second count are strictly within normal percentage. Repeated counts showing the trend or curve are of much greater value than a single count, although the latter in itself in well established infections may be diagnostic.

Early Counts. An early count to establish, relatively speaking, a base line of normal for the patient at the time is always advisable, and often imperative. Neutrophil percentage values of 40 or even 50, which are common, could rise, and eosinophil percentages of twelve or six could drop to 50 per cent, and yet be within the strict range of normal. It is under such conditions that the leukocyte count fails unless one has

taken an early count and charted the changing values (compare counts 1 and 2 in Chart 1).

Charting the Findings. To record repeated counts, nothing surpasses the use of a chart or diagram upon which one may visualize a changing record throughout the course of a disease. We use a blood report form which carries our modified Gibson chart, and upon which several complete blood examinations may be recorded. Here one may see at a glance, the changes from count to count and interpret the resistance units of disproportion indicated by a rising or falling line. The original Gibson chart[4] used a base line

as the starting point connecting 10,000, the normal extreme total count, which is recorded on the left side of the chart, with 75 per cent, the normal extreme neutrophil percentage, which is recorded on the right side. A rise in one per cent of neutrophils is met with an increase of 1,000 cells in the total count under normal conditions.[4] A horizontal line then indicates a resistance in proportion to the degree of infection. A rise of the neutrophil end of the line above that of the total count indicates that the infection is in excess of the resistance (Chart 1, line 5, and Chart 2, line 1). This is measured in the terms of minus units of disproportion for each point (one per cent) of rise. The greater the disproportion between these two ends of the lines, that is, the more sharp the rise in the line, with the neutrophil end being disproportionately high, the more severe is the condition and the more guarded should be the prognosis. To the reverse of this, where the total cell count end of the line is above the neutrophil end, the measurement is a plus unit of disproportion and indicates resistance in excess of the infection (Chart 1, line 2). A rising line of more than five units of disproportion in surgical conditions indicates the necessity of surgery, and the greater the number of units of disproportion, the more urgent is this need for immediate surgery. A falling line is not contraindicative to surgery, but does mean that surgery is not imperative, although it may be advisable. With such counts, all facts pertaining to the patient must be used in determining the question of operation.

Postoperative or Post-Infection Counts. Daily

Date 1934	3-22	3-23	3-24	3-26	3-27
Time	6PM	3PM	9PM	8AM	8AM
Count number	1	2	3	4	5
Coagulation time					
Leucocytes per c mm	12448		14304	25100	31290 13312
Differential count					
P.M. Basophils					
P. M. Neutrophiles	54.7	75	92.6	97.3	94
P. M. Eosinophiles	1.3	0.7			
Lymphocytes	40	23	7.3	2.7	6
Large Mononuclears			1.3		
Transitionals					
Myelocytes					
Mast cells	4				
Immature P.M.	3	7	10	20	16.5
Erythrocytes per c					
Hemoglobin					
Color index					
Anisocytosis					
Poikilocytosis					
Polychromatophilia					
Granular degeneration					
Plasmodium Malariae					
Wasserman					
Widal					
Culture					
Blood sugar					
Blood urea					
Blood N. P. N.					

3-23-34. Operation 6 P.M. Diagnosis: Mechanically obstructed appendix. Small amount free murky peritoneal fluid.
3-24-34. Chill and fever.
3-26-34. Pneumococci in peritoneal exudate. 3-29- death, general peritonitis.
Chart 1, Count 1, early base line of normal, 2 shows rise to 75% neutrophils indicating infection. Counts 3 and 4 are 14 and 38 hours postoperative showing infection present and increasing. Count 5 on 4th postoperative day, resistance broken - prognosis very bad.

postoperative counts and daily counts in strictly medical conditions, such as pneumonia, are of great value in prognosis, in determining when infection has been overcome, when convalescence is established, or when there is reinfection, spread of infection, new field of infection, or loss of resistance. Often the change in curve is the only indication of something happening in the course of the disease that demands investigation and correction (Chart 2, count 3). Even in the absence of clinical evidences of these changes the leukocyte picture cannot be disregarded. Often a wound infection or an infection in an entirely new field, such as pneumonia, hepatitis, or pyelitis, may be suspected before there are other findings.

After surgical procedures in acute infection, especially where the peritoneum or other large areas are involved, the postoperative counts taken during the first twenty-four hours often show a rise in the neutrophil percentage above the preoperative finding. This may be interpreted as the continuation of a rising curve due to the stimulated bone marrow from the infection prior to its removal. However, we believe that in some cases it is due to the increased toxic absorption through the vascular channels as a result of physical manipulation during operation. Attention is called to this because unless this rise has been carefully watched under such interpretation, it may be taken as a sign of increasing gravity, which we feel is not warranted unless the rise is very sharp or persists over several days (Chart 1, counts 3, 4 and 5).

The graph and record on Chart 2 demonstrate the full value to be obtained by the methods advocated. The count recorded as line 1 with an absence of eosinophils reveals a preoperative finding one and one-half hours before the removal of an acute suppurative appendix with perforation. This line showing 13 minus units of disproportion indicates an acute pyogenic infection of a marked degree, with resistance not in proportion to the infection. Line 2 represents the expected normal postoperative receding line, with the reappearance of eosinophils to two per cent on the third postoperative day. The record of count 3 on the fifth day called for investigation. This represents a rise from line 2 with a disproportionate rise in neutrophils and a drop in percentage of eosinophils. Spreading of the wound revealed a deep pocket of pus. The count represented by line 4 followed drainage of this focus of infection and the reestablishment of the convalescent curve.

General Facts. Emphasis should be made relative to leukocyte values in the following conditions:—

Where spontaneous drainage occurs throughout the course of infection or at irregular intervals, as in pyelitis with its alternating periods of retention and drainage, the blood picture is subject to modification at least to a marked degree in the total cell count. Pneumococcic infections notoriously give high values especially in the total cell count. In appendicitis one rarely sees a total cell count above 30,000, but in pneumococcic infections one commonly finds them above this value. Recently we had a case of lobar pneumonia complicated by pneumococcic pericarditis which gave a total white cell count of 63,000 with 96 per cent neutrophils. A peritoneal inflammation gives a

Date 1933	4-14	4-17	4-19	4-22	
Time	7A.M.	10AM	10AM	8AM	
Count number	1	2	3	4	
Coagulation time					
Leucocytes per c mm	17050		13000	15400	8740
Differential count P.M. Basophile					
P. M. Neutrophils	95	75	82	62	
P. M. Eosinophiles	0	2	0.7	1.3	
Lymphocytes	5	21	14	33	
Large Mononuclears	0	2	3	3.7	
Transitionals					
Myelocytes					
Unclassified					
Erythrocytes per c mm					
Hemoglobin					
Color index					
Anisocytosis					
Poikilocytosis		4-14-33. Operation 8:30 AM.			
Polychromatophilia		Diagnosis: Acute suppurative			
Granular degeneration		appendicitis with perforation			
		Chart 2. Count 1 - 1½ hrs.			
		preoperative. Counts 2-4			
Plasmodium Malariae		postoperative with count 2			
Wasserman		representing normal fall.			
Widal		Count 3 on 5th day called			
Culture		for investigation, conceal-			
Blood sugar		ed wound infection drained.			
Blood urea		Count 4 normal expectation			
Blood N. P. N.		of convalescence.			

Leucocytes per c mm   Neutrophils

higher total and differential count than does a localized purulent infection, such as is found in appendicitis, or walled off in an abscess. The literature abounds with statements to the effect that in acute appendicitis, pain is the only dependable finding, that the leukocyte count is at best only confirmatory, and absent in 20 per cent of the cases. This is not our experience. The most dangerous appendix is the acutely diseased one where pain ceases following perforation, thrombosis or marked necrosis. Too often the cessation of pain is mistaken for a quiescent condition of the disease, when in fact it is then in its most dangerous state. In these so-called silent, painless, highly malignant cases of appendicitis, the high and rising neutrophil percentage with a falling eosinophil value as an indicator of infection and of increasing gravity, surpasses everything and in fact often constitutes the only positive finding.

Delay. It is desired to emphasize the importance of delay in the mortality of one disease—acute appendicitis. In a survey of 5,121 cases of acute appendicitis, Bower[5] found that if a patient of good physical condition is operated upon within the first twelve hours, he is safe in at least 99 per cent of the cases, but at the end of the twenty-four hour period, the chances against recovery are one in thirty-nine, while in forty-eight hours it drops to one in seventeen, and after seventy-two hours, it is one in nine. Often the most important decision about a case, the type and extent of treatment, must of necessity be altered because of delay. The use and proper interpretation of the complete leukocyte picture is the best insurance against this costly delay.

Methods of Procedure. The opinions deduced and herein recited are based upon blood counts from 1,409 consecutive surgical patients seen in two local hospitals where the character of the lesion or lesions has been established or confirmed by histopathology. As in previous studies reported with my associate, Dudley A. Robnett, M.D., [6, 7, 8] the histologic diagnosis has been taken as final and interpretations of the blood pictures have been grouped into those cases showing acute inflammation on the one hand and those of non-acute, where evidence of acute inflammation was absent, on the other. The non-acute group includes normal organs, simple neoplastic processes, tissues removed for prophylactic purposes, or at "interval operations," and some taken out under a clinical diagnosis of "acute." When using this as a basis of measurement, some errors are inevitable. This is especially true where the tissue removed showed no inflammation and yet the blood picture indicated an infection. Such cases

are seen where symptoms point to the appendix, and upon its removal this organ was found free of acute inflammation, and later a pyelitis, pneumonia, or osteomyelitis was recognized.

Approximately 600 of these cases were of acute appendicitis, and of this number, our associates in surgery record a mortality rate of about one per cent,[8] which is much lower than we find reported in the literature. This low rate is not attributed to superiority of hospital facilities nor to unique surgical skill, but to the fact that our colleagues are using this simple blood procedure which permits clear-cut, sharp, frank and unequivocal interpretations. By its aid their cases are diagnosed early and operations are performed while the lesion is yet limited to or within the appendix.

In our studies, record is made only of those cases where an operation is performed. We have no means of accurately determining the wholesale numbers of patients who have been saved from operative procedures or where the operation has been made one of election by the fact that the blood picture was against there being an acute condition demanding immediate surgery. This is one side of the value of the blood findings not commonly taken into consideration.

SUMMARY

1. The leukocyte blood picture indicating infection, even in the absence of clinical evidence of such, cannot be disregarded. The blood picture, however, should not be used alone in making a diagnosis, but always in conjunction with complete clinical signs and symptoms.

2. Early counts are needed to establish the relative normal count for the patient.

3. The rising percentage of neutrophils is the best available guide to the presence of infection, but it does not show its location.

4. The total cell count in acute pyogenic infections is a guide to and of the patient's resistance.

5. The appearance of eosinophils after their absence, or a rise in percentage after their decrease, is often the first dependable evidence of convalescence.

6. A chart is useful in showing graphically a resistance curve or line and the variations from time to time throughout the illness.

7. The presence of young or immature neutrophils indicates a demand upon and the response by bone marrow to acute sepsis.

8. Single counts may be diagnostic. Wher they are not, repeated counts at two to three hour intervals are imperative if the blood findings are to constitute a deciding factor.

HISTORY

Cancers of the lung were known three centuries before our earliest statistic data were compiled. The earliest published reports were those concerning the Schneeberg miners. It was not recognized as such at this time and credit is given to Morgagni whose paper presented the first case in 1761. Bell is credited with having first diagnosed pulmonary neoplasm in life from the symptoms of dyspnea, cough, pain and stridor, having verified his case by autopsy, while Stokes was the first to diagnose a case by physical findings and give a complete description of its clinical manifestations. A summary of sixteen series by Breckwoldt[2] disclosed the fact that of 1050 cases 807 occurred in men, producing a ratio of 2.8:1. The age incidence as revealed by several series is fairly constant, closely approximating that of all carcinoma. Weller[3] in a large series (1,100) of microscopically verified cases found the peak to be between the ages of fifty-six and sixty.

ETIOLOGY

Coincident with the abundant literature relative to this subject there have been many theories propounded as to the etiologic agents.

The occupational causes are chiefly those of irritative substances such as radioactive, mechanical, thermal and chemical elements. While there has been no definite proof, the efforts of Schmorl, Saupe[4] and others in reviewing and studying the causes in the Schneeberg miners have been interesting. The nature of the mines, its ores, some of which were radioactive, were thought to be etiologic agents.

Laboratory experiments have produced within the lungs of rabbits and mice new growths following the insufflation of irritating substances. These could not be called definite malignant neoplasms however, because the cells did not assume the characteristics of a carcinoma.

Wolf established the theory that tuberculosis was a cause after finding thirteen of thirty-one cases associated with the disease. Ewing[5] gives his support to this as a cause and an impressive list of cases may be found in the literature in which carcinomas have been found in bronchiectatic cavities.

Cases are on record where external trauma has played its rôle as an etiologic agent. Three cases illustrating this as a factor are; a blacksmith who received a blow on the chest by a heavy piece of iron, a woman who struck her chest during a fall from a ladder, and a man who suffered chest injuries when he was caught in a power belt. All of these patients developed primary carcinoma of the lung.

Acute and chronic infections also are given as a cause. In 1919 the great influenza epidemic afflicted many individuals and since then some observers have noticed a definite increase in the incidence of lung neoplasms and have attributed this to the infection either directly or secondarily as a result of changes occurring therefrom.

The works of Slye, Lynch[3] and others cannot be neglected since their experimental data have shown that in succeeding generations the incidence of lung neoplasms may be determined by selective breeding.

SYMPTOMATOLOGY

The perpetual aphorism—diagnose cancer early—is always before us and applies in lung malignancies as well as neoplasms in other parts of the body. Particularly is this true since surgical and irradiation therapy may be the means of prolonging life. It is not the purpose of this paper to discuss this aspect, but a few of the more important symptoms will be briefly mentioned.

Cough is the most common symptom and it may be associated with or without sputum. The latter may or may not be blood tinged and if it contains blood without tubercle bacilli this finding affords the best early diagnostic evidence of lung malignancy. The cough varies in its severity and characteristics, depending upon whether it is due to a pleural irritation reflex or to an intrabronchial stimulus.

Pain is the next most common symptom although not one of the earliest. Probably the reason for its appearing secondarily is that many cases are well advanced before they seek medical aid. It varies in its intensity from a dull ache or soreness to a sharp, unbearable pain.

Dyspnea may be present early in the disease. Its severity is dependent upon the amount of involvement present. It is more likely to be present in the cases having peribronchial infiltration. This is attributed to a spasm of the vascular and lymphatic channels.

Other symptoms usually encountered are, weakness and loss of weight, fever, hoarseness and dysphagia.

PHYSICAL EXAMINATION AND SIGNS

Like the roentgen findings, these vary in their manifestations. Observation may reveal engorgement of the vessels of the neck. Cyanosis may be noticed. Clubbing of the fingers, although not a frequent sign, may direct attention of the examiner to the lungs. Inequality of the pupils and localized edema may point toward a mediastinal condition. Palpation often reveals axillary or supraclavicular glands in cases which are far advanced but which present relatively few symptoms. Tenderness over a rib, sternum or spine, shifting of the cardiac impulse, loss of respiratory excursion and inequality of the pulses may give important clues. Percussion and auscultation elicit dulness of varying degrees combined with diminished or absent breath sounds. Ewing very aptly states that no single factor is pathognomonic, but all combined form a clear picture.

PATHOLOGY

Weller[3] in a review of the literature found that bronchiogenic carcinoma greatly exceeded other neoplasms of the lungs and his own series showed a ratio of 10:1. No one site in the lung seems to be more prone to the development of a tumor than another, except that the right side has been slightly favored.

Gross pathologic classification is difficult but it has been generally conceded that there are two main types and possibly a third. The first is that which arises near the hilum; the second, or nodular type, is that which arises in the parenchyma of a lobe; and the disputed third type is a diffuse process often seen bilaterally and therefore considered as metastatic.

Metastases are common and are found in the following order of frequency: lymph nodes, liver, skeleton, lungs, brain, kidney, adrenal glands, pancreas and thyroid.

It is fitting to point out at this time that metastases to the central nervous system have frequently given rise to an erroneous diagnosis, usually of a primary brain tumor, whereas the real primary tumor has escaped detection.

Secondary changes in the lungs due to tumors depend upon the extent of involvement. One may find atelectasis from obstruction, or emphysema if the obstructor is of a ball valve type. Pleural effusion, the nemesis of roentgenologists, often masks the entire process. Other secondary changes which already have been mentioned are those affecting the vascular system and those made manifest by clubbing of the fingers.

DIAGNOSIS

Accurate diagnosis of a pulmonary neoplasm is difficult and requires all possible cooperation between the clinician, roentgenologist and bronchoscopist. The clinician suspects a lesion, the roentgenologist confirms the suspicion, whereas the otolaryngologist confirms the diagnosis if he is able to remove positive tissue at the time of bronchoscopy.

There are no definite roentgenologic criteria. The roentgenologist depends upon the fluoroscopic findings which are of value in determining the position and movements of the diaphragm, the effects of respiration upon the aerations of the lung fields and information relative to shifting of the mediastinal structures and heart. He must be able to visualize gross pathologic changes in order to interpret correctly varying densities in the stereoscopic and lateral films. The roentgenologic findings may offer no characteristic signs.

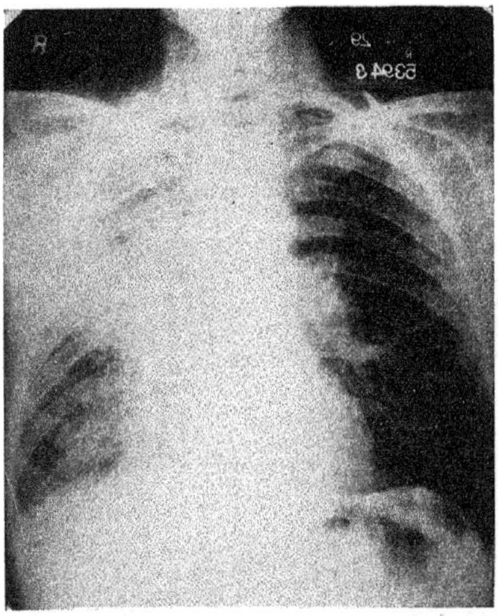

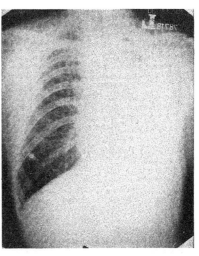

Fig. 1. Primary carcinoma of the lung located near the hilus with irregular projections extending toward the periphery.

Therefore the interpreter must come to his conclusions by deductions drawn from the various sized tumor masses, their position, density and shape, and the secondary changes of the thoracic cage and within it.

Primary findings produced by the mass itself may be sharply defined with smooth borders or may be exceedingly irregular with dendritic projections extending outward from a central dense zone. (See Fig. 1.) The origin of the tumor to a certain degree determines its manifestations, although one cannot say from the film whether the neoplasm has arisen from bronchial epithelium or alveolar epithelium. The bronchial epithelial tumors spread by way of the bronchi and toward the hilum, thus producing a density with irregular projections, and stenosis of the air passages with subsequent secondary changes. The carcinoma arising from the alveolar epithelium often produces a diffuse process affecting nearly the entire lobe and sometimes the pleura. In a majority of cases the tumors are well visualized because they

are within a space surrounded by air which affords good contrast media.

Secondary changes noted on the film are the result of obstruction and pleural irritation. (See Fig. 2.) Pleural changes are those of fluid and pleural thickening. Elevation of the diaphragm, narrowing of the intercostal spaces, shifting of the trachea, heart and mediastinal structures of the affected side, and widening of the inter rib spaces and compensatory emphysema on the opposite side, are secondary changes produced by the obstruction of the air passage causing an atelectatic condition of the lung in that region.

DIFFERENTIAL DIAGNOSIS

Pleural effusion should not be readily confused with a lung neoplasm but at times it masks the process causing confusion in interpretation. If the fluid is present and secondary changes are noted in the thoracic cage either on the side of the dense homogeneous shadow or on the unaffected side, a clue as to the basic pathologic process

Fig. 2. Primary carcinoma of the lung showing secondary changes produced by it.

is obtained and if confirmatory evidence is desired a thoracentesis should be resorted to. With removal of the fluid, its examination, and re-examination of the chest by x-ray, a positive diagnosis may often be made.

Primary neoplasms of the lungs at times become necrotic, (see Fig. 3) breaking down with the production of a vacuolization and a fluid level thus closely simulating a lung abscess, virtually an abscess within a neoplasm. To differentiate between these two, one must rely upon the history and clinical course plus progress examinations and if feasible, bronchoscopy.

Tuberculosis occasionally assumes characteristics not unlike a lung malignancy, particularly a tubercular lesion near the hilum and extending laterally into the lung field. The clinical course and progress examinations may offer no suggestions. The presence of tubercle bacilli does not necessarily differentiate the two since cases have been described where both have occurred in the same lobe. In cases where neoplasm or tuberculosis are unable to be differentiated, even though bronchoscopy is contraindicated in tuberculosis, this is the means of differentiation if suitable material can be obtained at the time for microscopic study.

Tumors of the pleura are rare but when they occur, and by the time that they are seen, symptoms are advanced and examination will reveal a massive pleural effusion which obscures the primary cause. After withdrawal of fluid from the chest and injections of air at the time of thoracentesis, these can be demonstrated very clearly in stereoscopic and lateral films, to be separated from lung tissue.

With a large area of increased density occupying the mediastinum, encroaching upon the lung field and closely related to the aorta, an aneurysm is immediately considered. This must of necessity be differentiated from a lung neoplasm. The physical findings and laboratory examination are of considerable aid. Added to this the visualization of intrinsic pulsation on screen examination, although lack of pulsation does not rule out aneurysm, plus a continuity of the shadow with that of the aorta on films taken in different projections, makes the diagnosis fairly certain.

Malignant lymphoma which necessarily includes the lymphoblastomas, leukosarcomas and Hodgkin's disease, is ordinarily thought to produce clear cut rounded shadows of increased density with sharply defined borders. (See Fig. 4.) At times these become irregular and hazy when the adjacent lung tissue becomes infiltrated, particularly near the hilum. Differentiation depends largely upon clinical and laboratory findings. Roentgen examination is helpful in that it reveals the position and the effects of the neoplasm upon the neighboring organs. This group rarely causes shifting of the mediastinal structures. They are more prone to surround an adjacent organ. Roentgen therapy offers another means of differentiation since this group is largely represented by radiosensitive

tissue, more sensitive than is a primary lung carcinoma.

Dermoid cysts are usually situated in the upper or middle anterior mediastinum and project asymmetrically from one side of the midline or the other. They are usually round or oval in shape and have smooth rounded surfaces, remaining well encapsulated and displacing organs rather than invading them.

The density of a malignant thymoma is significant in that its shadow is broader than it is long occupying the upper mediastinal region. It produces changes in the neighboring organs chiefly by pressure although extension into them has been noted.

Echinococcus cysts occur in the lower portion of the lung fields and are usually singular, but at

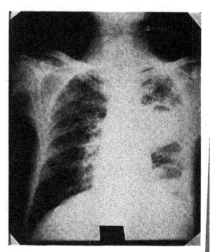

Fig. 3. Primary lung neoplasm with a cavity and fluid level suggesting a pulmonary abscess.

times can be multiple. When of the closed type they present sharply demarcated rounded dense areas surrounded by normal lung tissue. If rupture occurs the appearance depends upon the manner in which they drain, whether into a bronchus or into the thorax. They are differentiated by the history and complement reactions.

Benign tumors when small are not easily seen but they may produce changes, the result of obstruction. One sees mainly atelectasis and its associated findings. The bronchoscopist is called upon to determine the cause of the collapse and in doing so may be able to remove the obstruction

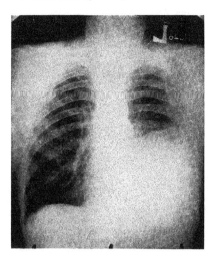

Fig. 4. Malignant lymphoma of the lung closely simulating carcinoma.

or part of it and have tissue at the same time for diagnosis. Lipomas, fibromas and chondromas may assume larger proportions and if so produce large well described areas of increased density.

Central pneumonia particularly when associated with a decompensated heart and of the unilateral type, may cause confusion. This produces a diffuse type of irregular densities simulating a diffuse carcinoma. The history offers the greatest aid for diagnosis.

Tuberculous mediastinitis is differentiated with difficulty. It produces a wide mediastinal shadow with a fairly sharp border and at times the mediastinal structures are shifted to the side of greatest involvement instead of the opposite side which is true in certain types of tumors.

It is apparent that even with the knowledge of the types of densities produced by various lesions a definite diagnosis by the roentgenologist is often difficult since many conditions present virtually the same type of findings on the roentgenograms.

CONCLUSION

1. To diagnose correctly neoplasms of the lungs there must be complete cooperation between the clinician, roentgenologist and bronchoscopist.

2. Roentgen findings do not always present features which are pathognomonic. The multiplicity of form can simulate almost any inflammatory or neoplastic disease of the lungs.

3. Since clinical and roentgenologic examinations offer no certainty in diagnosis and since accurate information can be obtained by microscopic examination of tissue, biopsies are indispensable to verify the diagnosis of malignancy in doubtful cases.

BIBLIOGRAPHY

1. Hruby, A. J., and Sweaney, H. C.: Primary carcinoma of the lung. Arch. Int. Med. lii:497-540 (October) 1933.
2. Theobald, R.: Zur Frage des Zunahme der Lungenkrebse. Ztschr. f. Krebsfarsch, xiii:128, 1926.
3. Weller, C. V.: Pathology of primary carcinoma of the lung. Arch. Path. vii:478-519 (March) 1929.
4. Schmorl, G.: Ueber den Schneeberger Lungenkrebs. Verhandl. d. deutsch. path. Gesellsch, xix:192, 1923.
5. Ewing, J.: Neoplastic Diseases. Second Edition, W. B. Saunders Company, Philadelphia, 1922.

THE NEWER TREATMENT OF GONORRHEA IN THE IMMATURE FEMALE*

JOSEPH BROWN, M.D., B.A., F.A.C.S.
Des Moines

Within the past decade the medical world has been almost bewildered by the rapidity of new physiologic truths, that have been propounded and experimentally proved in the field of endocrinology and especially in the field of menstrual physiology. From all this experimental work have come discoveries of vast clinical importance, not the least of which is the treatment of gonorrhea in the immature female.

It is not within the scope of this paper to give you the incidence or prevalence of gonorrhea in children, except to say that it occurs much more frequently than is generally supposed, and that children of the rich are as likely to contract the infection as children from the poorer sections of the community. Neither is it within the province of this paper to give you a resumé of the treatment of this condition as has heretofore been practiced, and is even now practiced except by a few. We all know that the treatment of gonorrhea in young girls is very unsatisfactory for the patient as well as for the doctor. Either our medication or our mode of treatment is wrong, for it is a matter of common knowledge that gonorrhea in a child before the age of puberty usually means treatment for from six months to two or three years.

About six months ago Lewis[1] of New Haven, published the results of a new treatment for gonorrhea in immature girls. It has been my pleasure within recent weeks to treat a number of cases by this newer method and the results have been not only interesting but, compared to the older methods, just short of miraculous.

This hormonal treatment of gonorrhea in young girls is based upon certain fundamental truths that have been established by those working with

* Presented before the Eighty-third Annual Session, Iowa State Medical Society, Des Moines, May 9, 10, 11, 1934.

the problem of gonorrhea in the female and by those working experimentally with the newer hormones. An understanding of these fundamental principles will clearly show why this newer treatment, as advocated by Lewis, is physiologically and clinically sound.

First, there is a vast difference in the histology of the female generative tract of the immature girl and that of the mature girl. That is, the histopathology of gonorrhea is much different before and after puberty. This is well shown by Schauffler and Kuhn[2] who, by a series of sections, demonstrated that the recesses or "harbors of infection" of the immature girl are confined entirely to the vaginal mucous membrane, which at this time consists of only three or four layers of epithelial cells and many rugae or folds of mucosa—the accessory glands are not yet developed—whereas, in the girl past puberty the "harbors of infection" are in the accessory glands of the generative tract—Bartholin-Skene's endocervical—and so forth, and not in the vaginal mucous membrane which is hypertrophied and multi-layered and does not have the rugae and plications characteristic of immaturity.

Second, it is an established fact that gonorrhea in the immature girl is confined almost wholly to the vaginal mucous membrane and seldom, if ever, affects the immature accessory glands or cervix.

Third, it is well known by those who have had the opportunity to observe many cases of gonorrhea in the female that gonorrhea of the vaginal mucous membrane, per se, is a rarity in the mature female or, if present, is of very short duration.

Fourth, Allen[3] when working with the female sex hormone, estrin, upon immature monkeys observed that injections of this hormone caused a vast hypertrophy of the vaginal mucous membrane. In fact, the immature mucous membrane of a few layers in thickness was rapidly converted to a multi-layered almost adult type of mucous membrane.

With the foregoing observations in mind we can easily understand the rationale of injections of female sex hormone (theelin) in the treatment of the distressing malady now under consideration. It seems quite reasonable to suppose that if we can convert the immature mucous membrane into an adult type of mucous membrane we will render the mucosa an unfit habitat for the Neisserian organism. What the actual biochemical changes are that go on within the many layers of the adult mucous membrane which render that type of membrane an unfit place for the gonococcus to live, we do not know, but it is an observation which every gynecologist has made and which he knows to be a fact. We now use that fact in the treatment of gonorrhea in immature girls. It is true that the glandular elements along with the endometrial tissues are developed by sufficiently large and sufficiently frequent injections of estrin but it is also a clinical observation that the gonococci die before the glandular elements are sufficiently developed to become in turn "harbors of infection."

Lewis reports eight cases thus treated, all with successful results. Today I have the privilege of reporting nine cases all brought to a final and successful conclusion by the intramuscular injections of theelin. Most of these cases were

TABLE OF NINE CASES TREATED WITH THEELIN

Name	Age	Duration of disease before treatment	Theelin begun	Total units	Daily injections	Smears 10 days	Smears 20 days	Smears 30 days	Genital reactions
L. W.	9*	8/1/29	11/10/33	600	12	neg.	neg.	neg.	none
D. B.	3	7/1/33	11/10/33	950	19	?	neg.	neg.	none
P.'M.	10	6/17/33	12/1/33	500	10	neg.	neg.	neg.	none
G. B.	2	8/21/33	12/4/33	2450	31	pos.	pos.	neg.	breasts labia
M. S.	7	10/21/33	12/8/33	1500	22	pos.	neg.	neg.	none
W. J.	9	6/14/33	12/8/33	400	8	neg.	neg.	neg.	none
B. T.	4	9/1/32	12/29/33	900	18	neg.	neg.	neg.	none
J. M	6	10/6/33	1/8/34	3400	39	?	neg.	?	breasts labia
D. L.	2	11/1/33	3/1/34	2000	25	pos.	V. neg. B. pos.	V. neg. B. pos.	slight breasts

clinic cases of the Broadlawns General Hospital, of Des Moines.[4] These patients had had the disease from two months to four and one-half years before beginning this hormonal treatment. Every patient had had regular, conscientious treatment—local of course—by successive crops of internes and attending men, but many who were coming to the clinic at the beginning of the service were left behind at the conclusion of the service— left with the ever present positive slide. In these cases treated with theelin it was noted that where there had been profuse vaginal discharge at the beginning of treatment the discharge was completely eliminated or greatly lessened five or six days after the beginning of the injections. In only four cases were more than twenty daily injections given. Of these nine cases, four or 45 per cent had negative slides within ten days; eight or 88 per cent had negative slides within twenty days; and there was not one single positive vaginal smear at the end of thirty days. Two of these cases require some explanation. One was a private patient and at the end of thirty days the laboratory report was returned as being suspicious for gonorrhea. The mother of the youngster, knowing the harmlessness of the treatment insisted upon a further course of two weeks treatment to be doubly secure. This was given and all slides have been negative including a recent followup examination some two months after the last injection. The other chanced to present an anomalous development of a left Bartholin gland. This is the only instance of Bartholin development in a child we have seen at the hospital or that I, personally, have ever seen at that age. I purposely did not give the gland (which was exuding pus almost in profusion) any treatment whatever to see what effect the injections of theelin would have on the glandular disease. After 15 daily injections a peculiar thing was noted; the smears from the interior of the vagina were negative for gonorrhea while the pus expressed from the infected Bartholin gland was positive. At the end of thirty days conditions were the same—the vaginal smear was negative and the Bartholin smear was positive. At this time I ordered mercurochrome injections of the Bartholin gland daily and after the third injection of the gland it was noted that the mercurochrome on injection came out through the vagina. The Bartholin gland had ruptured through the vaginal wall forming a fistulous tract. This tract was slit open, swabbed out with a surgical solution of mercurochrome and nothing else done. All slides have remained negative since. This case was interesting because it showed that the gonococcus was not again implanted upon the vaginal mucosa as long as the mucous membrane

was under the stimulating influence of theelin, and we felt that the Bartholin gland must be cleared up before the effects of the theelin wore off. Subsequent events have proved this to be correct.

Estrin, as we know, is a growth hormone which stimulates the growth of the entire sexual apparatus. As I have said above, the treatment is based upon this fact so we were not surprised to see a slight fulness of the labia and a slight enlargement, a nodule about the size of a bean, in each breast in those patients who had had the largest total number of units, but these precocious developmental changes returned to normal within two or three weeks after cessation of treatment. While it is possible, also, theoretically, to develop the endometrium by the injection of large amounts of theelin to the point where there is desquamation with a bloody uterine discharge, in no case of mine did such a phenomenon occur.

The procedure followed at the Broadlawns General Hospital is as follows: theelin, one ampule (fifty units) is injected intramuscularly daily, into the gluteal or deltoid regions. Vaginal smears are taken every second day. If at the end of ten days the slides are negative the one ampule dosage is continued for one or two more weeks. If at the end of ten days from the beginning of injections the slides are positive for the Neisserian organisms, the dosage is doubled and two ampules (one hundred units) are given daily until five or six consecutive slides have shown no gonococci.[*] The fact that there is a vaginal discharge sometimes present at the end of a course of treatment is of no consequence, for the microscope shows no specific organisms and no pus cells, but an abundance of squamous epithelium and detritus, which is merely the reaction of the growth hormone. In ten to fourteen days this reaction discharge has subsided and the vagina is clean. In no instance is any local treatment to the vaginal mucosa used.

These injections are wholly without danger if given with the ordinary aseptic precautions used in any hypodermic injection. The results are truly marvelous. In our clinic which was always burdened by cases of gonorrhea in young, uncooperative girls, we feel that such cases are no longer a source of anxiety, for we believe that at last we have found in theelin a specific treatment for gonorrhea in the immature female.

CONCLUSIONS

1. The hormonal treatment of gonorrhea in im-

---

[*] Since writing this paper we have begun to use the newer preparation, Theelin in oil (1000 international units) for its slower absorbtion, slower elimination, and higher potency (300 not units per ampule). We give one ampule every second or third day. We feel it has great possibilities but it is too early yet to report results with this oily solution.

mature females follows logically upon our knowledge of the newer physiology of the female generative tract.

2. The histopathologic differences between gonorrhea in the immature and adult female are shown.

3. Nine cases of gonorrhea, of varying duration, in immature girls were brought to a successful conclusion within twenty to thirty days after the beginning of treatment with injections of theelin.

REFERENCES

1. Lewis, R. M.: A study of the effects of theelin on gonorrheal vaginitis in children. Amer. Jour. Obst. and Gynec., xxvi, 593 (October) 1933.
2. Schauffler, G. C., and Kuhn, Clifford: Information regarding gonorrhea in the immature female. Amer Jour. Obst. and Gynec., xxv, 374 (March) 1933.
3. Allen, Edward: Reactions of immature monkeys (Macacus Rhesus) to injections of ovarian hormones. Jour. Morph. and Physiol., xlvi, 479 (December) 1928.
4. By courtesy of Superintendent Dr. Charles Sprague, Broadlawns General Hospital, Des Moines, Iowa.

802 Equitable Building

DIFFERENTIAL DIAGNOSES OF ACUTE APPENDICITIS IN THE FEMALE

JAMES H. WISE, M.D.
Cherokee

Since the days when appendicitis was termed typhlitis or inflammation of the bowels and treated mechanically with heat, great strides have been made in our knowledge of this condition. It is seldom, but yet too often, that cases of acute appendicitis are left undiagnosed until the patient's recovery is in great doubt. Most cases of subacute appendicitis with recurrent attacks of colic are usually operated upon before they cause any considerable lasting damage to health. On the other hand, appendicitis can prove a most deceptive ailment, disguising itself under symptoms so slight that they do riot alarm the patient 'nor raise great worry to the doctor unless he has made a very searching examination.

The pitfall of mistaking a subacute appendix, with recurrent attacks and intervals of quiescence, for a number of gynecologic diseases is now generally appreciated and guarded against. The confusion of gynecologic diseases and acute appendicitis would not be so frequent if a complete gynecologic examination were made as a matter of routine or, at least, in all possibly doubtful cases. Diseases in the female most frequently confused with acute appendicitis are acute adnexitis, extrauterine pregnancy, ovarian hemorrhages and hematomas, and finally, twisted ovarian tumors, rupture of ovarian cysts and torsion of tubes, hematometra and hematosalpinx. In the early stages, the differential diagnosis is very difficult because objectively demonstrable findings are missing, and if they were present, the extreme sensitiveness would forbid their palpation, especially in obese women. All the landmarks for sensitiveness and pain may be common to both diseases, and it is the exceptional case which must always be kept in mind. Sensitiveness toward the back and sacro-uterine ligaments in rectal palpation points to adnexitis, but does not exclude appendicitis, considering the many possibilities for an inflamed appendix hanging down in the pelvis. The same is true of dysuria, that is, difficult and painful micturition and other signs thought to be pathognomonic.

As a general rule in cases which I have personally observed, the general condition of the patient is better in adnexitis, although the fever is very high. In appendicitis the pressure pain at the McBurney's pressure point increases as palpation extends upward; in salpingitis it increases toward the true pelvis. Gastric and intestinal disturbances suggest appendicitis. Discharge or increasing discharge during the attacks suggests adnexitis. In adnexitis which is usually of gonorrheal origin, the temperature is very high from the beginning, and the pulse is rapid but full, while in appendicitis the temperature rises more slowly. When the infection arises during the menstrual cycle, one is more suspicious of salpingitis.

We have another rather small group of nongonorrheal cases which causes acute adnexitis. These are what we term septic infection where we have a history of operatively or artificially effected deliveries; a febrile puerperium, abortions or curettage after abortion, and intra-uterine interventions of all kinds point to adnexitis. In virgins and very young girls, appendicitis is more likely to be present than is adnexitis.

Of other gynecologic conditions somewhat less common to be differentiated are pedunculated ovarian tumors, rupture of ovarian cysts, and occasionally, torsion of the Fallopian tubes. Twisted pedunculated tumors are very often confused with appendicitis, not only in adults, but also in young individuals. Too often a healthy appendix is removed and the ovarian tumor is overlooked. If the torsion is not relieved spontaneously, the colic-like pains in the hypogastrium increase constantly. In the early stages the temperature is, if at all, only slightly increased. The pulse is usually more frequent when torsion has taken place, and sometimes severe collapse symptoms may appear. In the presence of palpatory findings, the diagnosis is easy. These tumors are easily overlooked unless a thorough gynecologic examination is made prior to operation, and unless a thorough exploration is made at the time of the operation.

The rare cases of tubal torsion are more frequently confused with ovarian tumors and extra-uterine pregnancy than with appendicitis. They, of course, necessitate an operation as well as appendicitis, but diagnosis is desirable before operating because of the choice of incision. Another gynecologic condition to be differentiated is that of extra-uterine pregnancy. The history here is of very marked importance. Delay in menstruation and irregular hemorrhage thereafter are indicative of extra-uterine pregnancy. An acute tubal rupture, which aways follows, is characterized by sudden collapse, tenderness of the lower abdomen and Douglas pouch with slight increase in temperature, increasing pallor as a sign of hemorrhage, nausea, vomiting, and thready pulse. The tenderness to pressure is most marked in the hypogastrium, and it decreases upward. There are usually slight labor-like pains repeated at short intervals. The abdomen is not so bloated nor the tension so great as it is in inflammatory disease of the peritoneum on examination. There are no positive gynecologic findings in the early stages, but in the later stages there is an enlargement of the uterus, a sponge-like bulging, and distinct pain on pressure in the pouch of Douglas. In extreme cases a post cervical puncture clarifies the situation. Another laboratory finding of note in these cases of ruptured ectopic pregnancy with abdominal hemorrhage is the extreme leukocyte count. Another form of hematoma is that caused by ovarian hemorrhage. The differentiation from acute appendicitis is very seldom possible before operation. Occasionally they are present simultaneously, and I think, they are usually caused by direct contact with the appendix.

Acute appendicitis during pregnancy is always a severe complication, and yet it is a frequent one. The mortality rate is fairly high due to the fact that acute appendicitis is not recognized early enough, and the operation is performed too late. The diagnosis is rendered difficult by the many possible displacements and abnormal postures of the appendix caused by the growing uterus. The cecum is crowded up high by the enlarging uterus which soon fills the small pelvis; encapsulation of exudates is rendered more difficult, and hence diffuse peritonitis easily results. The symptoms, such as discomfort, vomiting, and abdominal pain which are characteristic of appendicitis, can be elicited by pregnancy itself. The time of operation has a very important bearing on the prognosis. On the other hand, there is danger that an operation will injure the pregnant woman, although, according to most authorities the percentage of abortion is about ten per cent, wound infections and postoperative complications increase this percentage. Abortion, however, causes disturbance in the postoperative course and must be cared for as symptoms arise. Cases in which pregnant women have been operated upon for appendicitis, and the removed appendix found to have no signs of inflammation are known to every surgeon.

Pyelitis associated with pregnancy is common; it is usually located on the right side due to the physiologic inclination of the pregnant uterus to the right. These physiologic cases, of course, offer difficulties in recognition. They may have completely negative sediment findings. This pain need not involve the region of the kidney. Those women, however, with mechanical congestion in the right urinary tract, who feel intense pain upon pressure over McBurney's point (corresponding to the obstruction of the ureter) and yet have a normal urine, are often operated upon under the false diagnosis of appendicitis. These cases can be distinguished only by pyelography. A contrast medium can be administered intravenously without preparation of the intestine. The writer uses Neo Iopax, made by the Schering Corporation, as the contrast medium. The pyelogram in this type of case shows the obstruction in the renal pelvis, the calices and in the dilated ureter on the right side. The excretion on the left side is seen to be normal.

Especially in young women and girls, acute pyelitis is one of the most important diseases which, owing to difficulties in differential diagnoses, leads wrongly to the performance of an operation for appendicitis. If these diseases were typical, there is rarely a necessity for a mistake in diagnosis. It is the atypical case that gives us the difficulty. Some of the differential points are:

1. In pyelitis the fever is usually high and the urine shows a pyuria while in appendicitis there is slight fever or none, and negative urine, unless the appendix lies behind the cecum in contact with the ureter causing sufficient ureteritis; thus, there is the possibility of finding pus or even blood in the urine.

2. In acute pyelitis the pain is in the upper abdomen or back, often referred to the groin or labia, and tenderness may be anterior or posterior, while in appendicitis, the pain is first generalized over the abdomen or especially in the epigastrium, later localizing to the right lower quadrant, and tenderness is over McBurney's point.

3. In acute pyelitis there is a high leukocytosis, and pathology is slight in comparison with findings, but in appendicitis, there is slight or moderate leukocytosis, and pathology is marked in comparison with findings.

4. In pyelitis, the rigidity is usually posterior, and there is no rebound tenderness; in appendi-

citis tenderness is over McBurney's point and rebound tenderness is nearly always elicited.

This paper, although it does not cover all diseases to be differentiated, is written to emphasize the need of thorough and careful examination of every patient, no matter how trivial her complaint may seem. First impressions, though lasting, are not always correct; therefore let us avoid them!

THE FINLEY HOSPITAL CLINICO-PATHOLOGIC CONFERENCE

DIVERTICULOSIS AND DIVERTICULITIS OF THE COLON

LESTER G. ERICKSEN, M.D., Dubuque

In the routine x-ray examination of the gastrointestinal tract it is not uncommon to detect diverticula which may involve any portion of the alimentary canal. These are usually discovered accidentally and are of little clinical significance, particularly those in the stomach and duodenum. When they occur in the colon, however, they give a very definite symptom complex, easily recognizable, but often not appreciated by the physician taking the history and making the physical examination. It is for this reason that the following case is presented. It is typical in every respect of diverticulitis of the descending and pelvic colon.

CASE REPORT

Complaint: The patient, a white male, fifty-five years of age was admitted to The Finley Hospital March 4, 1934, with a complaint of "diarrhea for thirty hours; nausea and vomiting for twelve hours and considerable gaseous distention of the abdomen."

Past history: For many years the patient had been troubled with constipation requiring the frequent use of cathartics, and coarse foods such as bran, fruits and vegetables with a high content of cellulose. He had had several attacks similar to the present one. He had gained weight steadily for several years and attempts to reduce were unsuccessful.

Physical examination: On admission to the hospital the physical examination revealed the following pertinent points: the temperature was 98 degrees F.; the pulse was 96 per minute and regular; the blood pressure was 124 systolic and 82 diastolic; the respirations were 20 per minute and regular; the height was 68 inches and the weight was 215 pounds; the head, neck and chest were negative. The abdomen was distended and

tympanitic. There was tenderness in the left lower quadrant and a questionable mass could be palpated in this region. The blood and urine examinations were normal. The feces contained no occult blood.

X-ray report: Examination of the colon with a barium enema showed a marked diverticulosis involving the descending and pelvic colon (Fig. 1). There was little evidence of spasm at this time but this was probably due to the belladonna which the patient had been taking. The remainder of the colon was negative.

Treatment: The bran and coarse vegetables were prohibited. Vegetables of low residue and

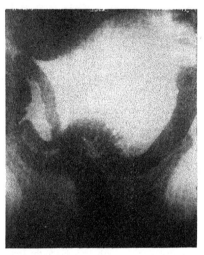

Fig. 1.   Roentgenogram showing multiple diverticula of the sigmoid.

fruit juices as well as the full diet usually used in chronic ulcerative colitis were substituted. The constipation was overcome by the use of agar and Russian oil. Belladonna was given in small doses to overcome the tendency of the colon to spasm.

DISCUSSION

What are the outstanding points in the history and physical examination of this patient which should lead one to suspect a diverticulitis? He was a stockily built man, who was obese and led a sedentary life. This is the type patient in which diverticula are usually encountered. Furthermore he gave a history of constipation of many years duration and of previous attacks similar to the present one. This is the usual story given by these patients and should lead the clinician to consider diverticulitis as the most probable diagnosis. There is one other condition which should be ruled out and that is malignancy. This is sometimes very difficult either by x-ray examination or at the time of operation. The fact that these diverticulitis cases sometimes degenerate into malignancy makes this problem doubly difficult. Each may form a hard tumor mass and gives the same appearance roentgenologically if the diverticulitis is advanced. Usually, however, one can make the differentiation. · In the case under discussion the absence of blood in the feces was a point against malignancy. ·

Diverticula of the large bowel may be congenital or acquired.[1] The congenital forms are pouches whose walls have the same structure as the bowel wall at the point of origin ; these are true diverticula. Acquired diverticula may be either true or false. The latter has no muscular coat and is the form under discussion. Diverticulosis of the colon is a fairly common condition. Thus Rankin and Brown[2] state that it occurs in five per cent of persons who have symptoms referable to the large bowel. They estimate that diverticulitis occurs in about 17 per cent of the cases of diverticulosis. In their series of 227 cases, an associated malignant condition was found in only four instances. In a series of 200 adult autopsies in The Finley Hospital there were three cases of congenital and eleven of acquired diverticula of the intestine which were divided as follows :

Diverticulosis:
  Congenital
    Duodenum 1
    Jejunum 2
  Acquired
    Descending colon.................... 9
Diverticulitis:
    Descending colon.................... 2
      (one of which was perforated)

In all of our cases of diverticulosis of the colon the patients were obese and had relaxed abdominal walls. They led sedentary lives and gave histories of constipation with the usual illogical attempts at treatment by cathartics of various types and diets containing large amounts of roughage. The latter probably accounted for some of the exacerbations as this diet is contraindicated in these patients. Spasmodic pain usually on the left side, low in the abdomen, and referable to the region of the rectum was also complained of by five of the eleven patients.

The etiologic factors are age, obesity, constipation, relaxed abdominal wall and possibly inherent weakness of the intestinal musculature. Men are affected nearly three times as frequently as women. Practically all patients are over forty, obese, constipated, and lead sedentary lives. Diverticulitis results from inability of the diverticula to empty themselves and is due to the invasion by bacteria. Abscesses or perforations may result and are the most serious complications. The treatment of diverticulosis may be medical or surgical. On a bland diet which keeps the bowel movements fluid, or at least soft, these patients are often comfortable. If attacks indicating persistent irritation or infection occur, surgery should be considered, especially in younger individuals. The ideal surgical procedure is resection of the affected portion, but this is not always possible. At times only a single diverticulum may require amputation ; at others an extensive resection is demanded. With the complication of infection with abscess formation or perforation, drainage should be instituted and later resection and anastomosis done.

Note : I wish to express my appreciation to Dr. L. E. Cooley for his clinical record.

REFERENCES
1. Masson, J. C.: Diverticulitis of the large bowel. Collected Papers of The Mayo Clinic, p. 160, W. B. Saunders Company, Philadelphia, 1921.
2. Rankin, Fred W. and Brown, Philip W.: Diverticulitis of the colon. Collected Papers of The Mayo Clinic, p. 202, W. B. Saunders Company, Philadelphia, 1930.

REPORT OF CASES FROM THE BROADLAWNS GENERAL HOSPITAL, DES MOINES

CECIL C. JONES, M.D., Des Moines, of the Section on Diseases of the Eye, Ear, Nose and Throat

The patient was a male Italian, thirty-eight years of age, who entered Broadlawns Hospital, April 1, 1934, complaining of a sore throat and swelling in the right parotid and superior cervical regions. The sore throat had developed on March 26 ; three days later the patient noted swelling and tenderness in the region of the right parotid gland, and the superior cervical regions with trismus. There was marked dysphagia. On questioning the patient admitted that in 1918 he had had a severe sore throat, with pain on the left side, which eventually "broke," draining a profuse amount of pus.

Examination of the throat showed the presence of marked trismus ; the opening between the teeth being only one centimeter. There was a large fluctuant swelling of the right posterior lateral pharyngeal wall in the region of the posterior pillar. Edema extended for several inches in all directions from the area of fluctuation. No pus was obtained from the parotid duct. No devitalized teeth or ulcers were found. Externally there was a massive tender red edematous swelling most marked at the lower border of the right parotid gland. It extended forward over the zygoma, above the right eye, and well over the temporal fossa. The swelling occluded the ear canal. It extended below to the clavicle, and the apex of the swelling was just behind the angle of the mandible. The general physical examination was negative; temperature, 103 degrees; pulse, 80; respirations, 28; white blood count, 21,200; polymorphonuclears, 83; lymphocytes, 16; and urine, negative.

Treatment on entrance consisted of hot normal salt irrigations, with hot boric dressings to the right parotid and superior cervical regions. On April 3, I saw this patient in consultation just after he had had a definite chill. At that time, the temperature was 104.6 degrees, and the previous findings were as described, except that they were more exaggerated. A diagnosis of pharyngomaxillary fossa abscess, secondary to lateral pharyngeal abscess, was made, and immediate external drainage was advised. A blood culture was requested. The treatment of hot packs and hot normal salt irrigations was continued; the lateral pharyngeal abscess was lanced, and drained foul pus; and on April 6, the patient died.

Not infrequently an acute lateral pharyngeal abscess or cellulitis, or a peritonsillar abscess, is complicated by extension into the pharyngomaxillary fossa by way of a retrograde thrombophlebitis. There are two retropharyngeal lymph glands lying on the face of the second cervical vertebra which become involved, and which are connected with the deep cervical lymph glands. However, an abscess may develop in the pharyngomaxillary fossa, secondary to infection, extending from the parotid gland or the mesial side of the mastoid tip. Anatomically the normal pharyngomaxillary fossa is only a potential space. It is cone shaped, with the skull about the jugular foramen as its base, and the hyoid bone as its apex. The carotid sheath enters the fossa at the apex. The fossa is bounded mesially by the superior constrictor, the muscle upon which the tonsil lies. The lateral boundary below is the internal pterygoid muscle which lines the inner surface of the ascending ramus of the mandible. · Above and laterally is the parotid gland which in this location is not covered by a fascia. The prevertebral muscles and fascia form its posterior wall. This potential space, the so-called pharyngomaxillary fossa, is the site of election for the collection of pus in the neck. True mid-line retropharyngeal infections, unlike lateral pharyngeal infections, do not drain into this space, but gravitate downward toward the mediastinum. A pharyngomaxillary fossa suppuration endangers life because it results in either a thrombophlebitis of the internal jugular vein, or an edema of the larynx. The treatment is always external drainage.

The symptomatology and physical findings warranting the diagnosis of pharyngomaxillary fossa suppuration are as follows:

1. Rule out other sources of a septicemia, such as a lateral pharyngeal cellulitis or abscess, or a peritonsillar abscess, in which symptoms do not subside after lancing. Quinsy or lateral pharyngeal abscess are usually the original diagnoses.

2. Marked trismus due to splinting of the internal pterygoid muscle.

3. Chills, temperature suggestive of a septicemia, and sweats following a sore throat.

4. The presence of a von Bezold's abscess, associated with signs of severe sepsis.

5. A positive blood culture.

6. External swelling may be entirely absent, but continued sepsis demands external drainage.

7. A parotid abscess with no external signs, and which is associated with edema of the lateral pharyngeal wall.

8. A septicemia following the extraction of a tooth.

————

The patient was a colored female, ten years of age, who was admitted to the Contagious Hospital, on December 8, 1933, with nasal diphtheria. At the time of admission the ears were negative, but on December 24, the nurse noted a profuse discharge coming from the left ear. On that day, the morning temperature was 99 degrees, and the evening temperature was 101.8 degrees. On December 25, the maximum temperature was 101 degrees, and on December 27, it rose to 102 degrees. Tenderness and edema over the left mastoid were present. Her temperature gradually subsided, and on December 30, she was discharged from the hospital, with a normal temperature, and no tenderness, redness or edema over the mastoid.

During the following week, the patient complained of pain in the left ear, which continued to discharge. This pain was behind the ear, and was accompanied by a headache, stiff neck, and photophobia, although she did not complain of pain in or behind the left eye. Projectile vomiting began at 3:00 A. M. on January 10, 1934, and she was admitted to Broadlawns General Hospital with a temperature of 105 degrees. During the afternoon she had a definite chill.

Examination showed the presence of a profuse purulent discharge from the left ear. The drum was bulging in spite of an ample opening. Redness, edema, and tenderness were present over the mastoid, with the helix pushed out and forward, characteristic of a cortical perforation. All reactions and rotations of the eyes were normal. No vestibular nystagmus was present, but a moderate ocular nystagmus was noticed. There was no paresis of the cranial nerves. The whole body was extremely sensitive to touch. All reflexes were exaggerated; there was a bilateral Kernig's sign, and still neck with opisthotonos. The white blood count was 29,100; the Schilling count showed an extreme shift to the left; the red blood count was 2,650; hemoglobin was 50 per cent; cerebrospinal fluid cells, 1,020, with globulin plus. No organisms were found in the smear or culture.

A diagnosis was made of acute diffuse suppurative meningitis, secondary to acute suppurative mastoiditis.

Since no organisms were found in the smear of cerebrospinal fluid, a left mastoidectomy was advised, with exposure of the dura of the middle fossa and sigmoid sinus throughout. This was performed under gas anesthesia on the evening of January 10. The dura was red and shreddy, and the lateral sinus appeared normal. The wound was left open, and iodoform packs and hot boric dressings were applied. Marked improvement followed until the fourth postoperative day, when the temperature reached 104.6 degrees. The cerebrospinal fluid was cloudy, the cell count ranging from 200 on January 11 to 2,676 on January 17, but it continued to be negative for organisms. However, on January 19, the cells were too numerous to count and streptococci were present. By this time the headache was so intense and diffuse, that pain localized in, about or behind the left eye could not be elicited. This suppurative streptococcic meningitis took its usual course, and at autopsy a classical perforation of the petrous apex was demonstrable.

In retrospect, I feel that this condition should have been diagnosed, the operation should have been performed, and the patient should have recovered, because the original x-ray film revealed a pneumatic type of mastoid development with cells extending far forward into the apex. The cerebrospinal fluid was negative for organisms, and although the diagnostic symptoms of pain in or behind the eye were masked by the meningeal symptoms, an x-ray of the petrous apex should have been made. In review, it would seem to us proper that every case of mastoiditis complicated by a serous meningitis or meningismus, and which on x-ray reveals either a pneumatic or diploic type of mastoid development, should have an x-ray of the petrosa, made according to Kopetsky's technic.

SPECIAL ARTICLE

A Report of Stewardship*

CHARLES B. TAYLOR, M.D., Ottumwa

President, Iowa State Medical Society, 1933-1934

I can think of nothing to offer that would be of value but a report. First I want it understood that nothing which I shall say is to be construed as a boast. I feel no boast in my heart. I do feel thankful that I have been well and able to meet most of the calls and perhaps have been able to accomplish something. I have kept my mind open for suggestions from others, and some of the things instituted have been the thoughts of others.

I was solicited so many times to be present at medical functions that I early made it a practice not to attend where the invitation was simply routine. This took me, with few exceptions, only to those meetings where it was thought that my presence might be of value. Many societies have no need of the president. They are well-organized, functioning concerns, and the presence of the president would be but incidental. In many other societies the president can be of decided value in acquainting members of his plans and the aims and purposes of the state organization. This is a function which should not be neglected by future presidents. I know from experience that one can quicken the society pulse and expose new sources of thought which will eventuate in a determined support of medical affairs.

I attended about fifty-five medical gatherings outside my own county, one of them being the Northwest Conference at St. Paul, Minnesota. I was invited and attended every meeting of the Board of Trustees and the Council. Attendance at these meetings is essential to an understanding of business problems of the state organization. To be an ex-officio member of these two boards might at sometime be of real help to a president, but if all presidents are treated with the same courtesy as I was, it would be of no value to have this official connection. Both boards take their work seriously and do their best in the interest of organized medicine.

The trustees and councilors should always be chosen with great care. Men differ greatly in their qualifications. One may be thoroughly scientific and gifted as a practitioner, but have no qualities

*Presented before the Eighty-third Annual Session, Iowa State Medical Society, Des Moines, May 9, 10, 11, 1934.

that would fit him for the position as trustee or councilor. A trustee must be the business man of the organization. Without business instinct a trustee would be of little value. A councilor should be a triumvirate within himself. He should be scholarly, so that he may direct the scientific programs of his district. He should be a political organizer, and, unless he is this, he is valueless as a councilor. A councilor's biggest task is to know that the machine is assembled, oiled, tank filled and moving. He must be more than a nice fellow and an intellectual practitioner. The third qualification demands that he is willing to sacrifice some of his own business for work in connection with state society affairs. No man can be a councilor who refuses to visit his counties in season and out of season, giving of his counsel and helping the local society to plan its activities, and, in addition, coördinating these county societies into a district society that has real vitality. Good councilors are few, but should be found and kept when their worth has been proved.

From years of experience in society work I have learned that many capable young men are left on the side lines for lack of an opportunity to break into the game. Some do not have the initiative or nerve to force recognition. To my thinking, these should be drafted—drafted while they are mentally capable of supporting the flag. Our past war showed that the men who were drafted made as good soldiers as did the volunteers. I have found a ready response from these men in medicine, and they are presenting many of the best programs in their societies, besides taking responsible positions in the organizational work. This activity by the younger men has elicited a like activity in the older men, many of whom are finding a new interest in the newer thoughts as presented by the younger men. The older man knows that he has much to give the younger man; the art and grace and poise accumulated throughout the years are some of the things that he can convey to his younger brethren.

I believe that our programs have grown too stereotyped. For years the informal discussion has given me the most benefit. That the program cannot become a free-for-all is evident. It must be a directed informal program if anything is to be accomplished. Our speakers in the conferences are instructed to present no formal papers. We hope, and have every reason to believe, that the speakers will know their subjects and will present them in an understandable way to their listeners. The chairmen of the various sections will regulate the starting and stopping of all discussions. Along with the discovery of the young men, the idea of sectional conferences is my pet. It is my hope that this type of program will furnish vastly more instruction; that the instruction will be given in a way to be more readily digestible; and that both teachers and listeners will benefit by the change. I stand or fall on this program. I want to stand. Our invited guests are outstanding men who are sure to please and instruct. I solicit for them your support and know that your courtesy will be rewarded. Your hospitality to these guests is assured in advance, because that is your way.

Since physicians as a class are gregarious animals, they naturally come together. To save black eyes and other damage to their persons, they organize. They set metes and bounds. They select leaders and draft rules for their conduct, and for the conduct of themselves. This is all very necessary. Man cannot live unto himself alone and do it well. Nor can he live with his neighbor without rules, implied or written. Emerson says: "Sanity of mind consists in variety and facility of association." Some few physicians in the state are living almost hermit lives. They occasionally see other physicians in consultation, but any regular meeting with a consistent interchange of views they have not.

County societies that are active furnish a meeting place; beyond the neighborhood the district meeting makes for a fine outing; but for the grand celebration the state society is it. It would be an economic and cultural gain if every active physician were to affiliate with his local and state societies. That should be our ultimate aim. Some sort of intellectual dynamite should blow hermits out of their seclusion. If you can find it here, take some home with you and use it. Our hope rests with strong, self functioning local societies. From these come our leaders and our everlasting strength.

If I could have had more ideas I would have done more. I have given my best service. I trust that something has been accomplished.

"A man's reach should exceed his grasp—Or what's a heaven for."—Browning.

STATE DEPARTMENT OF HEALTH

A SPECIAL ARTICLE ON SYPHILIS*

In a letter addressed to the Commissioner of Health, John McMullen, Assistant Surgeon General and Chief, Division of Venereal Diseases of the United States Public Health Service, desires that attention be directed to a special article dealing with syphilis which appeared in the April number of *Venereal Disease Information*. The title of the article is "Standard Treatment Procedure in Early Syphilis—A Resumé of Modern Principles." A group of prominent syphilologists prepared this article, the material for which "embraces the records of 75,000 cases of syphilis, of which 3,244 were examples of early syphilis followed for six months or more."

This special article discusses the following topics: "The Aims to Be Achieved," "Principles Governing the Control of Infectiousness," "The Individual 'Cure'," "Combined Arsenical and Heavy Metal Treatment and Its Functions," "The Control of Relapse by Treatment," "The Danger of the Rest Interval or Lapse," "The Dangers of Little Arsphenamine and the Short Arsphenamine Course," "Optimum Treatment," "Physician-Patient Relationship and Responsibility" and "Observation Throughout Life."

Under "The Control of Infectiousness in Syphilis," a series of 25 principles are tersely stated. These principles or conclusions are taken from "Modern Clinical Syphilology," by John H. Stokes. Conclusions 2, 5, 6, 7, 20 and 25 read as follows:

"Infectiousness is not a function of the serologic state of the patient. No serologic test has any value as a proof of infectiousness early or late.

"Infectiousness is controlled and syphilis will be extinguished, if ever, as a health problem, by treatment of the infectious person.

"The public health responsibility of the physician is therefore with the early months and years of the disease.

"Treatment to control infectiousness must be with the arsphenamines. No other drug will do.

"The great promoter and source of relapse is the short arsphenamine course (one to four injections) unsupported by other treatment.

"The child of the pregnant syphilitic woman should not be destroyed but protected in utero by treatment of the mother, before and after conception, and of the father if syphilitic, before conception."

* Reprints available to physicians upon request through State Department of Health.

The term "cure" is defined, for practical purposes as the "complete extinction of all symptoms and signs of the disease, with nontransmission of the infection over a lifetime or as close an approximation to it as present follow-up clinical material permits us to study." The outlook for apparent cure, based on a statistical study of the 3,244 cases followed for six months or over is indicated in the following table:

Stage of Disease	Average Results (Per Cent "Cure")	Best Methods (Per Cent "Cure")
Seronegative primary	71.4	83-86
Seropositive primary	53.3	64-70
Secondary	50.0	61-82

It will be seen from the above figures, that when treatment is not begun until after the development of the secondary eruption, there is "a possible loss of 21 per cent by average and 14 per cent by best methods, over the outlook prevailing when treatment is begun in the seronegative primary stage."

"It is apparent, therefore, that his duty to the individual patient, dear to the heart of the conscientious physician, even more than his duty to the public health, demands the earliest possible application of treatment."

The special article referred to and from which the above quotations have been taken contains information, which is useful, practical, and of fundamental importance to practicing physicians and health officers.

The State Department of Health will forward a copy of this article without charge to physicians who may desire to have it.

AMEBIC DYSENTERY

Evidence warrants a strong suspicion that amebic dysentery occurs sporadically among Iowa residents.

In 1933 prior to the Chicago outbreak, amebic dysentery was reported as the cause of death in two adults in Iowa. In ten other deaths the type of dysentery was not stated. A recorded death from this condition usually indicates the occurrence of several known or unrecognized cases.

As stated in an earlier issue of THE JOURNAL OF THE IOWA STATE MEDICAL SOCIETY several cases have been recognized by A. A. Johnson, M.D., of Council Bluffs. There are no known reasons why this disease should be unusually prevalent in that part of the state compared to other sections. It appears likely that these sixteen cases were found because over a period of years Dr. Johnson made it a practice to look for amebae in stool specimens of patients with suggestive intestinal disorders. An early diagnosis in such cases is particularly important since by means of it a distressingly chronic or dangerously acute colitis may be changed to the effectively treated amebic dysentery. Physicians need to have a more general awareness of the possibility of meeting this infection and a wider expertness in its clinical and laboratory diagnosis.

In this disease, laboratory examination must be made on freshly passed stool specimens. Arrangements are being made in some cities and states for ambulatory cases to go directly to the laboratories and there to provide the specimens which may be examined at once. The more severely ill are best examined in a hospital with adequate laboratory service.

Further studies of this disease have been stimulated as a direct result of the Chicago outbreak. The United States Public Health Service is sponsoring these studies under the direction of G. W. McCoy, M.D. A. V. Hardy, M.D., Iowa City, Iowa, has been appointed special agent for the service to make such studies in Iowa. The physicians of Iowa can help to further this work by keeping in mind the possibility of seeing cases of amebic dysentery and by reporting such cases promptly to the State Department of Health, Des Moines, Iowa.

ROCKY MOUNTAIN SPOTTED FEVER

This disease, known for years to affect certain areas in western Montana and the Rocky Mountain region, has extended its boundaries in a remarkable manner and has laid claim to a definite place in the list of newly recognized diseases in Iowa.

During the warm months of 1933, five cases of Rocky Mountain spotted fever were reported to the State Department of Health. The first case was recognized by Dr. C. N. Freligh, M.D., of Waucoma, and was reported by him on June 13, 1933.

The first case of spotted fever in 1934, was reported June 20, 1934, by R. E. Gunn, M.D., of Boone, Iowa. A field investigation was made by a representative of the State Department of Health on June 23 in the company of Dr. Gunn and Mr. R. E. Wells, Entomologist, United States Department of Agriculture. Mr. Wells, who is stationed at Ames, was formerly associated with Dr. R. R. Parker of Hamilton, Montana, in the study of Rocky Mountain spotted fever in that state.

The patient, a girl five years of age, had an onset of symptoms on June 17, with fever, headache, severe pain in the nose, irritability, vomiting and moderate diarrhea. On June 23 the patient's temperature was 105.5 degrees, she was irritable and showed a maculopapular rash on the arms, legs and chest. From the clinical standpoint, the condition was regarded as Rocky Mountain spotted fever. The Weil-Felix agglutination test on blood serum, which is an aid in diagnosis, is seldom positive within ten days after onset of symptoms.

Significant from the diagnostic as well as epidemiologic viewpoints, was the information elicited from the mother that she had discovered a tick on the child's head while washing her hair. There was no dog belonging to the household, and a history to the effect that the child had played with any dog could not be obtained. A goat and a pony belonging to the family were examined but no ticks were found on them. The patient's home is located in a part of the city devoid of trees and not likely to be tick infested. An interesting finding is the fact that the family had, however, taken supper and spent several hours in one of the city parks a few days before the tick was discovered and removed. It is possible that ticks are numerous in public parks as well as in rural, wooded areas.

Other cases of Rocky Mountain spotted fever may appear in widely separated localities in the state and it is desired that all recognized and suspicious cases be reported promptly to the State Department of Health.

PREVALENCE OF DISEASE

Disease—	May, 1934	April, 1934	May, 1933	Most Cases Reported From
Diphtheria	25	39	29	Woodbury
Scarlet Fever	235	243	104	Polk
Typhoid Fever	4	0	6	(For State)
Smallpox	23	26	104	Humboldt, Cerro Gordo
Measles	1432	976	319	(For State)
Whooping Cough	184	267	70	Montgomery, Black Hawk
Cerebrospinal Meningitis	6	9	4	Polk
Chickenpox	290	245	185	Linn, Dubuque
Mumps	280	313	414	Woodbury, Linn
Poliomyelitis	3	0	0	Scott
Tuberculosis	41	24	46	(For State)
Undulant Fever	7	8	18	(For State)
Syphilis	70	117	188	(For State)
Gonorrhea	133	131	176	(For State)

The JOURNAL of the Iowa State Medical Society

ISSUED MONTHLY

SUBSCRIPTION $3.00 PER YEAR

Address all communications to the Editor of the Journal,
1122 Bankers Trust Building, Des Moines

OFFICE OF PUBLICATION, DES MOINES, IOWA

Vol. XXIV   JULY, 1934   No. 7

GRANULOCYTOPENIA DUE TO AMIDOPYRINE

While the singular triad of symptoms now recognized as typical of granulocytopenia has been described for many years, the condition as a clinical entity was not recognized until 1922 when Schultz described this disease, stressing the acute febrile course with high mortality, the ulcerative lesions of the mucous membrane, particularly in the oral cavity, and finally a complete or almost complete disappearance of granulocytic cells from the peripheral blood. One year later Friedemann proposed the name agranulocytic angina. Although the number of cases reported during the ensuing twelve years has not been large, sufficient factual data have accumulated to support fully Schultz' contention of a distinct disease entity. These data have failed to furnish a satisfactory explanation of the etiology of this disease but do suggest that the causes may be multiple and that predisposing qualities or reactions must be present in the individual for the operation of certain known etiologic agents.

A primary or essential type is described which includes all cases of idiopathic or unproved origin. A second group of secondary or symptomatic cases are reported to result from a number of conditions, including those of chemical poisons, particularly arsphenamine, bismuth and benzol.

Recent studies, particularly those of Hoffman, Butt, and Hickey,[*] advance our knowledge regarding the etiology of many of these cases, carrying the consideration from the speculative into the experimentally proved field. Their work is doubly

[*] Hoffman, Arthur M., Butt, E. M., and Hickey, N. G.: Neutropenia following amidopyrine. Jour. Am. Med. Assn., cii:1213-1214 (April 14) 1934.

interesting since it not only offers positive confirmatory proof that granulocytopenia may result from chemical poisons, but also inasmuch as it incriminates the very commonly employed sedative, amidopyrine. Their observations of fourteen definite cases with thirteen fatalities present one constant and apparently significant finding in personal history. "All of these patients had received amidopyrine alone or in conjunction with codeine for the pain of arthritis, sciatica, bone tumor, and so on."

In spite of the inconclusive evidence resulting from the animal experimentation of Madison and Squier in 1933, Hoffman and his associates have and are conducting animal experiments with amidopyrine which they believe will substantiate their theses that granulocytopenia may result in susceptible individuals from the use of amidopyrine alone or in combination with other drugs.

Lending additional evidence to the correctness of this observation may be cited the report of Watkins of the Mayo Clinic last year, reviewing thirty-two cases of granulocytopenia observed in the clinic. Of this number "twenty-four had taken amidopyrine or a derivative of barbituric acid for various periods before the onset of the granulocytopenia." He further points out that inasmuch as the remaining group of patients in the series had been under medical observation for chronic illnesses, "it is possible that these patients may have received barbiturates or amidopyrine."

As a theoretic consideration it is not difficult to accept these observations, since amidopyrine contains the benzene radical and since Kracke has fully demonstrated his ability to induce the characteristic picture of this disease in rabbits by the subcutaneous injection of benzene.

While these observations point to a very definite hazard in the prolonged use of amidopyrine, pyramidon and the barbiturates, drugs all containing the benzene ring, the evidence is not submitted that the occasional use of these preparations is harmful, or in fact that the prolonged use of these drugs, in the absence of other factors, produces this disease syndrome. If other factors did not play an important rôle in the causation of symptoms, we might readily expect granulocytopenia to be a very common disease, inasmuch as many, if not most, of the modern sleeping and pain-relieving powders are formed by the combination of these drugs, or allied drugs containing the benzene ring. It would be very interesting and perhaps informing if those observing large groups of epileptic patients, or those afflicted with chronic ailments who daily take anti-spasmodic drugs of this group over months and years of time, would report the frequency with which granulocytopenia develops and determine if the percentage is sufficiently great in these groups to incriminate the anti-spasmodic drug used.

Pending additional observations in this regard it appears timely to repeat the warning sounded by Hoffman and his associates, that until the study is more complete "the use certainly of amidopyrine alone or in combination with other drugs should be restricted to patients having leukocyte counts several times a week."

HYPERGLYCEMIA A RESULT OF TOBACCO SMOKING

From the time when the brash servant of Sir Walter Raleigh interrupted the tranquility of this gentleman in his after dinner smoke, man has been busy explaining his indulgence in the burning aromas of the tobacco plant. If his digestion is poor, he explains that smoking brings relief. If he is over weight, smoking is sure to effect the desired reduction, or if perchance he is underweight, the aromas of burning tobacco are equally sure to add the needed pounds. If one is thirsty, it takes the place of a drink, and if one is hungry, a smoke serves the purpose of food. If one is nervous, it lowers nerve tension, or if sluggish, it provides the needed stimulation. And if one is drowsy, a smoke relieves fatigue. What a panacea man finds in this delightful habit.

Empirically one might conclude that gross exaggeration entered into these several claims, or that tobacco smoking, like opium smoking, led to weird delusions and fantastic dreams. Can it be that the habit so enslaves a man that he cannot interpret its reactions? It would seem far more likely that he interprets sensations and reactions correctly, but being denied a scientific basis for explanation becomes hopelessly lost in abstract reasoning and consequently ineffective in his logic.

While much scientific and more pseudo-scientific discussion has been voiced concerning the merits and demerits of this habit, the scientific viewpoint has often been rejected because of personal prejudice, and the pseudo-scientific reasoning been made ridiculous as propaganda. The approach in most instances is taken upon the ground of personal preference and usually in defense of one's own habits or tastes. The results of such investigations have been singularly valueless and usually a travesty on science.

Happily the truth, or at least a part of the truth, explaining some of these various reactions from smoking, has recently been discovered by a chance observation of two Yale University scientists, Drs. Howard W. Haggard and Leon A. Greenberg. These observers were quite innocently drawn into the tobacco question while investigating the problem of the "optimum meal time interval," a problem undertaken to determine how children, college students and industrial workers should be fed. Using the blood sugar concentration as a basis for food needs, they observed, as would be anticipated, that following a hearty meal the blood sugar concentration rose rapidly, but fell again to the fasting level within two to four hours, if another meal was not taken, and remained at this fasting level for many hours. In a few of the adults, but in none of the children, the blood sugar curve was freakish and showed marked rises and falls after it had reached the fasting level. The explanation for the freakish fluctuation in the sugar curve was not immediately apparent, but finally the observers surmised that tobacco smoking in these adults might furnish a proper explanation. Here the unsought King Nicotine crept into the picture. Subsequent investigation conclusively proved the correctness of these surmises.

With uncontestable regularity hyperglycemia resulted when the fasting individual indulged in tobacco smoking. While this hyperglycemia parallels closely the reaction which takes place following the ingestion of food, it was observed to be of shorter duration. Paralleling further the reaction produced by food, that produced by tobacco smoking could be reproduced and prolonged by repeating the smoking at the end of the hyperglycemic curve.

To explain this observation Drs. Haggard and Greenberg logically postulate that nicotine, or some other alkaloid in tobacco smoke, acts upon the adrenal glands, causing them to discharge an excessive amount of adrenalin into the blood stream. This, in turn, releases glycogen from the liver and muscles, and increases the sugar concentration of the blood. Hyperglycemia resulting from the ingestion of food has long been recognized as creating a state of well-being, in which the responses to stimuli are more prompt and more lasting than those observed when the sugar concentration is at the normal level. It becomes immediately apparent, then, that the hyperglycemia produced by tobacco smoking would probably induce the same physiologic response.

A smoke, then, may relieve fatigue and dispel hunger, or lower nerve tension, if the nervousness results from fatigue. In fact, it may be truly the panacea which it is claimed to be by those who are addicted to its use. Those opposed to the habit will find satisfaction in this same physiologic reasoning. If smoking destroys or dispels the reaction of hunger, it may be definitely harmful when permitted to replace the ingestion of needed food, or again one may reason that the constant over stimulation of those organs concerned in the hype glycemic reaction may prove definitely detrimental to the organism and predispose to malfunction or disease at a later period.

In any event this observation concerning the hyperglycemia of tobacco smoking is thought-provoking and opens the way for other researches in this field, where truly scientific observations have been so conspicuously absent.

THE PHYSICIAN AND THE IOWA SALES TAX

Apparently the provisions of the Iowa State Sales Tax are not entirely clear to all physicians and inasmuch as this act definitely defines "sales," it appears desirable to present in these columns a review of this law as it affects physicians.

The State Board of Assessment and Review rules that all returns must be made for the entire gross receipts of a business. No returns will be acceptable if they are made only upon cash receipts. They must include the receipts from all sources—cash, credit and things other than cash taken in as consideration.

In the event a merchant sells numerous articles to one purchaser a tax may be collected upon the total purchase price of the article sold. In no event may there be a tax collected upon each individual article. Physicians and surgeons primarily render professional services. They are users or consumers of such tangible, personal property as medicine, drugs, dressings, bandages, and the like, and buy them incidentally in the performance of professional services, irrespective of whether or not such items are billed separately to the patient. The person selling such articles to a physician or surgeon is making a sale at retail, and must pay a retail sales tax as to his gross receipts from said sales.

In some instances physicians prescribe and compound their own remedies, which they sell separately and apart from the rendering of service. In these instances they must pay a tax with respect to their receipts from such sales. Physicians and surgeons are likewise taxable as to receipts from sales of any other items of tangible property, such as proprietary medicines when sold separately and apart from the rendering of services.

It is apparent, then, that physicians will not be required to pay a sales tax on moneys received for the sale of professional services, but should pay a retail sales tax where moneys or other tangible property are collected for medicines or supplies incident to or independent of the professional service rendered.

INCREASED HOSPITAL BEDS FOR TUBERCULOUS PATIENTS

General hospitals are opening their doors to tuberculous patients, increasing facilities are being provided for the care of tuberculous children, and 6,863 new beds for the treatment of the disease have been added to the nation's public health armament despite the depression.

These are the outstanding facts revealed by a three years' survey of tuberculosis sanatoria throughout the United States just completed by the National Tuberculosis Association. The data have been compiled in the form of a sanatorium directory, listing facts about 659 institutions containing a total of 86,917 beds. There are now available for tuberculosis patients in the United States, 64 federal institutions containing 11,431 beds; 357 state, county and municipal institutions containing 56,540 beds; 73 private institutions containing 4,344 beds; and 165 semi-private institutions containing 14,202 beds. These figures do not include provisions made in day camps or in summer preventoria.

QUINTUPLETS

Mrs. Olivia Dionne of North Bay, Parry Sound, Ontario, created front page news during the last week in May by giving birth to quintuplets. General interest in this rare occurrence rose to such heights that the mother and five daughters were invited to exhibit themselves at the Century of Progress in Chicago.

Interest in medical circles centered about the person of Allen Ray Dafoe, M.D., the attending physician, and about the multiple birth as a medical curiosity. Every physician has been interested in Dr. Dafoe's efforts to keep ablaze the spark of life in these five tiny individuals, and when the doctor publishes his observations, as he no doubt will do, we as physicians will be interested in the details of his report.

Dr. Jeannette Dean-Throckmorton, Librarian at the Iowa State Medical Library, became interested statistically in multiple births and has furnished the following table taken from De Lee's Obstetrics of 1933:

Twins—once in 85 cases.
Triplets—once in 7,600 cases.
Quadruplets—once in 670,000 cases.
Quintuplets—once in 41,600,000 cases.

In a careful search of the literature she was able to obtain references to forty-one previous cases of quintuplets. Dr. De Lee in 1928 found references to thirty cases. The statistics will emphasize the rarity of this interesting phenomena.

SPEAKERS BUREAU ACTIVITIES

LABORATORY COURSE

Below is given a tentative outline of the practical laboratory course to be held in Des Moines durir the last two weeks in July. The work to be covered in this course is two-fold. In the forenoons, the will be demonstrations of the laboratory tests which have been found to be of real value to practitioner and in the afternoons an evaluation of these tests will be presented by Iowa physicians who are compete to appraise these laboratory procedures.

PROPOSED LABORATORY COURSE

Des Moines, Iowa—July 16 to July 28, 1934

	Laboratory Demonstrations 9:00 to 12:00 a. m.	Round Table Discussions 1:30 to 4:30 p. m.
Two mornings	HEMATOLOGY: Making of a slide and smear Red and white blood counts Hemoglobin Differential count Sedimentation tests Coagulation tests Blood typing and grouping	HEMATOLOGY—July 16 and 17 C. W. Baldridge, M.D., Iowa City F. H. Lamb, M.D., Davenport
One morning	IMMUNOLOGY OF THE BLOOD: Pneumococcus grouping Kahn's test Glutination test Schick test Allergy tests	IMMUNOLOGY—July 18 Julius S. Weingart, M.D., Des Moines M. E. Barnes, M.D., Iowa City
One morning	BLOOD CHEMISTRY: Blood sugars Blood ureas	BLOOD CHEMISTRY—July 19 D. J. Glomset, M.D., Des Moines Mrs. D. J. Glomset, Des Moines
One morning	URINALYSIS: Routine urinalysis Kidney function test Finding of red cells in urine	URINALYSIS—July 20 John L. Kestel, M.D., Waterloo
One morning	BACTERIOLOGY: Tuberculosis Diphtheria Gonococcus Pneumococcus Typhoid fever Simple bacteriologic stains	BACTERIOLOGY—July 21 I. H. Borts, M.D., Iowa City
One morning	GASTRIC ANALYSIS AND STOOL ANALYSIS:	GASTRIC ANALYIS AND STOOL ANALYSIS—July 23 J. T. Strawn, M.D., Des Moines
One morning	TISSUE EXAMINATIONS:	TISSUE EXAMINATION—July 24 F. P. McNamara, M.D., Dubuque
One morning	METABOLISM:	METABOLISM—July 25 H. W. Rathe, M.D., Waverly
One morning	ELECTROCARDIOGRAPHY:	ELECTROCARDIOGRAPHY—July 26 B. F. Wolverton, M.D., Cedar Rapids
Two mornings	X-RAY:	X-RAY—July 27 and 28 H. Dabney Kerr, M.D., Iowa City T. A. Burcham, M.D., Des Moines

Laboratory procedures are becoming increasingly important in the practice of modern medicine. bewildering number of new tests are brought forth each year. It is vitally important, therefore, for physician, who desires above everything else to give the best possible service to the sick, to be fam with those procedures that are pertinent to the proper practice of medicine and to be able to eval properly the results of these laboratory tests.

The course is scheduled to begin July 16, and those wishing to enroll should do so at once.

WOMAN'S AUXILIARY NEWS

Edited by the Press and Publicity Committee

MRS. OLIVER J. FAY, *Chairman,* 405 Thirty-seventh Street, Des Moines

THE NATIONAL MEETING

Officers of the Woman's Auxiliary to the American Medical Association met in a preconvention board meeting at 2:30 p. m., Monday, June 11, at the Hotel Carter in Cleveland.

Two important matters were discussed. The first was the recommendation of Mrs. James F. Percy of California for appropriations to the Corinne Jackson Freeman Memorial Fund. It was suggested that this fund be put at the disposal of each national president, to be used as a revolving fund at her discretion. The second matter of vital interest to all Auxiliary members was a report by Mrs. Willard Bartlett, of St. Louis, Missouri, on the First Twelve Years of the Woman's Auxiliary.

A very instructive talk was given by Dr. Junius Brainard Harris of Sacramento, California, on "The Technic of Putting a Bill Through a State Legislature." Dr. Harris was introduced by Mrs. Phillips Doane, of Pasadena, California, who is the chairman of the national legislative committee. Dr. W. W. Bauer of Chicago, Director of Health and Public Instruction for the American Medical Association, also presented a most worthwhile address, stressing the rôle which the Woman's Auxiliary could and should play in helping to maintain the high standards of public health, for which the medical profession is working.

Mrs. Rogers N. Herbert of Nashville, Tennessee, chairman of the Hygeia Committee, reported that one thousand copies of *Hygeia* had been placed in the public schools of Tennessee. This holds the record for being the largest group subscription of *Hygeia* ever placed.

The retiring president, Mrs. James Blake, of Hopkins, Minnesota, complimented Iowa on the outstanding work done this year, and asked me to bring that message to you.

Officers were elected for the coming year as follows:

President—Mrs. Robert W. Tomlinson, Wilmington, Delaware.

President-elect—Mrs. Rogers N. Herbert, Nashville, Tennessee.

First Vice President—Mrs. Rollo K. Packard, Chicago, Illinois.

Second Vice President—Mrs. Otis F. Lamson, Seattle, Washington.

Third Vice President—Mrs. J. B. White, Atlanta, Georgia.

Fourth Vice President—Mrs. William Lett Harris, Norfolk, Virginia.

Secretary—Mrs. Elmer L. Whitney, Detroit, Michigan.

Treasurer—Mrs. Eben J. Carey, Milwaukee, Wisconsin.

Board of Directors—Mrs. A. A. Herold, Shreveport, Louisiana; Mrs. F. N. Scatena, Sacramento, California; Mrs. M. L. Stevens, Asheville, North Carolina.

This report contains no mention of the social functions which were arranged for the visiting ladies, since I was unable to attend any. However, they were many, and varied, and everyone in attendance agreed that this meeting was decidedly worthwhile, and thoroughly enjoyable from every standpoint. For those present from Iowa, the high light of the convention was undoubtedly the reception held in honor of the President-Elect, Dr. Walter L. Bierring. The members of the Woman's Auxiliary are indeed proud of the recognition accorded Dr. Bierring, and wish for him unlimited success, confident that by reason of his outstanding ability and profound understanding of human nature, coupled with his innate charm and graciousness of manner, he will easily attain to that degree of fame which marks a true leader of men.

Mrs. E. L. Bower, Delegate.

Mills County

The Woman's Auxiliary to the Mills County Medical Society met in conjunction with that organization in Glenwood, Thursday, June 14. Mrs. I. U. Parsons of Malvern presented a report of the state meeting, and Mrs. T. B. Lacey of Glenwood reviewed a part of Dr. Palmer Findley's book on "Childbirth." Following the afternoon program, both societies met for lunch and enjoyed a social hour.

Twin Lakes Auxiliary

At a meeting held in Rockwell City Thursday, June 21, the following officers were elected to serve the Woman's Auxiliary to the Twin Lakes District Medical Society for the coming year: Mrs. M. J. McVay of Lake City, president; Mrs. Roy E. Parry of Scranton, secretary, and Mrs. W. E. Hart of Odebolt, treasurer.

Minutes of the Iowa State Medical Society
Eighty-third Annual Session
May 9, 10, 11, 1934—Des Moines

Wednesday Morning, May 9, 1934

The opening session of the Eighty-third Annual Session of the Iowa State Medical Society, held at the Fort Des Moines Hotel, Des Moines, May 9-11, 1934, convened at eighty-thirty o'clock, Dr. Charles B. Taylor of Ottumwa, president, presiding.

The invocation was offered by the Reverend Eugene Beach of Ottumwa.

The scientific session began with a symposium on arthritis, which included the following papers:

"General Considerations" by Dr. John C. Parsons of Creston.

"Eye, Ear, Nose and Throat Aspect" by Dr. J. K. von Lackum of Cedar Rapids.

"Orthopedic Phase" by Dr. Arch F. O'Donoghue of Sioux City.

Discussion on the symposium was opened by Dr. M. B. Call of Greene, followed by Dr. W. Eugene Wolcott of Des Moines; Dr. J. C. Hill of Newton; Dr. J. C. Parsons of Creston; Dr. J. K. von Lackum of Cedar Rapids and Dr. Arch F. O'Donoghue of Sioux City.

At the request of President Taylor, First Vice President William E. Ash of Council Bluffs, presided for the remainder of the session.

The following papers were presented:

"Papillary Cystadenoma of the Ovary" by Dr. C. W. Ellyson of Waterloo; discussed by Dr. J. H. Randall of Iowa City; Dr. W. J. Brackney of Sheldon, and Dr. C. W. Ellyson of Waterloo.

"Treatment of Pelvic Infections" by Dr. A. C. Page of Des Moines; discussed by Dr. W. H. Rendleman of Davenport; Dr. O. F. Parish of Grinnell; Dr. Lawrence D. Smith of Des Moines; Dr. E. D. Plass of Iowa City and Dr. A. C. Page of Des Moines.

President Taylor introduced Dr. C. G. Farnum of Peoria, the official delegate from the Illinois State Medical Society, who extended to those present the good will and good wishes of the Illinois Medical Society, and an invitation to attend the annual session of that society in Springfield, Illinois.

The Surgical Chairman, Dr. Lester D. Powell of Des Moines, introduced Dr. Verne C. Hunt of Los Angeles.

Dr. Oliver J. Fay of Des Moines presented a paper, "Shall Organized Medicine Survive?" which was discussed by Dr. Harold A. Spilman of Ottumwa.

President Taylor presented his presidential address, "A Report of Stewardship".

The meeting adjourned at eleven fifty-five o'clock.

Thursday Morning, May 10, 1934

The Thursday morning session convened at eight-twenty o'clock, President Taylor presiding.

Dr. Fred Smith of Iowa City, chairman of the Section on Medicine, introduced the medical guest speaker of the morning, Dr. R. Wesley Scott of Cleveland.

Dr. Scott presented a paper on "Syphilis as the Cause of Heart Disease" and conducted a medical clinic, illustrating cases of this type.

Dr. Lester D. Powell of Des Moines, chairman of the Section on Surgery, introduced the surgical guest speaker, Dr. Verne C. Hunt of Los Angeles.

Dr. Hunt presented a paper on "Surgical Lesions of the Stomach and Duodenum" and conducted a surgical clinic, illustrating these types of cases.

At the request of President Taylor, Second Vice President Frank H. Conner, of Nevada, assumed the chair.

The following papers were presented:

"The Significance of Urinary Findings in Nephritis," by Dr. F. P. McNamara of Dubuque; discussed by Dr. Julius S. Weingart of Des Moines.

"The Treatment of Gas Bacillus Infection," by Dr. William Jepson of Sioux City; discussed by Dr. W. A. Rohlf of Waverly and Dr. A. B. Deering of Boone.

President Taylor resumed the chair.

In the absence of Dr. Royal French, of Marshalltown, chairman of the Eye, Ear, Nose and Throat Section, Dr. Gordon F. Harkness, of Davenport, introduced the guest speaker of the section, Dr. John Shea, of Memphis, Tennessee.

Dr. Shea presented a paper on "The Relationship of Otolaryngology to General Medicine".

The meeting adjourned at twelve o'clock.

Friday Morning, May 11, 1934

The Friday morning session convened at eight-thirty o'clock, First Vice President Ash presiding.

Dr. Verne C. Hunt, of Los Angeles, presented a paper on "Surgical Aspects of the Gallbladder and Biliary Tract" and conducted a surgical clinic.

Second Vice President Conner assumed the chair.

Dr. R. Wesley Scott, of Cleveland, presented a paper on "Hypertensive Heart Disease" and conducted a medical clinic.

Dr. Walter L. Bierring, of Des Moines, State Commissioner of Health, presented a paper on "The Relation of the State Department of Health to the Practice of Medicine".

Dr. R. G. Leland, of Chicago, Director of the Bureau of Medical Economics of the American Medical Association, presented a paper on "Some Causes of Professional Unrest".

Secretary Robert L. Parker reported the transactions of the House of Delegates.

President-elect Thomas A. Burcham, of Des Moines, was introduced and thanked the Society for the honor bestowed upon him.

President Taylor presented the gavel to the incoming president, Dr. Gordon F. Harkness, of Davenport.

The meeting adjourned at eleven-fifty o'clock.

Section on Ophthalmology, Otology and Rhinolaryngology

Thursday Morning, May 10, 1934

The opening session of the Section on Ophthalmology, Otology, and Rhinolaryngology, held in connection with the Eighty-third Annual Session of the Iowa State Medical Society, at the Fort Des Moines Hotel, Des Moines, May 9-11, 1934, convened at nine-thirty o'clock, Chairman Royal F. French of Marshalltown, presiding.

Chairman French read his address, "Lacrimal Duct Stenosis". The following papers were presented:

"Cases of Non-Metallic Foreign Bodies in Trachea and Bronchi in Children," by Dr. H. E. Thompson of Dubuque; discussed by Dr. L. G. Ericksen of Dubuque; Dr. Snyder D. Maiden of Council Bluffs; Dr. James A. Downing of Des Moines; and Dr. H. E. Thompson of Dubuque.

"Strabismus—General Consideration," by Dr. J. B. Naftzger of Sioux City; discussed by Dr. George A. May of Des Moines; Dr. C. W. Rutherford of Iowa City; Dr. William W. Pearson of Des Moines Dr. Harold J. McCoy of Des Moines; Dr. James E. Reeder of Sioux City; and Dr. J. B. Naftzger of Sioux City.

Thursday Afternoon, May 10, 1934

The second session of the Section on Ophthalmology, Otology, and Rhinolaryngology, was called to order at two o'clock, Chairman Royal F. French presiding. The following papers were presented:

"Two Mastoids," by Dr. Carl E. Sampson of Creston; discussed by Dr. DeVoe Bovenmeyer of Ottumwa; Dr. Fred F. Agnew of Independence; Dr. Gordon F. Harkness of Davenport; and Dr. Carl E. Sampson of Creston.

"The Management of Allergic Manifestations of the Nose and Throat," by Dr. John J. Shea of Memphis, Tennessee, guest speaker for the section.

"Differential Diagnosis of Headaches," by Dr. Cecil C. Jones of Des Moines; discussed by Dr. T. R. Gittins of Sioux City; Dr. H. C. Payne of Pella; Dr. William W. Pearson of Des Moines; and Dr. Cecil C. Jones of Des Moines.

"Thrombophlebitis, Secondary to Throat Infections," by Dr. Sumner B. Chase of Fort Dodge; discussed by Dr. F. H. Reuling of Waterloo; Dr. George C. Albright of Iowa City; Dr. T. R. Gittins of Sioux City; Dr. H. M. Ivins of Cedar Rapids; Dr. H. C. Payne of Pella; and Dr. Sumner B. Chase of Fort Dodge.

The report of the nominating committee was presented, and Dr. Sumner B. Chase of Fort Dodge, was elected chairman of the section for the coming year. Working with him as co-chairman of the section, will be Dr. Abbott M. Dean of Council Bluffs.

Transactions House of Delegates
Iowa State Medical Society, Eighty-third Annual Session
May 9, 10, 11, 1934—Des Moines

The first meeting of the House of Delegates, held in connection with the Eighty-third Annual Session of the Iowa State Medical Society, in American Legion Hall, Plymouth Building, Des Moines, convened at four-five o'clock, President Taylor presiding.

President Taylor: Will you please come to order?

The first order of business is the roll call.

Secretary Parker: Mr. President, our roll call will consist of the proper filling out of these cards which will constitute the official registration. If the delegate is present, he should fill out that card; if he be not present, the alternate may be seated. Should the delegate return for a later session, it is proper that the alternate who is seated today give up his seat for the delegate later. But should a delegate be seated today and then have to leave, the alternate then is seated for the rest of the session. In filling out these cards be sure to designate whether you are a delegate, alternate or state officer. These cards will be collected later and will constitute the official registration.*

I *move* you, Mr. President, that, since a quorum is present by this official registration, we proceed with the regular order of business.

The motion was regularly seconded, put to a vote and carried.

President Taylor: We will proceed with the approval of the minutes of the Friday morning session of 1933.

Secretary Parker: I *move* you, Mr. President, that the minutes of the Friday morning session as printed in the July Journal of 1933 be approved.

The motion was regularly seconded, put to a vote and carried.

President Taylor: The next is the report of the Secretary.

Secretary Parker: Mr. President, before giving my report I wish to *move* that all reports as published in the Handbook be received by this body.

The motion was regularly seconded, put to a vote and carried.

---

* The official registration included 68 delegates, 10 alternates and 17 officers, or a total of 95.

Reports of Officers

REPORT OF THE SECRETARY

House of Delegates, Iowa State Medical Society:

The following report for the year 1933 is respectfully submitted:

The Secretary has "so far as it is in his power, used the influence of his office to aid the Councilors in the organization and improvement of the county societies and in the extension of the power and usefulness of this Society."

During the year we have visited every district and as many county societies as was possible. It is our impression that the morale of the profession over the state is much better and that there are more doctors interested in medical organization than ever before.

The stimulus to organized medicine caused by the reports of various foundations and lay organizations has done much to bring about an appreciation of what a truly organized profession can do.

The Secretary's office is just a part of the *office of the Iowa State Medical Society*. This office is yours and every member of the Society should acquaint himself with its activities.

The Secretary's work this year, as in the past,

because of the faithful cooperation of the Executive Secretary and other employees, has been a joy.

Membership

The paid membership of the Society on December 31, 1931, was 2,310; on December 31, 1932—2,213; and on December 31, 1933—2,163. Approximately ninety per cent of the doctors in active practice in the state belong to the State Society. Iowa ranks among the strongest state societies of the American Medical Association. A more detailed statement of membership follows. (Tables I and II.)

TABLE I

Active Members, 1933.........................2,163
Delinquent Members.......................... 192
Eligible Non-members........................ 321
Percentage of Eligible Physicians who are
　Members 81%
Ineligible Non-members 173
Physicians retired or not in practice.......... 110
100% County Medical Societies................ 13

Adair	Ida	Muscatine
Adams	Jackson	Poweshiek
Audubon	Marshall	Scott
Boone	Mills	Van Buren
Hamilton		

.TABLE II

County	1933 Membership	Delinquent Members	Eligible Non-Members	Ineligible Non-Members	Not in Practice	Percentage of Eligible Physicians Who Are Members
Adair	8	.....	.....	.....	1	100
Adams	7	.....	.....	.....	.....	100
Allamakee	7	5	2	2	.....	50
Appanoose	13	2	6	.....	.....	62
Audubon	9	.....	.....	.....	.....	100
Benton	16	.....	5	.....	1	76
Black Hawk	66	.....	2	3	2	97
Boone	23	.....	.....	.....	4	100
Bremer	15	.....	2	2	.....	88
Buchanan	11	?	?	?	?	?
Buena Vista	13	2	4	.....	1	68
Butler	10	.....	3	3	.....	77
Calhoun	15	4	1	.....	1	75
Carroll	18	2	2	.....	.....	81
Cass	21	2	1	5	.....	88
Cedar	6	4	8	.....	1	33
Cerro Gordo	42	.....	3	2	.....	93
Cherokee	16	.....	8	2	.....	67
Chickasaw	9	5	.....	1	1	64
Clarke	6	.....	2	.....	1	75
Clay	6	1	8	.....	3	40
Clayton	15	.....	6	2	3	71
Clinton	41	.....	6	2	4	87
Crawford	5	10	2	3	.....	29
Dallas-Guthrie	37	2	9	1	2	77
Davis	10	1	2	.....	.....	77
Decatur	8	2	5	.....	.....	53
Delaware	7	3	4	5	1	50
Des Moines	33	4	8	2	.....	73
Dickinson	10	2	.....	.....	.....	83
Dubuque	54	1	6	14	.....	89
Emmet	11	2	.....	.....	.....	85
Fayette	14	7	9	1	1	47
Floyd	15	1	.....	4	.....	94
Franklin	7	1	4	.....	.....	58
Fremont	10	2	3	.....	2	67
Greene	12	2	4	1	.....	67
Grundy	9	2	1	.....	.....	75
Hamilton	22	.....	.....	.....	3	100
Hancock-Winnebago	13	8	5	.....	2	50
Hardin	24	.....	1	1	2	96
Harrison	12	4	6	.....	1	55
Henry	7	8	6	.....	.....	33
Howard	9	1	1	.....	1	82
Humboldt	5	.....	5	.....	.....	50
Ida	11	.....	.....	.....	1	100
Iowa	12	1	4	1	3	71
Jackson	20	.....	.....	1	2	100
Jasper	30	3	1	.....	1	88
Jefferson	16	1	2	1	1	84
Johnson	109	.....	26	3	6	81
Jones	11	.....	.....	3	.....	73
Keokuk	10	6	3	5	2	53
Kossuth	14	2	3	.....	.....	74
Lee	39	3	1	4	3	91
Linn	100	.....	12	6	10	89
Louisa	13	.....	1	2	1	93
Lucas	14	.....	1	.....	2	93
Lyon	8	2	1	1	1	73
Madison	10	.....	1	.....	3	83
Mahaska	19	3	2	3	1	73
Marion	21	.....	2	2	1	91
Marshall	40	.....	.....	4	.....	100
Mills	12	.....	.....	1	2	100
Mitchell	6	2	7	2	.....	40
Monona	6	5	1	1	2	50
Monroe	6	.....	6	1	.....	50
Montgomery	11	4	3	1	2	56
Muscatine	27	.....	.....	2	2	100
O'Brien	12	3	2	2	.....	71
Osceola	7	.....	2	.....	.....	78
Page	19	2	7	2	1	68
Palo Alto	11	.....	2	.....	.....	85
Plymouth	12	5	8	.....	.....	48
Pocahontas	9	5	3	1	.....	53
Polk	213	9	19	24	4	88
Pottawattamie	53	1	11	8	2	81
Poweshiek	22	.....	.....	.....	.....	100
Ringgold	10	.....	1	.....	.....	91
Sac	15	1	1	.....	.....	88
Scott	91	.....	.....	14	1	100
Shelby	6	2	1	.....	3	67
Sioux	12	6	2	.....	1	60
Story	28	6	4	2	.....	74
Tama	25	.....	1	2	1	96
Taylor	11	2	1	.....	.....	79
Union	17	1	1	2	2	89
Van Buren	13	.....	.....	.....	.....	100
Wapello	44	3	3	3	5	88
Warren	9	3	1	1	1	69
Washington	23	.....	1	.....	.....	96
Wayne	10	1	3	.....	.....	71
Webster	37	6	1	1	.....	84
Winneshiek	15	2	1	.....	.....	83
Woodbury	117	3	9	9	4	91
Worth	5	2	2	.....	.....	56
Wright	21	.....	1	.....	.....	95
Total	2163	192	321	173	110	81%

The "Iowa Plan" of contract between the county medical society and the county board of supervisors for care of the indigent sick is receiving increasing notice from other states. During the present period when counties have been forced to lengthen their lists of county charges, the plan has offered a safeguard to the medical profession and a concrete working arrangement for the county boards. In those counties in which the contract machinery has been well established, it has simplified the new task undertaken by many counties, of caring for the unemployed, representing a large section of the population not on the indigent list, but requiring care through the present emergency.

More than half the counties in Iowa have some such arrangement; either an actual contract between the medical society and the local board, or an agreement as to a definite fee schedule. Table III shows the types of plan adopted in various counties.

TABLE III

County Societies Having Lump Sum Contracts

Benton (Belle Plaine)	Marshall
Boone	Ringgold
Calhoun	Scott (Davenport and
Clay	Davenport Township)
Guthrie	Story
Hardin	Tama
Johnson	Van Buren
Lee (Fort Madison)	Washington
Marion	Woodbury (Sioux City)

County Societies Having Fee Schedule Contracts

Black Hawk	Floyd	Jefferson
Buchanan	Hamilton	Louisa
Buena Vista	Henry	Sac
Cerro Gordo	Jasper	Wright

County Societies Having Agreement as to Fee Schedule, but no Contract

Cass	Humboldt	O'Brien
Clarke	Ida	Page
Davis	Jackson	Pocahontas
Decatur	Kossuth	Poweshiek
Delaware	Linn	Shelby
Emmet	Lyon	Sioux
Fayette	Mitchell	Wayne
Franklin	Monona	Winnebago
Fremont	Muscatine	Worth

For the financial report of the Secretary, you are referred to the annual audit, prepared by a certified public accountant, and published elsewhere in the handbook.

In closing, I wish to thank the other officers and the various committees for their support, and the 1933 House of Delegates for my election for another term.

Respectfully submitted,
Robert L. Parker, Secretary.

Secretary Parker: As regarding membership I wish to report that a year ago today we had 1817 paid-up members. Today we have 2063 paid-up members.

With that additional report I *move* that the Secretary's report as published in the Handbook be approved.

The motion was regularly seconded.

President Taylor: You have heard the report of the Secretary which seems to be a good one, almost 300 paid-up members in advance of this time last year. As many as favor this report as published in the Handbook with the supplementary report he has just given say "aye"; contrary "no." *The Secretary's report is accepted.*

We will now have the report of the Treasurer. Harold McCoy does not seem to be here. We will pass on to the report of the Council. Is the Chairman of the Council here? (Absent.) The Secretary is here.

REPORT OF THE CHAIRMAN OF THE COUNCIL
House of Delegates, Iowa State Medical Society:

In reviewing the reports of the Councilors of the various districts of the State Society for the year 1933-34, and as a result of visits made to meetings in the majority of the districts, the Chairman of the Council is impressed with the evidences of increased interest and activity. He is further greatly encouraged by the part played by the younger men in the organization, not only in the scientific programs, but also in the administrative functions of the county societies.

The reports of the several Councilors all show conscientious effort to promote the welfare of the individual county societies and consequently of the State Society. This is evidenced in a large degree in the increased interest in district meetings in nearly every district in the Society. It is reflected in the good fellowship and active participation of the members in those districts in which such meetings have been held.

These are chaotic times and many new and untried plans are being advocated throughout the length and breadth of our land, but the tendency of the medical profession in this state is in the main to keep its feet on the ground and progress slowly but definitely. The members of the State Society are alert to the significance of present-day trends as they may affect the medical profession, but are not ready to grasp at innovations until their worth has been tested.

Because of the economic conditions, there have been only two Council meetings during the year, both of which have been held in conjunction with meetings of the Board of Trustees, pursuant to the belief that affairs of the Society will be conducted more effectively by a closer cooperation and more thorough understanding between these two bodies.

Respectfully submitted,
Harold A. Spilman, Chairman

REPORTS FROM COUNCILOR DISTRICTS
First Councilor District

The following reports from officers of the various county societies in this district will show the activities of the district during the year:

Felix A. Hennessy, Councilor

Bremer County. The Bremer County Medical Society during the past year has held regular monthly meetings in conjunction with the staff of St. Joseph's Mercy Hospital.

On July 7 a heart and lung clinic was held at Waverly, conducted by Drs. Peck and Glomset.

During the year Dr. A. M. Stegeman left the county and Drs. P. J. Amlie and H. F. Turner moved into the county. Both have applied for membership and their applications are awaiting the required six months' residence prior to acceptance. Dr. R. H. Stafford was reinstated, following his application for membership and the withdrawal of previous objec-. tions.

James A. Whitmire, Secretary

Chickasaw County. The Chickasaw County Medical Society has held four meetings this year. We have had one guest speaker, Dr. Erwin von Graff, of Iowa City, who spoke to us on "The Dangers of Stump Cancer after Subtotal Hysterectomy."

We cooperated with the local unit of the Iowa Tuberculosis Association in carrying out the diphtheria immunization program throughout the county for immunization of children up to ten years of age.

Paul E. Gardner, Deputy Councilor

Clayton County. The Clayton County Medical Society held only one meeting during the year, the majority of the members preferring to attend larger group meetings. The Clayton County society participated in six group meetings of the four counties in northeastern Iowa. Some of the members regularly attended the meetings of the Study Club, which represents six counties.

We had one social meeting, a supper and boat excursion on the Mississippi, to which we invited the doctors and their wives from an adjoining county.

At the annual meeting it was decided to hold one or two meetings during the coming year, with papers to be read by the members of the society.

Participation of the medical profession in nonmedical activities was practically nil.

J. W. Hudek, Deputy Councilor

Fayette County. The following was the program of the Fayette County Medical Society for the year 1933:

June 6. Meeting of Allamakee, Clayton, Fayette and Winneshiek County Medical Societies at West Union. "Anemias", Frank Rohner, M.D., Iowa City; "Blood Morphology", Lester Larson, M.D., Decorah.

July 18. Postville. "Laboratory Methods", A. H. Sanford, M.D., Rochester, Minn.

August 8. West Union. "Functional Disturbances of the Stomach and Bowel", C. W. Baldridge, M.D., Iowa City; "Treatment of Peptic Ulcer with Metaphen", A. A. Schmidt, M.D., Postville.

September 5. Postville. "Female Sex Hormone", R. I. Theisen, M.D., Dubuque; "Cancer Survey in Iowa", Felix Hennessy, M.D., Calmar.

October 4. West Union. "Blood Dyscrasias with Special Relation to Coagulation", J. L. Kestel, M.D., Waterloo.

November 7. Waucoma. The Clayton and Fayette

County Medical Societies were the guests of Dr. and Mrs. J. M. Smittle. "Headaches with Special Reference to Migraine", Fred Moersch, M.D., Rochester, Minn.; "Treatment of Major Neuralgias", Dr. Long, Rochester, Minn.

December 7. Maynard. The Fayette County Medical Society members were the guests of Drs. Hall and Hall. Special business meeting. "Diagnosis of Chest", Otis Britt, M.D., Waterloo.

December 20. West Union. Special called business meeting with CWA directors.

C. C. Hall, M.D., Deputy Councilor

Floyd County. The Floyd County Medical Society has held a scientific meeting on the fourth Tuesday of each month during the past year. These meetings were preceded by a dinner and followed by a short business meeting. The speakers on these monthly programs were well known men from the State University Hospital and from the Mayo Foundation. During the winter months, when traveling was difficult, programs were furnished by men from our local ranks and from nearby county societies. Following each meeting the doctors met at the office of one of the Charles City physicians for light refreshments and cards. These very interesting and instructive meetings have been enjoyed not only by the members of the Floyd County Medical Society, but also by members of nearby societies.

J. B. Miner, Jr., Secretary

Howard County. The annual meeting of the Howard County Medical Society was held on December 6, at which time officers were elected for the coming year. We received one new member, Dr. T. J. Nereim, of Lime Springs.

A resolution requesting our secretary to make an effort to get one of the district meetings at Cresco was passed unanimously.

The Women's Auxiliary entertained the members of the society and guests at a dinner on March 10, at the home of Dr. George Kessel. Following the dinner and a scientific program, separate business meetings of the society and auxiliary were held.

Wm. A. Bockoven, Deputy Councilor

Mitchell County. The Mitchell County Medical Society has held regular meetings on the first Monday of each month during the past year. Two new members were received into the society this year: Dr. T. G. Walker of Riceville, and Dr. Theodore Blong of Stacyville.

John O. Eiel, President

Winneshiek County. The Winneshiek County Medical Society has completed a very satisfactory year. Seven meetings were held and were well attended, with a good spirit shown by the individual members.

The First Councilor District met in Decorah in November. This meeting was well attended and very instructive to all.

We have sponsored the formation of an Interprofessional Group, including physicians, dentists, veterinarians, pharmacists, nurses, and one Ph.D. from Luther College. This group will have three regular meetings each year and will supervise local health matters for the community. Dr. T. N. Stabo is president of the organization.

We have recently suffered the loss of three of our members: Dr. W. H. Emmons, Dr. Otto O. Svebakken and Dr. J. A. Juen. These men were very active in the county society and their loss will be felt by all members in time to come.

During the past year we have sponsored and given weekly fifteen-minute health talks over KGCA, the local radio station at Decorah. These talks, given by our members, were received by the surrounding community and an active interest in their presentation was shown by all. We are now outlining our program for the coming year.

We are glad to report one hundred per cent membership for 1934 and look forward to a successful year in medical society activities.

Edward F. Hagen, Secretary

Second Councilor District

On reviewing the work in the Second District for the past year, the most outstanding thing is the postgraduate course that was put on at Algona beginning in November, 1933. The men of Kossuth County promoted this course, driving to all the surrounding towns and gathering in sixty members to take the course. All the members of the Kossuth County Society deserve credit for this very constructive piece of work. The professors from the University who gave the course are to be complimented for the working up of such a thoroughly practical series of lectures. This is a line of work which we feel should be actively continued, for it is our firm conviction that our best means of combating irregulars is by becoming better doctors ourselves. It is beyond the reach of most of us to go to medical centers for postgraduate instruction, but we can all avail ourselves of these courses which are brought to us. We note that the fostering of postgraduate instruction is one of the chief objectives of the Massachusetts Medical Society and also of the Michigan State Medical Society, which has appropriated a large sum to foster this work.

On August 18, at the invitation of the Cerro Gordo County Medical Society, the doctors of the Second District, together with their families, had a most enjoyable picnic at Clear Lake. We had an afternoon of fun, then after a delicious picnic dinner supervised by the Woman's Auxiliary, we had an address by Dr. W. L. Bierring on the "Historical Sequence of Medical Events." Dr. T. A. Burke of Mason City, and Dr. S. S. Westly of Manly, gave us very enjoyable accounts of their European trip. We intend to make the Second District picnic at Clear Lake an annual affair.

We have continued the district meetings, following up Dr. Taylor's idea of using the younger men on the programs to give papers. On October 22, a meeting was held at Hampton which was well attended. The program consisted of papers on "The Management of Compound Fractures" given by Dr.

Burger, of Hampton; "Calcium Therapy in Preeclamptics" by Dr. Sage, of Eagle Grove, and "Nephritis in Children" by Dr. G. E. Harrison, of Mason City. Dr. Westly, of Manly, also talked on "The Medical Situation in Europe."

Another district meeting was held in Forest City on January 25, at which the program consisted of "Fracture of the Vertebra" by Dr. I. T. Schultz; "Edema" by Dr. W. C. Egloff, of Mason City, and "Rheumatic Fever" by Dr. C. V. Hamilton, of Garner.

We are having another meeting at Clarion on March 27. The program is to be "Colitis" by Dr. M. G. Bourne, of Algona; "Whooping Cough in Children" by Dr. Nelle T. Schultz, of Humboldt; Case History, "Cerebral Thrombosis" by Dr. B. L. Basinger, of Goldfield; "A Cold Potato" by Dr. C. B. Taylor, of Ottumwa.

We are finding that these programs are well attended and some very excellent papers are prepared and presented. There have also been some very good discussions.

The care of indigents has undergone some changes in the district. The Worth County doctors now have a contract on a fee basis. Cerro Gordo County has taken the contract on a fee basis with a maximum limit. The money is paid directly to the County Society and is used primarily for the advancement of scientific medicine in Cerro Gordo County. Thus far, we are finding it very satisfactory.

Membership in the district for 1933 remained about the same as in 1932. In only two instances did we hear any complaints on the ten dollar dues, but the loss in membership which we sustained in 1931 continued in 1932 because of financial stringency.

L. R. Woodward, Councilor

Third Councilor District

The Third Councilor District has been carrying on its activities during the past year with no great changes. There have been about the usual number of meetings in the nine different component societies. The matter of fees, especially those pertaining to the care of the indigent, has often been under discussion. Some counties are seriously considering adopting the contract plan with the boards of supervisors, which I feel is the best solution under present economic conditions. This question of the care of the indigent is, of course, a permanent one, and we will learn much in the way of handling such patients in the years to come.

Some counties are meeting quarterly, with good attendance. Only one county in the district is meeting monthly. The Northwest Iowa District meets semiannually and always has a good program and a good attendance.

The matter of State Society dues is still a question for discussion. Some of the doctors feel that dues of ten dollars are too high, while a majority of the profession think that we should make some sacrifice if necessary to maintain an efficient state organization.

There is evidence of increased interest in organized medicine all along the line. Doctors are giving more time and attention to the economic side of the practice of medicine. They are beginning to realize that this has been too much neglected in the past. I am unable to make a complete report of the district because up to date only a few of the counties have submitted their annual reports.

Clay County. The annual meeting of the Clay County Medical Society for election of officers was held January 9. There are fourteen physicians in the county, nine of whom have paid their 1934 dues. Dr. C. C. Jones, a graduate of Rush Medical College, located at Spencer in September and is now a member of the society.

A diphtheria immunization program was carried out in the schools of the county in February and March.

E. E. Munger, Deputy Councilor

Emmet County. The only meeting worthy of note for the year 1933 was the annual meeting on December 5, at which officers were elected for the coming year.

The Dickinson and Emmet County Medical Societies decided to hold joint scientific meetings during the year 1934, these meetings to alternate between the county seats, Spirit Lake in Dickinson County and Estherville in Emmet County. In accordance with this decision, three meetings have been held. There was lively discussion of all papers presented at these meetings and everyone seems to be taking serious interest.

The membership of the Emmet County Medical Society is one hundred per cent.

M. T. Morton, Deputy Councilor

O'Brien County. The first meeting of the O'Brien County Medical Society during the past year was held at Primghar on March 8, 1933. Another meeting was held at Primghar on March 21. The annual meeting for election of officers was called on December 26. A fourth meeting was held in Sheldon on April 9.

There were no deaths among the doctors in O'Brien County during 1933. Changes were made as follows: Dr. J. W. Myers, who had practiced in Sheldon for nineteen years, located in Postville in March and is practicing there. Dr. Ralph L. Irwin, formerly of Sioux City, has located in Paullina.

Walter R. Brock, Deputy Councilor

Palo Alto County. The Palo Alto County Medical Society has held six meetings during the past year. In addition, most of the doctors of the county attended the postgraduate course given at Algona in September and October. This course was one of the finest things which the doctors have done in a cooperative way.

The county society has immunized about 1,800 children against diphtheria during the past few weeks. This work was done in cooperation with the Red Cross. Fees for the work have been paid into the society, so that all doctors of the county will now be members of the County and State Medical Societies, since the understanding was that dues would be paid from these fees.

The cooperation among the doctors of Palo Alto County is very healthy, and we look to organized medicine to help us solve some of our problems.

Harold L. Brereton, Deputy Councilor

Pocahontas County. The Pocahontas County Medical Society has had five meetings during the past year. Half of our members attended the postgraduate course in Algona last fall. The society has reached an agreement with the county board of supervisors for the care of the indigent.

J. H. Hovenden, Deputy Councilor

Some complaints have been made in regard to certain doctors cutting fees far below the minimum fees regularly charged in their respective communities. We feel that this is bad ethics and we will endeavor to correct these practices as soon as time will permit.

On the whole, the Third Councilor District is in very healthy condition.

Frank P. Winkler, Councilor

Fourth Councilor District

As Councilor of the Fourth District I wish to report the following:

J. H. O'Donoghue, M.D., secretary of the Buena Vista County Medical Society, reports: Contract with the board of supervisors for care of county poor approved by all doctors in county. The professional meetings of this county are held in association with Plymouth, Ida and Cherokee counties, at Cherokee, under the caption of The Four County Association. Dr. J. H. Wise, Cherokee, is secretary of this association.

Walter A. Anneberg, M.D., secretary of the Carroll County Medical Society reports: The Carroll County Medical Society held two scientific meetings in 1933, and helped provide the postgraduate course held at Jefferson last fall. There has been very good cooperation and good feeling between the doctors in the county for the past year.

Dean Tipton, M.D., secretary of the Cherokee County Medical Society, reports: Activities for the year 1933 limited to regular monthly business meetings. Our society acts as a staff meeting for the Sioux Valley Hospital of Cherokee.

W. P. Crane, M. D., secretary of the Ida County Medical Society, reports: Several business meetings held during 1933 but no scientific meetings. Have one hundred per cent membership.

L. C. O'Toole, M.D., secretary of the Plymouth County Medical Society, reports: Monthly meetings held in conjunction with Sacred Heart Hospital Staff meetings. Interesting papers and cases have been presented by members.

J. R. Dewey, M.D., secretary of the Sac County Medical Society, reports: Society met seven times for business and scientific sessions. The funeral of Dr. F. H. McCray was attended by the society in a body and six members served as pallbearers. The care of the indigent sick was handled by county contract plan which was essentially fifty per cent of the 1930 fee bill. Negotiations now under way for renewal of contract which will eliminate some of the injustices and defects of the 1933 arrangement.

A joint meeting of deputy councilors of the Third and Fourth District was held in Sioux City, January 23, 1934, at the time of the Sioux Valley Medical Association meeting. Total of fifteen members present. Civil Works Administration was discussed. W. L. O'Keefe, Injury Clerk for the local Civil Works Administration, discussed the various forms necessary to complete the claims by employees of the federal government. This meeting was very much appreciated by those who attended, as a number of them stated they were not properly informed as to the necessary paper work to be carried out in accident cases employed on Civil Works Administration work. This permitted the deputy councilors to take this information back to their respective county societies. The federal government had instructed that those in charge of the disability work should select members of component county societies to take care of those injured where they did not have physicians holding federal appointments.

In addition I wish to report the results of the county contract plan in Woodbury County over a period of ten months, or the duration of the contract. Up to Feburary 15, 1934, our out-patient department took care of 4,379 new cases and 4,615 recurrent cases, a total of 8,994. Visits: new 5,649, recurrent 13,357, a total 19,006. Hospital medical cases 518, surgical cases 601, total 1,119. House calls 4,050. Obstetrical cases, 123 delivered in the home, 109 delivered in hospital. Practically the entire medical society agreed to do this work. We have developed a rotating service, and up to the present time a very high percentage of the men have stated that in their opinion, although not ideal, this method, namely, the county contract plan, has been the best way of solving the problem of the care of the indigent sick. James E. Reeder, Councilor

Fifth Councilor District

The meeting of the Deputy Councilors of the Fifth Councilor District of the Iowa State Medical Society was held in Des Moines on February 16, 1934. There were present:

Dr. Mark C. Jones, Councilor of Boone County.
Dr. P. W. Van Metre, Councilor of Calhoun County.
Dr. S. J. Brown, Councilor of Guthrie County.
Dr. E. J. Butterfield, Councilor of Dallas County.
Dr. B. C. Hamilton, Jr., Councilor of Greene County.
Dr. M. B. Galloway, Councilor of Hamilton County.
Dr. Ralph Parker, Councilor of Polk County.
Dr. E. B. Bush, Councilor of Story County.
Dr. Robt. L. Parker, Secretary of the State Society;
Dr. L. L. Leighton, President of the Webster County Medical Society, who substituted for Councilor Roland Stahr who was unable to attend; Dr. Harold Spilman, Chairman of the Council, as well as Mrs. McCarthy, Executive Secretary of the State Medical Society, and Miss Nelson, Secretary of the Speakers Bureau, were also present.

The subjects discussed in order were: membership, Federal Emergency Relief, legislation, Speakers Bureau, district meetings, cancer committee.

The importance of a full paid-up membership in consideration of our state representation in the national organization was stressed, as well as the registration by individual members in the American Medical Directory.

Rather a brief discussion of the possibilities in the way of legislation was indulged in. It was emphasized that while our own Legislative Committee has accomplished but little in the way of positive results the Committee did accomplish a great deal in preventing adverse legislation.

The work of the Speakers Bureau was presented by the secretary of this division in the central office, Miss Nelson. The extent of this work was related and marked commendation of the work and accomplishments of this division was quite apparent.

The district meetings throughout the state were mentioned and the type of meeting discussed. The report indicated that some of these were purely social while others were extremely scientific and some were a combination of the two. The conclusion seemed to be that the influence of the many activities of the state organization was being appreciated and amplified in the district meetings.

The Cancer Committee, of which Dr. Jepson is chairman, apparently has not received much encouragement from our state organization. At this meeting each Deputy Councilor was urged to have a cancer committee appointed by his society to gather the data and information required by the national organization directed in the state by Dr. Jepson.

The following counties in the Fifth District have contracts for the care of indigents: Boone, Calhoun, Guthrie, Hamilton, Story and Webster. It is apparent there is a lack of uniformity in these contracts in the different counties. The variability in the contracts relating to practice and surgery and the difference in the population of the different counties is such that it does not seem advisable to incorporate these contracts in this report. They are, however, available at the central office.

The second subject for discussion was delayed to the last—that of Federal Emergency Relief. The Federal Civil Works Administration Rules and Regulations No. 5, revised and published December 12, 1933, was before us while we were discussing the Civil Works Administration program in the Ninth District, the state being divided into districts in accordance with the Federal Administration.

Considerable discussion was indulged in along this line and the importance of filling out the government papers, as required, was specifically emphasized.

Dr. Harkness and Dr. Reeder had kindly supplied me with the Scott and Woodbury County Contracts

postgraduate course with one hundred twenty-five matriculants.

Regular scientific meetings have been held on the third Tuesday of each month and special or business meetings may be held on the first Tuesday of the month when required. These meetings have been most interesting. Good scientific programs have been arranged for the balance of the year.

The county society members have agreed to care for the injured CWA workers as they may be sent to physicians on order from the superior officers in charge.

A satisfactory percentage contract for the care of the indigent sick has been in operation for the past year.

A self-sustaining county medical bulletin, *The Voice*, has been published and mailed to the physicians in the surrounding territory for the past year. This entails considerable work, but is well worth it.

Grundy County. Dr. H. V. Kahler, Deputy Councilor, reports a reorganization of the Grundy County Medical Society and plans for regular meetings, including a joint meeting with the Sixth District in June at the Golf Club between Reinbeck and Grundy Center.

The rebirth of the Grundy County Medical Society was reported as a birthday present to State Secretary Robert Parker, as he spent most of his own birthday anniversary delivering this one hundred per cent Grundy County Society. Encourage this baby by being present at the June District-Grundy County social meeting.

Hardin County. Dr. E. O. Koeneman, Deputy Councilor, reports meetings held monthly at Eldora or Iowa Falls. All physicians of the county but two are members of the Society. One new member was added in 1933.

Outside talent is engaged for programs. Many of the members participated in postgraduate work at Waterloo, Ames and Marshalltown.

The poor are taken care of by a contract with the board of supervisors, supervised by a trained social worker. Hardin County claims the honor of being the first county in the United States to function under a contract, the first contract being entered into in 1905.

Iowa County. Dr. I. J. Sinn, Deputy Councilor, reports considerable difficulty in keeping the men in good standing. Iowa County seems to be near enough two larger medical centers to make a strong medical organization impossible.

Two meetings are held a year, one, a chest and lung clinic, and the other the annual business meeting.

A weekly noon medical luncheon club, in each locality where there is more than one physician, will go a long way in increasing interest in medical organization and meetings.

Jasper County. Dr. S. E. Hinshaw, Secretary, reports:

Strength of organization: All eligible physicians in county signed up for 1933; five did not pay dues or make any arrangements to do so; three physicians have an honorary membership, one of whom still attends most all meetings and takes an active part in society proceedings; one new member moved to the county during 1933.

Postgraduate work: Several of our members attended postgraduate lecture courses during the year; one member gave a series of radio talks sponsored by the Speakers Bureau of the State Society.

Special meetings: In September our county society held a joint meeting with the sixth district. This meeting was well attended, and a very interesting program followed a 6:30 dinner at the Hotel Maytag.

Method of caring for the indigent: By contract with the Board of Supervisors and the County Medical Society. All bills rendered at the regular fee, as printed in the State JOURNAL, and amount paid is one-half of the bill rendered.

Regular meetings: Are held the first Tuesday of each month. Visiting physicians are always welcome to meet with us.

Marshall County. Dr. R. S. Grossman, Deputy Councilor, reports regular monthly meetings held the first Tuesday of each month. Seven excellent scientific programs were put on by speakers from Chicago, Des Moines and Iowa City, and during September, October, November and December, the University of Iowa Faculty gave a splendid course on the "Fundamentals of Medicine."

Marshall county membership is one hundred per cent, all state and national dues are paid from the fund received from the county contract for indigent care.

Poweshiek County. Dr. C. V. Lawton, Deputy Councilor, acting for Dr. E. E. Harris, reports five meetings held in the past year, with good attendance and interest. Membership is one hundred per cent, and one new member, Dr. John R. Parish, was added during the year.

A satisfactory contract is held with the board for the care of the indigent sick.

Meetings of special interest were held with the Keokuk and Mahaska County Societies, at which state legislators were guests. Proposed legislative problems were discussed.

A great interest and a fine spirit exists in this one hundred per cent county society.

Tama County. Dr. A. A. Pace, Deputy Councilor, reports twenty-four members and one eligible nonmember. Six meetings were held in 1933, with good attendance. Five new members were received in 1933 and two were lost by death.

The society supported the Marshalltown postgraduate course, personally and financially. It paid the members' county and state dues from the society treasury, entertained its speakers, distributed $50.00 each to its members and left a substantial reserve in the treasury.

It carries a satisfactory contract with the Board of Supervisors, with extra fees for major and emergency cases requiring hospital care and for x-ray work.

There is a good feeling of fellowship among the members and a fine cooperative spirit.

I wish to thank the deputy councilors and county officers of the Sixth District for their prompt and cheerful cooperation during the past year.

C. W. Ellyson, Councilor

Seventh Councilor District

The appended reports of Deputy Councilors are offered as evidence that a reasonably high average of interest and activity has been maintained during the past year by the unit societies of the Seventh District. As I have gone about through the district, it has seemed that the zeal of the county societies and their members is improving and increasing. In spite of the hard times, the condition of the profession appears to be good. Is it not possible, that the financial difficulties in which most of us find ourselves, and the strain of living in these trying times, may merely be tending to cement the bonds of friendship with our colleagues, be teaching us to meet vicissitudes with courage and equanimity, and to rely more and more upon that ancient and honorable code, according to which physicians try to mold their lives?

Because of the scientific activity of the societies in the more populous counties, Clinton, Dubuque, Johnson and Linn, no district meetings have been held. The annual dinner of the county officers for the promotion of good fellowship and conviviality was attended by an enthusiastic group consisting of everyone invited.

Arthur W. Erskine, Councilor

Buchanan County. The Buchanan County Medical Society meets four times a year as a medical society. At these meetings we have an outside speaker and have a 6:30 dinner, paid for by one-fourth of the society membership. We also have eight meetings as a staff of the Peoples Hospital. At these meetings we usually have a short paper on a subject of interest to all, after which interesting case reports are discussed and also medical economics. Last year we had fifteen paid-up members. To date we have twelve paid-up with four more to pay.

The doctors of Independence have immunized about 150 children in the schools against diphtheria. We have also examined 300 school children for which we are paid at the rate of fifty cents a child. The money is used to buy instruments for the hospital.

According to an agreement between the Board of Supervisors and the Medical Society, the indigent patients may select their physicians. Calls are paid for at the rate of $1.50 each, plus mileage at 25 cents per mile one way when calls are made at a distance. The fees for obstetrical cases, fractures, consultations and special examinations are very low, but it is understood that the present agreement is merely temporary and will be revised as soon as the recovery program materializes. There is a good spirit of cooperation and harmony between the Board of Supervisors and the County Medical Society. It seems to us that it has been easier for the Society to arrange for local medical and hospital care for indigents since the service at the University Hospitals has been curtailed. The supervisors are recognizing the advisability of saving their quota of University Hospital beds for cases needing specialized or long continued care. Besides this agreement, the Peoples Hospital also has an agreement with the supervisors to furnish service amounting to 400 bed days for $1,200.00. Last year's agreement called for 450 days. This agreement also calls for payment for service in excess of 400 bed days at cost or not to exceed $6.00 a day.

The Society has functioned very well and the meetings have been very well attended.

C. W. Tidball, Deputy Councilor

Cedar County. The activities of the Cedar County Medical Society have been chiefly centered in attempts to follow outlines adopted by surrounding counties. There has been manifested a unanimous desire to cooperate on the part of members who attended our Society meetings. Affiliations of Cedar County physicians with adjoining county societies render a large membership and attendance locally a problem. However, I am glad to report that there have been no dissensions, and in fact, a fine spirit of harmony has been shown with the efforts of the representatives of the State Medical Society to bring about unity of purpose and to provide care for the indigents in a manner befitting the traditions of our profession.

E. J. Van Metre, Deputy Councilor

Clinton County. There are fifty-five physicians in the county. Forty-five are members of the County Society. This represents a gain of five new members in the past year. Five of the non-members are eligible.

Meetings are held the first Thursday of every month except the months of August and September, when no regular meetings are held.

The meetings are scientific in nature, a paper being given by an individual of note in his specialty. The meetings are well attended by the members of the Society and we have the pleasure of entertaining guests from Illinois and surrounding communities in Iowa.

The Medical Society administered diphtheria toxoid to the school children of Clinton. The Society received a fee for this work from the school board.

The fees obtained for examining state patients under the Perkins, Haskell-Klaus laws are turned into the treasury of the Society.

A modified New Jersey Plan for care of the county indigents was presented to the county supervisors. They rejected it and accepted the bid presented by a physician and his two co-workers. The same group had the contract last year.

R. T. Lenaghan, Deputy Councilor

Delaware County. The Society has held two meetings this year trying to get organized.

Membership, at present, consists of but three paid-up members, but we hope and expect at least a fair percentage of the men in the county to join soon and pay up their dues for this year.

Our first meeting was well attended and included an interesting discussion of diagnostic problems met in the every-day practice of some of our local men.

Our second meeting, while not so well attended, was large enough so that we could make some real advance with our greatest activity for the year. This is the problem of providing medical care for the indigent sick of the county. We have obtained the signatures of all the physicians in the county to a fee bill for these cases which we believe to be fair and just. It has been presented to the county supervisors who now have it under consideration. We are also asking for a monthly list of the indigents of the county so that we may know at the time of a call if it is a private or county case. This should be a real help if we are able to obtain it.

We feel that the fact that all the doctors in the county are working together on this fee bill problem so well is a good omen, and that this year we may be able to gather together the remains of our county society and rebuild it into a good live active group. At least we are going to try and will do our best to keep the faith and see it through.

J. I. Jones, Deputy Councilor

Dubuque County. Relief Work. In spite of the fact that the full force of the economic depression was felt in Dubuque County during 1933, the County Medical Society has "carried on" in a manner worthy of the highest ideals of the medical profession. As in past years the members have voluntarily aided the county physician in the great task of caring for the indigent and unemployed, most often without recompense and frequently at actual personal losses. In addition they have cared for those families who were without funds but who still retained enough American spirit and backbone to refuse to "go on the county." In many instances the only reward of the physician was the gratitude of the patient for whom he had cared. The writer believes that the real "forgotten man" of the present era is the family physician. Certainly his labor and sacrifices have not been generally appreciated by the public and especially by governmental employees. In spite of this injustice the members of the medical society are cooperating in every way with local, state and national relief agencies.

Meetings—Regular monthly meetings, 8; average attendance, 27; special meetings, 3; average attendance, 19; anniversary meeting 1; attendance, 100.

We had one public meeting which was addressed by Doctor Arthur J. Cramp, Director of the Bureau of Investigation of the A. M. A. Doctor Cramp spoke on "Pink Pills and Panaceas" and an audience of 500 was keenly interested in his exposure of the methods by which the manufacturers of "patent" medicines foisted their products on the gullible. The speaker also addressed the Rotary Club and criticized the far-reaching and exaggerated advertising claims made in radio broadcasts by the patent medicine interests. He stressed the need for greater control of radio advertising as well as the necessity of a revised pure food and drug act.

During the year a progressive group of officers and an active program committee united to make our meetings more interesting and more valuable from a scientific standpoint. Local men were encouraged to present papers at our meetings. This was done in the belief that our members would thereby receive the greatest benefits. Many excellent papers were prepared and were presented before meetings in neighboring counties as well as locally. In addition the following guests appeared on our programs during the year:

Dr. G. F. Harkness, Davenport, Iowa.
Dr. M. D. Ott, Davenport, Iowa.
Dr. H. E. Pfeiffer, Cedar Rapids, Iowa.
Dr. T. F. Thornton, Waterloo, Iowa.
Dr. C. W. Losh, Des Moines, Iowa.
Dr. Arthur C. Strachauer, Minneapolis, Minn.
Dr. Amos C. Fey, Galesburg, Ill.
Dr. Wm. R. Cubbin, Chicago, Ill.
Dr. James J. Callahan, Chicago, Ill.
Dr. F. H. Falls, Chicago, Ill.
Dr. F. L. Lederer, Chicago, Ill.

Other very valuable meetings which were unofficially conducted by the members of the county society were The Finley Hospital Clinicopathologic Conferences. These conferences were held each week and a total attendance of 696 members of the county society during the year indicates the interest in this type of meeting. Their great advantage lies in the fact that they represent actual clinical problems which are encountered in every-day practice. They also aid greatly in coordinating the activities of the various groups using the hospital—internists, surgeons, roentgenologist and pathologist. In many ways they are our most valuable meetings.

Notable Events. There were two especially notable events during the year. The first was that the members of the Society were invited to reorganize the medical staff of St. Joseph's Mercy Hospital. This was accomplished and undoubtedly will do much to advance medicine in Dubuque. The second notable event was the award of a silver medal to The Finley Hospital Laboratory for a scientific exhibit at the Milwaukee session of the American Medical Association. This was important because it indicates what can be accomplished by the hospitals in Iowa if the members of the medical profession unite to develop the scientific aspects of their local hospitals to the highest possible degree. The Finley exhibit was made possible only through the united efforts of the members of the County Medical Society.

In conclusion it can be said from a scientific viewpoint that the Dubuque County Medical Society has had one of its most successful years. While we have problems to be solved, the strength and unity manifested by the profession during the past year intensifies our faith in their solution as well as that of new problems which may arise in the future.

F. P. McNamara, Deputy Councilor

Jackson County. The Jackson County Medical Society has had a fairly successful year, and the outlook seems to be good for 1934. For the past year our membership has been diminished by two, one because of death, and the other because of the financial depression. The Society has held only three meetings instead of the usual four. Two were scientific, the third a business meeting. The meetings were fairly well attended, but there was a noticeable lack of interest. The Society has not been very active. An anti-diphtheria campaign was waged, the work being done by members of the Society without compensation. Our county indigent work is done by the members selected by the patients. If the work has been authorized by the supervisors, the bills are usually allowed, although they are cut from thirty to fifty per cent We have no county physician and no contract. Each year the supervisors advertise for bids on the county indigent work, but no one bids as the members perfer the present method on account of its providing for a division of the work and of the compensation.

G. C. Ryan, Deputy Councilor

Johnson County. Ten meetings of the Society were held during the year at which there was an average attendance of 61. At seven meetings the programs were given by members of the Society. At three meetings out-of-town speakers addressed the Society. They were Father Schwitalla, Dr. G. A. Bennett, and Dr. Lindberg.

The membership sustained a loss of twelve Senior and twenty Junior members. There was a gain, however, of twelve Senior and thirty Junior members. On December 31, 1933, the membership of the Society consisted of three life members, 87 active members, eight associate members, five non-resident members, two affiliates, and 31 Junior members.

George C. Albright, Deputy Councilor

Jones County. The Jones County Medical Society remains about the same from year to year.

The profession in our county numbers nineteen, twelve of whom are members of the county society. Of the seven non-members all except one are eligible.

Eight of our twelve county society members are non-resident members of the Linn County Medical Society which we attend for the scientific programs.

The Jones County Medical Society meets about twice a year, once to elect officers and once to hear our delegate's report.

One of our county society members holds a contract with the county supervisors to look after the sick at the County Poor Farm. The balance of the indigents are cared for by individual physicians who present their bills to the county supervisors as they do the work. The supervisors are anxious that the County Medical Society contract to do all the indigent work, but the Society has thought it best not to do this.

T. M. Redmond, Deputy Councilor

Linn County. Eleven scientific meetings of the Linn County Medical Society were planned for the year 1933-34. The following essayists appeared, or will appear, on the programs at these meetings: Drs. Edward H. Skinner, Kansas City, Missouri;

have contracts, and these two have satisfactory financial arrangements with the boards of supervisors. The Van Buren County Medical Society rewrote a contract for 1934, having lost the contract in 1933. Most contracts are based on a percentage of the standard fee bill. When a lump sum is contracted for, there is a tendency for the county board to load too much work on the doctors. Contracts based on a percentage of the fee bill are preferable. Every encouragement should be given county societies to secure equitable remuneration for indigent work.

There have been six deaths among the membership in 1933 and six new practitioners.

Every Deputy Councilor expresses himself as favorable to brief medical articles in the press; to the use of the radio, and to public medical addresses to lay audiences. Only two counties report any public medical addresses during the year, both locally arranged.

Trained social workers have replaced local overseers of the poor in a few counties; better arrangements have been made in others. An inter-professional group, composed of members of the five professions, has been organized in Washington County.

The quota plan of the University Hospitals is going to increase the burden of the county society membership, especially in the care of venereal diseases, and to a certain extent in surgery. This is well. The local physicians should care for practically all of the indigent patients, and be reasonably paid for it. Only those cases which are in need of special care in a hospital and which are suitable for teaching purposes should be sent to the University Hospitals.

The year 1934 holds the promise of increased work for the physician and the Society, greater opportunities for service to the profession, the physician and the public, and by effective organization, greater financial returns.

C. A. Boice, Councilor

Des Moines County. The Des Moines County Medical Society holds nine monthly meetings during the year, omitting the summer months. The interest in the meetings is good and the average attendance about fifty-four per cent. Programs are both home-made and imported.

The Society does not have a contract. A county physician is paid a fair fee for medical work and fifty per cent of the standard fee bill for obstetric work. All physicians are eligible to receive fifty per cent of the fee bill for surgery. In 1933 the medical costs for the indigent in Des Moines County were $46,615.77, of which the dentists received $1,371.00; drugs cost $4,364.37; hospital costs amounted to $28,204.20; and the doctors were paid $12,676.20.

Dr. A. B. George, of Burlington, died December 29. Dr. C. D. Jenkins located in Burlington.

There appears to be a definite improvement in financial affairs for the doctor. Twenty-five of our members have joined the credit bureau and are using its service. This free interchange of credit information is found effective.

J. T. Hanna, Deputy Councilor

Jefferson County. Bimonthly meetings are held. Imported talent is usually well received. The interest is good; much better than five years ago. A much better contract for care of the indigent has been effected. There were no deaths and no new practitioners in the county during the year. Better organization causes each to take better care of his own business.

Ira N. Crow, Deputy Councilor

Lee County (Fort Madison). The local membership is fourteen. Meetings are held regularly and the interest is good. Talent for the programs is imported. A contract has been in force for several years and is to be continued for 1934.

There were no deaths and no new practitioners during 1933.

It is recommended for the improvement of the profession that there be more cooperation among the doctors themselves, frequent talks along this line, less fee-cutting to discourage shopping, better ethics, adoption of fee schedules by societies, and a penalty for violation of the fee schedule, unless work is done for charity.

R. L. Feightner, Deputy Councilor

Louisa County. The Louisa County Medical Society has twelve meetings a year, all dinner meetings, to which the wives of the members are invited. Membership is complete, as usual, and interest good. Programs are both home-grown and imported. An improved contract on a fee schedule basis has been effected for the year 1934.

J. H. Chittum, Deputy Councilor

Muscatine County. The Muscatine County Medical Society has not held regular meetings, but there has been some improvement over former years. Programs have been furnished by local and outside talent.

The Society received $4,800.00 in 1933 for indigent care and did entirely too much work. The public in general believed that because the doctors were getting a stipulated amount, they should care for anyone who applied, and the board of supervisors, overseers of the poor, welfare and social workers acquiesced too readily in the practice. After several conferences, a percentage fee bill was agreed upon, which is fair to the doctors and the public.

There were no deaths, no new doctors, and no public lectures in 1933. No improvement in financial condition for the doctors has been apparent. We should preach and continue to practice ethical rational standards, ignoring and ostracizing, rather than fighting (personally, at least) the cultists and irregulars. By the slow method of education we are gaining in public favor, even though at times the outlook is discouraging and almost disgusting.

T. F. Beveridge, Deputy Councilor

Scott County. The Scott County Medical Society meets ten times a year, and programs are furnished by imported talent. A free meal and a good place to meet keeps the interest at a high level.

About $92,000.00 worth of indigent work was done in 1933, for which the Society was paid $18,500.00. A better contract is in force for 1934.

Dr. C. T. Haller died on February 28, and Dr. J. G. Rohrig on March 25. New physicians in the county are Drs. T. W. McMeans and James Roger, both of Davenport.

The Scott County Medical Society will ask to entertain the State Society at the annual session in 1935.

A. P. Donohoe, Deputy Councilor

Van Buren County. The Van Buren County Medical Society does not have regularly called meetings. Dinner is served to augment the attendance.

The Society has a new contract for 1934.

Continuation of plans so far instituted is recommended.

C. R. Russell, Deputy Councilor

Washington County. The Washington County Medical Society continues, as for the past five or six years, to have monthly meetings except during July and August. Talent for the programs is always imported and meetings are of a postgraduate nature, only one subject being discussed each time. Attendance averages about eighty-five per cent of the membership and interest is excellent.

For four years the Society has had satisfactory financial arrangements with the board of supervisors for care of the county indigent. The arrangement continues. All Society expenses, including dues, are paid from this fund.

Two members died during the year 1933: Dr. C. C. Tilden, of Kalona; and Dr. C. W. Stewart, of Washington. Dr. Stephen Ware located at Kalona and Dr. D. T. Yoder at Wellman during the year.

E. E. Stutsman, Deputy Councilor

Ninth Councilor District

The general tone of organized medicine in the Ninth Councilor District is good. There are some places which need a great deal of improvement. In general, there has been an increase in interest on the part of individual members of the component county societies. There were several meetings sponsored by county societies which included the district membership and these were very well attended.

The appended reports, received from Deputy Councilors, show the sincere efforts toward accomplishment for the development of organized medicine.

H. A. Spilman, Councilor

Appanoose County. We have twenty-one doctors in this county and all are eligible to membership, but only thirteen paid their dues last year. We had six meetings in 1933 with an average attendance of eight. At the last two meetings we did not have a quorum, consequently there were no officers elected for the year 1934. So far only two have paid their dues for this year. We do not have a contract with the board of supervisors for the care of the indigent sick.

We do not have a postgraduate course and to my knowledge no Appanoose County members have attended courses in other counties.

We have a Woman's Auxiliary.

C. S. Hickman, Deputy Councilor

for county and state society activities, however, has never waned. This Society can be counted upon one hundred per cent for anything concerning the State Society.

We do not have a contract with the board of supervisors for care of the indigent sick this year. The Society waived in favor of one of our members. The contract is for $2,400.00, or $600.00 more than the county has ever paid before.

We have had no postgraduate course this year, but are having one beginning in March.

We do not have a Woman's Auxiliary.

L. F. Catterson, Deputy Councilor

Marion County. Eight meetings of the Marion County Medical Society were held during the year, with an average attendance of ninety-five per cent. The October meeting was a joint meeting with the Marion County Veterinarian Medical Society, and was listed in the JOURNAL as the meeting of merit for October. Interest in the Society is keen. Eighty per cent of the membership attended the State Society meeting in Des Moines last May.

We have had no postgraduate course in this county. However, sixty per cent of the membership attended the course sponsored by Polk County in September, October and November, 1933.

Our Woman's Auxiliary was organized February 24, 1934.

A blanket contract for care of the indigent sick was signed March 3, 1934, for the sum of $3,000.00.

Corwin S. Cornell, Deputy Councilor

Monroe County. There were four regular meetings of the Monroe County Medical Society and two called meetings during the year. The meetings were well attended. Scientific programs have been furnished at the regular meetings. The annual meeting is held the second Thursday in December of each year, and is always preceded by a dinner for the members and their ladies.

We are working on a plan for a diphtheria prevention week in the near future and a smallpox prevention week later in the season. There is a splendid spirit in the Society and the members are very cooperative.

We do not hold a county contract for care of the indigent sick. We placed a bid with the board of supervisors for fifty per cent of the fee schedule recommended by the House of Delegates. This was not accepted, however, and the contract was given to one man for $1,200.00.

We have had no postgraduate course in this county. We have a Woman's Auxiliary.

T. A. Moran, Deputy Councilor

Wapello County. The Wapello County Medical Society has had nineteen meetings during the year, seventeen of them being regular meetings, and two special meetings. Of the regular meetings, three were dinner meetings to which the members of the Ninth Councilor District and the four counties east of Wapello County were invited. There was no charge for dinner at these meetings. The first meeting on September 19, was complimentary to Dr. C. B. Taylor,

President of the Iowa State Medical Society; the second meeting, on October 17, was complimentary to our Dean of Medicine, Dr. S. A. Spilman; another was in conjunction with Sunnyslope Sanatorium. All were well attended and seemed to be much enjoyed.

The percentage of really active members of the Wapello County Medical Society is about sixty-five to seventy per cent. The interest shown has been very gratifying.

We do not have a contract with the board of supervisors for care of the indigent sick.

We have not had a postgraduate course. A few of the members have attended meetings at various times at other places.

There is a Woman's Auxiliary to the Wapello County Medical Society.

Evon Walker, Deputy Councilor

Wayne County. During the past year the Wayne County Medical Society was inactive except for two meetings, in September and December, when we had local talent programs, with a marked increase in interest over former years. There were only three meetings during the year. About eighty per cent of the members attended each meeting.

We have a contract with the board of supervisors for care of the indigent sick, on the basis of seventy-five per cent of the standard fee schedule.

An Auxiliary to the Wayne County Medical Society was organized in January.

T. D. Englehorn, Deputy Councilor

Tenth Councilor District

There has been more than ordinary activity in the county societies, composing the Tenth District, this year. A district meeting was held at Creston, September 22, which was attended by fifty representatives from the county societies. We were fortunate in having our president, Dr. Taylor, with us; also the chairman of the Council, Dr. Spilman. Papers were presented and discussion led by the younger men of the district. A second meeting is contemplated under the auspices of the Adair County Medical Society.

Madison and Taylor Counties are very active, holding meetings monthly at the homes of the members. The programs are for the most part given by local men.

Clarke and Warren Counties are functioning well, each holding several meetings during the year.

James G. Macrae, Councilor

Adair County. Like all counties in the state, Adair has felt the effect of the depression and found that certain factors were operatng to the disadvantage of the medical profession beyond that which normally would accompany such conditions. As a society we felt that we were willing to do our rightful duty, but that for future welfare we could accomplish much by cementing our forces for a better working organization.

1. During the year we have established a precedent that upholds the present law as pertaining to indigent patients;

A decision was obtained in Judge Cooper's court by Attorney Carlson of the Iowa State Department of Health to the end that osteopaths cannot be employed as county physicians;

That if indigents demand a regular licensed physician they can secure one.

2. We have knit the Adair County Medical Society into a close unit, working harmoniously to prevent patients mulcting physicians by the practice of going the rounds without paying anybody.

3. The medical fraternal spirit existing in Adair County is at a peak never before existing and there is a unified spirit in all matters pertaining to County Medical Society welfare.

We intend to resume medical matters this year and everyone feels that it can be done in a better atmosphere than ever before.

A. S. Bowers, Deputy Councilor

Adams County. In addition to their regular quarterly meetings, the Adams County Medical Society held a Heart and Chest Clinic, August 2, with all members of the Society taking active part, and with the assistance of Drs. Peck and Kottke of Des Moines, and Miss Ruth Walker and Mrs. Dorothy Gerard.

Dinner was served at the I. O. O. F. dining room by the Rebekkahs to the members of the Adams County Medical Society and their wives and the following visitors: Drs. Kottke and Peck of Des Moines; Drs. Macrae, Beatty, Parsons, Stoll and Carl Sampson of Creston, and Dr. F. E. Sampson of Monterey Park, Calif.

After dinner, Dr. Peck gave an interesting talk on tuberculosis and Dr. Kottke gave an interesting talk on heart diseases. These papers were discussed by Drs. F. E. Sampson and James Macrae.

At the regular meeting of the Society on December 5, officers were elected for 1934.

J. H. Wallahan, Deputy Councilor

Decatur County. The most important event in the past year for the Decatur County Medical Society was the opening of the Decatur County Hospital for which the Society has worked unremittingly for fifteen years. The hospital was opened last August with an open air ceremony at which Drs. F. E. Sampson of Creston and W. A. Rohlf of Waverly were the principal speakers. The building is new and completely equipped in all respects. There are twenty-two beds. The superintendent is Miss Eva Green, R.N., formerly of the Iowa Methodist Hospital, Des Moines.

There are eight active members who have sponsored a program of six meetings, the last of which was attended by thirty-eight physicians. The Society has been very active in attempts to revise the laws in regard to the indigent. Recently the members conducted a fifteen hour course in first aid for CWA foremen.

J. E. McFarland, Deputy Councilor

Ringgold County. The Ringgold County Medical Society has done fairly well as regards meetings in the past year. We have used little foreign talent, and the meetings have been principally on call instead of at regular intervals.

We renewed our county contract, which has been quite satisfactory in the year past.

We have ten members out of a possible eleven. One physician operates a drug store and did not care to participate in the contract.

Harmony prevails in the ranks and the interest is greater than in previous years.

E. J. Watson, Deputy Councilor

Union County. The Union County Medical Society has met the first Wednesday in each month throughout the year· in conjunction with the staff of the Greater Community Hospital at Creston. In connection with the State Tuberculosis Association, a "heart and chest clinic" was held at the hospital in Creston in September. The Society also worked in conjunction with the Seal Sale Committee in making an opportunity available for the school children of Creston to have "Shick" tests. During the year a movie projector was bought by the Society for the showing of medical films at the Society meetings. An attempt was made to obtain a contract with the county board of supervisors for the treatment of the indigent sick by the members of the County Medical Society. This plan failed, however, and the contract again went to an individual.

There are sixteen members of the county Society, two doctors who are eligible for membership and three who are not eligible.

John C. Parsons, Deputy Councilor

Eleventh Councilor District

Meetings were held in the various county societies, ranging from one to nine meetings during the year. Two counties, Audubon and Cass, reported one hundred per cent membership in their county societies.

Several of the counties are working on contract plans for the care of the indigent sick.

At the program meetings, Medical Economics was an important point for discussion as well as scientific programs in most counties. At the present time all counties are working in cooperation with the CWA projects. Immunization campaigns and pre-school examinations were participated in by several of the societies. The county societies have also expressed their willingness to cooperate with the State Society and the Department of Health in carrying out the Child Health Program which is being planned at the present time.

The Councilor District held two district meetings; one on November 8 at Atlantic, which was very largely attended and the other at Shenandoah on March 21, which was also well attended. The aim of these meetings is to use the members of the various societies for the bulk of the programs; in other words to interest our own members in appearing on scientific programs. These programs as arranged and presented were very well received by the membership. The idea of district meetings of this type seems to meet everybody's approval and will undoubtedly be continued.

M. C. Hennessy, Councilor

Dr. Erskine: I *move* that the report of the Council and the Councilors as published in the Handbook be approved.

The motion was regularly seconded, put to a vote and carried.

President Taylor: Report of Council Committees. The next one will be the Speakers Bureau. Is Dan Glomset or the secretary, Dorothy Nelson, here? If not, we will pass on to the Board of Trustees.

REPORT OF THE BOARD OF TRUSTEES

House of Delegates, Iowa State Medical Society:

In submitting to you an account of its stewardship for the past year, your Board of Trustees wishes to express something more than a casual appreciation of the loyal support and active cooperation it has received from the Officers, the Council, and the Committees of the State Society. The troubled times through which we have lived have of necessity brought many special problems, and any degree of success which may have been attained in solving them is due primarily to the effective and wholehearted spirit of cooperation which has been so uniformly accorded us in our work. The Councilors have twice met jointly with the Board of Trustees, and these meetings have been so constructive and satisfactory that we hope they may be made a permanent institution.

We would again point out that the Board of Trustees is in no sense a legislative or creative body, but is strictly an executive one entrusted with the duty of carrying out the mandates of the House of Delegates. We have endeavored to fulfill this duty to the best of our ability, but the task becomes a difficult one when, as sometimes happens, the legislative acts are not sufficiently clear or specific. The difficulty is particularly great when an act authorizes certain expenditures, but fails to specify from what sources the necessary funds are to be obtained. As a specific instance we may cite the problem of providing relief for indigent physicians. It was evidently the intent of the House of Delegates to provide some measure of relief for the needy within the ranks of the profession, but when the original plan providing for the sale of seals to raise the necessary funds was found not to be feasible, no substitute source of revenue was provided. Recently the Committee on Indigent Physicians was called upon to provide relief for an indigent physician in urgent need and finding itself without funds, referred the matter to the Board of Trustees for action. In the belief that this case constituted an emergency, the Board provided for payment of twenty-five dollars monthly, to be continued until this current session of the House of Delegates. It believes that such action was within the spirit, but not within the letter of the law, and it is hoped that the House of Delegates may see fit to make more definite provisions for relief of the occasional case of indigency within the ranks of the profession.

A comparative financial statement prepared from

the auditor's reports of the past three years is presented herewith:

Total net worth January 1, 1931	$34,649.14	
(Including bonds—$25,000.00)		
Total income, 1931	$33,369.23	($7.50 dues)
Total expenditures	37,523.40	
Excess expenses over income	$ 4,154.17	
Less profit on sale of bonds	1,546.53	
NET LOSS FOR YEAR	$ 2,607.64	

Total net worth January 1, 1932	$31,879.50	
(Including bonds—$26,384.68)		
Total income, 1932	$36,735.68	($12.00 dues)
Total expenditures	33,988.56	
NET INCOME FOR YEAR	$ 2,747.12	

Total net worth January 1, 1933	$34,626.62	
(Including bonds—$34,601.53)		
Total income, 1933	$32,195.23	($10.00 dues)
Total expenditures	27,816.53	
NET INCOME FOR YEAR	$ 4,378.70	
Cash in banks December 31, 1932	25.09	
Treasury bonds	34,601.53	
NET WORTH JANUARY 1, 1934	$39,005.32	

INCOME—1932 and 1933

	1932	1933
Journal advertising	$ 5,486.16	$ 4,560.45
Reprints	774.48	956.15
Annual Session	880.00	1,323.50
Speakers Bureau	2,805.58	3,650.70
Miscellaneous	49.38	......
Dues	25,798.50	20,132.18
	$35,794.10	$30,622.98
Interest on bonds		1,130.63
Refund Legislative Committee		441.41
Interest savings account		.21
		$32,195.23

1933 income $3,598.87 less than 1932.

EXPENDITURES—1932 and 1933

	1932	1933
Journal and Reprints	$10,305.82	$11,026.40
Annual Session	1,065.59	1,913.61
Speakers Bureau	5,855.70	3,744.06
Miscellaneous	671.65	401.38
Rent and office supplies	2,161.33	2,053.59
Stationery and Printing	1,499.63	945.46
General Salaries	5,488.75	3,460.00
Trustees	257.11	182.77
Council	1,242.11	791.80
Medico-legal	1,695.66	1,956.60
Legislative	1,500.00	602.58
Medical Economics	202.73	54.15
Other Committees	410.43	113.78
County Society Services	729.91	520.80
	$33,984.42	$27,766.98
Plus Federal taxes and returned checks		60.35
Minus dividend on Iowa City account		10.80
		$27,816.53

Expenditures in 1933 $6,167.89 less than in 1932.

It will be seen that we have once more succeeded not only in living within our income but, by the practice of rigid economies and through the efficiency and wholehearted cooperation of the present office personnel, have actually succeeded in increasing our reserves. While it may be argued that there is no need for creating and maintaining a large reserve, the present surplus, representing as it does somewhat less than the gross income for a single year, can hardly be regarded as excessive. It serves as a cushion fund and must be maintained as protection against unforeseen and unpredictable emergencies. In this connection, our present budget system continues to demonstrate itself as a necessary and efficient means for regulating the expenses and expenditures of the Society, and aids in coordinating the legislative work of the House of Delegates and the executive work of the Board of Trustees. In instituting new activities, the expense involved should be considered and the funds from which these costs are to be defrayed should be specifically set out by the House of Delegates in order that the Board of Trustees may carry out the policies determined upon by the House of Delegates without appearing to usurp the rights and duties of the latter. (See Chapter IX, Section 3, of the By-laws.)

All the established activities of the Society have been carried on during the past year, and it has been our impression not only that we can ill afford to sacrifice or curtail any of these activities, but also that the membership as a whole desires that these activities be continued and perhaps in some fields even extended. The socialistic trend of the times constitutes a growing menace to the development of medicine as a free profession, and today as never before the profession needs a unified, active organization. To maintain our present activities in the face of rising costs means that we must maintain the present dues and continue to practice the rigid economies that have already been instituted, but the physician who is actively interested in the development of his profession, not only from the broad humanitarian but also the selfish standpoint of increased returns, is not concerned with the reduction of his Society dues. He desires only the assurance that these dues are wisely expended in the furtherance of his professional interest.

There is an obvious need for adjustment of the expense of carrying protective insurance. Under the present plan, the Society is called upon to pay the expense of legal services in malpractice suits brought against members not carrying commercial insurance, in all cases in which no criminal charge is involved. The cost of such services has been a considerable item, and inasmuch as some seventy-five per cent of the membership already carries professional insurance which provides for defraying the cost of legal defense as well as for payment of possible adverse judgments against the insured, this expense to the State Society seems an unjustifiable one. It seems unfair that the cost of defending malpractice suits against the uninsured twenty-five per cent of the membership should be borne by the seventy-five per cent who are paying for their own insurance also. A special hazard must also be considered in this connection. Among this uninsured twenty-five per cent of the membership, there may from time to time be included members who are uninsurable, i. e., members who have been refused medical protection by some standard insurance carrier because of unethical practices or because for other reasons the risk is considered unduly hazardous. We believe that there are few such men in the ranks of this Society, but these few constitute a grave ethical as well as financial problem.

In the work of the Society, it has frequently been necessary to seek legal advice, and in the past such legal services have been secured on a fee basis. The Legislative Committee in particular is often in need of legal services, and has felt the necessity of establishing closer relations between the profession and the legislature through some duly authorized representative of the Society. Accordingly Mr. Gerald O. Blake, an attorney who from time to time has been consulted in medico-legal problems, has been retained on a salary basis in the belief that this will make possible fuller service at a more readily predictable expense. Mr. Blake will render legal opinions, prepare all contracts and legislative bills, represent the Society in all legal matters, and act as its legislative representative.

In conclusion, your Board of Trustees would again point out that it is not within its scope to suggest or define the future policies of the State Medical Society: to do so would be to attempt to usurp the rights and duties of the House of Delegates—but it would reaffirm its sincere desire to carry out the instructions of the House of Delegates and to help in every possible way in the correlation of the work of the various committees and departments.

Oliver J. Fay, Chairman
E. M. Myers
John I. Marker

Dr. Fay: The Board of Trustees does not wish to make a further report. I *move* that the report as published in the Handbook be approved.

The motion was regularly seconded, put to a vote and carried.

President Taylor: Report of Delegates to the American Medical Association.

Dr. Fay: Exhibit A who is to be presented has just arrived at the hotel. I move you that you pass that report until Exhibit A arrives here.

President Taylor: Whom does that happen to be?

Dr. Fay: The President-Elect of the American Medical Association. Dr. Moore wants to present Exhibit A.

President Taylor: Will you waive this report until Exhibit A appears on the scene, Fred?

Dr. Moore: I shall be glad to do so.

President Taylor: Reports of Standing Committees of the House of Delegates. Report on Constitution and By-laws, Dr. Peck.

Reports of Standing Committees

REPORT OF COMMITTEE ON CONSTITUTION AND BY-LAWS

House of Delegates, Iowa State Medical Society:

Your Committee on Constitution and By-laws herewith submits its report in accordance with the provisions of the By-laws.

No amendments to the Constitution were presented for first reading at the 1933 session for final action this year.

The Committee met at the offices of the State Society, March 16, 1934, and unanimously agreed to propose the following changes in the Constitution for your consideration, pending final action in 1935:

Article IV, Sections 1, 2, 3, 4 and 5 be omitted in their entirety and in lieu thereof, enact the following: "This Society shall consist of members who shall be members of the component county medical societies who have been certified to the headquarters of this Society, and whose dues and assessments for the current year have been received by the secretary."

(Your Committee believes that, should this proposed amendment carry, the various classifications of membership, included in the present Article IV, should be defined in the By-laws instead of in the Constitution. Also that the method of selection and the requisite qualifications for life membership should be modified and changed. Therefore proposed amendments covering these points will be offered next year if this amendment carries.)

Article VII, Section 1. The word "daily" be deleted from line 2.

(It has been the custom for many years to hold but one session on Friday, the third day of our annual session. Thus we have long violated the provision of the Constitution which requires not less than two general meetings daily. This word should be omitted to conform with established custom.)

Article VIII, Section 4. That this section be omitted.

(This section was added at the time of the change to the President-Elect system. It has served its purpose and should now be deleted from the Constitution.)

Your Committee also proposes the following amendments to the By-laws of the Society:

Chapter VIII, Section 1. Omit the line "A Committee on Finance (3)" and substitute therefor "A Committee on Medical Economics (3)."

(Since the Board of Trustees requires an annual audit of the accounts of the Society by a certified public accountant, the functions of the Finance Committee have been taken over and there are no duties for the members of this committee to perform.)

(The Committee on Medical Economics has been a special committee of the Society for several years past. On account of its very important duties, it seems advisable that it should now be made a standing committee.)

Chapter VIII, Section 10. Omit this section which defines the duties of the Finance Committee, and substitute therefor this proposed section defining the dutes of the above Medical Economics Committee: "The Committee on Medical Economics shall consist of three members whose duty shall be to investigate matters affecting the economic status of the medical profession of the state and it shall report annually to the House of Delegates such recommendations as may in its judgment seem proper."

Chapter VIII, Section 11. Enact this new section as follows: "The Committee on Medical Education and Hospitals shall consist of three members, who shall serve in this State for the Council on Medical Education and Hospitals of the American Medical

Association and shall have referred to it all questions pertaining to hospitals and medical education."

(When this committee was made a standing committee of the Society in 1932, the matter of defining its duties was evidently overlooked and the adopton of this section simply corrects the omission.)

The chairman of the Medico-Legal Committee recommends modification of the provisions of the By-laws pertaining to medico-legal defense and proposes the following amendments:

Chapter I, Section 5. Omit in its entirety.

(Should Section 8 of Chapter VIII be amended as proposed, discontinuing certain features of medical defense, this section is superfluous and should be deleted.)

Chapter VIII, Section 8. To be amended to read as follows:

"The Medico-Legal Committee shall consist of three members, all of whom shall serve without pay. The term of service of each member shall be three years, provided that in the original organization of this committee the services shall be grouped by lot into three divisions with terms expiring in one, two and three years respectively. It shall be the duty of the members of this committee, severally and collectively, upon request, to investigate any claim of malpractice against a Society member, to adjust such claims in accordance with equity where possible, and if in their judgment, an adjustment is impossible, advise the defendant concerning the proper methods of procedure and assist in procuring such medical evidence as may be ethically justified in the furtherance of the defense."

John Peck, Chairman
Channing G. Smith
James C. Donahue

Dr. Peck: In addition to the proposed amendments as printed in the Handbook, the Committee was given this proposed amendment today by Dr. McManus of Waterloo. As it must be read, here it is:

"That Section 1, Chapter IX of the By-Laws be amended by striking out the first sentence which reads: 'A per capita assessment is authorized by the House of Delegates on membership of component societies and hereby made the annual dues of the Society,' and substituting therefor:

'An assessment of Ten Dollars per capita on membership of the component societies is hereby made the annual dues of this Society, except whenever the total net assets at the close of the fiscal year are more than $10,000, the assessment for the ensuing year shall be Five Dollars per capita."

I *move* that the report be accepted.

President Taylor: No action is to be taken on this change until Friday. Do you have a further report to make?

Dr. Peck: The President-Elect requests that the President-Elect be made a member of the Committee on Scientific Work. Therefore Chapter VIII, Section 2, should be amended as follows:

In line 3, after the word "Treasurer," insert the words "and President-Elect".

President Taylor: I am waiting for a motion to approve the report of the Committee on Constitution and By-Laws.

Dr. Peck: I will so *move*.

The motion was regularly seconded.

Dr. Albright: I rise for information. What effect will the approval of this report have upon the subsequent report of the Medico-Legal Committee? I refer to Chapter VIII, Section 8.

Dr. Peck: It has no immediate effect. You see these amendments have to lay over a day, so there will be no action on these today.

President Taylor: It has been moved and seconded that the report of the Constitution and By-laws Committee be approved. Those in favor say "aye;" contrary "no." *The report is approved.*

Is the Treasurer here yet?

REPORT OF THE TREASURER

House of Delegates, Iowa State Medical Society:

For a detailed report of the financial transactions of the Society for the year 1933, I refer you to the Auditor's Report, published herewith, but would make one correction. The audit shows, under "Investment Account," 3% per cent Treasury Bonds of a face value of $34,500.00 in the Iowa-Des Moines National Bank safety deposit vault. Of these bonds, $25,500.00 (face value) bear interest at 3% per cent; and the remaining $9,000.00 (face value) bear interest at 3 per cent.

The income for the year was $32,195.23, and of this amount $2,747.12 was an excess of income over expenditures for the year 1932. Expenditures for the year 1933 were $27,816.53, leaving $1,631.58 net income for the year, which, added to the 1932 saving of $2,747.12, shows a total of $4,378.70 surplus of income over expenditures for the two-year period.

There was a two-dollar reduction in annual dues for the year 1933, which, together with a slight loss in membership, reduced the dues income $5,666.32.

I feel that the Board of Trustees, the Secretary and the office personnel should be congratulated upon this good record.

Harold J. McCoy, Treasurer.

AUDITOR'S REPORT
December 31, 1933

Oliver J. Fay, M.D., Chairman,
Board of Trustees, Iowa State Medical Society,
Des Moines, Iowa.

Dear Sir:

In accordance with your instructions we have examined the books of account of the

IOWA STATE MEDICAL SOCIETY
DES MOINES, IOWA

for the year ended December 31, 1933, and submit our report thereon, together with the following statements:

Exhibit "A"—Cash Account for the year ended December 31, 1933.

Exhibit "B"—Income Account for the year ended December 31, 1933.

Schedule No. 1—Expenditures for the year ended December 31, 1933.

Schedule No. 2—Expenditures (Speakers Bureau) for the year ended December 31, 1933.

The following comments are made on the principal items included in the foregoing Exhibits:

CASH ACCOUNT

A detailed cash account for the year ended December 31, 1933, is given in Exhibit "A" showing the balance on hand at the beginning of the year, receipts and disbursements during the year and the balance in the respective bank accounts at December 31, 1933, a summary of which is as follows:

Cash in Banks, December 31, 1932.......$		25.09
Receipts		32,195.23
Total $32,220.32		

Expenditures:

Expenses, Schedule No. 1......$25,567.12		
Expenses, Speakers Bureau, Schedule No. 2		2,209.08
Bank Charges and Returned Checks		40.33
Total Expenditures		27,816.53

Cash in Banks, December 31, 1933........$ 4,403.79

Representing:

Iowa - Des Moines National Bank and Trust Company...$	1,811.31
Bankers Trust Company	2,584.25
Des Moines Savings Bank and Trust Company	8.23
	$ 4,403.79

All receipts as herein shown were traced to the respective depository accounts, and all disbursements therefrom were supported by cancelled checks.

The balances in the respective bank accounts were reconciled with their statements for December, 1933, and the balances shown thereon verified by communication with the banks.

Schedules No. 1 and No. 2, respectively, set out in detail the expenditures for the year ended December 31, 1933. All of these disbursements were supported by checks drawn by the Treasurer upon vouchers drawn by the Secretary.

Attached to and supporting the vouchers were invoices from various creditors duly approved by the Board of Trustees.

INCOME AND EXPENSE ACCOUNT
AND
INVESTMENT ACCOUNT

A detailed Income and Expense Account and Investment Account for the year ended December 31, 1933, is given in Exhibit "B" which shows an excess of income over expenses of $4,378.70, as compared with a net income for 1932 of $2,747.12.

The following is a summary of the aforesaid Exhibit "B," showing the comparative amounts for the year 1932:

INCOME:	1933	1932	Increase or Decrease
Receipts from Secretary $25,648.78	$32,041.13	$6,392.35	
Speakers Bureau.	3,650.70	2,775.58	875.12
Annual Session ..	1,323.50	880.00	443.50
Interest on Liberty Bonds	1,130.63	995.62	135.01
Interest on Savings Account ..	.21	43.35	43.14
Refund, Legislative Committee	441.41	0...	441.41
TOTAL INCOME $32,195.23	$36,735.68	$4,540.45	

EXPENSES:			
Schedule No. 1...$25,567.12	$29,626.13	$4,059.01	
Schedule No. 2...	2,209.08	4,362.43	2,153.35
Bank Charges and Return'd Ch'ks	40.33	0.....	40.33
TOTAL EXPENSES $27,816.53	$33,988.56	$6,172.03	

| TOTAL INCOME ......$ 4,378.70 | $ 2,747.12 | $1,631.58 | |

It will be observed that the Net Income has increased in the sum of $1,631.58 over the amount shown for 1932.

The Speakers Bureau Account is summarized as follows:

	1933	1932
Fees $3,650.70	$2,775.58	
Expenses 2,209.08	4,362.43	
Net Income or Loss$1,441.62	$1,586.85	

INVESTMENT ACCOUNT

The following are the transactions affecting this account for the year 1933: ·.

Income for the year 1933................$	4,378.70

Add:

Cash in Bank, Dec. 31, 1932...$	25.09
Treasury Bonds on Hand, Dec. 31, 1932	34,601.53
	34,626.62
Total Funds on Hand Dec. 31, 1933....$39,005.32	

Represented by:
Cash in Banks:
Iowa-Des Moines National
Bank and Trust Company.$ 1,811.31
Bankers Trust Company 2,584.25
Des Moines Savings Bank &
Trust Company 8.23

Total Cash in Banks......$ 4,403.79
3% Treasury Bonds (Face
Value $34,500.00) Cost.... 34,601.53

$39,005.32

The 3% Treasury Bonds of a face value of

$34,500.00 were submitted for our inspection.

Dues for 1934, collected during December, 1933, were deposited with the Bankers Trust Company (arrangement committee account) in the sum of $1,110.00 and are not included in the foregoing accounts.

We did not examine the Legislative Committee account in any manner whatsoever.

We desire to record our appreciation of the courtesies extended us during our examination, and we shall be glad to supply any additional information herein, if desired.

Respectfully submitted,
W. WIDDUP & COMPANY,
Certified Public Accountants,
Chartered Accountants.

Exhibit "A"
Cash Account
For the Year Ended December 31, 1933

	Total	Ia.-Des Moines Nat'l Bank & Trust Co.	Bankers Trust Company	Des Moines Savings Bank
CASH IN BANKS:				
December 31, 1932...............................	$ 25.09	$ 15.47	$ 1.60	$ 8.02
RECEIPTS:				
Dues	$20,132.18	$ 0...	$20,132.18	$ 0...
Advertising	4,497.68	0...	4,497.68	0...
Reprints	956.15	0...	956.15	0...
Miscellaneous	62.77	0...	62.77	0...
Total	$25,648.78	$ 0...	$25,648.78	$ 0...
Receipts, Speakers Bureau:				
Fees	$ 3,558.26	$ 0...	$ 3,558.26	$ 0...
Traveling Expense	92.44	0...	92.44	0...
Total	$ 3,650.70	$ 0...	$ 3,650.70	$ 0...
Annual Session	$ 1,323.50	$ 0...	$ 1,323.50	$ 0...
Interest on Treasury Bonds.......................	1,130.63	1,130.63	0...	0...
Interest on Savings Account......................	.21	0...	0...	.21
Refund, Legislative Committee...................	441.41	441.41	0...	0...
TOTAL RECEIPTS	$32,195.23	$ 1,572.04	$30,622.98	$ .21
TOTAL RECEIPTS, INCLUDING CASH IN BANKS	$32,220.32	$ 1,587.51	$30,624.58	$ 8.23
FUND TRANSFERS	$ 0...	28,000.00	28,000.00	0...
BALANCE AFTER TRANSFER OF FUNDS.........	$32,220.32	$29,587.51	$ 2,624.58	$ 8.23
EXPENDITURES:				
Expenses, Schedule No. 1.........................	$25,567.12	$25,567.12	$ 0...	$ 0...
Expenses, Schedule No. 2........................	2,209.08	2,209.08	0...	0...
Bank Charges and Returned Checks...............	40.33	0...	40.33	0...
TOTAL EXPENDITURES	$27,816.53	$27,776.20	$ 40.33	$ 0...
CASH IN BANKS:				
As at December 31, 1933.........................	$ 4,403.79	$ 1,811.31	$ 2,584.25	$ 8.23

Exhibit "B"
Income and Expense Account Including Investments
For the Year Ended December 31, 1933

INCOME:
Received from Secretary:
Dues $20,132.18
Advertising 4,497.68
Reprints 956.15
Miscellaneous 62.77

Total $25,648.78

INVESTMENT ACCOUNT:
Cash in Banks and Treasury
Bonds on Hand at December
31, 1932:
Cash in Banks........$ 25.09
Treasury Bonds, Cost.... 34,601.53
(Face Value $34,500.00)

Total $34,626.62

Exhibit "B"—Continued

Speakers Bureau:
Fees .... $ 3,558.26
Travel Expense........... 92.44
$ 3,650.70
Annual Session........................ 1,323.50
Interest from Liberty Bonds........... 1,130.63
Interest from Savings Account........ .21
Refund, Legislative Committee....... 441.41

TOTAL INCOME.............. $00,100.00

EXPENDITURES—EXPENSES:
Expenses, Schedule No. 1....$25,567.12
Expenses, Schedule No. 2.... 2,209.08
Bank Charges and Returned
Checks 40.33

TOTAL EXPENSES...........$27,816.53

EXCESS INCOME OVER EXPENSES:
For the Year ended December 31, 1933..$ 4,378.70

TOTAL CASH IN BANKS AND TREASURY
BONDS ON HAND:
As at December 31, 1933..............$39,005.32

REPRESENTED BY:
3¾ Treasury Bonds (Face Value $34,-
500.00) Cost......................$34,601.53
Cash in Banks:
Iowa-Des Moines National
Bank ....$ 1,811.31
Bankers Trust Company... 2,584.25
Des Moines Savings Bank &
Trust Company......... 8.23

Total Cash in Banks........... 4,403.79

TOTAL CASH IN BANKS AND
TREASURY BONDS (AS
Above) $39,005.32

Schedule No. 1
DISBURSEMENTS
For the Year Ended December 31, 1933

Date 1933	Check No.	Order No.	Drawn in Favor of	In Payment of	Distribution	Amount
1-7	2011	3961	Cash............................	Office Postage.............	Rent and Office Supplies.............	$ 10.00
1-19	2012	3962	Postmaster.....................	Post Cards................	Miscellaneous.............	20.00
1-19	2013	3963	W. B. Saunders Company......	Medical Dictionary........	Rent and Office Supplies.............	7.50
1-20	2014	3964	Postmaster.....................	Post Cards................	County Society Services.............	2.30
1-25	2015	3965	Iowa Press Clipping Bureau.....	December Clippings........	Journal Ptrg. and Engraving..........	17.30
1-25	2016	3966	Cash............................	Office Postage.............	Rent and Office Supplies.............	10.00
1-25	2017	3967	Robert L. Parker..............	January Salary............	General Salaries.............	50.00
1-25	2018	3968	Grace McDonald................	January Salary............	General Salaries.............	65.00
1-25	2019	3969	R. R. Simmons................	January Salary............	Journal Ptrg. and Engraving..........	100.00
1-25	2020	3970	Dorothy Nelson................	January Salary............	Speakers Bureau.............	115.00
1-25	2021	3971	Virginia Stewart..............	January Salary............	General Salaries and Journal..........	125.00
1-25	2022	3972	Dorothy McCarthy.............	January Salary............	General Salaries.............	150.00
1-25	2023	3973	N. W. Bell Telephone Company..	Telephone Service.........	Rent and Office Supplies.............	14.30
1-25	2024	3974	Bankers Building Corporation....	January Rent.............	Rent and Office Supplies.............	107.00
1-25	2025	3975	L. R. Brown...................	Dictaphone Machine.......	Journal Printing and Engraving.......	140.00
1-25	2026	3976	Iowa-Des Moines National Bank..	Safekeeping Rental........	Rent and Office Supplies.............	17.25
1-25	2027	3977	W. W. Bowen..................	Council Meeting...........	Council.............	10.00
1-25	2028	3978	C. W. Ellyson.................	Council Meeting...........	Council.............	15.50
1-25	2029	3979	A. W. Erskine.................	Council Meeting...........	Council.............	19.90
1-25	2030	3980	F. A. Hennessy................	Council Meeting...........	Council.............	20.90
1-25	2031	3981	James Macrae..................	Council Meeting...........	Council.............	7.00
1-25	2032	3982	James E. Reeder..............	Council Meeting...........	Council.............	20.00
1-25	2033	3983	Hal A. Spilman................	Council Meeting...........	Council.............	10.00
1-25	2034	3984	C. B. Taylor...................	Council Meeting...........	Council.............	9.60
1-25	2035	3985	F. B. Winkler.................	Council Meeting...........	Council.............	23.00
1-25	2036	3986	Multigraph Company...........	Multigraph Machine.......	Rent and Office Supplies.............	181.84
1-25	2037	3987	Western Union.................	Telegrams.................	Miscellaneous and Council..........	3.08
1-25	2038	3988	Remington Rand Co............	Adding Machine Ribbon....	Rent and Office Supplies.............	1.00
1-25	2039	3989	Zaisers.......................	Office Supplies...........	Rent and Office Supplies.............	5.35
1-25	2040	3990	Addressograph Company........	Changes on Plates........	Rent and Office Supplies.............	1.56
1-25	2041	3991	Central Engraving Co..........	Halftones.................	Journal Printing and Engraving.......	35.60
1-25	2042	3992	Wallace-Homestead Co..........	Printing..................	Journal Printing and Engraving.......	99.66
1-25	2043	3993	Dutcher, Walker & Ries........	Legal Defense.............	Medico—Legal.............	291.00
2-9	2045	4001	Wallace-Homestead Co..........	Printing..................	Journal Printing and Engraving.......	560.38
2-10	2046	4002	W. Widdup & Co...............	Audit for 1932............	Miscellaneous.............	100.00
2-15	2054	4003	Postmaster.....................	Journal Postage..........	Journal Printing and Engraving.......	100.00
2-23	2055	4004	LaVere Braucht Floral Co......	Hennessy Flowers.........	Miscellaneous.............	20.75
2-23	2056	4005	D. M. Electric Light Co.......	Bulbs for Office..........	Rent and Office Supplies.............	3.20
2-23	2057	4006	Capital City Printing Co.......	Signature Cut............	Legislative Comm.............	1.96
2-23	2058	4007	Iowa Press Clipping Bureau.....	January Clippings.........	Journal Printing and Engraving.......	14.52
2-23	2059	4008	Cash............................	Office Postage............	Rent and Office Supplies.............	10.00
2-23	2060	4009	Iowa-Des Moines National Bank..	Check Books..............	Rent and Office Supplies.............	2.50
2-23	2061	4010	Wallace-Homestead Co..........	Printing..................	Journal Printing and Engraving.......	476.59
2-23	2062	4011	Robert L. Parker..............	February Salary..........	General Salaries.............	50.00
2-23	2063	4012	Grace McDonald................	February Salary..........	General Salaries.............	65.00
2-23	2064	4013	R. R. Simmons................	February Salary..........	Journal Printing and Engraving.......	100.00
2-23	2065	4014	Dorothy Nelson................	February Salary..........	Speakers Bureau.............	115.00
2-23	2066	4015	Virginia Stewart..............	February Salary..........	General and Journal Salaries..........	125.00
2-23	2067	4016	Dorothy McCarthy.............	February Salary..........	General Salaries.............	150.00
2-23	2068	4017	L. R. Woodward...............	Council Meeting...........	Council.............	13.85
2-23	2069	4018	John I. Marker................	Meeting and Telephone....	County Society and Med. Econ........	11.20
2-23	2070	4019	C. A. Boice...................	Council Meeting...........	Council.............	12.40
2-23	2071	4020	Bankers Building Corp..........	February Rent............	Rent and Office Supplies.............	107.00
2-23	2072	4021	Esser-Frederick Co............	Dictionary................	Journal Printing and Engraving.......	6.35
2-23	2073	4022	Western Union.................	Telegrams.................	Misc. and Journal Printing..........	7.27
2-23	2074	4023	Zaisers.......................	Office Supplies...........	Rent and Office Supplies.............	16.15
2-23	2075	4024	Central Engraving Co..........	Halftones.................	Journal Printing and Engraving.......	67.95
2-28	2076	4025	Berkowitz Envelope Co.........	Envelopes.................	Journal Printing and Engraving.......	155.81
2-23	2077	4026	H. S. Hoyt....................	Advertising Commissions...	Journal Printing and Engraving.......	51.40
2-23	2078	4027	N. W. Bell Telephone Co.......	Telephone Service.........	Miscellaneous.............	30.00
2-23	2079	4028	F. A. Hennessy................	Council Meeting...........	Council.............	20.90
2-23	2080	4029	L. R. Woodward...............	Council Meeting...........	Council.............	13.75
2-23	2081	4030	F. P. Winkler.................	Council Meeting...........	Council.............	23.00
2-23	2082	4031	James E. Reeder..............	Council Meeting...........	Council.............	20.00
2-23	2083	4032	C. W. Ellyson.................	Council Meeting...........	Council.............	15.50
2-23	2084	4033	A. W. Erskine.................	Council Meeting...........	Council.............	11.90

Amount Forward...$ 4,686.57

Schedule No. 1—Continued

Date 1933	Check No.	Order No.	Drawn in Faver of	In Payment of	Distribution	Amount
				Amount Brought Forward		$ 4,686.57
2-23	2085	4034	C. A. Boice	Council Meeting	Council	11.40
2-23	2086	4035	H. A. Spilman	Council Meeting	Council	10.00
2-23	2087	4036	James G. Macrae	Council Meeting	Council	7.50
2-23	2088	4037	M. C. Hennessy	Council Meeting	Council	2.60
3-1	2089	4038	Postmaster	Postage	County Society Services	2.00
3-29	2090	4039	Iowa Press Clipping Bureau	February Clippings	Journal Printing and Engraving	14.00
3-29	2091	4040	Baldwin Studio	Glass Print (Dr. Shultz)	Annual Session	1.00
3-29	2092	4041	Des Moines Clean Towel	Towel Services	Rent and Office Supplies	3.75
3-29	2093	4042	N. W. Bell Telephone	Telephone SerVice	Misc. and Rent and Office	20.13
3-29	2094	4043	Robert L. Parker	March Salary	General Salaries	50.00
3-29	2095	4044	Grace J. McDonald	March Salary	General Salaries	65.00
3-29	2096	4045	R. R. Simmons	March Salary	Journal Printing and Engraving	100.00
3-29	2097	4046	Bankers Building Corp.	March Rent	Rent and Office Supplies	107.00
3-29	2098	4047	Dorothy Nelson	March Salary	Speakers Bureau	115.00
3-29	2099	4048	Virginia Stewart	March Salary	General and Journal Salaries	125.00
3-29	2100	4049	Dorothy McCarthy	March Salary	General Salaries	150.00
3-29	2101	4050	James E. Reeder	Travel Expense	County Society Services	12.20
3-29	2102	4051	J. C. Donahue	Med. Econ. Committee	Med. Econ. Com.	9.00
3-29	2103	4052	John I. Marker	Committee Expense	Med. Econ. Committee	21.40
3-29	2104	4053	E. C. McClure	Finance Committee Expense	Committees other	6.15
3-29	2105	4054	A. W. Bennett	Finance Committee Expense	Committees other	12.50
3-29	2106	4055	R. L. Barnett	Finance Committee Expense	Committees other	8.50
3-29	2107	4056	American Medical Association	Copies of Medical Ethics	Rent and Office Supplies	.75
3-29	2108	4057	C. Kranz Floral Co.	Herrick Flowers	Administrative Miscellaneous	10.00
3-29	2109	4058	Western Union	Telegrams	Misc. and County Society	3.46
3-29	2110	4059	Zaisers	Office Supplies	Rent and Office Supplies	15.40
3-29	2111	4060	Central Engraving Co.	Halftones	Journal Printing and Engraving	87.66
3-29	2112	4061	Wallace-Homestead Co.	Printing	Stationery, Journal and Reprint	1,020.86
3-29	2113	4062	L. R. Woodward	Phone Calls	Council	12.10
4-6	2126	4075	I. J. Sinn	Refund of Dues	Miscellaneous	10.00
4-8	2127	4076	Cash	Office Postage	Rent and Office Supplies	10.00
4-18	2128	4077	Wallace-Homestead Co.	Printing	Stationery, Journal and Reprints	267.83
4-24	2129	4078	Iowa Press Clipping Bureau	March Clippings	Journal Printing and Engraving	12.57
4-24	2130	4079	Robert L. Parker	Expense of Dinners	Other Committees	4.00
4-24	2131	4080	Cash	Office Postage	Rent and Office Supplies	10.00
4-18	2132	4081	Robert L. Parker	Travel Expense	County Society Services	11.50
4-24	2133	4082	N. W. Bell Telephone Co.	Telephone Service	Supplies—Trustees, Committee	39.00
4-24	2134	4083	E. B. Winnett	Salary	General Salaries	50.00
4-24	2135	4084	Robert L. Parker	April Salary	General Salaries	50.00
4-24	2136	4085	Grace J. McDonald	April Salary	General Salaries	65.00
4-24	2137	4086	R. R. Simmons	April Salary	Journal Printing and Engraving	100.00
4-24	2138	4087	Bankers Building Corp.	April Rent	Rent and Office Supplies	107.00
4-24	2139	4088	Dorothy M. Nelson	April Salary	Speakers Bureau	115.00
4-24	2140	4089	Virginia R. Stewart	April Salary	General and Journal Salaries	125.00
4-24	2141	4090	Dorothy C. McCarthy	April Salary	General Salaries	150.00
4-24	2142	4091	Capital City Printing Plate	Signature Cut	Other Committees	3.18
4-24	2143	4092	C. W. Ellyson	Joint Meeting	County Society Services	6.20
4-24	2144	4093	Western Union	Telegrams	Legislative and Speakers Bureau	2.86
4-24	2145	4094	Zaisers	Office Supplies	Rent and Office Supplies	77.15
4-24	2146	4095	Central Engraving Co.	Halftones	Journal Printing and Engraving	17.25
4-24	2147	4096	W. W. Bowen	Travel Expense	Misc., Council, Legislative, etc.	44.30
4-24	2148	4097	Dutcher, Walker & Ries	Legal Defense	Medico-Legal	574.18
4-29	2157	4106	Postmaster	Postage	Annual Session	16.80
5-1	2158	4107	R. N. Meng	Commission on adv.	Journal Printing and Engraving	42.15
5-16	2160	4108	Wallace-Homestead Co.	Printing	Annual Session, Journal and Report	661.90
5-23	2161	4110	Freeman Decorating Co.	Booths for Exhibitors	Annual Session	162.50
5-23	2162	4111	Lauren Crosten	Music for Banquet	Annual Session	20.00
5-23	2163	4112	Wallace-Homestead Co.	Printing	Annual Session and Journal	442.90
5-23	2164	4113	Mrs. Thos A. Burcham	Woman's Auxiliary	Annual Session	42.40
5-23	2165	4114	E. A. Baumgardner	Night Watchman	Annual Session	7.50
5-23	2166	4115	W. C. Finnoff	Travel Expense	Annual Session	57.75
5-23	2167	4116	Shrine Temple	Tables for Exhibits	Annual Session	12.00
5-23	2168	4117	C. A. Juber	Hauling Tables	Annual Session	5.00
5-23	2169	4118	Julia Ford Hill	Travel Expense	Annual Session	21.00
5-23	2170	4119	Wilson Floral Co.	Flowers for Banquet	Annual Session	25.00
5-23	2171	4120	Petty Cash	Office Postage	Rent and Office Supplies	10.00
5-23	2172	4121	S. Joseph & Sons	President's Gavels	Annual Session	28.00
5-23	2173	4122	R. N. Meng	Work on Exhibits	Annual Session	25.00
5-23	2174	4123	H. M. Richter	Guest Expense	Annual Session	28.99
5-23	2175	4124	Haas Sign Company	Signs	Annual Session	3.25
5-23	2176	4125	Hartzler Public Address	Amplifying System	Annual Session	35.00
5-23	2177	4126	Hotel Fort Des Moines	Hotel Expense	Annual Session	349.05
5-23	2178	4127	M. W. Bredimus		Annual Session	5.00
5-23	2179	4128	Wingate Costume Co.		Annual Session	3.75
5-23	2180	4129	Walter D. Abbott		Annual Session	20.00
5-23	2181	4130	L. A. West	Expenses for Smoker	Annual Session	7.25
5-23	2182	4131	Thomas Electric Co.		Annual Session	8.00
5-23	2183	4132	Hotel Fort Des Moines		Annual Session	200.35
5-26	2185	4133	Iowa Press Clipping Bureau	April Clippings	Journal Printing and Engraving	12.60
5-26	2186	4134	F. A. Hennessy	Phone Calls	Council	4.05
5-26	2187	4135	N. W. Bell Telephone	Telephone Service	Misc., Council, etc	22.45
5-26	2188	4136	Journal of the I. S. M. S.	Due Bill of Hotel Ft. Des M.	Annual Session	35.50
5-25	2184	4137	W. E. Sturges	Bond Premium	Adm.—Misc	87.50
5-26	2189	4138	Robert L. Parker	May Salary	General Salaries	50.00
5-26	2190	4139	Grace J. McDonald	May Salary	General Salaries	65.00
5-26	2191	4140	R. R. Simmons	May Salary	Journal Printing and Engraving	100.00
5-26	2192	4141	Dorothy Nelson	May Salary	Speakers Bureau	115.00
5-26	2193	4142	Virginia R. Stewart	May Salary	General and Journal Salaries	125.00
5-26	2194	4143	Dorothy C. McCarthy	May Salary	General Salaries	150.00
5-26	2195	4144	David P. Barr	Travel Expense	Annual Session	38.60
5-26	2196	4145	Bankers Building Corp.	May Rent	Rent and Office Supplies	107.00
5-26	2197	4146	Gordon F. Harkness	Trustees Meeting Expense	Trustees	38.80
5-26	2198	4147	E. M. Myers	Trustees Meeting	Trustees	9.96
5-26	2199	4148	P. A. Bendixen	Legislative Committee	Legislative Committee	37.20
5-26	2200	4149	Gordon F. Harkness	Travel Expense	Med. Economics Comm	18.25
5-26	2201	4150	W. W. Bowen	Travel Expense	County Service and Annual Session	25.20
5-26	2202	4151	American Medical Association	Copy of Law Rulings	Legislative Committee	1.00
5-26	2203	4152	Western Union	Telegrams	Misc. Departmental	.58
5-26	2204	4153	Central Engraving	Halftones	Annual Session—Journal	127.04
			Amount Forward			$11,953.22

Schedule No. 1—Continued

Date 1933	Check No.	Order No.	Drawn in Favor of	In Payment of	Distribution	Amount
					Amount Brought Forward	$11,955.22
5-26	2205	4154	Zaisers	Office Supplies	Rent and Office Supplies	12.65
5-26	2206	4155	Iowa State Medical Library	Postage	Other Committees	1.55
5-26	2207	4156	M. C. Hennessy	Expenses	Council	3.20
5-27	2208	4157	Yellow Cab Co.	Fares for Clinical Patients	Annual Session	7.65
5-31	2209	4158	H. A. Spilman	Travel Expense	County and Annual Session	36.10
5-31	2210	4159	C. A. Boice	Travel Expense	County and Council	13.48
5-12	2159	4109	E. F. Biddle	Projection Work	Annual Session	36.50
6-7	2223	4172	Master Reporting Co.	Reports on General Session	Annual Session	308.89
6-7	2224	4173	Wallace-Homestead Co.	Printing	Stationery, Journal and Reprints	522.66
6-23	2227	4176	Michigan State Medical Society	Copy of Survey	Miscellaneous	2.50
6-23	2228	4177	Iowa Press Clipping Bureau	May Clippings	Journal Printing and Engraving	12.63
6-23	2229	4178	Iowa Press Clipping Bureau	May Clippings	Legislative Committee and Engraving	12.63
6-23	2230	4179	C. B. Taylor	Travel Expense	Trustees and Other Committees	12.75
6-23	2231	4180	John I. Marker	Trustees' Meeting	Trustees	18.40
6-23	2232	4181	E. M. Myers	Trustees' Meeting	Trustees	4.80
6-23	2233	4182	H. A. Spilman	Trustees' Meeting	Council	10.00
6-23	2234	4183	Robert L. Parker	Travel Expense	Miscellaneous	46.00
6-23	2235	4184	Robert L. Parker	June Salary	General Salaries	50.00
6-23	2236	4185	Grace J. McDonald	June Salary	General Salaries	65.00
6-23	2237	4186	R. R. Simmons	June Salary	Journal and Engraving	100.00
6-23	2238	4187	Dorothy Nelson	June Salary	Speakers Bureau	115.00
6-23	2239	4188	Virginia Stewart	June Salary	General Salaries and Journal	125.00
6-23	2240	4189	Dorothy McCarthy	June Salary	General Salaries	150.00
6-23	2241	4190	D. M. Clean Towel Co.	Towel Service	Rent and Office Supplies	3.75
6-23	2242	4191	Royal Typewriter Co.	Ribbons	Rent and Office Supplies	4.00
6-23	2243	4192	French Way Cleaners	Cleaning Drapes	Rent and Office Supplies	5.00
6-23	2244	4193	Postal Telegraph	Telegrams	Journal Printing and Engraving	.76
6-23	2245	4194	Multigraph Co.	Type & Ribbons	Rent and Office Supplies	3.76
6-23	2246	4195	Addressograph Co.	New and Changes on Plates	Rent and Office Supplies	4.34
6-23	2247	4196	Thomas Electric	Cleaning Fan	Rent and Office Supplies	1.00
6-23	2248	4197	Western Union	Telegrams	Misc. Annual Session and Jour.	3.91
6-23	2249	4198	Zaisers	Office Supplies	Rent and Office Supplies	7.60
6-23	2250	4199	Central Engraving	Halftones	Journal Printing and Engraving	57.09
6-30	2251	4200	Robert L. Parker	Travel Expense	County Society Services	8.50
6-30	2252	4201	N. W. Bell Telephone	Telephone Service	Rent and Supplies, County and Session	23.70
6-23	2253	4202	Thos. A. Burcham	Freight Charges	Annual Session	18.00
6-30	2254	4203	Cash	Office Postage	Rent and Office Supplies	10.00
7-12	2255	4204	Wallace-Homestead	Printing	Council, Journal and Reprints	566.43
7-20	2260	4209	Wallace-Homestead	Envelopes	Stationery and Printing	163.20
7-20	2261	4210	Postmaster	Postage	County Society Services	22.04
7-24	2262	4211	Iowa Press Clipping Bureau	June Clippings	Journal Printing and Engraving	12.92
7-24	2263	4212	Old Dutch Ribbon Co.	Coupon Books	Rent and Office Supplies	9.00
7-24	2264	4213	Capital City Printing Co.	Signature Cut	Stationery and Printing	2.45
7-24	2265	4214	N. W. Bell Telephone Co.	Telephone Service	Rent and Supplies, Speakers Bureau	12.95
7-24	2266	4215	Iowa-Des Moines National Bank	Safety Box Rental	Miscellaneous	17.25
7-24	2267	4216	Robert L. Parker	Travel Expense	County Society Service	12.50
7-24	2268	4217	Bankers Building Corp.	July Rent	Rent and Office Supplies	107.00
7-24	2269	4218	Robert L. Parker	July Salary	General Salaries	50.00
7-24	2270	4219	Grace J. McDonald	July Salary	General Salaries	75.00
7-24	2271	4220	R. R. Simmons	July Salary	Journal Salaries	100.00
7-24	2272	4221	Dorothy Nelson	July Salary	Speakers Bureau	125.00
7-24	2273	4222	Virginia Stewart	July Salary	General and Journal Salaries	125.00
7-24	2274	4223	Dorothy McCarthy	July Salary	General Salaries	150.00
7-24	2275	4224	Zaisers	Office Supplies	Rent and Office Supplies	13.32
7-24	2276	4225	Central Engraving Co.	Halftones	Journal Printing and Engraving	37.84
7-24	2277	4226	Dutcher, Walker & Ries	2nd Quarter Expense	Medico-Legal	105.08
8-8	2278	4227	Wallace-Homestead	Envelopes	Stationery and Printing	35.28
8-10	2279	4228	Wallace-Homestead	Printing	Stationery, Journal and Reprints	707.48
8-15	2291	4240	Postmaster	Postage	Journal Printing and Engraving	100.00
8-16	2292	4241	Cash	Petty Cash	Rent and Office Supplies	10.00
8-25	2293	4242	Iowa Press Clipping Bureau	July Clippings	Journal Printing and Engraving	11.25
8-25	2294	4243	R. N. Meng	Advertising Commissions	Journal Printing and Engraving	35.10
8-25	2295	4244	Northwestern Bell Telephone	Telephone Service	Misc. Rent and Office Supplies	15.80
8-25	2296	4245	Cash	Postage	Rent and Office Supplies	10.00
8-25	2297	4246	T. B. Throckmorton	Flowers for Eiker	Miscellaneous	5.00
8-25	2298	4247	Robert L. Parker	Travel Expense	County Society Service	14.20
8-25	2299	4248	Bankers Building Corp.	Rent for August	Rent and Office Supplies	107.00
8-25	2300	4249	D. M. Electric Light Co.	Light Bills	Rent and Office Supplies	2.40
8-25	2301	4250	Robert L. Parker	August Salary	General Salaries	50.00
8-25	2302	4251	Grace J. McDonald	August Salary	General Salaries	75.00
8-25	2303	4252	R. R. Simmons	August Salary	Journal Printing and Engraving Salaries	100.00
8-25	2304	4253	Dorothy M. Nelson	August Salary	Speakers Bureau	125.00
8-25	2305	4254	Virginia Stewart	August Salary	General and Journal Salaries	125.00
8-25	2306	4255	Dorothy McCarthy	August Salary	General Salaries	150.00
8-25	2307	4256	Thomas Electric Co.	Repairing Fan	Rent and Office Supplies	1.00
8-25	2308	4257	American Medical Association	100 Apps. for Members	Rent and Office Supplies	.75
8-25	2309	4258	Zaisers	Office Supplies	Rent and Office Supplies	6.98
8-25	2310	4259	Central Engraving Co.	Halftones	Journal Printing and Engraving	72.27
8-25	2311	4260	Dorothy McCarthy	Travel Expense	Council	10.10
9-8	2312	4261	Wallace-Homestead Co.	Printing	Stationery, Journal and Reprints	591.63
9-26	2317	4266	Iowa Press Clipping Bureau	Clippings	Journal Printing and Engraving	14.20
9-26	2318	4267	Bankers Building Corp.	September Rent	Rent and Office Supplies	107.00
9-26	2319	4268	Pacific Carbon & Ribbon	Typewriter Ribbons	Rent and Office Supplies	4.50
9-26	2320	4269	N. W. Bell Telephone Co.	Telephone	Rent and Office Sub. and S. Bu.	24.00
9-26	2321	4270	Robert L. Parker	September Salary	General Salaries	50.00
9-26	2322	4271	Grace J. McDonald	September Salary	General Salaries	75.00
9-26	2323	4272	R. R. Simmons	September Salary	Journal Printing and Engraving	100.00
9-26	2324	4273	Virginia Stewart	September Salary	Speakers Bureau	125.00
9-26	2325	4274	Dorothy M. Nelson	September Salary	General and Journal Salaries	125.00
9-26	2326	4275	Dorothy C. McCarthy	September Salary	General Salaries	150.00
9-26	2327	4276	Dorothy Nelson	Travel Expense	Miscellaneous, Speakers Bureau	12.85
9-28	2331	4277	James G. Macrae	Council Meeting	Council	7.50
9-28	2332	4278	C. A. Boice	Council Meeting	County Service and Council	20.72
9-28	2333	4279	C. W. Ellyson	Council Meeting	Council	12.75
9-28	2334	4280	James E. Reeder	Council Meeting	Council	20.00
9-28	2335	4281	L. R. Woodward	Council Meeting	Council	13.85
9-28	2336	4282	M. C. Hennessy	Council Meeting	Council	14.55
9-28	2337	4283	A. W. Erskine	Council Meeting	Council	15.50
9-28	2338	4284	F. F. Winkler	Council Meeting	Council	15.50
			Amount Forward			$18,857.97

Schedule No. 1—Continued

Date 1933	Check No.	Order No.	Drawn in Favor of	In Payment of	Distribution	Amount
				Amount Brought Forward		$18,857.97
9-28	2339	4285	H. A. Spilman	Council Meeting	Council	19.15
9-28	2340	4286	Robert L. Parker	District Meeting	County Society Service	3.50
9-28	2341	4287	Robert L. Parker	Meeting Expense	County Society Service	23.00
9-26	2328	4288	Dess Powers	Hennessy Flowers	Miscellaneous and Council	21.00
9-28	2342	4289	Addressograph Co.	New Plates	Rent and Office Supplies	1.82
9-28	2343	4290	Koch Bros.	Ledger Dater	Rent and Office Supplies	1.20
9-28	2344	4291	Des Moines Slide Co.	Slides for Hennessy	Council	7.01
9-28	2345	4292	Western Union	Telegrams	Council and Speakers	3.90
9-28	2346	4293	Zaisers	Office Supplies	Rent and Office Supplies	26.75
9-28	2347	4294	Central Engraving Co.	Halftones	Journal Printing and Engraving	111.24
9-26	2329	4295	R. N. Meng	Advertising Commission	Journal Printing and Engraving	49.50
9-28	2348	4296	C. B. Taylor	Council Meeting	Trustees and Council	9.10
9-28	2349	4297	P. A. Bendixen	Council Meeting	Legislative Committee	22.90
9-28	2350	4298	E. M. Myers	Trustees' Meeting	Trustees	4.85
9-28	2351	4299	John I. Marker	Trustees' Meeting	Trustees	22.90
9-28	2352	4300	Gordon F. Harkness	Council Meeting	Trustees and Council	22.90
9-28	2353	4301	C. B. Taylor	Misc. Expense Travel	County Service and Committees	122.23
10-5	2354	4303	King Typewriter Ser. Co.	Typewriters	Rent and Office Supplies	122.50
10-10	2355	4304	Wallace-Homestead Co.	Printing	Journal Printing and Reprints	495.14
10-19	2356	4305	Cash	Postage, etc.	Rent and Office Supplies	10.00
10-25	2357	4306	Iowa Press Clipping Bureau	September Clippings	Journal Printing and Engraving	11.75
10-25	2358	4307	Old Dutch Carbon Co.	Coupon Books	Rent and Office Supplies	15.00
10-25	2359	4308	King Typewriter Service	Repairing Typewriter	Rent and Office Supplies	7.50
10-25	2360	4309	D. McCarthy	Travel Expense	County Society Service	1.75
10-25	2361	4310	Des Moines Clean Towel	Towel Service	Rent and Office Supplies	3.75
10-25	2362	4311	Cash	Postage, etc.	Rent and Office Supplies	10.00
10-25	2363	4312	N. W. Bell Telephone Co.	Telephone	Rent and Office, Council, Speakers	24.25
10-25	2364	4313	Robert L. Parker	October Salary	General Salaries	50.00
10-25	2365	4314	Grace J. McDonald	October Salary	General Salaries	75.00
10-25	2366	4315	R. R. Simmons	October Salary	Journal Printing and Engraving	100.00
10-25	2367	4316	Dorothy Nelson	October Salary	Speakers Bureau	125.00
10-25	2368	4317	Virginia Stewart	October Salary	General and Journal Salaries	125.00
10-25	2369	4318	Dorothy McCarthy	October Salary	General Salaries	150.00
10-25	2370	4319	Bankers Building Corp.	October Rent	Rent and Office Supplies	107.00
10-25	2371	4320	C. W. Ellyson	Travel Expense	County and Council	14.85
10-25	2372	4321	Robert L. Parker	Travel Expense	County Society	17.50
10-25	2373	4322	Multigraph Company	New Type & Ribbons	Rent and Office Supplies	3.06
10-25	2374	4323	Western Union	Telegrams	Miscellaneous and Council	2.29
10-25	2375	4324	Central Engraving Co.	Halftones	Journal Printing and Engraving	7.09
10-25	2376	4325	Zaisers	Office Supplies	Rent and Office Supplies	2.90
10-25	2377	4326	Dutcher, Walker, Ries	Medico-Legal	Medico-Legal	760.89
10-31	2378	4327	R. N. Meng	Advertising Commissions	Journal Printing and Engraving	67.95
11-13	2379	4328	Wallace-Homestead Co.	Printing	Journal and Reprints	524.10
11-15	2380	4329	Thos. A. Burcham	Committee on Public Policy	Legislative Committee	500.00
11-20	2395	4344	Iowa Press Clipping Co.	October Clippings	Journal Printing and Engraving	14.07
11-20	2396	4345	F. A. Hennessy	Telephone Calls	Council	2.05
11-20	2397	4346	Bankers Building Corp.	November Rent	Rent and Office Supplies	107.00
11-20	2398	4347	Robert L. Parker	Travel Expense	County Service	9.70
11-20	2399	4348	Northwestern Bell Telephone	Telephone	Misc. Rent and Office Supplies	15.85
11-20	2400	4349	Robert L. Parker	November Salary	General Salaries	50.00
11-20	2401	4350	Grace J. McDonald	November Salary	General Salaries	75.00
11-20	2402	4351	R. R. Simmons	November Salary	Journal Printing and Engraving	100.00
11-20	2403	4352	Dorothy Nelson	November Salary	Speakers Bureau	125.00
11-20	2404	4353	Virginia Stewart	November Salary	General and Journal Salaries	125.00
11-20	2405	4354	Dorothy McCarthy	November Salary	General Salaries	150.00
11-20	2406	4355	Zaisers	Office Supplies	Rent and Office Supplies	18.50
11-20	2407	4356	Central Engraving Co.	Halftones	Journal Printing and Engraving	25.70
11-20	2408	4357	Lessing Advertising Co.	Advertising Commission	Journal Printing and Engraving	12.60
11-27	2409	4358	Postmaster	Post Cards	County Society Service	7.18
12-10	2410	4359	Wallace Homestead	Printing & Engraving	Journal Reprints	583.30
12-14	2411	4360	Cash	Postage	Petty Cash	10.00
12-13	2412	4361	Wallace-Homestead Co.	Envelopes	Stationery and Printing	44.10
12-20	2413	4362	Iowa Press Clipping Bureau	November Clippings	Journal	14.42
12-20	2414	4363	King Typewriter Co.	Typewriter Keys	Rent and Office Supplies	7.00
12-20	2415	4364	Des Moines Electric Co.	Light Bulbs	Rent and Office Supplies	1.60
12-20	2416	4365	Des Moines Clean Towel	Towel Service	Rent and Office Supplies	2.50
12-20	2417	4366	N. W. Bell Telephone Co.	Telephone	Telephone and Telegraph	20.30
12-20	2418	4367	Robert L. Parker	December Salary	General Salaries	50.00
12-20	2419	4368	Harold J. McCoy	Treasurer's Salary	General Salaries	50.00
12-20	2420	4369	Grace J. McDonald	December Salary	General Salaries	75.00
12-20	2421	4370	R. R. Simmons	December Salary	Journal Printing and Engraving	100.00
12-20	2422	4371	Dorothy Nelson	December Salary	Speakers Bureau	125.00
12-20	2423	4372	Virginia Stewart	December Salary	General and Journal Salaries	125.00
12-20	2424	4373	Dorothy McCarthy	December Salary	General Salaries	150.00
12-20	2425	4374	Bankers Building Corp.	December Rent	Rent and Office Supplies	107.00
12-20	2426	4375	Robert L. Parker	District Meetings	County Society Services	42.60
12-20	2427	4376	Thomas A. Burcham	District Meetings	County Society Services	9.00
12-20	2428	4377	Earl B. Bush	Committee Expense	Other Committees	16.10
12-20	2429	4378	W. F. Amdor	Committee Expense	Other Committees	23.80
12-20	2430	4379	Frank P. Winkler	Travel Expense	County Society	11.00
12-20	2431	4380	Zaisers	Office Supplies	Rent and Office Supplies	11.50
12-20	2432	4381	American Medical Association	Application Blanks	Rent and Office Supplies	.75
12-20	2433	4382	Reliable Rug Cleaning	Repairing Office Rug	Rent and Office Supplies	2.50
12-20	2434	4383	C. W. Ellyson	Expense	County Society Ser. and Council	16.35
12-20	2435	4384	H. A. Spilman	Council Expense	Council	60.80
12-20	2436	4385	Multigraph Company	Re-inking Ribbons	Rent and Office Supplies	1.72
12-20	2437	4386	Addressograph Co.	New Plates & Repairs	Rent and Office Supplies	4.89
12-21	2438	4387	Central Engraving Co.	Halftones	Journal	48.69
12-21	2439	4388	C. A. Boice	Misc. Expense	County Society Ser. and Council	39.30
12-21	2440	4389	Gleysteen, Purdy & Harper	Medico—Legal	Medico—Legal Com.	126.45
12-21	2441	4390	M. C. Hennessy	District Meeting	County Society Service	20.40
12-21	2442	4391	Chas. B. Taylor	Misc. Expense as President	County Soc. Serv. Adm. Misc. Council, Other Comm., Trustees	96.59
12-21	2443	4392	John I. Marker	Trustees Meeting	Trustees	11.65
12-21	2444	4393	Gordon F. Harkness	Trustees Meeting	Trustees	11.65
12-21	2445	4394	Chas. B. Taylor	Trustees Meeting	Trustees	9.20
12-21	2446	4395	E. M. Myers	Trustees Meeting	Trustees	4.90
12-22	2461	4410	R. N. Meng	Adv. Comm.	Journal Printing and Engraving	10.00
			Bank Charges for 1933			9.22
			TOTAL			$25,567.12

Schedule No. 2
DISBURSEMENTS—SPEAKERS BUREAU
For the Year Ended December 31, 1933

Date 1933	Check No.	Order No.	Drawn in Favor of	In Payment of	Distribution	Amount
2-11	2047	3994	Dorothy M. Nelson	Travel Expense	Traveling Expense	$ 6.00
2-11	2048	3995	L. C. Kern	Travel Expense	Traveling Expense	13.50
2-11	2049	3996	John C. Parsons	Travel Expense	Traveling Expense	7.50
2-11	2050	3997	F. A. Hennessy	Post-graduate Course Expense	Post-graduate Courses	5.00
2-11	2051	3998	E. Von Graff	Travel Expense	Traveling Expense	10.24
2-11	2052	3999	M. E. Barnes	Radio Talks	Miscellaneous	5.00
2-11	2053	4000	M. E. Barnes	Travel Expense	Traveling Expense	5.90
4-1	2114	4003	M. E. Glomset	Radio Talks	Miscellaneous	16.00
4-1	2115	4064	Harry L. Alexander	Post-graduate Travel Expense	Post-graduate Course	50.00
4-1	2116	4065	C. Van Epps	Post-graduate Travel Expense	Post-graduate Course	10.00
4-1	2117	4066	P. C. Jeans	Post-graduate Travel Expense	Post-graduate Course	12.50
4-1	2118	4067	S. A. O'Brien	Travel Expense	Traveling Expense	8.60
4-1	2119	4068	Fred Moore	Travel Expense	Traveling Expense	13.50
4-1	2120	4069	M. E. Barnes	Travel Expense	Traveling Expense	13.25
4-1	2121	4070	C. S. Day	Travel Expense	Traveling Expense	4.00
4-1	2122	4071	T. U. McManus	Travel Expense	Traveling Expense	12.70
4-1	2123	4072	E. M. Myers	Travel Expense	Traveling Expense	10.00
4-1	2124	4073	A. J. Carlson	Travel Expense, Post-graduate	Post-graduate Course	35.00
4-1	2125	4074	D. J. Glomset	Travel Expense	Traveling Expense	93.65
4-25	2149	4098	Russell M. Wilder	Travel Expense, Post-graduate	Post-graduate Course	22.00
4-1	2150	4099	H. L. Beye	Travel Expense, Post-graduate	Post-graduate Course	27.50
					Traveling Expense	5.80
4-1	2151	4100	Rock Island Railway	Travel Expense, Post-graduate	Post-graduate Course	8.00
4-25	2152	4101	Harry L. Ulrich	Travel Expense, Post-graduate	Post-graduate Course	30.00
4-25	2153	4102	Frank C. Mann	Travel Expense, Post-graduate	Post-graduate Course	12.00
4-25	2154	4103	M. B. Galloway	Travel Expense	Traveling Expense	2.10
4-25	2155	4104	Joseph Brown	Travel Expense, Post-graduate	Post-graduate Course	18.00
4-25	2156	4105	A. H. Woods	Travel Expense, Post-graduate	Post-graduate Course	38.20
6-1	2211	4160	O. L. Tatum	Travel Expense, Post-graduate	Post-graduate Course	32.00
6-1	2212	4161	J. R. Dewey	Travel Expense	Traveling Expense	2.00
6-1	2213	4162	Paul Cannon	Travel Expense, Post-graduate	Post-graduate Course	35.00
6-1	2214	4163	J. D. Boyd	Travel Expense, Post-graduate	Post-graduate Course	22.85
6-1	2215	4164	C. Van Epps	Travel Expense, Post-graduate	Post-graduate Course	16.14
6-1	2216	4165	C. W. Baldridge	Travel Expense, Post-graduate	Post-Graduate Course	32.75
6-1	2217	4166	William Malamud	Travel Expense, Post-graduate	Post-graduate Course	13.00
6-1	2218	4167	R. A. Stewart	Travel Expense, Post-graduate	Post-graduate Course	15.50
6-1	2219	4168	E. D. Plass	Travel Expense, Post-graduate	Post-graduate Course	9.00
6-1	2220	4169	D. J. Glomset	Travel Expense, Post-graduate	Post-graduate Course	19.40
				Miscellaneous Expense	Miscellaneous	1.35
6-1	2221	4170	Business Office—Mayo Clinic	Travel Expense, Post-graduate	Post-graduate Course	70.50
6-1	2222	4171	M. E. Barnes	Miscellaneous	Miscellaneous	5.00
6-9	2225	4174	O. H. Plant	Travel Expense, Post-graduate	Post-graduate Course	11.90
6-9	2226	4175	M. J. Shapiro	Travel Expense, Post-graduate	Post-graduate Course	20.00
7-17	2256	4205	Mrs. Judd Shellitto	Refund on Course	Post-graduate Course	10.00
7-17	2257	4206	Mrs. Walter McCody	Refund on Course	Post-graduate Course	10.00
7-17	2258	4207	Frank A. Osincup	Refund on Course	Post-graduate Course	10.00
7-17	2259	4208	E. C. McMillan	Refund on Course	Post-graduate Course	10.00
8-11	2280	4229	Tom B. Throckmorton	Post-graduate Expense	Post-graduate Course	7.20
8-11	2281	4230	L. R. Woodward	Post-graduate Expense	Post-graduate Course	8.50
8-11	2282	4231	John C. Parsons	Travel Expense	Traveling Expense	7.30
8-11	2283	4232	Felix A. Hennessy	Travel Expense	Traveling Expense	8.50
8-11	2284	4233	L. C. Kern	Travel Expense	Traveling Expense	2.20
8-11	2285	4234	E. D. Plass	Travel Expense	Traveling Expense	9.00
8-11	2286	4235	M. E. Barnes	Radio Talks	Miscellaneous	5.00
8-11	2287	4236	H. W. Rathe	Radio Talks	Miscellaneous	12.00
8-11	2288	4237	D. J. Glomset	Travel Expense	Miscellaneous	20.00
8-11	2289	4238	D. M. Nelson	Post-graduate Travel Expense	Post-graduate Traveling Expense	13.00
8-11	2290	4239	Moses Barron	Travel Expense	Travel Expense	25.00
9-15	2313	4262	Andrew M. Woods	Travel Expense	Travel Expense	6.96
9-15	2314	4263	W. A. Rohlf	Travel Expense	Travel Expense	20.30
9-15	2315	4264	Capital City Plate Co.	Signature Cut for Multigraph	Printing	2.45
9-15	2316	4265	D. J. Glomset	Travel—Radio Expense	Travel Expense	43.00
9-28	2330	4302	Wallace-Homestead	Envelopes & Printing	Printing	17.64
11-18	2381	4330	C. W. Baldridge	Traveling Expense	Traveling Expense	6.00
11-18	2382	4331	George H. Keeney	Traveling Expense	Traveling Expense	5.60
11-18	2383	4332	D. J. Glomset	Traveling Expense	Traveling Expense	51.00
11-18	2384	4333	A. A. Schultz	Traveling Expense	Traveling Expense	17.90
11-18	2385	4334	Fred Sternagel	Traveling Expense	Traveling Expense	3.00
11-18	2386	4335	Gordon N. Best	Traveling Expense	Traveling Expense	3.00
11-18	2387	4336	M. E. Barnes	Radio Talks	Miscellaneous	5.00
11-18	2388	4337	Ray Rich	Radio Talks	Miscellaneous	10.00
11-18	2389	4338	Robert L. Parker	Travel Expense	Traveling Expense	9.70
11-18	2390	4339	Wallace-Homestead Co.	Printing & Stationery	Printing	22.40
11-18	2391	4340	W. W. Bowen	Travel Expense	Traveling Expense	5.65
11-18	2392	4341	H. W. Rathe	Travel Expense	Traveling Expense	7.00
11-18	2393	4342	Ben C. Hamilton, Jr.	Travel Expense	Traveling Expense	6.00
11-18	2394	4343	R. L. Barnett	Travel Expense	Traveling Expense	2.25
12-29	2462	4411	Coll. of Medicine Univ.		Post-graduate Courses	871.30
12-21	2447	4396	H. P. Moen	Traveling Expense	Traveling Expense	5.00
12-21	2448	4397	F. M. Smith	Trav. Exp. & Post-graduate	Traveling Expense and Post-graduate	36.10
12-21	2449	4398	H. B. Henry	Miscellaneous	Miscellaneous	3.00
12-21	2450	4399	F. Sternagel	Travel Expense	Traveling Expense	4.50
12-21	2451	4400	M. E. Barnes	Misc. and Trav. Expense	Traveling Expense and Misc.	8.95
12-21	2452	4401	P. W. Van Metre	Travel Expense	Traveling Expense	11.00
12-21	2453	4402	I. T. Schultz	Traveling Expense	Traveling Expense	7.20
12-21	2454	4403	E. M. Myers	Traveling Expense	Traveling Expense	10.80
12-21	2455	4404	F. A. Hennessy	Traveling Expense	Traveling Expense	26.15
12-21	2456	4405	M. D. Ott	Traveling Expense	Traveling Expense	7.00
12-21	2457	4406	R. A. Stewart	Traveling Expense	Traveling Expense	6.30
12-21	2458	4407	B. T. Broghammer	Traveling Expense	Traveling Expense	2.50
12-21	2459	4408	Ray Rich	Miscellaneous	Miscellaneous	5.00
12-21	2460	4409	D. J. Glomset	Traveling Expense	Traveling Expense	5.20

TOTAL .... $ 2,209.08

Dr. McCoy: I *move* that the report of the Treasurer as published in the Handbook be approved.

The motion was regularly seconded, put to a vote and carried.

President Taylor: Is anyone ready to report on the actions of the Council?

Dr. Spilman: We will withhold the report until later.

President Taylor: We are at the point where we should have a report from the Council, if the Council is ready to report.

Dr. Spilman: The Council is not ready to report.

President Taylor: Committee on Finance, Dr. McClure.

REPORT OF THE FINANCE COMMITTEE

A meeting of the Finance Committee was held in the central office of the Society on April 2, 1934. All members of the committee were present.

Twenty-five checks which were outstanding at the time the 1932 report of the committee was made, had in the meantime been cleared and were accounted for.

The committee reviewed the audit for the fiscal year 1933, including all bills with their corresponding orders and checks. Eleven checks were outstanding on December 31, 1933, when the books were closed for the year. These were listed and filed to facilitate the 1934 audit. The committee voted to accept the 1933 audit prepared by Mr. Widdup.

Notes for 1932 and 1933 dues in the amount of $424.00 are being held by the Secretary. Of this total, $70.00 is collectible for 1932 dues, and $354.00 is the amount of the notes held for 1933 dues.

Ernest C. McClure, Chairman.

Dr. McClure: I *move* that the report as printed in the Handbook be approved, and I hope you will all read it.

The motion was regularly seconded, put to a vote and carried.

President Taylor: Committee on Publication, Ralph R. Simmons. (Absent.) Is anyone ready to report on Publications? How about the Chairman of the Board of Trustees?

REPORT OF THE PUBLICATION COMMITTEE

House of Delegates, Iowa State Medical Society:

While the economic conditions of the past twelve months have not favored increased advertising as a source of revenue for the operation of the JOURNAL, we are happy to report a financial condition which we believe in these times does not require apology. We are advised through many channels that with the general up-turn in business noted in many if not most, industries, we may confidently expect greater returns from the sale of advertising space during the coming year.

Your Publication Committee, however, has appreciated that their function and responsibility is not one primarily of securing financial gain for this publication. As a house organ for the members of our Society, the JOURNAL has attempted to maintain a high standard in its several departments. By careful planning we have been able to print a score or more of original articles contributed by our members or distinguished authors from outside the state without in any way interfering with the priority rights which we have accorded papers read before the annual session of the State Society.

The section reporting the activities of the Iowa State Department of Health has been enlarged to reflect more accurately the many activities sponsored by this agency. A section devoted to the Woman's Auxiliary of the State Society has been edited each month by a board appointed by that body. Some additional space has been devoted to studies made on the history of medicine in Iowa. A most complete and painstaking history of medical practice in Lucas County has just been concluded.

Despite the several augmented activities of the JOURNAL careful planning has permitted the publication of this material without the added expense of over-sized publication.

In recounting the several accomplishments of the JOURNAL during the past year we would do so with modesty, since we fully appreciate the great service which has been rendered by the members of the Society in furthering the many projects attempted by your editor. It would, therefore, seem fitting and timely that appreciation should be expressed in this report to all who have through a hearty spirit of co-operation rendered the duties of the editor less arduous and more effective. We earnestly hope that the readers of the JOURNAL will continued to feel the responsibility for the success of this, their house organ, and through a continuation of their support, suggestions and constructive criticism, assist the editor and the committee in their efforts to make the JOURNAL OF THE IOWA STATE MEDICAL SOCIETY outstanding among publications of its kind.

Respectfully submitted,

R. R. Simmons, M.D., Editor and
Chairman of the Publication Committee.

Dr. Fay: I *move* that the report as published in the Handbook be approved.

The motion was regularly seconded, put to a vote and carried.

President Taylor: Committee on Public Policy and Legislation, Dr. Burcham.

REPORT OF THE COMMITTEE ON PUBLIC POLICY AND LEGISLATION

House of Delegates, Iowa State Medical Society:

The Committee on Public Policy and Legislation presents the following report covering activities for 1933-34:

The bill of major importance to the medical profession introduced in the Forty-fifth General Assembly, Extra Session, was Senate File 112 which passed both the Senate and the House. This changes the Perkins, Haskell-Klaus laws with special reference to the commitment of patients to the University Hospitals.

A detailed discussion of this bill was included in the three reports made by the Committee of Nine, which were published in the January, 1934, issue of the Iowa State Medical JOURNAL. The bill passed with the section containing the county quota plan, which is fully explained in letters sent to every member of the profession under date of February 26, 1934, and March 15, 1934, signed by John T. McClintock, M.D., and R. E. Neff, administrator of the University Hospitals.

As a matter of record and general information the bill as passed is given below:

H. F. 112

AN ACT to amend chapter one hundred ninety-nine (199), Code, 1931, by inserting after section four thousand eighteen (4018) a new section; to amend sections four thousand twenty-five (4025), four thousand twenty-six (4026) and four thousand twenty-eight (4028), Code, 1931; and to repeal sections four thousand ten (4010), four thousand twelve (4012), four thousand sixteen (4016), four thousand seventeen (4017), and four thousand twenty-one (4021), Code, 1931, and to enact substitutes therefor, all relating to the treatment of indigent persons.

Be It Enacted by the General Assembly of the State of Iowa:

Section 1. Section four thousand ten (4010), Code, 1931, is repealed and the following substituted therefor:

"When such complaint is filed, the clerk shall furnish the county attorney and board of supervisors with a copy thereof and said board shall, by the overseer of the poor or such other agent as it may select, make a thorough investigation of the facts as to the legal residence of the patient, and the ability of the patient or others chargeable with his support to pay the expense of such treatment and care; and shall file a report of such investigation in the office of the clerk, at or before the time of hearing."

Sec. 2. Section four thousand twelve (4012), Code, 1931, is repealed and the following substituted therefor:

"The county attorney and the overseer of the poor, or other agent of the board of supervisors of the county where the hearing is held, shall appear thereat. The complainant, the county attorney, the overseer of the poor or other agent of the board of supervisors, and the patient, or any person representing him, or her, may introduce evidence and be heard. If the court finds that said patient is a legal resident of Iowa and is pregnant or is suffering from a malady or deformity which can probably be improved or cured or advantageously treated by medical or surgical treatment or hospital care, and that neither the patient nor any person legally chargeable with his or her support is able to pay the expenses thereof, then the clerk of court, except in obstetrical cases and cases of crippled children shall immediately ascertain from the admitting physician at the university hospital whether such person can be received as a patient within a period of thirty days, and if the patient can be so received, the court shall then enter an order directing that said patient be sent to the university hospital for proper medical and surgical treatment and hospital care. If the court ascertain, excepting in obstetrical cases and orthopedic cases, that a person of the age or sex of the patient, or afflicted by the complaint, disease or deformity with which such person is affected cannot be received as a patient at the said university hospital within the period of thirty days, then he shall enter an order directing the board of supervisors of the county to provide adequate treatment at county expense for said patient at home or in a hospital. Obstetrical cases and orthopedic cases may be committed to the university hospital without regard to the limiting period of thirty days hereinbefore stated.

"In any case of emergency the court without previous inquiry may at its discretion order the patient to be immediately taken to and accepted by the university hospital for the necessary care as provided in section four thousand fourteen (4014), Code, 1931, herein, but if such a patient cannot be immediately accepted at the university hospital as ascertained by telephone if necessary, the court may enter an order as in certain cases above set forth directing the board of supervisors to provide adequate treatment at county expense for the said patient at home or in a hospital.

"On the date this act becomes effective the commitments of all persons then waiting for treatment at the university hospital are hereby cancelled. Should commitments be applied for on behalf of any of those said patients within six months thereafter, they may be committed without regard to the thirty day provision of the preceding paragraph and they shall have preference as to sixty (60) per cent of the beds of the university hospital available for the use of indigent persons."

Sec. 3. Section four thousand sixteen (4016), Code, 1931, is repealed and the following substituted therefor:

"If the physician appointed to examine the patient shall certify that an attendant to accompany the patient to the said hospital is necessary, and the university hospital attendant and ambulance service is not available, then the court or judge may appoint an attendant who shall receive not exceeding two dollars ($2.00) per day for the time thus necessarily employed and actual necessary traveling expenses by the most feasible route to said hospital whether by ambulance, train or automobile; but if such appointee is a relative of the patient or a member of his immediate family, or receives a salary or other compensation from the public for

his services, no such per diem compensation shall be paid him. The physician appointed by the court to make the examination and report shall receive therefor three dollars ($3.00) for each examination and report so made and his actual necessary expenses incurred in making such examination, but if said physician receives a salary or other compensation from the public for his full time services, then no such examination fee shall be paid. The actual, necessary expenses of transporting and caring for the patient shall be paid as hereinafter provided."

Sec. 4. Section four thousand seventeen (4017), Code, 1931, is repealed and the following substituted therefor:

"An itemized, verified statement of all charges provided for in the preceding section and in section two (2) hereof, in cases where the patient is admitted or accepted for treatment at the university hospital shall be filed with the superintendent of the *university hospital, and* ⟨illegible⟩ by the judge under whose order the same were incurred, they shall be charged on the regular bill for the maintenance, transportation and treatment of the patient, and be audited and paid in the manner as hereinafter provided.'

Sec. 5. Section four thousand twenty-one (4021), Code, 1931, is repealed and the following substituted therefor:

"Treatment of other patients. The university hospital authorities may at their discretion receive into the hospital for medical, obstetrical or surgical treatment or hospital care, patients not committed thereto under the provisions of this chapter; but the treatment or care of such patients shall not in any way interfere with the proper medical or surgical treatment or hospital care of committed patients.

"All of the provisions of this chapter except as to commitment of patients shall apply to such patients. The university hospital authorities shall collect from the person or persons liable for the support of such patients reasonable charges for hospital care and service and deposit the same with the treasurer of the university for the use and benefit of the university hospital. Earnings of the hospital whether from private patients, cost patients, or indigents shall be administered so as to increase as much as possible, the service available for indigents."

Sec. 6. Section four thousand twenty-five (4025), Code, 1931, is amended by adding after the period in line six (6) thereof the following:

"If the physician, surgeon or nurse is not in the regular employ of the state board of education, his or her compensation shall be paid by the county upon approval of the board of supervisors."

Sec. 7. Section four thousand twenty-six (4026), Code, 1931, is amended by striking out all of the section following the period in line seven (7) and inserting in lieu thereof the following:

"But he shall render separate bills showing the actual cost of all appliances, instruments, x-ray and other special services used in connection with such treatment, commitments, and transportation to and from the said university hospital, including the expenses of attendants and escorts.

"All purchases of materials, appliances, instruments and supplies by said university hospital, in cases where more than one hundred dollars ($100.00) is to be expended, and where the price of the commodity or commodities to be purchased are subject to competition, shall be upon open competitive quotations, and all contracts therefor shall be subject to the provisions of chapter sixty-two (62), Code, 1931."

Sec. 8. Chapter one hundred ninety-nine (199), Code, 1931, is amended by inserting after section four thousand eighteen (4018) thereof, the following:

"4018-f1. County Quotas. Subject to subsequent qualifications in this section, there shall be treated at the university hospital during each fiscal year a number of committed indigent patients from each county which shall bear the same relation to the total number of committed indigent patients admitted during the year as the population of such county shall bear to the total population of the state according to the last preceding official census. This standard shall apply to indigent patients, the expenses of whose commitment, transportation, care and treatment shall be borne by appropriated funds and shall not govern the admission of either obstetrical or orthopedic patients. If the number of patients admitted from any county shall exceed by more than ten per cent the county quota as fixed and ascertained under the first sentence of this section, the charges and expenses of the care and treatment of such patients in excess of ten per cent of the quota shall be paid from the funds of such county at actual cost; but if the number of excess patients from any county shall not exceed ten per cent, all costs, expenses, and charges incurred in their behalf, shall be paid from the appropriation for the support of the hospital."

Sec. 9. Section four thousand twenty-eight (4028), Code, 1931, is amended by adding at the end thereof the following:

"The superintendent of the said university hospital shall certify to the auditor of state on the first day of January, April, July and October of each year, the amount as herein provided not previously certified by him due the state from the several counties having patients chargeable thereto, and the auditor of state shall thereupon charge the same to the county so owing. A duplicate certificate shall also be mailed to the auditor of each county having patients chargeable thereto.

"The county auditor, upon receipt of such certificate, shall thereupon enter the same to the credit of the state in his ledger of state accounts, and at once issue a notice to his county treasurer authorizing him to transfer the amount from the poor or county fund to the general state revenue, which notice shall be filed by the treasurer as his authority for making such transfer; and he shall include the amount so transferred in his next remittance of state taxes to the treasurer of state, to accrue to the credit of the university hospital fund.

"The state auditor shall certify the total cost of commitment, transportation and caring for each indigent patient under the terms of this statute to the county auditor of such patient's legal residence, and such certificate shall be preserved by the county auditor and shall be a debt due from the patient or the persons legally responsible for his or her care, maintenance or support; and whenever in the judgment of the board of supervisors the same or any part thereof shall be collectible, the said board may in its own name collect the same and is hereby authorized to institute suits for such purpose; and after deducting the county's share of such cost shall cause the balance to be paid into the state treasury to reimburse the university hospital fund."

Another bill of interest to the medical profession was House File 146, known as the Hospital Lien Bill, which passed both the Senate and the House and is published herewith in full for your information:

H. F. 146

AN ACT giving the operator of a hospital in this state a lien upon all causes of action for damages accruing to a patient therein, or to the legal representatives of such patient, for the reasonable charges for hospital care necessitated by the injuries giving rise to such causes of action.

Be It Enacted by the General Assembly of the State of Iowa:

Section 1. Every association, corporation, county or other institution, including a municipal corporation, maintaining a hospital in the State of Iowa, which shall furnish medical or other service to any patient injured by reason of an accident not covered by the Workmen's Compensation Act, shall, if such injured party shall assert or maintain a claim against another for damages on account of such injuries, have a lien upon that part going or belonging to such patient of any recovery or sum had or collected or to be collected by such patient, or by his heirs or personal representatives in the case of his death, whether by judgment or by settlement or compromise to the amount of the reasonable and necessary charges of such hospital for the treatment, care and maintenance of such patient in such hospital up to the date of payment of such damages; provided, however, that this lien shall not in any way prejudice or interfere with any lien or contract which may be made by such patient or his heirs or personal representatives with any attorney or attorneys for handling the claim on behalf of such patient, his heirs or personal representatives; provided, further, that the lien herein set forth shall not be applied or considered valid against anyone coming under the Workmen's Compensation Act in this State. No such lien shall be effective, however, unless a written notice containing the name and address of the injured person, the date of the accident, the name and location of the hospital, and the name of the person or persons, firm or firms, corporation or corporations alleged to be liable to the injured party for the injuries received, shall be filed in the office of the clerk of the district court of the county in which such hospital is located, prior to the payment of any moneys to such injured person, his attorneys or legal representatives, as compensation for such injuries; nor unless the hospital shall also mail, postage prepaid, a copy of such notice with a statement of the date of filing thereof to the person or persons, firm or firms, corporation or corporations alleged to be liable to the injured party for the injuries sustained prior to the payment of any moneys to such injured person, his attorneys or legal representatives, as compensation for such injuries. Such hospital shall mail a copy of such notice to any insurance carrier which has insured such person, firm or corporation against such liability, if the name and address shall be known. Any person or persons, firm or firms, corporation or corporations, including an insurance carrier, making any payment to such patient or to his attorneys or heirs or legal representatives as compensation for the injury sustained, after the filing and mailing of such notice without paying to such hospital the amount of its lien or so much thereof as can be satisfied out of the moneys due under any final judgment or compromise or settlement agreement, after paying the amount of any prior liens, shall, for a period of one year from the date of payment to such patient or his heirs, attorneys or legal representatives, as aforesaid, be and remain liable to such hospital for the amount which such hospital was entitled to receive as aforesaid; any such association, corporation or other institution maintaining such hospital may, within such period, enforce its lien by a suit at law against such person or persons, firm or firms, corporation or corporations making any such payment.

Sec. 2. Every clerk of the district court shall, at the expense of the county, provide a suitable well-bound book to be called the hospital lien docket in which, upon the filing of any lien claim under the provisions of this act, he shall enter the name of the injured person, the date of the accident and the name of the hospital or other institution making the claim. Said clerk shall make a proper index of the same in the name of the injured person and such clerk shall be entitled to twelve cents (12c) for filing each claim, and at the rate of eight cents (8c) per folio for such entry made in the lien docket, and six cents (6c) for every search in the office for such lien claim.

Below you will find a list of bills introduced in the Senate and House which were of interest to the medical profession. A notation has been included as to the final disposition of each bill:

House File No. 67, introduced by Schroeder and Dreessen, and Senate File No. 22 by Chrystal, sought to provide methods for apportioning among the several counties of the state the cost of treatment of indigent persons at the hospital of the College of Medicine of the State University. House File No. 67 was referred to the steering committee and was not brought out for passage, while Senate File No. 22 was referred to the public health committee and was not recalled.

House File No. 91, by Fuester, was an act to repeal Section 4028, Code, 1931, and to enact a substitute therefor, relating to the treatment of indigent persons with special reference to the issuing of warrants and providing authority to the Board of Supervisors to collect the costs of caring for the indigents in case the patients or persons legally responsible for their care are ever in a position to pay such costs or any part thereof. This bill was later withdrawn.

On November 24, 1933, House Joint Resolution No. 2 was introduced by Mercer and Wolf, providing for the removal of restrictions on the public use and patronage of the State University Hospital during the present economic depression. This bill was referred to the steering committee and did not come out for passage.

Senate File No. 170, by Schmidt, and House File No. 219, by Beswick and Grell, were identical bills relating to the examination of indigent persons who are candidates for admission into the hospital of the State University and the fixing of the qualifications of such examiner. Senate File No. 170 was referred to the public health committee, which recommended indefinite postponement; while House File No. 219 was referred to the steering committee and not recalled.

Senator Schmidt introduced Senate File No. 171, which sought to repeal Chapter 149, Acts of the Forty-third General Assembly of Iowa, relating to contracts for the support of the poor, and to authorize the board of supervisors to contract for professional services for poor persons. Had this bill passed, it would have been impossible to enter into a contract with the board of supervisors for the care of the indigent sick. However the bill was referred to the committee on county and township affairs and the committee recommended indefinite postponement.

In like manner, Senate File No. 172, by Schmidt, and House File No. 222, by Beswick and Grell, sought to repeal the law as it now appears in Chapter 118, Code, 1931, and to enact a substitute therefor regulating the practice of Osteopathy and of Osteopathy and Surgery. Senate File No. 172 was referred to the public health committee, which recommended indefinite postponement of the measure, while House File No. 222 was referred to the steering committee and was not brought out for passage.

Representative Johnson introduced House File No. 7 seeking to legalize the practice of Naprapathy, but this bill was referred to the steering committee and did not reappear.

A bill creating a state board of Naturopathy, defining and regulating its practice, was introduced by Representatives Dreessen and Stanzel under House File No. 246, but it was referred to the steering committee and was not recalled.

Early in the session, this Committee presented a

basic science bill to the chairman of the Public Health Committee of both the Senate and the House, the bills to be presented at their discretion. However we were informed by members of both branches of the Legislature that bills of a controversial nature, with the exception of tax revision, poor relief and liquor bills, would not be considered at the extra session. They explained that it was their intention to concentrate on the emergency measures and as they adhered to their determination the basic science bills were not introduced.

Respectfully submitted,

Thos. A. Burcham, M.D., Chairman

Dr. Burcham: Mr. President, in addition to the report that is published in the Handbook, I think that this organization at this time should take action particularly in the instruction of the Legislative Committee as to proposed changes in the Medical Practice Act. At the meeting of the Councilors and the officers, along with the Legislative Committee of the Society last September, we all agreed on the basic science law as the one that would best solve our problems at this time. Therefore, in the extra session of the legislature, we introduced a bill, a basic science law, in the legislature. What happened to that bill is covered in the Handbook.

I think this Society, through the House of Delegates, at this time should instruct the Legislative Committee to use its efforts in trying to get a bill passed which embodies the basic science law. I have a sufficient number of copies to supply all of the delegates and all of the officers. If you so instruct the Legislative Committee, I want you to take this argument which has been prepared by the Legislative Committee, with Mr. Gerald Blake, and a copy of the bill, and discuss it before your county medical societies and get in contact with your senators and representatives and let us start out, before the session of the legislature, in trying to educate our representatives as to what we want. If this body wants the basic science law, I think you can so designate it at this time.

Dr. Bendixen: I *move* that the House of Delegates instruct the Legislative Committee to work on a basic science law and that it have the sanction of the House of Delegates for such a law.

President Taylor: You have heard the motion that we instruct the Legislative Committee to draft a basic science law, and that we give it our support.

The motion was regularly seconded.

President Taylor: Is there any discussion on this motion? This is a question you will want to discuss, I think.

Dr. Pearson: I think it would be well for Dr. Spilman, the Chairman of the Council, to say something along this line. The action which the Councilors took today might give us some idea of the strength we may develop in the ability to put this thing over.

Dr. Spilman: It has been strongly talked of during the past year that there should be developed in all of the counties throughout the state an interprofessional association which would look after the interests of the public health and measures designed along that line.

The Council passed a resolution today to appoint a special committee to study and work out, wherever possible in the various localities, the formation of these interprofessional societies or associations similar to that in Woodbury County, which was so successful in disciplining some legislators whose actions were inimical to the public welfare. I feel that that is the thing that every delegate and every member of the House of Delegates can take home and can work on actively, because by creating such associations you can have a powerful influence and a powerful force to bring to bear upon these legislators on these measures which are not particularly selfish, designed to protect our own interests, but are measures which are designed to protect the public along medical lines.

President Taylor: Is there any further discussion on the motion to the effect that we approve of the Legislative Committee drafting a basic science law? If not, as many as favor the motion say "aye;" contrary "no." *The "ayes" have it.*

Is the Council ready to report, Dr. Spilman?

Dr. Spilman: The report of the Chairman and the reports of the Councilors with those incorporated reports of Deputy Councilors are printed in the Handbook and, I believe, tell the activities of the Council during the past year.

President Taylor: Medico-Legal Committee, Frank Ely.

REPORT OF THE MEDICO-LEGAL COMMITTEE
1933-34

House of Delegates, Iowa State Medical Society:

The Medico-Legal Committee wishes to report that during the past year its work has been rather uneventful. The usual routine pertaining to advice of members concerning their legal difficulties has been followed.

Owing to the fact that more of our members are constantly buying commercial malpractice insurance, the Committee has not been called upon for assistance in as many cases as formerly. A more vindictive attitude on the part of claimants, owing to a reduction in their incomes and those of their legal representatives, has made some of our cases more difficult to defend. During the year, one malpractice case has been carried to the Supreme Court, and the costs of this appeal have been very heavy. Owing to this and other expenses, entailed in defense matters, the question has arisen in the minds of a number of our members as to the advisability of continuing our defense program. The following analysis of the situation is an attempt to show the reason why it is pertinent for us to consider whether continuation is practical and advisable.

These data are based on the number of members which were in good standing on January 1, 1934, and the cost of medical defense for the calendar year, 1933.

Total membership of State Society as of Jan. 1, 1934		2,163
Members insured with commercial insurance companies	1,598	
M.D.'s in insurance work and needing no insurance	24	
M.D.'s in state institutions, needing no insurance	41	
M.D.'s Life members but living out of state	16	
M.D.'s members, but uninsurable by insurance companies	34	
M.D.'s over 65 who have never carried insurance, therefore uninsurable, or who are retired (approximately)	230	
Total M.D.'s insured or who do not need insurance	1,943	1,943
Total M.D.'s covered by State Society Protection		220
State Society dues per member	$ 10.00	
Members depending on Society for protection	220	
Total dues paid by these $220 members	$2,200.00	
Cost of medical defense for these 220 members during the year 1933	1,931.60	
Balance	$ 268.40	

These 220 members paid the State Society $1.22 each for all other activities outside of Medical Defense.

It is only fair to state that the legal expense for the fiscal year ending in May of this year has been less than that for the calendar year, 1933. As previously stated, this is largely due to the increased number of members who have purchased commercial insurance.

The Medico-Legal Committee does not wish to exert its influence for or against discontinuance of our defense program, but is pleased to present, in an unbiased manner, the facts as they now stand.

Some questions of expediency have arisen with relation to this problem among which are the following:

(1) Will the abolition of Society malpractice defense weaken our position in the courts?

(2) Will the commercial indemnity companies impose on us in the event that our defense is discontinued?

(3) Will we lose ethical control of matters pertaining to defense and out-of-court settlement of threatened suis?

There is a majority and minority feeling among the three members of our Committee. Two believe that abolition of our defense activities is advisable if the majority of our members who carry commercial insurance do not wish to pay for the protection of the few. One believes that we should continue as we have in the past.

The Chairman's answer to the question above indicated is as follows. It is improbable that our power in court will be affected in any way if we cease to defend our members, because it has always been our policy to soft-pedal the Society's legal participation in such matters for fear of provoking the "doctors' trust" idea. The premium rates on malpractice policies issued by commercial companies depend very largely on the laws of the states in which they operate. In some states they are very high and in some low, depending on the statutory obstacles to be overcome. If any company treats us unfairly, we have the power to influence the discontinuance of approximately 1,598 policies and can at any time enact bylaws providing for both protection and indemnity by the Society itself.

As pertains to the possible loss of ethical control in the conduct of defense, and settlement of suits out

of court, it may be said that the members, themselves, should be as they now are, largely responsible for what is done. Every time a threatened suit is settled too easily, it breeds another group of claims. As matters now stand, a commercially insured member can settle a claim against him if he so chooses and is advised by his insuror to do so, but one defense company has been kind enough to consult the Chairman of the Medico-Legal Committee before out-of-court settlements have been made, and there is no reason to believe that this consideration will not be shown in the future.

The Medico-Legal Committee is neither strongly for or against defense discontinuance. The crux of the matter is just this as revealed by the statistical outline previously offered. In 1933, 220 members out of 2,163, or 10 per cent, were protected at Society expense. The 220 protected members paid into the Society $2,200.00, and it cost $1,931.00 to defend them, so that this minority actually contributed $1.22 per member to the activities of the Society other than legal protection. The cost per member for medical defense in 1933 was approximately ninety cents. It is to be supposed that ninety cents a year will not make or break any member; yet, in line with the times, there has been some complaint with regard to the medical defense expenditures. If we are obliged to carry many of our cases to the Supreme Court it is to be expected that our legal costs may be much higher. It so happens that some of our members forget to pay their commercial insurance premiums and find themselves without such coverage. The Society defense might be looked upon as memory insurance and it is up to the House of Delegates to decide whether it wishes to continue our defense features and pay for the same without grumbling, or abolish this feature of our activities.

Frank E. Ely, Chairman.

Dr. Ely: I feel a certain amount of responsibility to the House of Delegates. We have not spent a lot of money bringing members of the Committee to Des Moines, but most of our Committee meetings have been carried out by correspondence. When any very important subject has come up, the matter has been discussed through correspondence with the various members of the Committee.

You will note in the Handbook that the report really was signed by myself, and I take responsibility for some of the answers to some of the questions from the Chairman's point of view.

With regard to this matter of whether we shall or shall not discontinue our medico-legal defense features, there was a two to one vote of the Committee for discontinuing, but I want you to understand that the Committee does not feel at all strong in either direction. An attempt has been made to familiarize you with the situation. I want to tell you how this all arose.

There has been a lot of feeling that the medico-legal expense is very heavy. We have tried to keep it down. It isn't anywhere near what it used to be. We happened to have one case in the Supreme Court that was very costly this year. It is a question of whether the case should have gone to the Supreme Court or not. But in order to quiet criticism with regard to the expense of continuing the defense features, we thought it was very much better to lay the whole matter right before you as plainly and as concisely as possible and let you decide whether you are going to continue to defend a few members who do not carry commercial insurance. As far as I am concerned, it is neither here nor there. One of the members of the Committee will speak on this question when the changes in the Constitution and By-laws are discussed. I shall be very glad to have him give his views.

There is just one possible argument that I can see in favor of our continuing our defense feature, and that is that possibly we may have a little more leverage with the commercial insurance companies if we continue it than if we do not. Whether that is more of an imaginary idea than not, I do not know. I think we would get along all right without it and we would get along all right with it.

As you will notice by my wording of the report in the Handbook, we are spending a small amount per member to keep the insurance feature going, and if a man happens to forget to pay his commercial insurance premium, he would be very glad, of course, to be able to fall back on the Society for his defense. So do not think that the Medico-Legal Committee is in any sense of the word, trying to dictate, but we are just trying to talk turkey to you so that you can know, if the expense of our defense goes up, that you have voted to continue it and therefore you will have to be contented with paying the bill.

I *move* that this report be approved.

The motion was regularly seconded.

Dr. Albright: Inasmuch as I will not be here Friday, and inasmuch as I am the dissenting member on this, I should like to present my views to the House of Delegates.

The first thing I want to say is that the House of Delegates will hunt a long time before they will find a man who is as devoted to his work and who is as conscientious in his work and who has been as fair to all the members of the Committee, who has been willing to assume responsibility and has been backed up by the Committee as well as Dr. Ely.

However, the question of totally dispensing with the protection feature of our Society, it seems to me, goes a good deal deeper than the .phase that Dr. Ely has put forward, and that is, will it give us additional leverage with the commercial insurance companies if we retain it?

Ever since I have been a member of the medical profession, the thing that has been outstanding to me is the solidarity of the medical profession. A member of the firm of lawyers who is at present the attorney for the State Medical Society said to me, "I wish that there were some way that the legal profession could have the fine solidarity that exists in the medical profession." That is the viewpoint

of the legal profession. To me the greatest feature of the indemnity insurance or the defense features of the State Medical Society is the feeling of unity that it gives to the men in the Society.

The second thing that is almost equally as important is the feeling our patients have before they file suit. Very frequently when a suit is threatened, they are told by their attorney that it will be an uphill business to get a verdict because the medical profession stands together on this proposition, and they realize that.

Then, you know how it is if you have an automobile accident. The first question they ask is, "Are you carrying insurance?"

"Yes."

"All right, then we will put in a bill for so much, and a bill for so much of this and so much of that."

It doesn't make any difference to you so long as the insurance company is paying it. If you were paying it, you would not think of putting in a bill for that amount. I think the same thing will be true if we abandon our defense features in the Medical Society and turn them over completely to the commercial insurance company.

The actual expense of the members of the Medical Society for maintaining medical defense is about ninety cents per member, as Dr. Ely's report shows. Ninety cents a member is pretty cheap insurance for this unity of the profession among themselves, for their unity against influences from without, and I am very, very much opposed to dropping it. Commercial insurance can be carried, yes, but it does not have the same effect upon the medical profession as would the maintenance of this feature. If the medical defense feature is dropped, I doubt very much that our dues will be decreased one cent; perhaps they would, but I doubt it. So I am opposed to this change.

Dr. Bellinger: I happen to be another member of the Medico-Legal Committee. Personally I have concurred in the viewpoint that Dr. Ely has taken. However, the argument that the other member of our Committee has put up is very plausible, very reasonable.

As Dr. Ely has stated, to cut down expense, our Committee has not held a meeting on this matter under discussion. We have discussed the matter through letters. Personally, I felt that the majority of the members of the Iowa State Medical Society carried commercial insurance. With these times that we are going through, and whether they will get better or not only the future will tell us, the defense department of this Society possibly will grow in the extent of expense.

This insurance has been up before this Society for discussion during the past several years; in fact, I think it was before the Society at the meeting at Marshalltown. It is a subject to which the House of Delegates should give deep consideration. We would not wish to offer any motion here for a change in this defense if it is not accepted by a great majority of the delegates represented by the medical profession of this state.

Personally, I have felt that inasmuch as the majority of us were carrying commercial insurance and the expense is liable to increase to the Society, the best thing for this Society is to accept the change along the line that we have made in our report. That is all I have to say, but I do ask that the delegates take deep consideration and analyze this subject thoroughly before any change is made.

President Taylor: I think it has been a very fine thing that these two arguments have been brought forward at this particular time. This will be considered, as you know, in the By-law change which will come up at the Friday meeting. Is there any further discussion? If not, all in favor of the approval of the report of the Committee on Medico-Legal Defense will signify by saying "aye;" contrary "no." It is carried.

Committee on Necrology, Dr. Erskine.

REPORT OF THE COMMITTEE ON NECROLOGY

House of Delegates, Iowa State Medical Society:

Sixty-three of our colleagues have died since the last report of this committee. The youngest was thirty-one years of age, the oldest, eighty-five. One of the sixty-three deaths was before the age of forty; twenty-four were between forty and sixty; and thirty-three between sixty and eighty, and five over eighty.

Twenty-three died after a long illness; six of heart

disease or arteriosclerosis; seven died of cerebral hemorrhage, and six deaths were accidental. There were three postoperative deaths, and one each from leukemia, cancer, peritonitis, acute infection and uremia.

May we stand, honoring our dead, while their names are read?

Harold A. Spilman, Chairman
Arthur W. Erskine, Secretary

January 1, 1933 to April 1, 1934

Name	Place	Age	Date	Cause
Allen, Manning L.	Tama	70	Mar. 11, 1933	Prolonged illness
Armitage, George Ira	Murray	62	Sept. 10, 1933	Prolonged illness
Armstrong, Charles Herman	Preston	53	Nov. 11, 1933	Prolonged illness
Brown, Cecil W.	Clinton	57	Jan. 8, 1934	Prolonged illness
Bush, Fred Wilson	Van Horne	63	April 12, 1933	Prolonged illness
Cady, Clinton Colfax	Alden	63	July 27, 1933	Cerebral hemorrhage
Caldwell, James W.	Steamboat Rock	80	Mar. 14, 1933	Prolonged illness
Carpenter, William Edwin	Tama	63	Sept. 27, 1933	Prolonged illness
Chalmers, Francis Edward	George	58	Aug. 1, 1933	Cancer
Clark, Charles Bryant	Cedar Rapids	62	June 24, 1933	Subarachnoid hemorrhage
Condon, Joseph Redmond	Des Moines	52	Oct. 12, 1933	Cerebral hemorrhage
Davenport, Frank Douglas	Winterset	69	May 22, 1933	Angina pectoris
Deschler, Joseph Jordan	Glidden	76	Mar. 31, 1933	Prolonged illness
Deitz, Charles Frederick	Neola	68	April 21, 1933	Prolonged illness
Dilley, Harry Horace	Des Moines	41	Dec. 13, 1933	Uremic poisoning
Emmons, William Henry	Decorah	65	Sept. 9, 1933	Heart
Ferris, Lewis Henry	Melbourne	52	Sept. 16, 1933	Prolonged illness
Frear, Edwin D.	Danbury	79	Mar. 19, 1934	Prolonged illness
George, Abel Benson	Burlington	55	Dec. 29, 1933	
Gethman, Charles Christian	Eldora	70	Sept. 5, 1933	Prolonged illness
Grimes, Eli	Des Moines	66	Jan. 14, 1934	Cancer
Haller, Julius Theodore	Davenport	55	Feb. 28, 1933	Burns from automobile accident
Hennessy, Albert Vincent	Council Bluffs	48	Jan. 15, 1933	Accidental
Herrick, John Francis	Ottumwa	69	Feb. 23, 1933	Leukemia
Hickman, Mack	Indianola	58	Jan. 26, 1934	Prolonged illness
Hill, Leslie Grant	Estherville	67	Feb. 24, 1934	Prolonged illness
Hinkle, George Wesley	Harvard	83	May 13, 1933	Senility
Johnson, Norman Willis	Quasqueton	60	Sept. 17, 1933	Cerebral hemorrhage
Juen, Joseph A.	Ossian	59	Mar. 11, 1934	Cerebral hemorrhage
Kelleher, George Francis	Postville	46	Oct. 23, 1933	Automobile accident
Keppler, Fred Albert	Dubuque	31	Feb. 2, 1933	Following operation
King, T. W.	Lamoni	53	Mar. 28, 1934	
Lass, Daniel George	Ocheyedan	75	Feb. 4, 1933	Cerebral hemorrhage
Luckey, John Eddy	Vinton	66	June 29, 1933	Prolonged illness
McCrary, Delbert W.	Lake City	66	Jan. 9, 1934	
McCray, Frank Herbert	Schaller	67	Jan. 14, 1934	Prolonged illness
McCray, Walter R.	Charles City	58	May 15, 1933	Following operation
Martin, Worley George	Rippey	57	June 6, 1933	Heart
Merritt, William H.	Pleasantville	81	May 31, 1933	Prolonged illness
Moore, Robert A.	Silver City	79	Oct. 9, 1933	Prolonged illness
Pascoe, Henry R.	Carroll	56	July 7, 1933	Cerebral hemorrhage
Pond, Issi Otto	Perry	60	Mar. 15, 1934	Coronary Thrombosis
Reynolds, John William	Creston	59	Mar. 14, 1934	Heart
Rice, Earl	Ames	66	Oct. 30, 1933	Heart
Rohrig, John George	Davenport	50	Mar. 25, 1933	General Peritonitis
Sanders, Charles W.	Northwood	74	Mar. 28, 1934	
Schmidt, Arthur Albert	Postville	52	Jan. 22, 1934	Throat infection
Shellito, Judd Campbell	Independence	44	April 16, 1933	Automobile accident

Singleton, Eustace	Marshalltown	69	Nov. 29, 1933	Myasthenia gravis
Smith, John Christopher	Stacyville	45	Dec. 28, 1933	Essential hypertension
Stewart, Charles Walker	Washington	68	Nov. 12, 1933	Accident
Svebakken, Otto O.	Decorah	59	Jan. 12, 1934	Automobile accident
Thomas, Samuel W.	Melcher	85	Mar. 6, 1934	Prolonged illness
Thompson, Daniel Whitfield	Council Bluffs	49	Aug. 13, 1933	Prolonged illness
Tilden, Charles George	Kalona	61	Mar. 17, 1933	Following operation
Valenta, Joseph A.	Cedar Rapids	62	Mar. 17, 1934	Heart
Van Werden, William	Des Moines	70	April 18, 1933	Prolonged illness
Weston, Burton French	Mason City	64	Nov. 18, 1933	Acute endocarditis
Wilder, Carleton Victor	Atlantic	82	Feb. 13, 1934	Diabetes mellitus
Wiley, Edward B.	Grinnell	75	Mar. 5, 1934	Prolonged illness
Witt, Max Brauch	Clarinda	74	Jan. 29, 1933	Cerebral hemorrhage
Yenerich, Charles Otis	Rockford	45	Oct. 14, 1933	Prolonged illness
Zinn, George	Klemme	66	Jan. 29, 1934	Coronary Thrombosis

Dr. Erskine: Will you please stand?

The members stood in silent tribute as the names of the deceased members were read by Dr. Erskine.

Dr. Erskine: I *move* that the report be approved.

The motion was regularly seconded, put to a vote and carried.

President Taylor: Committee on Medical Education and Hospitals, Dr. Erskine.

REPORT OF THE COMMITTEE ON MEDICAL EDUCATION AND HOSPITALS

House of Delegates, Iowa State Medical Society:

The Committee on Medical Education and Hospitals was made permanent at the suggestion of the late Dr. B. L. Eiker, who believed that such a committee could serve a useful function as a liaison between those in control of medical education, the Legislature and the State Medical Society. The work of the committee in the past year has been almost entirely submerged in that of the committee commonly known as the "Committee of Nine." Although the medical members of the Committee of Nine tried by means of conciliation, compromise and cooperation to secure such changes in the indigent laws as have been approved by the Iowa State Medical Society, their efforts ended in failure. The reasons for the failure of the Committee of Nine seem to have been a mutual mistrust of motives and a lack of confidence in integrity. It becomes apparent that the usefulness of the Committee on Medical Education and Hospitals is ended. Your committee respectfully requests that it be discharged.

Arthur W. Erskine, Chairman.

Dr. Erskine: I *move* that the report as published in the Handbook be approved and that the request that the Committee be discharged, be granted.

The motion was regularly seconded.

Secretary Parker: This Committee is a Standing Committee of the House of Delegates. The personnel of this Committee, of course, can be discharged, but that Committee still stands because it is a Standing Committee of the House of Delegates. The President-elect appoints the membership of the committee with the approval of the House of Delegates at the Friday morning session.

President Taylor: I will ask for some further information on that. Is that correct? Wasn't there

a modification suggested that this Committee be made a permanent committee by the Committee on Constitution and By-laws? I am asking for information.

Dr. Fay: Mr. President, Dr. Erskine is perfectly right in his desire to be relieved of a committee in which conciliation, compromise and cooperation have meant absolutely nothing. This work that Dr. Erskine has been doing over the last number of years has been a monumental piece of work. It is a work which has analyzed the relationship of our institution at Iowa City and the medical profession of the state of Iowa. This Committee had its conception in the brain, I think, of the late Dr. Eiker. Did it not, Dr. Erskine.

Dr. Erskine: Yes.

Dr. Fay: Arguments for that Committee were put before the House at that time. The idea was that it be a permanent committee corresponding to one of somewhat the same name and function of the American Medical Association. The work of harmonizing the University Medical Department at Iowa City and the Iowa State Medical Society is not complete, and, therefore, a committee which would connect these two things and try to work them out should be continued. Whether Dr. Erskine as an individual should be continued on that committee or not is a thing of his personal feeling. However, as a man trained and as one who understands the art of conciliation, compromise and cooperation, he should be retained upon that committee because he knows more about this than anybody else. He was on the famous, or infamous, Committee of Nine and worked not only hours but days trying to get a report that would be acceptable to all of us. You failed, Art, and so did I, but that does not mean that the committee should be discontinued. I do not think it is within the power of this meeting to do away with the committee because it is a standing committee, and the President-elect has the right to put this in. If you will look at your By-laws you will see it has to be continued as a committee.

But I wish to offer at this time, or would like to have the chairman offer at this time, some expression of thanks to Dr. Erskine, and Drs. Bert Eiker and A. V. Hennessy, now dead. They have never had any recognition, not even so much as thanks for the work they have done on this committee.

I therefore *move* you, Mr. Chairman, that the living chairman and the two dead men be offered the thanks of this organization for the monumental work they have done in the past.

Dr. Spilman: I *second the motion.*

President Taylor: You have heard the motion that the House of Delegates render its thanks to this committee or to the originators of this idea, Drs. Eiker, Hennessy and Erskine. So many as favor this motion will signify by saying "aye;" contrary "no." *It is carried.*

Dr. Parker will read a record that went into the Society's proceedings in 1932.

Secretary Parker: Friday morning session, May 6, 1932, under unfinished business: "Dr. Suchomel moved that the Medical Education and Hospitals Committee be made a Standing Committee of the Society. The motion was seconded and carried."

President Taylor: So, Dr. Erskine, that solves the matter as to the discontinuance of the Committee. They may discontinue you but not the Committee.

Dr. Erskine: Perhaps the motion was not made correctly. If the House of Delegates can make a committee, they can also discontinue a committee.

I *move* you, Mr. President, that the Committee on Medical Education and Hospitals be discontinued.

President Taylor: That would be a modification of the By-Laws.

Bob says it is in the By-Laws. Is that right?

Dr. Erskine: No, I don't think so.

Secretary Parker: Mr. Chairman, the Standing Committees of the House of Delegates are listed under that one head in the By-Laws.

Dr. Erskine: I should like to have the Secretary read the section in the By-Laws that says the Committee on Medical Education and Hospitals is a Standing Committee of the House of Delegates.

Secretary Parker: Mr. Chairman, our Constitution and By-Laws has not been reprinted since 1930, but the matter of record was made from this resolution in 1932. Chapter VIII of your By-Laws, under Committees, says: "The Standing Committees shall be as follows: Committee on Scientific Work, Committee on Public Policy and Legislation, Committee on Publication, Committee on Necrology, Committee on Nominations, Committee on Arrangements,

Medico-Legal Committee, Committee on Constitution and By-Laws, the Finance Committee," and then was added "Medical Education and Hospitals Committee." That is to be in the revised Constitution and By-Laws.

Dr. Suchomel: The amendment to the list of committees of the House of Delegates read by the Secretary, covering the Committee on Medical Education and Hospitals, was offered at the 1931 session here in Des Moines and laid over for a year and was finally acted on at Sioux City.

President Taylor: I think the ruling will be, Dr. Erskine, that this Committee is a part of the permanent committees now, and a change would have to be offered by the Constitution and By-Laws Committee in order to change the status of the Committee. That would be my ruling.

Dr. Bush: What is the status of the motion where he asked to be relieved? I ask for a rising vote on that.

President Taylor: If I understand it correctly, I rule that he cannot be relieved, that the motion he made was out of order, because it would be a constitutional change. Dr. Erskine has just asked if a change in the By-Laws may be offered right now and acted upon next Friday. I have given him that privilege. He may write it up if he sees fit and present it some time during this session unless there is some objection to taking that step.

Dr. Peck: If you will note the report of the Committee on Constituton and By-Laws, this matter may be voted upon Friday and very easily settled at that time, because that motion of Dr. Suchomel's at Sioux City in 1932 was a simple resolution, and there had never been an amendment prepared to cover that point in the By-Laws. That has been done this year, and it appears in that report. So if you wish to dispense with the Committee on Medical Education and Hospitals, it will be very easily done Friday morning in that way.

President Taylor: Does that satisfy you, Dr. Erskine?

Dr. Erskine: Yes.

President Taylor: Reports of Special Committees of the House of Delegates. Medical Library Committee, Dr. Hennessy of Calmar.

Dr. Hennessy: The Librarian will make the report.

Reports of Special Committees

REPORT OF THE MEDICAL LIBRARY COMMITTEE

Report of the Iowa State Medical Library for the past twelve months. Submitted to the Iowa State Medical Society, April, 1934.

Requests for literature...................................... 3,013
Pieces of literature loaned................................. 12,179
Pieces of literature borrowed from other libraries........ 42
Letters written 1,350
Cards written 1,245

Visitors in the Library..................................... 2,216
Telephone calls coming in (long distance ?)............... 700

Cards made for new acquisitions—book file........ 2,615
                              journal file ... 118
                              reprint file 8,476
                                                ———————
                                                11,209   11,209
Periodicals received by subscription regularly.......135
                         by gift 77
                                                ———————
                                                 212   212
Accessioned volumes in the Library June 30, 1933.........17,036
    (Increase of 1,323 since July 1, 1932)

library have that $700 back? Then, second and last, I want you to remember that the medical library is yours. If you have a paper to prepare or a rare or unusual case, the more rare the better, let me look up all similar cases for you or make a bibliography, and the library is yours. As I look at you, I have faith that you are going to do this, because I feel as if already I have been among friends all day.

I thank you, Dr. Hennessy, for this courtesy, and I thank you, Mr. President. (Applause.)

President Taylor: Do you have any further report to make, Dr. Hennessy?

Dr. Hennessy: No.

President Taylor: Committee on Medical Economics, Dr. Cornell of Knoxville.

REPORT OF THE MEDICAL ECONOMICS COMMITTEE

House of Delegates, Iowa State Medical Society:

During the current year the Medical Economics Committee has had no matters referred to it that necessitated a meeting.

Most of the current economic problems are those pertinent to the National Recovery Act and its program, particularly the various projects of the Federal Emergency Relief Administration, and provision has been made for the various medical phases of the same.

In the matter of fees for services to CWA employees under the U. S. Employees' Compensation Commission, the regulations state that "the commission will settle all reasonable charges for fees not in excess of these charged patients in the same income class as the injured person." It is quite gratifying to this committee to know that the minimum fee bill for compensation cases as drawn up by it and adopted by the House of Delegates in 1933, is being used as a standard.

Rather recently one or two new collection agencies have sought advertising space in the State JOURNAL. When it was explained that the standardization tests previously drawn up by this committee and still in force must be met and in addition that the approval of the members of the present committee must be secured, they immediately lost interest.

Two members of the Medical Economics Committee attended the Northwest Medical Conference held at St. Paul in February. Many valuable ideas and much new information pertinent to the field of Medical Economics were obtained.

This committee, though only in its infancy (1929 marked its inception), has done its best to render a worth while service to the brethren of Organized Medicine. It is quite cognizant of the fact that a united effort is essential for settling differences among ourselves and solving our mutual problems, and, last but not least, for showing the laymen that we are united to supervise and direct our own economic affairs.

Corwin S. Cornell, Chairman

Dr. Cornell: I *move* that the report of the Medical Economics Committee as printed in the Handbook be approved.

Dr. Spilman: I *second the motion.*

The motion was put to a vote and carried.

President Taylor: Committee on History, Dr. Walter Bierring.

REPORT OF THE HISTORICAL COMMITTEE

To the House of Delegates:

During the past year interesting and valuable data pertaining to the developing of medical practice in Iowa have been published in the department of the History of Iowa Medicine in the JOURNAL.

The History of Medicine in Lucas County by Drs. Tom Morford Throckmorton and Tom Bentley Throckmorton has been completed and represents a most complete and accurate historical account of medical events in this county.

Similar histories are being prepared in Black Hawk, Jackson and Des Moines counties which will be published during the coming year. The publication of the history of the State Board of Health begins in the May JOURNAL and will be completed in two succeeding issues.

The committee will appreciate any biographical data, photographs or other information regarding Iowa physicians of the pioneer period.

Walter L. Bierring, Chairman
Frank M. Fuller
Tom B. Throckmorton
John T. McClintock
Henry B. Young

Dr. Bierring: If the other members of the Committee are agreeable, I should like to *move* that the report as printed in the Handbook be approved.

The motion was regularly seconded, put to a vote and carried.

President Taylor: Committee on Military Affairs, Dr. Suchomel.

REPORT OF COMMITTEE ON MILITARY AFFAIRS

House of Delegates, Iowa State Medical Society:

Your Committee on Military Affairs has done a bit of investigating of the activities of Medical Department Reserve Officers in the State of Iowa. There are a large number of Medical Reserve Officers in this state, and due to the decrease in appropriations for active duty training in the various summer camps, very few are given the opportunity for field training. The War Department does, however, give the Medical Reserve Officer an opportunity to keep abreast with recent changes and developments in Medico-Military affairs.

We are all acutely aware of the general unrest throughout the world, and it would not surprise anyone if the needed spark to start another world war might be applied at any time. Our experiences in the last World War proved to us that we were unprepared, not only in the combat branches but in medical equipment, as well. Most of the Medical Reserve officers who hold commissions as a reward, in part, for their World War service, have not turned a hand in keeping abreast with the developments in their branch of service. There is as much difference between the organization and tactics of the Medical Department today and that of the World War, as there is between night and day. Chemical warfare and mechanization have influenced the organization and tactics of all branches of the service. We are enabled to keep up to date with these changes, through the Extension Courses offered by the War Department to every Reserve Officer. The Office of Medical Instructor of the Seventh Corps Area informs your committee that of all of the reserve officers in the Medical Department in the State of Iowa, only 111 are enrolled in extension courses. These are distributed at follows: Medical, 53, Dental 37, Veterinary 9, Medical Administrative 7, Sanitary 3, and Civilian 2. These 111 officers have completed 2,887 hours of credit as follows: Medical, 1,081, Dental 996, Veterinary 176, Medical Administrative 318, Sanitary 316, Civilian 20.

Your committee recommends to the Reserve Officers who are members of the Iowa State Medical Society, that they avail themselves of the opportunities to keep abreast of the times, and at the same time renew their eligibility for promotion.

The Military Surgeons Club of the Iowa State Medical Society met at the Hotel Fort Des Moines, on May 10, 1933. There was a total attendance of 54. Our guest speaker was Major Harding Polk, Cavalry, U. S. A., who spoke on the subject: "The Need for National Defense." Dr. Earl Bush of Ames was the toastmaster of the evening. We were also honored by the presence of Major General Matt Tinley of Council Bluffs, Iowa. Election of officers for the year 1933-34 resulted as follows: Chairman, Thos. F. Suchomel, Captain, Medical-Reserve, Cedar Rapids; vice chairman, Harold A. Spilman, Lieutenant-Colonel, Medical-Reserve, Ottumwa; secretary-treasurer, A. C. Conaway, Colonel, Medical-Reserve, Marshalltown. The Club then passed a resolution, endorsing the National Defense Act of 1920, and urging the Senators and Representatives from Iowa to support an increase in the Regular Army to 165,-000 men and 14,000 officers, and a continuance of the Reserve Officers Training Corps, and the Citizens Military Training Camps. The next meeting of the Club will be held in Des Moines, Iowa, May 9, 1934.

Thomas F. Suchomel, Chairman

Dr. Suchomel: I *move* that the report as printed in the Handbook be accepted.

Dr. Spilman: *I second the motion.*

The motion was put to a vote and carried.

President Taylor: Committee on Child Health and Protection, Dr. Fred Moore.

of local committees to whom these questions should be referred. It was suggested that this Committee might be the county society's Committee on Child Health and Protection. The name is not so important except that it may indicate that the Society is alert and responsive to the layman's interest in child health. This could be made quite worth while for publicity purposes and the value of favorable publicity for organized medicine should not be overlooked. More important is the appointment of such committees and notification to the offices of the State Health Department and the Iowa State Medical Society of the personnel so that the references can be made directly and without loss of time. This gives your County Medical Society opportunity to review proposed programs for your own communities, to approve, make suggestions for modifying, or disapprove them. It gives your county society a voice in determining economic and other arrangements which are developed for medical and health education activities in your own counties. It gives you a voice in the selection of medical men who may be invited into your community by lay groups and gives you some control over the conditions under which such visitors appear.

Reports from the State Department indicate that the plan is working with satisfaction. Reports from some of the doctors in communities where the requests have been referred indicates that the doctors have found satisfaction in it. Two weeks ago the chairman of the committee appeared before the Central Division of the State P. T. A. which was in session at Ames, to advise them of this plan. One of the women on the program described the procedure followed in her home community in the conduct of the summer round-up examinations in conjunction with the P. T. A. The procedure which she described conformed exactly to that which is advised by this Committee. The handling of the medical phases of the program was placed in the hands of the local medical society and judging from her report, was done entirely to their satisfaction. I asked her to state how this plan had been determined. Was it suggested to them from outside or was it arrived at from within? She told her audience that it was entirely from within, arrived at only after numerous and painful efforts in which the medical profession was not consulted except that it was requested to provide service. She seemed to feel that their troubles had disappeared when they asked the medical profession to join them in the solution of their problem. Finally they have arrived at the point where they consult the local county society, tell them their desires, discuss with them the desirability of their objectives, how they shall be attained, and the basis of participation by the doctors. These are some of the objectives which this Committee is fostering in the development of projects in child health and protection.

To further this end the Committee and the office personnel of the State Society have taken every opportunity to present this plan before county and district societies, parent-teacher organizations, educational groups, etc. The Farm Bureau organization sent announcements to this effect to sixteen hundred township chairmen in the state.

Literature of the Bureau of Child Health and Health Education

The Committee has given much consideration to the publications of the Bureau. After consultation with the Commissioner of Health, Dr. W. L. Bierring, and his assistants, Drs. Kinnaman and Swift, it was agreed that the Committee would review all the publications that the Bureau has for distribution and offer criticism and advice to the State Department regarding them. The State Department agreed to distribute only those which receive the approval of the Committee, provided that these may bear the stamp of approval by the Committee of the Iowa State Medical Society on Child Health and Protection. This of course was very acceptable.

Twenty-seven pieces of literature have been submitted by the Bureau to the Committee. These vary in length from a leaflet to pamphlets of forty to fifty pages. Each member of the Committee read all of these, presented his criticism on details and his general reactions to the publications as a whole. All comments were passed from one member of the committee to another. Finally each member of the Committee prepared his individual ballot on all the literature classifying each piece in one of three groups as follows:

To be distributed upon request,
To be distributed upon request of physician only,
Not to be distributed in present form.

This ballot was prepared and presented to the Bureau with all the individual comments of the Committee,—the unexpurgated comments. The Bureau appreciated this service and is guided by it. Of the twenty-seven items of literature the majority of the Committee regarded:

Twenty-one as suitable for distribution upon request,

Four as suitable for distribution upon request of physician,

Two as not suitable for distribution in present form.

This was accomplished insofar as was possible by correspondence. Finally the Committee was called together with the members of the State Department for an afternoon session in Des Moines. All were present. The meeting was very satisfactory and made it possible to iron out many details which otherwise would have been quite impossible. Perhaps the subject best known to the members of the House is the "prenatal letters." The Committee voted unanimously that they should be distributed upon request of physician only. The State Bureau has been operating on that basis since the Committee reported to the Bureau.

One of the stumbling blocks was the form for consent for immunization which the Bureau was using in promotion of immunization campaigns. This was revamped so that it places emphasis on the personal responsibility for having this done by the parents' own physician. It is a "double-barreled" arrangement in which the parent may indicate his choice,—private physician or group immunization. In either choice the right of the physician to compensation for his services is recognized. The Committee does not believe it possible to state a consent slip in such manner as would be applicable to all the various arrangements for immunization that may be arranged within the borders of the state, or wholly acceptable to all the varying points of view of the different people involved. For example, take the person who would have all school children immunized under direction of school authorities and compare his point of view with that held by sound medical opinion that immunization against smallpox should be completed within the first six months of life and protection against diphtheria in the second six months. No consent slip could be equally satisfactory to both such persons or groups.

The State Bureau has certain literature from the Federal Children's Bureau for distribution. The Committee voted this for distribution upon request because it is available to anyone who makes request for it from the Washington offices. Dr. Kinnaman objects to this with apparent propriety. He regards the action of the Committee as inconsistent if it fails to criticize the Federal bulletin with the same standards as those applied to the State Bureau. He makes the pertinent criticism that the Committee is unfair in its attitude and action if it disapproves a statement in a state publication and permits tacit approval of the same statement in Federal publications. He has expressed himself as ready to forward the Committee criticisms on Federal publications to the Children's Bureau and omit distribution of any that do not have the approval of the Committee. Action of the Committee sometime during this session will determine if it possesses the jewel of consistency.

Drs. Swift and Kinnaman advised the Committee that the State Department of Health contemplates requesting at the next session of the state legislature, restoration of sufficient funds in the Department budget to provide free Wassermann testing for practitioners. The Committee expressed itself as favorable to such a request. If the State Department does include such funds in its next budget, the Committee urges that the House of Delegates and the Council support the Department in such asking.

The Committee feels that its activities overlap those of the following committees: (1) Speakers Bureau, (2) Medical Economics, (3) Public Relations, and (4) Newspaper Publicity. Even so, it believes that its accomplishments have been worth while. The Committee is unanimous in the opinion that all activities of these several committees should be closely coordinated through the Council. It is only by so doing that the most desirable ends can be accomplished through organized medicine.

The Committee requests the advice of the House of Delegates and recommends that the activities in which it has been engaged shall be continued.

Fred Moore, Chairman
J. D. Boyd
H. E. Farnsworth
L. F. Hill
E. D. Plass

ture was so classified. The prenatal letters, to which many members of the profession have taken exception, have since been distributed only upon the request of the physician, and we hope that that is a satisfactory solution for that particular problem.

The activities of this Committee overlap, necessarily, with the functions and influences and activities of the Speakers Bureau and Public Relations and Medical Economics Committees. This Committee feels that there was very great value last year in tying the activities of this Committee into the Council. You know it is a Committee of the House of Delegates; still by action last year we were associated with and made responsible to the Council. That has been very helpful because it helps to unify the objectives and procedures of the various committees and keep them from going off at cross-purposes.

There is one paragraph of this report to which I want to call your attention particularly, on page 46:

"Drs. Swift and Kinnaman advised the Committee that the State Department of Health contemplates requesting at the next session of the state legislature, restoration of sufficient funds in the Department budget to provide free Wassermann testing for practitioners. The Committee expressed itself as favorable to such a request. If the State Department does include such funds in its next budget, the Committee urges that the House of Delegates and the Council support the Department in such asking."

I read that paragraph particularly because in submitting this report to you and recommending its adoption, I should like a ruling from the Chair, first, to know whether or not, if the report is adopted in its present form, that is equivalent to the support of the House of Delegates in such a budget action by the Department of Health.

President Taylor: I would rule, Dr. Moore, that, unless there are objections, the House of Delegates will accede to your request and that it will become a part of your report. Are there any objections? Now would be the time to register them.

Dr. Spilman: Is that for all Wassermanns?

Dr. Moore: That is a detail to be worked out. They were contemplating including money in their budget for that purpose. That would come up before another meeting of this Society, so that is the primary reason for bringing this out at this time.

Question: Where it is contemplated that the work be done, in the various laboratories?

Dr. Moore: That would be another detail to be worked out by the State Department.

Dr. Spilman: Is that to replace the present charge of one dollar that is made?

Dr. Moore: Yes. Formerly we had that service. Then it was taken away. We pay one dollar for each test we ask for. I take it that is equivalent to asking for the restoration of the former service.

Mr. President, I submit the report and *move* its adoption.

The motion was regularly seconded.

President Taylor: You have heard the report with the recommendation that this special report be included in what has already been printed. Are there any remarks?

Dr. Harkness: Do you think, Dr. Moore, that it will cut off all local clinical laboratories and they will have no opportunity to do Wassermanns, that this will be free for all people?

Dr. Moore: I suppose it would undoubtedly take some revenue away from them.

Dr. Harkness: I sometimes wonder if we do not overlook small groups in our profession. If we as a large group were affected we would be up in arms if they were going to take the money away from us. There are not very many clinical pathologists or men running clinical laboratories, but it should be our purpose to protect the minority just the same as the large group. It seems to me we ought to be a little bit slow about advocating free Wassermanns for everybody without any restrictions at all.

Dr. Moore: May I add, Mr. Chairman, that the discussion in the Committee on this particular thing, I will frankly say, did not consider the thing from any other point of view except that of the general public health and the desirability of having more Wassermann tests made than are made at the present time. The discussion was wholly in the interest of finding prevalent syphilis, that it might be brought under treatment. The feeling was that much more of it is found with that privilege than is found without it.

Dr. Swift: The thought back of that was this, that one of the functions of the State Health Department is to render a service to the physicians that they cannot render themselves. The idea was that, due to the fact that the doctor may have to go down in his own pocket to pay one dollar for a Wassermann, it prevented a great many Wassermanns that would otherwise be made.

We had in mind, of course, the Wassermann for the indigent patient, with the idea that ten per cent of our syphilis in the state of Iowa is congenital, and with free Wassermanns it might be possible, in the course of time, to have a Wassermann on every pregnant woman, which would assure her the possibility of treatment and a clean baby.

Under present conditions, charging one dollar for a Wassermann, they have fallen off at the state laboratory. The idea, of course, was primarily that if a doctor felt a patient should have a Wassermann he could have that without cost to himself. That was the idea of the proposition.

Dr. McNamara: This has been up before the American Clinical Pathologists repeatedly. If it is all right to do laboratory work in state medicine, why not all medicine? I am trained to do Wassermanns. We cannot even pay to feed the sheep we have to use in doing the Wassermann test, simply because we are in competition with the state laboratory. If they can find out where syphilis is and can correct it by free Wassermanns, we are for it, but

can they do it? You cannot find out where syphilis is in this state because it is kept dark, every doctor here knows it. Give us at least what it costs to do the Wassermann. The state thought it cost one dollar, but then the Wassermanns dropped off.

If you are going to give it for nothing, why not go all the way down the line and have state medicine, which we are all opposed to. That is the first wedge in state medicine. If it is good for laboratory work, then it is good for everything in medicine. I admit that as a public health measure it is perfectly good, if you have a full-time health director and he checks on indigent patients, or any patient as a public health measure, then there should be a place available where he can have the work done for nothing, as it is in our county. But if it is a private patient, and it is a diagnostic procedure and the patient is able to pay, he should pay for his Wassermanns just the same as for a nose and throat examination. (Applause.)

Dr. Moore: Mr. Chairman, I should like to ask a question by way of information. It seems to be readily conceded that since charging one dollar for the Wassermann at the state laboratories the number of Wassermanns done has decreased. Would it be fair to ask the men who are doing laboratory work if, with the decrease of Wassermanns done in the state laboratory, there has been an increase in income to them for Wassermanns in their own private laboratories?

Dr. Harkness: We do all of ours at home. Every indigent patient is given a Wassermann test. Every case that comes into our clinic has a Wassermann. Our own men get the benefit of it.

Dr. Hanna: I can say the same thing for Des Moines County. We are supporting a laboratory down there. We feel that all this work is necessary to keep the laboratory working in order to maintain good laboratory work. Personally I am opposed to the inclusion of free Wassermanns.

Dr. Bush: I wonder how many counties there are in the state that maintain laboratories. I think there are about thirty-five county contracts.

Secretary Parker: There are more than that.

Dr. Bush: Thirty-nine. About five or six are on a large enough scale so they can have a laboratory. The other twenty-eight or twenty-nine of us pay one dollar each for each indigent patient. It comes out of our pockets, because we have agreed to do that. It seems to me there should be a happy medium. My bill last month was eight dollars. That comes out of my pocket. Two-thirds of that was for indigent patients. If we get a flat rate, that is included. I personally would like to see us keep the laboratories running. I think it is essential for the organization, but I am getting tired of this dollar stuff. Personally, I think that about twenty-eight or twenty-nine of these county men who have these contracts are likewise situated.

It would seem to me that there should be some way worked out so that we fellows who do not have laboratories at hand could be remitted that dollar. With the man who is favored and given a lot of county work, that can run into quite an item during the year. I do not know that it is going to hurt me much, but I get tired of paying seven or eight dollars every month when I feel that it should be done free because it is indigent work that I am doing, and I do not have any other facilities to get it.

President Taylor: Let the county pay for it.

Dr. Bush: We do not have control of the supervisors as you fellows seem to have. We do not seem to be able to do that.

Dr. Hanna: Get control.

Dr. Bierring: Mr. President, may I have the privilege of the floor for a moment to say that perhaps this was premature. I think the Committee has the best of intention in proposing this, but I believe we should confer with Dr. Barnes, who is the Director of the State Hygienic Laboratory. Possibly if you referred this in some way, either to a committee or to your Legislative Committee, I am sure there will be a full conference to determine whether this is practical or not, and you will be advised of it through the columns of the JOURNAL so that you will have an opportunity to decide it yourselves before the next legislative session.

I believe there is something to be said for both sides. The state has no idea of going into state medicine. I think we proved that during the past year when we changed all the methods with reference to publicity and immunization programs. But we do feel that if this may help the preventive program on congenital syphilis this is one way of doing it. If that is the only way you can get Wassermanns made, it is a proper form of preventive medicine to be conducted on a community or large basis.

President Taylor: I think the only thing to do, if there is no further discussion on this question, is to vote first on the question as proposed by Dr. Moore, as to whether we approve of his report as published in the Handbook and include in that his supplemental report that all Wassermanns in the state be done free. If you vote down that report, then we can take up the further question of accepting his report as published and do whatever you see fit with the other. That will be my ruling. Is there a second to the motion?

Dr. Moore: I was going to suggest that we simply change it in this manner: Move the adoption of the report with the exception of that paragraph referring to free Wassermann testing.

I move the adoption of the report with the exception of that paragraph referring to free Wassermann testing and that that be referred to the Committee on Medical Economics.

Dr. Hanna: I second the motion.

President Taylor: You have heard the motion. As many as favor say "aye;" contrary "no." It is approved.

Woman's Auxiliary Committee, Dr. Junger of

Soldier. (Absent.) Is there anybody on that Committee who is ready to report? If not, we will pass to the Committee on Superannuated Physicians, Dr. Amdor of Carbon.

REPORT OF THE COMMITTEE ON SUPERANNUATED PHYSICIANS

House of Delegates, Iowa State Medical Society:

The Committee on Superannuated Physicians was established by resolution adopted at the Annual Session of the House of Delegates in 1930, and instructed to formulate one or more plans for affording adequate aid to superannuated members of our profession in good standing in this Society. At the 1931 session the House of Delegates voted to adopt the plan suggested by the then chairman of the committee, the late Dr. W. L. Hearst; namely, that each member of the Society be sent one hundred printed seals and asked to contribute in return one dollar toward a fund for the aid of indigent physicians. This plan, however, was never carried out, and in its 1932 report, the committee expressed the opinion that the proper source for aid to indigent members of the organization would be the American Medical Association. The matter has been discussed at annual meetings of the American Medical Association, but no affirmative action has been taken. We cannot, therefore, expect financial assistance for our needy members from the national Association.

Your committee has been somewhat embarrassed during the past year by the receipt of three requests for aid, and the absence of any designated fund, or instructions for raising such a fund, to meet these emergencies. In one instance, which seemed to the committee of sufficient urgency to require emergency action without the customary constitutional provision, we asked the Board of Trustees to assist us by appropriating the sum of twenty-five dollars per month for the relief of a truly needy physician. The Board of Trustees, recognizing the emergency, consented to assume the responsibility of appropriating this amount from the reserve fund of the Society, up to the month of May, or until such time as definite action could be taken by the House of Delegates. The total amount thus expended, from January to May, has been $100.00. At this time we would ask the House of Delegates to approve this request of your committee and the action of the Board of Trustees in granting the appropriation.

On July 21, 1933, your committee sent a letter to each county society secretary, asking for a report of any indigent member of the Society.

On November 9 a questionnaire was sent to the secretary of each state medical association, in an effort to ascertain what other associations were doing for their indigent members. Of the forty-two replies received, only five states reported any provision for such aid. The Louisiana State Medical Society has a small fund accumulated from the surplus of the Entertainment Fund for the Annual Sessions. While the Massachusetts State Medical Society has not entered into a program of caring for its needy members, there is an independent organization, called the Massachusetts Medical Benevolent Society, which is able to help ten to twenty physicians or their families each year. The New Hampshire Medical Society two years ago voted to reserve fifty cents of each member's annual dues for a benevolent fund until the income reaches a size practical for use. The Medical Society of the State of Pennsylvania has a Benevolence Fund, inaugurated in 1905 by an allotment of fifteen cents from each member's dues. Only the earnings of the Fund are at present available for distribution and the Committee on Benevolence has solicited subscriptions and legacies to be added to the principal. The West Virginia State Medical Association sets aside one dollar from each member's dues toward its Indigent Fund. It is apparent from the replies received that the great majority of state medical associations have made no provision for their needy members.

Your committee respectfully requests that the House of Delegates at this present Annual Session decide in the first place, whether it wishes to continue its present policy of providing financial aid to indigent physicians. In this connection we would suggest that the recently enacted Iowa Old Age Pension Law might well receive attention in your discussion of the subject. In order that the House of Delegates may go on record as approving or rejecting the present policy, we would ask your careful and thorough consideration of the following resolution:

RESOLVED: That the Iowa State Medical Society continue its present policy of providing financial aid to indigent members of the Society.

In the event that the House of Delegates approves the foregoing resolution, we would ask that you further consider definite means of providing funds for the use of the Committee on Superannuated Physicians. Your present committee is unanimous in the opinion that a fund, if provided, should be established by appropriation from Society income, and not by solicitation of added contributions from members. In compliance with Chapter IX, Section 3 of the by-laws ("All motions or resolutions appropriating money shall specify a definite amount, or so much thereof as may be necessary for the purpose indicated, and must be approved by the Board of Trustees before being presented for final action to the House of Delegates"), we have suggested to the Board of Trustees that not more than $500.00 be appropriated annually for this purpose (based upon approximately twenty-five cents of each member's dues). The Board of Trustees has approved this amount. We present for your approval or rejection the following resolution:

RESOLVED: That an amount not to exceed $500.00 be appropriated annually by the Board of Trustees from the current year's income of the Society, to be used at the discretion of the Committee on Indigent Physicians for providing aid to needy members of the Society.

In formulating a plan for distribution of this fund, your committee is agreed that recipients of Society aid should be only those indigent members of the profession who have been affiliated with and have actively supported organized medicine; but that no definite age limit should be set, or no definite requirements made as to duration of membership. We submit for your approval the following proposed plan:

Upon receipt of a request for aid for an indigent physician, a standard comprehensive questionnaire shall be sent to the secretary of the county medical society of the physician's membership. The questions contained therein shall be answered, not by one member or officer of the county society, but by vote of the society. If, when the questionnaire has been answered, it is the consensus of the county society that the physician in question is entitled to aid from the State Society, the completed questionnaire and a formal request for aid shall be submitted to the Committee on Superannuated Physicians. Careful consideration of all aspects of the case shall be given by the committee and a favorable decision shall require unanimous vote of the committee. The committee having so voted, shall decide the amount of financial aid suitable in the case, and shall request the Board of Trustees to approve and appropriate that amount from the established fund.

W. F. Ambor, Chairman

Dr. Amdor: Mr. President, the first part of this report is purely a record of history. I believe I had better read this:

"Your Committee has been somewhat embarrassed during the past year by the receipt of three requests for aid, and the absence of any designated fund, or instructions for raising such a fund, to meet these emergencies. In one instance, which seemed to the Committee of sufficient urgency to require emergency action without the customary constitutional provision, we asked the Board of Trustees to assist us by appropriating the sum of twenty-five dollars per month for the relief of a truly needy physician. The Board of Trustees, recognizing the emergency, consented to assume the responsibility of appropriating this amount from the reserve fund of the Society, up to the month of May, or until such time as definite action could be taken by the House of Delegates. The total amount thus expended, from January to May, has been $100. At this time we would ask the House of Delegates to approve this request of your Committee and the action of the Board of Trustees in granting the appropriation."

I so move, Mr. President.

Dr. Spilman: I second the motion.

President Taylor: You have heard the motion. So many as approve the request of the Committee and the action of the Board of Trustees authorizing the payment of $25 a month for four months, a total of $100, which was not covered by any regulations, will signify by saying "aye;" contrary "no." The action has been approved.

Dr. Amdor: Some of the rest of this is a matter of record of other state societies that I won't read.

"Your Committee respectfully requests that the House of Delegates at this present Annual Session decide, in the first place, whether it wishes to con-

matically be cut out of the old age pension. Is that right?

President Taylor: Has anybody an answer to that?

Member: This is only $500 for the whole state.

Dr. Bendixen: It is $500 at the present time. What is going to be the limit in the future? The next thing I should like to know from Dr. Amdor is whether or not we are going into the insurance game. There is no limit if you start on something like that. To start with, I do not think it is legal.

Secretary Parker: Chapter IX, Section 3, of the by-laws says: "All motions or resolutions appropriating money shall specify a definite amount, or so much thereof as may be necessary for the purpose indicated, and must be approved by the Board of Trustees before being presented for final action to the House of Delegates."

Therefore, I *move* that this resolution is out of order.

The motion was regularly seconded.

President Taylor: No motion is necessary. It is ruled out of order according to that.

Dr. Erskine: Mr. President, the report of the Committee says the Board of Trustees has approved this amount.

President Taylor: I am not ruling on that; that has already been voted. I am ruling on this motion of allowing $500 to be used in the future for indigent physicians.

Dr. Erskine: Mr. President, your Committee says in its report that the Board of Trustees have approved the $500.

Dr. Harkness: Isn't the only solution to this to refer this to the Board of Trustees? They will meet between now and Friday before the House of Delegates takes final action.

Dr. Erskine: Did they or didn't they approve it?

President Taylor: We have not approved the report of this Committee as yet. We have been discussing all sorts of things and ruling some things out of order because they were illegal, as I believe, one of those things being the fact that it was not properly presented.

I will call at this time for a motion to approve or disapprove the report of this Committee.

Dr. Amdor: I *move* that the Committee's report as published in the Handbook be approved.

The motion was regularly seconded.

President Taylor: You have heard the motion that we approve the report of the Committee as published in the Handbook? Is there any discussion on this approval? That includes everything in that report.

Dr. Erskine: That approves this thing that you just ruled out of order?

President Taylor: If we approve of this report, my ruling would be that we approve of the report as is, whatever is in there. It is up to you to approve the report or not, as you see fit.

Dr. Sternberg: Is it possible to have that report read again? I don't know what is in that report.

Dr. Fay: Mr. President, this thing has taken a very peculiar angle. The Board of Trustees individually agreed to approve a $500 appropriation. Dr. Myers was going to present that before this House and make the statement very clearly (and I will do that for him now) that in approving that amount it does not mean that we approve of the scheme of appropriating $500. Do you get the distinction?

If the House of Delegates sees fit to continue this Committee, to go into the insurance business, to do all the things suggested in that report, certainly the Board of Trustees would approve the $500 appropriation. But what Dr. Amdor wants to know and what this House of Delegates ought to know is, what are you doing? Are you going into the insurance game and take care of these people? How many of them are you going to take care of? Who is going to determine whether they are indigent or whether they are not? Who is going to determine how much you shall pay, how long you shall continue to pay it, and whether dependents are going to come in? This Committee has had a request from a doctor who had been taking care of his father, also a physician, for ten years. He found it hard to continue with it. You ruled that down, didn't you, Dr. Amdor? You have that sort of thing coming in.

What Dr. Amdor wants to know is whether or not it is the sense of this organization, first, to enter into the insurance game for superannuated physicians. You can conceive of a man twenty-five or thirty, with a broken back, who has done a lot of work, and who might need to come into the thing and be helped by the Society, if you preferred to do it.

Lest you misunderstand what my own attitude is, I don't think you want to get into this insurance game. That is what I personally think. Just the same, the Board of Trustees will approve the $500 if that is the will of the House of Delegates which is the ruling board of this Society. Do I make myself clear? You ought to straighten out this thing. Dr. Amdor ought to know. Is this one of the standing committees that has to be acted upon?

Secretary Parker: It is a special committee.

Dr. Fay: You can dispose of it now, is that the idea?

Secretary Parker: Yes.

Dr. Fay: You ought to determine whether you want the Committee to continue. If you do continue it, you ought to go into the details of whom you are going to help and what you are going to pay them. I don't know whether $25 a month is enough. We in the Board of Trustees looked at this as an emergency, that it was the right thing to do for this man who had a right to hope for something so long as that was on our books. But, for heaven's sake, dispose of it. Don't leave Amdor up in the air.

President Taylor: I still insist that the only thing we can do is to approve or disapprove of this report.

If we approve it, we accept whatever resolution and recommendation they make. If you disapprove it, then it is another story.

Dr. Amdor: Understand, this Committee neither approves nor disapproves. This is the report we put in there, and we want the action of this House, as Dr. Fay stated. I made that motion simply to get it before the House, if it was in order.

President Taylor: As many as favor the approval of the report of the Committee on Superannuated Physicians as published in the Handbook signify the same by saying "aye;" contrary, "no." *The report is disapproved;* therefore everything in it is disapproved.

Dr. Fay: Is it proper at this time, then, to *move* that this Committee be dismissed and that we are not in the insurance game?

President Taylor: Yes.

Dr. Fay: I *make such a motion,* that the Committee be discharged and that the superannuated physician idea be discontinued.

Dr. Amdor: I *second the motion.*

Dr. Wurtzer: I believe Dr. Amdor had a motion before the House to accept that last paragraph in his report.

President Taylor: The whole report has been thrown into the discard. As many as favor the discontinuance of this Committee will signify the same by saying "aye;" contrary "no." *The Committee is discontinued.*

Dr. Bendixen: I think a resolution should be made that the Board of Trustees be reimbursed $100, and that would be sanctioned by the House of Delegates in this report.

Dr. Fay: That has already been taken care of.

President Taylor: Are there any other special committees to report?

Dr. Kern: This is the report of the special committee appointed to investigate the Monroe County situation.

Dr. Kern read the report of the committee.

REPORT OF SPECIAL COMMITTEE APPOINTED TO INVESTIGATE MONROE COUNTY SITUATION

House of Delegates, Iowa State Medical Society:

Your committee was created by action of the House of Delegates in session on May 11, 1933. Its function was designated in the following motion, made by Dr. L. R. Woodward, seconded by Dr. H. A. Spilman and carried:

"Moved, that the matter of the Monroe County situation be referred to a committee of three members of the House of Delegates, appointed by the President, with authority to settle the Monroe County situation, and that its decision be accepted as final."

The President, Dr. W. W. Bowen, appointed the following members of the House of Delegates to serve on the committee: Dr. L. C. Kern, Waverly, chairman; Dr. E. B. Bush, Ames, and Dr. R. M. Sorensen, Cumberland. Dr. Sorensen was later called into Civil Conservation Corps service, and Dr. C. B. Taylor, then President, appointed Dr. W. F. Amdor, of Carbon, to replace Dr. Sorensen on the committee.

The committee met at the call of the chairman at the Iowa State Medical Society office on August 21, 1933. By telephone and correspondence a meeting was arranged at Albia, with the Monroe County Medical Society and with Drs. F. N. Bay, T. E. Gutch and G. A. Jenkins, on September 20.

Your committee, with Dr. Sorensen as their guest, met at the Hotel Clark in Albia at noon on September 20. The committee at that time discussed the advisability of employing a stenographer and agreed that the services of a stenographer would not be needed.

In accordance with previous arrangements, your committee, with Dr. Sorensen, met with five members of the Monroe County Medical Society, (Drs. T. R. Castles, S. T. Gray, C. N. Hyatt, T. A. Moran and Burk Powell) and with Drs. F. N. Bay, W. S. Chester, T. E. Gutch and G. A. Jenkins, at the office of Dr. Burk Powell in Albia at 2:00 p. m.

The meeting was called to order by Dr. Kern. It was noted that a stenographer was present. Dr. Bush asked Dr. Kern who the young lady was and what her purpose in the meeting might be. Upon inquiry, Dr. Kern was told that she was the stenographer of the Monroe County Medical Society. A motion was made, within the committee, by Dr. Bush, to the effect that the committee meet with the members of the Monroe County Medical Society, and with Drs. Bay, Chester, Gutch and Jenkins, with Dr. Sorensen present as the guest of the committee, and that all others withdraw from the room. The motion was unanimously carried and the stenographer was asked to leave. Dr. Gray, the President of the Monroe County Medical Society, stated that if the above motion prevailed, the members of the Monroe County Medical Society would withdraw. Dr. Kern then polled the committee vote and ruled to uphold the motion as carried. The members of the Monroe County Medical Society withdrew.

The meeting of the committee was adjourned, to meet again on call of the chairman.

The committee asked permission of the Board of Trustees to employ legal counsel, and their request being granted, met in the offices of the Iowa State Medical Society on January 17, 1934, in consultation with Mr. Gerald O. Blake, attorney. His written opinion is herewith submitted, together with an opinion from Dr. William C. Woodward, Director of the Bureau of Legal Medicine and Legislation of the American Medical Association.

From these opinions it is apparent that the appointment of the committee, being contrary to the provisions of the Constitution and By-laws of the Iowa State Medical Society, was illegal and that any action which it might take would be void and could not be recognized.

Your committee therefore feels that in submitting this report of the foregoing facts it has fulfilled its obligation and duties to the House of Delegates, and that your committee must be considered as automatically discharged.

L. C. Kern, Chairman
E. B. Bush
W. F. Amdor

Des Moines, Iowa.
April 30, 1934.

Dr. L. C. Kern, Committee Chairman,
Iowa State Medical Society,
1122 Bankers Trust Building,
Des Moines, Iowa:

I desire to acknowledge receipt of your request as to the legality of the committee appointed by the House of Delegates under the following motion:

"Dr. Woodward moved that the matter of the Monroe County situation be referred to a committee of three members of the House of Delegates, appointed by the President, with authority to settle the Monroe County situation, and that its decision be accepted as final. Dr. Spilman seconded the motion. Carried."

Under the provisions of Article V of the Constitution, the House of Delegates shall be the legislative and business body of the Society and under the provisions of Section 3 of Chapter XII of the By-laws the sole power to grant or revoke charters to county societies is vested in the House of Delegates.

The Council is designated the Board of Censors of the Society by the provisions of Section 3, Chapter VII of the By-laws and shall hear appeals of members refused membership or who are expelled or suspended from county societies, and at such hearing may hear oral or written evidence and in the event the matter cannot be adjusted through compromise or conciliation, the Council may take such action as it deems necessary relative to reinstatement or may reallocate the member to another society and such decisions would be final. This authority does not extend to the extent of revoking a Society's charter or directing that it be done by the House of Delegates, who, as previously stated, are the sole authorities in whom is vested the power to grant or revoke charters.

It is apparent that provisions of Section 3, Chapter VII of the By-laws and Section 3 of Chapter XII appear to be in conflict, but a thorough examination of the duties and obligations of the two bodies definitely determines that while the matters concerning ethics and conduct are questions for the Council, the extremely vital question of granting or revoking charters is vested in the House of Delegates.

It then becomes necessary to ascertain what authority the committee herein appointed might have under the Constitution or By-laws of the Society. Section 9 of Chapter IV of the By-laws authorizes the appointment of Committees for special purposes by the House of Delegates, but it is apparent that such committees are to act only in an advisory capacity and could not be delegated power which rests solely in the House of Delegates.

Therefore, in view of the wording of the motion hereinbefore set out, I am of the opinion that the appointment of this committee is contrary to the provisions of the Constitution and By-laws and any action taken by the Committee would be void and of no effect.

Trusting this answers your inquiry, I am

Yours truly,
GERALD O. BLAKE,
Attorney at Law.

Chicago, Illinois.
April 21, 1934.

Dr. L. C. Kern, Committee Chairman,
Iowa State Medical Society,
1122 Bankers Trust Building,
Des Moines, Iowa.
My dear Dr. Kern:

Your letter of April 5 was duly received, but the pressure of work prevented an earlier reply. I am sorry.

I.

The By-laws of the Iowa State Medical Society, as revised May 8-10, 1929, in defining the duties of the Council, say:

"It shall hear and decide all questions of discipline affecting the conduct of members, or of a county society, upon which an appeal is taken from the decision of an individual Councilor. Its decision in all such cases shall be final." Ch. VII, Sec. 3.

I can see nothing in that language that authorizes the Council to determine what action the House of Delegates shall take if a decision of the Council is not acquiesced in by the parties to a controversy adjudicated by the Council. Certainly there is nothing in that language authorizing the Council to direct the House of Delegates to revoke the charter of a recalcitrant county medical society. The most the Council can do or should do in case of recalcitrancy is to report the facts to the House of Delegates, with or without recommendation.

The revocation of the charter of a county society is an exclusive function of the House of Delegates under the By-laws:

"The House of Delegates shall have authority to revoke the charter of any component county society whose actions are in conflict with the letter or spirit of this Constitution and By-laws." Ch. XII, Sec. 3.

While the By-laws authorize the House of Delegates to revoke a charter when certain stated conditions are found to exist, it is not compel the House to do so. In event of the continuing of an offense by a county society, after notice to desist and to repair any harm that may have been done has been given, the

House of Delegates could hardly do otherwise than to revoke the charter of the offending society, but certainly the House would be acting within its legitimate discretion if it first served notice on the offending society and gave it an opportunity to conform to the requirements of the Iowa State Medical Society.

II.

I can find no authority for the appointment by the Iowa State Medical Society of a committee to review the action of the Council, *without first amending the By-laws*. The By-laws, as has been pointed out above, give the Council jurisdiction to hear and decide all questions of discipline affecting the conduct of a county society, upon which an appeal is taken from the decision of an individual Councilor, and make the decision of the Council in all such cases final. The appointment of a committee to hear and decide any such question of discipline and to render final judgment would be in derogation of the By-laws, and therefore void.

Authority to amend the By-laws is limited by the By-laws themselves as follows:
"These By-laws may be amended at any Annual Session by a majority vote of all the delegates present at that session, after the amendments have laid upon the table for one day." Ch. XIII.

The resolution under which a committee to review the action of the Council was appointed was adopted at a special session of the House of Delegates, not at an annual session. While the record does not show that, before undertaking to divest the decision of the Council of the finality inherent in it under the By-laws, the House of Delegates undertook to amend the By-laws to enable the House so to do, even if any such action was taken, it was void and of no effect, because the session of the House of Delegates was a special session and the By-laws can be amended only at an annual session.

In anticipation of the possibility that the resolution for the appointment of a committee of review was passed under a *suspension* of the By-laws, it may be stated that any such action would be of at least doubtful validity. If it should be conceded that under ordinary parliamentary procedure for the suspension of the By-laws they could be suspended and action taken entirely inconsistent with such By-laws and continuing beyond the period of suspension, the safeguards of the By-laws with respect to amendments would be meaningless, and the By-laws themselves playthings in the hands of two-thirds of the members present at any meeting, whose votes might suspend the By-laws and impose on all members of the Society, without notice, such conditions as two-thirds of the voting members at the meeting might desire.

III.

If your committee of review were a legally constituted committee, membership on it would not deprive of their votes in the House of Delegates those members of the committee who were in fact members of the House of Delegates and normally entitled to vote. Any rule that deprived such members of their votes would, in effect, deprive county societies of their normal representation in the House of Delegates. There is no reason for making one rule with respect to the voting powers of the members of a committee of review, such as the Society undertook to create, and another rule with respect to the voting power of all other committees—and I assume that it has not been the custom of the Iowa State Medical Society to deny to every member of each and every committee the right to vote on the report of that committee when it came before the Society.

IV.

In my judgment, the appointment of your committee of review is only a meaningless gesture, and the report of your Council is still before your House of Delegates. The fact that your Council has exceeded its authority in directing the House to take certain action may well be ignored and the term "direct" be construed to carry a meaning within the authority of the Council, namely, "recommended."

Yours truly,
WM. C. WOODWARD,
Director, Bureau of Legal Medicine and Legislation,
American Medical Association.

Dr. Kern: I *move* that this report be accepted and the Committee be discharged.

The motion was regularly seconded.

President Taylor: Are there any remarks? Being an illegal committee, as has been definitely told us by authoritative sources, I take it for granted that this is almost a love's labor lost in discharging the committee, but I shall put the motion.

Dr. Harkness: Why was the Committee illegal?

President Taylor: Do you want these opinions? They are long.

Dr. Harkness: Can't you give them to us in a few words?

President Taylor: Dr. Kern can give them to you in a few words.

Dr. Kern: Dr. Taylor and Members of the House

of Delegates: Mr. Blake calls attention to the fact that all special committees must be appointed from the membership and not from the members of the House of Delegates, for this reason: If we submitted a report and it came to a vote we would not be allowed to vote on our own work, and, therefore, our counties would be deprived of their legal right of representation in this House of Delegates. That is practically the basis of the opinion given by Dr. Woodward. That is the thing in a nutshell, because the Constitution and By-laws distinctly state that. They are long opinions.

President Taylor: Does that satisfy you, Dr. Harkness?

Dr. Harkness: I could not hear them.

President Taylor: I will let you read them. As many as favor the acceptance of the report and the discharge of the Committee signify the same by saying "aye;" contrary "no." *It is carried. The report is accepted and the Committee is discharged.*

Memorials and Communications. By the way, we have not yet had a report from the Delegates to the American Medical Association. Dr. Fred Moore.

REPORTS OF THE DELEGATES TO THE AMERICAN MEDICAL ASSOCIATION

Report on Education and Scientific Problems

Various subjects of scientific and educational interest were considered during the Milwaukee session with the emphasis largely upon educational problems.

The House of Delegates adopted the report of the Council on Medical Education and Hospitals on Essentials of an Acceptable Medical School. This report designated certain minimal criteria, which are of general interest: "Nominations for faculty positions should originate in the faculty." In the preclinical sciences there should be at least ten teachers of professional rank and at least one full-time assistant for each twenty-five students in a class in each preclinical department. The school should own or control a general hospital, which "should have a daily average of not less than two hundred patients who can be utilized for clinical teaching". There should be additional facilities for "children's diseases, contagious diseases, and nervous and mental diseases". The school should own or control a well ordered dispensary or out-patient department with an average daily attendance of at least one hundred patients (visits)". "At least fifteen maternity cases should be provided for each senior student". "The number of students to whom an adequate medical education can be given by a college is related approximately to the laboratory and hospital facilities available and to the size and qualifications of the teaching staff". "Facilities should be provided for at least fifty necropsies during each school year."

The competition offered to practicing physicians in some localities by local-medical schools was recognized and a resolution adopted requesting the Council on Medical Education and Hospitals to submit a plan (a) to restrict the amount of clinical material used by medical schools to the amount needed for teaching and research, and, (b) to restrict competitive practice by schools of medicine.

A resolution was offered which would have restricted staff appointments of hospitals approved for interne training to members in good standing of their local county medical societies. The Reference Committee on Medical Education regarded this resolution as an expression of opinion in favor of a standard which should be striven for, and as such approved it, recognizing at the same time that it may not be desirable at present to make it a hard and fast rule.

The problem of an over-supply of physicians was given consideration under two resolutions. In the first instance, no action was taken upon a request to study "the actual yearly need of medical men for our country." On the other hand, a resolution was adopted requesting the Council on Medical Education and Hospitals to study "the medical matriculates and graduates for the purpose of determining annual quotas of admissions for students".

The only suggestion which referred to the curricula of medical schools concerned the advisability of introducing "some training in basic business principles such as will enable graduates to conduct successfully the business of a medical practice". In another similar resolution, this suggestion was broadened to include information on "medical ethics and on the relationship of physicians to patients and to the fundamental purposes and activities of county, state and national organizations". Both were adopted.

The Council on Medical Education and Hospitals was also requested "to (a) evaluate and compare the merits of the curricula of approved medical colleges and those alleged colleges operated by the cults; (b) study a plan to abolish the State Board examinations and in lieu of such examinations to accept a certificate of an approved medical college as to the candidate's training and graduation."

Consideration was given to the function of the American Medical Association through its Council on Medical Education and Hospitals in the general movement for the designation of specialists by certificating boards. After considerable discussion the Council on Medical Education and Hospitals was authorized to express its approval of such special examining boards as conform to standards of administration formulated by the Council, and the Board of Trustees was urged to use the machinery of the American Medical Association, including the publication of its Directory, in furthering the work of such examining boards as may be accredited by the Council. Since these authorizations were given last year, considerable progress has been made in aligning the Council on Medical Education with the various certificating boards, and there is every reason to believe that a completely harmonious cooperation can be developed.

Another item of business, which is of general medical significance, was the adoption of a resolution asking Congress to appropriate $2,000,000 for the construction of new buildings to house the Army Medical Library and Museum adjacent to the Army Medical School and the Walter Reed Hospital.

From the scientific angle there was relatively little of general interest. However, a resolution was adopted sanctioning the appointment of a committee to cooperate with other interested national organizations in securing blood Wassermann tests on all pregnant women with the hope that the treatment of luetic women during pregnancy will reduce the incidence of congenital lues. It was stated that ten per cent of all syphilitic infection is congenital in origin.

Your delegates offered a resolution asking for the appointment of a special committee of five on "The Study of Contraception", the committee to report to the 1934 Executive Session of the House of Delegates. The resolution specifically stated that the appointment of this committee should not be construed as an endorsement of birth control on the part of the A.M.A. This resolution was referred to the Reference Committee on Hygiene and Public Health, which reported, "Your committee is of the opinion that it is proper and desirable that the House of Delegates should have in its possession full and accurate knowledge and information in regard to the subject of Birth Control, which may be used for guidance in such further action as it may wish to consider. The Committee, therefore, recommends the adoption of the resolution." After discussion of a motion to adopt the report, it was laid on the table by a vote of 66 to 46.

E. D. Plass.

Report on Economic, Business and Organization Problems

I have been asked to report on matters of economic, business and organization character, and beg leave to submit the following report:

I. I wish to commend the masterful address of our President, Dr. E. H. Cary. The work which he has done and the principles which he enunciated are so thoroughly in accord with the best thoughts of organized medicine that I urge a perusal of this splendid document by each member of the Society. It appeared in the *Journal of the American Medical Association* June 24, 1933, page 2017. He reviewed the year's accomplishments, calling attention to the successful issues attained: (1) the right of the physician to use his own judgment in prescribing alcoholic liquors; (2) the defeat of Sheppard-Townerism and the substitution of state and local agencies for Federal bureaucracy; (3) the step taken in further control of narcotics through uniform state legislation; (4) the activities of the legislative committee in regard to veterans' care, which, without doubt, exerted marked influence in the recent executive orders affecting the hospitalization of cases not having service origin; (5) endorsement of the Minority Report of the Committee on the Costs of Medical Care and emphasis on the soundness of the principles enunciated; (6) recognition of the need for unity of spirit and professional desire in our county and state societies as a necessary corollary to successful action through our national Association.

II. I endorse the views of the President-Elect in

his interpretation of the attitude the medical profession should take in regard to the care of the veterans.   To this end we would call attention to his
suggestion that after all, the personal contact of the
doctor with his representative in the legislature is
one of the most vital factors in influencing legislation along this line.   The President-elect has well
touched on the cost of medical care and emphasized
an important phase sometimes overlooked in the high
cost of hospital construction, which greatly increases
the cost without increased benefits to the patient.   I
also commend his attitude against questionable forms
of insurance for the care of the sick.   He likewise
admirably states his conviction that merging of hospitals in many communities would lead to better
service to all parties concerned.   He deals with the
limitation of specialism and the simplification of
medical practice, which we believe should provide
for a more satisfactory relationship of medical practice in the light of changes now in progress, especially in medical education.

III. Rules and order of business:

A resolution was adopted: that constituent associations elect their delegates far enough in advance
so that the names of all delegates may be properly
listed in the Handbook of the House of Delegates and
that copies of this resolution be sent to the secretaries
of all constituent associations.

IV. The Reference Committee on Medical Economics presented the following report:

"Your committee has carefully reviewed the report
as published in the Handbook and concurs with the
Bureau that 'the problems that presented themselves
were not all the result of current social and economic
conditions, but were, in some instances, the culmina-
tion of long standing and gradually developing practices.   The schemes which were promulgated in the
guise of cures for certain alleged faults in the administration of medical service represent a rapid
extension of commercialism into the provision of
medical services.'

1. "Your committee appreciates the special consideration that has been given to contract practice and
agrees that this type of medical work is constantly
changing.   It recommends that the study of contract
practice be continued, and the action of county societies in dealing with these problems be based on
the recommendations of the Judicial Council:

"By the term 'contract practice,' as applied to
medicine, is meant the carrying out of an agreement
between a physician or a group of physicians as principals or agents and a corporation, organization or
individual, to furnish partial or full medical services
to a group or class of individuals for a definite sum
or for a fixed rate per capita.

"Contract practice *per se* is not unethical.   However, certain features or conditions if present make a
contract unethical, among which are: (1) When there
is solicitation of patients, directly or indirectly.   (2)
When there is underbidding to secure contracts.   (3)
When the compensation is inadequate to assure good
medical service.   (4) When there is interference with

"Gentlemen: I cannot better indicate to you how this man is esteemed at home than to tell you that our democratic administration, the first we have had in forty years, lean and hungry for pork, turned to this life-long republican and asked him to accept the appointment of Commissioner of Health for the purpose of reorganizing the State Department of Health in conformance to the needs of the public and the standards of organized medicine.

Gentlemen. I am pleased to place in nomination the name of Walter L. Bierring."

Fred Moore

Dr. Moore: Mr. Chairman and Members of the House: It is rather an uncommon privilege for a member of a state society to have the opportunity to promote the candidacy of one of its own members for the highest office which organized medicine in the United States has to offer. It is a rarer privilege to do it and win.

It was a real privilege to promote the candidacy of one from the rank and file of the practitioners of medicine, and that was the real basis on which we offered a member of our own organization. It was a very happy delegation from Iowa when a member of our Society was chosen as President-elect of the American Medical Association.

If you hear more or less kidding about the situation, I think you should be entitled to know just what some of the things refer to. We were organized, perhaps, as a racing stable. We had our horse; we had our trainer; we had our stable boys, and we had our carriers. We had plenty of competition. The rival candidates were Dr. Heckel of Pittsburgh, who has rendered long service to the American Medical Association as Trustee, Dr. Harvey Cushing of Boston, whose reputation is known to all of you, and General Cummings of the U. S. Public Health Service.

We are very pleased to give you this final account of our stewardship. Before presenting Exhibit A, the President-elect of the American Medical Association, I want to make this one statement, that we have not contracted or bought on the installment plan, and any delegate from this Society who goes to the American Medical Association in the future is under no obligations to any delegation from any other state, other than that of good fellowship and good friendship. The President-elect!

The members arose and applauded President-elect Bierring of the American Medical Association.

Dr. Bierring: Mr. President, Officers, Members of the House of Delegates of the Iowa State Medical Society: There are times when it is difficult to say what is in your heart, and you have been so gracious to me in the many years of happy association that I have had with you that there is nothing I can say to you that will, in any sense, give you an idea of how appreciative I am of this further expression of your confidence. That it is pleasing to Iowa is to me the greatest satisfaction.

I suppose, if I might digress into a lighter vein, since there was to be a derby, you had to have a horse, but it takes an awfully good jockey rider to win, and it takes a lot of preparation in the way of currying and other essentials to make him get under the wire. I sort of feel that these essentials and necessaries were mighty well taken care of, and that is where I feel that my friends here in Iowa did so much. It seems an unusual responsibility. One hesitates even to think about what it means in this particular period in the history of our association, but I sort of have the feeling that if I have your sympathy and your good feeling at all times I will do the very best I can to make you feel that you have not been mistaken in your choice.

I feel that what it means to the State Society of Iowa, what it means to the profession of Iowa is a thing that ought to be of greatest gratification to all of us, that someone who was born in the state, who was educated in it and who was educated in it and who had all his experience in it, and that is all he had to offer—if that was enough to make these horsemen win, why I think it was something very unusual.

Again I say in all humility, I thank you. (Applause.)

President Taylor: Is there any new business?

Dr. Suchomel: At the last minute the Linn County Medical Society instructed its delegates to present this matter to you. As you know, there has been a considerable amount of practice of medicine going on in the press that has had detrimental effects on the laymen in general. I wish to present this resolution, together with the information attached:

"Whereas, practice of medicine is being conducted through the lay press by means of syndicated health articles recommending certain types of practice and condemning others, and

"Whereas, the information contained in these syndicated articles is largely misleading and detrimental to the welfare of the layman, be it therefore

"Resolved, that the House of Delegates, through its Committee on Public Policy and Legislation, seek to obtain cooperation of the press in having syndicated articles censored by competent authority before publication."

Mr. President, I *move* the adoption of the resolution.

The motion was regularly seconded, put to a vote and carried.

The meeting adjourned at six o'clock.

Friday, May 11

The second session convened at eight-ten o'clock, President Taylor presiding.

President Taylor: The first order of business is the roll call.

Roll was called. *Motion was made* that Dr. E. E. Morton of Cass County be seated as a delegate. *The motion was regularly seconded, put to a vote and carried.*

Secretary Parker: The roll call at present consists of: Officers, 11; delegates, 48; alternates, 8,

making a total registration of 67. A quorum is present, Mr. President. I *move* that we proceed with the regular order of business.

The motion was regularly seconded, put to a vote and carried.

President Taylor: We will now have the reading of the minutes.

Secretary Parker: Mr. President, I would like permission of the Chair to have the Executive Secretary read the minutes.

There being no objection, an abstract of the minutes of the previous session was read by Mrs. McCarthy, Executive Secretary.

President Taylor: You have heard the minutes of the previous session. Are there any objections to the minutes as read? (There were no objections.) If not, they will stand approved as read.

Secretary Parker: Mr. President, the corrected roll call at this time shows a total of 75—14 officers and 61 delegates and alternates seated.

President Taylor: We will have the report of the Committee on Nominations, Dr. E. B. Bush, Secretary.

Dr. Bush: Mr. President: The following candidates were placed in nomination.

President-elect: Thomas A. Burham, Des Moines, F. M. Tombaugh, Burlington, L. R. Woodward, Mason City.

First Vice President: F. B. Dorsey, Jr., Keokuk.

Second Vice President: J. C. Hill, Newton.

Trustee: Oliver J. Fay, Des Moines.

Third District Councilor, Frank P. Winkler, Sibley.

Eighth District Councilor: C. A. Boice, Washington.

Delegates to A. M. A.: T. F. Thornton, Waterloo, Vernon L. Treynor, Council Bluffs.

Alternate Delegates: R. H. Lott, Carroll, F. P. McNamara, Dubuque.

Meeting Place for 1935: Davenport.

Time: Wednesday, Thursday and Friday of the second week in May, 1935.

The Nominating Committee offers the following resolution for the consideration of the House of Delegates:

"Resolved, that the Iowa State Medical Society assure the Convention Bureau of Des Moines its support in extending an invitation to the American Society for the Study of Goiter to hold its annual meeting in Des Moines at some future date."

President Taylor: You have heard the report of the Nominating Committee. We will now prepare for the election of these officers. You understand that it is perfectly legitimate that any additional nominations may be made for any one of these offices named by the Nominating Committee. Nominations from the floor are in order. Are there any further nominations?

Dr. Fred Moore (Des Moines): Mr. President, I would like to urge continuous representation—by continuous representation, I mean continuation of personnel in representation of this Society in the

President Taylor: I declare them elected.

Now we have a contest. Three names have been presented for delegates to the A. M. A.; T. F. Thornton of Waterloo, Vernon L. Treynor of Council Bluffs, and E. D. Plass of Iowa City.

Dr. T. U. McManus (Waterloo): There has been no contest or question raised at all regarding the nomination of Dr. Thornton. The only nomination made was that of Dr. Plass as against Dr. Treynor.

President Taylor. That is correct.

Dr. McManus: I *move*, unless you rule me out of order, that the secretary be instructed now to cast the unanimous vote of this House for Dr. Thornton.

The motion was seconded.

Dr. Moore: Mr. President: In nominating Dr. Plass from the floor I did not mean to precipitate a contest between any two particular delegates. It was my purpose to present Dr. Plass' name as a candidate and give the reasons for so doing.

President Taylor: You have heard the motion. There is a motion before the House.

Dr. E. B. Bush (Ames): Mr. President, I *offer a substitute motion* that we vote for two men for delegates.

The motion was regularly seconded, put to a viva-voce vote and was apparently lost. On a standing vote *the motion was lost.*

President Taylor: We are ready for the original motion as presented by Dr. McManus.

Dr. John T. Hanna (Burlington): I rise to a point of order. I am wondering how the nomination of one man as a delegate to the A. M. A. can be set off against the one or the other of the names presented by the Nominating Committee. I wish the Chair would explain, please.

President Taylor: The House of Delegates is the authoritative body and it would be my ruling that the House of Delegates can do just what it pleases in this matter; you can call for a vote by ballot if you see fit. Otherwise, I will declare that Dr. Thornton has a right to come into a class by himself by virtue of this vote that has just been taken. If you want a vote by ballot on Dr. Thornton or on that substitute motion, I will be very glad to give it.

Dr. Hanna: The nomination added one name to the two, as I understand it.

President Taylor: That is correct.

Dr. Hanna: The third entry was the candidate running against either of the other two, or, rather, against the one singled out. How that one was singled out, I cannot understand.

President Taylor: By the House of Delegates, would be my ruling. Unless you want to ballot on it to verify it.

Dr. Walter E. Baker (Des Moines): Mr. President, could we have the reading of Dr. Moore's original motion?

Dr. McManus: Mr. President, in the interest of harmony, with the consent of my second, I will *withdraw the motion.*

The seconder of the motion gave his assent and *the motion was withdrawn.*

President Taylor: The field is open. We will vote for the three candidates now running as delegates for the A. M. A., Drs. T. F. Thornton, Vernon L. Treynor, and E. D. Plass. There are now eighty registered delegates and officers.

Ballots were distributed, collected, and counted by the tellers and Secretary Parker.

Secretary Parker: Mr. President, I beg leave to report on this last ballot: Dr. Thornton, 67; Dr. Treynor, 49; Dr. Plass, 38.

President Taylor: According to the ballot Drs. Thornton and Treynor are the delegates to the A. M. A.

We will now elect the alternate delegates to A. M. A.

Dr. Suchomel: Mr. President, I *move* the by-laws be suspended and the secretary be instructed to cast a unanimous ballot for these names, as presented, for alternates.

The motion was regularly seconded, put to a vote, and carried.

Secretary Parker: Mr. President, the vote is so cast.

President Taylor: Dr. R. H. Lott of Carroll and Dr. F. P. McNamara of Dubuque are the alternate delegates to the A. M. A. I declare them elected.

The next order of business will be to select the meeting place for our 1935 meeting. Davenport and Dubuque are the two places on which you are to vote.

Dr. William C. Goenne (Davenport): Mr. President: As one of the delegates from the Scott County Medical Society, and also representing Davenport, Iowa, I wish to tell the delegates that I am just awfully sorry, and feel it is unfortunate that we could hold our yearly meeting in only one city.

Davenport and the members of the Scott County Medical Society have all the respect and all regard for Dubuque's desire to hold the meeting there next year. There has always been a very friendly spirit between the members of the Iowa State Medical Society located in the two cities, and it is just unfortunate that at this time we are both desirous of having our next year's meeting in the eastern part of the state.

Naturally, living in Davenport I am somewhat like the man from Los Angeles who, when he did not know of anything else to speak about, always spoke about Los Angeles.

It is my purpose this morning, in a few words, to tell you what we have in Davenport. We have gone to a great deal of trouble and made surveys as to the facilities we have there to take care of the State Medical Society meeting. We have three first class hotels that are absolutely fireproof in every way, shape and form. There are approximately 600 rooms so that as far as hotel facilities are concerned they are very adequate to take care of any number of men that come.

Further than the three first class hotels we have two that are not first class but are really good hotels. Across the river at Rock Island we have the Fort Armstrong hotel and at Moline we have the LeClair

hotel, so that so far as housing facilities are concerned Davenport is well situated.

In regard to the meetings, the Black Hawk hotel is very adequate to take care of all the meetings that we may possibly have. If it is not adequate we have a Masonic Temple there that is more than adequate. There are plenty of rooms. We have made a survey, have placed chairs in the rooms to see whether the rooms would be crowded or not. The mezzanine floor or the lobby could very well be used for registrations and for the exhibits. There is a director's room that could be used for committee meetings that will accommodate twenty people. We have two rooms that will accommodate sixty—they will possibly take care of ninety, but sixty in comfort. We have two more rooms that will take care of 100 people in comfort and if necessary we can seat 150.

We have two more rooms that will seat 200 people comfortably and if necessary will take 250. We have one large room that will comfortably seat 300 people, and if necessary we can seat 350.

Further than that we have an auditorium that will seat 3,000.

So far as roads are concerned, Davenport is situated on the River Road. It is very easy for anyone who wishes to drive to get there on the hard pavement. Further than that, the Lincoln Highway is situated about thirty miles north so you can use the Lincoln Highway.

I really believe that Davenport is as well situated as any city, and if you do feel you would like to come there, I can assure you, you will be very hospitably received and well taken care of. (Applause.)

Ballots were distributed, collected, and counted by the tellers and Secretary Parker.

Secretary Parker: Mr. President, the result of the ballot is: Davenport 42, Dubuque, 38. There are eighty registered votes, and Davenport has the majority by one vote.

President Taylor: Davenport gets the next convention.

Is Dr. Harkness here? If so, I want him to come to the front. He is from Davenport. I want to introduce to you gentlemen your very soon to be President Dr. Gordon Harkness, the handsome gentleman who now stands before you. (Applause.)

President-elect Gordon F. Harkness: So far as the conventions and the meetings of the Iowa State Medical Society are concerned "you ain't seen nothin' yet." Wait until you come to Davenport! That is all I can say. I talked myself out last night, and I expressed last year my appreciation of the honor you have given me. I can only say that I hope, that I pray, for the cooperation and the support you have given the past presidents of our Society, and I assure you that I will do my utmost to carry out my part. I can do no more. (Applause.)

President Taylor: I think I can speak for the entire organization that it will give Dr. Harkness every support in the world at its command.

Study of Goiter by the House of Delegates would carry considerable weight. For that reason he asked us to present this resolution. I *move* the adoption of the resolution.

The motion was regularly seconded, put to a vote and carried.

President Taylor: To my way of thinking it should have come up as New Business, but it doesn't make any particular difference. The resolution is adopted.

We are ready for reports of Committees.

The report of the Speakers Bureau Committee was not approved the other day. Have you anything further to add?

ncil Committees

stands for clinic. When written together, it means that these meetings were held jointly. The letter "L" designates the lay meetings held in that county; "D" the district meetings held in the district of which that county is a constituent part. The letters "PG" show the number of physicians in the various counties who attended the Speakers Bureau postgraduate courses.

Under the heading "Speakers" the various letters and figures indicate the number of speakers sent out from the various counties to talk at different types of meetings. The letter "S" means that a doctor from that county was asked to address a scientific group; "L" a lay group; "I" an inter-professional group; "PG" a lecture on one of the Bureau postgraduate courses; and "R" to prepare a radio talk. Where there are two sets of figures following a letter, the first indicates the number of speakers used from that county and the second is the number of talks given during the year by those speakers. The letter "C" shows that that doctor conducted a clinic; "SC" means that he conducted a clinic and took part in a scientific meeting as well.

The Speakers Bureau feels that this table shows an excellent distribution of services and speakers throughout the state and that the total figures indicate a busy and successful year for the Bureau. A total of 420 speakers was used to carry out the activities of the Bureau, 131 of whom gave scientific talks, 69 conducted clinics, 118 gave lectures on postgraduate courses, 66 addressed lay audiences and 46 prepared radio talks to be broadcast over WOI and WSUI on the weekly broadcasting period of the Speakers Bureau. Fifty-two scientific meetings were held; ten of which were district meetings, three were group meetings—Iowa Heart Association, Upper Des Moines Medical Society, and the Southwest Iowa Postgraduate Group, and the rest were county medical society meetings. Thirty-one clinics were held, twenty-six of which were chest clinics and five were baby clinics—four in connection with county or township fairs. Postgraduate courses were held in seven centers—Waterloo, Mason City, Ames, Algona, Jefferson, Des Moines and Marshalltown—with the following enrollment respectively: 100, 40, 44, 50, 04, 75, and 55, or a total enrollment of 415 members.

COUNTY	MEETINGS					SPEAKERS				
Adair	SC			D						
Adams				D		S				
Allamakee		L		D(2)						
Appanoose				D(3)						
Audubon										
Benton				D(2)	PG(2)					
Black Hawk		L	I	D(2)	PG(47)	S(2)	L		I(2)	R(2)
Boone	SC	L					L(1)(2)			R
Bremer	SC			D(2)	PG(14)	S-SC	L(2)			R
Buchanan	S	L(2)			PG(4)		L(1)(2)	PG		
Buena Vista		L								
Butler		L		D(3)	PG(2)					
Calhoun					PG(6)		L			
Carroll					PG(4)					R
Cass	S	L(2)							I	
Cedar	S									
Cerro Gordo	S	L(3)		D(3)		S(3)	L(4)			R
Cherokee		L								
Chickasaw	SC			D(2)	PG(8)					
Clarke				D						
Clay					PG(2)					
Clayton		L	I	D(2)	PG(1)					
Clinton	S									
Crawford										
Dallas-Guthrie		L(2)			PG(1) PG(10)		L			R
Davis	SC			D(3)						
Decatur	SC(2)	LC(2)		D		S				R
Delaware	S									
Des Moines	SC(2)		I			S			I	
Dickinson	SC				PG(3)	S				
Dubuque	S					S(2)				
Emmet					PG(3)					
Fayette		L		D(2)	PG(8)	S	L			
Floyd	SC	L		D(2)	PG(9)		L(1)(2)			
Franklin				D(3)		S				
Fremont	SC									
Greene	SC				PG(12)					
Grundy				D(2)	PG(2)(4)					
Hamilton							L			R
Hancock-		L		D(3)	PG(3)					
Winnebago		L		D(3)	PG(2)	S				
Hardin		L		D(2)	PG(2)					
Harrison	SC									
Henry				D(2)						
Howard										
Humboldt	SC	L(4)		D(3)	PG(6)	S(2)	L			
Ida										
Iowa	SC			D(2)			L(1)(2)			
Jackson		L	I	D(2)	PG(1)			PG	I	
Jasper										
Jefferson										
Johnson	S					S(9)(14) SC(2)	L(4)(5)	PG(16)(94)		R(2)
Jones		L								
Keokuk	SC			D(3)						
Kossuth	SC	LC	I	D(3)	PG(14)	S(2)			I	
Lee		L								
Linn						S(3) SC	L			R(2)
Louisa										
Lucas				D(3)						
Lyon										
Madison	SC	L		D			L			R(2)
Mahaska				D(3)						
Marion				D(3)			L			R
Marshall	S			D(2)	PG(36)(4)	S	L			R
Mills										
Mitchell		L		D(2)						
Monona										
Monroe		L		D(3)						
Montgomery	SC	L	I							
Muscatine		L								
O'Brien		L					L			
Osceola										
Page							LC			
Palo Alto	SC				PG(8)		L			R
Plymouth		L					L(3)			
Pocahontas					PG(6)					
Polk		L(10)	I(2)		PG(56)	S(16)(24) SC(5)(45) C(3)(2) S-SC	L(10)(16) LC(4)	PG(5)(6)	I	R(16)(17)
Pottawattamie		L(5)		D(2)	PG(2)	S	L(2)			R
Poweshiek				D						
Ringgold										
Sac	SC	L					L			
Scott	S(3)	L				S(4)		PG		R(2)
Shelby	SC									
Sioux	SC									R(4)
Story		L(4)C			PG(2)					
Tama	SC	L		D(2)	PG(10)(4)	S				
Taylor	SC(2)	L		D						
Union	C			D		S	L-LC			
Van Buren	SC									
Wapello			I	D(3)		S(5)(6)	L		I	R
Warren				D		S(1)(2)	L(1)(2)			R
Washington	S									
Wayne	SC			D(3)						
Webster						S	L(5)(6)			
Winneshiek	SC	LC		D(2)	PG(1)				I	
Woodbury		L	I			S(2)-SC	L		I	R(2)
Worth	SC			D(3)		S(1)(2)				
Wright		L		D(3)	PG(9)	S	L			
Out of State						S(3)		PG(15)(16)		

three of the courses were Bureau courses, given by men from Iowa, the College of Medicine, and by men from outside the state. The course given in the other centers was a double header course given by the faculty members of the College of Medicine of the University of Iowa. Fifty-eight lay meetings were held to which the Bureau was asked to send speakers. These meetings represented the following organizations: · Colleges, Parent-Teacher Associations, Kiwanis Clubs, Rotary Clubs, Women's Clubs, Lions Clubs, Community Meetings, Cosmopolitan Clubs, County and Township Fairs, Community Clubs, Commercial Clubs, Citizens' Clubs, Pre-medic Clubs, and Woman's Auxiliary Meetings. Speakers were sent to ten inter-professional group meetings, which represents the nine district meetings and the state meeting of the Iowa Pharmaceutical Association.

In addition to these activities, the Speakers Bureau has cooperated with the Program Committee in the arrangements for the annual meeting, and with the Committee on Child Health and Protection and the Woman's Auxiliary in their educational work.

The financial report of the Speakers Bureau for the year 1933 is as follows:

INCOME

Fees		$3,558.26
University Courses	$1,759.00	
Bureau Courses	1,799.26	
Traveling Expenses (Refund)	92.44	
		$3,650.70
Minus $50.00 returned check	50.00	
		$3,600.70
Allowance from general budget	1,000.00	
		$4,600.70

EXPENDITURES

Salary		$1,440.00
Telephone and Telegraph	75.71	
Radio Talks (read)	53.00	
Miscellaneous	21.35	
Traveling Expenses	585.62	
Committee	$244.97	
Speakers	340.65	
Printing and Stationery	55.34	
Postgraduate Courses		
Traveling Expenses of Lecturers	1,513.04	$3,744.06
SURPLUS		$856.64

The Speakers Bureau is the boomerang of the State Society. Whatever energy is expended in its activities comes back in increased returns. Its scientific program makes its return in a better trained profession; its lay education program makes its return in increased confidence and reliance on the doctor. The Bureau is the service committee of the Council and of the Society, or more properly speaking, it is the Educational Committee. It can do no more than it is asked to do; its activities are expanded or curtailed by the demands of the profession and the laity. The Bureau can do nothing by itself—its activities are made possible by the cooperation of the individual members of the Iowa State Medical Society and to all who have so contributed the Bureau expresses its appreciation.

D. J. Glomset, Chairman

Dr. Daniel J. Glomset (Chairman): Mr. President: I wish to report the activities during this part of this year. This is a supplemental report.

In addition to furnishing speakers for medical societies and lay organizations and continuing our regular broadcasting schedules over radio stations WOI and WSUI, the Speakers Bureau has been engaged in three main activities to date in 1934.

First, the Bureau organized postgraduate courses in three centers. One course on General Therapeutics was given at Creston. The total enrollment for this course was 64 physicians; 49 of these took the entire course and 15 attended individual lectures. A course on Neurology and Psychiatry was given at Oskaloosa, where 36 doctors took the complete course and 9 doctors attended some of the lectures. The third course was given at Mt. Pleasant and covered the subject of infectious diseases. Nineteen doctors enrolled for the full course and 6 others attended intermittently. In the three courses a total of 134 doctors took advantage of this postgraduate medical education.

The second major activity of the Bureau was in cooperating with the Woman's Auxiliary in sponsoring a Health Essay Contest in the public high schools in Iowa. Two hundred essays were submitted from high schools throughout the entire state. Twenty-three prize winning essays were selected—representatives from the State Department of Health, State Department of Public Instruction, State Parent-Teachers Association, the Woman's Auxiliary and the Speakers Bureau acting as judges. A first, second and third prize of $15.00, $10.00 and $5.00, respectively were awarded. The other twenty essayists were given $1.00 each. The Bureau helped to finance these prizes and in addition awarded the winner of first place a trip to Ames to read the winning essay over the radio station WOI.

Finally, the Bureau has, whenever possible, aided the Program Committee in making arrangements for the present meeting.

Our income and expenditures to date balance.

Dr. Glomset read the prepared report and *moved* the adoption of the report as given in the handbook, and also the adoption of the supplementary report. *The motion was regularly seconded, put to a vote and carried.*

President Taylor: The report of the A. M. A. delegate was not approved. Is there an auxiliary report? Has anyone anything to say on that?

Dr. Moore: Mr. Chairman, I *move* that the reports be received and approved.

The motion was regularly seconded, put to a vote and carried.

President Taylor: The reports are approved. The Medical Library report was not approved. Is there a further report on that?

No further report was given.

Dr. Felix A. Hennessy (Chairman): Mr. President, I *move* that the report be approved.

The motion was regularly seconded, put to a vote and carried.

President Taylor: Dr. Peck, will you please give the report of the Committee on Constitution and By-laws?

Dr. John H. Peck: Mr. President, there is no

further report other than the one made the other day.

President Taylor: But you have some amendments to the By-laws. Shall the Secretary read these?

Dr. Peck: In addition to the report published in the handbook the supplementary report was turned over to the Secretary. There were some amendments that were proposed at that time. The Secretary has that.

President Taylor: I would like to ask our Executive Secretary to present those amendments and we will act upon them right now.

Executive Secretary McCarthy read the proposed amendment, Chapter VIII, Section 1.

Dr. Arthur W. Erskine of Cedar Rapids requested the reading of the present By-law now proposed to be amended and asked for discussion on the proposed amendments.

The present By-law now proposed to be amended was read. *Motion was regularly made and seconded that the proposed amendment be adopted.*

Secretary Parker: If this amendment is adopted it will do away with the Committee on Finance, so the question is now, do you want to do away with the Committee on Finance?

President Taylor: Are you ready for the question?

President-elect Harkness: I would like to say a word about the Committee on Finance. I have served on our Board of Trustees. We have had a Chairman of the Committee on Finance for a number of years who has been a most sincere man in everything he has done on that Committee. Your Board of Trustees is the most powerful committee we have in the Society. They are practically all-powerful between meetings. I believe that you cannot have too many checks on such a powerful committee. It is true they have an audit. If they are doing right they have nothing to fear. If they do not do right your extra checks all help.

But there is another purpose that your Finance Committee serves. Sometimes a committee may be doing the very best they can. They may be doing all right, but there develops an undercurrent of criticism against that committee, and your Committee on Finance serves a very useful purpose in that field.

I will give you a specific instance of two years ago when Dr. McClure was chairman. He very sincerely offered some criticism of the Board of Trustees and their expenditures. If we had had no committee to turn to, to clear this matter up there might have been an undercurrent of criticism that would go on without the Board of Trustees being able to vindicate or substantiate their position. Dr. McClure was asked to come to a meeting of the Board of Trustees. He was shown just what we were doing. This is absolutely no criticism of Dr. McClure; he was doing his duty. But we said to him, "Mac, we are here for constructive suggestions, if you have anything to give us."

When he was with us and saw what we were

doing, he did not have any suggestions. He agreed with us. In other words, we wiped out any undercurrent of criticism. It is a small committee, it doesn't make a great deal of work, but there may come a time when it is a very useful check to this Society. For that reason I stand opposed to the elimination of the Committee on Finance.

President Taylor: Is there any further discussion?

Dr. Oliver J. Fay (Des Moines): Mr. President: Speaking for the Board of Trustees, I wish to say we welcome such a committee as we have had over the years. I think it would be wrong to eliminate this Committee on Finance.

I agree with the chairman that the Board of Trustees does need to be checked, and so does every other organization that has the handling of money. I would be opposed to taking out this committee.

The motion was put to a vote and lost.

Dr. Lee R. Woodward (Mason City): I think it is a bit unfortunate that this should be tied up together so that to save the Committee on Finance we have to kill the Committee on Medical Economics.

President Taylor: We have not had that read yet.

Secretary Parker: Mr. President, may I explain? The purpose of this amendment was to do away with the Committee on Finance and substitute as a standing committee in its place, the Committee on Medical Economics. By defeating this amendment you have left the Committee on Medical Economics a special committee of the House of Delegates, where it has always been.

President Taylor: We will proceed with the next proposed amendment.

Executive Secretary McCarthy read "Chapter VIII, Section 11. Enact this new section as follows:"

President Taylor: You have heard the amendment as read.

Dr. James A. Downing (Des Moines): Mr. President, you haven't any committee in your By-laws to function as a special committee, and you are defining the duties of that committee in your By-laws.

Secretary Parker: Mr. President, this committee by Dr. Suchomel's resolution, adopted in 1932, has been made a standing committee, but we have not revised the Constitution and By-laws since 1930. This Committee on Medical Education and Hospitals, according to my interpretation is now a standing committee, and as other committees, is appointed by the President.

President Taylor: Dr. Erskine, have you a word on this?

Dr. Erskine: To clarify the record, is the present Committee on Medical Education and Hospitals a permanent committee of the House of Delegates by resolution, or by an amendment to the By-laws?

President Taylor: Dr. Peck, can you explain?

Dr. Peck: Mr. President: Dr. Downing's point was well taken. When you voted down the amendment to Chapter VIII, Sec. 1, you did leave out the line "A Committee on Medical Economics," and if you do adopt Chapter VIII, Section 11, which simply defines the duties of the Committee on Medical Edu-

you give us some idea of what this legal committee is costing?

Dr. Ely: What is it, Mrs. McCarthy?

Executive Secretary McCarthy: About $2,000 last year.

Dr. Fay: Formerly this defense feature cost six and seven thousand dollars a year. You ought to think very clearly on what you are proposing to do. There are a lot of arguments that you heard here day before yesterday about this defense feature which gives the idea, at least to lay people and some other people that the medical profession stands solidly together. They do not. You and I know that, but there won't be much of a malpractice claim if you don't have some doctor chipping into the thing and helping with it.

Members of the Iowa State Medical Society are said to be refused insurance because of this thing. None of you read the report of the Board of Trustees, of course. We could not expect you to read it. I think you want to be very, very careful what you are going to vote on. If you pass this amendment, you take out the defense feature. Personally, I think it would be wrong to take it out, but that is for the House of Delegates to decide. That defense feature is worth something.

Dr. Bush: Mr. President, I would be opposed to any change that would take away from me the privilege that is at present our protection. I am sincere in that.

As a unit here today, most of us if asked to go on the stand by reason of this very By-law would not like to do it. You cannot get us to go on the stand unless the thing is bona fide. Take that away and make it a matter of dollars and cents—God knows we are all after the dollars now, what few we have a chance to get—I don't know what is going to happen. We will go from county to county, from city to city. It is bad enough now. In my judgment this would take down that little bond we have holding us together today. I think it is fifty cents a year, isn't it?

Dr. Ely: It is ninety-one cents.

Dr. Bush: It is cheap at ninety-one cents.

Dr. Clyde A. Boice (Washington): I merely want to add my voice to the statements already made. I think it would be very unwise to do away with this malpractice defense. I am absolutely opposed to a procedure which will compel our members to pay $21 a year to some commercial company in order to get protection.

For many years I have traveled over one section of the state. I know the feelings of the general practitioner in southeastern Iowa, and I am opposed to any action of this Society which is going to compel them to spend $21, at least, to get protection which we are furnishing very satisfactorily at ninety-one cents apiece.

Dr. William W. Pearson (Des Moines): Mr. Chairman: Within the past year I had a little experience. It did not amount to much, but I was impressed by one feature. That is, the fact that we have one man in the state who is especially qualified through years of training to handle cases of this type. The average lawyer cannot very well match his skill against the man—this man Dutcher, of Iowa City. He has had such experience that he is invaluable, and if we were to drop him out of the organization, or something of that kind, I think that would interfere very materially with the success of the defense of the ordinary medical practitioner.

Dr. James E. Reeder (Sioux City): Mr. President: I am inclined to believe this protection should not be dropped for the simple reason that it does not carry indemnity. I had a little experience in Nebraska a short time ago. I had to testify. One of our colleagues had a little difficulty. In the state of Nebraska they can ask in open court, "Do you carry insurance?" And you have to state. While in Iowa, fortunately, the law protects us. We do not have to make that statement. Therefore, where there is knowledge of such protection, I really think it encourages these suits, because they feel, or the supposition is, that protection is had and the insurance company is going to pay it.

They feel it is not going to be much out of the doctor's pocket. That was brought out in this particular case. This doctor admitted he had insurance. There happened to be a bunch of farmers on the jury and the final conclusion which came to me later was: "Well, the doctor doesn't have to pay that. The insurance company pays it, and the poor fellow is about to lose his farm," and they gave him a couple of thousand dollars.

I know a lot of men in the state do not carry commercial insurance. They depend upon the support of the Society, and I feel where this information is handed out in a prospective malpractice suit, that it discourages the individuals. They may know, perhaps, that the doctor does not have any property, in a material way which they can collect in case they should get judgment. I really think we would make a mistake, at such a nominal charge or cost of ninety-one cents a member, in discouraging, or dropping the support of our members through the medical defense of our State Society.

Dr. Peter A. Bendixen (Davenport): Mr. President: I am thoroughly opposed to the abolition of this medical defense. I have occasion to get into quite a number of suits and quite a number of legal affairs with the insurance companies, and there are so many friendly suits, especially in the present day of the automobile. I have only had one occasion within the last year in which there was a friendly suit against a dentist. A dentist pulled a tooth, fractured a jaw, and the dentist said, "You know I am protected by insurance, and I think he ought to get something out of it."

There is a friendly suit. Under that condition, with the protection by the medical profession, in which you have a certain moral obligation that you do not want to appear, I think you have a permanent tie. I think also, the Committee ought to stand, with its functions as it has in the past.

Question was called, *the motion was put to a vote and lost*, by a unanimous negative vote.

President Taylor: Dr. Peck, will you now read the proposed changes which we have to vote on yet in order to complete this part of our program?

Dr. Peck: This proposed amendment is the one that Mrs. McCarthy read first. Chapter 1, Section 5. It was proposed to omit that chapter in its entirety.

Dr. Peck read Chapter 1, Section 5.

Dr. Peck: Inasmuch as you voted down the proposed amendment to Chapter VIII, Section 8, of course you want to vote down this proposed amendment. As stated in the handbook, if we had amended Section 8 of Chapter VIII, as proposed, this section 5 would have been superfluous. However, we did not amend Section 8 of Chapter VIII, therefore, this Chapter 1, Section 5 should be retained.

Mr. President, I *move* that we reject this proposed amendment.

The motion was regularly seconded, put to a vote and carried.

Dr. Peck: There were two other amendments which were offered too late to get them into the handbook.

One is proposed by Dr. McManus of Waterloo, that Section 1, Chapter IX of the By-laws be amended by striking out the first sentence, which reads: (Read) He proposes to substitute therefor "An assessment of ten dollars per capita on membership of the component societies is hereby made the annual dues of this Society, except whenever the total net assets at the close of the fiscal year are more than $10,000, the assessment for the ensuing year shall be five dollars per capita."

Dr. McManus: Mr. President: I am still supporting that amendment in substance. I have had a conference with our secretary and I am yielding to his request and asking that that amendment be withdrawn. I would like for the House to vote that down and present the five dollar dues proposition later as a motion. But I am asking the voting down or the withdrawal of the amendment.

Dr. Ely: Dr. Taylor, may I help you with that? The dues for the ensuing year are fixed by this House for the ensuing year. What Dr. McManus wishes to do is to withdraw this proposed amendment. Then when it comes time for the dues that will come up later.

President Taylor: Dr. McManus, do you move that this proposed amendment be withdrawn.

Dr. McManus: I so *move*.

The motion was regularly seconded, put to a vote and carried.

Dr. Peck: The second amendment which was not printed in the handbook was a request that the President-elect be made a member of the Committee on Scientific Work. At present the Committee on Scientific Work is the President, Secretary, and Treasurer, and of course they call in the section chairmen and the Speakers Bureau, and such other people

Mr. Blake: Mr. President and Members of the House of Delegates of the Iowa State Medical Society: This Iowa Liquor Control letter that was read by Dr. Parker is more or less in the way of a "racket," as one doctor expressed it to me yesterday.

There are two kinds of permits authorized under the Liquor Control Commission. One is an individual permit which each individual in the state of Iowa will have to secure in order to buy liquor for his own consumption.

In addition to that, they are asking you doctors if you dispense any liquor medicinally to have it done in a compound, and before you can buy that liquor to place in the compound, or in the medicine, you must first secure this three-dollar permit. That does not authorize you to resell liquor as a beverage in any form that it can be used as a beverage.

That would only be of benefit perhaps to those physicians who compound their own medicines and who are not in a position where they can send their patients to the liquor store.

I asked the attorney for the Liquor Commission yesterday about it, and he said, "Prescribe and furnish liquor, is the purpose of this three-dollar permit."

I said, "You don't mean to tell me that it is going to cost these doctors three dollars in order that they prescribe liquor to their patients?"

"Oh, no," he said, "I guess they can prescribe it, but if they want to purchase it, it would cost them this three-dollar permit."

The only benefit I can see to this three-dollar permit (this is just my personal opinion) would be where some of you gentlemen wanted to include liquor of any character in some compound. If you want to prescribe whiskey, or wine, or whatever you thought your patient needed, you of course could send him to a liquor store, and under his own individual permit he could get whatever he wants. Those of you who want this permit and subscribe for it, paying in your three dollars, do not have to go and get your liquor if you do not want to. You can send your permit in here to Des Moines and into a central store, if there isn't a store located in your town or city, and the Liquor Commission will deliver it to you.

There may be some questions some of you want to ask. If so, I will try to answer.

Question: What effect will that have on hospitals?

Mr. Blake: It applies to hospitals.

Question: What about alcohol used for laboratory purposes and sterilization? Would you have to have a permit?

Mr. Blake: That would be their ruling.

Question: Is alcohol specified in the bill? I thought it was left out.

Mr. Blake: They would so hold alcohol is included.

Question: Can you buy alcohol at liquor stores under the personal permit—not professional—for any use, unspecified use?

Mr. Blake: I assume if they had it on hand you could. Under the law as it now stands there is an awful lot left to the man whom they term "vendor" or chief clerk, in each liquor store. He tells you about what you can have and what amount, and that sort of thing.

One thing I did overlook, however, there are no reports necessary under this new law, so it rather invalidates itself if a doctor buys five gallons of whiskey for his own use and it is used for whatever purpose he wants to use it. There are no reports made either under the special permit or the other one.

Question: Can you prescribe alcohol or combinations of alcohol in the hospital or in your office without a permit?

Mr. Blake: You can prescribe it, yes.

Question: Can I buy, without this permit, five gallons of alcohol on my individual permit?

Mr. Blake: So far as I know, you can.

Question: Can I use that for any purpose I want in my profession?

Mr. Blake: It is only for your own consumption. There are no reports necessary, so you can use your own judgment on that.

Question: Where hospitals have tax-free permits, does it affect them? Are those permits cancelled?

Mr. Blake: Any state permits will be cancelled.

Question: I mean federal.

Mr. Blake: Of course the state cannot affect any federal permit.

Question: What about the administration in emergency cases?

Mr. Blake: That, of course, would be a question that is more of a common sense ruling than anything else. I do not think there would ever be any question about that sort of thing.

Question: By June first this expires as I understand this?

Mr. Blake: Yes.

Question: You pay three dollars a month this time?

Mr. Blake: Yes.

Question: As I understand it the hospital holds a federal permit to withdraw alcohol for hospital purposes. Can a hospital in Iowa have alcohol shipped from a distiller over in Peoria into the state of Iowa under their tax permit?

Mr. Blake: I would believe not.

Question: Why?

Mr. Blake: For the simple reason that while the state of Iowa cannot do away with the federal permit, you understand the handling of liquor comes under the police bar of the state, and the federal government cannot authorize anything which is prohibited under the statutes of this state.

Question: Then they would have to pay this fee?

Mr. Blake: I am afraid they would.

Question: Isn't it true that you have to have the stamp of the state of Iowa on all liquor or else it is illegal?

Mr. Blake: Yes. The possession of any liquor not stamped with the Iowa State Liquor Control stamp is considered illegal.

the Society of any state in the Union. But at that, only eighty-one per cent are members of our State Society.

For many years we have accumulated funds under the wise guidance and leadership of our trustees until now we have $39,000 in our treasury.

President Taylor: Doctor, I hate to say anything to a Past President, but I wish you would make a motion and then talk to the motion.

Dr. McManus: I am getting to a motion. If we reduce our fees from the ten dollar rate to five of course it will make a deficit. It will make a deficit but our membership will be increased to what it was before the fees were raised. It would make that deficit equal to $2,800. But I believe it is worth it. I believe we should go to Davenport next year with a membership of 2,500, and that is within the range of possibility.

And for that purpose, for the purpose of boosting our membership, I *move* that the membership dues be five dollars for the ensuing year.

The motion was seconded.

President Taylor: You have heard the motion. Is there any discussion?

Dr. Fay: Mr. President, I would like to have you invite Dr. Harkness to tell you something of the budget system and expenditure of money that is now carried on by the Board of Trustees.

The reason I ask that is because he is the father and the mother and the grandfather of the budget system.

President Taylor: Dr. Harkness, will you respond?

President-elect Harkness: Mr. President and Members: On this question of dues, I am very glad that Dr. McManus withdrew his amendment because I think it is up to the House of Delegates each year to decide what they want to do, and the officers are to abide by the decision of the House of Delegates; whatever the House of Delegates decides we must carry on.

If you reduce the dues you should also instruct your officers not to reduce activities of your Society. In other words, give them specific directions that you are going to go into your accumulated funds to carry on.

Or, if you do not want to do that and you want your Society to do less work, have less activities, that is up to you.

Finally, I think we have only gotten started. There are many more things that we can do. I cannot conceive of membership in the State Society, or of any man in his professional life where he does not get ten dollars worth from that membership. There are men who object to it, and yet those same men will go out and in recreation spend a good deal more than that.

I doubt very much whether reduction of dues is going to increase membership very much. It may. We made up our budget this year and the budget was made up on a basis of a $3,000 deficit. Our membership has increased. We may not have that deficit, but at least we planned our activities for

this year expecting and willing not to be disappointed
if we were in the red $3,000 at the end of the year.

The only thing I have to say is, it is for you men
to decide what you want to pay, but if you do reduce
the dues, be specific to your officers as to whether
you want to go on and build up your activities, make
your Society of some real worth to you in your own
locality, but do not reduce the dues and then walk
out on your officers without letting them know what
you want to do.

At the present time our budget is based on a
$3,000 deficit. If you reduce your dues it is going
to be more than that, of course.

Dr. G. P. Reed (Davis City): Mr. President:
I held for the five dollar fee last year. A great many.
people do not understand. I mean a great many of
you doctors in the city do not understand the condition in the small country towns.

We are in worse condition than we have been at
any time since I have been practicing medicine.
There isn't a doctor in our county who is making one
penny a year above his expenses. It is far worse
than it has ever been, and I know three doctors who
are absolutely unable to take out insurance. I mean
absolutely unable to pay their fees here and their
insurance and their taxes. They are in arrears and
you do not understand it.

I have mine to pay so far as that is concerned, but
I am only talking for the poor fellows who cannot,
and they are just as loyal as anybody.

Let's reduce it to five dollars and I think we can
get three more members in our county. But they
say they just do not have that much money to spend.

Dr. W. E. Sperow (Carlisle): Personally, in our
county we haven't a full membership, but it is not on
account of the ten dollar dues. I do not think our
membership would be any more if dues were $2.00,
and also our experience has been that if we had a
little heavier activity ten or fifteen years ago, some
of us would not have chiropractic competition today
legalized and making it so darned hard to get the
ten dollars.

Dr. Fay: I do not believe that reduction of these
dues to five dollars or two dollars would have any
effect on getting membership. When our distinguished president was in the house thirty-one years
ago, and our distinguished townsman, Dr. Priestley,
was president, the question of dues was discussed.
They were then $3.00. They made a proposition at
that meeting to have them $1.50. Can you remember
it, Mr. President? And Linn County was there pro-
testing at the same time about the University Hospital.

You would not increase your membership at all
by reducing the dues. You need ten dollars to carry
on, and if the Iowa State Medical Society is not
worth ten dollars to every member of it, it is not
worth a single cent. And the thing you want to keep
in mind all the time is to get these fellows interested.
Get them doing things to keep at work.

Do as you have done, Mr. President. You got
this big crowd here because you put them to work,

The original motion made by Dr. McManus was put to a vote and lost.

President Taylor: The substitute motion that was voted for the ten dollars dues has been accepted and the dues for 1935 will be ten dollars.

Is there anything further under New Business?

There was nothing further under New Business.

President Taylor: Dr. Harkness, do you want to make your Committee appointments here, or at the general session? It has been customary to make them here.

President-Elect Harkness: The Committee appointments have to be approved by the House of Delegates.

The only reason why I would like to read them is just to make a few remarks. I have spent a good deal of time going over these appointments. There has been a feeling over the state that there was a concentration of appointments in too few localities. Other counties and districts thought they were not being represented.

I have taken the Councilors into my confidence and I have worked with each Councilor in the district. Some of these men I do not know personally. These appointments were made on the advice of men who do know them, but I am making these appointments in an attempt to try and bring new blood into the activities of our Society. They may be "duds," I don't know. I am taking a chance and I surely do not want any "duds."

These are the appointments, and I have tried to distribute them according to our Councilor Districts. There are not enough appointments to recognize every county organization.

President-Elect Harkness read the prepared list of appointments.

STANDING COMMITTEES OF THE HOUSE OF DELEGATES

Committee on Constitution and By-laws

W. R. Brock, Chairman..................................Sheldon
John H. Henkin...Sioux City
W. A. Sternberg....................................Mount Pleasant

Committee on Finance

Ernest C. McClure, Chairman...........................Bussey
Leslie L. Carr...Clermont
A. S. Bowers..Orient

Medico-Legal Committee

Frank A. Ely, Chairman....................Des Moines, 1935
George C. Albright..............................Iowa City, 1936
F. Earl Bellinger..........................Council Bluffs, 1937

Committee on Public Policy and Legislation

Fred Moore, Chairman................................Des Moines
Ransom D. Bernard..Clarion
Peter A. Bendixen...Davenport

Committee on Medical Education and Hospitals

Arthur W. Erskine, Chairman................Cedar Rapids
T. J. Irish...Forest City
B. J. Dierker..Fort Madison

SPECIAL COMMITTEES OF THE
HOUSE OF DELEGATES

Committee on Child Health and Protection

R. H. McBride, Chairman............................Sioux City
E. D. Plass...Iowa City
H. E. Farnsworth..Storm Lake
Lee F. Hill...Des Moines
James F. Gerken...Waterloo

Historical Committee

Walter L. Bierring, Chairman.................Des Moines
Frank M. Fuller..Keokuk
T. B. Throckmorton.......................................Des Moines
John T. McClintock...Iowa City
Henry B. Young...Burlington
William Jepson...Sioux City

Committee on Medical Economics

T. F. Thornton, Chairman...............................Waterloo
James C. Hill..Newton
James C. Donahue...Centerville

Medical Library Committee

Con R. Harken, Chairman...................................Osceola
H. A. Tolliver...Charles City
Jeannette Dean-Throckmorton....................Des Moines

Committee on Military Affairs

T. F. Suchomel, Chairman.........................Cedar Rapids
Harold A. Spilman..Ottumwa
Arnold L. Jensen....................................Council Bluffs

Woman's Auxiliary Advisory Committee

Aldis A. Johnson, Chairman.................Council Bluffs
W. E. Baker...Des Moines
Charles F. Snopek..Cresco
W. T. Peters...Burt
T. I. Wigim...Muscatine

President-Elect Harkness: I offer these to you for your approval.

Dr. Ely: I *move*, Mr. Chairman, they be approved.
The motion was regularly seconded, put to a vote and carried.

President Taylor: Is there any further business?

Dr. L. A. Thomas (Red Oak): I think there seems to be a lack of understanding of our By-laws. There have been so many amendments made since the last pamphlet was printed that I *make a motion* the Secretary be instructed to have pamphlets printed of the By-laws as now amended.

The motion was seconded.

President Taylor: I think that is a very good suggestion. Is there any discussion?

There was no discussion and *the motion was put to a vote and carried.*

Dr. Frank M. Fuller (Keokuk): Mr. President: Dr. Bierring is very anxious, as Chairman of the Committee on History of Medicine in Iowa, to have as many men responding to the request he has made as possible, for historical data to be sent to the Committee for publication.

I merely mention this because he has emphasized the fact that the history of medicine in Iowa will rapidly go into oblivion as the men now living go out of existence. I am requesting, for Dr. Bierring, that

SOCIETY PROCEEDINGS

Adair County

The Adair County Medical Society held its mid-year meeting at the Hotel Greenfield, in Greenfield, Tuesday, June 5. Following a six-thirty dinner a short business session was held by members and the councilor of the district, Dr. James Macrae of Creston. An invitation was extended by the society to hold the next district meeting with the Adair County Medical Society. The evening was devoted to papers and lantern slides relating to Infections of the Upper Respiratory Tract, given by the guest speakers, Ralph H. Parker, M.D., George A. May, M.D., and C. C. Walker, M.D., all of Des Moines.

A. S. Bowers, M.D., Secretary

Appanoose County

The following officers were elected to serve the Appanoose County Medical Society, at a meeting held in Centerville, Thursday, June 21: Dr. F. B. Leffert of Centerville, president; Dr. C. T. Slavin of Moravia, vice president; and Dr. E. A. Larsen of Centerville, secretary and treasurer.

Black Hawk County

Members of the Black Hawk Medical Society met Tuesday, June 19, at Wameso Lodge, and a symposium on Gastric and Duodenal Ulcer: Experimental and Clinical Aspects, was presented by Walter L. Palmer, M.D., associate professor of medicine, University of Chicago; and Lester R. Dragstedt, M.D., professor of surgery, University of Chicago. Discussion was opened by Drs. J. E. Brinkman, H. J. Hartman, and W. O. Preece, all of Waterloo.

Bremer County

The regular meeting of the Bremer County Medical Society was held at Mercy Hospital in Waverly, Monday, May 14. Dr. L. C. Kern of Waverly, reported on the proceedings of the House of Delegates.

James E. Whitmire, M.D., Secretary

Cerro Gordo County

Donald P. Abbott, M.D., professor of medicine, Rush Medical College, Chicago, addressed members of the Cerro Gordo County Medical Society, Thursday, June 21, on Indigestion, the Diagnosis of Stomach Disorders and Their Treatment.

Clinton County

Thursday evening, June 7, the members of the Clinton County Medical Society met at the Country Club for a dinner. This was followed by a scientific program furnished by Howard R. Hartman, M.D., of the Mayo Clinic, who spoke on Lesions of the Small Intestine other than Peptic Ulcer, and Joseph Mayo, M.D., also of the Mayo Clinic, who gave a brief address on the subject of Secondary Anemias. The program was very much enjoyed by all the members.

Mr. W. D. Little of Davenport, a representative of the sales tax division of the Iowa Board of Review, instructed the society in regard to regulations governing the collection of sales tax, insofar as they apply to physicians.

The society will have its annual picnic in September, and the next regular meeting, Thursday, October 4.

E. V. Donlan, M.D., Secretary

Hardin County

Julia Cole, M.D., of the State University of Iowa College of Medicine, furnished the scientific program for the Hardin County Medical Society at a meeting held in Iowa Falls, Tuesday, June 26. Dr. Cole spoke on The Diagnosis and Treatment of Bronchial Asthma.

F. N. Cole, M.D., Program Chairman

Jasper County

The Jasper County Medical Society met in Newton, Tuesday, June 5, and the following program was presented: Astronomy Through the Camera, Dr. D. W. Morehouse, president of Drake University, Des Moines; The Art of Mysticism, Mr. Carl C. Burgess, Newton; Glomerular Nephritis, Daniel J. Glomset, M.D., Des Moines; Eye Changes in Nephritis and Hypertension, C. S. O'Brien, M.D., Iowa City; Hypertensive Nephritis, Martin I. Olsen, M.D., Des Moines; The Basic Science Law, Fred Moore, M.D., Des Moines; and a Report on Membership, Robert L. Parker, M.D., Des Moines, secretary of the state society.

Johnson County

Wednesday, June 6, members of the Johnson County Medical Society held a meeting at the Jefferson Hotel in Iowa City, and were addressed by Frank L. Love, M.D., of Iowa City, on the Relation of the Practitioner to the Military Medical Service; and by William H. Gibbon, M.D., also of Iowa City, on Congenital Cystic Disease of the Lung.

Lee County

One hundred and thirty-five physicians from southeastern Iowa and from Illinois and Missouri, braved the heat to attend the summer meeting of the Lee County Medical Society, held at the Country Club near Keokuk, Thursday, June 28. The afternoon program consisted of: Premature Detachment of Normal Implanted Placenta, Frederick H. Falls, M.D., of Chicago, discussion opened by L. H. Harris,

M.D., of Iowa City; and Angina Pectoris, Joseph A. Capps, M.D., of Chicago, discussion opened by W. M. Fowler, M.D., of Iowa City. A fried chicken dinner was served at six-thirty after which the following papers were presented, closing the session: An Analysis of One Thousand Consecutive X-Ray Examinations of the Stomach from the Clinical and Roentgenologic Viewpoint, David S. Beilin, M.D., of Chicago, discussion opened by P. B. Goodwin, M.D., of Peoria; and Surgery of Gastric and Duodenal Ulcers and Cancer of the Stomach, Nelson M. Percy, M.D., of Chicago, discussion opened by H. L. Beye, M.D., of Iowa City. The next quarterly meeting will be held at Fort Madison.

C. A. Boice, M.D., Councilor

Linn County

Officers elected by the Linn County Medical Society at the business meeting held Thursday, June 7, are: Dr. T. Frank Hersch of Cedar Rapids, president; Dr. John R. Gardner of Lisbon, president-elect; Dr. H. R. Hess of Cedar Rapids, vice president; Dr. Ernest G. Kieck of Cedar Rapids, secretary; and Dr. Emma J. Neal of Cedar Rapids, treasurer.

Marshall County

The Marshall County Medical Society held its regular monthly session, Tuesday, May 29, at the Elmwood Country Club. The following scientific program was arranged by Dr. Fred L. Wahrer, and was attended by more than one hundred local and county physicians: Prevention and Treatment of Tuberculosis of the Lung, Benjamin Goldberg, M.D., assistant professor of medicine, University of Illinois College of Medicine, discussion opened by John H. Peck, M.D., Des Moines; and Electrosurgical Removal of the Gallbladder, Max Thorek, M.D., surgeon in chief, American Hospital of Chicago, discussion opened by E. J. Harnagel, M.D., Des Moines.

Mills County

Thursday, June 14, the Mills County Medical Society met at the State Institution at Glenwood, and the following program was presented: Delegate's Report of the State Meeting, I. U. Parsons, M.D., of Malvern; Basic Science Necessary for State Licensure, H. B. Dye, M.D., of Glenwood; Treatment of Cervicitis, Ward A. DeYoung, M.D., of Glenwood, and Medical Economics, M. S. Campbell, M.D., of Malvern.

Monroe County

The regular meeting of the Monroe County Medical Society was held Thursday evening, June 14, in Dr. C. N. Hyatt's office at Albia. S. T. Gray, M.D., delegate to the state convention, presented a report of the business transacted at the last annual session, after which there was a general discussion of the fundamental science law as outlined by the Committee on Public Policy and Legislation.

T. A. Moran, M.D., Secretary

Ringgold County

The Ringgold County Medical Society held a meeting at the court house in Mount Ayr, Friday, June 22. The following papers were presented: Some Odds and Ends of General Practice, Con. R. Harken, M.D., of Osceola; and Complications in Acute Appendicitis, Fred A. Bowman, M.D., of Leon. The papers were discussed freely. John C. Parsons, M.D., of Creston, explained the fundamentals of the proposed basic science law.

J. W. Hill, M.D., Secretary

Scott County

Tuesday, June 5, the Scott County Medical Society held a dinner meeting at the Lend-A-Hand Club in Davenport. A. B. Kuhl, Sr., M.D., of Davenport, presented an address on Medical Economics, after which there was a general discussion of certain phases of county contract work.

Des Moines Valley Medical Association

The Sixty-first Annual Meeting of the Des Moines Valley Medical Association was held in Ottumwa, Tuesday, June 19. The morning session, which was held at the Ottumwa Hospital, was featured by addresses by two physicians from the Mayo Clinic, Rochester; John Pemberton, M.D., spoke on Carcinoma of the Thyroid Gland, and Paul A. O'Leary, M. D., discussed Newer Concepts in the Treatment of Syphilis. After a twelve-thirty luncheon at the Ottumwa Country Club, the afternoon session convened at the St. Joseph Hospital, where the two following papers were presented: The Untoward Effects of Some Commonly Administered Drugs, C. W. Baldridge, M.D., of Iowa City; and The Clinical and X-Ray Findings of Some Interesting Cases, M. H. Goldman, M.D., of the United States Veterans' Hospital at Knoxville.

Sixth Councilor District Meeting

The joint meeting of the Grundy County Medical Society and physicians from the Sixth Councilor District was held Thursday afternoon and evening, June 28, at the Grundy County Golf and Country Club, two miles west of Reinbeck. An afternoon of amusements, consisting of golf, bridge, horseshoes, etc., was followed by a six-thirty dinner, after which the evening program was presented. Speakers were secured through the Speakers Bureau of the Iowa State Medical Society, and were: M. E. Barnes, M.D., of Iowa City, who addressed the group on The Application of Preventive Medicine to the Public Milk Supply; and R. D. Bernard, M. D., of Clarion, who spoke on The Proposed Basic Science Law. The meeting proved successful and enjoyable in spite of the intense heat, and the most profitable evening program was attended by sixty-five physicians and guests.

C. W. Ellyson, M.D., Councilor.

Southwestern Iowa Postgraduate Medical Association

The Southwestern Iowa Postgraduate Medical Association met Thursday, June 7, at the Hotel Lin-

INTERESTING NEWS
In Brief

It is now reported that there are more than 100,000 lepers in India.

———

Undulant fever causes illness in about 3,000 persons annually in France.

———

The rate of increase in population during 1933 was twice as great in Japan as in the United States.

———

Careful bacteriologic studies indicate that urinary antiseptics are most efficacious when fluids are restricted.

———

The death rate from tuberculosis among Indians is quoted as seven or eight times that of the general population.

———

During the spring months of this year twenty-five cases of psittacosis, with nine deaths, were reported in and around Pittsburgh.

———

Spices and condiments in moderate amounts really help digestion by stimulating part of the digestive apparatus to greater activity.

———

The unpalatable star fish and red sponge, among the most abundant of sea life, are being studied for their food and vitamin contents.

———

Dr. Dean Lewis of John Hopkins Medical School states that "the general practitioner has actually fared better during the depression than the specialist."

———

Under the guidance of Dr. Theobald Smith, a group of leaders interested in tropical diseases have recently formed the American Academy of Tropical Medicine.

———

Experiments conducted by Dr. C. M. Jackson of the University of Minnesota would indicate that females stand a diet deficient in protein much better than males.

———

Gamma ferric oxide injected into the blood stream is aiding Yale University scientists in their study of the hemoglobin content of the blood, and the deposit of iron in the body.

———

A prophylactic serum against yellow fever has been developed in the Rockefeller Institute for Medical Research and is said to give at least two years complete protection against this disease.

———

Incident to the study of the migratory habits of mosquitoes, the United States Department of Agriculture, by observing marked specimens, have determined that some mosquitoes live as long as 104 days.

From the University of Paris comes the statement that the daily ingestion of small quantities of aluminum, such as might result in the use of cooking utensils, is not dangerous and does not induce cancer, as some have feared.

———

Sounding a warning against the imperfectly cleaned soda fountain or bar glass, public health authorities state that about 92 per cent of all communicable diseases are transmitted through the secretions of the nose and mouth.

———————

PERSONAL MENTION

Dr. Zella White Stewart of Iowa City returned recently from a southern hemisphere cruise, having visited the South Sea Islands, New Zealand, Australia, the Dutch East Indies, India, South America and Africa.

———

Dr. Fred A. Bowman of Leon spoke before the Leon Rotary Club Monday, June 11, on "Abdominal Pains."

———

Dr. John C. Bennett, formerly of Hudson, has located in Waterloo for the practice of medicine, where he will be associated with his uncle, Dr. G. G. Bickley.

———

Dr. Howard I. Down of Sioux City was elected president of the Morningside College Alumni, at a meeting held Monday, June 4.

———

Dr. H. R. Sugg of Clinton addressed the Clinton Rotary Club at a meeting held in the Lafayette Hotel Monday, June 18. His subject was "Why People Die."

———

Dr. Roger James, who has practiced medicine in Davenport for the past year and a half, has located in Bennett.

———

Dr. J. S. Newton, who recently completed a term as assistant surgeon at the Ohio Soldiers and Sailors Hospital, has located in Keota for the practice of medicine. Dr. Newton is a graduate of the State University of Iowa College of Medicine.

———

Dr. and Mrs. H. H. W. Kruse of Rockford left recently on a European trip. They will visit Germany, Switzerland and Holland, with Dr. Kruse taking postgraduate work in Berlin and Munich.

———————

MARRIAGES

Miss Rose Stanek and Dr. J. C. Petrovitsky, both of Cedar Rapids, were married at the home of Mrs. W. E. Andre in Cedar Rapids on Saturday, June 9.

The bride and groom left immediately after the ceremony for a brief stay at their summer home near Hackensack, Minnesota.

———

At eight o'clock, Saturday morning, June 16, in St. Cecelia's Cathedral in Omaha, Miss Wyliette Heald of Omaha became the bride of Dr. Eugene B. Floersch of Council Bluffs. The young couple left in the afternoon for a trip to California, after which they will return to Council Bluffs, where Dr. Floersch is engaged in the practice of medicine.

———

Friday, June 8, the marriage of Miss Hazelle Petersen and Dr. George Elvidge, both of Perry, took place at the Congregational Church. For the past four years the bride has been a nurse at the local Kings Daughters Hospital, while the groom has been practicing medicine for several years in Perry.

———————

DEATH NOTICES

Bocken, Herman, of Harlan, aged forty-seven, died June 10, of complications following a heart attack and pneumonia. He was graduated in 1911 from the University of Nebraska College of Medicine, Omaha, and at the time of his death was a member of the Shelby County Medical Society.

Gustin, Plomer Julius, of Bedford, aged thirty-eight, died May 27, of a self-inflicted gun shot wound. He was graduated in 1927 from the University of Nebraska College of Medicine, Omaha, and was formerly a member of the Taylor County Medical Society.

Hogle, Kate Anna Mason, of Mount Vernon, aged seventy-four, died June 2, following a prolonged illness. She was graduated in 1885 from Northwestern University Woman's Medical School, Chicago, and at the time of her death was a life member of the Linn County and Iowa State Medical Societies.

———————

RADIO BROADCASTS

The schedule for the radio talks of the Iowa State Medical Society has been changed. These talks will now be heard over WSUI, Iowa City, on Thursdays from 7:45 to 8 p. m. During the months of July, August and September, station WOI, Ames, will broadcast our health messages on Mondays, from 5:30 to 5:45 p. m. The schedule of talks for the coming month is as follows:

July 5- 9—Hot Weather Hints.
        G. W. Harris, M.D.
July 12-16—A Few Facts About Cancer.
        W. E. Sanders, M.D.
July 19-23—Vacations.
        C. B. Taylor, M.D.
July 26-30—A Few Facts About Quacks.
        M. B. Call, M.D.
Aug. 2- 6—Swimming Hazards.

HISTORY OF MEDICINE IN IOWA

Edited by the Historical Committee

DR. HENRY B. YOUNG, Burlington
DR. FRANK M. FULLER, Keokuk
DR. JOHN T. McCLINTOCK, Iowa City

DR. TOM. B. THROCKMORTON, Des Moines
DR. WALTER L. BIERRING, Des Moines
DR. WILLIAM JEPSON, Sioux City

History of the Iowa State Board of Health

FREDERICK J. SWIFT, M.D.,
Deputy Commissioner—State Department of Health
Des Moines, Iowa

(Conclusion)

Dr. Guilford H. Sumner served as Secretary of the Iowa State Board of Health from 1910 to 1913, and as Commissioner of Health from then until December, 1921, when, because of failing health, he felt it necessary to resign from this position. Thus ended a very remarkable career in public health administration.

Dr. Rodney P. Fagen was appointed as successor to Dr. Sumner and served from January 2, 1922, to June 30, 1924. Dr. Fagen was born in Des Moines, Iowa, February 14, 1886, a descendant of the early pioneers of Polk county. His medical education was received at the Drake Uni-

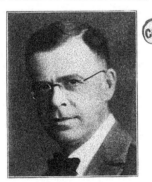

RODNEY P. FAGEN, M.D.
Commissioner, 1922-1924

versity Medical School, from which he was graduated in 1912. During the World War he had a long and honorable service in the Medical Corps of the United States Army, reaching the rank of Lieutenant Colonel.

During his term of office in the State Department of Health the Division of Vital Statistics, which had been established six months previously, was developed to a high degree of efficiency. Iowa was accepted in the United States Registration Area for deaths in 1923, and births in 1924.

REORGANIZATION

The Fortieth General Assembly, at the regular session, appointed a committee known as the Code Commission to revise the Code of Iowa. This Commission prepared bills No. 260 and 262 to rewrite, resectionize, and rechapterize all the laws relating to public health. Bill No. 260 provided for the consolidation of officers of the State Board of Health, State Hotel Inspector, Board of Medical Examiners, Podiatry Examiners, Osteopathic Examiners, Chiropractic Examiners, Nurses Examiners, Dental Examiners and Optometry Examiners into one department, to be known as the State Department of Health. It also provided that the State Board of Health should consist of the commissioner of public health, the members of the executive council and five health officers, to be appointed by the Governor; these appointments to be made prior to the second Tuesday in January of each odd numbered year for a period of two years or until the successor was appointed and qualified; not more than one such health officer to be appointed from any one congressional district.

Under the reorganization plan, the position of Secretary of the State Board of Health was changed to Commissioner of the State Department of Health, and Dr. Rodney P. Fagen was the first Commissioner of Public Health to be so named under the new law.

Dr. Don M. Griswold was appointed Commissioner of Health to succeed Dr. Fagen, serving from July 1, 1924, to June 30, 1926. Dr. Griswold was a native of Michigan, received his education at the Michigan Agricultural College, and was graduated from the Medical Department of

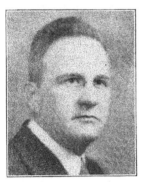

DON M. GRISWOLD, M.D.
Commissioner, 1924-1926

the University of Michigan. He was with the International Health Board of the Rockefeller Foundation for several years, a part of this time being spent in South America and the West Indies. During the World War he served as epidemiologist at a number of training camps in this country. During the five years preceding his appointment as Commissioner of Health, he was professor of preventive medicine and public health, at the College of Medicine of the State University of Iowa. Dr. Griswold is at present associated with the New York State Department of Health.

With the reorganization of the State Department of Health in 1926, when all of its activities were placed in charge of a Commissioner of Health, the medical profession unanimously approved the wisdom of Governor John Hammill in asking Dr. Henry Albert to return to Iowa in the service of the state.

Dr. Albert was a native son, born in Scott County, October 11, 1878. After completing a high school course at Reinbeck, Iowa, he received the degrees of B.S. in 1900, M.S. in 1901, and M.D. in 1902 from the State University of Iowa. He was appointed professor of pathology and bacteriology at the University of Iowa in 1903, and director of bacteriological laboratory, State Board of Health in 1904, continuing in both positions until 1922, when because of a throat affection he

obtained a leave of absence and accepted an appointment as director of the state hygienic laboratory and professor of bacteriology in the University of Nevada, at Reno, where he remained until 1926.

During his term of Commissioner, the division of public health engineering was established, stream pollution control was instituted and a complete survey of public water supply of the state was inaugurated. The divisions of child health and health education, public health nursing, nursing education, and law enforcement, were also established during this period. At the very height

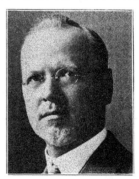

HENRY ALBERT, M.D.
Commissioner, 1926-1930

of his usefulness, Dr. Albert succumbed to an acute appendicitis on the morning of April 4, 1930, and this closed the life's work of Iowa's greatest health commissioner. The words of tribute by Dr. Bierring at the time were most fitting. "He passed from our midst at the threshold of still greater opportunities for service, yet measured by its accomplishment his life encompassed far more than the brief span of years would imply. His happy sunny nature enlivened every circle in which he moved, and he left a bit of cheer and sunshine all along Life's pathway. The spirit of his fine fellowship will linger with us as long as memory lasts."[1]

Following the death of Dr. Albert, Dr. D. C. Steelsmith, Deputy Commissioner, was appointed Commissioner of Health until July 1, 1933. Dr. Steelsmith also was a native of Iowa, and an alumnus of the College of Medicine of the State University, Class of 1902. He later completed his training in public health in Boston, receiving a certificate of Public Health (C.P.H.) at Harvard University and Massachusetts Institute of Technology School of Public Health. Previous

Dr. Lanpher quietly but with unerring instinct and accuracy exposed the course and indicated the measures whereby the disease in question could be controlled. Little publicity attended these efforts. In fact, very few of his reports were ever published. Yet few men in the state have rendered a more real and definite service to large groups of our people than did Dr. Lanpher during the few years in which he labored in Iowa. In his untimely death, the State Department of Health has lost a most gifted and valuable staff member, and the state has lost one of its most useful public servants."[2]

Governor Clyde L. Herring appointed Walter L. Bierring, M.D., of Des Moines, Commissioner of Health for the term beginning July 1, 1933.

REFERENCES

1. Journal of the Iowa State Medical Society, xx:231 (May) 1930.
2. Journal of the Iowa State Medical Society, xxii:613 (December) 1932.

REUNION OF KEOKUK GRADUATES

The fourth reunion of the alumni of the College of Physicians and Surgeons, Keokuk Medical College, Keokuk Medical College and College of Physicians and Surgeons and the Keokuk Dental College, was held in Keokuk, Iowa, on Monday, June 18, 1934. Three previous reunions had been held in 1927, 1928, and 1930.

According to the latest list of alumni it is noted that 747 graduates of the three medical schools are now living. The attendance was 375 including graduates, members of families and friends. The registration of alumni was about two hundred. At this year's reunion the oldest graduates attending were Dr. F. M. McCrae, Eddyville, Iowa, class of 1874; Dr. J. C. Boice, Washington, Iowa, class of 1876; Dr. I. F. Harter, Stronghurst, Illinois, class of 1877; and Dr. O. A. Geeseka, Mt. Pleasant, Iowa, class of 1878.

The banquet and social session which followed a business meeting was held at the Keokuk Country Club. Dr. J. M. Trigg of St. Louis, president of the Alumni Association, presided, and addresses of welcome were given by Dr. F. B. Dorsey, Sr., and Dr. Robert M. Lapsley. It was the largest and most representative gathering of Keokuk medical graduates since the merger with Drake University in 1908.

The oldest living graduate is Dr. J. B. Wright, 1540 S. E. 35th Place, Portland, Oregon, born in Virginia on January 16, 1835, who was graduated in 1876, and is still practicing medicine. Each time that a reunion was held he has sent an interesting letter. Herewith is submitted a copy of his letter for this occasion, which may be of interest to the readers of the JOURNAL, coming as it does from a physician who will soon reach the century mark in age.

Bruce L. Gilfillan, M.D., Secretary-Treasurer,
Alumni Association of All Keokuk Medical Schools.

Portland, Oregon.
May 18, 1934.

My Dear Doctor Gilfillan:

Your invitation to the next Medical College reunion at Keokuk, as Secretary, is at hand.

I appreciate your kind remembrance and invitation, and would love to mingle with the fraternity and enjoy the good eats you promise, and shake hands with the veterans, but am too old and feeble to undertake such a long journey.

I was born in Virginia, January 16, 1835, under the administration of Andrew Jackson, but Jackson never mentioned that important matter in his message to Congress, but I never held any grudge against him on that account. My father was a Whig and had never voted for him, and Jackson was a Democrat, and just doted on Democrats. Doubtless if my father had notified him of my arrival, he would have thought father was a Democrat, and said "bully" there's another Democrat.

I always had an ambition to be somebody. When I was a kid I sometimes got into a scrap with the negro boys with whom I played, and sometimes got the worst of it. When I was a small kid I heard about Barnum's big animal show and aspired to be a showman. I had a small dog to begin on, but he wouldn't do. I wanted a dog with his tail curled up his back, and then I could give his tail another curl, so that when he walked, his tail would lift his hind feet off the ground, and maybe he could stand on his head, and Barnum's mule would be a poor show in comparison. This little incident may have had much to do in shaping my career. It naturally lead to the study of anatomy and physiology in a practical way and later in life caused me to seek the association of those similar inclinations. Anyway I never regretted or forgot the trend of my ambition, and maybe it explains why I was found in Keokuk in 1858 with my matriculation ticket, No. 24.

Just consider me with you in spirit on the memorable June 18, 1934. Goodbye. I must now go to the polls and vote to nominate a ticket for the state election next November.

Yours truly,
J. B. Wright, M.D.,
1540 S. E. 35th Place.

OBITUARIES

HERMAN BOCKEN, M.D.

1887-1934

Herman Bocken was born in Harlan, Iowa, and with the exception of his college years, lived in this place until his untimely death which occurred June 10, 1934, from an attack of lobar pneumonia.

He attended and was graduated from the Harlan High School, later attending the University of Nebraska College of Medicine, receiving his medical diploma from this institution with the class of 1911. Dr. Bocken established his practice in Harlan, Iowa, shortly after his graduation and continued until only a few days before his death. For several years, as president of the Shelby County Medical Society, the doctor was always interested in progressive medicine. He was instrumental in establishing the present Harlan Hospital, and was active in medical and surgical practice over Shelby County. Dr. Bocken was local surgeon for the Northwestern Railroad Company, Shelby County coroner for many years and at the time of his death, a member of the Harlan board of school directors, an active member of the local Kiwanis Club and the Harlan Community Club.

At the funeral, which was held from St. Michael's church, fourteen of Dr. Bocken's medical associates from Shelby and neighboring counties, were honorary pallbearers. He is survived by his wife, two

sons, one of whom is a medical student, his parents, two brothers and one sister.

There can be no question but that devotion to duty and his continued answering of calls when his health had begun to suffer, contributed largely to the lack of resistance that made him a rapid victim of pneumonia. His medical friends and a host of loyal patients extend every sympathy to the bereaved widow, sons, aged parents and brothers and sister.

A. L. Nielson, M.D.

ALVAH NEGUS, M.D.

1865-1934

Dr. Alvah Negus of Keswick, died April 15, 1934, at the age of sixty-seven after a long illness. He was a member of the Keokuk County Medical Society, and active so long as his health permitted. He was graduated in 1906 from the State University College of Medicine and located in Keswick, after purchasing the practice of Dr. Ira F. Cameron.

Dr. Negus enlisted in the service early in 1917, and was sent to Ft. Riley where he was assigned to the contagious disease hospital. Here he had as many as sixty patients at one time, and as he had very little help, he carried the entire responsibility and was required to do most of the detail work. It was my privilege to meet the doctor the few times he was able to attend society meetings. A splendid general practitioner, loved and admired both by the laity and the doctors.

C. A. Boice, M.D.

NURSES ARE AIR STEWARDESSES

Four years ago this month the public was surprised by an announcement that women were to become regular members of airplane crews. Today on the fourth anniversary of their sky profession there are 100 planes carrying stewardesses or hostesses instead of the eight with which the United Air Lines inaugurated the experiment which has proved that woman has her place in the air. All of the stewardesses are registered nurses. Nurses are chosen because they have been institutionally trained and show an aptitude in dealing with the public. Twenty-four years is the average age, and preference is given to girls who are not more than five feet, six inches in height, and weigh not more than 125 pounds. Statistics show that there are ten applicants for every available position.

THE AMERICAN COLLEGE OF PHYSICIANS TO MEET IN PHILADELPHIA

With a view of appraising physicians generally of the meeting dates for the 1935 medical session of the American College of Physicians, and also to prevent conflicting dates with other societies that are now arranging their 1935 meetings, officers of the American College of Physicians have requested attention to the following announcement. "The American College of Physicians will hold its Nineteenth Annual Clinical Session in Philadelphia, April 29-May 3, 1935."

THE JOURNAL BOOK SHELF

BOOKS RECEIVED

THE BASIS OF PASSIONAL PSYCHOLOGY—By Dr. Jacobus X, French Army Surgeon. Privately printed, American Anthropological Society, 70 Fifth Avenue, New York City, 1934. Price, $4.00.

EXTERNAL DISEASES OF THE EYE, by Donald T. Atkinson, M.D., consulting ophthalmologist to the Santa Rosa Infirmary and the Nix Hospital, San Antonio, Texas. Octavo of 704 pages, illustrated with 479 engravings. Lea & Febiger, Philadelphia, 1934. Price, $7.50.

I KNOW JUST THE THING FOR THAT!—By J. F. Montague, M.D., medical director, New York Intestinal Sanitarium, The John Day Company, New York, 1934. Price, $2.00.

LOVE—A TREATISE ON THE SCIENCE OF SEX ATTRACTION—By Bernard S. Talmey, M.D. Fifth edition, newly revised and enlarged, with 52 illustrations. Eugenics Publishing Company, New York, 1933.

MEDICAL CLINICS OF NORTH AMERICA—Volume xvii, No. 4. Cleveland Clinic Number, per clinic year, July, 1933, to May, 1934. Octavo of 253 pages with 53 illustrations. W. B. Saunders Company, Philadelphia and London. Price, paper, $12.00; cloth, $16.00, net.

MEDICAL CLINICS OF NORTH AMERICA, Volume xvii, No. 5, New York Number, March, 1934. Per clinic year, July, 1933, to May, 1934. Octavo of 324 pages with 32 illustrations. W. B. Saunders Company, Philadelphia and London, 1934. Price, paper, $12.00; cloth, $16.00.

MEDICO-MILITARY SYMPOSIUM, 1934—Conducted under the auspices of the Kansas City Southwest Clinical Society and the Medical Department, Seventh Corps Area, United States Army, at the General Hospital, Kansas City, Missouri, March 12-17, 1934. Brown-White, Publishers, Kansas City, 1934.

THE 1933 YEAR BOOK OF GENERAL THERAPEUTICS—Edited by Bernard Fantus, M.S., M.D., professor of therapeutics, University of Illinois College of Medicine. The Year Book Publishers, Chicago, 1934. Price, $2.25.

THE 1933 YEAR BOOK OF NEUROLOGY AND PSYCHIATRY—Edited by Peter Bassoe, M.D., clinical professor of neurology, Rush Medical College; and Franklin G. Ebaugh, M.D., professor of psychiatry, University of Colorado School of Medicine. The Year Book Publishers, Chicago, 1934.

THE 1933 YEAR BOOK OF UROLOGY—Edited by John H. Cunningham, M.D., associate in genito-urinary surgery, Harvard University Postgraduate School of Medicine. The Year Book Publishers, Chicago, 1934.

SURGICAL CLINICS OF NORTH AMERICA, Volume xiv, No. 1, Philadelphia Number, February, 1934, to December, 1934. 225 pages with 62 illustrations. W. B. Saunders Company, Philadelphia and London, 1934. Price, paper, $12.00; cloth, $16.00.

SURGICAL CLINICS OF NORTH AMERICA, Volume xiv, No. 2, New York Number, April, 1934. Per clinic year, February, 1934, to December, 1934, 293 pages with 71 illustrations. W. B. Saunders Company, Philadelphia and London, 1934. Price, paper, $12.00; cloth, $16.00.

BOOK REVIEWS

MODERN DRUG ENCYCLOPEDIA AND THERAPEUTIC GUIDE

By Jacob Gutman, M.D., Phar. D., F.A.C.P., Consulting physician, Manhattan General Hospital, New York. Paul B. Hoeber, Inc., 76 Fifth Avenue, New York, 1934. Price, $7.50.

This volume presents all of the popular, non-pharmaceutical preparations, and other remedies found useful in the treatment of disease, describing the composition, uses and administration of the drugs. Inasmuch as many of the preparations described are available from only one manufacturer, the name of the pharmaceutical house is cited.

The second chapter is devoted to effective combinations where two or more fully defined constituents are commonly used. Another chapter deals with preparations of undeclared composition covering some 346 drugs. Other chapters deal with the biologicals, allergens, foods and beverages, and miscellaneous products not logically grouped under the preceding classifications. The closing section of the volume is a therapeutic guide which will prove beneficial as a reference index to the preceding chapters.

The volume is definitely encyclopedic in its scope, and if used in conjunction with the United States Pharmacopeia, will give information on all useful drugs and remedies. It would appear that there is a definite place for a volume of this sort and that it should be enthusiastically recieved by the medical profession.

THE COLLECTED PAPERS OF THE MAYO CLINIC AND THE MAYO FOUNDATION

Volume xxv. Papers of 1933, edited by Mrs. Maude H. Mellish-Wilson and Richard M. Hewitt, M.D. Octavo of 1,230 pages with 210 illustrations. W. B. Saunders Company, Philadelphia and London, 1934. Price, $11.50.

Maintaining the high standard established through the years of the publication of these studies, the volume for 1933 presents in a not too voluminous form the results of the studies and researches of this outstanding organization.

During the year of 1933 the staff of the Mayo Clinic produced 443 papers. Of these 114 are reproduced in this volume in their entirety, 21 are abridged, 40 are abstracted, and only the titles given of the remaining 268.

As in the past the selection of papers for inclusion in this volume has been determined on a basis of those which appeared to be of greatest practical interest to the general practitioner, diagnostician and general surgeon. Space does not permit a detailed discussion of even the most outstanding of the papers presented.

The high standards of the Mayo Clinic and the thoughtful editorship of the volume assure its character. Suffice it to say that a more distinguished collection of original papers dealing with the newer and more worthwhile phases of medical practice cannot be found.

MEDICAL CLINICS OF NORTH AMERICA

Volume xvii, No. 1. Cleveland Clinic Number, per clinic year, July, 1933, to May, 1934. Octavo of 253 pages with 53 illustrations. W. B. Saunders Company, Philadelphia and London. Price, paper, $12.00; cloth, $16.00 net.

This number, produced by the Cleveland Clinic, seems to the reviewer to be distinctly worthwhile. A number of the contributions are pertinent and of practical value to any reader.

Certain of the diseases now occupying the attention of the profession because of their present little understood nature are given attention. Notable among these are the anemias and arthritis. Dr. John analyzes diabetes occurring in children and in adults past fifty years of age. A number of charts are offered depicting the blood sugar curve as the patient progresses in his treatment. The result of his study shows that the insulin requirement for the elderly patient diminishes in direct contrast to the situation in the group of younger patients. He feels that the disease in the aged must present certain essential differences as it is less progressive and more easily controlled. Infection is the constant enemy in the other group. A child who is only mildly diabetic and not requiring insulin can pass into coma in twenty-four hours. The author feels that the handling of youthful diabetic patients has made great strides and that before long these patients will be reasonably secure in their hope for a useful life.

The articles on ulcerative colitis, renal tumors and albuminuria offer viewpoints of considerable interest.   F. R. H.

THE 1933 YEAR BOOK OF NEUROLOGY AND PSYCHIATRY

Edited by Peter Bassoe, M.D., clinical professor of neurology, Rush Medical College; and Franklin G. Ebaugh, M.D., professor of psychiatry, University of Colorado School of Medicine. The Year Book Publishers, Chicago, 1934.

Considerable progress has been registered during the past year in the field of neurology and psychiatry, and several phases of this important group of diseases have been productively studied. New observations have been made in the field of epilepsy and migraine. The St. Louis epidemic of encephalitis brought to light a new group of clinical characteristics which has centered much attention upon this disease during the past year. Sympathectomy has received great attention in many conditions, and its known indications and contraindications are faithfully discussed in this volume.

In psychiatry the trend in the literature is to a closer relation between the various fields of medicine and psychiatry; a trend most useful to both subjects. Forensic psychiatry and child psychiatry have received special consideration.

THE BASIS OF PASSIONAL PSYCHOLOGY

By Dr. Jacobus X, French Army Surgeon, privately printed, American Anthropological Society, 70 Fifth Avenue, New York City, 1934. Price, $4.00.

A number of very readable and enlightening books have recently appeared dealing with the sex instinct and discussing both the normal and abnormal physiology and psychology concerned. For the most part these books discuss the subject from either the physical or psychical side alone, and little or no attempt has been made towards the correlation of the two.

In this volume Dr. Jacobus presents a correlated study tracing the development of the sexual instinct from the lowest forms of mammalian life to the human being. The conclusions which he draws from his various studies form, perhaps, the most valuable aspect of the work. These conclusions are in many instances contrary to the popular teachings, but in each instance seem to follow logically the factual presentation of the chapter.

The volume is evidently prepared for the advanced student, and should not be confused with the many elementary and more superficial discussions of this subject prepared for the occasional reader in this field. Because of the controversial nature of the material presented and the somewhat arbitrary conclusions of the author, the volume will be thought-provoking and distinctly worthwhile to the physician.

THE 1933 YEAR BOOK OF GENERAL THERAPEUTICS

Edited by Bernard Fantus, M.S., M.D., professor of therapeutics, University of Illinois College of Medicine. The Year Book Publishers, Chicago, 1934. Price, $2.25.

The past year has been a productive one in the field of therapy, and the advances reviewed in this edition of the Year Book are particularly useful to the physician who would apply the latest and best in therapeutics in his practice.

The discussion of the newer treatments of anemia is particularly timely and helpful. Therapy in this group of diseases has been so signally advanced as to make it appear that a new nomenclature would be required on this therapeutic basis. Additional studies in the field of convalescent prophylactic serum, particularly in poliomyelitis and scarlet fever, are noteworthy. The office treatment of varicose veins of the legs, of hemorrhoids, and of hernia will interest every practitioner. Oral cholecystography has been advanced to equal the intravenous method.

The general scheme of the volume remains unchanged and a more extensive description of the volume seems unnecessary, inasmuch as it has been for many years outstanding in its particular field and comes again as an old friend to the attention of the practicing physician.

The JOURNAL
of the
Iowa State Medical Society

Vol. XXIV   Des Moines, Iowa, August, 1934   No. 8

ORATION IN MEDICINE

The Education of a Physician

George B. Crow, M.D., Burlington

According to Justice Cardoza, "There is in each of us a stream of tendency, whether you choose to call it philosophy or not, which gives coherence and direction to thought and action. None of us can escape that current. All our lives, forces which we do not recognize and cannot name, have been tugging at us—inherited instincts, traditional beliefs, acquired convictions; and the resultant is an outlook on life, a conception of social needs, 'a sense of the total push and pressure of the cosmos,' which when reasons are nicely balanced must determine where choice shall fall."

In order, then, to reach a proper understanding of the motivating factors in the life of any man, it would be necessary to consider the many and diverse influences which have played upon him. The biologist would want to know his ancestry, the sociologist would study his environment, while the psychologically inclined physician would look for the sum total of these—the physical state and mental reactions of the individual. Possibly future biographers may note that the irascible character of this man was due to a duodenal ulcer or an irritated gallbladder, while the superb diplomacy of another was incident to a proper balance of calcium and potassium ions in the tissues; this, in turn, being dependent on a proper functioning of the endocrine glands.

If an understanding of any man is difficult there are added difficulties when we approach the study of that peculiar type of individual, the physician. It is true he belongs to the genus homo, species sapiens, but popular opinion would provide some sort of subclass for him. He is not as other men. We would like to believe all the wonderful things Robert Louis Stevenson said of him, but we know him too well. Some may approach the

Presented before the Eighty-third Annual Session, Iowa State Medical Society, Des Moines, May 9, 10, 11, 1934.

high pedestal on which that charmer of our boyhood days placed us, but few can maintain such an exalted plane. The physician is a constant enigma, a man of many moods, a mass of contradictions. Under certain circumstances he is dogmatic and domineering, under others as soothing as oil. At times he appears utterly heartless and, again, on rare occasions, he will be found soft as putty. To his family and friends he may be alternately morose and exuberant without discernible reason. His long suffering wife has, we hope, some understanding of and forgiveness for these vacillations of spirit.

Now if this man is not as other men, what made him different? Surely not heredity or early environment. During that period the current of his life did not differ, on the whole, from that of his associates. We must look, then, to his medical education for the things that have changed him. Let us examine some of the factors which enter into a doctor's education. The current of his life is now definitely changed. He even enters a new stream; a stream that curiously courses the world about him and at the same time reaches into new and totally strange fields.

Into this stream, will come first, rivulets of highly technical and painfully acquired knowledge regarding the gross and minute structure of the human body, and how it functions in health; then other rivulets of fact and belief about the changes produced in that body by all the external and internal agencies that may assail it. Our embyro doctor is likely to be impatient with this stage of his education. He will be unable to understand fully the need of this basis for the study of disease, to visualize its later application. He wants to come in personal contact with disease and its many manifestations in the living body, but by and by he will see sick people. He will first hear the history, the subjective evidence of disease, and the sequence of its appearance, but this will usually come to him second hand, and something will be lost in the telling. The facts may all be there but the relative values of symptoms may be missed; and the pieces of this jig-saw puzzle must be fitted together to complete the picture. We grant that in some diseases and from some patients an adequate history may be obtained in the classroom, but in many other cases the complete story from the patient and the ability of the doctor to evaluate its parts can come only when that story is told in private to the particular doctor chosen by that particular patient, and that story may be the key necessary to unlock that particular problem. This is not a criticism of this aspect of teaching; the class method cannot be otherwise. The effectiveness of teaching will depend largely upon the ability of the teacher to transmit his first hand impressions to his students.

Following this will come the search for objective evidences of disease; an explanation of the symptoms which he has just heard. This search may end quickly or may necessitate the employment of several of the vast number of physical, biochemical and bacteriologic procedures which have gained recognition as aids in diagnosis.

Before the advent of the machine age in medicine, physicians had to depend solely upon their special senses and reasoning powers in making diagnoses. Because of that very necessity of depending upon themselves they developed a "clinical sense," a skill in interpretation of symptoms and observation of physical signs which is probably far less common today. The medical student of today is required to spend so much time in getting a fragmentary acquaintance with the innumerable laboratory tests that little time is left for acquiring even the beginning of this "clinical sense." He runs the further risk of becoming so imbued with the importance of these technical details that he may not place them in the auxiliary position where they belong. Some have entered practice feeling completely helpless unless all these aids were at their constant command. Recently in one of our large medical schools a teacher was gravely pointing out, while the students solemnly wrote down, the technical radiologic procedure for the recognition of ulcer appearing after gastroenterostomy. Too much of that sort of thing will leave our young graduate in the predicament recalled in the childhood rhyme of

"Old Dan Tucker (who) went to town
   To buy a pair of trousers,
But old Dan Tucker didn't see the town
   For there were so many houses."

The vast majority of graduates will become general practitioners. Therefore, the primary object of the schools should be to train men for the kind

of work most of them will be forced to do, and for which they can find time and physical equipment. Most cases of diabetes can be adequately managed without determination of the respiratory quotient and without frequent blood sugar readings. Few cases of nephritis are benefited by estimating the amount of retained nitrogen in the blood. These added data are always interesting and sometimes helpful, and the man in general practice should understand in a general way their significance. The point to be stressed is that he should not feel helpless without them.

The undergraduate school can do little more than teach the basic principles, and establish habits and methods for further study. There will be some attention given to prognosis in general, and somewhat more to treatment in particular. Somewhere in this process the student must learn the natural history of disease; the typical course of the more common diseases with the more common variations from the typical. Only in this way can disease be recognized in its varying presenting stages; only in this way can its future manifestations be predicted.

Thus far our young doctor-to-be has led a sheltered life. In college and hospital, pilots were ever at hand to point out hidden rock and snag, to steer him away from reef and bar. The tributaries to his stream of knowledge have, we hope, had their headwaters mainly in fact with only a minimum of tradition and belief to muddy the current.

However, the day comes when he goes out on his own. Here a thousand confusions await him; the solution of problems, the very existence of which were scarcely known to him. Fortunate for him if he has some stable older physician to guide him. According to tradition he "enters private practice." Does he? He does not. How can he enter something which for him does not exist? He must be a magician and create something out of nothing. Tradition tells him he must not use the printed page to tell the world how good he is, and for once, we believe, tradition is right. So he sits down with his books and his thoughts, and holds onto his courage as best he can. In time there will come to him the "deadbeat" and the disgruntled, with, perhaps, an occasional hard nut that the other fellow failed to crack. Here is his chance. If he cracks it his reputation is made and practice will enter unto him; but if he be wise he will also be humble. He will realize that the study of disease never ends. According to an ancient Greek philosopher nothing is certain but change. Dr. Henry Christian has recently phrased this in another way by stating "there is nothing static in this world, we are either learning or forgetting, progressing or retrogressing."

To keep step with that progress our young doctor must do more than make resolutions; he must do more than study recent textbooks and journals. He must also attend medical society meetings and clinics where he gets something that cannot be transferred to the printed page—the inspiration that can come only through the personality of the teacher.

Still something more must be learned; something which he will not find in books and journals and which he will get in only a limited way from clinics and consultants—the ability to make a reasonably accurate prognosis. This involves a broadly inclusive comprehension of the action of the disease and the reaction of the patient. In his early years of practice William Mackenzie apprenticed himself to Dr. Briggs, an old general practitioner of Burnley, Scotland. Dr. Briggs had little so-called scientific education; yet he constantly astonished young Mackenzie by his ability to foresee what would happen in the many cases they saw together. As Mackenzie put it, Dr. Briggs knew "the face of disease." In time the young apprentice came to realize that the old doctor in looking at a patient saw much more than that patient; he unconsciously visualized his experiences with hundreds of other similar cases. No doctor can quickly acquire this faculty, but careful study and observation will hasten the process.

To the doctor will come rather frequently a type of patient which he has seen only casually during his college days, a type that will be a source of much worry and possibly even of irritation. Following the promulgation of Virchow's cellular pathology, medical men for some time were loath to believe in the existence of disease without demonstrable structural change. We are seeing an ever increasing number of patients with a multiplicity of complaints, but without detectable organic defects to explain them. Nevertheless many of these individuals exhibit unmistakable evidence of deranged bodily function. Careful inquiry will often reveal that such patients are out of harmony with their world or with themselves. The problems of life have become too great for them, and they subconsciously take the by-path of physical reaction to escape emotional conflict. We put them through the diagnostic mill, find no evidence of organic disease and dismiss them. They try another doctor with the same results. Finally, in despair, they go to the quack who at least has sufficient gumption to make a show of sympathy and understanding. The discerning old family doctor who knew the intimate affairs of his patients almost as well as his own, probably never

psychoanalyzed these patients nor said to himself, "Here is an instance of changed personality;" but he did put his finger on the trouble, and quietly guided the confused sufferers to such stability as was for them possible. There are, of course, some conflicts which cannot be removed; some problems which cannot be solved; but we can let the patient know the nature of their problem, and perhaps stop their search for the unattainable.

The above reference is an indication of the complexity of the doctor's postcollegiate education. He will find that the practice of medicine brings to him a more intimate relation with humanity than any other calling. There will be revealed to him life, raw and naked, the joys and the sorrows of mankind, the physical and mental anguish of his patients, the weaknesses and the frailties of human nature, as well as courage and force of character where often it is unexpected. The sick must unreservedly place themselves in his hands if he is to give them the best service. Their life, and sometimes their honor will be in his hands. It is the physician's duty to protect these to the utmost; to take no unfair advantage of the fears and weaknesses of those who do unreservedly place themselves at his disposal. This may all appear trite; wholly unnecessary; but a re-affirmation of, and a new pledge to, our creed can do no harm, for to the doctor will come temptation. In the midst of his worries about how to pay the grocer and the landlord there will come opportunities for financial gain which are commonly condemned. Perhaps he will hear whispers that the established men in his community are resorting to these condemned practices. We hope that he will even then hold to the creed, and continue to worry about his unpaid bills.

What about the relations between the doctor and his fellow physicians? What rules shall guide him? We have a code of ethics which attempts to help us, but unfortunately we find different interpretations of that code, especially as it applies to the course one should follow when a patient leaves one doctor to consult another. That should not be a difficult problem. Common courtesy and common sense should solve it. We cannot escape the fact that the patient has the right to choose his medical adviser. It follows that he has the right to change advisers. We occasionally meet a physician who seems to feel that a lost patient is a stolen patient. Patients that can be stolen are not worth keeping. The unwilling patient is a liability and not an asset. We have heard tales about a kind of doctor who seeks by innuendo or open disparagement to belittle the qualifications of his confrère. If his mouthings are given credence he will, in the end, suffer as much as the one maligned; for whatever tends to undermine confidence in a part of the profession will react in the same degree on the whole of it. There is also the patient who for one reason or another, or without reason, flits from one doctor to another. These people do not realize that the best type of medical service will never be theirs. Their interim physician knows that he does not have their full confidence, and no physician can give his best without that confidence. Furthermore the physician brings to his more constant patients an accumulated fund of knowledge about them which, in the management of a given disease. may be invaluable.

Any discussion of the education of a physician. should include some reference to the specialist— the man who limits his work to one or a few types of diseases, or to diseases affecting a restricted anatomic field. There is no question as to the need for men with special skill in such fields. The scope of medical knowledge has become too extensive for any one man to be familiar with all of it. Concentration of effort provides not only opportunity for greater skill but for advancement of knowledge as well.

While we admit the need for men with such specialized training we must admit also a limited need for their services. There is apparently a well founded conviction that during the last two decades these special fields have become overcrowded. Several reasons have contributed to this. By limiting his field, a man may have the satisfaction of knowing all that is known about a few things. The specialist can expect better remuneration for his services and he also escapes much of the drudgery inherent in general practice. The attitude of the public has also helped to swell the ranks in the specialties. John Citizen has become strangely obsessed with the belief that his family doctor is capable of managing only minor ailments. Dr. George Morris Piersol, in his recent presidential address before the American College of Physicians, expressed his carefully considered opinion that only fifteen per cent of all illness actually needs the services of specialists; that the other eighty-five per cent could be properly cared for by the general practitioner. This would seem to imply, however, that the general practitioner has an obligation to keep himself fitted to do the work that rightfully belongs to him. Dr. Piersol also believes that professional standards in the various specialties should be established with, perhaps, special licensing boards to pass on the qualifications of applicants. What fee is the specialist entitled to? It is commonly conceded that the man who has spent extra time and extra money to equip himself in a special field is entitled to extra remuneration. The specialist should constantly re-

other sensory modalities, it is safe to assume that this critical function is also there, residual.

Clinicians make a distinction between what is known as central pain and that of peripheral origin. It is well known that vascular, degenerative, or neoplastic lesions in, or impinging upon, one optic thalamus may cause a hemiplegia, associated with an intractable form of pain in the paretic side. This is the best illustration of a condition in which we recognize so-called central pain. It is highly probable that other structures in the central nervous system, when attacked by pathologic processes, may cause central pain and yet our knowledge concerning this is very incomplete. What we now know about this type of pain throws little light on the subject of headache, because in the illustration just mentioned, the discomfort is referred to one side of the body and not to the head.

In an attempt to elaborate on my subject, I shall endeavor to assemble certain fragments of anatomic, physiologic, and neurosurgical evidence which I believe point definitely to the important rôle which the blood vessel born sympathetic nerves play in the production of the less explainable forms of headache. The neurosurgeons have learned the following facts during their operations on the head under local anesthesia (the patients being conscious) :

1. That the scalp can be readily anesthetized with novocaine but that an excessive amount needs to be injected in the region of the temporal artery.

2. That the calvarium is apparently insensitive to surgical attack.

3. That invasion of the dura causes little or no pain with the exception that novocaine needs to be applied over the middle meningeal artery when it is clipped and cut.

4. The brain tissues proper, especially those of the cerebrum, are insensitive to puncture and incision.

From the above observations, it would appear that the intracranial areas, which are, when traumatized, capable of producing pain, are in the immediate vicinity of blood vessels. One or two brain surgeons have told me that severe stretching of the tentorium occasionally causes pain.

The following clinical observations, other than surgical, which seem to bear out the neurovascular relationship to intracranial pain, are these: First, a paretic patient, whose brain is thoroughly peppered with treponema, although he suffers some discomfort referable to the head, seldom has severe headache, whereas the vicious headache of meningovascular syphilis is well recognized; and second, leptomeningitis, involving as it does, the most vascular covering of the brain, the pia, causes

the most atrocious form of headache known to
medicine. I now wish to call your attention to a
few anatomic points for which I must depend on
Gray's Anatomy. The authority just cited indicates that the dura mater is supplied by the following nerve mechanisms; the trochlear nerve, the
Gasserian ganglion, and its trigeminal divisions,
the vagus, the hypoglossal, and the sympathetic
nerves. In speaking of the trochlear nerve, the
following quotation is offered. "It gives off a recurrent branch which passes between the layers
of the tentorium, dividing into two or three filaments which may be traced as far back as the wall
of the lateral sinus. In the outer wall of the cavernous sinus it receives some filaments from the
cavernous plexus of the sympathetic." Inasmuch
as the trochlear nerve is essentially motor, it
would seem probable that its sensory function is
subserved by fibers of communication from the
sympathetic nerve. The Gasserian ganglia and
their trigeminal divisions have a predominant sensory rôle which might be expected to play a part
in intracranial pain. The vagus nerve, owing to
its wide distribution and varied functionings, may
also be thought of as having something to do with
headache. The hypoglossal nerve would not impress one as being a pain transmitting mechanism,
yet since it has no apparent motor function within
the cranial cavity, its representation there indicates that it has something to do with sensation,
possibly pain.

Two things must be born in mind with regard
to the nerves found in the dura. First, tic douloureux, which probably has its seat in the Gasserian ganglia, and finds expression through the trigeminal divisions, seldom if ever produces headache. Second, every nerve heretofore mentioned
is associated by way of various ganglionic connections with the sympathetic nerve. Quoting from
Gray's Anatomy, "There is no positive evidence
that nerves are present in the arachnoid." In
speaking of the pia, the same authority states
"The nerves of the pia accompany the arteries
and are derived chiefly from the sympathetic. A
few fibers are derived from certain cranial nerves
also which are probably of the afferent variety."
From the data thus far assembled, it would seem
that there is strong evidence upon which to base
the hypothesis that the nerve mechanism chiefly
involved in the transmission of the pain impulses
of headache, is the sympathetic nerve. Since I am
attempting to incriminate the blood vessel born
sympathetic fibers of the brain, I must remind you
that recent anatomic investigations have proved
that the brain as a whole is much more richly supplied with blood vessels than was previously believed, and that sympathetic vasomotor fibers are

is certainly less dangerous than the use of most intravenous dyes, and to my mind, a much more rational form of therapy.

Immunotransfusions are of even more recent origin than unaltered blood transfusions. First used by Sir Almroth Wright[1] in 1909, they apparently received little attention and subsequent thought in this country. He successfully treated a case of streptococcic septicemia with nonspecific immunotransfusion. At this time, Sir Almroth Wright set forth several very important principles in the treatment of septicemias. Some of these are still strictly adhered to; others are apparently forgotten or neglected. He pointed out that adequate surgical drainage of the infected focus, whenever possible, was extremely important. By this, we assist the organism in overcoming the conveyance of bacteria or bacterial toxins to the blood stream. Where drainage is impossible, rest and immobilization of the affected part are essential. Second, he found it possible to produce nonspecific bactericidal agents by inoculating blood, in vivo or in vitro, with different types of killed organisms. He also discovered that such inoculated blood, after six to eight hours, had definite curative effects in septicemias. Third, he stressed the use of specific immunotransfusions, whenever possible, in preference to nonspecific immunotransfusions. Last, an observation made often since, that unaltered blood transfusions are of no value in septicemia and may even be harmful.

In 1923, Colebrook and Storer[2] reviewed the work of Sir Almroth Wright and described their technic of immunotransfusions. In 1932, Brody and Crocker[3] reported a case of septicemia treated with specific immunotransfusion. In 1933, Stephenson[4] reported a case treated with nonspecific immunotransfusions following a procedure suggested by Brody.

I wish to report two cases of streptococcus hemolyticus septicemia treated with nonspecific immunotransfusions. The first case is one of a gunshot wound, complicated by bacillus Welchii infection, which later developed streptococcic hemolyticus septicemia.

CASE REPORT

Mr. C. P., twenty-one years of age, was accidentally shot below the right knee on November 13, 1932. Due to impassable roads it was seven hours before the patient finally reached the hospital. The patient was in extreme shock from the loss of blood and exposure. He was pulseless and no blood pressure reading could be obtained. A citrate blood transfusion of 500 c.c. was given. Antitetanic serum was also given. A normal salt solution was administered subpectorally. His condition was somewhat improved the next morning, his blood pressure now being 60 systolic and 40 diastolic. The red cell count was 2,140,000, and the leukocyte count 19,000. Amputation was delayed in the hope that the patient's condition would improve. On the morning of November 15, beginning gangrene of the foot was present. The next day, a light brownish drainage with a very pungent odor was found. There was no crepitation, but from the character of the drainage a diagnosis of bacillus Welchii infection was made. A portable x-ray plate showed gas in the tissues with multiple gun shot fractures of both bones of the leg just below the condyle of the tibia. He was given the first 10,000 units of gas bacillus antitoxin in the right thigh. The wound was saturated with hydrogen peroxide. A second blood transfusion of 700 c.c. was given. During the night his temperature rose to 105 degrees and his condition became critical. The following morning, a guillotine amputation at the junction of the lower and middle thirds of the thigh was performed. Following this there was a drop in temperature to below normal. The laboratory reported bacillus Welchii infection. On the morning of November 19, the infection was again very evident and the patient's condition was again critical. Since amputation appeared to be the only hope, he was subjected to the second amputation at the junction of the middle and upper thirds of the thigh. The shock following this was very severe. All the muscle planes were opened. A second 10,000 units of antitoxin was given in the right lumbar region. The wound was irrigated with potassium permanganate solution. It was evident that the infection had spread beyond the point of amputation, but the patient's condition permitted no further work. The following morning, his temperature, which had dropped during the day, again rose and the infection was again very evident. His condition appeared hopeless.

Needles were now placed about the upper stump and Dakin's solution injected through these into the stump every hour of the day and night. The right groin and lower abdomen were also infiltrated. On November 21, 10,000 units of antitoxin, the third dose, was given, this time intravenously. A third blood transfusion of 500 c.c. was given. The following day there was less drainage and the pungent odor was absent. The toxemia had greatly decreased. Irrigations were continued. On November 25, a fourth intravenous dose of antitoxin was given; a parotitis developed. Two days later the patient became rational, his condition was much improved and the gas bacillus infection appeared to be checked. The muscles now had a brick red appearance. Secondary infection evidenced itself, and hot boric dressings

were applied to the stump. Extreme pain developed in the chest and left shoulder, also in the epigastrium. A few days later, and for several days after, tarry stools were passed. On December 9, the fourth blood transfusion of 500 c.c. was given. Abscesses formed in the stump. The next day the red cell count was 3,310,000 and the leukocyte count was 15,000. His condition was less favorable. Five days later a fifth blood transfusion of 500 c.c. was given. The drainage had now become greenish in color. His condition showed no change, and on December 28, he had his first chill. An x-ray examination revealed the presence of an osteomyelitis of the lower portion of the stump. The infected portion was removed and the muscle planes again opened. The shock and weakened condition of the patient were so severe that no hopes of recovery appeared possible. The following day, there was some improvement but the chills continued. A diagnosis of septicemia was made. The pain in the chest and left shoulder required morphine. Following the chills, which lasted from twenty-five to thirty minutes, his temperature would reach from 103 to 105 degrees. Vaccine treatment was begun and continued over a period of ten days, but very little benefit was derived. The chills continued daily or every second day. On January 16, the first blood culture was taken and reported positive for streptococcus hemolyticus. The patient was extremely weak, and apparently unable to overcome the infection, and hopes for his recovery waned. His red cell count now was 2,740,000 and the leukocyte count was 10,500 with evidence in the Schilling hemogram of very little resistance. It was at this time, that we decided to try immunotransfusions. To tide the patient over and while preparing a specific donor, we decided to use nonspecific immunotransfusions.

At midnight of January 22, the first donor was given fifty million of dead typhoid bacilli intravenously. About one and a half hours later, he chilled for about fifteen minutes and his temperature rose to 102 degrees. About eight hours later, 250 c.c. of blood were taken by the citrate method. The brachial vein of the patient was then exposed and blood again taken for culture and reported positive. He was then given his first nonspecific immunotransfusion without any reaction. The chills continued but the temperature decreased. Slight improvement was evident. The red cell count the following day, was 3,310,000 and the leukocyte count was 10,000. On the night of January 25, the second donor was given fifty million dead typhoid bacilli intravenously. After about two hours he had a short chill and his temperature rose to 101.8 degrees. About eight hours later 400 c.c. of blood were withdrawn. A third

CASE REPORT

Mr. F. W.; thirty-three years of age, became ill on January 3, 1934, with a streptococcic throat infection, and entered the hospital on that date. The following day, a generalized exanthematous rash developed. This condition suggested scarlet fever, but was finally proved to be of toxic origin. After four days, the patient left the hospital. On January 8 and 9, his condition improved but on January 10, some pain was felt in the left side of his throat and a swelling appeared. By January 12, his throat, badly swollen, made swallowing painful; an abscess which had formed, was lanced, and some relief was obtained. On January 13, chills followed his bath and his temperature rose to 101.8 degrees. The patient was seen on the following evening. His temperature registered 103 degrees and the pulse rate was 90 per minute; the urine was negative; the leukocyte count was 15,300; the entire body, particularly the hands and back, were scaling; the left side of the throat, in the region of the posterior pillar was still slightly swollen; and there was a bilateral cervical adenopathy, more evident on the right. A precordial systolic murmur was audible. The lungs were negative. There were no abdominal symptoms or findings. A tentative diagnosis of an endocarditis or septicemia was made. A blood culture was taken on January 15. On this day, a chill occurred lasting about one hour. His temperature rose to 104.6 and his pulse to 100. He continued to feel chilly, while his temperature remained between 103 and 104 degrees during the two following days.

On January 17, the blood culture was reported positive for streptococcus hemolyticus. He now returned to the hospital. The red cell count was 3,660,000; the hemoglobin was 65 per cent; the leukocyte count was 15,700; and the Schilling hemogram showed segmented cells 33, band forms 59, juveniles eight, lymphocytes nine, and one large mononuclear. The patient was immediately typed and donors secured for nonspecific immunotransfusions. Every effort was made to locate a possible focus, but without success. On the night of January 17, the first donor was given fifty million of Lederle's triple typhoid vaccine intravenously and in the morning 300 c.c. of blood were withdrawn using the citrate method. The next day the patient was given his first nonspecific immunotransfusion. In the meantime the organism was subcultured and attempts were made to prepare a vaccine in preparation of a specific donor. Following the transfusion, his temperature dropped to 100 degrees, but by evening had risen to 104.4 degrees. The patient perspired profusely; the systolic murmur became more pronounced and a gallop rhythm was audible. The blood pressure dropped to 90 systolic and 50 diastolic. An endocarditis was feared. A chest plate showed general cardiac hypertrophy. On January 19, his condition seemed improved and his temperature had dropped to 98 degrees. The red cell count was 4,510,000; the hemoglobin was 75 per cent; the leukocyte count was 10,800; and the Schilling hemogram showed 30 segmented cells, 35 band forms, one juvenile, 28 lymphocytes, and six large mononuclears. By evening his temperature rose to 103.4 degrees and he became slightly irrational. Early the next morning the second donor was given 75 million of Lederle's triple vaccine, intravenously. Six hours later, the patient was given his second nonspecific immunotransfusion of 300 c.c. The patient's condition was improved and the gallop rhythm was absent. His temperature the following morning was 98.4 degrees and his pulse 88 per minute. The blood pressure was 100 systolic and 70 diastolic. The highest temperature on this day was 101.4. The patient was further improved on the following day, but still perspired freely. The leukocyte count was 14,900, Schilling hemogram showed 48 segmented cells, 29 band forms, no juveniles, 21 lymphocytes and two large mononuclears.

The temperature again rose to 103.4 degrees in the afternoon. About 4:00 A. M. on January 22, another donor was given fifty million triple typhoid vaccine, intravenously. Six hours later, 350 c.c. of blood were withdrawn and the patient given his third nonspecific immunotransfusion. Before the transfusion the condition of the blood was as follows: red cell count 4,260,000; leukocyte count, 10,900; Schilling hemogram showed 50 segmented cells, 24 band forms, two juveniles, and 16 lymphocytes. The highest temperature for this day was 100.6 degrees. We decided to repeat the transfusion the following day instead of allowing two days to lapse. The fourth transfusion was 300 c.c. and the highest temperature was 99 degrees with the patient showing definite signs of improvement. On January 24, the fifth transfusion of 300 c.c. was given and the temperature remained at 99 degrees. A blood culture was taken and reported negative. The following day another culture was reported negative, and perspiration had decreased. By evening his temperature rose to 101 degrees due to a flare-up of the throat infection, which subsided slowly. During the nonspecific therapy, we were unable to subculture sufficient organisms to make a vaccine for specific therapy. The throat infection continued to cause some distress, and on February 4, another exacerbation occurred with increased temperature and

pulse, as well as a leukocytosis of 15,000. The temperature gradually rose to between 103 and 104 degrees with profuse perspiration resulting in extreme weakness. By February 11, a large external abscess had formed on the right anterior lateral side of the neck. Under local anesthesia, this was incised, and profuse thick yellow greenish pus wa drained. There was immediate relief from pain in swallowing which had become acute and most distressing.

From then on the patient slowly improved. The temperature remained between 100 and 101 degrees for about one week and then slowly returned to normal. Perspiration became less, strength increased, and the patient began to gain the weight he had lost.

Comment

For most of us, the treatment of septicemia has always been attended with great difficulties. It is a common attribute of physicians to strive for some specific form of treatment for the diseases he encounters. In so doing, he is likely to be led astray. This has been well illustrated in the use of the new chemicals and various other forms of therapy alleged to be of value in the treatment of septicemia. The maintenance of an intelligent skepticism·is a prerequisite of every good and reliable physician.

Distinctions are still made between septicemia and bacteremia. In the former the blood contains multiplying organisms while in the latter, the bacteria are being transported into the blood stream from some focus, the bacteria, however, not multiplying in it. This distinction, I believe, may lead us into difficulty, as well as to a useless search for some possible focus, when other forms of therapy should be under way. True enough, in many cases there is a constant slow feeding of organisms into the blood stream from some infected focus. With the removal of this focus or the stopping of this influx by surgical procedures, the septicemia will often disappear. Unfortunately, this is, however, not always the case. In many cases the original focus has been drained but the septicemia persists and rapidly overcomes the patient. Hence, I believe it possible for the organisms, after once having gained entrance to the blood stream, to multiply in it, without the presence of a feeding focus. It is in these cases, where the surgeon has done all he can and the septicemia persists, that nonspecific and specific immunotransfusions become our anchor of hope.

The bacteria that exist in the blood stream in septicemia are usually staphylococci and streptococci, or both. The most common organims are the hemolytic streptococci and the streptococcus

3. Where anemia is present, the degree, depending on the duration and perhaps the virulence of the septicemia, it will be improved by the addition of red cells.

4. Unlike nonmodified blood, where we have no additional immunizing properties, we are adding blood with greatly increased immunizing properties in addition to normal leukocytes.

Disadvantages of this method:

1. Several compatible donors are needed and this necessitates typing many individuals.

2. The treatment can be carried out only in a hospital having adequate laboratory facilities.

It may be said by some, that unaltered blood transfusions would be as valuable. This has been fairly well proved untrue. If the anemia is very marked, there will be some response from the increase in red cells. However, blood transfusions were used for these cases for years and the results did not warrant continuance. By some it is even claimed to be harmful; at least, it is generally admitted to be of no definite value. In my first case, the patient had had five nonmodified transfusions and still developed septicemia. In the Brody and Crocker case, the patient had been given five nonmodified transfusions of 150 c.c. each, and another of 50 c.c., without affecting the septicemia. On the contrary, one specific immunotransfusion immediately overcame the septicemia. This evidence indicates that additional immunizing properties are essential in these cases.

I do not want to give the impression that specific or nonspecific immunotransfusions are a panacea for all septicemias. To my mind, they have definite indications. Herein lies the danger as in many other forms of therapy. Immunotransfusions are likely to be used where they are not indicated and if the result is unfavorable, the operator misconstrues the value of the treatment and pronounces it a failure. If we wish to have a scientific basis for our opinion and work, it is absolutely essential that a positive blood culture be obtained. The organism must be subcultured to determine definitely what organism is present. From this we can decide whether results can be expected. This type of therapy is of no value in streptococcus viridans, hence, it is not indicated. In septicemias resulting from pneumococcus or colon bacillus, it should be given a trial. Whether it is of value in these cases is not known. I believe that the remarkable results obtained in these two cases and in the case reported warrant a trial of this form of therapy in all cases of streptococcus hemolyticus septicemia. I would urge its early use.

SUMMARY

Two cases of streptococcus hemolyticus septicemia have been discussed and the results obtained with nonspecific immunotransfusions were reported. I believe this to be a most valuable form of therapy and hope for its further use to determine more fully its true value. Until then we may maintain an intelligent skepticism.

BIBLIOGRAPHY

1. Wright, A. E.: Prospects in the field of therapeutic immunization. Lancet (London), i:489-501, 1919.
2. Colebrook, L., and Storer, E. J.: Immunotransfusions. Lancet (London), ii:1341-1344, and 1394-1398, 1923.
3. Brody, W., and Crocker, W. J.: Specific immunotransfusion in the treatment of septicemia. Jour. Am. Med. Assn., xcviii:2191-2193, 1932.
4. Stephenson, Ruth: Nonspecific immunotransfusion in hemolytic streptococcus septicemia. Jour. Am. Med. Assn., c:100-102, 1933.

THE ROENTGEN RAY DIAGNOSIS OF NON-OPAQUE FOREIGN BODIES IN THE BRONCHI*

EDWIN L. RYPINS, M.D., Iowa City

Non-opaque foreign bodies in the bronchi are of especial interest because approximately 90 per cent of them occur in children under two years of age. Thus, the history obtained is less likely to prove of value as an aid in diagnosis. Also, infants are very prone to aspirate foreign bodies without knowledge of the parents. The vegetal foreign bodies, (peanuts, beans, peas, corn, wheat seeds, oats, etc.) are of particular importance because they are very apt to produce violent inflammatory reaction, in addition to lung suppuration, if they are not ultimately removed. Only a very small percentage of such foreign bodies are apt to be expelled spontaneously.

If a healthy child who is playing in a normal fashion, suddenly chokes, with or without cyanosis, the possibility of a foreign body should be considered. Furthermore, a history of the child playing with corn or peanuts, and then developing respiratory difficulty, is also of great value. The main difficulty in arriving at a diagnosis of a nonopaque foreign body in the bronchi comes in not considering the possibility, no matter what chest findings are presented.

Foreign bodies in the bronchi may cause any one of three types of obstruction.

1. Ball valve—where air may pass obstruction on both inspiration and expiration.

2. Stop valve—where no air either enters or leaves, and atelectasis quickly develops.

3. Check valve—where air passes into the lung on inspiration, but is trapped there.

This latter type is the one most commonly found, when non-opaque foreign bodies lodge in

*Presented before the Eighty-third Annual Session, Iowa State Medical Society, Des Moines, May 9, 10, 11, 1934.

a bronchus. Air readily passes the obstruction on inspiration due to the fact that there is an inspiratory widening of the bronchial lumen. On expiration the bronchial lumen narrows, and the air does not pass out. This, of course, results in emphysema of the involved side noted on expiration. A vegetal foreign body may cause such changes within from four to six hours. It is extremely important that such a foreign body be removed as soon as possible, as it tends to swell, due to the bronchial secretions, and thus causes complete atelectasis, with lung suppuration, and eventually death.

Since definite changes will occur at the two phases of respiration, films are so taken. A crying child can be exposed at the end of the expiratory phase of the cry, and at the instant of deep inspiration. Due to the emphysema at expiration the heart will be displaced away from the affected side, there will be increased transparency of the affected lung, and depression and partial fixation of the diaphragm on the affected side. As Manges has well shown, the heart diameter is shorter at expiration than at inspiration when a foreign body is present, but just the reverse is normally found. Also, the narrow diameter of the chest is found on expiration.

Case 1. The patient, eighteen months of age, was eating a peanut candy bar, forty-eight hours before entrance, when he suddenly choked. He was hung up by his feet, and struck on the back. The patient expectorated a considerable amount of chewed candy and peanuts. He wheezed for several hours, and had an occasional dry cough. Bronchoscopic examination revealed considerable edema and swelling of the opening of the right upper bronchus (See Figures 1 and 2.) Some thick tenacious secretion was aspirated from the right upper bronchus, along with several small pieces of peanut. This case illustrates how the foreign body may shift. It was undoubtedly in the left bronchus when the films were taken, but was removed from the opposite bronchus.

Case 2. Thirty-six hours before entrance the brother of the patient, two years of age, placed a handful of corn on a table. The baby was seen to take some in her hand. A short time later the mother found the baby coughing, wheezing, and blue in the face. Bronchoscopic examination revealed a kernel of corn impacted in the upper right main bronchus. This was removed. (See Figure 3.)

CONCLUSIONS

1. The possibility of non-opaque foreign bodies should be kept in mind in any child who presents pulmonary symptoms.

2. Since vegetal foreign bodies occur for the

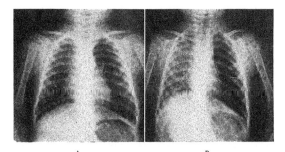

A   B

Figure 1.   Case 1—Before removal of non-opaque foreign body.   (A) Inspiration.
(B) Expiration.   This shows left sided emphysema present on expiration, with some
cardiac shift to the right.

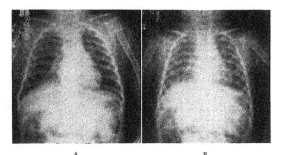

A   B

Figure 2.   Case 1—After removal of non-opaque foreign body.   (A) Inspiration.
(B) Expiration.

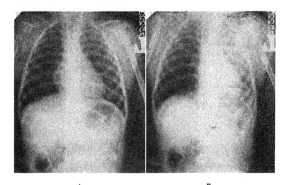

A   B

Figure 3.   Case 2—Before removal of non-opaque foreign body.   (A) Inspiration.
(B) Expiration.   This shows expiratory emphysema on the right side, with cardiac
shift to the left.

most part in infants and give rise to violent reactions, an early diagnosis is imperative.

3. Non-opaque foreign bodies in the bronchi are very apt so to alter the normal physiology of respiration, that indirectly they can be diagnosed by means of the roentgen ray.

BIBLIOGRAPHY

1. Allison, R. G., and Phelps, K.: Non-opaque foreign bodies in the air passages. Radiology, x:157-159 (February), 1928.
2. Vallar, D. H.: Vegetal foreign bodies in the bronchi. Canadian Med. Assn. Jour., xxvii:277-278 (September), 1932.
3. Jackson, Chevalier, Coates, G. M., and Jackson, C. L.: The Nose, Throat and Ear, and Their Diseases. W. B. Saunders & Co., Philadelphia, 1930.
4. Sneller, Charles: Factors in the roentgenological diagnosis of non-opaque foreign bodies in the bronchi. Illinois Med. Jour., lxii:410-414 (November), 1932.
5. Manges, W. F.: Roentgen diagnosis of non-opaque foreign bodies in the trachea. Am. Jour. Roent., xiii:429-437 (May), 1925.
6. Pepper, O. H., and Tucker, G.: Peanut in Left Lower Lobe Bronchus. Medical Clinics of North America. W. B. Saunders Co., Philadelphia, x:117-120 (July), 1926.

ROENTGEN VISUALIZATION OF THE LIVER AND SPLEEN, WITH THORIUM DIOXIDE SOL*

L. G. ERICKSEN, M.D., Dubuque

When Radt announced his work on the visualization of the liver and spleen roentgenologically with a colloidal suspension of thorium dioxide[1] (now marketed under the trade name of Thorotrast) in 1929, he struck a very interested and sympathetic audience in the medical profession as a whole. Up to this time we had only been able to outline these organs by indirect methods. Now the time seemed at hand whereby we could visualize their structural detail. It required little thought to realize the value of this procedure in such diseases of the liver and spleen as metastasis, primary tumors, cysts, abscesses, cirrhosis and the differentiation of abdominal masses. In the short time allotted one cannot take up the use of the procedure in detail and for a more complete report on its various applications in the field of medicine I refer you to a previous publication.[2] I will confine myself to its use in the preoperative diagnosis of metastasis to the liver, the field wherein it is most valuable.

Until Radt's contribution, many an abdomen was opened only to be closed again without further surgery because of metastasis to the liver. It is a well known fact that carcinoma of the stomach metastasizes to the liver at an early stage. Too often a malignant growth of the stomach, which is easily resectable from the standpoint of the local lesion, will prove inoperable because of liver metastasis when the abdomen is opened. The operative treatment of carcinoma of the rectum is a very formidable undertaking. How often has a

*Presented before the Eighty-third Annual Session, Iowa State Medical Society, Des Moines, May 9, 10, 11, 1934.

patient uselessly been put through this distressing experience only to die a short time later of metastasis to the liver. Nevertheless, no surgeon wishes to deny a patient the benefit of an operation that may cure him of a disease the result of which is otherwise uniformly fatal. It is little wonder, then, that this new diagnostic aid has been so welcome. In the department of surgery at the University Hospital, University of Minnesota, this procedure is now a routine in all preoperative cases of malignancy of the gastro-intestinal tract and in other primary malignancies when indicated, and has proved valuable in preventing needless surgery in many cases.

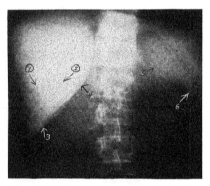

Figure 1. Arrow 1 indicates the vascular channels of the liver; arrow 2, the gallbladder fossa; arrows 3 and 4, the border of the liver; and arrows 5 and 6, the splenic border.

The patient is given a total of .8 c.c. of thorotrast per kilogram of body weight in three doses on successive days intravenously. The thorium particles are phagocyted by the cells of the reticuloendothelial system in the liver and spleen. These thorium particles are radio-opaque and thus a shadow of these organs is cast on the x-ray film. Not sooner than twenty-four hours following the last injection, a fourteen by seventeen film is taken of the abdomen with the patient in the prone position, using the Potter-Bucky diaphragm and exposing the film a little heavier than for the routine abdomen film. In the normal case, the liver and spleen will show up as homogenous, dense shadows (Figure 1). Metastatic areas, abscesses, cysts or other tumors will show as areas of rarefaction in the liver giving it a mottled appearance (Figure 2). If these areas are numerous, the problem is very simple. It is not possible to differentiate from a roentgenologic point of view between abscesses in the liver and metastasis. Both will appear as ragged areas of rarefaction while cysts have a sharper, more circumscribed border. One must, however, be careful of shadows cast by overlying gas in the bowel. If there are confusing bowel shadows overlying the liver, a cleansing enema should be given. The constancy of the rarefied areas as to location and size in the series of films taken is also very helpful. Occasionally the vascular channels of the liver stand out exceptionally well, as in Figure 1. These, however, have a radiating character and are linear and sharply defined. An area of rarefaction is usually seen in the gallbladder fossa, probably owing to the large ducts in this region.

The interpretation of the films in the field of malignancy requires much experience but may become very accurate. In a series of 142 clinical patients to whom we have given thorotrast, we have been checked either by autopsy or postmortem examinations in 61.

Table Showing Correctness of Diagnosis

Autopsy .... 21 cases
Operation .... 40 cases

	Correct	Error	Question of Error
Positive diagnosis	14	1	1
Negative diagnosis	42	3	

You will note from the above table that one of the errors made on the positive side was questionable. The two errors that were made on the positive side were made by misinterpreting either vascular striation or thinning out of liver between the intercostal spaces as metastasis. On the negative side there were 45 cases, three of which were in error. One of these was an extremely small metastasis, so small that it was only picked up on the microscopic examination. Another was a case in which the examination was very unsatisfactory because of the condition of the patient while the third was a definite error. The latter was a case of primary tumor which infiltrated the whole liver, yet no defect was seen on the film. The probable explanation is that the cells of this particular type of tumor absorbed the thorotrast. If a doubt arises in one's mind as to whether metastasis is present or not, it is better to err on the negative side and give the patient the advantage of an exploratory laparotomy, since the mortality rate would be 100 per cent without the operation. Until, through much experience, we feel entirely confident in our diagnostic ability, we feel this to be the best attitude to take.

There have been some scattered reports in the literature of damaging effects on the liver and spleen, disturbances of blood count and the like, but most investigators have yet to discover that thorotrast produces any damaging effects when used in doses necessary for diagnostic visualization. Our observations on microscopic sections removed two and three years following administration of the thorotrast show most of the particles still remaining in the reticulo-endothelial cells, but no apparent celluar damage. This agrees with other recent reports. The fact that the particles remain in the body for so long a time has been considered as objectionable to the use of the procedure, but so far no observations have been made of harmful effects of this delayed elimination. We have found that this has one advantage. A patient who has been given the preparation may show no evidence of metastasis to the liver on the first examination; with the subsequent development of a metastasis, the roentgen studies may be obtained without further injection. We have had several such patients.

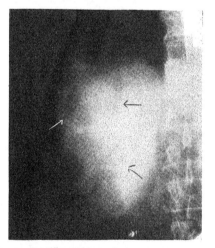

Figure 2. Arrows indicate large areas of metastasis.

Thorium, however, is a very slightly radioactive metal and the fact that it remains in the tissues such a long period of time brings up the danger of latent effects. Whether this effect of the radioactivity is enough to do the patient any harm is very doubtful since some elimination does take place. Thus far, no harmful effects whatever have been observed over a period of about four years in cases which have been followed. We know, however, that it is possible for the deleterious effects to be delayed for as long as nine or ten years. With these facts in mind, the utilization of this method should be cautiously restricted until sufficient time has elapsed to permit a final conclusion as to the actual dangers involved. It is fortunate that the cases in which this diagnostic aid is of most value are those in which the eventual mortailty rate is very high whether the procedure is used or not. Also, the age of the patient is usually advanced. We believe it is wise, until time has eliminated the possibilities of danger from

ANALYSIS OF 142 CASES

Diagnosis	Positive	Negative	Total
Carcinoma of stomach	18	30	48
Carcinoma of colon	4	12	16
Carcinoma of rectum	7	9	16
Carcinoma of breast	7	5	12
Carcinoma of ovary	2	2	4
Primary hepatoma	3	0	3
Tumors, miscellaneous	10	14	24
Cirrhosis of liver	4	1	5
Diseases, miscellaneous	4	10	14

latent radioactivity, to confine the treatment to this group. In other types of cases, the dose we have used for outlining the liver and spleen is one-third to one-fourth the average dose and we do not believe this amount could cause any harm. We have observed no contraindications to the use of the procedure and have experienced no serious reactions following the injections. The following table will give an idea as to the type of case in which we have used it to advantage.

REFERENCES

1. Radt, Paul: Eine Methode zur rontgenologischen Kontrast-darstellung von Milz und Leber, Klin. Wchnschr, viii :2128-2129 (November 12), 1929.
2. Ericksen, Lester G. and Rigler, Leo. G.: Roentgen visualization of liver and speen with thorium dioxide sol. Jour. Amer. Med. Assn., c:1758-1764 (June 3), 1933.

INDICATIONS FOR THYROID SURGERY*

T. E. DAVIDSON, M.D., Mason City

There is no field of surgery in which the indications for operative interference are any more definite than they are in abnormalities of the thyroid gland. One would not hesitate for one moment to remove an acute or moderately inflamed appendix, or a diseased gallbladder, and the same should be true with a diseased thyroid gland. Surgical treatment of pathologic conditions of the thyroid gland is a reasonable procedure and there is no doubt now that operations can be performed even in severe cases, with a mortality rate that is very slight and result in vast improvement in the patient's health.

Every physician should be goiter conscious. Anyone can make a diagnosis of a case of exophthalmic goiter with a classical text book picture of rapid loss in weight, rapid pulse, excessive perspiration, stimulation and excitable behavior, moist flushed skin, ravenous appetite, with or without the typical eye changes. Even a case of

*Presented before the Eighty-third Annual Session, Iowa State Medical Society, Des Moines, May 9, 10, 11, 1934.

adenomatous goiter with or without hyperthyroidism can ordinarily be diagnosed, but it is the atypical case with indefinite symptoms or an unexplained tachycardia above 90 that causes trouble.

I want to call to your attention here the apathetic type of thyrotoxicosis in which many of the outward signs of hyperthyroidism are lacking; for instance, the eye changes and the excessive stimulation and excitability are absent, but the tachycardia, loss of weight and strength, and enlargement of the thyroid gland are present. These patients have gone from one physician to another, with their conditions remaining undiagnosed. Recently I saw one of these patients in crisis just before he died. If his condition had been recognized earlier, surgery might have saved his life. It is also a significant fact that on practically every thyroid service, there are now more preoperative than postoperative deaths. It should be remembered that every patient who dies from hyperthyroidism, either with or without operation has at some stage of the disease represented a perfectly safe operative risk.

There are an infinite number of different grades of severity of hyperthyroidism. I have in mind a patient with a basal metabolism of plus 17, slightly above normal, who tired easily, with a tachycardia of 90, loss of strength and weight, and a palpable thyroid gland. He regained his normal activities after a thyroidectomy. Then there are occasional clinical curiosities such as a patient with marked toxic hyperthyroidic symptoms with no appreciable enlargement of the thyroid gland. On the other hand, very large goiters may cause no subjective symptoms. The size of the goiter has no constant ratio to the amount of damage it may be causing. We sometimes find a case of unilateral exophthalmos instead of the common bilateral type. Many patients with hyperthyroidism consult an eye specialist before having a general examination.

It has been my good fortune to perform thyroidectomies three times for thyroid disease in pregnancy without interrupting the pregnancy in a single case. The risk is so slight that thyroidectomy should always be performed rather than let the patient go to term with the burden of a toxic goiter. We should always bear in mind that the basal metabolic rate is elevated from 20 to 30 points in a normal pregnancy and a rate much higher than this would be necessary, together with the other signs of hyperthryroidism, before a diagnosis of toxic goiter complicating pregnancy could be made.

Diabetes is frequently complicated with thyroid disease and every physician should consider hyperthyroidism in a case of diabetes. Because of the

goiter, however, does not cure a hypertension which was present before the goiter appeared.

Patients with coronary disease and angina pectoris, complicated with hyperthyroidism, regardless of severity, are relieved of their symptoms by thyroidectomy. Blumgart, et al., gave reasons for believing that patients with a normal metabolism who suffer from congestive heart failure or angina pectoris might show striking improvement if the metabolic rate were significantaly lowered by subtotal thyroidectomies.

Thyroid patients easily contract infection and the clinical evidence of infection is increased by the presence of thyroid disease. Also, any intercurrent infection adds to the severity of a hyperthyroid state. I have always made it a rule to remove the thyroid gland first, and the foci of infection later. Cholecystitis is very commonly associated with thyroid disease of the toxic nodular type in patients past forty years of age. A patient with gallbladder disease should be checked very carefully for hyperthyroidism. If there is any doubt, the goiter should be removed first unless the case is an emergency one. As the nodular goiter is not influenced materially by medical treatment, usually develops toxicity and is responsible for tracheal pressure, I advocate surgical removal early, when the body has attained its full development, say between the ages of twenty-five and thirty or earlier, if the goiter shows evidence of toxicity.

Th diffuse colloid goiter of earlier life which remains stationary in size or continues to enlarge and does not respond to iodine or thyroid extract should be removed surgically.

Operative interference in postoperative occurrence of hyperthyroidism should depend largely upon the size of the regenerated gland and the length of time following the operative procedure. I believe further surgery is indicated in those that recur within a short time after operation, due to the inadequate removal of the thyroid gland, and in which a large portion of one or both lobes can be felt. Sometimes the hyperthyroidism returns after a period of one year or more of complete remission of symptoms. In this case, the remaining gland has regenerated but little, and is scarcely palpable, and I believe that iodine and x-ray treatments will do as much for the patient as anything, and there are no postoperative complications.

Thyroiditis is not an indication for surgery unless an abscess forms. Occasionally, this condition will cause the thyroid gland to become so hard and brawny that it cannot be differentiated from malignancy except by histologic section, and in such cases biopsy is indicated for diagnosis.

Let me suggest, then, that every patient who

comes to the physician with a history of loss of weight, nervousness, and tachycardia, whether he has the appearance of hyperthyroidism or not, be carefully examined and watched for a possible diseased thyroid gland, bearing in mind the fact that every case of thyroid disease is a law unto itself and should be studied in every detail.

The basal metabolic rate is a valuable adjunct to a careful clinical examination of the patient and at least three readings should be made, in "the doubtful group" before the determination of the rate will be of much value. Occasionally it will be necessary to give Lugol's solution for a week or ten days to a case of neurocirculatory asthenia in order to differentiate it from a case of mild hyperthyroidism. In a case of hyperthyroidism, the general condition of the patient will improve. The pulse rate will decrease and the nervousness will improve. This will not be true in a case of neurocirculatory asthenia. Before doing this, however, I place the patient on heavy doses of some sedative, preferably luminal, for a day or two, and give him a grain of codein one hour before the metabolic rate is taken. In the majority of instances, the test will be normal or below.

At present, I believe surgery is the treatment of choice for pathologic conditions of the thyroid gland and will result in more cures and less invalids than the medical treatment which means years of treatment and invalidism. There are many patients with mild hyperthyroidism who are practically invalids; this class would be benefited by thyroidectomy.

Mosser reports that after an interval of three to five years 96 per cent of the patients who had been operated upon were relieved of hyperthyroidism, and four per cent had a definite recurrence. Clute and Veal have published similar results from a consecutive series of patients who had been followed for five years. There is reason to believe that if every patient with hyperthyroidism or enlargement of the thyroid gland, were operated upon early enough, the operative mortality should be even lower than it is at the present time.

The deduction I wish to make is that we must eliminate the term "simple goiter" after maturity. There is no such thing as a harmless simple goiter. When there is demonstrable disease in the thyroid gland, it requires treatment, preferably surgery. The advisability of early operation has been repeatedly demonstrated in studying the end results. The percentage of disability varies directly with the duration of the disease.

Case Report

CONGENITAL ABSENCE OF A LUNG*

JAMES E. DYSON, M.D., Des Moines

Failure of a lung to develop normally can apparently be due to abnormalities in the formation of the anlage of the lung or to regressive changes in the anlage which had a normal beginning. As pulmonary vessels are absent to the side of the missing lung, the failure of the circulatory development may be the primary factor in the causation of the lung abnormality. Different explanations of this condition have been offered by Furst[1] and also by Klebs[2]; but so many case reports list other anatomic defects that it seems most probable that it is an agenesis. If absence of a lung is due to regressive changes there will be a rudimentary lung and pulmonary vessels.

Ellis[3] in 1917 reviewed eighteen cases briefly and reported the case of an eight year old boy who died from acute endocarditis and had an absence of the left lung. Levy[4] in 1920 found twenty-one reported cases and presented one more, a forty-nine year old man, who had died of general septicemia from genito-urinary infection and terminal pneumonia. At autopsy he was found to have an absence of the left lung, left bronchus and left pulmonary vessels. The heart occupied the left chest. The lateral and posterior surfaces of the pericardium were adherent to the wall by firm connective tissue. No traces of visceral pleura were found.

Finner[5] in 1932 reviewed twenty-four cases in the literature and pointed out that of these twenty-four cases three were stillbirths, three were infants who survived only a few minutes or hours, seven others were infants under six months, and the remaining eleven ranged in age from eight to sixty-five years. The left lung was absent in eighteen cases and the right lung absent in six. In the majority of cases the opposite lung was enlarged. In seven of the reports it is described as unilobular. In one of Theremin's cases[6] where the single lung was on the right side only two lobes were present. Ellis' case[3] exhibited a left lung which was comprised of five lobes. The pulmonary artery was absent on the defective side in all cases. Finner[5] reported a case of absence of the right lung in a twenty-two months old boy, who died from a peanut in the trachea. In this case there was complete absence of the right lung, bronchus and pulmonary vessels.

I wish to report another instance of this very

*Read before the Iowa Lutheran Hospital Staff Meeting, March 16, 1934.

unusual condition. As absence of the lung has never been diagnosed during life, this case was also found at the postmortem examination. The infant gained well and seemed very slightly handicapped by the deformity. She did not, however, withstand a slight respiratory infection and died promptly from an interstitial pneumonia of the one and only lung.

The patient, a female infant, was born eight months prematurely, on November 22, 1932. Her weight at birth was four and one-half pounds. The mother was seventeen years of age, and father twenty. Feeding was given by gavage for ten days. The infant was referred to the Iowa Children's Home for care at the age of six weeks.

Her weight on January 14, 1933, was six pounds. The feeding was citric acid milk. Examination showed a fairly well nourished infant of normal color, normal temperature and pulse,

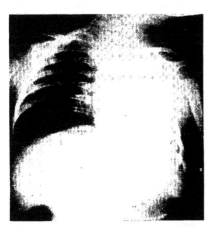

Figure 1. X-ray picture showing a total collapse or absence of the left lung.

with a slightly increased respiratory rate. Externally the chest was somewhat flattened on the left side anteriorly and had diminished respiratory movement. The abdomen was normal and diaphragm action was normal. The entire left chest was flat to percussion; no breath sounds could be heard. The heart was of normal width but entirely to the left of the mid-line.

My first impression was that this was a massive atelectasis of the newborn. Because of the lung collapse I considered two other conditions, paralysis of the diaphragm[7] and a foreign body in the

bronchus.[8] X-ray films showed a normal diaphragm and no foreign body in the bronchus. The pictures also showed a total collapse or absence of the left lung and a shift of the mediastinum, heart and thymus to the left.

On January 19, 1933, the weight was six pounds, fifteen ounces; color was normal, and nutrition was improved.

On February 16, 1933, the weight had increased to eight pounds, six ounces. A Kahn test was negative.

On March 16, 1933, the weight was nine pounds, five ounces; the skin appeared slightly cyanotic; a few coarse râles were present in the right chest; the temperature was normal.

On April 14, 1933, the weight was ten pounds; bronchial râles were present. The patient had had a cold since April 8. The temperature remained normal.

The patient was sent to the State University Hospital at Iowa City on April 27, 1933, and the following report was received from Ernest Ekermeyer, M.D., of the Children's Hospital on May 3, 1933.

"Physical examination at the time of admission showed her to be fairly well developed and fairly well nourished. She had some difficulty with breathing and appeared slightly cyanotic. Examination of the chest showed it to be symmetrical. There were some lag movements in the left chest. Most of the chest seemed hyper-resonant to percussion. Breath sounds over the left lung were suppressed and fine râles could be heard on that side. The remainder of the examination seemed negative."

"Laboratory examination showed: urine negative; red blood count, 3,950,000; white blood count, 6,100; hemoglobin, 78 per cent; blood Wassermann and Kahn tests were both negative. Intradermal tuberculin tests were negative. X-ray examination of the chest was reported as follows: stereoscopic films of the chest show evidence of a marked shift of the heart and mediastinum toward the left side, with a marked decrease in the intrathoracic volume of the left chest and no evidence of any aerated lung on the left side. The findings suggest a complete collapse or atelectasis. There is a compensatory emphysema of the right lung."

"It has been our impression that this baby has a congenital atelectasis of the left lung. We have considered the possibility of a foreign body also. We plan to have a bronchoscopic examination done. This has been postponed temporarily because the baby has been having a low grade fever associated with upper respiratory infection."

May 10, 1933. "During the past week she has had an upper respiratory infection with bilateral otitis media. On May 6 it was necessary to do bilateral myringotomy. The white blood count was 12,000. X-rays of the mastoids were reported negative."

May 15, 1933. "Became suddenly worse with temperature of 104 degrees, and very rapid labored breathing, became cyanotic and died."

A postmortem examination was performed by M. T. Bates, M.D., whose report I quote as follows: "The body is that of a well developed, well nourished, white female measuring 55 cm, age, six months. There is a yellowish discharge in both external auditory canals. Nasal passages clear. The peritoneal cavity contains no free fluid or adhesions. The appendix lies in the right lower quadrant and is free. The diaphragm on the left extends to the third interspace and on the right to the fourth rib. The mesenteric lymph nodes vary in size from B.B. shot to pea size.

"Pleural cavities: The right pleural cavity contains no free fluid and no adhesions. The left is practically entirely obliterated by adhesions be-

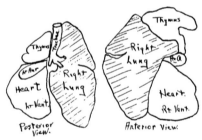

Figure 2. Sketches made at the time of autopsy.

tween the chest wall and the pericardial sac. In the upper portion, the space ordinarily occupied by the apex of the left lung is occupied by the thymus. There is a marked shifting of the mediastinum to the left. The pericardial cavity contains five c.c. of straw-colored fluid. The heart is markedly shifted to the left and is also rotated to the left. The myocardium of the left ventricle measures one centimeter and of the right ventricle three centimeters. No congenital anomalies of the heart are found.

"On removing the chest plate, after first clasping the trachea, the right lung is found to extend to the left of the mid-line for a distance of about four centimeters. The left lung is not visible.

The heart and pericardial sac lie entirely to the left of the mid-line, the pericardium being adherent to the chest wall laterally, anteriorly and posteriorly, so that the pleural cavity is completely obliterated. There is no evidence of a left lung. The mediastinum is shifted to the left and presents a thymus which is somewhat enlarged and lies slightly to the left of its ordinary position and also with a lateral extension in the usual location of the apex of the left lung. On opening the trachea, it is found to end blindly, the blind ending being a direct continuation of the course of the trachea. There is no evidence of even a rudimentary branch to the left. There is one main bronchus to the right lung, which subdivides to give a branch to the upper lobe. The right lung presents only two lobes. The fissure between the two lobes is short and incomplete. The right lung is somewhat pale in color and crepitant throughout. On cut section it appears normal and presents no definite evidence of a gross pneumonia. Further inspection of the aorta reveals no congenital anomalies. The pulmonary artery is continued to the right lung with no evidence of a subdivision for the left lung.

"The spleen weighs ten grams, and there are two accessory spleens at the hilus. The surface of the spleen is purplish in color. The capsule is smooth and only a moderate amount of pulp scrapes away. The gastro-intestinal tract and pancreas are normal. The liver weighs 175 grams and is brownish-red in color. The ducts are patent. The gallbladder is thin-walled and there are no stones present. The right kidney weighs 20 grams. The capsule strips easily, leaving a smooth surface which shows persistence of fetal lobulations. The cortex measures four millimeters. The pelvic mucosa appears normal. The left kidney weighs 20 grams and is similar to the right. The adrenal glands are normal. The bladder is thin-walled and the mucosa is smooth. The genitalia are of the normal female infant type. The aorta presents no congenital anomalies. The thymus appears somewhat enlarged, but its anterior posterior diameter does not seem to be increased. The brain weighs 650 grams. On gross inspection it presents no abnormalities. Both middle ears show pus. There is no gross evidence of mastoid infection.

"Gross summary: This is evidently a case of congenital absence of the left lung in an infant of six months. During the last few days of life she developed bilateral otitis media. Both ear drums were punctured and adequate drainage was maintained. It was felt that her reaction was considerably out of proportion to the local findings in the ears, and clinically it was felt that she possibly had a pneumonia. On gross examination at post-

REPORT OF CASES FROM THE BROADLAWNS GENERAL HOSPITAL, DES MOINES

FRANK W. FORDYCE, M.D., and

DANIEL F. CROWLEY, M.D.

The patient, a colored female, forty years of age, was first seen in the out patient department in September, 1933, complaining of tumor masses in the thyroid and abdominal regions, a weight loss of twenty pounds and irregular menstrual periods. The mass in the abdomen had been present for five years during which time it had increased to three times its original size. The general health had remained good. For the past two years she had noted a profuse, grayish white discharge which persisted for several days following each menstrual period. Four months before her first entry, the patient noticed that the menstrual periods which had been of three days' duration and regular, became longer in duration and more profuse; also bleeding for a day or so occurred between periods. The mass in the neck had been present for some time, probably fifteen to twenty years. It never had been painful and had formed gradually. The patient had had no symptoms of increased metabolism.

Physical examination: The patient's skin was hot and moist; the eyes normal. Examination of the neck revealed a rounded, cystic, elastic mass in the region of the isthmus of the thyroid gland. Both lateral lobes were enlarged. The chest was essentially negative except for a visible precordial impulse and a palpable thrill over the conus arteriosus. The heart was enlarged to the anterior axillary line in the sixth interspace. The right border was three centimeters to the right of the mid-line in the fourth interspace. Sounds were snapping in character and a loud systolic murmur was present at the apex along the left border of the sternum and in the aortic area. Abdominal examination revealed a hard, nodular mass about the size of a six months' pregnancy. On vaginal examination the uterus was found to be an integral part of the mass. The extremities presented a fine tremor.

Laboratory examination: The urine was negative, and the Kahn test was negative. The basal metabolic rate was plus 52 on September 27, and plus 38 on October 4.

The patient was admitted to the ward on September 26, 1933, and on October 9, 1933, an encapsulated adenoma was removed from the left lateral lobe of the thyroid gland. The postoperative course was good and the patient was discharged nine days later. She remained at home for two weeks at the end of which time she returned to the hospital for a hysterectomy. The postoperative course was good and the patient was discharged two weeks after the operation. For a time she returned to the out patient department for observation, but she was not seen from December 8, 1933, until May 16, 1934. At this time she complained of backache and a marked increase in weight. The possibility of an endocrine imbalance due to thyroidectomy was investigated, but ruled out; her complaints being explained on the basis of an artificial menopause due to hysterectomy. The backache was found to be of the static type.

Clinical diagnosis: Leiomyomata of the uterus; hyperthyroidism. The pathologist reported a leiomyomata of the uterus with myomatous polyps of the uterine cavity, and cystic hemorrhagic adenoma of the thyroid gland.

This case is reported to emphasize the importance of a careful examination of the patient for hyperthyroidism, when a goiter is present with some other pathology which brings the patient to the hospital.

The basal metabolic rates were plus 52 and plus 38, which showed definitely that this patient had a hyperthyroidism and if the hysterectomy had been performed first, a thyroid crisis might have been precipitated. By performing the thyroidectomy first, this patient was restored to a somewhat normal level. The subsequent postoperative course following the hysterectomy justified our assumption.

                                        F. W. F.

————

The patient was a white female, married, twenty-eight years of age, with an entrance complaint of periodic vomiting which had become constant during the last twenty-four hours. After a brutal attack by her husband a severe pain developed in the lumbar region radiating to the lower right quadrant. Two days later the patient began vomiting and continued to do so for twenty-four hours. These episodes were followed by a repetition of her abdominal pain and vomiting. Three days previous to her entrance, the patient had been unable to retain any food or water.

Past history: The patient had vomited some blood in 1928. She had had no operations, but had what was termed typhoid pneumonia at the age of five years. She also had diphtheria, scarlet fever and measles. The patient presented a history of

vomiting when she eats potatoes, beans and cabbage, while at the same time, oranges or other fruit juices are retained. Menstruation began at fifteen years of age; the periods occurred every 25 to 26 days and lasted five days. The onset was accompanied by cramps and pain. After the birth of her only baby eight years ago, the periods became more profuse and irregular. She never had any discharges of any kind.

Family history: Husband living and well, but had Neisserian infection ten years ago. The mother has tuberculosis. Two sisters and two brothers are living and well; another sister has heart trouble.

Physical examination: The head, face and neck were negative. No râles were evident upon examination. The heart was not enlarged; sounds were clear; rhythm was regular; and the rate was 90. The abdomen was somewhat distended and was markedly rigid over most of the right side with extreme tenderness at McBurney's point. In 1928, the patient had a bilateral salpingitis and also a gastric ulcer. Vaginal examination revealed a marked fixation of the uterus with a large mass which was very tender on the right side. The reflexes were normal. Appearance of the skin was normal.

The patient entered the hospital on May 16, at which time the temperature appeared to be normal. However, the next day she developed a temperature of 101 degrees which continued and ranged from 100 to 103 degrees during the fifteen days between the time of entrance to the hospital and the day of operation, at which time the temperature had reached 104 degrees. During these fifteen days, the patient had periodic attacks of vomiting which continued for several hours each time. All efforts to obtain bowel movements were inadequate. The abdomen became enormously distended and the patient gave the appearance of suffering from a paralytic ileus or definite intestinal obstruction. Repeated catheterized specimens of urine were negative. The white blood count was 11,600 and the hemoglobin was between 60 and 65 per cent. Slides from the vaginal smear were negative and the Kahn test was negative. The preoperative diagnosis was an intestinal obstruction resulting from a bilateral salpingitis associated with a pelvic peritonitis.

On June 2, 1933, an exploratory laparotomy was decided upon with the intention of doing an ileostomy. The patient was given a spinal anesthetic, and a right rectus incision was made. An enormous amount of straw colored fluid escaped from the abdomen. Upon examining the parietal peritoneum it was found to be studded with small bead-like masses and our first impression was that we were dealing with a definite case of peritoneal tuberculosis. Upon further exploration of the small intestine and the pelvic organs we were inclined to change the diagnosis. There were many loops of small intestine packed in the pelvis which were kinked and completely obstructed as far as the lumen was concerned. This was due to a massive growth upon the peritoneal surface but it showed no involvement of the muscular coat of the bowel. The entire pelvic organs were examined and found to be covered with enormous quantities of these massive growths. Both tubes were occluded at the end, both ovaries showed definite inflammation due to the same new growth formation. The uterus was slightly enlarged and retroflexed in the cul-de-sac. After complete exploration of the intestines and pelvic organs, an ileostomy was done and the abdomen closed with drainage.

After the operation, the temperature dropped to 100 degrees where it remained until the fourth postoperative day. The gas distension was greatly relieved, but no gas or fecal material passed through the external outlet.

The patient died on the fourth postoperative day from exhaustion. The postoperative diagnosis was that of an extensive rapidly growing adenocarcinoma of indefinite origin. The autopsy findings were practically the same as the operative findings. It was found that the entire pelvis and pelvic organs were covered with these new growths. The entire small intestine was examined at autopsy and while there were many obstructions in the bowel due to kinking and formation of new growths on the peritoneal surface, there was no involvement of the muscular coat.

The diagnosis at autopsy was adenocarcinoma of indefinite origin. Microscopic sections were made from the ovaries, the omentum, the diaphragm, and the surface of the small intestine, all of which revealed evidence of an adenocarcinoma. A definite focus from which the carcinoma sprang was undetermined. The final diagnosis, however, was multiple metastases of adenocarcinoma of unknown origin.

The rapid development of so extensive a carcinoma is most unusual. There was no history or evidence of a previous carcinoma. The whole course of the illness was only four weeks and the extent of the metatases found at autopsy was quite remarkable.

D. F. C.

THE FINLEY HOSPITAL CLINICO-PATHOLOGIC CONFERENCE

AORTIC STENOSIS WITH CALCIFICATION OF THE CUSPS

J. C. KASSMEYER, M.D., Dubuque

The case to be described is an unusually good example of aortic stenosis with calcification of the cusps occurring in a young man. It presents many of the physical signs and symptoms which Christian[1] considered characteristic of this particular lesion. The condition is not rare, as evidenced by the fact that it has been encountered in eleven (5.5 per cent) of our 200 adult necropsies. Until recently it was only detected at the postmortem examination but since Christian called attention to the clinical signs it has been diagnosed in two cases in this hospital. In each instance the roentgenologist has confirmed the diagnosis by fluoroscopic studies.

CASE REPORT

Chief complaint: The patient, a white man thirty-five years of age, was admitted to The Finley Hospital, February 15, 1931, with a complaint of "difficulty in breathing, pain in the abdomen with eructations of gas."

Past history: He had had measles when a child and an attack of pleurisy several years ago. He did not remember any other illnesses. When in the army during 1918 and 1919 he was told that he had heart disease, but he did not know when it had developed. During the last ten years he noticed that he became short of breath comparatively easy, but he had been able to continue his work as an automobile mechanic. Four months ago the heart became decompensated and he remained in bed six weeks after which he felt well.

Family history: Negative.

Present illness: Two months ago he developed a severe attack of bronchitis and this caused a recurrence of his decompensation. One week ago his dyspnea became more severe; he was unable to sleep; had pain in the region of the stomach, did not desire to take food, and had been troubled with eructations of gas ever since.

Physical examination: The patient was a well developed man weighing 150 pounds. He breathed with considerable difficulty and appeared very ill. The temperature was 98 degrees; the respirations were 26 per minute and of the Cheyne Stokes type. The pulse was 90 per minute and of poor volume.

There was a suggestion of a plateau. Systolic blood pressure was 100 and the diastolic 60 mm. of mercury. His color was ashen gray and his eyes bulged moderately. The pupils were equal and reacted normally. The blood vessels in the neck were engorged but did not pulsate. The head and neck were otherwise unremarkable. Scattered râles were heard over the base of each lung. The heart was tremendously enlarged and the apex beat was in the seventh interspace. The left border was just inside the mid-axillary line. There was a systolic thrill over the cardiac region which was most marked in the aortic region. There was a systolic murmur at the apex which was transmitted to the back. There was a soft blowing diastolic murmur heard in the aortic area which was transmitted over a considerable portion of the cardiac area. The edge of the liver was smooth, firm, somewhat tender to pressure, and extended five centimeters below the costal border on the right. There were no other abdominal findings. There was a slight edema of the ankles.

Course in hospital: The patient gradually became more and more cyanotic. The dyspnea became more pronounced and there was evidence of fluid in the abdomen. The temperature gradually fell from 98 to 96.8 degrees. Several blood pressure readings were made and are as follows: 100/60; 110/60; 100/50. He died forty-eight hours after admission.

Clinical diagnosis: Chronic aortic endocarditis with stenosis; cardiac hypertrophy with decompensation.

Abstracted necropsy report: The body of a well developed and well nourished white man was remarkable externally only because of moderate edema of the ankles. The peritoneal cavity contained 1500 cc. of clear, straw-colored fluid; the right and left thoracic cavities contained 1500 and 300 cc. respectively; the pericardial sac contained 150 cc. The heart was enormous in size, weighing 895 grams. The left ventricle was very large and the wall measured 15 mm. in thickness. The other heart chambers were dilated. There were small thrombi in the right auricle and several fresh infarcts were found in each lung. Aside from the hypertrophy of the left ventricle the most interesting feature was the condition found in the aortic cusps. They were greatly thickened, fused together and were stony hard due to calcification (Figure 1). The aortic orifice was represented by a slit five millimeters in length and averaging two millimeters in width. The aorta was thin, smooth and elastic. The other organs showed only chronic and acute congestion.

Anatomic diagnosis: Primary:

1. Chronic aortic endocarditis with fusion and calcification of the cusps (stenosis and regurgitation).

2. Dilatation and hypertrophy of the heart; chronic and acute passive congestion of all the viscera; anasarca.

3. Thrombosis of the right auricle; pulmonary infarcts.

GENERAL DISCUSSION

The etiology of calcification of the aortic cusps is in doubt. Two theories have been advanced to explain the condition: first, that it is due to a

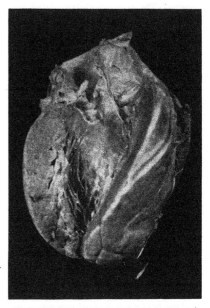

Fig. 1: Photograph of the heart showing the dilatation of the left ventricle; hypertrophy of the myocardium; and fusion and calcification of the aortic cusps. Note the smooth aorta without evidence of arteriosclerosis.

metabolic disturbance and a part of the arteriosclerotic process that goes with age, and second, that it is the end result of inflammatory disease of the cusps (aortic endocarditis). The latter theory seems more probable, as frequently the process is limited to the aortic valve, and as the lesion occurs sometimes in individuals well below the age when arteriosclerosis is usually encountered. On the other hand a history indicating endocarditis is obtained in a goodly percentage of cases. Clawson[2], who has made an extensive study of this condition, obtained a history of rheumatism in 40 per cent of 93 cases which came to necropsy. Christian also reported that eleven of twenty-one patients gave definite histories of rheumatic fever. He believes that a "rheumatic etiology" seems most probable. The lesion has been encountered three times as frequently among men as in women. The diagnosis is made by a recognition of the following characteristics listed by Christian:

1. Occurrence chiefly in males, relatively late in life.

2. Slow progression of the lesion with symptoms of decompensation appearing late, though not necessarily prolonged after their development.

3. The presence of a systolic thrill and harsh, loud systolic thrill in the aortic area, with or without a diastolic murmur of aortic insufficiency.

4. Often a characteristic pulse with a normal or decreased pulse pressure.

5. Enlargement of the heart.

6. Roentgenographic demonstration of calcification in the region of the aortic valve.

7. A history of rheumatism early in life.

The prognosis varies according to the stage of the disease. Many of these patients live for years with a fully compensated heart. Apparently the myocardium hypertrophies to overcome the mechanical disability caused by the narrowed valve orifice. At this time their only symptom may be shortness of breath. Decompensation is usually precipitated by overwork or some infectious disease. Usually these patients die within a year as decompensation supervenes. The general treatment is that of cardiac decompensation from other causes.

REFERENCES

1. Christian, Henry A: Aortic stenosis with calcification of the cusps. Jour. Am. Med. Assn., xcvii:158-161 (July 18) 1931.
2. Clawson, B. J.: Nonsyphilitic aortic valve deformity. Arch. Path. xii:889-899 (December) 1931.

COLLECTION AGENCIES

From time to time, warnings have appeared in the columns of this publication against specific collection agencies whose representatives were soliciting accounts from physicians throughout the state.

It seems necessary at this time to issue a general warning against any collection agency which has not been investigated and approved by the Medical Economics Committee of the Iowa State Medical Society. This function is one of the most important duties of this committee and it is hoped that the members of this society will realize the true value of such a service. The Committee makes a thorough investigation of the policies and principles of each and every company requesting the same, and if the organization

meets with the approval of your committee, cards of approval are issued for each representative of the agency to carry. Ask to see this card the next time you are solicited. If the agent does not have this card it may be that the company has not yet applied for approval, but it is also likely that the policies and practices adopted by the organization have not met with the approval of the committee conducting the investigation.

Only by cooperating with the State Society to this extent can you be assured of honest, fair-minded treatment in the collection of your accounts.

AMERICAN JOURNAL OF DIGESTIVE DISEASES AND NUTRITION

In March of this year the *American Journal of Digestive Diseases and Nutrition* made its first appearance. This journal, published under a distinguished editorial council, brings to its readers clinical and investigative original contributions in the field of digestive diseases and nutrition, together with editorials, book reviews, abstracts and monographs in this and allied realms.

Since it is the only journal published in this country limiting its scope to these specialties, it will, no doubt, fill a particular need and be enthusiastically welcomed by physicians whose interests lie in these specialties.

The first number presents several articles on amebic dysentery, discussing parasitology, symptomatology and treatment. Other outstanding articles have to do with the diagnosis of peptic ulcers and the problems in plastic surgery of the colon.

The JOURNAL OF THE IOWA STATE MEDICAL SOCIETY welcomes this newcomer, the *American Journal of Digestive Diseases and Nutrition*, to the field of medical journalism and recommends it to its readers.

PHYSICIANS WANTED

The following letter has been received at the State Society office and we are herewith calling your attention to this need.

Fort Des Moines, Iowa
July 3, 1934

Journal, Iowa State Medical Society,
Ralph R. Simmons, Editor,
Des Moines, Iowa

Dear Dr. Simmons:

The Civilian Conservation Corps in Iowa urgently needs the services of approximately ten (10) graduates of medicine who have completed their internships. The grade and pay is that of a first lieutenant in the United States Army. If you know of any eligibles please direct them to this office.

Sincerely,
J. H. Whiteley,
Major, Medical Corps,
District Surgeon.

Office of the District Surgeon
Iowa District C. C. C.

STATE DEPARTMENT OF HEALTH

MOTTLED ENAMEL OF TEETH IN IOWA

Mottled Enamel of Teeth:

What is the appearance of mottled teeth of the type related to certain water supplies? Here is a girl, twelve years of age, all of whose teeth show a moderately severe grade of the enamel defect. The teeth are nearly perfect in form and alignment; however, the enamel, instead of being smooth and translucent, has an opaque, white appearance not unlike the broken surface of a piece of china. Brown stains in pitted areas on the surface of the front teeth are very noticeable. Unfortunately, the areas of brown discoloration cannot be removed by cleaning and nothing can be done to the enamel; the defect is permanent in character. In localities such as Ankeny, a severe grade of mottled enamel affects practically 100 per cent of the children who through infancy and early childhood drink the water from the deep well which provides the city water supply.

Development of Knowledge Regarding Mottled Enamel:

Mottled enamel of teeth was first described by J. M. Eager of the United States Marine Hospital Service, in 1902. His description was based on cases seen in Naples. In 1910, H. A. Fynn of Denver, described this dental defect among children in Colorado Springs. In 1930, Frederick S. McKay, D.D.S., listed thirteen states in this country in which mottled enamel was known to occur. He stated that the defect was also found in Holland, Italy, Spain, North Africa, China, Mexico and the Argentine. H. Trendley Dean, D.D.S., dental surgeon of the United States Public Health Service, completed a nationwide survey in 1933, reporting 125 localities in this country which represent endemic areas giving rise to mottled enamel.

Although certain water supplies were for years regarded as being the cause of mottled enamel, the causative factor was not discovered and announced until 1931. H. V. Churchill was first to demonstrate by chemical means, the presence in certain water samples, of fluorine in amounts varying from two to 13.7 parts per million. Smith and Smith, working in Arizona, announced in 1931 that the mottled enamel defect was due to the presence of fluorine in water supplies. The source of the fluorine which appears in water is regarded as being in certain types of granite and in other rock (or coal?) formations far below the surface.

Fluorides and Mottled Enamel in Iowa:

The attention of workers in Iowa was directed to the subject of fluorine and the associated mottled enamel defect by R. W. Kerr, assistant engineer of the Kansas State Board of Health, following a survey made in that state. Mr. A. H. Wieters, director of the Division of Public Health Engineering of the Iowa State Department of Health did much toward stimulating the state-wide survey which has been made in Iowa during 1933 and 1934. Mottled enamel was first reported in Iowa by Ostrem, Nelson, Greenwood and Wilhelm as affecting school children at Ankeny, (population 712), Polk county, twelve miles north of Des Moines. This was in 1932. Early in 1933, publicity was given to experimental work of an extensive nature, which had been carried out with rats and dogs, by Nelson and his assistants at Iowa State College, Ames, Iowa.

Following the report of mottled enamel at Ankeny, the Iowa State Department of Health began a state-wide survey to determine the number of areas in the state in which mottled enamel occurs. This work has been carried out in cooperation with the Iowa State Dental Society, the Bureau of Dental Hygiene, dentists, local health officers, research workers and others interested in this subject. In March of 1933, routine analysis was begun for the presence of fluorine, of all water specimens forwarded to the State Hygienic Laboratories at Iowa City. Arrangements for this work were made by M. E. Barnes, M.D., director of the State Hygienic Laboratories. The laboratory work has been done under the direction of Jack Hinman, Jr., chief of the water division. An effective method of discovering endemic areas of mottled enamel was found to be that of looking for clinical evidence of the defect among school children in those counties in which water supplies were reported as containing fluorine. Up to and including the first quarter of 1934, the water supply of 367 cities and towns was found to be free from fluorine. In sixty-five water supplies, less than two parts per million of fluorine were reported. Twenty-two supplies were reported as containing two parts per million, and twenty-nine supplies more than two parts per million. There were sixty water supplies on which analysis had not as yet been made.

In addition to Ankeny the following localities have been found to be endemic areas giving rise to mottled enamel:

Town	County
luxley	Story
laxwell	Story
Jevada (very mild)	Story
lanson	Calhoun
ituart	Guthrie-Adair
)akland	Pottawattamie
)ayton	Webster
iowrie (mild)	Webster
Juncombe	Webster
tratford	Hamilton-Webster
ledfield	Dallas
)gden (very mild)	Boone

It is expected that Altoona (Polk county) and ireenfield (Adair county) will prove to be endemic reas, although sufficient time has not as yet elapsed) establish the fact.

There are different grades of mottled enamel rang-ig from severe to very mild. A water supply con-aining two parts per million of fluorine apparently auses a mild type of mottling, whereas the Ankeny rater with nine parts per million causes the severe orm. Fluorine disturbs calcium metabolism and ffects the enamel rods as well as the substance which inds these together. In the mild type of the enamel ystrophy, part of the enamel may appear normal, ut the cusps of permanent teeth have a pearly ap-earance. This dental defect does not manifest itself ntil six or seven years after a water supply contain-ig fluorine has been used.

'revention of Mottled Enamel:

It has been found possible to remove much of the uorine from water containing this element. The rocess is not practical at this time due to the pro-ibitive expense. The solution to the problem in localities lacking a surface water supply is difficult. 1 municipalities like Ankeny, with ready access to n abundant surface water supply, failure to effect change in the city water is condemnatory. It is ow known with certainty, that each month of delay ibjects helpless children to a hazard, which although ifferent in nature from typhoid fever, represents a rmanent physical defect of distressing character.

POLIOMYELITIS

There is at present no increased incidence of polio-yelitis in Iowa. Press reports have called attention an unusual outbreak of this disease, beginning in the Los Angeles area and later involving other urban centers in California. The weekly bulletin of the California State Department of Health, dated June 30, reported a total number of 1,333 cases for the state from January to June 23, 1934. The health officers weekly statement issued by the United States Public Health Service, reported 316 cases of polio-myelitis for the forty-eight states and the District of Columbia, for the week ending July 7, 1934. Among the 316 cases, 200 or 64 per cent, occurred in California. Reporting of cases in California is very thorough. Most of the cases are said to be mild in character and it is expected that the fatality rate will be low.

Although statistical proof of the value of immune serum in preventing paralysis is as yet lacking, most authorities prefer to use serum. Relatively large amounts (50 to 100 c.c.) are more effective. Sher-man[1] recently reported on 71 patients in Brooklyn which he treated by direct transfusion, using from 150 to 400 c.c. of blood. Through a community survey, there was access to 130 donors who repre-sented all blood groups. The nine symptoms in order of frequency in Sherman's series of cases were:

1. Fever, thirty-eight.
2. Nausea and vomiting, thirty-two.
3. Headache, twenty-nine.
4. Neck rigidity, fifteen.
5. Drowsiness, ten.
6. Restlessness, seven.
7. Gastric distress, five.
8. Pain in neck, five.
9. Tremors, five.

Cell counts in spinal fluid examinations varied from 40 to 1,100.

Smellie[2] stresses the value of immune serum (20 c.c.) as a prophylactic measure for contacts, in the presence of an outbreak.

A pamphlet entitled "Practical Suggestions on Poliomyelitis" was prepared in connection with the poliomyelitis exhibit in Milwaukee in 1933. This pamphlet dealing with recent phases of diagnosis and treatment, can be obtained from the American Medi-cal Association, 535 North Dearborn Street, Chicago, Illinois.

REFERENCES

1. Sherman, Irving: Am. Jour. Dis. Child., v:533-547 (March), 1934.
2. Smellie, James M.: Arch. Dis. Child., viii:75 (February), 1933.

PREVALENCE OF DISEASE

	June, 1934	May, 1934	June, 1933	Most Cases Reported From
iphtheria	34	25	22	Lee, Linn
carlet Fever	139	235	49	Lee, Polk
yphoid Fever	5	4	9	(For State)
nallpox	3	23	45	Boone, Cerro Gordo, Polk
easles	679	1,432	194	(For State)
hooping Cough	141	184	89	Woodbury, Black Hawk
erebrospinal Meningitis	4	6	2	Monroe
iickenpox	123	290	80	Linn, Dubuque
umps	94	280	128	Linn, Woodbury
liomyelitis	1	3	3	Bremer
iberculosis	39	41	32	(For State)
)cky Mountain Spotted Fever	1	0	2	Boone
ndulant Fever	7	7	24	(For State)
'philis	121	70	215	(For State)
inorrhea	161	133	224	(For State)

The JOURNAL of the Iowa State Medical Society

ISSUED MONTHLY

SUBSCRIPTION $3.00 PER YEAR

*Address all communications to the Editor of the Journal,
505 Bankers Trust Building, Des Moines*

OFFICE OF PUBLICATION, DES MOINES, IOWA

Vol. XXIV   AUGUST, 1934   No. 8

CONSTITUTIONAL AND HEREDITARY FACTORS IN DIABETES

Since the discovery of insulin, interest in the disturbed carbohydrate metabolism, designated as diabetes mellitus, has been greatly intensified, and our knowledge of this condition signally advanced. Many of the old conceptions of this disease have been disproved, whereas others have been demonstrated as correct.

Two factors in the etiology of the disease are particularly interesting, since with each there has been a great diversity of opinion expressed in the literature and also since in each instance proof either supporting or opposing their significance is very difficult to obtain. These factors are: first, the influence of over-nutrition; and second, the importance of an inheritable familial tendency to this disease.

The idea is widespread among laymen that like gout, diabetes is a disease of the wealthy with their opulent diets. Although this idea is not founded on facts, there is no doubt that well-to-do people contract the disease much more frequently than do the poor. This may be due to the fact that wealthy people do no manual labor, or it may result from a tendency toward obesity and the degenerative diseases. That over-nutrition is an important

factor in the development of diabetes is substantiated by many observations, particularly those made during the World War, which showed that as nutrition grew worse the morbidity of diabetes decreased. Certainly degenerative diseases, particularly arteriosclerosis, are important predisposing factors.

Joslin[1] reports that fat men are nineteen times more liable to the disease than thin men, and both Joslin and v. Noorden state that obesity is associated with diabetes in 40 per cent and 35 per cent respectively of the cases which they have observed. Sugar is discovered in some obese patients as soon as their weight exceeds a certain definite point. It would appear then that over-nutrition has established itself in a very firm etiologic relationship to this disease, although evidence submitted by other investigators would indicate, particularly in young individuals, that obesity is of very minor importance. Obesity is ordinarily considered as a familial characteristic, and if we admit an etiologic relationship between obesity and diabetes, we prepare the way for the acceptance of the constitutional or hereditary predisposition of definite etiologic significance.

Further supporting this idea may be cited the prevalence of diabetes among the Semitic races, reaching some 40 per cent in v. Noorden's series of 27,000 cases. So important is the hereditary factor that Cecil in his recent textbook of medicine begins his definition of diabetes mellitus by this significant statement, "Diabetes mellitus is an inheritable constitutional disease." If we concede, then, that the tendency to this disease is inheritable, it immediately opens the question of how this inheritability behaves. Does the tendency toward diabetes follow the laws of Mendelian inheritance as a dominant or a recessive characteristic? The thought that this tendency behaves as a dominant characteristic has apparently been successfully disproved, since a careful investigation of the family history in a rather large number of diabetic patients did not produce satisfactory evidence to support the theory of dominancy.

Confirming the earlier suggestion of White and reiterated by Allen, Pincus and Hoyt[2] have recently collected the family histories of 523 diabetic patients appearing at the Joslin Diabetic Unit from July to October, 1932. This study indicates the potentiality for developing diabetes as an inherited characteristic which follows the Mendelian law as a recessive characteristic. Of the diabetic patients studied, 22.94 per cent gave history of diabetes other than parents, as contrasted with 10.42 per cent in a non-diabetic group. It is seen that there was reported in the diabetic cases a significant excess of families with diabetic blood relatives (other than parents and siblings) as compared with the controlled families. The diabetic patients were divided into three main groups: first, both parents non-diabetic; second, one parent diabetic; and third, both parents diabetic. The first group included 440 cases and the second, 81 cases. Pincus and Hoyt conclude from their data that diabetes follows the Mendelian expectation.

In a statistical study conducted by a large insurance company, 2,002 individuals were exposed to risk presenting a family history containing two or more cases of diabetes. The actual death experiences in this group were 24, as compared with an expected death of 18.24, giving a ratio of actual to expected deaths of 13.3 per cent plus or minus 18.

Dingman[3] quotes eight prominent authorities on diabetes who, as a result of an analysis of their individual case records, state that a family history of diabetes in blood relatives was obtained in percentages varying from 18 to 46 per cent with the different observers. These observations would appear as conclusively demonstrating the inheritability of the tendency toward diabetes, and the work of Pincus and Hoyt would apparently fix this inheritance as a definite Mendelian characteristic.

However, the problem is not so simple, and in considering the question of heredity one must bear in mind that members of the same family share similar environmental influences and have similar dietary habits. For this reason much difficulty has been experienced in separating the truly hereditary traits from those environmental influences which may or may not be of significant importance in the consideration of this problem. Few go so far, however, as Buchanan to conclude that: "So far as the data collected are reliable there is not the slightest evidence to justify the statement that diabetes mellitus is at times hereditary."

Explaining, perhaps, the difference in the widely dissimilar viewpoints expressed above, Otto May in reporting his studies on family histories in a series of 1,143 cases, deduces that there are two types of diabetes insofar as inheritance is concerned. The first, or inherited type, with an incidence in early life runs to a more rapid termination. The second, a non-inherited type, with an incidence in middle or late middle life runs a comparatively mild course and shows but slow progression. In youth the disease is more likely to be inherited and be due to a developmental impairment of the pancreatic cells, while in middle age the cause is often, in his opinion, due to over-eating or over-drinking with little physical exercise, so that the carbohydrate metabolism breaks down under the overload.

It is interesting to note also that in Otto May's analysis of his group of inherited cases when the diabetic family history was on the male side the age at death of the diabetic applicant averaged 38.3 years, while, when the history occurred on the mother's side, the age at death averaged 49.3—a difference of eleven years. It would appear, therefore, that the hereditary factor is more manifest in the male, and that the death from diabetes of a father or brother is more ominous than the death of the mother or sister. While May's material for analysis was not large, his observations were borne out by the figures obtained at the Registrar's general office for England in 1926.

From these several statistical studies it appears proved that in the genesis of diabetes certain constitutional and hereditary factors are of great importance. Obesity of itself may predispose to the disease, but when obesity is associated with a family history of diabetes, it constitutes a considerable hazard. A tendency toward the disease is definitely inheritable, and it appears likely that this tendency follows the laws of Mendelian inheritance as a recessive characteristic, particularly when diabetes manifests itself in youth.

REFERENCES

1. Joslin, E. P.: The Treatment of Diabetes Mellitus, Fourth Edition, Lea and Febiger, Philadelphia, 1928.
2. Pincus, Gregory, and White, Priscilla: On the inheritance of diabetes mellitus—an analysis of 675 family histories. Am. Jour. Med. Sc., clxxxvi:1 (July) 1933.
3. Dingman, H. W.: Insurability—Prognosis and Selection. The Spectator Co., Chicago, 1927.

SURGEONS VIEW SICKNESS INSURANCE PLANS

A plan characterized by the American College of Surgeons as one "looking to a more adequate medical service to the whole community" and censured by the American Medical Association as "confusing to the public mind" and "harmful to the profession," was publicized in the lay press under the sponsorship of the American College of Surgeons, on the first day of the Cleveland session of the American Medical Association.

The proposed plan of the College violates in many respects the official attitude of the American Medical Association and apparently justifies the resolution "that the House of Delegates of the American Medical Association expresses condemnation of such tactics and of this apparent attempt of the Board of Regents of the American College of Surgeons to dominate and control the nature of medical practice." It is not our purpose in this article to condemn or approve the attitude of the American College of Surgeons in this matter. This will be properly settled by committees from the two organizations. We do believe, however, that the more thoroughly the problems dealing with the future practice of medicine are studied, the more surely we will arrive at a proper solution of the problem of adequate medical care. It is from the standpoint then of stimulating thoughtful consideration among our readers and also to acquaint them with the substance of the resolutions adopted by the American College of Surgeons that we review these recommendations.

At a meeting of the Board of Regents of the American College of Surgeons held on June 10, 1934, a report was presented by the Medical Service Board, announcing the principles which, in the opinion of the Board, should govern payment plans for hospitals and medical service to individuals of moderate means. While no specific plan was recommended or suggested, *the Board viewed as desirable some scheme directed toward this end.*

They affirm the interest of the American College of Surgeons in a plan looking toward a more adequate medical service to the whole community, and express their desire to cooperate with other agencies to this end. They believe that it is the duty of the medical profession to assume leadership in this movement and to take control of all measures which may be instituted to accomplish this purpose. They believe that encouragement should be given to the trial of new methods and practices designed to meet these needs, and a careful evaluation of their success should be the duty of the medical profession before they are offered for general adoption. All such new and experimental methods of practice must be conducted strictly in accordance with the accepted code of ethics of the medical profession, so that the interests of the patient and of the community may be protected.

The College recognizes for immediate study four groups of the population for whom more adequate medical service should be made available, as follows:

1. The indigent.

2. The uneducated and prejudiced members of the community.

3. Those who because of limited resources are unable to meet the cost of serious illness and hospitalization.

4. Those living in remote districts where adequate medical service is not obtainable.

The care of the indigent sick should be a direct obligation upon the community and (unless otherwise compensated by intangible benefits such as staff and teaching appointments, opportunity and experience), physicians fulfilling this public service should receive remuneration. The College

should work in cooperation with other medical groups in order to dispel the ignorance and credulity of the public, and to bring the people to a proper realization of the protective and curative resources of modern medicine.

The American College of Surgeons recognizes that the periodic pre-payment plan, providing for the costs of medical care of illness and injury of individuals and of families of moderate means, offers a reasonable expectation of providing them with more effective methods of securing adequate medical service.

Periodic pre-payment plans providing for the costs of medical service may be divided into two classes:

A. Payment for medical service.

B. Payment for hospitalization.

It is suggested by the Board that plans for the payment of hospitalization alone without provision for payment for medical service, may be considered the first project to be undertaken in the average community.

"The American College of Surgeons believes that certain general principles can and should be established, the observance of which will tend to obviate known difficulties and dangers which may threaten the success of these special forms of medical service. These principles are as follows:

A. Periodic pre-payment plans for medical service should be free from the intervention of commercial intermediary organizations operating for profit. After deduction of the clerical costs of operation of the fund and such accumulation of reserve as may be legally imposed, the full amount paid by the contributors should be available for medical and hospital services.

B. In the interest of the patient, the organization of plans for the periodic payment of medical and hospital costs must be under the control of the medical profession. The medical profession must act in concert with the hospitals and such other allied services as may be involved in the individual project, together with a group of citizens representative of the whole community and of industry who are interested in the successful operation of the plan.

C. The principle of free choice of the physician and hospital by the patient must be assured to the end that the responsibility of the individual physician to the individual patient shall always be maintained. When hospitalization is required, this choice must of necessity be limited to the physicians and surgeons who hold appointments on the staffs of the hospitals participating in the plan or to those physicians and surgeons who are acceptable to the hospital. It is further recommended

Reporting on the proposals received for bringing about an increased employment of the handicapped, the commission declared some to be acceptable while others, although good, obviously did not come within the scope of the National Recovery Administration. Of the latter character was mentioned the suggestion that the Federal Government and other governmental agents should set the example to business and industry by adopting regulations which would make certain the allocation of a fair proportion of public positions to the handicapped worker. Also meritorious, although outside the province of the NRA, except insofar as it relates to sheltered workshops, was the proposal that the handicapped not absorbable by industries be encouraged to produce well selected and standardized articles that could be marketed in the government purchase fields.

While the two suggestions outlined above were rejected by the Administration, three very concrete recommendations made by the Commission were found desirable and the National Recovery Administration is advised to "call to the attention of all coded industries . . . as socially desirable measures for their codes, either in a mandatory way or as recommended practices, the following:

"A. Every employer should, whenever the nature of the disability or the individual personality does not negate such a step, rehire in suitable employment persons who have received permanent injuries in their employ.

"B. Employers should in the ordinary course of expansion call back on an equal basis with others, handicapped workers who have been in their employ within the last four years.

"C. Employers should endeavor to have a suitable proportion of handicapped workers, whether substandard or fully efficient, in the ranks of their employees in order to make certain of a fair distribution of opportunity to work. This proportion in all probability would be as large as two per cent and might even be close to five per cent."

THE INDUSTRIALIZED COMMUNITY AND TUBERCULOSIS

In the recent annual meeting of the National Tuberculosis Association in Cincinnati, especial attention was given to the problem of tuberculosis among the industrial class. It was pointed out at this meeting that tuberculosis kills about 75,000 people annually, a number greater than the total number of American soldiers who died in action or of wounds in the World War. It was stated that tuberculosis stands seventh as the cause of death among the general population, but that among men in industry tuberculosis ranks in second place. While this observation would lead to the conclusion that the industrialized community favored tuberculosis, other observations cited in the discussions of this meeting would indicate the contrary.

During the last few years, the mortality from tuberculosis, even in the industrial community, has been distinctly lowered, whereas it is common knowledge that there has been a rapid industrial development during the same period. Statistical studies made in Chicago, St. Louis and Cincinnati lead to the conclusion that "A regular job with a regular pay check is the best insurance against tuberculosis that a man has for himself and his family." These observations closely paralleled those made by other investigating bodies which indicate that tuberculosis and other nutritional diseases increased with unemployment and its attending privations, and decreased as reëmployment was restored.

. It would appear, then, that the following conclusion may safely be drawn: the more highly industrialized a community, the lower the tuberculosis rate.

THE BULLETIN OF THE AMERICAN SOCIETY FOR THE CONTROL OF CANCER

Reliable statistics would indicate that the death rate from cancer in the total population of the United States has increased about eighty-four per cent in the past thirty years. That some of this increase is the result of more accurate means of diagnosis cannot be doubted, but the fact remains, apparently conclusively demonstrated, that cancer *per se* is actually more prevalent today than it was thirty years ago. These facts demand that the modern physician become cancer-conscious and that malignancy be searched for and recognized, so that proper therapeutic management may be instigated at a time when cure is possible.

It is for these reasons that we take pleasure in calling the attention of our readers to *The Bulletin of The American Society for the Control of Cancer*, which we can recommend as an outstandingly useful instrument in this field. It contains a number of short, practical articles written by distinguished authorities in the field of cancer therapy and cancer research. It offers at a subscription price of only $1.00 per year, an easy and practical way for a physician to keep abreast of cancer control progress. Readers unfamiliar with this publication may receive a complimentary copy upon request from the American Society for the Control of Cancer, 1250 Sixth Avenue, New York City.

THE OPEN FORUM

To the Editor of THE JOURNAL,

Dr. Fay's article "Shall Organized Medicine Survive?" pleases me so much that I must comment on it. I agree with him in every respect, except in seeking for the cause of the changed public attitude toward the members of our profession. Dr. Fay blames shifting economic conditions. He sees in the sociologist a brain trust agent reaching out for the control of our cherished interests. To me, in looking back over a period of forty-five years in general practice, the change is fundamentally one in the attitude of the average physician toward his work. Dr. Fay mentions that we, as a fellowship, are unusually ready to admit our shortcomings, and because that is true I make this assertion.

Our younger physicians, influenced by the ideals of the age in which they matured, are too prone to keep an eye on the clock, too ready to count the cash returns, and the reaction of the public in general is the natural one of considering the physician on the same footing with the grocer and the butcher. The tendency to shop around for an operation or a confinement is akin to scanning the Friday night papers for the best Saturday bargains, a manifestation of our commercial age. Only when we as physicians give service compatible with our highest ideals, service that cannot be bought and paid for in cash alone, then only will we receive from our patients that allegiance which is the only true recompense for our labors.

In other words, I am asking for an increase of individualization in service to offset the leveling tendencies of a socialistic age. It is imperative that we impress our young physicians with the importance of the *art* of medicine to balance the science of it. Take as an example the practice of obstetrics, so often under discussion. We will lower the death rate of these mothers and their babies not so much by furnishing more scientifically trained physicians, but by teaching well trained physicians intelligently to wait on Nature and not to oppose her; to observe the patient and minister to her particular needs, not to classify the case, follow the accepted rules in the book and get home in time for golf or the bridge club. Common sense and self-abnegation may be hard to teach in any college curriculum, but they are the fundamentals of the art of our profession, and the two qualities of mind and heart which will never be subject to regulations or state control. If we make these ideals a live issue instead of a dead letter, organized medicine not only must live, but it cannot die.

July 14, 1934   GEO. B. MAXWELL, M.D.

| SPEAKERS BUREAU ACTIVITIES | WOMAN'S AUXILIARY NEWS |

POSTGRADUATE WORK

The proposed laboratory course which was outlined on the Speakers Bureau page last month was cancelled. Although many doctors indicated interest in the course and many commendatory letters were received regarding the outline, a sufficient number did not enroll to enable the Bureau to carry out its plans. This is the first summer that an attempt has been made to conduct postgraduate study during that season in addition to the usual courses given in the fall and spring. The failure of this experiment may indicate that such courses are not feasible during the summer and vacation period, or it may be that the excessively hot weather this particular summer did not give the experiment a fair chance.

Since so many enthusiastic comments were made about the idea of a laboratory course, however, it is very probable that such a course will be given some time in the future. It has been suggested that instead of making it a two weeks' concentrated course, it be given on the usual schedule of one meeting a week for a period of ten weeks.

Plans for the usual fall postgraduate courses, under the supervision of the members of the faculty of the College of Medicine of the State University of Iowa, are now under way. One of the courses given by the University last year—that on the diagnosis and treatment of common internal disorders—will be repeated this fall at the request of the Speakers Bureau, since it was so enthusiastically received by those taking the courses last fall. The new course for this fall will be a surgical course, planned on the same basis as the medical course—diagnosis and treatment.

RADIO BROADCASTS

WOI—Mondays, 5:30 to 5:45 p. m.

WSUI—Thursdays, 7:45 to 8:00 p. m.

July 30-August 2—Facts About Quacks, M. B. Call, M.D.

August 6- 9—Swimming Hazards, American Medical Association.

August 13-16—First Aid to Medical Terms.

August 20-23—Plastic Surgery, R. J. Lynch, M.D.

August 27-30—The Nurse, Janet Sinclair, R.N.

CONVENTION NOTES

The following recommendations presented at the twefth annual meeting of the Woman's Auxiliary to the American Medical Association, are of especial interest to all auxiliary members, and it is hoped that the suggestions contained therein may be carried out.

Recommendations of Public Relations Committee
Mrs. David S. Long, Chairman

1. That the auxiliary support, through individual members in various communities, the policy of the National Congress of Parents and Teachers to encourage summer round-up examinations in the office of the family physician in preference to organized clinics; the latter to be supported only when the former is impractical, and then only in cooperation with the medical society.

2. That the county chairmen of public relations, when authorized by the county medical society, select material from the Hygeia news sheets for local publicity.

3. That regional or county health institutes be promoted and to be dignified with a printed or typed program.

Recommendations of Press and Publicity Committee
Mrs. Robert E. Fitzgerald, Chairman

1. It is again recommended to the attention of the auxiliary women that the Bulletin of the American Medical Association is available to the wives of all fellows of the American Medical Association. Those members of the American Medical Association who are not fellows have the opportunity of subscribing to the Bulletin at a cost of fifty cents a year. It then follows that the auxiliary section of the Bulletin is available to practically all auxiliary women. It is recommended that members make it a point to read this periodical and that county presidents take steps to call the attention of all county members to the Bulletin.

2. It is recommended that there be a quarterly News Letter sent to the president, president elect, and chairman of press and publicity of each state.

SOCIETY PROCEEDINGS

Davis County

The Davis County Medical Society held its annual picnic Wednesday, July 11, at the Bloomfield Country Club. Dr. Gordon F. Harkness of Davenport, president of the State Society, was the guest speaker for the occasion, and delivered his address immediately after the noon luncheon. J. C. Donahue, M.D., of Centerville, spoke on Fracture of Cervical Vertebrae, and Postmaster John J. Ethell of Bloomfield, addressed the group on The Doctor and the Postmaster. Following the program the guests were entertained at golf, croquet, and bridge.

Floyd County

The Floyd County Medical Society held its regular monthly meeting at the Cedar Valley Hospital, Tuesday evening, June 26. After a six o'clock complimentary dinner, J. B. Miner, Jr., M.D., read a paper on Clinical Types of Nocturnal Dyspnea. The following case reports were presented: Infection of the Petrous Portion of the Temporal Bone, F. H. Fillenwarth, M.D.; Bladder Diverticulum, C. W. McQuillen, M.D.; Diverticulitis of the Sigmoid, H. A. Tolliver, M.D.; Tumor of the Sigmoid, R. A. Fox, M.D.; and Paroxysmal Tachycardia, C. H. Cords, M.D.

J. B. Miner, Jr., M.D., Secretary.

Hamilton County Annual Meeting

Officers elected at a recent meeting of the Hamilton County Medical Society are: Dr. T. F. Desmond of Webster City, president; Dr. E. W. Slater of Jewell, vice president; Dr. D. W. James of Kamrar, secretary and treasurer; and Dr. G. T. McCauliff of Webster City, censor.

D. W. James, M.D., Secretary.

Linn County

Paul J. Hanzlik, M.D., professor of pharmacology and toxicology at Leland Stanford University, California, addressed a combined meeting of the Linn County Medical Society, the Cedar Rapids Dental Association and Cedar Rapids druggists, Thursday, July 26. He spoke on the recent advances in pharmacology and therapeutics, and his talk included a discussion of many new drugs on the market.

The next meeting of the society will be held Wednesday, September 12, at which time Dr. Dean Lewis of Johns Hopkins University Medical School will be the guest speaker.

Sac County

The Sac County Medical Society met in regular session at the Lakewood Park Hotel in Lakeview, Thursday, July 26, for a dinner and business meeting. Twelve members were present. Following the dinner, a business meeting was held at which many matters of mutual interest were discussed. The injustices of any method of handling the care of the indigent sick, the basic science law proposed in the last session of the House of Delegates, the registration of births, the Sac county quadruplets, and the heat, were all thoroughly covered in a discussion entered into by every member present. Dr. L. F. Eaton of Schaller was admitted to membership.

J. R. Dewey, M.D., Secretary.

Austin Flint-Cedar Valley Society

The annual meting of the Austin Flint-Cedar Valley Medical Society was held at Clear Lake, Wednesday, July 11. The following addresses were given during the afternoon session: Surgery of the Biliary Tract, Howard K. Gray, M.D., of Rochester, Minnesota; Toxemias of Pregnancy, William E. Brown, M.D., of Cedar Rapids; The Present Status of Poliomyelitis, Roland Stahr, M.D., of Fort Dodge; and Poisoning from Commonly Used Sedatives, C. W. Baldridge, M.D., of Iowa City. Those in attendance at the six-thirty banquet were addressed by C. H. Plattenberg, lecturer for the University of Wisconsin extension department, on The Physician, the Banisher of Fear. New officers elected at the business session are: Dr. M. J. McGrane of New Hampton, president; Dr. T. J. Irish of Forest City, vice president; Dr. R. A. Fox of Charles City, secretary; and Dr. W. E. Long of Mason City, treasurer.

Iowa-Illinois Central District Medical Society

Thursday, July 26, the annual meeting of the Iowa-Illinois Central District Medical Society was held at the Outing Club in Davenport. The following program was arranged by the Speakers Bureau of the Iowa State Medical Society: Allergy, Harry L. Alexander, M.D., of St. Louis, Missouri; The Value of Theophylline in the Treatment of Arteriosclerotic Heart Disease, H. W. Rathe, M.D., of Waverly; Diets and Disease, Clifford J. Barborka, M.D., of Chicago. O. H. Wangensteen, M.D., of the University of Minnesota, was the speaker of the evening after the six-thirty banquet, and took for his subject, Diagnostic and Therapeutic Considerations in the Management of Acute Abdominal Lesions.

INTERESTING NEWS
In Brief

Chemists have been able to prepare on a commercial scale pure Vitamin C in the form of ascorbic acids from paprika.

———

Contrary to the general belief the disease-bearing type of mosquitoes are practically unknown in the Florida Everglades.

———

A diet containing an excess of phosphorous and a minimum amount of calcium is said to be helpful in the prevention of industrial lead poisoning.

———

A French scientist states that the races of man were set in their present form, at least the white and black, as far back as the Aqridnaciana, 30,000 years ago.

———

Researches conducted at the University of California Medical School point to a Vitamin C deficiency as an important factor in the causation of rheumatic fever and rheumatoid arthritis.

———

Convalescent serum may be protected from deterioration by a new method of processing, which involves freezing the serum at 100 degrees below zero Fahrenheit and sealing in a vacuum after the water has been removed.

———

According to announcements just received in this country, twenty-eight Jewish physicians were dismissed from various hospitals in Vienna, and many others were given notice that their contracts would not be renewed.

———

Outstanding among the exhibits presented before the recent meeting of the American Heart Association was that on coronary disease prepared by Drs. Fred M. Smith and W. D. Paul of Iowa City and H. W. Rathe of Waverly, Iowa.

———

Dr. E. C. McCollum of John Hopkins University is credited with the statement "there is little reason to doubt that at least one new soluble vitamin remains to be discovered, and probably at least two more water soluble vitamins exist."

———

By attenuating the virus of psittacosis a vaccine has been developed at the Rockefeller Institute for Medical Research, which is said to prevent this disease. The vaccine is now being tried by the United States Public Health Service, where eleven cases have developed among laboratory workers.

———

Anthropologic studies conducted at the Smithsonian Institute upset the generally accepted idea that characteristic features attained in adult life are permanent in the individual. Their studies show that every feature, teeth, hair, bones and body cells change without cessation from the beginning of life before birth to the oldest age.

———

The State University of Iowa spent a total of $3,383,593.62 during the fiscal year ending June 30, 1933, and ended the year with an excess income of $122,065.48. The increase in the net income of the University Hospitals amounted to $76,362.82. During the previous fiscal year, the hospital operated at a deficit of $15,067.31.

———

Substantiating the observations of other scientists on the effect of alcohol on the nerve structures, Dr. C. C. Speidel of the University of Virginia Medical School states that little or no perceptible harm is done to nerves by mild daily drinking of alcoholic beverages, but permanent damage is done by alcohol consumed on a "spree."

———

Invention of the centrifuge microscope, one of the most powerful of the newer tools for scientific research, will be rewarded by the presentation of the Wetherill Medal of the Franklin Institute to Alfred L. Loomis, banker-scientist of Tuxedo Park, New York, and Professor E. Newton Harvey of Princeton University.

———

In a paper read recently before the Society for Experimental Biology and Medicine at the University of Minnesota, it was reported that common salt may prove to be an effective treatment for diabetes. Records of reported cases showed that the sugar losses were definitely reduced by a 200 to 300 per cent increase over the normal average salt ration.

———

A new drug, one of the chemicals known as dinitro compounds, can be used to take off any amount of weight desired, when used properly, Dr. Edward L. Bortz of Philadelphia, declared in a paper presented recently before the American College of Surgeons. The drug works on the principle of putting the body under a "forced draft," and thus "burns the fat off."

PERSONAL MENTION

Dr. A. F. Barfoot of Decorah, addressed the local Child Study Club, Tuesday, June 19, on the subject of "Nervous Fears."

———

Dr. Erwin von Graff, former professor of obstetrics and gynecology at the State University of Iowa College of Medicine, has located in Des Moines, where he is engaged in the private practice of medicine.

———

Dr. Leonard A. West of Des Moines, spoke on 'Aviation and Medicine," at a meeting of the Winterset Rotary Club, held Thursday, June 21.

———

The following physicians have located in various towns and cities in Iowa during the past month:

Dr. Joseph D. Fitzgerald, who was graduated in 1930 from Creighton Medical School, and who practiced in Cincinhati for two years, has taken over the practice of the late Dr. Lee Prescott in Sloan; Dr. Leland S. Lewis, who was graduated in 1932 from Rush Medical College, will be associated in practice with Dr. D. J. Townsend at Lohrville; Dr. R. E. Almquist, for the past six years surgeon for the United States Steel Corporation at Gary, Indiana, has purchased the equipment and practice of the late Dr. I. O. Pond at Perry; Dr. R. E. Mailliard, formerly of Lincoln, Nebraska, has located for the practice of medicine in Storm Lake; Dr. Wilbur W. Hayne, who was graduated in 1933 from the State University of Iowa College of Medicine, and who just completed his interneship at Broadlawns Hospital in Des Moines, will be associated with Dr. William Woodburn of Boone; Dr. R. F. Martin, formerly of Madison, Wisconsin, has taken over the practice of the late Dr. James F. Taylor of Sioux City; Dr. Emil M. Christensen, formerly on the staff of the Danish-American Hospital in Chicago, has moved to Vinton, and has established himself in the offices occupied by the late Dr. J. E. Luckey; Dr. William Johnson, who was graduated in 1933 from the State University of Iowa College of Medicine, and served a year's interneship at the Cook County Hospital, has returned to his home in Alden, where he will be associated with his father, Dr. Jonathan Johnson; Dr. Wayland R. Hicks, formerly of the faculty of the State University of Iowa College of Medicine, has entered private practice in Sioux City; Dr. John F. Hardin, formerly of St. Joseph, has located in Bedford, where he will take over the practice of the late Dr. P. J. Gustin; Dr. R. J. Carlson, a graduate of the State University of Iowa College of Medicine, has moved to Hawarden from Omaha, where he was resident physician for the Covenant Hospital; Dr. C. D. Oelrich, a recent graduate of the State University of Iowa College of Medicine, will start practicing medicine in Sioux Center; Dr. Frank R. Ford, a graduate of the Tulane University School of Medicine, is taking over the practice of the late Dr. Karl Fauth of Wellsburg, coming direct from Nashville, Tennessee, where he has been examining physician at the Veteran's Hospital; Dr. W. H. Gibbon, formerly of the faculty of the State University of Iowa College of Medicine, has entered private practice in Sioux City, where he will be associated with Dr. H. M. McCuiston; Dr. Robert E. Britt, who was graduated in 1929 from Creighton Medical School, and served his interneship at Highland Hospital, Oakland, California, is opening an office in Burlington; Dr. R. M. Minkel, who was graduated in 1932 from the State University of Iowa College of Medicine, and interned at the Vassar Hospital in Poughkeepsie, New York, and the Craig Hospital and Sanitarium in Beacon, New York, is now located for the practice of medicine in Swea City.

MARRIAGES

Mrs. Belle Sunderlin of Spencer, and Dr. B. A. Smillie of Gilmore City, were married Monday, June 18, in Boone, Iowa. The couple will make their home in Gilmore City, where Dr. Smillie has been practicing for several years.

The wedding of Miss Opal Sarchet Morrison and Dr. Melvin G. Bourne, both of Algona, took place, Saturday, June 16, at the home of the bride's aunt in Algona. After the honeymoon trip through several western states, they will return to Algona, where Dr. Bourne has been practicing for three years.

DEATH NOTICES

Allen, Paul Edward, of Cherokee, aged fifty-one, died July 2, following an extended illness of streptococcic infection. He was graduated in 1910 from the State University of Iowa College of Homeopathic Medicine, and had long been a member of the Cherokee County Medical Society.

Folsom, Shirley Dan, of Muscatine, aged forty-six, died suddenly on July 22, from acute dilatation of the heart. He was graduated in 1917 from the Hahnemann Medical College and Hospital, Chicago, and had long been a member of the Muscatine County Medical Society.

Harrison, Edward Wesley, of Winfield, aged sixty-six, died suddenly July 6, after a heart attack. He was graduated in 1894 from Keokuk Medical College, and had been a member of the Henry County Medical Society.

Hejinian, Aram Garabed, of Anamosa, aged seventy, died July 5, after an illness of two months. He was graduated in 1893 from Rush Medical College, Chicago, and at the time of his death was a Life Member of the Jones County and Iowa State Medical Societies.

Patrick, Russell A., of Marshalltown, aged thirty-two, died June 22, from a short illness of Bright's disease. He was graduated in 1932 from the State University of Iowa College of Medicine, and at the time of his death was a member of the Marshall County Medical Society.

Runyon, William Darrow, of Sioux City, aged forty-seven, died June 23, after a long illness. He was graduated in 1909 from the State University of Iowa College of Medicine, and had long been a member of the Woodbury County Medical Society.

Taylor, James Fitz, of Sioux City, aged sixty-seven, died July 2, following a heart attack. He was graduated in 1892 from Bellevue Hospital Medical College, New York City, and at the time of his death was a member of the Woodbury County Medical Society.

Vorwerk, Anthony H., of Burlington, aged sixty, died suddenly July 26, of heart disease. He was graduated in 1897 from the State University of Iowa College of Medicine, and at the time of his death was a member of the Des Moines County Medical Society.

HISTORY OF MEDICINE IN IOWA

Edited by the Historical Committee

DR. HENRY B. YOUNG, Burlington
DR. FRANK M. FULLER, Keokuk
DR. JOHN T. MCCLINTOCK, Iowa City

DR. TOM. B. THROCKMORTON, Des Moines
DR. WALTER L. BIERRING, Des Moines
DR. WILLIAM JEPSON, Sioux City

Pioneer Physicians of Page County

J. F. ALDRICH, M.D., Shenandoah

ORGANIZATION OF PAGE COUNTY

When one speaks of the characteristics of the men and women of a community, he is mentioning the things of value to be preserved for future generations. Nature had provided boundless prairies, beautiful streams and small stretches of woodland, and it was now for men of courage, strength and endurance to occupy the land of plenty. The "prairie schooner" was the means of family transportation.·

Page county takes its name from a distinguished Mexican war veteran, Captain Page. The county is bounded on the west by the most southwesterly county of the state, Fremont county; on the east by Taylor county; on the north by Montgomery county; and on the south by portions of two Missouri counties, Nodaway and Atchison. Some of the details of the surveying work in laying out townships was done before the state boundary line difficulty was settled. The line as it now stands was established by the commissioners appointed by Act of Congress for that purpose in 1851. The county is well supplied with living streams of water and a fertile soil, and is, therefore, well adapted for stock raising.

The early settlement of Page county can be traced to those pioneers who left their homes in Pennsylvania, Ohio, Virginia, Kentucky, Indiana, Tennessee, North Carolina, Illinois, Missouri, and New York and even industrious natives of Germany and the British Isles, who came to the new West for the purpose of making homes for themselves. The first white man actually to make settlement in the county was George W. Farrens who came from Jackson county, Missouri, in the spring of 1840, to what is now Buchanan township.

The third general assembly appointed William Hudson organizing sheriff for Page county and thus this county became one of the organized counties in 1851. The first district court convened at the house of Philip Boulware on September 22,

1851, with A. H. Farrens, a brother of the first settler, as clerk. Clarinda became the seat of justice in 1853. After three defeats at the polls of bond issues for court house purposes, the board of supervisors decided to act on its own initiative and let a contract for a partially efficient building for work and records. In December, 1887, the present structure was completed and accepted, having a total cost of $86,500.

I wish to call attention in the following pages to a few of the courageous men who served the settlers of the early days in Page county. King Solomon chose wisdom rather than riches and dispensed knowledge rather than riches. The first essential of the success of these pioneer physicians was their perseverance in the face of the few facilities they had at that time.

The medical profession has been given one of its most glowing tributes by the genial literary invalid Robert Louis Stevenson in his tropical Samoan home. He wrote: "There are men and classes of men that stand above the common herd; the soldier, the sailor, and the shepherd not infrequently; the artist rarely, and rarer still, the clergyman; the physician almost as a rule. He is the flower (such as it is) of our civilization; and when that stage of man is done with, and only remembered to be marveled at in history, he will be thought to have shared as little as any in the defects of the period, and most notably exhibited the virtues of the race. Generosity he has, such as is possible to those who practice an art—never to those who drive a trade; discretion, tested by a hundred secrets; tact, tried in a thousand embarrassments; and, what is more important, Herculean cheerfulness and courage. So it is that he brings air and cheer into the sick room, and often enough, though not so often as he wishes, brings healing."

So wrote the man who knew much of physicians throughout his life of physical frailty, and knowing them well was eminently fitted to pronounce judgment upon them as a class. It is true, as a rule, that the standing of the doctor among his fellowmen is exceptionally good. Wind your way from town to town in any part of our country, or through most European countries, and you will not fail to find the doctor reckoned among the leading citizens of the place. Not even the clergyman holds the honored place in the affections of the people to the same degree as does the family doctor. The chosen confidant to whom the hidden secrets are revealed, and who never fails this sacred trust; the one first sought at the hour of birth and when the angel of death hovers near, he comes closer to the heart and soul of each one of us than does any other member of the community.

· The doctor in literature is not always depicted as a lovable character; for instance the "Dr. Sawbones" of Dickens fame. So also we meet the resourceful "Dr. Watson" as the inseparable companion of Sherlock Holmes, and S. Weir Mitchell's "Dr. North" and his friends, to say nothing about genial old "Dr. McClure" in Beside the Bonnie Briar Bush.

PHYSICIANS WHO LOCATED IN CLARINDA

Unfortunately not every doctor in actual life is the paragon of virtue that Stevenson would leave you to believe. However, there are many among our pioneer physicians who have measured up to this standard.

Dr. Alexander H. Farrens, who was one of the earliest settlers in Buchanan township, was possibly the first doctor to practice the healing art. He was recognized as a natural physician and surgeon, and seemed to know just what to do with the meager drugs and appliances at hand. He died in March, 1858.

Dr. James L. Barrett is thought to be the first thoroughly schooled medical practitioner in Page county, and located in Clarinda in 1855. He began the study of medicine in 1838 but the exact number of years of his practice is not known. He was born in Kentucky, reared in Indiana, and labored in Iowa.

Dr. James H. Conine who had read medicine at Columbus, Ohio, after a few years of work decided to move westward because of failing health, and finally arrived at Clarinda in April, 1856. He established a drug store and gradually drifted out of the practice of medicine. Health conditions caused him to seek other climates and he finally died at Dallas, Texas, on September 3, 1874.

Dr. H. C. Brandt came to Clarinda in the summer of 1855 to look after some land interests. He was possessed of a most thorough education, having studied in the best medical schools of Europe. After a number of years in which he divided his time between Clarinda and his home town in Indiana, he removed to Kansas City, Missouri, where he spent the remaining years of his life.

Dr. Albert Heald came to Clarinda in 1859. He was afflicted with tuberculosis but continued to practice until his death in 1863.

Dr. Samuel H. Kridelbaugh located in Clarinda in 1855. He, like Dr. A. H. East, served in both the legal and medical professions. He was also a newspaper editor and writer of some note; was given the honor of, or was conspicuous in, organizing the first medical society known as the Southwestern Iowa Society on February 10, 1866. The early records were destroyed by fire but the society continued its activities until 1880.

Dr. M. Enfield was a graduate of Rush Medical College in 1873 and came direct to Clarinda, where he practiced until his death, the exact date of which is not known.

Dr. J. K. Rickey came to Clarinda in the eighties from Keokuk, and practiced in Clarinda for over fifty years.

Dr. A. G. Wall located in Clarinda subsequent to the war, but some time later removed to his native state of Pennsylvania to practice.

Dr. P. W. Lewellen was attracted to Page county because of its farming lands, but decided to practice here and became prominent in medicine and politics. In 1878 Dr. Lewellen was elected to the state senate from Page and Fremont counties. For several years he was a member of the State Board of Health and Trustee of the Mt. Pleasant Insane Hospital, and when the Hospital for the Insane was established in Clarinda he was chosen as its superintendent.

During the winter of 1856 and 1857, Dr. A. H. East, who had lived in the county three or four years, was admitted to the bar and began practicing that profession. The truth of the old adage, "Law is a jealous mistress and will not be content with divided affections," was again apparent, and his clients had more faith in him as a physician than as a legal adviser. During the Civil War he received an appointment as surgeon and upon his return, he entered the medical profession, rendering service until his death on September 19, 1872.

Dr. W. D. Van Sandt first made his home in Clarinda in 1858. He was associated with Drs. J. L. Barrett, A. H. Farrens and his brother-in-law, Dr. Albert Heald.

Dr. W. C. Stillians was a young practitioner who lived to practice only a few years.

Dr. W. H. Pittman, who arrived in Clarinda in 1886, had attended lectures at Cincinnati Medical College in 1872, University of Tennessee Medical

work. He died at an early age, lamented by all who knew him.

Dr. James G. Williams practiced in Clarinda only a short time, after which he moved to Braddyville in 1870. He had attended the Keokuk Medical College, but was graduated from the St. Louis Medical School in 1856, and practiced in Keokuk county until 1870. He became prominent politically, professionally, and financially, before his death in 1896.

Political activities were first evident at the election in 1879, when Dr. E. Eckerson was defeated for coroner. This is the first instance of a doctor being considered for this office. Dr. Lewellen had held the office during 1873, but he had been appointed. In 1893 Dr. George A. Pruitt was a candidate, but failed to receive the required number of votes. Dr. W. C. Fischer received a like reception in 1899, but in 1901 Dr. C. C. Parriott was successful. In 1903 it became a three cornered contest with Drs. C. C. Parriott, M. Enfield, and Mary Finley participating.

Records of the Clarinda Cemetery show the following doctors: Geo. Kridelbaugh, Allen Farrens, John Kridelbaugh, Albert Heald, A. H. East, J. H. Cameron, J. H. Conine, J. C. Holmes, J. L. Stillians, Sam'l H. Kridelbaugh, J. L. Barrett, Dr. Jeffrey, J. K. Rickey, H. L. Cokenower, W. L. Van Sandt, M. Enfield, S. H. Millen, P. W. Lewellen, Dr. Shaw, P. Herren, W. C. Philips, and T. E. Powers.

Clarinda's fraternity at present in 1934, consists of F. K. Burnett, E. L. W. Brown, J. F. Benning, F. H. Clark, E. T. Farrens, D. H. Killingsworth, R J. Mathews, J. W. Sellards, C. C. Parriott and W. W. West.

PHYSICIANS WHO LOCATED IN SHENANDOAH

Transferring our attentions now to the west side of the county we find that Dr. B. M. Webster was the first pioneer physician to locate in Shenandoah. He was graduated from Rush Medical College and came first to Manti, Fremont county, one of the stopping places of Mormon treking. From 1870 to 1875 he remained in Shenandoah, and then removed to Essex where he remained until 1888, combining the banking business with a medical practice.

Dr. H. P. Duffield, another Rush graduate, established himself in Shenandoah about this time.

Dr. G. J. Ross, later of Sioux City, was the next arrival. He was from the Cincinnati Eclectic School, and was associated with Dr. E. S. Whiting who was from the same school.

Dr. J. W. Humphrey came next to Shenandoah.

Dr. E. K. Bailey, who was graduated from the

Chicago Medical College in 1877, began practice at Hepburn, but soon removed to Shenandoah.

Dr. D. L. Allen came to Shenandoah in 1881 as a graduate of the Long Island Medical School. He had tuberculosis and remained only a short time when he moved to Princeton, Kansas, where he died in 1884 at the age of thirty-six years.

Dr. F. E. Stevens, a homeopathic graduate from Iowa City, came next to offer service. .

Dr. Bolton, another homeopathic physician, stayed a few months, leaving for further western fields.

Dr. Geo. L. Hester came to Shenandoah in 1884, and later removed to Glenwood, Iowa, where he is now practicing.

Dr. Wright came from Canton, Illinois, to Shenandoah in 1880. He had been in army service during the rebellion and had become a moral and physical wreck, finally ending his own life with a revolver.

Dr. R. H. Sutton next located in Shenandoah in 1888 and took the place of Dr. G. J. Ross in a partnership with Dr. E. S. Whiting. He formerly lived in Le Harpe, Illinois. He retired from practice because of ill health and died in California.

An "Indian doctor," William Crawford, who lived in Shenandoah from 1880 to 1889, had traveled much among the Indians. He had no medical standing but was fairly successful in his efforts. Contemporaries reported him as a very careless uncouth man.

Dr. Tilford L. Putman was born in Princeton, Missouri, on February 8, 1850, his parents being Green M. and Mary E. (Kelsey) Putman. The father was a native of Fulton county, Illinois, while the mother came from Greencastle, Indiana. The doctor's father and mother had died in 1897 and 1899, respectively, and are buried in the Locust Grove Cemetery near Shenandoah, Iowa. Tilford L. attended the country schools of Fremont county and the Southern Iowa Normal at Bloomfield, Iowa. For four years he taught in country schools and used his leisure hours in reading medicine as a preparation for matriculation in Rush Medical College of Chicago from which school he was graduated with honors in the class of 1885. His first location was Riverton, Iowa, in Fremont county, where he stayed for six years. He removed to Shenandoah in October, 1891. Postgraduate work was done in 1895, 1897, 1900 and 1909. He enjoyed a very extensive general and surgical practice until his death on August 26, 1926. Dr. Putman was married to Miss Jessie D. McKean on March 25, 1886, to which union one son Lynn J. was born who followed his father's footsteps and became a graduate of the medical department of the University of Maryland. The doctor was

active in many social, civic, and lodge affiliations. Through the efforts of Dr. Putman the Shenandoah City Hospital was founded as the first private or civic hospital in the county in 1905. This institution subsequently gave way to the Hand Hospital which was a beneficent gift to the community through the solicitous efforts of the doctor dealing with a long time friend and patron. He served as local surgeon to both the Wabash and Burlington railway systems for many years; and belonged to all the current active medical societies in his territory.

Dr. W. A. Parrette, a graduate from the University of New York in 1897, practiced in Greenfield, Iowa, and then at Shenandoah in 1909, and thence in various places. He gave special attention to eye, ear, nose and throat difficulties.

Dr. Charles E. Kellogg was born October 7, 1863, in Clinton county, Iowa, of parents who migrated from Massachusetts and Pennsylvania. The doctor acquired his academic education at Mt. Vernon, Iowa, and Dixon, Illinois schools. He was graduated in 1893 from the College of Physicians and Surgeons of Chicago with special honors and located at Northboro for about fifteen years before moving to Shenandoah. After several years of a lucrative practice here, he retired and moved to Santa Ana, California, where his parents had lived for some time after their retirement from active farm life.

Dr. George L. Smith was born in Rutland, Vermont, on September 19, 1852. He secured his medical education at the College of Physicians and Surgeons of Keokuk, from which institution he was graduated in 1882. Aside from his medical practice he was intensely interested in the geology of southwestern Iowa and became assistant geologist for the State University. He died in 1929.

Some of the other doctors who found Shenandoah a field of service were: F. L. Brockett, Dr. Caldwell, J. Fred Driver, C. F. Perkins, Thomas Reynolds, B. B. Sandy, Dr. Baker, Dr. Shrader, Mark L. Smith, A. C. Armitage, F. J. Van Meter, F. E. Stevens, R, P. Jensen, Dr. Teter, H. E. Marr, Dr. Hatfield, T. W. Stone (also practiced in Essex), J. B. Hamlin, J. O. Weaver, C. L. Jones (now of Gilmore City, Iowa), A. W. Parker and Lynn J. Putman (now of Elgin, Illinois).

Those who are practicing in Shenandoah in 1934 are: J. F. Aldrich, J. Edward Adamson, M. O. Brush, B. S. Barnes, H. McK. Bunch, E. J. Gottsch, J. D. Kerlin, Wayland H. Maloy, W. F. Stotler and A. O. Wirsig.

PHYSICIANS WHO LOCATED IN ESSEX

Dr. A. M. Stearns was graduated from the St. Louis Medical College in the class of 1877 and after a brief sojourn in Kansas, located in Essex in 1878 where he spent the remainder of his life, although he retired from active practice some time before his death.

Dr. E. Eckerson came from Buffalo, New York, to Essex, and practiced from 1878 to 1889, when he removed to Denver because of his health.

A popular "Dr." G. W. Wright was not a regular graduate but had a hankering for relieving suffering humanity and hung on for some time.

Dr. W. H. C. Moore took medical courses at Michigan University and Rush Medical College, graduating from the latter institution in 1867. After four years of practice elsewhere he located in Essex.

Dr. W. T. West, a graduate of the Keokuk Medical College in the class of 1884, came to Shenandoah in 1887 as pastor of the Christian Church where he labored until January, 1890, when he located in Essex for the practice of medicine.

Dr. John Emil Swanson located in Essex in 1903. He attended medical lectures at Keokuk, but was graduated from the University of Illinois School of Medicine in 1899. He succeeded Dr. W. F. Stotler when he removed to Shenandoah for practice.

Dr. J. N. Page practiced in Essex from 1873 to 1877. A homeopath by the name of Goodrich was the only one of that school to enter the community and he stayed only one year. Dr. O. M. Burhans first began practice in Essex in 1871. After his graduation from Rush Medical College in 1878, he again resumed the practice of medicine in Essex. Others who have come and gone at Essex are Drs. W. T. Stone, A. W. Parker, C. C. Parriott (now of Clarinda), W. F. Stotler (now of Shenandoah), and Dunlap T. C. Goodrich from 1875 to 1877.

The present medical needs of Essex are provided for by Drs. O. W. Okerlin and Carroll Nelson.

PHYSICIANS WHO LOCATED ELSEWHERE IN THE COUNTY

Dr. H. W. Scales was a native of Indiana and received his medical degree at the Ohio Medical College of Cincinnati in 1879. He located in Yorktown from 1882 until 1890 when he removed to Boonville, Indiana, where he practiced for fourteen years. He returned to Yorktown in 1904 and remained until his death in 1916.

Others who have practiced in Yorktown are J. F. Benning and C. C. Parriott both of whom are now in active practice in Clarinda; and Dr. S. L. Claybaugh, who later moved to Gravity, Iowa. No physician is in Yorktown at present.

Dr. William G. Johnson, a product of Mt. Vernon, Iowa, was given a medical degree at Northwestern University Medical School in 1908. He went to Uruapam, Mexico, as medical director of the National Mexico Packing House, but the climate proved detrimental to his health and he located in Coin for several years.

Dr. A. H. King was born in 1851, received his medical degree from Keokuk Medical School, and located in 1879 at Snow Hill or Coin, where he practiced until his death on March 23, 1928.

Dr. J. A. Gillispie was a graduate of Des Moines College in 1888. He practiced in Coin only a few years, before journeying further west.

Dr. S. L. Claybaugh practiced at Coin, Northboro, Yorktown, and finally at Gravity in Taylor county. F. R. Brockett, J. W. Coin, J. C. Burton, F. H. King and E. R. Monzingo have served Coin.

Dr Edward Luke has been the only physician for many years at Coin.

Northboro has been served at various times by Drs. Wm. L. Freeman, C. V. Beaver, J. Whittier, C. E. Kellogg and J. R. Thompson. There is no physician there at the present time.

Dr. J. W. Holliday came to Blanchard in 1882, but later moved to Tarkio, Missouri. Dr. G. A. Pruitt came in 1884, and the following physicians came some time during the eighties. Drs. Rogers, J. M. Livingstone, J. W. Chambers, M. Carter, Dr. Allan, R. W. Robb and A. W. Davies, who later located at College Springs. Dr. G. A. Reutter serves the town at present.

Dr. S. E. McClymonds practiced in College Springs during the prosperous years of the Amity College there. Only an osteopath remains there now, since Dr. A. W. Davies has retired.

The following have practiced at Hepburn: Drs. Case, Bailey (later of Shenandoah), Williams, Jackson, Beaver (later at Northboro), Oliver, McColm (later at New Market), Sams, Dodds and Mrs. E. J. Carlson.

Braddyville was served by Dr. A. F. Large, A. M. Sherman (now of California) and James G. Williams. Dr. R. A. Hawthorne is located there at present.

Dr. J. D. Elliott was a long time resident of Hawleyville.

Dr. J. F. Benning first practiced at Shambaugh as a graduate of the University of Nebraska in 1904, then at Yorktown and finally at Clarinda.

Dr. Richard Wallace is the only physician who made his home at Norwich, according to our records.

THE JOURNAL BOOK SHELF

BOOKS RECEIVED

THE BUSINESS MAN AND HIS HEALTH—By Jesse Feiring Williams, M.D., professor of physical education at Teachers College, Columbia University. McGraw-Hill Book Company, New York and London, 1932. Price, $2.00.

CORRECTIVE PHYSICAL EDUCATION—By Josephine Langworthy Rathbone, M.A., instructor in physical education, Teachers College, Columbia University, New York City. 292 pages with 153 illustrations. W. B. Saunders Company, Philadelphia and London, 1934. Price, $2.50.

THE DANGEROUS AGE IN MEN—A Treatise on the Prostate Gland by Chester Tilton Stone, M.D., Ridgewood, New Jersey. The Macmillan Company, New York, 1934. Price, $1.75.

A DOCTOR STUDIES CRIME—By Perry M. Lichtenstein, M.D., formerly resident physician, City Prison, Manhattan (Tombs). D. Van Nostrand Company, 250 Fourth Avenue, New York, 1934. Price, $3.00.

INDUSTRIAL TOXICOLOGY—By Alice Hamilton, M.D., Boston, Massachusetts, Harper's Medical Monographs. Harper and Brothers Publishers, 49 East 33rd Street, New York City, 1934. Price, $3.00.

THE LABORATORY NOTEBOOK METHOD IN TEACHING PHYSICAL DIAGNOSIS AND CLINICAL HISTORY RECORDING—By Logan Clendening, M.D., professor of clinical medicine, University of Kansas. C. V. Mosby Company, St. Louis, 1934. Price, fifty cents.

MEDICAL CLINICS OF NORTH AMERICA—Volume xvii, No. 6. Chicago Number, Index volume. Octavo of 266 pages with 38 illustrations. Per clinic year July, 1933, to May, 1934. W. B. Saunders Company, Philadelphia and London, 1934. Price, paper, $12.00; cloth, $16.00.

THE MERCK MANUAL OF THERAPEUTICS AND MATERIA MEDICA—Sixth edition, compiled and published by Merck and Company, Inc., Rahway, New Jersey, 1934.

A PRIMER FOR DIABETIC PATIENTS—A Brief Outline of the Treatment of Diabetes with Diet and Insulin. By Russell M. Wilder, M.D., professor of medicine, The Mayo Foundation. Fifth edition, reset and revised, 172 pages. W. B. Saunders Company, Philadelphia and London, 1934. Price, $1.75.

POSTURES AND PRACTICES DURING LABOR AMONG PRIMITIVE PEOPLES—By Julius Jarcho, M.D., New York City. With 130 illustrations. Paul B. Hoeber, Inc., New York, 1934. Price, $3.50.

THE SPASTIC CHILD—A Record of Successfully Achieved Muscle Control in Little's Disease—By Marguerite K. Fischel. C. V. Mosby Company, St. Louis, Missouri, 1934. Price, $1.50.

SURGICAL CLINICS OF NORTH AMERICA—Volume xiv, No. 1. Philadelphia Number, February, 1934. Per clinic year February, 1934, to December, 1934. Octavo of 226 pages with 62 illustrations. W. B. Saunders Company, Philadelphia and London, 1934. Price, paper, $12.00; cloth, $16.00.

THAT HEART OF YOURS—By S. Calvin Smith, M.D., Sc.D. Illustrated. J. B. Lippincott Company, Philadelphia, London and Montreal, 1934. Price, $2.00.

TROUBLES WE DON'T TALK ABOUT—By J. F. Montague, M.D., F.A.C.S., New York Intestinal Sanitarium, 139 East 36th Street, New York City. Second edition, revised and enlarged; illustrated. J. B. Lippincott Company, Philadelphia and London, 1933. Price, $1.00.

BOOK REVIEWS

ALCOHOL, ITS EFFECTS ON MAN

By Haven Emerson, M.D., professor of public health practice, Columbia University. D. Appleton-Century Company, New York and London, 1934. Price, $1.00.

This small volume has been prepared by a well known authority, and is based upon a large volume of clinical and statistical material which has been analyzed by Dr. Emerson and other scientists who have contributed to the factual evidence reported in this volume. The volume is the outgrowth of a larger and more comprehensive volume published in 1932 by this author, entitled "Alcohol and Man."

Since forty-six states now require the teaching of the effects of alcohol and other narcotics on the human system in all schools, supported wholly or in part by public funds, the author has attempted in this volume to present the essentials of the subject in such a form as to make them fully appreciated both by the teachers and the students in our schools.

While the volume fully answers all of the usual questions concerning the effects of alcohol upon the human body, it does so without creating the impression that the author is a propagandist either for or against the beverage use of alcohol. Because of its authoritativeness, its lack of bias, and its soundness from a scientific viewpoint, the volume may well be recommended not only to the medical profession and to the teachers in our public schools for whom it was written, but also to that great mass—the public— who are now eager for scientific information on this subject.

MEDICAL CLINICS OF NORTH AMERICA

Volume xvii, No. 5, New York Number, March, 1934. Per clinic year, July, 1933, to May, 1934. Octavo of 324 pages with 32 illustrations. W. B. Saunders Company, Philadelphia and London, 1934. Price, paper, $12.00; cloth, $16.00.

The opening paper in this number is by Harlow Brooks and reports a clinic in which he showed three cardiac cases. One was a case of heart block; another a case of myocardial failure and the third, a case of hypertensive disease. The presentation of these cases and the discussion is in the usual lucid manner of this clinician.

There is a group of three papers by workers in the Rockefeller Institute on various phases of kidney disease which put forth the latest information from research laboratories in the investigation of this disease.

Held and Goldbloom offer a paper on perforated peptic ulcer in which they discuss their subject rather exhaustively, including differential diagnoses. However, they fail to mention scarcely any pitfall into which one might drop in the diagnosis of this particular emergency.

The tannic acid treatment of extensive burns is well represented by Dr. Stanley-Brown, who reports a series of fifty-five cases observed in the Fifth Avenue Hospital with only six deaths, all of these being children under the age of five years. The remaining articles which appear in the volume are of interest.—F. R. H.

of ergot, marketed without adequate declaration of the composition and without adequate standardization under a nondescriptive proprietary name with unwarranted therapeutic claims; the report on diampysal, another pyridine derivative proposed for use in bacterial infections, convincing evidence for the therapeutic value of which is lacking; the report on euphydigital, an irrational mixture of digitalis and a theophylline preparation marketed under an uninforming, proprietary name, with exaggerated and unwarranted claims for its therapeutic value; the report on guphen, stated to be the guaiacol ester of phenylcinchoninic acid, marketed with unwarranted therapeutic claims under an uninforming, proprietary name and having no proved advantage over its constituents administered separately; the report on niazo, a pyridine compound of unsubstantiated value as a urinary antiseptic; the report on omnadin, a preparation recognized for use for nonspecific lipoprotein therapy practically as a cure-all; and the report on a group of endocrine preparations of the Rovin Laboratories variously unacceptable as being of indefinite composition and of undemonstrated therapeutic value.

In view of answers to a questionnaire, the Council reaffirmed its previous decision concerning the limitations of intravenous use of barbital compounds; namely, that these preparations should be administered intravenously only in a limited number of conditions in which administration by other routes is not feasible. The report carefully details these conditions.

MEDICINE, A VOYAGE OF DISCOVERY

By Josef Lobel, M.D. Translated from the German. Farrar & Rinehart, Inc., New York, 1934. Price, $3.00.

This volume has been prepared for the layman, but since it is so rich in philosophy, so accurate in factual discussion, and so humanly interesting and delightfully readable, it will appeal to every physician. The subtitle of the book is especially descriptive of its content.

Beginning with a discussion of medicine, its aims and purposes, its accomplishments and triumphs, the author proceeds to discuss those various elements which enter into its composite, rightly considering biology as a necessary background for the study of medicine. The various concepts of biology are discussed, and those advances and discoveries distinctly of service in the development of medical science are particularly stressed.

In his discussion of anatomy he presents a panoramic view of the development of anatomy, introducing such instances as that of Burke and Hare, who supplied the great Professor Knox with anatomic specimens.

In his chapter devoted to physiology he recounts in a fascinating fashion the work of Beaumont and his observations through the peep-hole in the stomach of Alexis St. Martin. In the same interesting fashion he reviews pathology, pharmacology, bacteriology, neurology, surgery and endocrinology. His closing chapter, entitled "Medicine," recapitulates and inter-relates the various truths developed in the earlier chapters.

Of his closing sentences the following are quotable. "True medicine is still in the cradle. But was not Hercules still in his cradle when he strangled the serpent? Medicine, too, has given the quietus to more than one serpent."

MAN INTO WOMAN

An Authentic Record of a Change of Sex. Edited by Niels Hoyer, translated from the German by H. J. Stenning, with an intro-duction by Norman Haire, Ch.M., M.D., with eighteen illustrations. E. P. Dutton & Company, 286 Fourth Avenue, New York City, 1933.

This book recounts the story of the miraculous transformation of the Danish painter, Einar Weg-ener, from an individual having all male attributes into one possessing female attributes. Incredible though the story seems, the transformation is sup-ported as a fact by documentary evidence from Pro-fessor Warnekros of Dresden.

At twenty years of age this individual married and carried on the functions of a husband, psycho-logically and physically. Diagnosed later as a neu-rotic or a homosexual individual, he began to have the emotional reactions and the psychic personality of a female. This change in personality took on such importance that he finally undertook a series of operations designed to remove male sex characteris-tics and replace them with female organs. The last operation performed upon this individual was de-signed to create the external genitals of a female and aid the individual, who had now been supplied with the female organs of generation, to become a mother. Death from heart disease terminated the experiment.

Physicians interested in the psychology of sex will be interested in the confessions of this individual. Any reader would be interested in the story as a thrilling narrative.

MODERN CLINICAL SYPHILOLOGY

By John H. Stokes, M.D., Duhring Pro-fessor of Dermatology and Syphilology, Uni-versity of Pennsylvania. Second edition, revised and entirely reset; 1,400 pages with 973 illustrations and text figures. W. B. Saunders Company, Philadelphia and Lon-don, 1934. Price, $12.00.

The first edition of this excellent work appeared in 1926 and immediately assumed a position of pre-eminence in this particular field.

This new edition, which is largely rewritten and expanded, assumes almost encyclopedic proportions and is without doubt second to no other volume on this subject in the English language. The author has faithfully adhered to his avowed purpose in pre-paring this volume on syphilology, providing a work for the uninitiated student and practitioner, a refer-ence work for the expert and near-expert, and finally to provide a reference work for all physicians and research workers interested in this branch of medicine. The present text discusses all of the newer advances in the treatment of syphilis with a comparative appraisal of the various arsphenamines, together with sections on acetarsone and tryparsa-mide. In the field of cardiovascular syphilis, the striking advances which have been made in treat-ment during the past few years are carefully and critically reviewed by the author.

It would appear to the reviewer that every physi-cian would demand access to this volume, since the author has so constructed the work that the physician may obtain either a thumb-nail epitomization or a most minute and detailed account of any particular phase of the subject desired. Bibliographic citations appear superfluous inasmuch as the author has so thoroughly and competently sifted the material gleaned from the world's literature and presents in the text the worthwhile and lasting developments. An extensive and carefully prepared cross index provides easy and immediate access to the material required.

I KNOW JUST THE THING FOR THAT

By J. F. Montague, M.D., Medical Direc-tor, New York Intestinal Sanitarium. The John Day Company, New York, 1934. Price, $2.00.

This volume written for the laity has been pre-pared by a well recognized authority in gastro-enterology. The author discusses various ailments of the alimentary tract, stressing particularly certain popular conceptions and misconceptions regarding functional and organic disorders of this system.

If he has erred in this book, it is the reviewer's opinion that the error has been committed in in-cluding too much, an error of commission rather than omission. In our opinion a more detailed discussion of fewer subjects would prove more useful to the average layman who requires a general survey of his subject. At any rate, those patients suffering from functional disorders may be saved many dollars and hours of anxiety by reading this discussion of various symptoms resulting from deranged functions of the digestive system. The author discusses things to do and things not to do, stressing always the value of consulting one's personal physician, as a background for all treatments.

A healthy and often subtle current of humor ex-tends throughout Dr. Montague's writings, making them pleasant reading, as well as informative study.

The JOURNAL

of the

Iowa State Medical Society

VOL. XXIV   DES MOINES, IOWA, SEPTEMBER, 1934   No. 9

SURGICAL CLINICS*

FIRST DAY

THE APPLICABILITY OF CERTAIN SURGICAL PROCEDURES FOR RECURRENT PEPTIC ULCER

VERNE C. HUNT, M.D., Los Angeles, California

The inability of the internist to procure relief of symptoms in all cases of duodenal and gastric ulcer by adequate medical management, and the relatively high incidence of one or more of the complications of hemorrhage, pyloric obstruction and perforation, require the institution of surgical treatment in many of these cases.

The complication of acute perforation of ulcer is recognized by all as an absolute indication for surgical intervention. High grade pyloric obstruction incident to chronicity and cicatricial pyloric stenosis, is too often procrastinated with by enthusiastic exponents of medical management. It is not my purpose to dwell particularly upon the indications for surgical treatment of duodenal and gastric ulcer, except to emphasize certain considerations which may be termed relative indications. The complication of repeated hemorrhage from ulceration in the duodenum or stomach is one which occasions much concern and question regarding surgical intervention. Hemorrhage from such lesions occurs sufficiently often to merit well planned methods of procedure. The slowly developing anemia from continued loss of blood over a period of weeks usually provides no great emergency, but the large, massive shock producing hemorrhage at times provides a situation as acute as perforation. It has been stated frequently that acute, massive hemorrhage is rarely fatal and that the effects of such loss of blood may be readily compensated by transfusion. Allen and Benedict have recently reviewed the subject of hemorrhage in 1804 cases of duodenal ulcer treated at the Massachusetts General Hospital. There was a history

* Presented before the Eighty-third Annual Session, Iowa State Medical Society, Des Moines, May 9, 10, 11, 1934.

of gross bleeding, or where bleeding occurred in amounts recognizable macroscopically, in 34 per cent of the cases. Acute massive hemorrhage to produce prostration and shock occurred in 138 cases, or 22 per cent of those in which bleeding was observed. The hemorrhage was fatal in twelve cases without operative interference, and eight others were operated upon without success. The mortality rate in the cases of massive hemmorhage was 14.5 per cent. Most of us have observed massive fatal hemorrhage from gastric or duodenal ulcer, and have had brought to our minds the question, how often and how much shall a patient bleed before surgical intervention is instituted? To my mind, repeated small hemorrhages are often enough, and one or more massive hemorrhages is too much. Either type of hemorrhage is a sufficient and just indication for direct surgical attack upon the known or suspected bleeding lesion, after sufficient rehabilitation of the patient to insure relative safety for a surgical procedure.

In the absence of complications requiring more or less urgent surgical treatment there is a relatively large group of ulcers where definite chronicity over a period of years has been established, and in which the medical management may not have been particularly successful, by virtue of impossible or incomplete cooperation of the patient, or other influences over which the physician may have little control. This group comprises those cases in which surgical treatment may or may not be instituted, dependent upon many factors, among which the degree of disability is perhaps the most important. The attendant risk of surgical procedures and the surgical skill available to the patient are factors that must be reckoned with, for the mortality rate of medical treatment of benign, uncomplicated ulcers is nil. It is well known that the mortality rate of conservative surgical procedures for uncomplicated duodenal and gastric ulcer is likewise extremely low in the hands of the experienced, skillful surgeon. Then too, the problem of postoperative recurrence is one which must receive due consideration. These general principles are applicable whether the lesion is on the duodenal or gastric side of the pylorus. The relationship of gastric carcinoma to gastric ulcer provides perhaps greater urgency for surgical treatment in cases of gastric ulcer than in duodenal ulcer, in the absence of perforation, hemorrhage or gastric retention. I do not wish to open for discussion the question of gastric carcinoma developing upon an old gastric ulcer, except to state that there is some apparent recent concurrence of opinion that such degeneration occurs in a small percentage of cases. Newcomb, working in the Department of Pathology of St. Mary's Hospital in London has reported an incidence of nearly four per cent malignant degeneration in gastric ulcer. Gömöri, of Budapest, stated recently that cancer secondary to gastric ulcer is not the rarity it is believed to be. In 64 cases of chronic peptic ulcer and 26 cases of carcinoma of the stomach carefully studied by him, six cancers were secondary to ulcer, an incidence of 6.6 per cent. Whether gastric carcinoma is always a malignant lesion from its inception or whether it may have developed on an old gastric ulcer is a question of much scientific interest. Of greater importance in the relationship of ulcer to carcinoma is the clinical differential diagnosis. The differentiation between a benign gastric ulcer and an early gastric carcinoma, as determined by competent roentgenologic examination, is not always easy nor entirely accurate. There are many lesions of the stomach, as determined by roentgenologic examination, in which only an exploration and microscopic study of the lesion will determine the accurate diagnosis. The therapeutic test, advocated by Lahey and others, possesses considerable merit when such observation is conducted by competent observers. However, its adoption has too frequently allowed an operable lesion to become inoperable during the period of such observation, largely through failure to adhere strictly to the principles of the therapeutic test.

So far as the relative indications for surgical procedures in uncomplicated duodenal and gastric ulcer are concerned, they present no particular difficulties to the internist and surgeon when each is familiar with the excellent results that may be obtained in many cases by adequate medical management, and the large percentage of cures that occur following the institution of surgical procedures. When each is cognizant of the deficiencies under certain circumstances of his own and the others' procedures of management, the interests of the patient are most likely to be best served. To quote Eusterman, "Neither the physician nor the surgeon should entertain any conceit concerning the virtues of his particular mode of treatment under all cir-

cumstances. The former should be mindful of the invariably permanent effectiveness of timely operative interference in the case of acutely perforated ulcer, of advanced cicatricial stenosis, of chronic penetrating, calloused, resistant lesion, or of chronic hemorrhagic lesions, when his own efforts may have proven unsuccessful, even in less formidable cases. On the other hand the surgeon must be mindful of reactivation, or recurrences in more vulnerable situations, which, although proportionately few when the patient is in competent hands, may frequently have far more serious import than the lesion for which the operation was originally done."

Recurrent Ulcer

The most common types of recurrence following surgical procedures for ulcer are those occurring subsequent to gastro-enterostomy. Such recurrences have developed usually in the suture line of the anastomosis as gastrojejunal or marginal ulcer, or in immediate proximity to the stoma either in the stomach or jejunum. In my experience gastrojejunal or marginal ulcers have accounted for 76 per cent of the recurrences; jejunal ulcer has accounted for fifteen per cent, gastric ulcer for six per cent, and the remainder have been miscellaneous recurrences or reactivation of the original lesion. The precise incidence of such recurrences is not easily determined. In published reports it has varied from 3.5 per cent (Wilke) to 34 per cent (Lewisohn). It is obvious that the incidence is higher among the Semitic and Teutonic races than among the Anglo-Saxons. It is probable that the true incidence of recurrence following gastro-enterostomy, when this procedure has been judiciously applied, is not more than five per cent. The relatively high incidence of recurrence in the experience of certain surgeons has, in my opinion, served as an unjust indictment of an operation which, when skillfully applied in carefully selected cases, has achieved results within a mortality rate unsurpassed by any subsequently designed operative procedure. It was in the cases of old, chronic, stenosing lesions about the pylorus with obstruction, that the operation of gastro-enterostomy in its earliest development achieved the results upon which its reputation was made. Departure from the more or less strict indications for surgical treatment of ulcer has broadened the applicability of the operation of gastro-enterostomy not only to many uncomplicated ulcers in patients who have not had the opportunity of adequate medical management, but also to patients in whom hyperchlorhydria, with its associated symptoms in the absence of intrinsic organic disease of the stomach or duodenum, became the occasion for gastro-

investigation, that in the dog the pyloric mucosa apparently plays only a minor part, if any, in gastric acidity. More recently Shapiro and Berg have shown in the experimental animal that, even following double vagotomy and subtotal gastrectomy, which is considered the most radical procedure to alter the different phases of gastric secretion, only a temporary diminution in acidity occurred. Subsequently the secretion of acid returned to its original preoperative level, with variation in the rate of recovery of normal gastric secretion. They concluded that there is no experimental proof or convincing clinical evidence to support the hypothesis that subtotal gastrectomy, even combined with vagotomy, is the operation of choice for the surgical cure of peptic ulcer in man on the basis that it provides for a permanent lowering in the secretion of hydrochloric acid and thus prevents the development of recurrences and jejunal ulcers.

On the other hand Steinberg, Brougher and Vidgoff have demonstrated that after the antrum is removed, the free acidity of the contents of the stomach is considerably reduced, or is entirely absent. Steinberg has furthermore stated that the biggest factor in the reduction of acidity is the neutralization of the contents of the stomach by the influx of alkaline contents of the duodenum or jejunum, and the rapid emptying of the stomach.

Various types of operations for duodenal and gastric ulcer have been devised, with or without excision of the lesion, either to neutralize gastric acidity by relatively conservative procedures, or by more radical procedures to modify gastric secretion by partial gastrectomy, thereby eliminating a large portion of acid producing mucosa as well as removing the so-called hormone-elaborating portion of the stomach. We know that some of the various surgical procedures in the treatment of ulcer are followed by excellent results and few recurrences. Even so, no surgical procedure has yet been devised which provides complete assurance against reactivation or recurrence of ulcer.

Surgical Procedures

A predisposition to recurrence exists in some individuals, and recurrences have repeatedly developed in the same individual irrespective of the surgical procedure. Fortunately the incidence of predisposition to repeated recurrence is extremely small. Such predisposition may seldom be recognized preoperatively. However, sufficient clinical evidence is at hand to serve as a guide to the future applicability of the certain surgical procedures for duodenal or gastric ulcer. Prevention of recurrences is possible through proper selection of patients, through rather strict adherence to surgical indications for surgical treatment of duodenal and gastric ulcer, and through utilization of such a surgical procedure which under the circumstances is best suited. Few have subscribed to the radical operation of partial gastrectomy as the one of choice in the treatment of duodenal or gastric ulcer; first, because of its relatively high mortality rate as compared to the conservative procedures and secondly, because little if any greater assurance against recurrence is provided. It is not to be inferred that radical partial gastrectomy may not be utilized to advantage in certain gastric ulcers. In my experience partial gastrectomy, with restoration of gastrojejunal continuity by a posterior Polya or Billroth No. II procedure, has been used in fifteen per cent of gastric ulcers. That such radical procedure is applicable to duodenal ulcer is most questionable. The semi-radical exclusion operation, with the various modifications, principally by Finsterer and Devine, of the original Von Eiselsberg operation, has a definite but small field of applicability, not as a procedure of choice at any time, but as one of necessity in dealing with perhaps the one combination of circumstances, namely, an inaccessible, bleeding duodenal ulcer. Objection to the various exclusion operations has arisen because of the relatively high incidence of recurrence, which has occurred particularly when part of the pars pylorica has been excluded with the duodenum. No single surgical procedure, whether conservative or radical, with or without excision of the lesion, is suitable to all cases. When either neutralization or reduction of gastric acidity or both, with or without excision of the lesion, and an adequate anastomotic stoma are accomplished, the purposes of surgery are achieved, and the incidence of recurrence is very low. So far as the anastomotic stoma is concerned, it should be of such size and situation to provide more rapid emptying of the stomach than existed preoperatively. It is my opinion that any surgical procedure which does not hasten the food from the stomach by virtue of too small a stoma, or is followed by mechanical dysfunction with duodenal or jejunal stasis, provides a situation highly predisposing to recurrence.

Postoperative reactivation and recurrences are particularly resistant to medical treatment and are often subject to formidable complications of hemorrhage or perforation. A positive diagnosis of gastrojejunal or jejunal ulcer usually justifies early surgical intervention. Recurrences following the direct surgical procedures for duodenal ulcer, in which some type of pyloroplasty has been done, present no great problem when secondary operations are necessary. Usually they may be surgically approached as an original lesion utilizing the most suitable and appropriate procedure. It is the

recurrences that follow gastro-enterostomy, partial gastrectomy and the exclusion operations which often tax the ingenuity of the surgeon. In general it may be stated that conservative surgical procedures have much to commend them as secondary operations over more radical methods. To be specific, to increase the height of the gastric resection, when an anastomotic ulcer has developed following partial gastrectomy, has not always reduced the existing predisposition to recurrence and has made each succeeding operation more formidable. To increase the height of gastric resection when a gastrojejunal ulcer has developed is at times not only the procedure of choice, but the only available method. Balfour has called attention to the advantages of restoration of the gastroduodenal continuity when such an anastomotic lesion has followed partial gastrectomy.

Ulcer developing in or about the stoma following gastro-enterostomy usually requires excision of the recurrent ulcer and disconnection of the gastro-enterostomy. For a period of years partial gastrectomy was widely used and still possesses usefulness in certain ulcers in or about a gastro-enterostomy, particularly in those cases in which the duodenum is inaccessible or is entirely unsuitable for any type of pyloroplasty. However, in cases in which the gastro-enterostomy has served its purpose with resultant healing of the primary lesion, and the duodenum is accessible and suitable for some type of pyloroplasty, the conservative operation of excision of the gastrojejunal or jejunal ulcer, disconnection of the gastro-enterostomy, and some type of plyoroplasty including removal of the major portion of the pyloric sphincter, has been productive of most gratifying results. Extensive involvement of the jejunum by gastrojejunal or jejunal ulcer such as to require its partial resection is rarely encountered.

Perforation of gastrojejunal or jejunal ulcer is usually a protective perforation to mesentery or transverse mesocolon. Perforation onto the transverse colon usually results in gastrojejuno-colic fistula, fortunately an infrequent occurrence. Wilke has recently stated that the mortality rate of the one stage surgical procedures for such complicated lesions is 40 per cent, and has advocated a two stage operation. As a rule, the condition of the patient should determine the method of procedure. The gastrocolic fistula provides a seriously contaminated stomach which should preclude all but the most conservative procedures. In a recent case of a bleeding gastrojejunal ulcer with a large gastrojejuno-colic fistula, excision of the ulcer, closure of colon, disconnection of gastro-enterostomy and pyloroplasty was accomplished as a one stage operation with no undue postoperative reaction or complication, and the patient gained thirty-seven pounds in the eight weeks following operation.

It should be emphasized that the diagnosis of gastrojejunal or jejunal ulcer justifies early surgical intervention. The advent of complications, hemorrhage, perforation and gastrojejuno-colic fistula, increase the technical difficulties and risk of operation. The patient in whom postoperative reactivation or recurrence of ulcer has occurred has thereby exhibited a predisposition to recurrence. The prospects of cure following secondary operations for such recurrences may be greatly enhanced by cooperative medical management and elimination of predisposing factors.

727 West Seventh Street.

REFERENCES

1. Balfour, D. C.: Reconstructive operations for jejunal ulcer. Ann. Surg. xciv:489-492 (October), 1931.
2. Eusterman, G. B.: Practical reflexion on certain gastroenterologic problems and trends. Jour. Am. Med. Assn., xcix: 791-795 (September 3), 1932.
3. Gömöri, G.: Carcinoma arising from chronic gastric ulcer. Surg., Gynec. and Obst., lvii:439-450 (October), 1933.
4. Priestley, James T., and Mann, Frank C.: Gastric acidity with special reference to the pars pylorica and pyloric mucosa. Arch. Surg., xxv:395-403 (August), 1932.
5. Newcomb, W. D.: The relationship between peptic ulceration and gastric carcinoma. Brit. Jour. Surg., xx :279-308 (October), 1932.
6. Shapiro, Philip F., and Berg, Benjamin N.: Return of gastric acidity after subtotal gastrectomy and double vagotomy. Arch. Surg., xxviii:160-179 (January), 1934.
7. Steinberg, M. E.: Exclusion operation for duodenal ulcer. Amer. Jour. Surg., xxiii:137-147 (January), 1934.
8. Steinberg, M. E., Brougher, J. C., and Vidgoff, I. J.: Changes in chemistry of the contents of the stomach following gastric operations. Arch. Surg., xv:749-761 (November), 1927.
9. Wilke, D. P. D.: Jejunal ulcer. Ann. Surg., xcix:401-409 (March), 1934.

SECOND DAY

THE COMMON DUCT IN RELATION TO SURGICAL CONDITIONS OF THE BILIARY TRACT

The common duct has assumed increasing importance in the surgery of the biliary tract during recent years. Before one may clinically suspect involvement of the common or hepatic ducts in disease of a part or all of the biliary tract the symptom of jaundice must have occurred previously, or be present at the time. It is noteworthy, however, that intrinsic pathology in the ducts may exist without jaundice, and furthermore, that not all instances of jaundice indicate obstruction in the common or hepatic ducts. Lahey has recently stated that in 37 per cent of the patients in whom he had removed stones from the common or hepactic ducts, no jaundice was present either at the time of operation or at any time in the past history. Judd and Marshall, following the study of a large series of cases in which stones had been removed from the common duct, noted that there was an absence of jaundice previously or at the time of operation in 26.5 per cent of the cases. Likewise, malignant disease of the biliary tract does not produce jaundice until it has progressed sufficiently to produce obstruction. So called catarrhal jaundice and hemolytic icterus should not by virtue of the presence of jaundice be confused with intrinsic disease of the biliary tract.

Inasmuch as jaundice directs attention to the common duct the clinical diagnosis of common duct involvement is dependent upon whether the jaundice is obstructive or non-obstructive. To differentiate between these two types of jaundice, it is most important to determine, by use of the duodenal tube, the absence or presence of bile in the duodenum, and the amount and nature of the bile. The most frequent cause of obstructive jaundice is the presence of one or more stones in the common or hepatic ducts, in which case the diagnosis is usually suggested by the history of repeated typical biliary colic. The next most frequent cause of jaundice is cholecystitis with stones, with extrinsic pressure of a large stone impacted in the neck of the gallbladder producing obstruction to the free passage of bile through the common duct to the duodenum. When present, the distended palpable gallbladder suggests the diagnosis of carcinoma of the head of the pancreas producing jaundice, accompanied or unaccompanied by pain. The diagnosis of primary carcinoma of the extrahepatic ducts or of the gallbladder is usually not made until an exploratory operation is performed, or at necropsy. Stricture of the common duct has occurred with increasing frequency with settlement of the old controversy of cholecystostomy versus cholecystectomy in favor of cholecystectomy.

So far as the various tests are concerned, particularly the icteric index and the van den Bergh test, their usefulness is somewhat limited, and they may be employed only as aids in making a clinical diagnosis of the type of jaundice, and in deciding what to do about it. They are chiefly of interest as a matter of record of the trend of jaundice and are not reliable as the sole means of differentiating between obstructive and non-obstructive jaundice. The differential diagnosis of the various causes of obstructive jaundice at times becomes a most complex problem, and there is an element of error in the clinical diagnosis, which in the past has apparently not been entirely avoidable, as proved at operation or necropsy. Experience has proved that in the absence of contraindications, and after sufficient rehabilitation of the patient, particularly directed to restoration of the glycogen reserve in the liver and reduction of coagulation time of the blood and of the bleeding time to within normal limits, practically all cases of obstructive jaundice should be explored surgically.

The operability of malignant disease of the biliary tract and carcinoma of the head of the pancreas is extremely low, although palliative operations for relief of the obstructive jaundice at times may be instituted with temporary benefit. Common duct stones, postoperative strictures of the common duct, and perhaps those cases of jaundice due to chronic pancreatitis are highly amenable to surgical procedures, and it is to these conditions that I wish to confine the discussion.

Common and Hepatic Duct Stones

Calculous disease of the biliary tract is a condition frequently encountered. When confined to the gallbladder the operation of cholecystectomy may usually be accomplished within a low mortality rate and with gratifying results. However, when the bile ducts become involved, usually as the result of the passage of stones from the gallbladder into the ducts or the formation of stones within the ducts in the presence of cholangitis, the problem becomes more complex insofar as the effects of common duct obstruction and the technical difficulties of surgical procedures are concerned.

Stones in the extrahepatic ducts seldom occur in the absence of primary calculous disease of the gallbladder. When stones are present in the ducts and absent in the gallbladder, the gallbladder usually has contracted down and extruded its stones through the cystic duct into the common duct, or the stones have passed into the intestinal tract by way of a cholecyst-duodenal fistula. Such cholecyst-duodenal fistulae are not infrequently encountered. Some years ago I reported a case in which such fistulous communication existed between the gallbladder and a large duodenal diverticulum in which many gall stones were densely impacted. Not a few instances of intestinal obstruction have occurred following the extrusion of a large stone through a cholecyst-duodenal fistula into the intestinal tract. Unquestionably a coëxisting or postoperative cholangitis with partial obstruction to adequate bile drainage from the common duct into the duodenum predisposes to intraductal calculous formation. Such formation is not infrequently encountered coincident with postoperative stricture of the duct.

The incidence of common and hepatic duct stones is most variable. In recent years we have properly been led to believe that the incidence is greater with increased diligence in the search for stones and the recognition of preoperative suggestions of their presence. Some time ago, in a review of a series of cases of gall stone disease that I had operated upon, it was noted that the common duct had been opened in 13 per cent of the cases. Exploratory choledochostomy was productive of stones in a little more than half of these, or 7.3 per cent of the series. Judd, in 1931, stated that stones were removed from the common or hepatic ducts in 13.2 per cent of a large series of cases of gall stone disease. Lahey recently reported that in his experience there had been an increase in the number and incidence of common duct stones from eight per cent previous to 1926, to 21 per cent in 1932. That diligence in the search for stones and the recognition of indications for choledochostomy are important is attested through opening the common duct in 48 per cent of Lahey's recent series of cases productive of the high percentage of stones in the common duct, whereas the common duct was incised and explored in only fifteen per cent of the cases productive of the lowest incidence of common duct stones. Crump demonstrated in 1,000 consecutive autopsies on subjects between eleven and ninety-four years of age that gall stones were found in 325 cases, and that stones were found in the ducts in seventy-eight, or 24 per cent of the cases having stones. These figures have been quoted in the literature and are misleading as to the incidence of stones in the common and hepatic ducts, for Crump has included those cases in which stones were impacted in the cystic duct. From a review of the published tables in Crump's original article the true incidence of stones confined to the common and hepatic ducts cannot be determined. It is of interest to note, however, that in more than fourteen per cent of the cases having gall stones, there were associated stones at the ampulla of Vater.

Multiplicity of stones in the common and hepatic ducts may account for their incomplete removal, with postoperative recurrence of biliary colic and jaundice. Migratory stones, particularly when there have been recurrent attacks of obstructive jaundice over a period of years with subsequent huge dilatation of the hepatic and intrahepatic ducts, into which stones can recede, may elude all attempts at removal. Stones high in the hepatic or intrahepatic ducts may readily escape detection by the use of the ordinary scoops and instruments designed for the removal of stones. The wax tipped bougie possesses little value as a detector of stones.

My purpose in discussing the subject of common and hepatic duct stones is to direct particular attention to the suction method alluded to by Lahey, which greatly facilitates the removal of stones impacted at the ampulla and those that are high and inaccessible by virtue of intrahepatic dilatation of ducts. I have had made, from more or less pliable metal, a series of tubes of various sizes with straight and bell shaped ends (Figure 1), that may be attached to the suction apparatus and inserted into an exploratory incision of the common duct. The suction method has served on a number of occasions to remove stones impacted at the ampulla which otherwise could have been removed only after considerable trauma or by transduodenal incision. The migratory stone receding high in dilated hepatic ducts, which so frequently eludes the scoop, may be readily removed by suction. On a

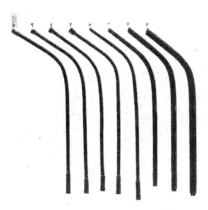

Fig. 1. Series of metal suction tubes, varying from six to nine millimeters in diameter.

number of occasions when I was certain that all stones had been removed by the scoop the suction method has been productive of one or more stones. Likewise, on several occasions recently, incision of the common duct and exploration by scoops has been unproductive of stones only to have one or more appear upon introduction of the suction tube.

The increasing frequency with which stones have been found to exist in the common or hepatic ducts justifies exploration of the common duct by incision, not only in those cases where stones may be palpated in the common or hepatic duct, but also in those cases where one or more small stones are impacted in the cystic duct to its junction with the hepatic duct, in all cases with an antecedent history of jaundice or in which jaundice is present at the time of operation, and in all those cases in which undue dilatation of the common duct is observed.

Stricture of the Common Duct

While stricture of the hepatic or common ducts may develop as the result of inflammatory processes within or without the ducts in the absence of any previous operation upon the biliary tract, the vast majority result from direct surgical injury in the performance of the operation of cholecystomy. The anomalies of the cystic, hepatic and common ducts, as well as those of the hepatic and cystic arteries, are well known.

The operation of cholecystectomy invokes the fundamental principle of accurate visualization of the cystic, common and hepatic ducts before dividing any ductal structures. This may be ideally accomplished in most cases by performing cholecystectomy from below upward. Elevating the neck of the gallbladder provides exposure and facilitates such dissection as is necessary to visualize all ductal structures. In recent years there has been a growing tendency to operate upon cases of acute cholecystitis early, before subsidence of the acute inflammatory process. It is in such cases that difficulty may be encountered in providing adequate exposure of the ducts, by attempting removal of the gallbladder in the usual way. Also in the obese individual with a deep seated gallbladder and with the liver situated high under the costal margin, such attempt at exposure may be entirely inadequate. In such cases and in those of acute cholecystitis, removal of the gallbladder from above downward favors elevation of the gallbladder away from the liver and out of the wound, and facilitates exposure and visualization of the ducts.

Immediate recognition of injury, either complete division or excision of a segment of common or hepatic duct, provides opportunity for immediate anastomosis or plastic repair, which as a primary procedure greatly enhances the prospects of a satisfactory end result. Primary repair has not always obviated postoperative stricture formation with resultant partial, intermittent or complete obstruction and jaundice. Unrecognized surgical injury with retraction of the distal and proximal segments of the common duct, when it has been divided, or the subsequent complete cicatrical occlusion of the duct following surgical injury with the resultant prolonged jaundice, biliary cirrhosis and hepatic functional insufficiency constitutes a situation to be dealt with by secondary surgical procedures. During the course of secondary operations for such strictures or segmental deficiencies of the duct it is seldom possible to restore the continuity of the duct by end to end anastomosis. The multiple stage operation, establishing in the first stage an external biliary fistula, possesses merit chiefly in decompressing a liver in which bile retention has been present over a long period of time, affording recovery of hepatic function to the degree that the liver may possess. However, subsequent implantation into the duodenum of the external biliary fistulous tract has not been followed by many satisfactory results, but rather by recurrent jaundice and the necessity for subsequent operation. Good results have not been obtained in all cases following any type of anastomotic or reconstructive procedure, but operations designed for some type of anastomosis between the proximal hepatic duct and the duodenum have proved most gratifying in their end results. Hepatic and renal insufficiency contribute largely to a conservative mortality rate of about fifteen per cent for such secondary operations for stricture and traumatic ductal deficiencies. Hepaticoduodenal anastomosis is best accomplished over a tube so fashioned as to become anchored in the hepatic duct and extending into the duodenum as a permanent or semi-permanent structure to maintain patency and obviate stricture formation at the site of anastomosis. I have never known just how long such tubes have remained in place. Unquestionably some remain permanently and others pass on through the intestinal tract within relatively short periods of time. Recently, I saw a necropsy specimen in which such a tube had remained in place for eight years. In but one of my personal cases has it been possible to learn the length of time that the tube remained.

The patient, a female, thirty-nine years of age, had had a cholecystectomy elsewhere for cholecystitis without stones on July 8, 1930. According to the history, a postoperative biliary fistula per-

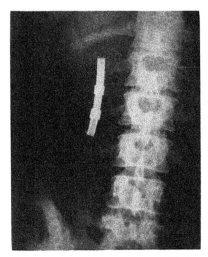

Fig. 2. Tube in stoma of hepaticoduodenostomy, immediately after operation.

sisted for weeks with subsequent closure, and the development of jaundice some months later. Upon admission to St. Vincent's Hospital March 30, 1931, the patient was deeply jaundiced and the liver edge was palpable at the level of the umbilicus

or about twelve centimeters below the right costal margin. The coagulation time of the blood and the bleeding time were not unduly prolonged. A diagnosis of postoperative stricture of the common duct was made, and after adequate preoperative

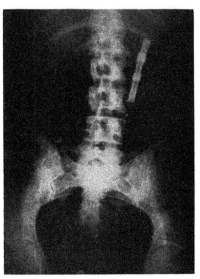

Fig. 3. Tube has just passed out of the hepaticoduodenostomy stoma, and is situated high in the jejunum (twelve hours after an attack of biliary colic), five months and ten days after operation. Two days later the tube had passed from the intestinal tract.

preparation, exploration of the common duct was accomplished on May 5, 1931. The proximal hepatic duct was greatly dilated and when opened drained approximately 400 c.c. of bile under tremendous pressure. Hepaticoduodenostomy over a Sullivan tube was made. Convalescence was uneventful and the patient was dismissed from the hospital on the fourteenth postoperative day, at which time the jaundice had practically entirely disappeared. Before the patient left the hospital a film was made to determine the presence of the tube. (Figure 2.) The patient's general condition continued to improve and she had remained entirely well until October 16, 1931, approximately five and one-half months after operation, when, after an alleged dietary indiscretion, an attack of pain in the upper right quadrant of the abdomen occurred, accompanied by nausea and vomiting; in other words a typical biliary colic. The urine was dark colored the next morning. She was not seen during this attack. However, the next day when she was seen at the office there was a slight icteric tinge of the sclera, suggesting recurrent obstruction to the common duct. The liver had receded under the costal margin and its edge was not palpable. A flat film of the abdomen was immediately made (Figure 3) which showed the tube inverted end for end, occupying a position to the left of the spine, interpreted as corresponding to a high loop of jejunum into which the tube had passed. A film two days later showed that the tube had passed out of the intestinal tract. It seemed therefore entirely regular to assume that the attack of biliary colic was produced by the passage of the tube from the stoma of the hepaticoduodenostomy. Thereafter the patient remained entirely well until November 10, 1933, two and a half years after opera-

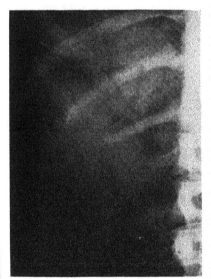

Fig. 4. Air in the biliary tract two years and six months after hepaticoduodenostomy, indicating patency of the stoma.

tion, when she had a very mild biliary colic. A flat film of the abdomen at that time showed air in the common and hepatic ducts indicating patency of the hepaticoduodenostomy stoma. (Figure 4.) The patient has been seen in the office within the past two weeks and has remained perfectly well, except for the two minor attacks described. It is now three years since the operation.

This case is presented for three reasons: first, the exact time that the tube remained in the he-

paticoduodenostomy stoma is known; five months and ten days; second, permanent retention of the tube is not necessary to insure patency of the hepaticoduodenostomy stoma; and third, the common and hepatic ducts are depicted by their air content.

It is worthy of emphasis that secondary operations for stricture or postoperative ductal deficiencies should be instituted before serious damage to the liver has occurred.

727 West Seventh Street.

A STUDY OF NEONATAL DEATHS AT THE UNIVERSITY HOSPITAL*

JOHN H. RANDALL, M.D., Iowa City

From time to time many authors have published data showing the most important factors in the causation of neonatal deaths. It is the purpose of this paper to review the results of a statistical study of neonatal deaths which have occurred at the University Hospital, Iowa City, Iowa, from July 1, 1926, to January 1, 1934, and to emphasize again the various causes of death during the neonatal period.

In this series we have classified as neonatal deaths only those cases in which the baby weighed 1,500 grams or more. Any baby weighing under 1,500 grams was considered not to have reached the period of viability. In all cases death occurred within the first seven days of life. Those babies who were born with the fetal heart still beating but who did not breathe, and those babies who made only feeble attempts to breathe were excluded. On this basis 56 neonatal deaths occurred in the above mentioned years. The number of live births during this period was 3,234, making the neonatal death rate 17.3 per thousand live births. Others have published similar findings. Lyon and Bemis found the neonatal death rate in 6,000 consecutive deliveries at the Woman's Hospital in New York City to be 17.8 per thousand deliveries. Quigley, in 1,960 consecutive private deliveries, had 23 neonatal deaths, or 11.7 per thousand deliveries.

Twenty-six in our series of neonatal deaths were full term babies and thirty were premature. Forty-eight or 85.7 per cent of the babies were autopsied very carefully so that the exact cause of death could be determined. In referring to Table I we find that the most common cause of death was intracranial hemorrhage. In many cases there was a noticeable tear in the dura particularly the tentorium, while in others only an extensive subdural or intraventricular hemorrhage could be found. In all cases in which intracranial hemor-

* Presented before the Eighty-third Annual Session, Iowa State Medical Society, Des Moines, May 9, 10, 11, 1934.

rhage is given as the cause of death it was felt that the hemorrhage in itself was sufficient to explain the death and that the other findings were only incidental. Since all babies were not autopsied the

Table I

ANALYSIS OF THE NEONATAL DEATHS AT THE UNIVERSITY HOSPITAL

July 1, 1926, to January 1, 1934

Cause of Death	Autopsied	Not autopsied
Intracranial hemorrhage	21	4
Prematurity	14	3
Congenital malformation	8	1
Asphyxia	2	0
Syphilis	1	0
Infection	1	0
Atelectasis	1	0
Total	48	8

cases in Table I are divided into two groups, namely those autopsied and those not autopsied. In the group not autopsied the cause of death is only a clinical impression and if these cases had been subjected to a careful postmortem examination other more important causes of death might have been disclosed.

Sixteen of the patients who died of hemorrhage were mature babies and nine were premature. Seven of the premature and six of the mature babies were delivered spontaneously. Premature babies have poorly ossified skulls and are very susceptible to intracranial injury. They are vulnerable babies and should be spared all stress and strain incident to a rapid delivery or to unnecessary operative procedures during birth. We would emphasize the importance of slow and careful delivery of the head even in what appears to be a perfectly easy and natural birth.

The common symptoms which were manifested soon after birth in the cases of intracranial injury were: difficult resuscitation, poor muscle tone, pale asphyxia, shallow respirations and a weak cry. The later symptoms were attacks of cyanosis, drowsiness, irritability and refusal to nurse. Erbenfest maintains that death from this particular cause rarely manifests itself conclusively in symptoms and clinical findings and can be discovered in the majority of cases only by means of an exhaustive postmortem study. In a large series of necropsies done on babies dying within the first few days of life, he found that fatal lesions within the cranium are discovered in about 25 per cent of the

cases, while in another 25 per cent definite evidence of some damage is present which, however, cannot be positively accepted as responsible for death.

Prematurity was found to be the second most important etiologic factor in the causation of neonatal deaths. In our series fourteen cases were autopsied in which it was felt that the underlying cause of death was prematurity, although the postmortem examination in all but two of these revealed accessory causes of death. Seven babies of this group were demonstrated to have had pulmonary atelectasis, four had infections, and one had intra-abdominal hemorrhage as the result of trauma to visceral organs.

Seven of the cases of full term neonatal deaths which were autopsied had one or more congenital malformations which were of such a nature that death was unavoidable. From the autopsied group six other full term spontaneously delivered babies died during the neonatal period, five from intracranial hemorrhage and one from asphyxia. The patient dying from asphyxia was found dead in its crib. Of the cases of congenital anomalies the following may be listed: achondroplasia associated with hydrocephalus; absence of a kidney in

Table II

FULL TERM NEONATAL DEATHS AT THE UNIVERSITY HOSPITAL

Cause of Death	Spontaneous	Forceps	Breech Extraction	Version and Extraction	Cesarean Section
Intracranial hemorrhage	6	2	5	3	0
Congenital malformations	8	0	0	0	0
Asphyxia	1	0	0	0	0
Atelectasis	0	0	0	0	1

PREMATURE NEONATAL DEATHS

Cause of Death	Spontaneous	Forceps	Breech Extraction	Version and Extraction	Cesarean Section
Intracranial hemorrhage	7	0	0	2	0
Prematurity	14	0	1	0	2
Syphilis	1	0	0	0	0
Asphyxia	0	1	0	0	0
Congenital malformations	0	0	1	0	0
Infection	1	0	0	0	0

can only be determined by a thorough postmortem study.

2. Prematurity is an important predisposing factor in the causation of neonatal deaths. Premature births should be prevented as much as possible.

3. Congenital malformations account for most of the neonatal deaths of full term babies who are delivered spontaneously.

BIBLIOGRAPHY

1. Browne, F. J.: Neonatal death. Brit. Med. Jour., ii:590-593 (September 30), 1922.
2. Ehrenfest, H.: Relation of birth trauma to neonatal mortality and infant morbidity. Am. Jour. Dis. Child., xliii:426-430 (February), 1932.
3. Quigley, J. K.: Stillbirths and neonatal deaths in 1,960 consecutive private cases. New York State Jour. Med., xxix:319-321 (March 15), 1929.
4. Lyon, E. C., Jr., and Bemis, G. C.: Study of neonatal deaths occurring in 6,000 consecutive deliveries. Am. Jour. Obst. and Gynec., xxi:373-380 (March), 1931.

INTRACRANIAL HEMORRHAGE*

Roy E. Crowder, M.D.

Sioux City

It is only recently that intracranial hemorrhage has become a recognized factor in stillbirths and neonatal deaths and as such, given the attention it merits. Beneke, in 1911, realized that the usual method of autopsy did not show the relation of the hemorrhage to the brain structures and so devised another method of approach. Since that time we have come to know the frequency with which the condition is met in these cases.

There are several classifications of intracranial hemorrhage which may be used to illuminate the relation between the anatomic lesion and the symptoms, but I feel that Ehrenfest's is as workable as any, and is less confusing. His classification is as follows:

1. Cephaloma internum.
2. Subarachnoidal hemorrhages.
3. Dural hemorrhages.
   (a) Supratentorial.
   (b) Infratentorial.
   (c) Mixed type.
4. Brain Hemorrhages.
   (a) Ventricular.
   (b) Diffuse or circumscribed.

Cephaloma internum, is a diffuse or circumscribed hemorrhage, over the lateral lobe of the brain under the periostium and is usually due to an injury to the middle meningeal artery. It is found rather infrequently and only when there has been a very definite bone injury during the birth.

Subarachnoidal hemorrhages are usually small hemorrhages in the subarachnoidal space. These

---

* Presented before the Eighty-third Annual Session, Iowa State Medical Society, Des Moines, May 9, 10, 11, 1934.

hemorrhages while frequent are much less fatal than those occurring in the dura.

Subdural hemorrhages are the most frequent causes of death in the newborn from intracranial hemorrhage. They are divided according to their relation to the tentorium into the supratentorial and infratentorial, and the mixed types.

In order to understand the mechanism and development of these hemorrhages, it is necessary to recall the anatomy of the dural septa. They are the falx cerebri, the tentorium cerebelli and the falx cerebelli. The falx cerebri arises from the crista galli and passes upward and backward, as a sickle-shaped structure, to insert into the upper leaf of the tentorium cerebelli. Enclosed between the superior edges is the longitudinal sinus; its free margin extending down into the sagital sulcus of the brain between the two hemispheres.

The tentorium cerebelli is attached laterally along the lateral sinus from the petrous portion of the temporal bone and the anterior surfaces of the occipital bone. Its two leaves, fusing at its inner margin, surround the midbrain. The falx cerebelli, which divides the two halves of the cerebellum, extends downward from the lower leaf of the tentorium to the foramen magnum.

These structures are simply thickenings of the dura which invest the entire surface of the brain and are continuous with the dura of the spinal cord. Its outer layer forms the periosteum of the cranial vault on the inner surface and its inner layer is in intimate contact with the brain surface. The falx cerebri and the tentorium are so placed that they are supporting structures tending to hold the cranial bones in more or less normal relationship to one another during the process of moulding at birth.

Due to the peculiar hinge arrangement of the bones of the vault of the skull on those at the base, any pressure applied to opposite sides of the skull at the same time causes an elongation upward of the vertical diameter. This elongation puts a strain on the falx cerebri which is in turn transmitted to the upper leaf of the tentorium by its insertion into it.

This leaf, being thin, gives way and causes a rupture of the blood vessels contained between the two leaves with a consequent escape of blood and the formation of a hematoma. If the hematoma is located above the tentorium we have sypmtoms of intracranial pressure which are: marked restlessness of the infant, a high pitched cry, failure to nurse properly, increased tension of the anterior fontanel, together with a spasticity of the extremities.

If the hematoma is located below the tentorium we have another group of symptoms which are:

marked apathy, moaning cry, interference with the respiratory center, as evidenced by irregular breathing, cyanotic spells, and rigidity of the neck muscles. Symptoms of the intracranial pressure appear late, if at all, and when present are usually evidence of a mixed type, that is a hematoma both above and below the tentorium. With either of these groups of symptoms, blood in the cerebrospinal fluid is confirmatory evidence. However, we may find blood in small quantities in the cerebrospinal fluid without any clinical evidence of an intracranial hemorrhage.

Ventricular hemorrhages are the result of the same mechanical factors as those of the dura, except that the vein of Galenus or its branches is ruptured, which allows the blood to enter the ventricles. Profuse oozing may be found in those infants born of mothers who are toxic or septic, due either to increased fragility and permeability, or to small thrombi causing stasis of the capillaries in the choroid plexus.

The predisposing causes to intracranial hemorrhage are: prematurity, blood dyscrasias, malpositions, such as occipitoposterior, parietal bone, brow, face and breech, and too rapid expulsion of normal presentations.

Since the development of the dural septa does not begin until late in the fifth month of fetal life one can readily see that they could be and are more easily torn by a minimum amount of trauma during the last trimester. The more premature an infant, the more possibility there is of damage being done to the septa, even in a fairly normal expulsion.

In the malpositions there is a very definite pressure applied to the opposite sides of the skull, which causes undue tension on the septa. Too rapid expulsion does not allow the slow stretching of the elastic fibers in the septa with the consequent gradual moulding of the head.

The immediate cause of a hemorrhage is the undue pressure applied to diametrically opposite sides of the skull, more particularly to the lateral sides, or to the anterior and posterior surfaces. This may be due to faulty application of forceps or too tight squeezing of the head with the forceps properly applied, and undue traction made upon them.

Of the abnormal presentations, the breech and occipitoposterior positions are the most frequent, the mechanism of injury being similar in both instances. In the former, the occipital bone comes to lie over the promontory of the sacrum and the frontal bones against the symphysis, causing an anteroposterior compression with a shortening of the anteroposterior diameter and an increase in the vertical diameter. In the breech presentation,

TREATMENT OF BURNS*

N. M. WHITEHILL, M.D., Boone

The treatment of burns is as old as the history of medicine, but the more recently acquired knowledge of physiology, metabolism and biochemistry, together with the advances in internal medicine and surgery have, during the last decade, placed the treatment on a more rational and scientific basis, and the older methods based on the understood pathology of the time, have been very largely discarded.

Statistics show that 45 per cent of the lethal burns occurring annually in the United States are in children under six years of age, the average age being three years. It is of interest to note that during the first three years of life, the highest death rate obtains in boys, while from the fourth to the ninth year the mortality is nearly double that for girls. At all ages, the morbidity is greater among boys. The most frequent cause of burns at this age is the spilling of hot water on the body or direct contact with flame.

The study of the systemic effect of various degrees of thermal trauma began during the war with the investigation of the effect of the lethal gases used at that time, many of which produce systemic changes in the body similar to the burns caused by contact of the body with flame, steam, electricity, etc. In 1923, Underhill published the results of his study on the systemic effect of burns. This study came following the disastrous New Haven Theatre fire in November, 1921. A severe burn of the body is followed by shock, differing very little from surgical or traumatic shock, and the treatment is practically the same; that is, heat, morphine, fluids, stimulants, etc. Like the inhalation of the lethal gases, a marked concentration of the blood is bound to follow, due in the case of the gases, to an acute edema of the lungs with an outpouring of fluid from the circulation, and in the case of burns to edema, blebs and the increased vascularity in the region of the burn. This resulting blood concentration, according to Underhill and his group of workers, is the primary cause of the high mortality rate in burns, and on the relief and prevention of which depends a great part of the treatment.

Experimenting with burned animals injected with trypan and methylene blue, it was found that the dyes passed readily from the blood into the fluid of the burned area, but that absorption of the dyes from the burned area back into the blood, did not occur during the first twenty-four hours. Lethal doses of strychnine injected into and around

* Presented before the Eighty-third Annual Session, Iowa State Medical Society, Des Moines, May 9, 10, 11, 1934.

the wound were not followed by strychnine poisoning. By the same token he reasoned, that if these dyes and strychnine were not absorbed from the burned area, there was no evidence that any indefinite toxin arising from the burned tissue could be absorbed from this area and produce the symptoms so constant in severe burns. About the second day, fluid oozes from the burned surface, blebs are formed, and the surrounding area becomes vascular, forming an ideal culture media for the growth of organisms. Sepsis, albuminuria, delirium, toxemia, extreme exhaustion and the characteristic odor follow. Blood examination at this time shows a marked concentration from loss of fluid. There is destruction of cells from heat and toxins, loss of chlorides and lowered blood pressure and temperature.

From animal experimentation we know that a burn covering one-sixth of the body area, gives a fluid loss of 75 per cent of the total blood volume in twenty-four hours. Applying these findings to a man weighing 150 pounds, and having a blood volume of 5,000 c.c., we find that he would lose about 3,500 c.c. of fluid in twenty-four hours. Underhill found that a blood concentration of 40 per cent above normal produced death in a short time; and that a concentration of 25 per cent above normal is extremely dangerous. These findings would clearly indicate the importance of blood concentration in the treatment of burns.

For the prevention and replacement of this fluid loss, liquids by mouth, and normal saline solution with dextrose, intravenously and subcutaneously, should be given freely to maintain the water and mineral balance, support the heart and circulation, restore normal blood pressure, and thus help to eliminate the poisons and decrease their toxicity.

In 1930, Frior of Johns Hopkins University, reported the results of his study of burns from the standpoint of a bacteriologist. He found, by taking cultures from the wound, that during the first twelve to eighteen hours after the burn, the field was practically free from organisms. After this time, in all severely burned cases, the streptococcus hemolyticus (and other organisms) could be grown from cultures, and signs of sepsis and toxemia due to the infection of the wound from these organisms developed similar to streptococcus infections in other wounds.

Local treatment should consist in the cleansing and protection of the burned surface, and in the prevention of the growth of organisms that develop rapidly in the secretions that form on the field. To this end, Davidson in 1925, brought out the tannic acid treatment of burns on the theory that the coagulating and styptic properties of a two per cent tannic solution renders the toxic substances less absorbable, forming a crust over the surface, thus preventing infection and loss of fluid. Tannic acid also acts as an analgesic, and the pain is markedly lessened, so that after the first twenty-four hours, narcotics are seldom necessary. The suffering is lessened, the treatment is more easily carried out either in the hospital or at home, and the patient is more quickly placed in a proper condition for the skin grafting that may be necessary later.

In 1912, Churchman proved the value of a one to one thousand solution of gentian violet, a coal tar derivative, as a specific against gram positive organisms. This solution has been used intravenously for septicemias with no report of gentian violet poisoning. Since that time, a gentian violet spray of the above mentioned solution has been used in the treatment of burns in much the same way as the tannic acid solution. The advantages claimed for the gentian violet treatment over that of tannic acid is its more potent germicidal effect, the fact that it forms a lighter and more flexible coating over the burned surface, and because the presence of infection beneath the eschar is more easily detected than in the tannic acid treatment. However, the gentian violet, while more potent as a germicide, does not have the styptic and coagulating properties of tannic acid. After cleansing the wound a fresh solution of tannic acid, two to three per cent, should be applied hourly until a firm eschar is formed.

This study of the systemic effect of burns, the preservation of the normal circulating volume of the blood, the maintenance of the normal blood pressure, and the normal distribution of oxygen to the tissues, together with improved local treatment has, during the past decade, placed the treatment of burns on a more rational basis, and the results are shown in the decreased mortality.

The time allotted to the treatment of burns does not permit the discussion of the many methods in use, nor the details in carrying out those just mentioned, to say nothing of the tedious after care in the way of skin grafting, and the prevention and correction of deformities. Certainly, we can say that real advancement has been made during the last decade in treating this most dangerous and distressing form of accident.

THE CLINICAL SIGNIFICANCE OF HEMORRHAGE FROM THE BOWEL*

WILLIAM H. RENDLEMAN, M.D.

Davenport

The presence of blood in the stools, or blood from the bowel without stool, calls for a thorough examination to determine its source and nature. The methods of determining this information constitute the aim of this discussion.

The intelligent patient will be able to give a history which may be of much help in locating the source of the hemorrhage. We know that blood described as bright red comes from the rectum or anus, and that blood which comes in spurts at the end of defecation or appears only on the toilet paper indicates bleeding from the anal canal, probably hemorrhoids, fissure, or varicose veins. The blood streaked stool and mucus streaked with blood also indicate a lesion of the terminal colon. The tarry, foul, sticky stool is characteristic of an upper bowel lesion.

A history of colic, flatulence, and constipation alternating with diarrhea points to an obstructive lesion. Tenesmus and frequent diarrheal bloody stools mixed with mucus, preceded by a history of repeated attacks of diarrhea with or without blood, leads to the suspicion of ulcerative colitis or dysentery. The vomiting of blood accompanied by tarry stools at once points to the stomach or duodenum as the source of hemorrhage. The patient's story will usually determine whether the pathology is in the stomach or bowel. This is particularly true in peptic ulcer but is not so certain in malignancy.

Anemia is an extremely important finding in gastro-intestinal diseases. The chronic loss of a small amount of blood from a hemorrhoid or the continuous passage of occult blood from a carcinoma of the stomach or cecum will produce an anemia which may be seriously considered as pernicious. I have had cases in which I made a tentative diagnosis of pernicious anemia after the blood counts and x-ray examinations were complete, but remained doubtful until a digital examination disclosed a rectal carcinoma as the cause of the anemia. A severe grade of anemia, often closely resembling the primary type, may be the only finding in a silent carcinoma of the stomach or bowel. In anemia of unknown origin repeated examinations of the stools are important and the finding of occult blood significant.

The gastro-enterologist must have at his command, chemical and microscopic facilities, a proctoscope, and an x-ray machine. The procedure after taking a careful history is to make a complete physical examination, including a digital examination of the rectum. The value of the digital examination is enhanced by having the patient in a squatting posture with instructions to strain. Internal hemorrhoids are palpated with difficulty. A bivalve speculum is a valuable aid to anal inspection. If the desired information is not obtained by these simple procedures, a proctoscopic investigation, preferably on a table designed for the purpose, is carried out. With the head low and the hips high, the sigmoid is carried up and the pressure of air from the outside balloons the bowel, making distention with the air bulb less necessary. The bowel should have been emptied previously with a cleansing enema. While the patient is on a meat free diet, several stools are examined for occult blood, pus, mucus, and parasites. When nothing in the terminal portion of the colon and anus is found to account for the hemorrhage, it becomes necessary to resort to the x-rays. This consists in the use of the fluoroscope following an opaque meal through the alimentary tract. The stomach and duodenum are examined for ulcer and carcinoma. At intervals the meal is followed through the bowel, the operator noting any filling defects, dilatations, abnormal haustral markings, narrowing or obstruction of the lumen and delay in passage. The barium enema furnishes the best view of the colon. This is carried out after the bowel has been emptied with a physic. The double contrast enema, the injection of air after the enema has been expelled, offers an advantage in looking for polyps and diverticulae. With the aid of the barium meal and enema one notes filling defects and their relation to a palpable tumor, dilation of the proximal colon, often present in distal obstruction, absence of haustral markings as in chronic dysentery, abnormal position and fixation of the bowel, prolonged retention in certain portions like the cecum, and retention of barium in diverticulae. X-ray films are made only for record and occasionally to improve detail.

The commonest cause of bowel hemorrhage is hemorrhoids. These as well as fissures and irritated veins may be diagnosed by inspection of the anal canal. A vein as a source may be overlooked unless bleeding is present at the time of inspection.

The diagnosis of carcinoma of the rectum, and often of the sigmoid, may be made with the proctoscope and sigmoidoscope, and the majority of those of the rectum by the finger alone. Above the rectum the diagnosis becomes more difficult and requires all the ingenuity and equipment at the

* Presented before the Eighty-third Annual Session, Iowa State Medical Society, Des Moines, May 9, 10, 11, 1934.

command of the examiner. The symptoms vary with the location. In the left half of the colon the lumen is narrower, consequently obstructive symptoms predominate. Pain, colic, flatulence, and constipation beginning after the age of forty should always excite suspicion of malignancy. Indeed, obstructions in patients above forty years of age without evidence of hernia or adhesions are best considered malignant until proved otherwise by operation. Metastasis from this portion of the bowel is slow and in a large percentage of deaths from perforation or obstruction the carcinoma remains local. When located in the right half of the colon, the picture is somewhat different. Here the lumen is larger and obstruction rare. An exception to this is found in involvement of the ileocecal valve producing obstruction of the ileum. The tumor grows larger before symptoms appear and becomes ulcerated and infected. Toxemia and anemia develop as a result of absorption and loss of blood. Anemia, loss in weight and strength, and a low grade of fever are thus the earliest symptoms. Any symptoms of indigestion are likely to be referred to the epigastrium. The diagnosis of carcinoma in any portion of the bowel is facilitated by examination with the fluoroscope and barium enema. A filling defect or a complete obstruction to the passage of the enema may correspond in location to a palpable tumor. If symptoms of obstruction are present, the barium meal should not be given because of the danger of converting a partial into a complete obstruction. Needless to say, the fluoroscopic examination should first rule out ulcer and carcinoma of the stomach. Of great importance in the diagnosis of carcinoma of the bowel is the finding of occult or visible blood in the stools.

Polyps, usually in the sigmoid, are important because of loss of blood and their malignant potentialities. Most reliance in their diagnosis is placed on the sigmoidoscope and the double contrast enema. Exploratory laparotomy is usually necessary to clear the diagnosis.

Ulcerative colitis may be due to tuberculosis, ameba, Shiga's bacillus, Bargen's diplostreptococcus, or to unknown causes. The symptoms are not characteristic. As a group diarrhea and tenesmus are more prominent than in other lesions of the bowel; more mucus and pus are present in the stools; and hemorrhage is less noticeable. When ulcers are in the rectum, the proctoscope gives the best diagnostic aid.

In amebic dysentery the punched out umbilicated ulcers are separated by normal mucosa. When the cecum is involved, the x-ray shows narrowing due to inflammatory thickening of the bowel wall, and an irregular outline from the deep ulcers. The ileocecal valve is patent. The final diagnosis rests on finding cysts and motile amebae in the mucus removed from an ulcer or in the fresh stool.

In chronic ulcerative colitis the mucosa between ulcers is congested, is finely granular in appearance, bleeds easily, and no amebae are found in the stools. The bowel, as shown by the x-ray, is narrow, and the haustra are gone, giving it the smooth "gas pipe" appearance.

A tuberculous ulcer, when present in the rectum, is larger, more liable to be solitary, is diffuse, and has a white pearly appearance. Tuberculous colitis is more likely to involve the cecum and lower ileum, where a mass may be felt. The fluoroscope will show an irregular filling and the barium does not remain as long as it does in other parts of the colon. Blood in the stool is not as common as mucus and pus. The finding of tuberculosis in the lung is the best proof that the lesion in the colon is tuberculous. Without this finding the diagnosis must remain in doubt.

There is another group of bowel diseases associated with hemorrhage which may be classed as surgical emergencies. These are intussusception, thrombosis of the mesenteric artery, and ulcer of Meckel's diverticulum. In intussusception occurring in young children there is a bloody mucoid discharge associated with tenesmus and distention. There should be no delay in laparotomy. Embolism and thrombosis of the superior mesenteric artery present a picture of sudden, severe abdominal pain and distention with passage of blood. The diagnosis is usually not made, but the symptoms are so urgent as to leave no doubt about the inadvisability of delayed operation. A bleeding ulcer of Meckel's diverticulum presents an almost impossible diagnosis. Unexplained, continuous, or frequently repeated loss of blood, whether from Meckel's diverticulum or from other causes, offers a plausible excuse for exploratory laparotomy. This method of diagnosis, much too often employed, still has an important place in abdominal diagnoses, especially in cases of acute abdominal pain. Unfortunately for the patient and the good name of the profession, it too often takes the place of study and the application of well proved methods of diagnosis.

Cirrhosis of the liver should be considered in any massive hemorrhage. Varicose veins about the cardiac end of the stomach may rupture, producing the greatest loss of blood of any alimentary lesion. The history of alcoholism, the large liver, the tarry stools with hematemesis, and the negative findings when the stomach is x-rayed usually suffice to make the diagnosis.

Rectal strictures due to syphilis or tuberculosis may ulcerate and cause bloody stools. The location is such as to be easily discovered with the proctoscope.

Diverticulitis not often a source of bleeding is best determined with the x-ray. After the bowel is emptied the diverticulae remain filled with barium. The enema may show a narrowing of the lumen or complete lack of filling which is differentiated from carcinoma by the greater length of bowel involved and by the lack of the abrupt shoulders in the filling defect of carcinoma.

There are many general conditions associated with bloody stools the diagnosis of which is evident from their characteristic symptoms and findings. The commonest of these are leukemia, severe anemias, acute nephritis, purpura, hypertension, typhoid, and various poisons.

The correct diagnosis of bowel hemorrhage implies a close study of the symptoms and the application of all physical, proctoscopic, laboratory, and x-ray methods at our disposal. By these means we are usually able to determine the location and cause, the prime necessities for successful treatment.

THE DIAGNOSIS AND SURGICAL TREATMENT OF PYLORIC OBSTRUCTION IN INFANTS*

HOWARD I. DOWN, M.D., Sioux City

Organic obstruction of the pylorus in infants is due, in the majority of instances, to congenital hypertrophic stenosis. This condition was first described by Beardsley in 1787, but it was not until the beginning of the present century that the underlying pathologic condition was understood and a rational form of surgical treatment advocated. The essential pathology of the condition is an hypertrophy of the circular muscle layer of the pylorus, and, due to this hypertrophy, a redundancy of the normal mucous membrane. The results following the release of the obstruction by severing the muscle by the Fredet-Rammstedt technic, are among the most gratifying in the entire field of gastric surgery.

It is not my purpose, in discussing this subject, to present anything new in regard to the disease or its treatment; nor do I propose to present any statistical data pertaining to any particular phase of the condition. I wish to review the diagnostic features of the disease, and to discuss certain phases of its treatment that seem to me to be worthy of emphasis.

Our knowledge concerning the etiology of hypertrophic stenosis is meager. The condition occurs

* Presented before the Eighty-third Annual Session, Iowa State Medical Society, Des Moines, May 9, 10, 11, 1934.

more frequently in males than in females in the proportion of about four to one. It is most frequently found in the first child in the family, although it may occur in two or three members of the same family. The condition is congenital, as evidenced by the fact that premature infants, and infants a few days old, have been found to have well developed tumors. This type of tumor is formed by the hypertrophic condition of the circular muscle of the pylorus, and while it shades off into the normal tissue on the gastric side, it stops abruptly on the duodenal side. Some observers believe that this hypertrophy is a response to increased resistance at the pylorus as a result of spasm, but it seems more logical to believe that it is a primary hypertrophy, and possibly hyperplasia, of the muscle.

The time of the onset of symptoms varies from shortly after birth to eight or ten weeks of age, the average being about three weeks of age. Up to the time symptoms begin, the infant has usually been perfectly well. MacHaffie has reported a case in which the symptoms began a few minutes after birth, and in which projectile vomiting was present in twenty-four hours time. At the time of operation, thirty-four hours after birth, a well developed, firm, gristle-like tumor was found.

Vomiting is the first and most outstanding symptom. At first it may be intermittent, small in amount, and there may be nothing unusual in its character. It soon becomes more or less continuous, and projectile in type. The vomitus consists of food and mucus, and at times, some blood. It does not contain bile. As the vomiting progresses the infant loses weight, becomes dehydrated and emaciated. Constipation is practically always present. There may be a small amount of formed fecal material consisting of mucus, bile, and intestinal secretions, with little or no food elements, the so-called starvation stool; or there may be small liquid, foul smelling slimy stools. The association of constipation with vomiting in an infant should at once suggest the possibility of some type of upper intestinal tract obstruction.

The physical signs of importance, aside from the varying degrees of emaciation and dehydration, are visible gastric peristaltic waves and a palpable tumor. The peristaltic waves are seen in the upper abdomen, and pass from left to right. They are best observed after a feeding, and while not pathognomonic of the condition, they are certainly helpful in establishing the diagnosis. Palpation of the pyloric tumor, when possible, is conclusive evidence of the disease. It is of value, in feeling for the tumor, to have the stomach empty, and the infant relaxed with a pacifier or his ordinary feeding. The tumor is more easily felt in those infants who have lost considerable weight. The tumor is sometimes very difficult to feel, and those who see a large number of cases will be able to palpate it more readily than those who see only an occasional case. Bolling considers it the most important sign of the disease and was able to palpate it in all but one of 454 cases. Donovan states that it can be felt in all cases if a painstaking examination is made. Strauss, on the other hand, pays little attention to it, and hence, reports palpation of the tumor in only a relatively small percentage of cases.

There has been considerable discussion regarding the value of the x-ray examination in the diagnosis of hypertrophic stenosis. Strauss is perhaps its most enthusiastic supporter. He uses it routinely, not only as a diagnostic agent, but also as a means of determining the type of treatment to be employed. He stresses the importance of observing the infant under the fluoroscope after a barium feeding, with the patient turned far on the right side. In his experience, those cases in which 80 per cent of the barium passes through the pylorus within four hours will respond to medical treatment, while those in which only 50 per cent of the barium passes through the pylorus within four hours will require operation. Ladd, on the other hand, uses the x-ray only in the borderline cases. He considers its routine use unnecessary for diagnostic purposes, and in fact is of the opinion that following its use the early postoperative feedings are less apt to be retained. The consensus of opinion seems to be that x-ray examination is not necessary in the average case, but that it is useful as a diagnostic aid in the occasional case.

The diagnosis of congenital hypertrophic stenosis of the pylorus, when the condition is well developed, is not difficult and can be made from the history and physical findings. Congenital stenosis or atresia of the duodenum or upper jejunum may present symptoms very similar to those of pyloric stenosis, but the fact that in these cases the symptoms usually date from birth, and the fact that the vomitus will at some time or other contain bile, will suffice to make the differentiation. Congenital retroperitoneal hernia, while a comparatively rare condition, may give rise to symptoms not unlike those of pyloric stenosis. The vomitus, however, will contain bile, and the tumor, if palpable, will be much larger and softer than the tumor of pyloric stenosis. Early in the course of pyloric stenosis it may be necessary to differentiate it from simple pylorospasm. This spasm may be dependent upon or associated with some local or general disease process. It may be associated with tetany. In these cases the diagnosis is best made by placing the infant on a treatment aimed at relaxing the spasm, and observing the effects after a few days.

The indication in the treatment of congenital hypertrophic stenosis is to remove the obstruction and allow food to pass through the pylorus. It is difficult to see how this obstruction, when due to a well developed tumor, can be relieved by any but surgical measures. There have undoubtedly been cases of hypertrophic stenosis which have been cured by medical means, and it may be that in those cases the element of spasm was important in the production of symptoms. In such cases one would expect that treatment with thick cereal feedings, gastric lavage, and physiologic doses of atropine, would produce beneficial results. Since the risk of operation is dependent upon the condition of the child at the time of operation, and this, in turn, is due mainly to the duration of the symptoms, one should not increase the risk of operation by persisting in medical treatment in the absence of material improvement in the symptoms.

One cannot predict, prior to trial, whether or not a given case will respond to medical treatment. While some men of wide experience believe that surgical treatment is indicated as soon as a definite diagnosis is made, I believe that there are patients who can safely be tried on medical treatment, particularly, if this treatment can be supervised by a pediatrician. Patients seen early in the course of the disease, and those seen later in the disease, in whom the symptoms are not severe, and in whom dehydration and emaciation are not present, and who have not lost much weight, should have the benefit of a trial on medical treatment. If, after a week or ten days, there is no improvement, as shown by a decrease in the vomiting, gain in weight, or increase in the bowel movements, surgery should be undertaken. Patients seen late in the disease, and those who are markedly dehydrated and emaciated should not be placed on medical treatment, but should be prepared for and given surgical treatment.

Obstruction of the pylorus, whether it is in the infant or the adult, is not a surgical emergency. Since this fact has been appreciated, and patients have been prepared for operation, the mortality rate in these cases has been materially decreased. In obstruction of the pylorus, as in other high intestinal obstructions, the loss of fluid and gastric secretion through vomiting produces marked changes in the chemistry of the blood and tissues. These changes, consisting of a decrease in the chloride and an increase in the plasma hydrogen ion concentration due to retention of the bicarbonate ion, predispose to postoperative shock and collapse. A few days treatment, prior to operation, aimed at correcting these changes will do much to avoid such complications. The administration of fluids, such as glucose, glucose and saline, or Ringer's solution, into the vein, or the administration of glucose or glucose and saline into the subcutaneous tissues, is the most important part of the treatment. Blood transfusion is valuable, and in some clinics where a good many of these cases are seen, it is routinely given to patients who are bad risks. Strauss, for example, who has published the lowest mortality rate, considers it the most vaulable part of the treatment. Many of his patients have been transfused twice prior to, and once after operation.

The history of the surgical attack on congenital hypertrophic stenosis of the pylorus is interesting, and illustrates the fact that in this, as in other phases of gastric surgery, the simplest and most conservative type of operation is usually superior to the more complicated procedure. This is particularly true when one is dealing with patients who are poor operative risks. Divulsion of the pylorus through a gastrotomy, gastrojejunostomy, and pyloroplasties of the Heinicke-Mikulicz and Nicoll types, were the operations that were employed up to 1908. Gastro-enterostomy was the operation most frequently employed. While the mortality from these operations was high, yet many patients were cured. In 1908 Fredet stressed the fact that the essential pathologic feature of the condition was hypertrophy of the circular muscle layer of the pylorus, and that the mucosa, while normal, was thrown into redundant folds. He therefore advocated a submucous pyloroplasty, which consisted of splitting the muscle down to the mucosa by a straight incision, and suturing the muscle ends. Rammstedt, in 1912, published his modification of this operation, which consisted of splitting the muscle as had Fredet, but leaving the wound open, or if necessary, covering it with omentum. This procedure, known as the Fredet-Rammstedt operation, has become almost universally accepted as the operation of choice in these cases. It is simple in principle, it corrects the pathologic condition, as postmortem studies show, and it can be applied by anyone with experience in abdominal surgery.

The operation is so well known that I will not attempt a description of its technic, but shall emphasize certain factors relative to the operative procedure which seem worthy of emphasis.

1. Ether is the anesthetic of choice in the average case. At times local infiltration may be advantageous, particularly if the surgeon is proficient in its use.

2. The child should be kept warm on the operating table, either by wrapping the body in flannel, or by the use of warm water bottles, or both.

3. The abdominal incision should be a right rectus incision placed so that the right lobe of the liver will extend beneath it for most of its length. This will help to prevent postoperative evisceration.

4. Because of the fact that the tumor stops abruptly at the duodenal end, and because the duodenal wall is very thin, the incision in the pylorus should begin on the stomach side, and extreme care should be used at the duodenal end to prevent perforation of the mucosa. The use of blunt forceps to separate the edges of the muscle after the initial incision has been made will help to avoid this complication. While perforation of the mucosa, if recognized and properly repaired, is not a serious complication, yet it is to be avoided. since its repair prolongs the time of operation unnecessarily. If perforation does occur, it should be closed immediately with a purse-string suture of fine silk, and this should be reenforced with a tag of omentum. Lamson has suggested that a triangular flap cut from the adjacent pyloric muscle be used to reenforce the silk suture.

5. The mucosa should bulge throughout the entire length of the incision to assure the operator that all of the constricting muscle fibers have been divided. Some patients have been operated on twice because all of the obstruction had not been relieved.

6. Hemorrhage is usually not to be feared if the incision in the pylorus is properly placed. The most avascular portion should be chosen. If there is bleeding one can control it with warm packs, or if necessary by the use of silk purse string sutures.

7. The postoperative care is important, and when possible, should be directed by the pediatrician. Fluids should be given rectally in the form of retention enemata, by subcutaneous injection, and if necessary by the intravenous route. After the effects of the anesthetic have worn off, small quantities of glucose water may be given by mouth, and the amount gradually increased. At the end of six hours small amounts of breast milk or formula feeding may be added to the water. At the end of three or four days the infant should be on a full diet schedule.

SUMMARY

Obstruction of the pylorus in infants is manifested clinically by vomiting, constipation, visible gastric peristaltic waves, and a palpable pyloric tumor. The x-ray is helpful in establishing the diagnosis in certain cases. The indication in the treatment is to remove the obstruction, and if this cannot be readily accomplished by medical means, surgery is indicated. Patients seen late in the disease, who are markedly dehydrated, should be immediately prepared for operation, and operated upon without trial on medical treatment. Preoperative preparation of the patient will do much to reduce the mortality rate. The Fredet-Rammstedt procedure is the operation of choice. It is simple in principle, is readily performed, and is curative, in that it adequately corrects the underlying pathologic condition.

BIBLIOGRAPHY

Boone, F. H.: The non-operative treatment of congenital hypertrophic pyloric stenosis. Canada Med. Assn. Jour., xxvii: 253-256, (September), 1932.
Clopton, M. B., and Hartman, A. F.: Fredet-Rammstedt operation for congenital pyloric stenosis. Surg., Gynec. and Obst., xlvii:527-530, 1928.
Donovan, E. J.: Congenital hypertrophic stenosis in infants. Ann. Surg., xcv:174-182, (February), 1932.
Goldbloom, A., and Spence, R. C.: Prognosis in operated cases of hypertrophic stenosis of the pylorus. Amer. Jour. Dis. Child., xix:263-268, 1920.
Ladd, W. E.: Congenital hypertrophic pyloric stenosis. Boston Med. and Surg. Jour., cxcvi:211-216, (February 10), 1927.
Lamson, O. F.: Congenital hypertrophic pyloric stenosis: treatment of accidental perforation of mucosa during Rammstedt operation. Surg., Gynec. and Obst., lvii:398-399, (September), 1933.
MacHaffie, L. P.: An early case of congenital pyloric stenosis. Amer. Jour. Dis. Child., xxxiv:699, 1927.
Mazies, M. and McArthur, C.: Cell and plasma chloride in pyloric stenosis in infants. Amer. Jour. Dis. Child., xli:35-44, (January), 1931.
Richter, H. M.: Congenital Hypertrophic Stenosis of the Pylorus. Abt. Pediatrics., iii:453-474.
Strauss, A. A.: Clinical observations of congenital pyloric stenosis. Jour. Am. Med. Assn., lxxi:807-810, 1918.
Wollstein, Martha: Healing of hypertrophic pyloric stenosis after the Fredet-Rammstedt operation. Amer. Jour. Dis. Child., xxiii:511-517, 1922.

REPORT OF CASES FROM THE
BROADLAWNS GENERAL
HOSPITAL, DES MOINES

JULIUS S. WEINGART, M.D., JOSEPH BROWN, M.D., FRANK W. FORDYCE, M.D., Hospital Staff Committee.

REPORT OF CASE NO. 71481

The patient was a colored girl who had jumped from a third story window and had suffered a compound fracture of the right leg. She entered the hospital May 22, 1933. Roentgenograms showed a comminuted fracture of the fibula, and a fracture at the internal malleolus of the tibia. The broken fibula had pierced the skin, and was contaminated with soil. The wound was cleaned, and painted with tincture of iodine and alcohol. An injection of 1,500 units of tetanus antitoxin was given. She was placed in the hospital, where she had a slight fever for about three days. Nine days after the injury a cast was applied, with an opening for the dressing of the wound. Six days later she was discharged. Two days after this she was brought to the hospital in a serious condition. She complained of stiffness and soreness of the neck and jaws, and had had some jerky movements of the arms and legs. These had begun during the previous day.

When seen by the writer, this being his first contact with the patient, about two hours after her second admission, she presented the typical features of tetanus. She had a temperature of 102.4 degrees, which rose to 107 degrees before death. This occurred in about twenty-four hours, in spite of vigorous therapeutic measures. Thus death from tetanus was the result of an accident eighteen days before, in spite of the fact that a prophylactic dose of the anti-serum had been given. The case is recited here as a salutary warning. It must be remembered that all antitoxins are excreted rather rapidly. They remain only two or three weeks in the body. Many previous cases of tetanus after an injection of prophylactic serum have been reported, and while most of these are modified, that is, milder, the danger of late severe tetanus must be kept in mind. In cases where there is gross contamination of a wound by garden soil or manure, it is wise, not only to give the prophylactic dose, but to repeat it in ten to fourteen days, and even oftener, if the wound is not yet healed.

REPORT OF CASE NO. 15367

This patient was a young man, twenty-one years of age, who had been employed as a sorter in a bag manufacturing company. About a year before, he had been injured in his upper anterior chest region by a fall against a stair post. He entered the hospital on May 17, 1933, with an infected sinus just to one side of the manubrium sterni. This had been present for seven months. The patient said that it would partially heal up, and then become sore and drain pus for several days. At this admission he stayed in the hospital for a week. Roentgenograms showed no evidence of osteomyelitis of the sternum or clavicle. He left without a definite diagnosis, for the classification on discharge, "infected sinus of the chest" cannot be considered especially illuminating. He came to the Out-patient Department for numerous dressings. It must be admitted that there was considerable effort to arrive at a diagnosis. Among other things, a culture of the pus was taken and it is not surprising that this showed a growth of staphylococci.

He again entered the hospital on January 30, 1934. He said he had had two episodes of trouble with his draining sinuses, for now another one had developed at a somewhat lower level. It is a matter of common experience that laboratory examinations are most apt to prove useful when a shrewd clinical guess has been made previously. The patient was presented at the Friday morning clinic and his case discussed. The possibility of ray-fungus infection was suggested by one of the staff. A direct examination of the pus from the sinuses was then made. This showed numerous masses of Actinomyces bovis.

Such an oversight for nearly a year may be excusable on the ground that the lesion was in a rather unusual situation. However, the lesson to be learned is obvious.   J. S. W.

THE FINLEY HOSPITAL CLINICO-PATHOLOGIC CONFERENCE

CARCINOMA OF THE GALLBLADDER

L. H. FRITZ, M.D., Dubuque

E. M. BENCH, M.D., Galena, Illinois

Primary carcinomas of the gallbladder constitute five to six per cent of all carcinomas, according to Kaufmann. In the vast majority of cases the patients give histories indicating many years of gallbladder disease and the malignant growths are associated with gall stones. Therefore as a practical method of cancer prevention it would seem logical to remove the diseased gallbladders before the carcinomas have developed. It has been estimated by Rolleston and Slade that four to eighteen per cent of cholelithiasis cases result in carcinoma. The following case illustrates the usual course of gallbladder disease ending in malignancy.

CASE REPORT

Chief complaint: The patient, a white woman seventy-four years of age, was admitted to the Finley Hospital, September 15, 1931, with a complaint of "severe pain in the upper right side of the abdomen."

Family history: Irrelevant.

Past history: For a number of years she had had frequent attacks of gastric and intestinal distress accompanied by eructations of gas which came on after eating. She had never been jaundiced but had been constipated for some time. She had had several normal pregnancies and all her children were well.

Present illness: The morning of the day of her admission, the patient, while shopping, had a sudden attack of severe pain in the right upper abdominal quadrant. The pain was so severe that morphine was given to relieve it. Her physician made a diagnosis of cholelithiasis and sent her to the hospital.

Physical examination: The patient's temperature was 97 degrees; her pulse was 100 and the respirations were 20 per minute. She was markedly cachectic, seemed actually ill and in shock. Pathology of the head and neck was negative. The chest was very thin, with prominent ribs. The breath sounds were short and an occasional râle was heard at the base of each lung. The heart was small and the pulse was rapid. On auscultation no unusual sounds were heard. The abdomen was scaphoid. The skin was loose and slightly yellow in color. A hard, tender and slightly movable mass could be felt in the right upper quadrant, and a notch was felt at the middle of the lateral border, about the size and shape of a kidney which has rotated. Two fingers could be placed between the upper border of the mass and the costal margin. The liver could not be felt, and

there were no other masses in the abdomen. The extremities were emaciated. The nervous system was negative. The blood vessels were sclerotic. The urine showed a moderate trace of albumin, an occasional hyaline and granular cast; a specific gravity of 1.016. The white blood count was 14,000; 85 per cent being polymorphonuclear leukocytes. The red blood count was 3,660,000, and the hemoglobin was 64 per cent

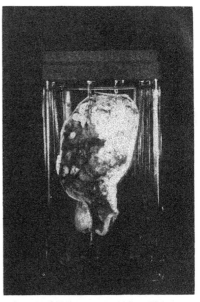

Fig. 1. Photograph of the gallbladder. Note the carcinoma in the lower third. The gall stones have been removed.

(Sahli). A pyelogram of the right kidney was essentially negative. A flat film of the abdomen showed an enlarged gallbladder with a thickened wall.

Preoperative diagnosis: Acute hydrops of the gallbladder; chronic cholecystitis.

Operative note: The gallbladder was markedly enlarged. It contained considerable cloudy fluid and many stones of various sizes. The common and hepatic ducts were large but free of stones.

Postoperative diagnosis: Chronic cholecystitis and cholelithiasis.

Pathologic report:

Grossly: The specimen is a moderately large gallbladder which has been emptied of considerable blood and what appears to be pus as well as numerous facetted stones. The wall is thickened and the mucosa is dark red and granular. The stones evidently were in the upper portion of the viscus and the cavity is partly divided by a shelf-like projection of thickened epithelium extending into the lumen approximately one centimeter in its thickest portion. This area feels hard and resembles a neoplastic growth. (Figure 1.)

Miscroscopically: The sections were taken from the junction of the relatively normal mu-

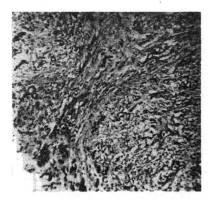

Fig. 2. Microphotograph showing the carcinoma cells sweeping through the thickened wall of the gallbladder.

cosa and the shelf-like projection. Each area shows well marked fibrosis and round cell infiltration of the outer coats. The mucosa above the thickened area appears relatively normal but as this area is approached it becomes more and more irregular. Finally large and small masses of epithelial cells can be seen extending down into the wall. The cells are rich in chromatin and mitotic figures are moderately numerous. (Figure 2.)

Anatomic diagnosis: 1. Chronic and acute cholecystitis and cholelithiasis.

2. Carcinoma of the gallbladder.

Subsequent course: The patient made an uneventful, immediate recovery, but died one year later of abdominal metastases.

GENERAL DISCUSSION

The clinical picture of carcinoma of the gallbladder is much the same as that of chronic cholecystitis and cholelithiasis. The usual complaints are indigestion, belching, constipation, and distress or pain in the region of the gallbladder. The pain is often referred to the back, to the right shoulder, or to the stomach. It has no relationship to meals or to the character of the food. Two important signs that should suggest malignancy, and both of which were present in our case, are the presence of a mass in the region of the gallbladder and the occurrence of cachexia. Jaundice may be an early or late symptom depending upon the site of origin of the carci-

noma and the location of metastases. If the tumor or the metastases cause obstruction to the main bile ducts, jaundice will occur. However jaundice does not necessarily occur and we have had three such cases which came to necropsy. One was in a woman who died suddenly. The carcinoma of the gallbladder was associated with gall stones and she had extensive metastases throughout the peritoneal cavity, but there was no obstruction to the bile ducts.

The etiology of carcinoma of the gallbladder like that of cancer in general is unknown. Nevertheless the frequent association of stones with the malignant change which has been reported in from 75 to 100 per cent of the cases must be recognized as an important etiologic factor. The stones set up the local irritation which precipitates the carcinomatous growth, whatever the underlying cause may be. It is for this reason that cholecystectomy should be considered as a prophylactic measure in all patients with cholelithiasis if they are able to stand operation. These tumors metastasize rather quickly to the liver, bile ducts, regional lymph nodes and to the peritoneum. After metastases have occurred, only palliative measures can be carried out. With the growth confined to the gallbladder there is no reason why cures should not result. Better still is the possibility of prevention. With highly accurate roentgenologic diagnoses of gallbladder disease, and modern surgery with its low mortality rate, the most logical attack on this type of cancer is removal of the diseased gallbladder before the malignant change occurs. The period of time from the beginning of symptoms of gallbladder disease until the cancer develops is probably a long one, i. e., months to several years. During this time the carcinoma may be prevented by removal of the gallbladder.

Case Report

AN INTERNAL HERNIA THROUGH A BROAD LIGAMENT

HENRY H. HAMILTON, M.D.

BEN L. KNIGHT, M.D.

Cedar Rapids

We are reporting this case, since a review of the available literature fails to reveal this particular type of internal hernia.

A married white woman, twenty-eight years of age, was injured in an automobile accident in Missouri in May, 1933. Her injuries were mainly of an internal nature. Six weeks after the accident she was told that an operation was necessary to save her life. She was operated upon in St. Louis, Missouri, and according to her story her appendix and left ovary were removed. She made an uneventful recovery and felt well until January 12, 1934.

On that day she had a sudden sharp abdominal pain while lying in bed. This persisted intermittently until on·January 14, 1934, she vomited for the first time. This was repeated several times throughout the day, and at no time was the vomiting fecal in nature. She was seen on the morning of January 15, complaining of severe abdominal cramps. Tenderness was noticeable throughout the entire abdomen on palpation, but there was neither rigidity nor distention. Her temperature was 98 degrees and her pulse was 96. The white blood count was 18,100. She had had no bowel movement for over twenty-four hours.

The patient was taken to St. Luke's Hospital with a diagnosis of obstruction, probably paralytic in nature. No results were obtained from the five enemas she received throughout the day. She also received six doses of pitressin. The following morning, January 16, her white count was down to 12,700, but she appeared to be definitely septic. It was felt that an exploratory laparotomy was warranted, since the abdomen was becoming distended. Under an ether anesthesia, a mid-line incision was made, about one-half inch to the left of her previous incision.

On opening the peritoneum a considerable amount of thin yellowish fluid gushed forth. The entire small bowel was enlarged to a diameter of about three inches. The distended bowel was followed down into the right pelvis where we encountered a strong band about one-half inch thick running in a vertical direction. This was a fold of mesentery which was adhered to an opening in the right broad ligament. This opening was large enough to admit the tip of the index finger, and through it, from anterior to posterior, was herniated about four feet of darkened and collapsed small bowel. This was carefully pulled out and the opening sutured. Hot towels were placed about the darkened bowel for a few minutes when it was returned to the abdomen and the abdomen was closed without drainage. The patient made an uneventful recovery.

We do not feel capable of saying whether or not the opening in the broad ligament was a result of the previous operation.

ANNUAL FALL CLINICAL CONFERENCE OF THE KANSAS CITY SOUTHWEST CLINICAL SOCIETY

The Kansas City Southwest Clinical Society announces the dates of the Twelfth Annual Fall Clinical Conference to be held from October first through October fourth, at Kansas City, Missouri. All scientific sessions will be held in the President Hotel, starting each morning at 8:30 and continuing throughout the day.

The guest speakers who will participate in the conference are: Dr. Walter L. Bierring, of Des Moines, President of the American Medical Association; Dr. Hugh Cabot, Professor of Surgery, University of Minnesota Graduate School of Medicine; Dr. Joseph B. DeLee, Professor of Obstetrics and Gynecology, University of Chicago; Dr. Morris Fishbein, of Chicago, Editor, Journal of the American Medical Association; Dr. Lee Forrest Hill, of Des Moines, member of the American Academy of Pediatrics; Dr. Samuel Iglauer, Professor of Otolaryngology, University of Cincinnati, College of Medicine; Dr. Samuèl Levine, Associate Professor of Medicine, Harvard University Medical School; Dr. Philip Lewin, Associate Professor of Orthopedic Surgery, Northwestern University Medical School; Dr. H. O. Mertz, Clinical Professor of Genito-Urinary Surgery, Indiana University School of Medicine; Dr. George Pfahler, Professor of Radiology, University of Pennsylvania, Graduate School of Medicine; Dr. Fred W. Rankin, Past Professor of Surgery, University of Louisville; Reverend Alphonse Schwitalla, Dean of the St. Louis University School of Medicine, and Dr. H. O. Woodruff, Woodruff Clinic, Joliet, Illinois.

Two hours will be allotted each morning to sectional lectures pertaining to pertinent medical subjects, presented by members of the society. Four of these lectures will run concurrently each morning on non-conflicting subjects. The public meeting will bring as speakers, Reverend Schwitalla, Dr. George Pfahler and Dr. Morris Fishbein. This meeting will be open to the public, with admission by ticket only, and will be one of interest to the layman as well as the physician. The local medical societies will cooperate with the Clinical Society in presenting the Tuesday evening scientific session, with Dr. Fred Rankin and Dr. Samuel Levine making the addresses.

An evening of entertainment for the visiting doctors and their families has been arranged at the William Rockhill Nelson Gallery of Art. The Alumni and President's dinner will be the closing feature of the conference. Two of the guest speakers will make addresses each day before the Round Table Luncheon on non-medical subjects which promises to afford a few minutes relaxation from scientific thoughts. Many features of entertainment are being planned by the local women's committee for the visiting women. A special registration desk will be available where they may obtain information relative to the women's programs.

STATE DEPARTMENT OF HEALTH

AN UNUSUAL OUTBREAK OF GASTRO-ENTERITIS

An outbreak of unusual character and affecting at least thirty persons, occurred at Harlan in Shelby county, May 5 to 7, 1934. Symptoms of onset were sudden, with nausea, vomiting and purging. Fever was absent. Twenty-two persons became sick on one day, Saturday, May 5. Illness lasted a number of hours, the patients being much improved on the second day. In one case illness was of rather serious character, the patient showing signs of shock during the hours following acute onset.

Inquiry showed that there was but one common factor to account for illness in this group of patients. All had used milk supplied by a local dairyman whose product was regarded as the best obtainable in the city. Ten persons became sick within three hours after drinking some of this milk at one of the cafes. Three members of one family made ice cream from the milk and were ill soon after eating it. The short period of time between ingestion of the milk, and onset of symptoms, indicated that the untoward effects were due to toxic rather than bacterial action.

What was the nature of this toxin or chemical substance? The dairyman himself suggested the possibility that the cases of illness might be due to a "caked" udder in a heifer which had calved two weeks before. Milk from this heifer was not used until two days prior to the outbreak. The bottled milk was allowed to stand over night on a basement floor, at a temperature not below 70 degrees. It was this milk, delivered the following day, Saturday, May 5, which apparently gave rise to the trouble. The weather at the time was very warm. Bacteriologic examination at the State Hygienic Laboratories, of milk from the heifer and of some of the milk known to have been used by the patients, showed the presence of large numbers of staphylococcus aureus. Broth was inoculated with this organism and incubated to develop a toxin. Although experimental animals failed to react following intraperitoneal injection of the broth filtrate, there is little doubt but that staphylococcus toxin was the inciting factor in causing the cases of gastro-enteritis. The part played by staphylococcus toxin in producing this type of milk poisoning, was first demonstrated by Barber in 1914. In recent years other reports in medical literature have demonstrated the rôle of staphylococcus toxin and of udder infection in causing acute gastro-intestinal symptoms in man.

A. L. Nielsen, M.D., local health officer, and attending physicians, assisted the State Department of Health in the study of this unusual epidemic of gastro-enteritis.

MILK-BORNE TYPHOID FEVER IN WATERLOO

Following the reporting of a number of cases of typhoid fever from Waterloo, an investigation was made by the State Department of Health, with the aid of J. E. Ridenour, M.D., city health officer and physicians who attended cases of illness.

Clinical and Epidemiologic Findings: The patients complained of severe headache, abdominal discomfort, loss of appetite, fever and malaise. Several "drooped" for a week before a physician was called. Visits were made to eleven homes in which twenty-two patients had developed symptoms of typhoid fever. Four patients had onset of symptoms on July 15, all becoming sick over a period between July 4 to July 25. Of the twenty-two patients, eleven were colored and eleven white; sixteen were males and six females. The youngest patient was three years of age, the oldest forty-six.

A Common Source of Infection: Sanitary surroundings in the different homes varied greatly. In several instances there were no modern conveniences, including sanitary toilets for excreta disposal, and public water supply. In other homes, sanitary conditions were good, there being access to the city water supply, sewer connections and effective screening to exclude flies. Although members of one family were not acquainted with some of the other families, it is significant that all of the homes were located in one section of the city. Of greater significance was the fact that these homes formed part of a milk route, all obtaining this food product from the same source.

The Milk Supply: The milk suspected of causing infection was distributed in raw form by a young man who had worked up a milk route about two months before the outbreak occurred. He supplied about sixty families, all of the milk coming from the same dairy farm. In the beginning, the milk was bottled after being brought to the city, but later bottling was done in a milk house at the dairy farm.

Conditions at the Dairy Farm: A visit to the dairy farm, the milk supply of which was incriminated in this outbreak of typhoid fever, showed that the dairy barn and milk house were in fairly good condition.

An outdoor privy was found to be very insanitary, flies having ready access to the interior and fluid contents covering the surface of the ground immediately back of the toilet.

Past History of Typhoid Infection: No history of a former attack of typhoid fever was obtained from the dairyman's family. It was learned, however, that relatives, an elderly woman and her daughter, were spending part of the summer at the dairy farm. Further inquiry revealed that both of these women, visitors from another part of the state, had had typhoid fever some years ago.

Demonstrating a Typhoid Carrier: The visitors had arrived at the dairy farm June 10, less than a month before onset of illness of any of the cases of typhoid fever. Neither the mother nor her daughter had helped with the milking or handling of utensils used in the milk house. These women, as well as members of the dairyman's family, prepared specimens which were forwarded to the State Hygienic Laboratories. Isolation of typhoid bacilli from the bowel discharges demonstrated that both of these women were typhoid carriers.

Control Measures: The milk supply concerned was stopped as soon as cases of typhoid fever were diagnosed. Patients were isolated, contacts immunized by attending physicians, and instructions given to those attending the sick, relative to prevention of secondary cases in homes. Adequate nursing care was provided. Sanitary conditions at the dairy farm were improved so as to minimize the hazard of fly-borne disease. The carriers left the dairy farm and have been placed under supervision.

COMMENT

This milk-borne outbreak of typhoid fever illustrates one of the common as well as the most dangerous hazards attending any raw milk supply, namely that of contamination by specific organisms from a typhoid carrier. Fortunately the urban families using this particular milk supply were few in number as compared with the total population. Much credit for the non-occurrence of major outbreaks of epidemic disease belongs to those in the milk industry who provide the public with carefully pasteurized dairy products, giving adequate attention at the same time to improvement of the quality of milk at its source. Further efforts to prevent milk-borne disease are dependent upon action taken by official bodies, such as adoption of a standard milk ordinance and provision for adequate personnel and facilities to ensure a safe public milk supply.

HEALTH TALKS AT THE STATE FAIR

Through a cooperative arrangement with the Speakers Bureau of the Iowa State Medical Society, talks on health subjects were featured in connection with the exhibit of the Iowa State Department of Health at the State Fair. A ten minute address was given each afternoon at 2:30, beginning August 23 and ending August 31.

Names of the speakers who cooperated and the titles of their talks follow:

August 23—Jack V. Treynor, M.D., Council Bluffs, Iowa, "Tonsils and Health."

August 24—R. O. Hughes, M.D., Ottumwa, Iowa, "The School Child and Health."

August 25—C. T. Ostrem, D.D.S., Ankeny, Iowa, "Pyorrhea and Its Relationship to Preventive Dentistry."

August 27—E. E. Shaw, M.D., Indianola, Iowa, "Serving the Public Health."

August 28—Douglas N. Gibson, M.D., Des Moines, Iowa, "Prevention and Treatment of Common Accidents."

August 29—R. D. Bernard, M.D., Clarion, Iowa, "Proposed Basic Science Law in Iowa."

August 30—J. F. Gerken, M.D., Waterloo, Iowa, "Important Features on Care of Preschool Child."

August 31—J. C. Hill, M.D., Newton, Iowa, "The Doctor's Relation to the Indigent."

NINTH ANNUAL MEETING OF THE IOWA PUBLIC HEALTH ASSOCIATION

The Ninth Annual Meeting of the Iowa Public Health Association will be held in Des Moines, Iowa, during the latter part of the month of October. Public health workers and health officers should plan now to attend that meeting. In the past a number of health officers have been authorized to attend such meetings by their local boards of health with expenses paid. Notice of the time and place of the meeting together with a complete program will be printed on these pages in the October issue of the JOURNAL OF THE IOWA STATE MEDICAL SOCIETY.

PREVALENCE OF DISEASE

	July '34	June '34	July '33	Most Cases Reported From
Diphtheria	14	34	21	Pottawattamie,Benton
Scarlet Fever	73	139	42	Polk
Typhoid Fever	8	5	5	(For State)
Smallpox	8	3	11	Cerro Gordo
Measles	168	679	29	(For State)
Whooping Cough	98	141	192	Woodbury, Boone
Cerebrospinal Meningitis	1	4	4	Wapello
Chickenpox	38	123	29	Boone, Linn
Mumps	41	94	46	Linn, Polk
Poliomyelitis	2	1	1	Johnson, Madison
Tuberculosis	49	39	47	(For State)
Rocky Mountain Spotted Fever	2	1	2	Adams, Lee
Undulant Fever	6	7	23	(For State)
Syphilis	111	121	176	(For State)
Gonorrhea	195	161	228	(For State)

The JOURNAL of the Iowa State Medical Society

ISSUED MONTHLY

RALPH R. SIMMONS, Editor.....................Des Moines

PUBLICATION COMMITTEE

RALPH R. SIMMONS, Editor.....................Des Moines
ROBERT L. PARKER, Secretary..................:.Des Moines
OLIVER J. FAY, Trustee.......................Des Moines
JOHN I. MARKER, Trustee......................Davenport
EDWARD M. MYERS, Trustee.....................Boone

SUBSCRIPTION $3.00 PER YEAR

Address all communications to the Editor of the Journal, 505 Bankers Trust Building, Des Moines

---

OFFICE OF PUBLICATION, DES MOINES, IOWA

Vol. XXIV   SEPTEMBER, 1934   No. 9

A STANDARD FOR INDUSTRIAL MEDICINE

Industrial medicine and traumatic surgery as special fields of practice employ more physicians in the United States than medical teachings, and require a greater personnel than that employed in public health activities. It has recently been estimated that nearly nine per cent of all practicing physicians are engaged for full time work in the industrial field. An equal or greater number engage in this practice for part of their time. Many consider that the rapid development of industrial medicine is largely responsible for the growing tendency toward a socialized plan of medical care. Every one engaged in medical practice feels directly or indirectly the influence of industrial medicine on the general scheme of medical practice. For these reasons it seems timely and appropriate that the American College of Surgeons should recognize the problems of industrial practice and should consider a program for the protection and guidance of this group. That this program should have received publicity through the lay press as a pronouncement of the College before its consideration by the appropriate committees of the American Medical Association is unfortunate.

At the early summer meeting of the Board of Regents of the American College of Surgeons this problem received positive attention when the Board endorsed and approved a report of the Medical Service Board, setting forth a minimum standard for industrial medicine and traumatic surgery, as outlined in the following paragraphs:

MINIMUM STANDARD FOR INDUSTRIAL MEDICINE AND TRAUMATIC SURGERY

A. That the industry shall have an organized medical department, or service, with competent medical staff including consultants and adequate emergency dispensary and hospital facilities and personnel to assure efficient care of the ill and injured.

B. That membership on the medical staff shall be restricted to physicians and surgeons who are (a) graduates of scientific medicine holding the degree of Doctor of Medicine, in good standing and licensed to practice in their respective states or provinces; (b) competent in the field of industrial medicine and traumatic surgery; (c) worthy in character and in matters of professional ethics, that in the latter connection, the practice of the division of fees under any guise whatsoever be prohibited.

C. That there shall be a system of accurate and complete records filed in an accessible manner —a complete record being one which includes identification data; cause of illness or injury; nature and extent of illness or injury; detailed description of physical findings; special examinations such as consultations, clinical, laboratory and x-ray; tentative or provisional diagnosis; treatment; prognosis with estimated period of disability; progress of illness or injury; final diagnosis; condition on discharge; end results; and such additional information as may be required by statute for Workmen's Compensation claims or for other purposes.

D. That all patients requiring hospitalization shall be sent to institutions approved by the American College of Surgeons.

E. That the medical department shall have general supervision over the sanitation of the plant and the health of all employees.

1. Physicians and surgeons, qualified as in paragraph two of the above Minimum Standard may properly be employed on a full time or a part time basis by industrial organizations to provide medical and surgical service for their employees, as follows:

a. To provide emergency service and first aid in injury or disease, and to provide adequate medical or surgical care for industrial injuries and diseases. Medical and surgical care of the families of employees, and of employees themselves, except for emergency and industrial injuries and diseases, should be provided by the industrial physician only in remote districts where other adequate medical service is not available.

b. To provide pre-employment and periodic physical examinations.

c. To study the hazards of the particular industry and to cooperate with other agencies in effecting such measures as may be needed for the prevention of injury and disease.

d. To keep accurate records such as may be required by local Workmen's Compensation laws, and so complete as to serve for scientific investigation of industrial hazards with a view to their further prevention. These records are privileged communications, subject always to due process of law.

2. The sale of a contract by an industrial organization to an individual physician or group of physicians for medical and/or hospital service for its employees encourages commercial competition, and is to be condemned.

3. Unethical practices in publicity, advertising, solicitation, and competition, either of a professional or of a financial nature, must be eliminated.

4. The accepted code of ethics of the medical profession, which is designed to protect the best interests of the patient, should apply to industrial medical service as to all other forms of medical practice.

An analytic study of the proposals outlined above in the Minimum Standard reveal little to be criticized. The plan on the whole seems sane and workable, and represents an effort to establish and maintain a high standard of professional service in this field. The Committee is to be particularly commended upon their effort to maintain a standard of medical ethics entirely in keeping with modern thought and practice. Especially commendable is their recommendation that "medical and surgical care of the families of employees and of the employees themselves, except for emergency and industrial injuries and diseases, should be provided by the industrial physician only in remote districts where other adequate medical service is not available." This section striking directly at the increasing tendency of medical bodies to extend rather than restrict medical service in the industrial program would return the medical and surgical care of employees and their families for extra industrial injuries or illnesses to the private practitioner. Since the growing tendency experimented with in industrial medicine and in the activities of the Veteran's Bureau has definitely failed to bring benefit either to the community served or to the profession as a whole, this recommendation appears timely and worthy of hearty endorsement.

It would appear unfortunate that recommendation number four "That all patients requiring hospitalization should be sent to institutions approved by the American College of Surgeons"—should appear, since it implies that the classification of hospitals as made by the American College of Surgeons excels that made by other official organizations. The American Medical Association, at much labor and expense, continuously conducts a thorough investigation of all hospitals, and annually advises the entire profession through the medium of the JOURNAL of their findings. It would seem, then, that this official classification would be more accurate and useful than that set up by an association representing members of a limited specialty.

It will be hoped that other influential bodies will give these problems the thoughtful consideration which they deserve, and on a basis of their separate investigations either subscribe to these or outline other principles for the guidance of those engaged in industrial medicine, and allied forms of contract practice.

EXCESSES IN EXERCISE

Youth has often been referred to as the playtime of life. It is during the period of youth, adolescent and young adult life that growth and development take place, and it is during this period that active vigorous physical exercise is physiologically desirable and required. With maturity and the acquisition of sedentary habits, vigorous exercise is ordinarily much restricted or eliminated from the daily schedule of living. With increased business or professional cares the working day is more and more filled with necessary duties, so that exercise becomes neglected, or if not neglected, a matter of duty hastily crowded into a day already too full.

When the individual is vigorous and healthy the need for exercise is easily denied. As the years advance and time begins to take its toll, minor or major physical impairments appear, which usually demand a reckoning. One promptly assumes that the impairments or infirmities noticed are the result of the lack of exercise—that all work and no play is not only making Jack a dull boy, but also a sick boy. Then it is that the obese, flabby business or professional man "takes up golf" or enlists in a gymnastic course at the local Y. M. C. A. Unless tempered in his ambitions by a knowledge of the damage which may result from excessive activities, he may immediately plunge into that vigorous exercise which he once enjoyed and performed with utmost ease, only to find that the physical machine rebels. Lucky is he if this rebellion declares itself in no more than physical exhaustion or muscular pain. Too often a strain is thrown upon the cardiovascular system, which leaves an indelible imprint. Athletes are not made at forty or fifty or sixty years of age. In fact, they are rarely made after thirty-five years of age. Ask your golf or tennis professional, or consult a boxing instructor to verify this statement. Life may begin at forty in many things, particularly the intellectual and the cultural phases of life, but in only the very rarest of instances does the athletic life begin at forty.

Temperance in exercise should be the keynote at this time, and the physician should realize the folly of advising exercise except where proper and due limitations are outlined. A brisk or even a leisurely stroll for an hour may do the middle-aged person, unaccustomed to exercise, a vastly greater good than a set of tennis or even a round of golf. Bear in mind in prescribing exercise as a therapeutic measure that exercise is very likely to be overdone. Be as specific in this regard as you would in outlining a diet or directing the use of a medicine.

Excesses in exercise may be just as harmful to the individual as excesses in eating or drinking, and the definition of excess in any of these regards must be measured in terms of individual endurance.

INVITATION TO WISCONSIN

The State Medical Society of Wisconsin extends a very cordial invitation to members in adjoining states to be guests at its Ninety-third Anniversary Meeting to be held at Green Bay on Wednesday, Thursday and Friday, September 12 to 14. All sessions will be held in the Columbus Community Club, Green Bay.

Morning programs will be devoted to section meetings and clinical presentations, with general sessions each afternoon. The president's address will be given at a smoker Wednesday evening, September 12, while Drs. Olin West, Secretary of the American Medical Association and Dean Lewis, Baltimore, will address the annual dinner on Thursday evening, September 13.

SIXTH ANNUAL MEDICO-MILITARY SYMPOSIUM AT THE MAYO CLINIC

The 1934 Medico-Military Symposium for Medical Department Reserve Officers of the army and navy will be held at the Mayo Clinic, from October 7 to 20, both dates inclusive.

This is the Sixth Annual Inactive Duty Training Course to be held at the Mayo Clinic and will follow the plan which has proved so satisfactory in past years; that is the morning hours will be devoted to clinics on subjects selected by the student officers, and the afternoon and evening hours will be given over to work in medico-military subjects. The program will be under the personal supervision of Colonel Kent Nelson, M.C., U.S. Army, Corps Area Surgeon, Seventh Corps Area, and Captain J. B. Mears, M. C., U. S. Navy, District Medical Officer, Ninth Naval District.

The general motif of the medico-military part of the symposium will be "Public Health and its Relation to National Defense." The problem of administration in military service presents features not dealt with in private practice. In the great field of sanitation as applied to military service, the medical officer has a distinct specialty. This course offers valuable and interesting training for the medical officer in all the components of our national defense. A splendid program of a thoroughly practical nature has been carefully compiled and the speakers selected for their ability to present authoritatively the subjects assigned to them.

Application for this course of Inactive Duty Training should be made either to the Corps Area Surgeon, Seventh Corps Area, Omaha, Nebraska, or to the District Medical Officer, Ninth Naval District, Great Lakes, Illinois. In the application should be stated the character of the work the candidate desires to follow in the morning hours. All student officers are expected to attend and participate in the afternoon and evening sessions. Each applicant should understand that the invitation to accept this course of study without charge is extended by the Mayo Clinic; that the project is without expense to the government and that one hundred hours' credit will be given those who take and complete the course. While it is desirable to attend the entire course, those whose time will not permit this may join or leave at any time and will receive credit for the hours spent in training. Uniforms are optional.

INTER-STATE POST GRADUATE MEDICAL ASSOCIATION OF NORTH AMERICA

The first International Assembly of the Inter-State Post Graduate Medical Association of North America to be held east of the Alleghenies is to take place in the public auditorium of Philadelphia, Pennsylvania, November 5, 6, 7, 8 and 9, 1934, with pre-assembly clinics on November 3 and post-assembly clinics on November 10 in the Philadelphia Hospitals. The public auditorium is located in the university area and across the street from the Philadelphia General Hospital, thus assuring the assembly close access to an abundance of clinical material.

The aim of the program committee with Dr. George W. Crile, as chairman, is to provide for the medical profession of North America an intensive postgraduate course covering the various branches of medical science. The program has been carefully arranged to meet the demands of the general practitioner, as well as the specialist. Extreme care has been given in the selection of the contributors and the subjects of their contributions. The Philadelphia County Medical Society will be host to the assembly and has arranged an excellent list of committees who will function throughout the assembly. A most hearty invitation is extended to all members of the profession who are in good standing in their state or provincial Societies, to be present and enjoy the hospitality of Philadelphia, "the City of Brotherly Love."

A list of distinguished teachers and clinicians who are taking part on the program will be found on page xvii, advertising section of this JOURNAL. Special reduced railroad rates will be in effect on all lines.

SPEAKERS BUREAU ACTIVITIES

TWO COURSES OFFERED IN POSTGRADUATE WORK

The postgraduate work to be offered by the Speakers Bureau this fall consists of two courses, both given by the faculty of the College of Medicine of our State University. One of the courses is a medical course, which was given in four centers last fall and which was so universally liked that the Bureau asked the University to repeat it this fall. The other course is a surgical one—outlined on the same plan, which seemed so highly approved, that is, stressing diagnosis and treatment.

Instead of combining these two courses into a "double-header" and offering them together, as has been the custom in past years, each course is to be given in three different centers. This will permit offering this extension work in more centers, thus reaching more doctors, and it will demand less time of the doctors who wish to take advantage of this opportunity for postgraduate work and yet are too busy to take both courses.

Below is given an outline of the two courses:

A Course in Internal Medicine Pertaining Particularly to Diagnosis and Treatment

By Department of Internal Medicine, College of Medicine, State University of Iowa

1. Gastro-intestinal disorders.

2. The discussion of the clinical significance of the so-called digestive form of distress. The diagnosis of peptic ulcer, gastric malignancy, gall bladder disease and gastro-intestinal neuroses (irritable colon, spastic constipation, etc.), and treatment of each.
   4 hours   Fred M. Smith, M.D.

3. Diabetes: Diagnosis and treatment.
   2 hours   W. D. Paul, M.D.

4. The differential diagnosis and treatment of diseases of the lungs causing chronic cough and dyspnea with particular emphasis on bronchial asthma.
   2 hours   E. L. DeGowin, M.D.

5 and 6.
   Heart Disease: Classification, the diagnosis of organic heart disease and the treatment of congestive failure.
   4 hours   H. M. Korns, M.D.

7. Diseases of the kidneys: Classification of nephritis, the distinguishing features of each type and treatment.
   2 hours   W. M. Fowler, M.D.

8 and 9.
   Diseases of the blood forming organs: Classification, diagnosis of each form, and treatment.
   4 hours   C. W. Baldridge, M.D.

10. Diseases of the thyroid gland: The diagnosis of hyperthyroidism (toxic adenoma and Graves' Disease) and hypothyroidism—treatment.
    2 hours   James A. Greene, M.D.

A Course in Surgery Pertaining Particularly to Diagnosis and Treatment

By the Department of Surgery, College of Medicine, State University of Iowa

1. Urologic Diagnosis in Relation to Abdominal Diagnosis.
   N. G. Alcock, M.D.

2. Diagnosis of Surgical Conditions in the Right Upper Quadrant of the Abdomen.
   H. L. Beye, M.D.

3. Diagnosis and Treatment of Vaginal and Uterine Relaxations.
   J. H. Randall, M.D.

4. Minor Infections of the Hand—Traumatic Lesions of the Tendons and Nerves—Problems in the Diagnosis and Treatment of Acute Appendicitis.
   F. R. Peterson, M.D.

5. Tuberculosis of Bones and Joints.
   Arthur Steindler, M.D.

6. Causes of Hoarseness—Acute and Chronic Suppurative Otitis Media with emphasis on Treatment.
   D. M. Lierle, M.D.

7. Practical Points in the Treatment of the Common Fractures.
   H. L. Beye, M.D.

8. Contractures and Ankylosis.
   Arthur Steindler, M.D.

9. Management of Diseases of the Thyroid Gland—Management of Breast Tumors—Diagnosis and Treatment of Lesions in and about the Rectum and Anus.   F. R. Peterson, M.D.

10. Treatment of Urogenital Malignancies—The Problem of the Enlarged Prostate Gland.
    N. G. Alcock, M.D.

These courses are to start the latter part of September and will be given one evening a week in each center, for a period of ten weeks, from 7:00 to 9:00 p. m. The fee for either one is ten dollars. The medical course is to be offered in three centers in the eastern section of the state and the surgical course in three centers in the central part. Not all of the centers in which the work is to be given are definitely settled, as yet. Humboldt has asked to be one of the centers for the surgical course and the Fort Madison Medical Society voted to have the medical course given there.

The other centers must be determined at once. If the doctors in your community are interested in the course to be given in your section of the state, write the Bureau immediately.

WOMAN'S AUXILIARY NEWS

Edited by the Press and Publicity Committee

MRS. OLIVER J. FAY, *Chairman*, 405 Thirty-seventh Street, Des Moines

Health—Our Greatest Asset and How to Maintain It*

MILDRED MAUER, Minden, Iowa

Health is the condition of our bodies resulting from the normal performance of all the life functions. Health is the foundation of happiness. There is nothing equal to good health to give joy to life. Life seems more worth living and the little irritations which sometimes occur are forgotten when you have good health. To be able to say truthfully that you have good health and that you feel fine today, is one of the most satisfying assets anyone can have.

Health is mental as well as physical. Good health not only means freedom from disease and physical defects but also lack of worry, the idea of success, and a feeling that life is worth living. To be healthy means that you are getting out of life the best there is. Nearly everybody can have good health if he is willing to try to reach the goal.

Some immediate advantages of having good health are that you will always be happy and pleasant and you'll be able to do your work well. You'll enjoy sports and will always be lively and full of pep. If you have good health, which everyone should try to have, you will be able to gain more friends. Nobody likes a friend who is laggy and always tired.

Your body is almost like an engine or car. Nerves in your body carry impulses back and forth just as wires do in cars. An engine is kept in good running order by having it repaired and by keeping it well oiled; while you must keep your body in good health by eating the proper foods, that is, foods that have a great amount of food values in them; and by taking exercise. Most people pay more attention to their cars to see that they are in good order than to their bodies. If they would just reverse their practices they would gain far more in the long run.

To be and to keep healthy you must eat the proper foods. Food is like coal. It is a form of energy. Your body is a living machine for taking this energy and changing it into heat, motion, and thought. Since it is a "living" machine it can turn the fuel it takes into growth and repair for the body. The eating of *proper* foods and their good digestion are most important. The most essential foods for your body are those containing plenty of minerals and vitamines besides caloric values. The life and alertness of your body will depend not on the amount of food you consume but upon the kind of food—its power to build and repair your body, to make your body strong and able to resist invading disease germs.

Milk is the best single food because it supplies almost every element necessary for growth and energy. To make sure you are not getting disease germs from the milk it should be properly pasteurized. Simple foods should compose your diet. Whole grain cereals and breads, fruits and vegetables in abundance, with a moderate supply of meats and proteins will usually insure a healthy body.

Your teeth may blight your health. Therefore look to their care with great diligence. One defect in the foods which we eat is that they require so little chewing that the teeth are not exercised enough to keep in a healthy condition. If you can obtain coarse, rough foods in your diet you are both fortunate and wise. But to insure good sound teeth you should brush them at least twice daily with a stiff brush. Visit your dentist twice a year and let him clean your teeth and protect them against dental decay. A stupid American habit very destructive to teeth is the unwise eating of candy. The food value in candy is high, but partaking of the sweets between meals only lessens your appetite and also leads to decay in your teeth. For the sugar left in the crevices of the teeth turns to acid which in turn dissolves the enamel surface and allows decay to begin. The mouth is the first step in digestion and therefore

---

* This essay was awarded second place in the recently conducted health essay contest. The essay which took first place has been read over Radio Stations WOI and WSUI.

a healthy body must have a clean, healthy mouth.

Water is of prime importance to life. Plenty of water used inside and out makes a clean body inside and out. Water makes up seventy-eight per cent of the body's weight and is present in nearly all foods. It does not build body tissues or provide energy, but it helps the secretions within the body which are needed for life itself. It behooves you to drink water often and in ample amounts to maintain the body content, to avoid faulty elimination, and to provide the body need.

Your body requires exercise to make good circulation of its life-bringing blood to all its tiny cells. Muscles will become stronger because more blood reaches each muscle cell to bring food and to carry back waste materials. The only force the blood in the veins has is that provided by exercise which works the vessel walls and pushes the blood along. The heart itself is strengthened by exercise for the same reasons the other muscles are, and it can thereby be more efficient. Exercise in open air and in the sunshine is best for your body. You will be sure of getting the best air it is possible for you to get; you can get more oxygen into your lungs, which is the great force for assimilation of food. Direct sunshine brings health-giving rays important to bones, and important in providing disease resisting vitamines. Direct sunshine has proved itself a cure for several diseases. For those who can not get sunshine, cod-liver oil has proved a wonderful substitute.

After a day's schedule of work, exercise, and recreation, should come adequate, restful, and deserved sleep. You cannot expect your heart to go at top speed for hours upon end without rest. During sleep your heart gets its only rest; and although it does not stop working it is resting. Sufficient sleep for your body demands should be one of your most important health habits.

One of the biggest mistakes in our American life is over-indulgence. Over-eating especially is a habit often formed while young. To break it you should form the new habit of quitting your meal when you are comfortably satisfied. Eating too much causes indigestion, sluggishness, and obesity.

Even though you are in fairly good health you should visit the doctor at least once a year and the dentist twice a year. Then if anything is wrong with your body or teeth you will find it out before it is too late and too much damage has been done. Diseases may often be checked at their very onset. Both time and money, as well as the supreme factor, health, will be saved.

A mentally healthy person has good mental health habits as well as physical ones. He is able to look the world in the face without fear. He is able to meet the problems of life with pretty good success, and to do it without too much strain or worry. You must form the habit of facing future problems without worry. As a rule the greatest per cent of what you fear will never happen. You must control your temper, have a feeling of good will toward your fellow man, and have a certain trust in the world of man and God.

The two most important things everyone seeks to attain are happiness and success. Before you can hope to attain these, you must have a healthy body and a sound mind. Few people succeed with an unhealthy body, and none with an unbalanced mind. It is up to the owner of the mind and body to get his wish.

SOCIETY PROCEEDINGS

Cerro Gordo County Host to Second District

A combined meeting of members of the Cerro Gordo County Medical Society and physicians of the Second Councilor District was held Tuesday afternoon and evening, August 14, at Clear Lake. The afternoon session was addressed by Fred Moore, M.D., of Des Moines, and R. D. Bernard, M.D., of Clarion, on the merits of the basic science law that is now in force in a number of states. The law proposed for the state of Iowa was thoroughly discussed, and favorable adoption of its principles was voted by the organization. H. D. Fallows, M.D., of Mason City, chairman of the Cerro Gordo County fact finding committee, reported on his committee's work. More than one hundred physicians, wives, and guests were present at the six-thirty picnic dinner served by the Woman's Auxiliary to the Cerro Gordo County Medical Society, after which Oliver J. Fay, M.D., of Des Moines, delivered the address of the evening, speaking on Observations on the New Economic Decalogue as Presented at the Last Meeting of the American Medical Association.

Dallas-Guthrie Society

The annual meeting of the Dallas-Guthrie Medical Society was held at Woodward, Tuesday, August 2. Dr. E. M. Myers of Boone presided as toastmaster during the dinner program, at which Dr. Walter L. Bierring of Des Moines, president of the American Medical Association, was present as an honored guest, delivering an address in the nature of a eulogy to Dr. M. N. Voldeng, superintendent of the

State Hospital at Woodward, who has given nearly fifty years of service to organized medicine. The afternoon session, which began at two-thirty, consisted of the following papers: Problems of the State Society, Thomas A. Burcham, M.D., of Des Moines, president elect of the Iowa State Medical Society; Diagnosis and Surgical Treatment of Carcinoma of the Breast, Stuart W. Harrington, M.D., of The Mayo Clinic, Rochester; and Presentation of Clinical Cases by the Woodward State Hospital staff, M. Nelson Voldeng, M.D., A. L. Smith, M.D., Grace Sawyer, M.D., and R. A. Foster, M.D.

Jackson County

The annual Mississippi catfish dinner of the Jackson County Medical Society was held Thursday, August 2, at the Bellevue State Park. The scientific program was furnished by two physicians from the State University of Iowa College of Medicine; Dean M. Lierle, M.D., speaking on Otolaryngology From the Standpoint of the Practitioner, and Nathaniel G. Alcock, M.D., talking on The Resection Method in the Treatment of Diseases of the Prostate. A social hour after the meeting was held at the home of Dr. E. L. Lampe.

Council Bluffs Medical Society

Dr. J. L. Stech was elected president of the Council Bluffs Medical Society, at the annual meeting held Wednesday, August 22, at the Hotel Chieftain. Other officers are: Dr. C. A. Hill, vice president; Dr. Harriett Hamilton, secretary, and Dr. M. C. Hennessy, treasurer.

New Officers—Iowa-Illinois Central District Medical Society

Newly elected officers of the Iowa-Illinois Central District Medical Society, named at a meeting held in Davenport, Thursday, July 26, are: Dr. J. C. Souders of Rock Island, Illinois, president; Dr. Howard A. Weis of Davenport, vice president; Dr. James Dunn of Davenport, secretary; Dr. F. E. Bollaert of East Moline, Illinois, treasurer, and Drs. Harry Lamb of Davenport and Carl Wahlberg of Moline, censors.

INTERESTING NEWS
In Brief

In some unexplained fashion infants up to about five months of age are capable of providing their own supply of Vitamin C.

A recent survey indicates that one-fifth of the beds in general hospitals in this country are used for patients with chronic diseases.

The first full-blooded Indian woman to become a public health nurse has begun her work among her own people on the Navajo Reservation.

It has been estimated that the death rate in the New York City slum area was six times greater sixty-five years ago than it is today.

The publicity accorded the Canadian quintuplets has brought out the statement that ancient writers mentioned quintuplet births in Egypt, Greece and Rome.

Although rare in this country, the tropical disease of dengue fever has appeared in epidemic form in Miami, Florida, this past summer, with a toll of some eighty cases.

The state of Baden, Germany, has published a warning of punishment for persons who ridicule subjects of sterilization operations, of which 572 have been performed since January 1, 1934.

Researches suggesting the possible existence of a heretofore unknown vitamin, have been conducted at the University in Copenhagen. This new vitamin is related to Vitamin C and is described as the antihemorrhagic factor.

For his outstanding service to American chemistry in his researches on blood hemoglobin and the chlorophyll of plants Harvard's newly elected president, Dr. James Bryant Conant, has been awarded the annual medal presented by the American Institue of Chemists.

The Federal Communications Commission has returned the application of Norman Baker of Muscatine, Iowa, for a permit to construct a radio station in that city, with the explanation that the state of Iowa had filled its quota of radio stations and that further permits could not be granted.

A graduate research student at the California Institute of Technology, has recently devised a new radio knife for surgery, which is said to have all the advantages of the present electric high-frequency surgical knives without the use of bothersome electric wire connections.

PERSONAL MENTION

Dr. W. S. Balkema, after concluding a year's practice in Newton, has moved his home and office to Sheldon.

Dr. Carl V. Lendgren, formerly of Eddyville, has accepted a position in the Hamlin Clinic at Estelline, South Dakota.

Dr. M. J. Brown of West Liberty has moved to Wellman, where he will be associated in the practice of medicine with Dr. A. L. Braden. Dr. Brown was graduated in 1933 from the State University of Iowa College of Medicine, and served his internship at the City Hospital in Akron, Ohio.

Dr. H. N. King, psychiatrist for the past four years at the United States Veterans Hospital in Knoxville, has been transferred to the Mount Alto Hospital in Washington, D. C.

Dr. Clarence Sears has located in Mechanicsville for the practice of medicine, having been graduated in 1932 from the State University of Iowa College of Medicine, and served a two years' internship at the General Hospital in Youngstown, Ohio.

Dr. T. J. Pfeffer, who has practiced medicine in DeWitt for the past three years, has accepted a position on the staff of Kings County Hospital in New York City. Dr. T. J. Nereim is moving from Lime Springs to DeWitt to fill the vacancy created by Dr. Pfeffer's appointment.

Dr. Peter A. Bendixen of Davenport, was elected president of the Association of Chicago, Milwaukee, St. Paul and Pacific Railway Surgeons, at a meeting held in Chicago, Tuesday, August 21.

Dr. Edward H. Paulus, a recent graduate of the State University of Iowa College of Medicine, who has spent the last two years interning at the University of Michigan Hospital in Ann Arbor, has located in Iowa City for the private practice of medicine.

Dr. H. J. Patchin, formerly of Cambridge, has located in Maxwell, where he will continue the practice of medicine.

Dr. C. A. Carroll, who has practiced for the past year in Manchester, has moved to Fort Collins, Colorado.

Dr. Haven McClurg, a graduate of the State University of Iowa College of Medicine, has located in Keosauqua, where he will be associated with Dr. E. E. Sherman. Dr. McClurg served his internship at the Western Reserve Hospital in Cleveland, Ohio.

Dr. A. E. Putz, formerly of Granville, has moved his office and family to Sheldon, where he will continue in the practice of medicine.

Dr. W. H. Jenks, who has practiced for some time in Tipton, has left that city to make his home in Phoenix, Arizona.

Dr. E. B. Woods is leaving Valley Junction for Augusta, Georgia, where he has accepted a position as assistant professor in obstetrics and gynecology at the University of Georgia Medical School. Dr. Fred Sternagel of Williamsburg is assuming Dr. Woods' practice in Valley Junction, coming direct from Williamsburg where he has been practicing for the past five years.

Dr. H. C. Yates of Mt. Vernon, announces the association of Dr. E. N. Hesbacher of Des Moines, in the practice of medicine with him. Dr. Hesbacher is a graduate of the State University of Iowa College of Medicine, and has just completed his internship at the Butterworth Hospital in Grand Rapids, Michigan.

Dr. C. A. Conklin, formerly of Garden Grove, has moved to Des Moines, where he will establish a practice in the Highland Park district.

Dr. Charles McLaughlin, Jr., son of Dr. C. U. McLaughlin of Washington, left New York recently for a trip to Edinburgh, Scotland, where he will spend several months with Dr. P. D. Wilkie, professor of surgery at the University of Edinburgh. Dr. McLaughlin also plans to work in the Royal Infirmary and Laboratory of Research Surgery of the University.

Dr. L. J. Leech of West Branch, newly chosen state G. A. R. commander, was the guest of honor at a celebration held in West Branch, Friday, August 3. Nearly two thousand people gathered to hear the musical program and special tributes paid to this eighty-eight year old Civil War veteran.

MARRIAGES

The wedding of Miss Helen Anderson and Dr. George D. Callahan, both of Iowa City took place Wednesday, August 22, at St. Patrick's Church in Iowa City. Dr. Callahan has just recently located in Iowa City for the practice of medicine, coming from Grinnell, where he had practiced for several months. After a short wedding trip to Chicago and Kansas City, Dr. and Mrs. Callahan will be at home in Iowa City.

DEATH NOTICES

Castles, Thomas Ralph, of Albia, aged fifty-two, died July 27 at the Iowa Methodist Hospital in Des Moines after a year's illness. He was graduated in 1907 from the Northwestern University Medical School, Chicago, and at the time of his death was a member of the Monroe County Medical Society.

Dougherty, John Philip, of Sioux City, aged fifty-seven, died August 11 afer a short illness of pneumonia. He was graduated in 1904 from the University of Illinois College of Medicine, Chicago, and at the time of his death was a member of the Woodbury County Medical Society.

Garrett, John Milton, of Fort Dodge, aged sixty-five, died suddenly August 18 of heart disease. He was graduated in 1892 from the Marion-Sims College of Medicine, St. Louis, and at the time of his death was a member of the Webster County Medical Society.

RADIO BROADCASTS

WOI—Mondays, 5:30-5:45
WSUI—Thursdays, 7:45-8:00

September 10-13—The Nervous Child, Martin D. Ott, M. D.
September 17-20—Gall Stones, J. M. Burger, M. D.
September 24-27—The Problem of Sweets for Children, Gail McClure, M. D.
October   1- 4—The Story of Anesthesia, John Russell, M.D.

HISTORY OF MEDICINE IN IOWA

Edited by the Historical Committee

DR. HENRY B. YOUNG, Burlington   DR. TOM. B. THROCKMORTON, Des Moines
DR. FRANK M. FULLER, Keokuk'   DR. WALTER L. BIERRING, Des Moines
DR. JOHN T. MCCLINTOCK, Iowa City   DR. WILLIAM JEPSON, Sioux City

Notes on Medical Licensure in Iowa

Licensure to practice medicine in Iowa came about in the late eighties. Prior to that time any person could announce himself as a physician, hang out his shingle, and begin the practice of the healing art. Naturally, in many instances, abuses sprang up as a result of indifference on the part of the public, and of those physicians who had obtained diplomas from reputable medical colleges. Charlatanism flourished like a green bay tree in many localities. Both the public and the reputable physician could do nothing legally to prevent the quacks from extolling their wares. When some of the sister states underwent a thorough house-cleaning by passing Medical Practice Acts, many of their undesirable practitioners found refuge on the prairie soil of Iowa, and continued to carry on their nefarious trade. In time, matters became so chaotic that the Iowa Legislature was forced to protect the people as well as the legitimate practitioner against these undesirable personages; hence a Medical Practice Act was passed.

The first meeting of the State Board of Medical Examiners was held July 8, 1886. At that time it was estimated that there were more than three thousand physicians in the state. The legal demand that these physicians comply with the law by registering with the Board, met with a great deal of indifference on the part of many members of the medical profession. Some physicians, who had been graduated from well known medical colleges, felt resentful that they should ,be obliged to register. Was not their diploma sufficient evidence of their fitness to practice medicine? One physician, a graduate of the Jefferson Medical College of Philadelphia, was highly incensed that he should be questioned by the State of Iowa concerning his fitness to practice the healing art. In substantiation of his claim, he pointed out to the Board of Examiners that his diploma,—transcribed in Latin on genuine sheepskin—if properly translated, would reveal to its several august members that "to him by virtue of this Diploma, we (the Faculty) have conceded and made valid, most

willingly and most fully, the several laws, honors, and privileges pertaining to the degree of Doctor in the Art of Healing *Among Us and Everywhere throughout the World.*"

However, the Iowa State Board of Medical Examiners took a firm stand on its prerogatives. It warned the physicians of Iowa that they must —willingly or otherwise—register and be certified. The following notice was sent out through the pages of the *Iowa State Medical Reporter,* September, 1886.

NOTICE TO PHYSICIANS

Iowa State Board of Medical Examiners
Office of the Secretary

Des Moines, Iowa, Oct. 11, 1886.

A meeting of the Iowa State Board of Medical Examiners will be held in this city at the Board of Health rooms, beginning at 2:00 o'clock P. M., Tuesday, Nov. 9th prox., for the purpose of verifying diplomas, receiving and voting upon applications for certificates to practice medicine, examining applicants and attending to such other business as may come before it.

All physicians who expect to continue the practice of medicine in this state after the first of January next and all midwifes who have commenced practice since April 3, 1886, should not fail to file their applications before November 9th. It is not probable that another meeting will be held, and a failure to procure a certificate will be a source of great embarrassment as well as expense. Blanks and all needed information will be promptly and cheerfully furnished by   J. F. Kennedy, Secretary.

In time the law became generally observed. Within five years after its passage, "the State Board of Medical Examiners had issued certificates to 3,871 applicants, unconditionally rejected 175, and compelled 86 to come up for examination. Of this latter number about fifty per cent ultimately passed, some of them after several trials. One persistent individual failed twice in succession, left the state for two years, came back and failed twice more, went away to a recognized college and was graduated; came back and passed on his diploma in triumph." Who could say that Iowa had no attractions as a field in which to practice medicine?

Undoubtedly it was just·such happenings as the one mentioned which aroused the ire of some of the "regulars." *The Vis Medicatrix*, the official organ for the Journal of the Iowa State Medical Society, edited by the late Dr. Woods Hutchinson in the April issue, 1892, published a paper which I feel may well be reproduced for its historical value concerning medical licensure and certification of physicians in Iowa. The author of this paper evidently had no intention of mincing words or of handling the situation with silk gloves. In the parlance of the pugilistic ring, he also made no effort "to pull his punches." The rabbit punch was then unknown, but many an individual, if he lived, knew how it felt to be kicked by a Missouri mule. As to whether the author had ever been the recipient of such a blow, I have no knowledge; however, I leave it to the readers of his paper as to whether or not his pen was not mightier than an angry mule's hoof.   T. B. T.

WHAT SHALL WE DO TO BE SAVED?

OSCAR BURBANK, M.D., Waverly

This is a question as old as the religious faith of our fathers, nor has the intensity of its interest diminished during these twenty centuries. It no longer relates exclusively to the hereafter, but concerns·all the affairs of the present life. It has become the great question of every party, political or religious, and permeates every occupation of labor. The organization of every profession, of every trade, of every occupation, into societies with set laws, rules and obligations, shows plainly enough the drift of popular thought at this time. The avowed object of all these dissimilar associations is for mutual protection, a more fraternal feeling, a general discussion of fair wages, mutual improvement, and efficiency in the various vocations of life.

All the labor movements and strikes are only vast currents of common thought moving in one direction, guided by the common instinct of self preservation.

The medical profession is no exception to the general tendency for every occupation to organize for its own salvation, as the county, city, state, national and other medical societies bear witness. Looking over the advertising columns of the medical colleges we find the general tendency is for a fuller and more perfect medical education in those whom they graduate. The polyclinic schools, schools for practitioners of medicine, are so many fingerboards pointing to the want of medical efficiency. All sorts of medical associations are clamoring for a higher state of knowlege and efficiency in the new-comers, and under this pressure many states have made laws to examine into the qualifications of all new doctors coming into the state, but I have never heard of any law unfavorable to the old medical snags that lie hidden in

th stream of medical life to wreck whoever is so unfortunate as to run against them.

In the river we blow up snags with dynamite, but in our profession we silently wait for the old man with the scythe. Is this honest and fair? Is it right that a man who has quacked it for a dozen years shall, on that account, and on that alone, be legally adjudged a legal practitioner of medicine, while another man with all the qualifications for his business must be examined by the state board or step down and out?

Some years ago Minnesota and Illinois enacted Medical Practice Acts, with state boards of examiners, with the happy result, to them, of unloading a part of their incompetent practitioners upon the state of Iowa. We petitioned the legislature, asking for laws unfavorable to this class of medical men, but the legislators replied substantially that it was not the business of an Iowa legislature to create a *privileged class*, and they did not.

In looking over the medical directory of Iowa for the year 1883 and 1884, I find there were 1,727 men with diplomas and 1,034 who had none. About five quacks to eight diplomas. What about these diplomas, and who granted them? Some were granted by the Hahnemann institutions, some by the Eclectic, some by the Physio-medical, and a few by the Buchanan institution. If to these we add the M.D. belonging to the liars (this word has no reference to a musical instrument) it will be about fair to assume that half of the doctors were never entitled to a diploma.

In my time, I have seen hung up in physicians' offices sheepskins upon which were inscribed the righteousness of the name therein mentioned and certified to by learned professors. Now what this part of the sheep's anatomy had to do with the doctor's qualifications for the practice of medicine after more than forty years of trying to find out, I freely confess I cannot understand. Many years ago a doctor died in our place leaving his diploma behind. Some years after this an old medical snag consulted me in relation to purchasing this diploma. I inquired of him what use he could make of a diploma, if he would use it to make an infusion, or an extract, or pills, or powders. I soon found out that he had no idea what a diploma was. He seemed to think it contained the essence of all medical knowledge, a sort of little god on wheels, that would be handy to consult when shadows fell across his way.

If this old quack could have lived until the Medical Practice Act of Iowa was passed he would have added one more to the legal practitioners of medicine in Iowa. If ever the legislature of Iowa passed an act that did not mean anything, and was not intended to mean anything, the Medical Practice Act is one.

When the Medical Practice Act of Illinois went into effect on May 1, 1882, of the 8,951 practitioners of medicine in the state, 2,725 quit the business or left the state, giving Iowa her share of the dump. The Medical Practice Act of Iowa made medical ignorance respectable, by making it legal, so nobody quit the business or left the state. These fellows are asking us, "what are you going to do about it?"

If the medical act means anything it is that time sanctifies a wrong, for if five years of charlatanry had just ended when the act went into effect, that time, in the judgment of an Iowa legislature, constituted a legal qualification. This is a free country, and class legislation is offensive. Does the legislature believe what it practices? Look at the sanitary laws. If a contagious disease exists in a house, the house is flagged with a red flag, a danger signal. Here the individual right yields to the public good; but when one of these unqualified medical men goes about the country, more dangerous than any contagious disease, what Iowa legislature ever thought of flagging him? A pile of manure in a back alley, or even on your own lot, causes a visit from the health officer. Here, again, personal rights yield to the public good. The dunce has as good a natural right to the head of his class as any other member of the class, but if he gets there he will have to win the position. Every aspirant for legal fame must be examined. No five years of being the oracle in his vicinity admits him to practice. Our school teachers must pass a satisfactory examination before they can teach the humblest child. These examinations must be repeated yearly, beside the institute attendance of about a month, all involving cost to the teacher, and all for the public good.

Why should the medical profession be an exception to the general rule? Can it be that the representatives of the people regard it as a grand humbug from A to Z?

Is it any use to groan because the people give their patronage to unqualified practitioners of medicine? When we have groaned and scolded and resolved, who has cared or paid any attention to it, and why should they until the regular profession of medicine can demonstrate to the public their superior claim upon public confidence?

With humility and becoming modesty I venture to suggest a remedy which I think no legislature of Iowa would regard as class legislation. It is a square deal all around. With this idea clearly before them, I think no legislator will refuse his vote to a Medical Practice Act, whose object clearly is the public safety, and treats every medical man alike. It is to do unto others as you would have them do unto you. Some centuries before the Christian era this idea was propounded in the Roman senate, and later it reappears in the gospels. It has lost nothing of its beauty or intensity as it has rolled down the ages. It is still a yard wide, dyed in the wool, and warranted not to fade.

My plan is to legally organize an able board of state medical examiners, who shall examine every medical man and pass judgment upon his qualifications for the practice of medicine, letting nothing influence the results except the answers to the questions. Whoever passes, give him a diploma, and whoever cannot pass, let him step down and out, until he can.

In my opinion the trade-marks upon too many doctors' signs would disappear, for then they would be prouder of their State Board diplomas than of the flaunting lie that now disgraces their signs, and if a doctor had a peculiar notion as to how a medicine wrought a cure, or how much or how often it should be taken, it would be regarded as his private judgment and nobody's business but his own. The fact that a doctor holds a diploma from an able state examining board is at least a public guarantee that he is fairly up in medical science, and I think the medical profession would not refuse him consultation because he was a crank in materia medica or anything else. Under such a rule or law the state of Iowa would secure a more efficient medical service than any state ever had.

I would give everyone a year, or some reasonable time, to prepare for the examination, and if in that time he cannot win his diploma it should be evidence that he was so ignorant and incompetent that justice and the public safety require him to step down and out. I would lead the old medical fossil out into the stream of medical science as it flows today, giving him a fresh baptism in its pure waters, renewing his faith in medical works.

If the public good requires school teachers to be examined every year, I am of the opinion that the public safety also requires every physician to be examined at stated times. I have several certificates over fifty years old, saying that I was qualified to teach a common town-school. Would your superintendent of public instruction permit me to teach school on such a certificate?

I have a diploma over forty years old, granted by the medical department of Harvard University, Massachusetts, but is that any evidence that I am up with the science of medicine, and qualified for its duties today?

I well know that my suggestion, by some men having diplomas hanging in their offices, as a sort of fetish, will be viewed with holy horror. To them it is wellnigh irreverent to call in question the soundness of the hoary custom and sanctified precedent that allows one to fall back in dignified silence upon an old diploma which today means nothing, instead of answering the question which this marching age with its battle cry of onward, asks of every man. "Are you posted" in your special line of work? Having presented these suggestions, I again ask you "What Shall we do to be Saved?"

JOURNALS SOUGHT BY MEDICAL LIBRARY

Dr. Jeannette Dean-Throckmorton, librarian of the Iowa State Medical Library, is anxious to secure old copies of the blue backed journals, which were issued when Dr. E. E. Dorr was editor of the IOWA MEDICAL JOURNAL. In this connection it is well to remember that the Medical Library welcomes any and all contributions of old journals and books. It is true that the Medical Library exists to serve the members of the Iowa State Medical Society, and it deserves and has a right to expect our loyal support. This obligation can be filled, in a measure, by responding to the appeals which come to us from our librarian.

THE JOURNAL BOOK SHELF

BOOKS RECEIVED

THE DANGEROUS AGE IN MEN—A Treatise on the Prostate Gland by Chester Tilton Stone, M.D., Ridgewood, New Jersey. The Macmillan Company, New York, 1934. Price, $1.75.

INDUSTRIAL TOXICOLOGY—By Alice Hamilton, M.D., Boston, Massachusetts. Harper's Medical Monographs. Harper and Brothers Publishers, 49 East 33d Street, New York City, 1934. Price, $3.00.

THE LABORATORY NOTEBOOK METHOD IN TEACHING PHYSICAL DIAGNOSIS AND CLINICAL HISTORY RECORDING—By Logan Clendening, M.D., Professor of Clinical Medicine, University of Kansas. C. V. Mosby Company, St. Louis, Missouri, 1934. Price, 50c.

MEDICAL CLINICS OF NORTH AMERICA—Volume xvii, No. 6. Chicago Number, Index volume. Octavo of 266 pages with 38 illustrations. Per clinic year July, 1933, to May, 1934. W. B. Saunders Company, Philadelphia and London, 1934. Price, paper, $12.00; cloth, $16.00.

THE MERCK MANUAL OF THERAPEUTICS AND MATERIA MEDICA—Sixth edition, compiled and published by Merck & Company, Inc., Rahway, New Jersey, 1934.

POSTURES AND PRACTICES DURING LABOR AMONG PRIMITIVE PEOPLES—By Julius Jarcho, M.D., New York City. With 130 illustrations. Paul B. Hoeber, Inc., New York, 1934. Price, $3.50.

A PRIMER FOR DIABETIC PATIENTS—A Brief Outline of the Treatment of Diabetes with Diet and Insulin. By Russell M. Wilder, M.D., professor of medicine, The Mayo Founda-

tion. Fifth edition, reset and revised, 172 pages. W. B. Saunders Company, Philadelphia and London, 1934. Price, $1.75.

THE SPASTIC CHILD—A Record of Successfully Achieved Muscle Control in Little's Disease—By Marguerite K. Fischel, C. V. Mosby Company, St. Louis, Missouri, 1934. Price, $1.50.

SURGICAL CLINICS OF NORTH AMERICA—Volume xiv, No. 3, Mayo Clinic Number, June, 1934. Octavo of 221 pages with 70 illustrations. W. B. Saunders·Company, Philadel-phia and London, 1934. Price, paper, $12.00; cloth, $16.00.

TEST TUBE BABIES—A History of the Artificial Impregnation of Human Beings. By Dr. Hermann Rohleder. The Pan-urge Press, 70 Fifth Avenue, New York City, 1934. Price, $3.50.

A TEXTBOOK OF GYNECOLOGY—By Arthur Hale Curtis, M.D., professor and head of the department of obstetrics and gynecology, Northwestern University Medical School. Second edition, reset; 493 pages with 300 original illustra-tions. W. B. Saunders Company, Philadelphia and London, 1934. Price, $6.00.

THAT HEART OF YOURS—By S. Calvin Smith, M.D., Sc.D. Illustrated. J. B. Lippincott Company, Philadelphia, Lon-don and Montreal, 1934. Price, $2.00.

TROUBLES WE DON'T TALK ABOUT—By J. F. Montague, M.D., F.A.C.S., New York Intestinal Sanitarium, 139 East 36th St., New York City. Second edition, revised and en-larged; illustrated. J. B. Lippincott Company, Philadelphia and London, 1933. Price, $1.00.

BOOK REVIEWS

THE BUSINESS MAN AND HIS HEALTH

By Jesse Feiring Williams, M.D., professor of physical education at Teachers College, Columbia University. McGraw-Hill Book Company, New York and London, 1932· Price, $2.00.

It is estimated that over 50 per cent of America's 126 million population are indoor workers. It is quite worthwhile then that some active investiga-tions regarding their special requirements for health should be conducted.

Of these factors perhaps none are greater than the effort of the city dweller to obtain the amount of physical exercise which he feels is required. Dr. Williams exhibits a keen appreciation of these prob-lems and a sympathetic understanding of the in-door worker's viewpoint. He discusses exercise in modern life, the usefulness and place of hobbies, when and how to take a vacation, and the mental hygiene necessary for health. He discusses the prob-lems of the retired business man and how he may prevent the degeneration of ennui.

The entire book is written in a delightfully pleas-ant style that carries the reader swiftly along through the pages of his very practical discussion. We fully believe that any physician who will read or even partly read this small volume will agree that it is not only safe, but highly desirable to place the volume in the hands of every adult indoor worker.

CORRECTIVE PHYSICAL EDUCATION

By Josephine Langworthy Rathbone, M.A., instructor in physical education, Teachers College, Columbia University, New York City. 292 pages with 153 illustrations. W. B. Saunders Company, Philadelphia and London, 1934. Price, $2.50.

This book has been prepared for students of phys-ical education and physical therapy, and presents in small compass the basic knowledge necessary for reconstructive physical education. In the opening chapters of the volume the author reviews the neces-sary anatomy and physiology of muscles and joints, and properly stresses the blood supply and innerva-tion of these parts. She then proceeds to a dis-cussion of the treatment necessary for each type of underdevelopment or faulty development.

Appreciating that the technic for applying these corrective exercises may vary and be subject to con-troversy, the author, with commendable insight, has stressed the physiologic and psychologic principles which underlie the treatment of the given condition, and has emphasized the mental and emotional factors to be studied and corrected.

Recognizing that many of the physical defects for which reconstructive exercises are demanded, oc-cur in the early developmental period of a child's life, the author has devoted a full chapter to the dis-cussion of the responsibility of the school in preventing and correcting physical defects, particularly those of a postural character.

The volume is commended to the attention of the physician since this reconstructive work should be carried out under his direction, and for this reason it is essential that he be familiar with a reliable text, not only one for his own use, but one that may safely be placed in the hands of his patient or his patient's nurse.

A DOCTOR STUDIES CRIME

By Perry M. Lichtenstein, M.D., formerly resident physician, City Prison, Manhattan (Tombs). D. Van Nostrand Company, 250 Fourth Avenue, New York, 1934. Price, $3.00.

Digressing from the traditional practice in the handling of medical criminology, Dr. Lichtenstein presents in this volume those factors in criminal behaviorism which may be detected in the growing child, since it is his conviction that more can be done to regulate and control crime by prevention than will ever be accomplished by punishment. His discussion of the various problems involved in this study is exemplified by many individual citations taken from his years of contact with criminals as prison physician.

His chapter on moral defects not only shows unusual insight into the problems of criminology, but also points the way toward the recognition of a moral defect in the behavior of the growing child.

The volume has not been prepared for the advanced criminologist, but rather for the lay student and the general public. Any physician will be well repaid in the reading of this revealing study of criminals.

SURGICAL CLINICS OF NORTH AMERICA

Volume xiv, No. 1, Philadelphia Number, February, 1934. Per clinic year, February, 1934, to December, 1934. 226 pages with 62 illustrations. W. B. Saunders Company, Philadelphia and London, 1934. Price, paper $12.00; cloth, $16.00.

There are two outstanding articles in this number. The first deals with postoperative pulmonary atelectasis. Here the author presents a critical analysis of thirty-two cases occurring during the past ten and one-half years in his practice. Of these, twenty-three occurred in males and nine in females. Fifty per cent developed following operation on the stomach or biliary tract. Of the postoperative cases, 83 per cent developed during the first three postoperative days. Thirty of the cases were treated conservatively, two were subjected to bronchoscopy and three died.

A second outstanding group of three articles discusses foreign bodies in the gastro-intestinal tract. These articles discuss the subject from the standpoint of the surgeon, the internist and the roentgenologist. These discussions demonstrate the need for cooperation between these three specialists for the successful management of these cases.   F. W. F.

SURGICAL CLINICS OF NORTH AMERICA

Volume xiv, No. 2. New York Number, April, 1934. Per clinic year February, 1934, to December, 1934; 200 pages with 71 illustrations. W. B. Saunders Company, Philadelphia and London, 1934. Price, paper, $12.00; cloth, $16.00.

In this number there are some very interesting and practical articles. Among them may be mentioned Dr. Keyes' presentation of the management of cases of urinary retention due to prostatic disease. Because of the practical nature of this clinic it will be appreciated by both the general practitioner and the specialist.

Ludwig's angina is discussed, and several cases are reported. The treatment presented is radical in that it involves the resection of the submaxillary gland. Justification of the treatment appears established in the good results reported.

The treatment of peptic ulcer is presented with special reference to the operation of gastro-enterostomy.

Two unusual cases of common duct obstruction are reported, the one due to a very large stone and the second due to echinococcus daughter cyst.

A closing section presents a very interesting report of an analysis of the deaths occurring in the gynecologic service of the Woman's Hospital during the year 1932.   F. W. F.

TUBERCULOSIS IN THE CHILD AND THE ADULT

A discussion of pathologic anatomy, physiology, immunology, diagnosis and treatment. By Francis M. Pottenger, M.D., clinical professor of medicine, University of Southern California School of Medicine. Illustrated. C. V. Mosby Company, St. Louis, 1934. Price, $8.50.

This new work on tuberculosis has been prepared by an outstanding authority and reflects his experiences and observations in a very large number of cases. He stresses particularly childhood infections and their relationship to the problems of prevention and active tuberculosis in the adult. He discusses the reactions of the body toward infection, emphasizing the importance of a knowledge of these reactions and the part that immunity plays not only in the outcome of the disease but in its symptomatology and diagnosis.

He maintains that the proper choice of methods for treatment should be based solely upon maintaining an adequate natural and specific resistance, and in bringing about mechanical conditions within the chest which are favorable to cure.

Because of its clearness in description, its thorough treatment of the subject and its authoritative background, we predict an immediate popularity for this work. Because of the fundamental handling of this problem and the careful analysis of essentials, the book will have on especial appeal for the general practitioner.

The JOURNAL

of the

Iowa State Medical Society

Vol. XXIV Des Moines, Iowa, October, 1934 No. 10

MEDICAL CLINICS*

FIRST DAY

LATENT SYPHILIS AS A CAUSE OF HEART DISEASE

R. Wesley Scott, M.D., Cleveland, Ohio

Had I known that syphilitic heart disease was as rare in this state as my friends here tell me it is, I might have selected another subject for discussion this morning, but even if it is unusual in Iowa, latent syphilis as the cause of heart failure is by no means rare in other parts of the country. For example, data from the registration area indicate that syphilis is responsible for from ten to fifteen per cent of deaths from organic heart disease at the present time.

During the past fifteen years at the Cleveland City Hospital we have had a series of more than three hundred autopsied cases in which syphilis was the chief etiologic factor responsible for death from heart failure, and it is the pertinent clinical and pathologic data of this material that I propose to consider this morning.

Only a few years ago it was taught in many quarters that syphilis frequently invaded the myocardium, causing characteristic degenerative changes—the so-called syphilitic myocarditis—which was responsible for deaths from heart failure. Many instances of sudden death or cases of obscure heart failure were thus ascribed to syphilitic involvement of the myocardium. This view, sponsored particularly in this country by the late Dr. Warthin, is not widely held at the present time because it fails to check with the facts observed both by the clinician and by the pathologist.

A study of the material mentioned above shows clearly that latent syphilis is an important etiologic factor leading to heart failure only when it involves the root of the aorta. This vessel may be seriously involved from syphilis even with aneurysmal dilatation, but so long as the process spares

* Presented before the Eighty-third Annual Session, Iowa State Medical Society, Des Moines, May 9, 10, 11, 1934.

the valve area there is no cardiac enlargement and no clinical evidence of heart failure.

It is a well known fact that the aorta is the most frequently involved viscus in the body in tertiary lues. For example, upward of 80 per cent of all patients with latent syphilis show post-mortem evidence of syphilitic aortitis. In some cases the disease is clinically silent and appears as an accidental autopsy finding; in others a widened aorta is found during life with or without free aortic regurgitation. In those cases of latent syphilis presenting the well known signs of aortic insufficiency we may be quite sure that the syphilitic process has extended to the root of the vessel and in this situation it assumes great significance so far as the heart is concerned. Here are located the three leaflets which seal the aortic orifice during cardiac diastole, thus preventing a regurgitation of blood back into the left ventricle. Here also are the mouths of the two coronary arteries which supply the heart wall with blood. The chronic inflammatory process of syphilis extends to the aortic leaflets and distorts them in such a way that they are no longer able to close the orifice during diastole and we have the clinical picture of aortic insufficiency. The same process also narrows, and in some cases, completely closes, the mouths of the coronary arteries. In a few instances the media at the orifice is undermined, and the ring is dilated so that even normal leaflets are unable to seal the opening. Thus we see that the ravages of syphilis at the root of the aorta produce aortic insufficiency either by involvement of the valve or by ring dilatation, or by both, and in addition, narrow or completely close the mouths of the coronary arteries. In the face of such handicaps therefore, the remarkable fact is not that the heart ultimately fails, but that it is able to carry on as long as it does in some cases.

In order that we may more clearly appreciate the variety of clinical pictures seen in patients with syphilitic heart disease it is necessary to mention a few of the more important postmortem findings observed in a large series of cases. The most consistent finding is, of course, the involvement of the aorta by syphilis—so-called syphilitic aortitis. In younger subjects this lesion is usually evident grossly whereas in those patients above fifty years of age, simple intimal arteriosclerosis often obscures the gross picture of syphilis and the diagnosis must be established by microscopic examination. In patients presenting the well known clinical signs of free aortic regurgitation the aortic leaflets are involved or the ring is dilated. A variety of distortions are seen in the architecture of the aortic valve but all are of such a nature as to cause functional insufficiency. Uncomplicated syphilis does not produce aortic stenosis. In some hearts the valves are attacked several millimeters below the normal site, in others they are shrunken in size to mere fibrous cords.

The earliest sign of syphilitic involvement of the aortic valve, and from the standpoint of gross diagnosis the most significant, is a separation of the commissures. Normally adjacent aortic leaflets have a common site of origin from the intima of the aorta, called the commissure. In my experience, a syphilitic valve invariably shows a lesion at its commissure which appears widened in the gross specimen. At this point the question may be asked: how does syphilis spread from the aorta to the aortic valve? Histologic studies of our material have led to the following conclusion concerning the evolution of syphilitic aortic insufficiency. The earliest lesion is found in the adventitia of the aorta and affects chiefly the smaller vessels, the vasa vasorum, and is of the nature of an obliterative endarteritis with perivascular infiltration. A similar process appears in the region of the commissures where it involves the smaller vessels normally found extending from the aorta and supplying the lateral margins of the aortic leaflets. As a result of this progressive vascular disease, degenerative and later chronic inflammatory changes appear which ultimately lead to a fusion of the lateral margins of the leaflet with the adjacent aortic intima. Thus we have the gross appearance in the late case of a widened commissure. Such a process may be years in developing, but finally the body of the valves shrink, they are no longer able to close the orifice, and an anatomic defect now becomes a functional handicap to the heart. The ostia of the coronary arteries are often involved in the syphilitic inflammatory process and appear narrowed or even completely obliterated. So much then for important anatomic changes produced by syphilis at the root of the aorta—a vital spot

as far as the functional integrity of the heart is concerned.

Clinical Data: The pertinent clinical facts observed in a large series of cases of syphilitic heart disease may be considered. In our own series males predominated in the proportion of six to one, and negroes outnumbered white in the proportion of three to one. The youngest patient with a fatal case of heart failure was twenty-nine years of age, the oldest seventy-six, with the peak incidence falling between forty and fifty years of age. Because of its importance in diagnosis, the physician should keep in mind the interval which may elapse between the acquisition of a primary syphilitic infection and later death from heart failure. The shortest interval in our series was five years, the longest forty-four years, with an average of twenty years. Thus we see that syphilis may exist as a progressive chronic inflammatory process in the aorta, clinically silent for a long period of time in some cases. During this period the patient may have no symptoms, may lead a perfectly normal life and have a healthy family of children, and not until the later decades of life will there be any evidence of organic heart disease. However, as time goes on the process at the root of the aorta spreads to the aortic valve which finally becomes incompetent and we then have the appearance of the signs and symptoms of heart failure.

Symptoms and Clinical Course: The symptoms and clinical course observed in a large series of cases vary widely. In the majority of patients seen in a large municipal hospital, congestive heart failure is often present at the time of admission and the clinical picture is dominated by the signs and symptoms of progressive myocardial failure. Substernal pain and nocturnal dyspnea, alleged early symptoms of syphilitic aortitis, are uncommon except in those cases showing a marked narrowing of the coronary orifices. The first symptoms complained of in our patients were palpitation and breathlessness on exertion. Many patients paid little or no attention to these symptoms but continued to work, often at hard labor. Medical advice was seldom sought until the dyspnea became marked or until frank signs of congestive heart failure appeared. The rather sudden onset of symptoms and the progressive nature of heart failure in many cases were conspicuous features. Fairly typical of our experience with this group of cases is the following account. A well developed male between thirty-five and forty-five years of age observes that he is no longer able to carry on his usual work because of breathlessness and palpitation. He has never had rheumatism and is quite unaware of any pre-existing heart disease. His symptoms gradually increase in severity over a period of months until he is finally forced to stop work because of dyspnea and often edema of the lower extremities. In this condition he is admitted to the hospital presenting the cardinal signs of congestive fail- ure, an over active enlarged left ventricle and the peripheral vascular signs of aortic insufficien- cy. The patient may gradually fail in spite of all treatment; or he may make a temporary re- covery, only to fail again in a few weeks or months. Some patients may lose their edema, be fairly comfortable walking about the wards, but another period of decompensation soon ensues. We believe that a cardiac breakdown with frank signs of congestive heart failure marks the be- ginning of the end in the vast majority of people with syphilitic aortic insufficiency.

Physical Signs: The outstanding physical signs presented by this group of patients were those of aortic insufficiency, jumping peripheral arteries showing the typical water hammer pulse. The left ventricle which bears the brunt of the burden in aortic valve disease is more or less dilated and thickened and the maximum apical thrust is dis- placed downward and outward. Except in se- verely decompensated cases, palpation over the area of the left ventricle usually reveals a more vigor- ous impulse than normal. Over the anatomic site of the aortic valve, as well as in the second right intercostal space, one usually hears a to and fro murmur. In some the systolic element may be louder than the diastolic. This may lead one to suspect the presence of aortic stenosis, but with the exception of the rare case in which syphilis is complicated by an old rheumatic aortic valvulitis or other type of bacterial endocarditis, the un- complicated case of syphilis does not show a nar- rowed aortic orifice at the postmortem table. The diastolic murmur is sometimes so harsh as to be accompanied by a palpable thrill. This has oc- curred in instances of ruptured valve leaflets which may flap in the regurgitating blood stream much as a sail flaps in the breeze and thus produce the thrill. Often one hears the typical presystolic Flint murmur which may be occasionally accom- panied by a thrill. The intensity of the thrill and the drum roll character of the murmur may suggest mitral stenosis, but if the diagnosis of syphilitic aortic insufficiency rests on reasonably secure grounds the interpretation of the Flint murmur offers little difficulty, because a combina- tion of mitral stenosis and syphilitic aortic insuffi- ciency is quite rare.

Diagnosis of Syphilitic Aortic Insufficiency:

Since incompetence of the aortic orifice is caused by an extension of the inflammatory process from the aorta to the valve area, the diagnosis of syphil- itic aortitis is of paramount importance in de- termining the etiologic diagnosis in a case of aortic insufficiency. As so often happens in chronic dis- ease, success in the therapy of syphilitic heart disease depends on an early diagnosis. This is frequently difficult and in many instances im- possible. One often sees clear examples of syphil- itic aortitis at the postmortem table that were clinically silent. Many patients never consult the physician until the disease has produced some structural defect in the aorta or at the aortic ori- fice. In the majority of cases studied in this series symptoms of syphilitic aortitis other than those of aneurysm or myocardial failure were sel- dom noticed. If we are to recognize syphilitic aortitis before it has changed the gross architec- ture of the vessel, the diagnosis must be largely in- ferential particularly in patients who have no other symptoms. We must bear in mind certain facts emphasized above: *first*, that latent syphilis more often involves the aorta than any other viscus; *sec- ond*, that syphilis may be present in the aorta for many years, yet the patient may show no signs or symptoms of the disease; *third*, the fact that the in- dividual is the parent of normal children does not exclude the existence of aortic syphilis; *fourth*, a positive blood or spinal fluid Wassermann test is of value in some cases and it may be the only positive objective evidence of syphilitic aortitis; but a negative reaction does not exclude the dis- ease, as more than ten per cent of proved cases have a negative Wassermann reaction during life. An excellent rule to follow in the diagnosis of syphilitic aortic insufficiency and one that rarely fails is this: free aortic regurgitation appearing out of a clear sky in an adult with a negative his- tory of heart disease, is syphilis until proved other- wise. Exceptions to this rule occur, but they are rare.

Treatment and Prognosis: The management of a case of syphilitic aortic insufficiency depends largely on the condition of the heart at the time the patient first comes under observation. Too often frank signs of congestive failure are present and such patient should be treated as any other case of cardiac decompensation. With a definite improvement in the circulation, antisyphilitic treat- ment may be started with mercury or bismuth and the oral administration of iodides. If a diag- nosis is established before cardiac failure appears more intensive, antisyphilitic treatment may be in- stituted. In addition to mercury and bismuth, intravenous arsenicals may be used, but cautiously, beginning with small weekly doses such as 0.05 grams of arsphenamine and increasing to 0.1, 0.15, 0.2, etc., until ten to twelve injections have been given. The intensity of the treatment will, of course, depend on the age and physical condition of the patient. If the patient has sound kidneys and no evidence of myocardial insufficiency one is safe in employing fairly intensive measures. Any medication tending to allay the syphilitic process in the aorta and prevent its spread to the valve area or retard the development of aneurysm may add years to the patient's life.

The prognosis depends on the capacity of the myocardium to carry on in the face of serious handicaps, a leak at the aortic orifice and narrowed coronary ostia. These lesions may progress rapidly in some cases and lead to death from progressive heart failure in spite of all treatment. In early cases with less serious coronary involvement the heart muscle may meet the demands of increased work for several years before congestive failure appears. However, the prognosis after frank cardiac decompensation is usually gloomy. Many patients never recover from the first breakdown and those that do are virtually invalids the rest of their lives.

SUMMARY

Latent syphilis is a significant cause of heart disease only insofar as it involves the root of the aorta. In this situation, a vital spot, as far as the heart is concerned, the inflammatory process may extend to the valve leaflets, or dilate the aortic ring and cause free aortic regurgitation. The ostia of the coronary arteries may be obstructed and seriously impair the blood supply to the heart wall. Aortic insufficiency appearing insidiously in an adult with a negative cardiac history is due to syphilis in the vast majority of cases. The question of management of syphilitic heart disease depends on the early diagnosis and proper treatment of syphilitic aortitis.

SECOND DAY

HYPERTENSIVE HEART DISEASE

The subject I have chosen this morning is, as all of you in the general practice of medicine know, one of the most important problems with which we deal.

If one follows a large series of patients with a persistent elevation of both systolic and diastolic blood pressure through to the end, the following facts appear. In the first place, sooner or later, the majority will develop signs and symptoms of myocardial insufficiency and die of congestive

heart failure. In my own series about 60 per cent of people with hypertension die of heart failure; about 20 per cent die of a cerebral accident, either thrombosis or hemorrhage, and around 10 to 15 per cent die of uremic poisoning. As a rule, a postmortem examination of the heart shows an enlargement and more or less dilatation of the left ventricle. The normal weight of the adult human heart is about 300 grams. The hypertensive heart at the postmortem table is, as a rule, above this, varying from 450 to 800 or 900 grams. Most of the increase in weight is due to a thickening of the left ventricle, that chamber of the heart which bears the brunt of the burden of hypertension. In addition, one finds varying grades of coronary arteriosclerosis in these patients. This may have been manifested during life by angina pectoris or by an attack of coronary thrombosis. On the other hand, many patients with hypertension die without having had anginal attacks or coronary thrombosis.

. In the light of these facts, what may we learn about the management and treatment of people with hypertension, particularly those suffering from myocardial insufficiency? The informed clinician should anticipate ultimate cardiac failure in his patient with persistent hypertension. He should say to himself, "The heart is bearing the brunt of the burden. It hypertrophies; it dilates; it does its best to keep the individual a going concern as long as possible. Sooner or later, however, it reaches the end of its string and fails."

Time was when such failures were thought to be due to an inflammatory process in the myocardium; hence, the slipshod diagnosis of chronic myocarditis was frequently made, and the clinicians who believed that focal infection caused myocardial damage often subjected their patients to unnecessary surgical procedures of various sorts in the hope of finding some focus of infection responsible for the heart failure. Fortunately this practice is waning because there is no sound experimental or clinical evidence to show that focal infection is responsible for the degenerative changes in the vascular system accompanying chronic hypertension.

The question of hypertension must at once appear as paramount in a consideration of hypertensive heart disease. Let us for a moment consider the problem of hypertension through the eyes of the physiologist. To him, our cardiovascular apparatus is designed, in the first place to convert a pulsating stream into a steady flow, and in the second place, to maintain this steady flow through microscopic blood vessels, where the real business of life takes place. The large arteries in our bodies act as conduits conveying blood from the central pumping station into the periphery where it can be used. Blood in the larger arteries is of no more use to us than water in the main in the middle of the street. It must be piped into the faucet if we are to use it. So it is in our circulatory apparatus. Unless the blood reaches the microscopic structures which we call the arterioles and capillaries, we cannot utilize it. Therefore, the chief function of the circulatory apparatus is to maintain a steady flow of blood through the small vessels. These vessels, billions of them, offer a resistance, naturally, to the flow of blood. If you put a million nozzles on the end of the main you must have a pressure in the main if you wish to sprinkle the lawn. Likewise we must have a pressure in our mains if the resistance afforded by the billions of small microscopic blood vessels is to be overcome.

The fact that blood in the mammalian system in arteries is under pressure was first discovered by a clergyman, Stephen Hales, in the seventeenth century. He placed a cannula in the carotid artery of a mare and saw that the blood rose several feet above the level of the heart and that this blood pulsated with each heart beat. It was nearly two hundred years after this fact was established before we had an apparatus to determine the blood pressure during life. After the introduction of the sphygmomanometer in the nineties of the last century it was discovered that the blood pressure of some people was too high; in others too low. In spite of the fact that we have been taking pressures for over thirty years, there is still much that we do not know about hypertension. If one studies the vascular system of patients dying of hypertension, whether their route out has been the cardiac one, the cerebral one, or the kidney one, the thing that impresses the student is that the patient's vascular system is more or less seriously diseased, and definite lesions are often found at the end of the stream in the microscopic vessels.

For the last ten years at the Cleveland City Hospital we have been interested in the small vessels of people dead of hypertension. We found lesions in the small vessels of many of the viscera, particularly in the kidneys, as well as in the small vessels of the skeletal muscles. Whether or not the lesions in the small vessels are the cause or the result of hypertension is not known at the present time.

The future of the average patient with hypertension who has this deterioration of his vascular system, as we said, depends on the heart, the cerebral arteries and the renal arteries. The hypertensive heart fails for two chief reasons; first, because it carries a much greater load than a normal heart.

sooner or later it becomes exhausted, and ultimately fails; and second, because the blood supply to the heart wall is often impaired by coronary arteriosclerosis. Indeed, the associated coronary disease is frequently the most important factor determining the clinical picture. Thus some hypertensive patients may have anginal seizures or attacks of coronary thrombosis. Others run a progressive down-hill course from congestive failure and at autopsy one finds extreme myocardial fibrosis secondary to more or less severe coronary disease. In many patients, therefore, the capacity of the heart to meet the demands of an elevation in blood pressure, the period of time that the patient is able to carry on, depends chiefly on the state of the coronary arteries. Since this factor is a variable one, one sees at one extreme patients with hypertension able to lead fairly active lives for many years; at the other, individuals who succumb rapidly to heart failure. With the onset of failure, the left ventricle, as well as the other heart chambers, undergoes more or less dilatation. The mitral ring is widened and a relative mitral insufficiency results which is manifested by a blowing systolic murmur at the apex, so commonly heard in failing hypertensive hearts. Contrary to a prevalent conception, there is no actual inflammation, chronic myocarditis, of the heart muscle in uncomplicated cases. Such changes as are found microscopically, patchy areas of fibrosis and slight infiltration with lymphocytes and plasma cells, are secondary to the associated coronary disease. In a word, the pathologic findings in the hypertensive heart are those of an organ which has withstood a long siege. It often doubles, and in some instances trebles, its normal weight in an attempt to maintain an adequate circulation in the face of great odds. Sooner or later, its reserve is exhausted and we see the appearance of peripheral circulatory failure. Under these circumstances it is not necessary to invoke a chronic inflammatory process in the myocardium to explain the heart's exhaustion. The wonder is, not that the average hypertension heart fails, but that it carries on as long as it does.

As long as the heart is able to meet the demands of an elevated blood pressure, there are no symptoms of hypertensive heart disease. True, the heart hypertrophied from whatever cause, does not possess a normal reserve, but for all ordinary exertion the patient may be quite unaware of any cardiac insufficiency. The most common symptom of early failure is dyspnea on exertion. A slight swelling of the ankles toward evening often ascribed by the patient to age or overweight, is frequent. Another early symptom of left heart failure, is attacks of nocturnal dyspnea sometimes called cardiac asthma. These attacks vary widely in severity. In mild ones the patient may be awakened by a paroxysmal cough, or a sensation of smothering. He may sit up in bed, bring up a little viscid mucus, and fall asleep again. In severe attacks, the dyspnea may be extreme, the breathing noisy, the face ashen or cyanotic. Paroxysmal coughing may bring up the characteristic pink, frothy sputum of pulmonary edema. The physician must be con-. stantly on the lookout for these earlier manifestations of heart failure because a correct diagnosis and proper therapeutic managament at this stage may spare the patient a more serious breakdown.

Therapy: We may consider the management of the patient suffering from hypertensive heart disease under two headings; first, the treatment of the patient before signs and symptoms of heart failure develop; and second, the management of the case after failure appears. During that period, varying from months to years, in which there are no cardiac symptoms, the informed physician is guided by certain fundamental concepts. For example, he knows that the heart is bearing the brunt of the burden, and that its capacity to withstand the strain will in the majority of cases determine the patient's expectancy. Therefore, all therapeutic endeavors are directed toward sparing the heart. Factors known to influence blood pressure, such as mental or emotional strain, obesity, excesses of all kinds, are controlled within reasonable limits. Often the hopeful assurance on the part of the physician, a vacation, a simple sedative insuring a few nights sleep, or even in these times, a rise in the market, may be responsible for an appreciable fall in blood pressure, which is still too often regarded as a specific effect of some medicine. It is needless to say that the heart burdened by hypertension must be spared the load of undue physical exertion, and so a curtailment in the patient's activities is indicated. The most reliable guide for this is the amount of exertion that the patient can do without undue breathlessness or fatigue. If the patient is living within these limits and controlling the factors mentioned above as influencing blood pressure, he is doing all that is known at present to prolong his days. We have as yet no cure for hypertension.

With the development of myocardial insufficiency, we may again be guided by modern concepts in the diagnosis and treatment. Aware of the extra load the heart has been carrying, its exhaustion is anticipated. Therefore, such early manifestations as dyspnea on exertion, mild attacks of cardiac asthma and puffiness about the ankles, should be ascribed to heart failure rather than to bronchitis, asthma or kidney disease. At this stage a period of bedrest is of paramount importance. Sedatives to guarantee sleep, with moderate doses of digitalis and caffeine are useful. If auricular fibrillation is present, the ventricular rate should be brought to normal and maintained with adequate digitalis dosage. Sooner or later many hypertensive patients develop congestive failure and the management of this complication differs in no fundamental way from that of advanced heart failure from other causes. Unfortunately the older concept of the renal origin of hypertension still survives to influence the diagnosis and treatment in such cases, and a failing heart is frequently neglected because dropsy and an albuminous urine are regarded as evidence of kidney disease rather than chronic passive congestion from heart failure. Both before and after the stage of heart failure, the patient with hypertension is too often regarded as having, or destined to develop, renal insufficiency. How frequently the first advice given the patient concerns a dietary restriction! Protein is thought to be harmful, particularly that in the form of red meat. Eggs are given sparingly, but a little white meat and fish are usually permitted. Since the vast majority of hypertensive patients have no inability to utilize protein, over-zealous attempts at protein restriction are not only contraindicated but may do actual harm. There are no reliable clinical or experimental data to prove that the ingestion of a normal amount of protein in food has any influence on blood pressure or on the kidneys in hypertension.

ARTERIOSCLEROTIC HEART DISEASE: THE RELATION BETWEEN ANGINA PECTORIS AND CORONARY OCCLUSION*

B. F. WOLVERTON, M.D., Cedar Rapids

From the time of Heberden's[1] classic account of angina pectoris in 1768, until the appearance of Herrick's first writings on thrombosis of the coronary arteries in 1912[2] and 1919,[3] attacks of cardiac pain were grouped together under the common name of angina pectoris. Stress was laid only on the symptoms, particularly the pain, while the underlying pathology and pathologic physiology were only vaguely surmised. Since Herrick's clear separation of cases of anginal pain due to acute occlusion of a coronary artery or branch by a thrombus, interest in the whole group of cases exhibiting cardiac pain has increased tremendously, resulting in a great deal of investigation and much new

*Presented before the Eighty-third Annual Session, Iowa State Medical Society, Des Moines, May 9, 10, 11, 1934.

knowledge. In recent years more and more emphasis has been placed on the pathology and pathologic physiology, and an attempt has been made to interpret the clinical manifestations in relation to the condition in the heart. It is now a fairly well established fact that angina pectoris and coronary thrombosis represent special manifestations of sclerosis of the coronary arteries

The clinical syndrome resulting from coronary thrombosis has been so well and so frequently described that it need not be repeated here in detail. It occurs about four times as often in men as in women, rarely before the age of forty and with increasing frequency during each succeeding decade of life. The incidence is much greater among business and professional men than among laborers and those of similar occupations. The onset is usually sudden and painful, although in exceptional cases it may be neither. The pain, when present, may be agonizing or so mild as to require direct questioning to bring out its occurrence. It does not end abruptly, in a few minutes, but lasts for hours or days. It is commonly located in the region of the sternum and may radiate to either or both shoulders or arms, to the neck, jaw, or upper abdomen. The pain may be so severe in a distant part that the sternal or precordial pain receives little notice by the patient. The distress may be described as other than pain, sometimes as pressure, aching, or tightness. The blood pressure usually (but not always) falls to a level lower than its customary one. Shock is shown by pallor, perspiration, anxious expression and soft pulse. Vomiting is not uncommon. The heart rate is usually increased, but may be normal or slow. Heart block, sudden auricular fibrillation or ventricular paroxysmal tachycardia may occur in the attack or later. The heart sounds are usually distant and of poor quality, but they are sometimes apparently normal. The myocardial infarction resulting from the arterial occlusion gives rise to a variable grade of fever during the few days after the accident, as well as a polymorphonuclear leukocytosis. If the infarction involves the visceral pericardium anteriorly, a pericardial friction rub may be heard on the second or third day. If the endocardium is involved, a mural thrombus forms over this area, and may give rise to single or multiple embolism. A toxic psychotic state frequently occurs and increases the difficulty in management of the patient. Electrocardiograms taken at various intervals show changes in the great majority of cases which are characteristic of acute heart muscle injury. The most important of these, in early cases, are elevation of the RT or ST segment in Lead I, with a corresponding depression in Lead III or vice versa.

Later this segment returns to the normal level and the T wave becomes deeply inverted in the lead previously showing elevation of the RT or ST segment. Bundle-branch block, auriculoventricular block, and arrythmias as before mentioned, may result from myocardial infarction. It is extremely important to remember that, as in many other conditions, no one symptom or sign is invariably present. Any one or several of the common symptoms, physical or laboratory signs may fail to be distinctive.

The clinical picture of angina pectoris, exclusive of acute coronary occlusion, is similar, yet strikingly different. The character and distribution of the pain—and pain is the essential feature of the angina syndrome—is like that occurring in coronary thrombosis, since in both instances, the pain is caused by a relative deficiency in blood supply to an area of heart muscle. The essential difference lies in the fact that the deficiency lasts for only a few seconds or minutes in angina pectoris, while in coronary thrombosis the interference with coronary blood flow remains. In angina pectoris, as soon as the temporary deficiency in blood supply is relieved, the heart presumably resumes its previous status; after coronary thrombosis there remains an infarct of the myocardium which may soften and rupture, give rise to serious embolism, or, at best, after healing, never contributes to the work of the heart as did the heart muscle it replaced. In angina pectoris we have a temporary condition; in coronary occlusion a permanent one.

The typical clinical picture of angina pectoris which we carried from medical school was that of an elderly gentleman stopping suddenly, as he walked along the street, standing pale and rigid as if transfixed by the agonizing vise-like pain which gripped his heart and radiated into his shoulder and arm; with fixed gaze and in silence, scarcely daring to breathe, he waited for the attack to end, either in relief or sudden death, then passed on to live in dread of the next attack which was sure to come. We see a few cases of that type, and no one could fail to recognize them. Much more common, however, is the man, or surprisingly often nowadays, the woman, who states, or admits on questioning, that on several occasions during the past few weeks or months there has been a sensation of constriction or pressure or weight across the front of the chest as a result of a certain type of exertion which did not previously cause distress. The sensation may or may not be referred to various areas distant from the sternum or precordium, but the reference of distress or lack of it is not of prime importance in making a diagnosis. The essential feature is the fact that the sensation is induced by exertion regardless of character or distribution. It is far more important to recognize that such a symptom constitutes the angina syndrome and that it is caused by coronary sclerosis, than so to designate only the classical and extreme type. At best, we recognize only a fraction of all the cases of coronary sclerosis that come under our observation. It is only by eliciting a history of the mildest types of angina pectoris and identifying the smallest coronary thromboses, that we can hope to reduce to a minimum the number of cases of coronary sclerosis that escape detection.

These mild cases, if unrecognized, are ripe material for the accident, coronary thrombosis. Fitzhugh and Hamilton[4] have shown that many fatalities due to coronary thrombosis are avoidable. When consulted by patients exhibiting even the mildest forms of angina pectoris, it is our responsibility to place them on a regime which, so far as possible, protects them against acute coronary occlusion. Every physician who sees many cases of coronary thrombosis, encounters instances in which the accident might have been avoided or delayed had the antecedant anginal history been elicited and its significance appreciated. Such individuals frequently show no abnormal findings on physical examination, and may even have normal electrocardiograms, but the lack of substantiation in these respects in no way weakens the diagnosis of coronary heart disease with angina pectoris. In some cases there may be an associated arterial hypertension, the heart sounds may be poor in quality, and the electrocardiogram may show significant changes; there may even be a systolic heart murmur due to sclerosis of a papillary muscle, of the mitral ring or relative mitral insufficiency due to dilatation; but it is often difficult to discover a single objective finding to indicate cardiac impairment. The history alone is sufficient proof of the diagnosis regardless of the presence or absence of objective findings, provided the patient is truthful. A malingerer could claim that he suffers from anginal symptoms, and no one could disprove the existence of coronary sclerosis on the basis of a lack of objective findings. His deception could be exposed only by detection in the act of undergoing strenuous exertion with apparent comfort. Another fact of medico-legal importance is that an insurance applicant might withhold a history of angina pectoris and pass his physical examination successfully.

Not infrequently, a patient is seen during or after an attack of pain in whom it is difficult to say whether or not myocardial infarction has occurred. It is very important that a decision on this point be made since in the one case, a long period of bed rest must be imposed, while in the other it is unnecessary. An abrupt onset during exertion or intense emotional stress, duration of a few seconds or minutes, absence of fall in blood pressure; absence of fever, pericardial friction rub, leukocytosis or electrocardiographic changes characteristic of acute myocardial injury appearing during the next few days, point to absence of infarction. As many sources of information as possible should be utilized, since any one or more of the usual evidences of coronary occlusion with myocardial infarction may be absent. When the features of the acute attack are not distinctive, the safer course is tentatively to regard it as due to coronary occlusion, and to keep the patient at bed rest for a few days while the late signs of infarction are sought. Frequent observation of temperature, blood pressure, leukocyte count, search for pericardial friction rub, and serial electrocardiograms will settle the question in a few days. If the diagnosis of coronary thrombosis cannot be established, bed rest need not be enforced longer unless other considerations require it. In doubtful cases the patient should never be taken from his bed to an electrocardiographic laboratory. If he cannot be transported without effort on his part, or a portable instrument brought to the bedside, it is better to forego this method of study and rely on other means to make the diagnosis.

Differentiation between pain of myocardial origin and acute abdominal surgical conditions, pleuritis, pulmonary infarction, neurocirculatory asthenia, and other extracardiac conditions will not be considered here. It should be remembered, however, that coronary thrombosis may be painless and masquerade as cardiac asthma (paroxysmal cardiac dyspnea).

It is not uncommon to observe cases in which the onset of the anginal syndrome dates from an attack of coronary thrombosis. This fact might suggest the possibility that an unrecognized infarction may be a necessary antecedent of a series of attacks of angina of effort. Such a theory would assume that thrombosis of a small coronary branch, giving slight and indistinctive symptoms, would reduce the available blood supply to a small island of myocardium which would, then suffer from relative ischemia at a certain level of activity, and thus give rise to anginal pain. While this is undoubtedly true in some cases, it happens much oftener that patients first notice the slightest discomfort on exertion, then gradually experience an increasing distress with succeeding attacks until they become sufficiently alarmed or inconvenienced to consult a physician. In addition, patients are occasionally seen whose angina of effort is termi-

the rapidly acting nitrites in hyper-susceptible individuals with coronary disease, and even the routine use of nitroglycerin and amyl nitrite in severe forms of angina pectoris has recently been criticized. Many surgeons do not appreciate the desirability of a careful cardiac examination before operating electively on patients past forty years of age. "Acute dilatation" of the heart occurring after operation is usually coronary thrombosis or an arrhythmia resulting from organic changes in the heart. The practitioners of all branches of medicine must keep in mind the necessity of preventing, as far as possible, the occurrence of coronary occlusion.

SUMMARY

1. Any person with sclerosis of the coronary arteries may develop mild or severe anginal pain or may remain symptom-free.

2. Coronary thrombosis may occur as an accident, usually preventable or postponable, in individuals with coronary sclerosis, whether or not they have angina pectoris.

3. Angina pectoris should be regarded as a danger signal requiring a warning against indiscretions which may precipitate coronary thrombosis.

4. When acute coronary occlusion does occur, proper treatment depends on its differentiation from anginal pain without myocardial infarction.

REFERENCES

1. Heberden, William: Some account of a disorder of the breast: Med. Trans. Royal Coll. Phys., ii:59, 1786.
2. Herrick, James B.: Clinical features of sudden obstruction of the coronary arteries. . Jour. Am. Med. Assn., lix:2015-2020 (December 7), 1912.
3. Herrick, James B.: Thrombosis of the coronary arteries. Jour. Am. Med. Assn., lxxii:387 (February 8), 1919.
4. Fitzhugh, G. and Hamilton, B. E.: Coronary occlusion and fatal angina pectoris. Jour. Am. Med. Assn., c:475-480 (February 18), 1933.

THE DIAGNOSIS AND TREATMENT OF RENAL TUBERCULOSIS*

LAWRENCE E. PIERSON, M.D., Sioux City

A well known urologist once made the statement that he knew of no lesion in the urinary tract, which is accompanied by such variations in clinical symptoms or offers greater difficulties of diagnosis than renal tuberculosis.

With such an introduction, it is needless for me to attempt the description of a typical case history. One patient may scarcely be aware of urinary symptoms save for the occasional passing of bloody urine, while another patient complains of a constant desire to void, with severe tenesmus and pain. By far the greater percentage of these patients complain of "bladder trouble," which is their

*Presented before the Eighty-third Annual Session, Iowa State Medical Society, Des Moines, May 9, 10, 11, 1934.

description of frequency, nocturia, dysuria, hematuria and terminal tenesmus. A number of them have been under treatment, but the distress has become progressively worse.

Any patient who presents himself with such a story deserves a complete urologic investigation, always with the possibility of renal tuberculosis in mind. Such an investigation should include, physical, laboratory, cystoscopic and x-ray examination. Pulmonary, glandular or bone tuberculosis may each serve as the origin of a renal infection. Rectal or vaginal examination may reveal a nodular ureter. Palpation of the prostate, seminal vesicles and epididymis may reveal evidence of infection in these structures.

The demonstration of tuberculous bacilluria in a patient is not as simple as we sometimes consider it to be. A single observation, even under the most exacting technic is not sufficient, since the excretion of the bacilli is not always a constant process. Periodic showers of bacilli, at irregular intervals is the usual event, especially in the early stages of the disease. Tuberculous bacilli may be absent in renal tuberculosis, during the early closed stage, before ulceration into the pelvis occurs, or in the later stages with occlusion of the ureter, and occasionally even in the absence of ureteral obstruction. Hence, repeated search is absolutely essential to determine accurately the presence or absence of tuberculous bacilli.

Location of the source of tuberculous bacilli is possible only by means of cystoscopy. Such an examination is often impossible under ordinary anesthesia of the urethra, because of the severe cystitis characterizing such an infection. Caudal block or spinal anesthesia is most efficient for satisfactory examination. Only rarely does the patient come for examination before the bladder has become involved. Such involvement produces changes in the bladder which are characteristic in appearance. Submucous hemorrhagic spots, especially located around the ureteral openings are always suspicious. Ulceration and tubercle formation render these suspicions positive evidence, and later stages result in transformation of the ureteral orifice into a "golf hole" appearance which is practically pathognomonic of tuberculosis.

Ureteral catheterization in suspicious tuberculous cases has been a much debated question. However, in view of the fact that renal tuberculosis precedes bladder tuberculosis, it hardly seems logical to fear the possibility of transmitting such infection to the kidney from the bladder. Most authorities agree that renal tuberculosis is bilateral from the start directly through the blood stream. Consequently it is logical to assume that both kid-

neys are simultaneously infected. That kidney which has the most efficient drainage through its ureter will be more able to retard development of the lesion, while its mate being relatively handicapped will become progressively worse with extension of the infection through the cortex and medullary portions of the kidney. Finally the process ulcerates into the renal pelvis, and the heretofore closed lesion develops into an open or pyelitic type of infection. With its onset, the invasion continues to the bladder and the symptoms of urinary tuberculosis arise.

Examination of renal specimens reveals the relative amount of pus as well as the tubercle bacilli in each kidney and the relative excretion of dyes, such as phenolsulphonephthalein, will produce evidence of the difference between both kidneys in their excretion power.

One of the greatest sources of information through the use of ureteral catheters is the retrograde pyelogram, obtained by injecting radioopaque solutions into the renal pelvis and ureter. In the early or closed stage, no structural deformity is present, consequently a normal pyelogram is obtained. It has been stated that a normal pyelogram will rule out tuberculosis in 90 per cent of the cases. The truth of this statement becomes apparent when we realize that these patients have no incentive to seek medical relief until the lesion erodes into the pelvis and ureter with secondary bladder involvement.

Such ulceration and cavitation is made evident only by means of pyelography. Its earlier stage is represented by a fuzzy or "moth eaten" appearance at the periphery and its progress can be accurately outlined by a series of subsequent pyelograms. Changes in the ureter are similarly shown.

During recent years, intravenous urography has been developed, and some have predicted that it would replace cystoscopy and ureteral catheterization, but such a destiny has failed to materialize. In the early or closed type of lesion, parenchymatous involvement has restricted normal excretion to such an extent that the dye fails to accumulate fast enough in the pelvis or ureter to show any detail. Consequently, early changes in the pyelogram will easily be overlooked. Also, in later ulcerative stages, the rate of excretion is more and more restricted, consequently preventing a sufficient accumulation of dye to outline the cavities— cavities which could easily be seen with a retrograde injection. Occasionally, in the presence of ureteral obstruction, sufficient dye will accumulate to show outlines of a cavernous pyelitis. However, in the majority of cases, complete reliance on intra-

THE DIAGNOSIS AND CLINICAL SIGNIFICANCE OF AURICULAR FIBRILLATION*

LAURENCE E. COOLEY, M.D., Dubuque

Auricular fibrillation is one of the most frequent irregularities of the heart that is seen by the physician. I will limit my discussion today to a few points in the diagnosis and the relationship of this disease to other disease processes in the body.

The diagnosis of auricular fibrillation can usually be made by a simple clinical examination. When we see irregular pulsations in the neck vessels, we become suspicious of auricular fibrillation. The pulse heightens our suspicion. It is totally irregular as to rate, force and rhythm. There is no relationship between the various beats as felt at the wrist. The heart examination should confirm or exclude the diagnosis of auricular fibrillation. Inspection and palpation of the apex beat reveal no definite rhythm. Auscultation will make the diagnosis certain in almost all cases. There is also that total lack of rhythm, that is, there is a lack of regularity of the force, of the rate, and also of the rhythm. There is a difference in the rate at the apex and the rate to be felt at the wrist. This is known as the pulse deficit and is due to a failure of some of the weaker beats of the ventricle to overcome the aortic pressure and be transmitted to the wrist.

In the differential diagnosis of auricular fibrillation, we must consider a number of different irregularities. The first and simplest is sinus arrhythmia, which occurs most frequently in young individuals. It is particularly likely to occur with deep breathing. Holding the breath will usually stop this arrhythmia. Extrasystoles may occasionally give rise to some difficulty in differentiating from auricular fibrillation. However, there are usually a number of regular beats in between the extrasystoles, and there is always a compensatory pause after the extrasystole. Multiple extrasystoles from many foci may give rise to an irregularity which is impossible to differentiate clinically. We therefore must call upon the electrocardiograph to make the differentiation. Partial heartblock with many drop beats will give rise to an irregularity which often cannot be differentiated clinically, and we must also call upon the electrocardiograph in such a case. Auricular flutter, where the ventricular rate is irregular, which occurs not infrequently, will also give rise to an irregularity which is hard to differentiate clinically.

If the patient with auricular fibrillation is well

---

* Presented before the Eighty-third Annual Session, Iowa State Medical Society, Des Moines, May 9, 10, 11, 1934.

enough, you can have him exercise. If auricular fibrillation is present exercise will not diminish the irregularity but it will often accentuate it. In the other types of irregularity which I have mentioned, the irregularity will often disappear with exercise. The electrocardiogram is the final court of judgment, and we must rely upon the electrocardiogram for the difficult cases.

In considering the clinical significance of auricular fibrillation, we should first speak of the etiologic factors. In from ten to fifteen per cent of the cases, they are non-cardiac in origin. In the non-cardiac group the etiology is given as being due to poisons of many different sorts, including tobacco, alcoholic excesses, infectious diseases, and food poisonings, as well as trauma and surgical operations. There are a few cases in which excitement or some abnormality of the nervous mechanism of the heart seems to be the only cause of auricular fibrillation. In the non-cardiac cases, this is usually not serious. It is usually also of the paroxysmal type. If we are able to remove the cause, we are able to terminate the fibrillation. However, fibrillation does temporarily lower the efficiency of the heart, especially when the ventricular rate is rapid. Stewart and Cohen have demonstrated this in normal dogs. They induced fibrillation in these dogs and were able to show a definite decrease in the volume output of blood per minute from the heart.

Among the cardiac conditions associated with auricular fibrillation, we list the three common conditions, that is, first, rheumatic heart disease; second, hypertension and coronary artery disease; and, third, thyrotoxicosis. In the old rheumatic heart disease, the characteristic signs of valvular lesions will often be obliterated by the fibrillation. The presystolic murmur and the diastolic murmur and thrill will often disappear when auricular fibrillation occurs. Also, auricular fibrillation often initiates cardiac decompensation in cases of rheumatic heart disease. Therefore, we should always think of rheumatic heart disease as the cause of cardiac decompensation and auricular fibrillation. Stroud and his associates have shown that the prognosis of rheumatic heart disease is much poorer when the auricular fibrillation occurs before the age of twenty-five. Auricular fibrillation associated with hypertension or coronary artery disease occurs not infrequently, and I believe the prognosis is always more serious. Thrombi are prone to form in the incompletely contracting auricles. Thrombi break off at intervals. Winchester and others have reported a number of cases where embolic phenomena have been observed in connection with auricular fibrillation. I recently saw a patient who had had a number of embolic phenomena, including temporary loss of consciousness, slurring of speech and occlusion of the popliteal artery, renal infarction, and finally hemiplegia and death due to a clot found in the left auricle. I believe that this patient would be living today if he had not had auricular fibrillation.

Paroxysmal auricular fibrillation in this group may also be of serious consequence. The following case will illustrate that. A salesman, forty-seven years of age, was awakened one night with acute dyspnea. When seen thirteen hours later, his heart rate was 200 and was totally irregular. There was a marked pulmonary edema, and the liver was tender and swollen. Fortunately, we were able to terminate the attack promptly. There is a question in my mind as to whether this patient would have lived for any length of time if this very rapid and irregular heart rate had continued.

Another condition may occur in paroxysmal auricular fibrillation which may be illustrated by the following case. A young girl, twenty-eight years of age, gave a history of very severe precordial pain radiating down the left arm and lasting for forty-eight hours. There was a marked dyspnea and a definite cyanosis accompanying it. A diagnosis of coronary thrombosis was made. The patient had a number of similar attacks after this first very severe attack. When seen one week after one of these attacks there was nothing to be found clinically. The heart was normal. The electrocardiogram was normal. The blood Wassermann test was negative. I believe that this patient's angina was due to the extremely rapid heart rate which occurred with every attack. I do not know whether this patient had a paroxysmal auricular fibrillation or paroxysmal tachycardia. There have been cases reported, however, where a definite angina has been induced by paroxysmal auricular fibrillation. White and Camp and many others have reported such cases. I do not think we are justified in condemning this patient who is only twenty-eight years old, with a diagnosis of coronary thrombosis.

We have all seen cases of auricular fibrillation which have occurred with the onset of thyrotoxicosis, or we have also seen cases where, immediately after operation, the auricular fibrillation has been induced. I believe that the prognosis in these cases is much more serious. We should also remember that cardiac decompensation with auricular fibrillation may be caused by an unsuspected thyrotoxicosis. In two cases which I recently saw, the substernal adenomatous goiters were found to

compensated. I do not know how long it will last. The case was hypertension. What the cause back of that is, I will not attempt to say.

THE DIAGNOSIS AND TREATMENT OF BRONCHIAL ASTHMA*

JULIA COLE, M.D., Iowa City

The diagnosis of bronchial asthma may be considered under two heads: first, the diagnosis of the condition as such, which involves its differentiation from other forms of dyspnea, and second, the etiologic diagnosis which must be attempted before one can proceed to any rational therapy. The criteria which we employ in differentiating bronchial asthma from other conditions attended by dyspnea are of two sorts: those concerned with the clinical picture of the asthmatic attack and those related to the personal and family histories of the patient.

In the attack of bronchial asthma we have a type of dyspnea characterized by wheezing with prolonged expiration. Auscultation usually reveals sonorous and sibilant râles, and accentuates the wheezing character of the breath sounds, especially of expiration. Cough in the majority of cases is not present early in the attack, and if present is short, dry and ineffectual. As the attack subsides the cough often becomes more pronounced and productive. Adrenalin relieves the dyspnea partially or completely and the subjective relief is accompanied by an increase in vital capacity measured on the spirometer. Between attacks, at least in the early years of asthma, there is freedom from respiratory embarrassment and examination of the chest at such times is negative. After years of asthma and with the establishment of the common complications of chronic bronchitis and emphysema there may be more or less constant respiratory difficulty, but it is of importance that at some stage in the history of a case of true bronchial asthma the patient has paroxysmal attacks of dyspnea with freedom from respiratory distress between attacks. From a laboratory viewpoint the sputum in bronchial asthma may show Curschman spirals and Charcot-Leyden crystals but of much more importance probably is the presence of eosinophiles. A blood eosinophilia may be found also.

Turning to the personal and family histories of the patient we find that the onset of bronchial asthma is usually in early life, often in childhood and occurs uncommonly after thirty-five years of age. In a large percentage of cases there is a

*Presented before the Eighty-third Annual Session, Iowa State Medical Society, Des Moines, May 9, 10, 11, 1934.

history of allergic disease. Of greatest importance is the possible incidence of hay fever or of eczema which are recognized generally as of probable allergic etiology. There are other conditions, however, less firmly established as allergic but regarded as at least presumptively so. Among these are vasomotor rhinitis, migraine, urticaria, and periodic gastro-intestinal upsets. The history in a case of suspected bronchial asthma should always include an inquiry into the possible incidence of these conditions. A third feature found in a majority of cases is a tendency to develop protein sensitivity.

The family history in fifty per cent or more of cases of bronchial asthma shows an incidence of allergic disease. Again the conditions about which we inquire especially are asthma, hay fever, and eczema, but we are interested also in migraine. vasomotor rhinitis, urticaria and periodic gastro-intestinal upsets.

The diagnosis of bronchial asthma, then, involves the application of the criteria discussed above and which may be summarized briefly as follows. The patient has paroxysmal attacks of dyspnea with freedom from respiratory embarrassment between attacks. The seizure is characterized by wheezing with prolonged expiration and is relieved by adrenalin. Cough is more pronounced as the attack subsides than at the onset. Sputum eosinophilia usually is found. Blood eosinophilia may be present. The age of onset generally is before thirty-five years. Often there is a past history of allergic disease and in a majority of cases there is also a family history of allergy.

All of these features may not be present in every case just as every patient with pernicious anemia may not complain of a sore tongue or of diarrhea. Taken together, however, they constitute a clinical picture which a given case must approximate fairly closely in order to be considered bronchial asthma.

The conditions which may simulate bronchial asthma are:

1. Cases in which there is pressure on the trachea or bronchi due to inflammatory, neoplastic or aneurysmal masses usually in the mediastinum. In such cases respiratory difficulty may be present and because the respirations may be wheezing in character the patient is sometimes considered asthmatic. The respiratory difficulty in such cases. however, is usually not paroxysmal. There is not the prolongation of expiration seen in bronchial asthma. · Adrenalin does not relieve the dyspnea. Sputum eosinophilia is not present. The personal and family histories may or may not be positive for allergic disease. Differentiation here is chiefly on the basis of the difference in the type of respiratory difficulty. confirmed usually by x-ray.

aged or elderly people with rather marked emphysema in whom a careful history shows that the patients probably have had bronchial asthma. In some instances an allergic basis can be demonstrated and an appropriate eliminative regime may result in a definite improvement, a much more marked improvement than one would expect considering the amount of emphysema present. On the other hand, if the past history was that of chronic bronchitis, there is no reason to submit the patient to the tedium and expense of an allergic study.

Having decided that the patient has bronchial asthma, only part of the diagnostic task is finished. There still remains the etiologic, or what Walzer terms the specific, diagnosis to be made and here one enters a field of controversy. The last twenty years have seen much progress in the study of asthma as an allergic disease, that is, as a manifestation of protein hypersensitiveness, but we still do not know whether or not all bronchial asthma is allergic. This is, in fact, probably the major problem today in the study of asthma. There seems to be rather general agreement among clinicians who have studied large numbers of cases of bronchial asthma that forty to sixty per cent of them are allergic. Concerning the remainder there is much dispute. One group of workers is of the opinion that all bronchial asthma is allergic, and that as our methods of testing for sensitivity are refined, a larger and larger percentage of cases will be shown to belong to the allergic group. Such workers incline to the opinion that where infection seems to play a part in precipitating attacks, the underlying mechanism is sensitivity to bacterial proteins.

The opposite viewpoint is that in bronchial asthma we have a disease in which heredity plays an important, in fact, a deciding part. What is inherited, however, is, according to this opinion, not primarily a capacity for the development of protein sensitivity, but rather a tendency toward so-called "shock reactions" on the part of certain tissues. These shock reactions may be precipitated in some patients by antigen-antibody reactions, that is, by protein sensitivity, but in many patients they are provoked by other influences. The workers who subscribe to this viewpoint seem to be of the opinion that foci of infection in the respiratory tract play a part in asthma, not through the medium of bacterial allergy, but rather because of local irritation.

The details of this argument cannot be given here. From a practical viewpoint, what can and should be done to attempt to determine the etiology in a given case of bronchial asthma? Obviously an effort should be made to determine whether or not the patient belongs to the indisputably allergic group. This is not necessarily a problem for the specialist, the allergist. Much can be done by the general practitioner, either with or without equipment for skin testing. Careful history taking is of the greatest importance. A thorough history may obviate the need for skin tests or may so limit the number of probable etiologic agents that skin testing can be confined to a few materials. Is the asthma seasonal or perennial? If seasonal, the obvious and probably correct interpretation is that it is a pollen asthma and an inquiry into the dates of onset and cessation of symptoms will give a clue as to the pollens which are responsible for the condition. If the asthma is perennial, the problem becomes more difficult, but again a thorough history may give valuable information. If the patient is a farmer who has his asthmatic attacks only around stock, that is a rather clear hint that animal danders are of importance; if a woman, who has attacks only when she is doing her baking, wheat flour as an inhalant may be the offender. If no definite hints can be secured by careful questioning of the patient, there are certain statistical probabilities established by clinics which have had long experience with asthmatics. Thus a large percentage of asthmatics is found to be sensitive to feathers and a trial elimination of feathers is always worthwhile. The same is true of face powder. Even in the case of foods much may be learned from elimination diets if skin tests are not available. One possible method of procedure is to put the patient on orange juice alone for a few days and then to add foods one at a time, observing any reactions that may take place. If no information has been gained through the history and common sense elimination of materials known to be powerful antigens, then skin testing should be resorted to if available.

If investigation along these lines fails to show sensitivity to foods or inhalants, one must conclude that the patient belongs to the group which for the present we shall have to call non-allergic, and it is necessary in such cases to search for other factors which may be instrumental in bringing on attacks. Walzer, concluding his discussion of the specific diagnosis in bronchial asthma states that "one obtains the best therapeutic results when one considers asthma as a symptomatic expression of a constitutional disturbance and seeks to find any abnormality in the body which might share in the basic, secondary or contributory etiology of such a condition."

It is impossible to discuss all of the conditions

which have been cited as contributing to the production of asthmatic attacks. However, a few deserve special mention.

1. Infection in the upper and lower respiratory tract. Anyone who has taken histories on large numbers of asthmatics knows that in many cases the first attack followed a severe respiratory infection and that subsequent attacks often coincide with periods of recurrent infection. As I have said, there is disagreement as to whether infection in such cases has its effect through the medium of bacterial allergy or of local irritation. Whatever the mechanism, if sensitivity to foods or inhalants has been ruled out, infectious foci should be investigated.

2. Occasionally mechanical factors causing obstruction to breathing may be of importance. One must always be guarded in assigning significance to such conditions. Especially in the case of nasal polypi it is quite possible that they are the effect of an allergic condition toward which treatment should be directed.

3. Psychic factors. The importance of psychic factors in bringing on specific attacks of asthma and in determining their severity cannot be overemphasized and occasionally psychic factors seem to play a chief etiologic role.

In summary, then, of the etiologic diagnosis of bronchial asthma one may say that in no other condition is it more important to consider the patient as a whole, that in possibly forty to sixty per cent of cases an allergic basis will be demonstrated, but that in the remainder one will have to search for other precipitating factors.

It is obvious from the above discussion that treatment in bronchial asthma can hardly be separated from diagnosis. Many of the steps taken to arrive at a specific diagnosis, such as elimination diets, may in turn become therapeutic measures. Treatment is of two general types: first, that directed toward alleviation of the asthmatic state; and second, treatment of individual attacks.

Treatment of the asthmatic state is dependent on one's conception of the etiology in a specific case. If it is allergic asthma, sensitivity may be to pollens, foods, drugs, animal epidermals or miscellaneous inhalants. In pollen asthma, desensitization is usually very successful. Again this is something which can be carried out by the general practitioner, convenient equipment for injections of graduated doses of pollen extracts being available from most of the large drug houses. In the event of sensitivity to foods, drugs, epidermals and miscellaneous inhalants, avoidance of the offending protein is the best procedure. A clear understanding of what elimination implies is necessary. If

the patient is sensitive to feathers, not only should he himself discard feather pillows, there should be no feather pillows in the room with him, or if present they should be covered with rubber or oilcloth. If he is sensitive to wheat he should avoid not only gross amounts as in bread and pastries, but also flour used in small amounts in cooking as in gravies and cream sauces. A misunderstanding or neglect of such simple rules of elimination often defeats efforts at treatment.

Treatment of the non-allergic cases presents greater difficulties. If the asthma seems dependent on infection in the upper respiratory tract, appropriate treatment is indicated. It should be emphasized again, however, that operative work on the foci of infection is not justified until an effort has been made to rule out an allergic basis for the asthma. There are two reasons for this. In the first place if the asthma is allergic, removal of possible foci of infection will not help, and in the second place what seems to be chronic upper respiratory infection may be merely an expression of an allergic state and may itself respond to an antiallergic regime. All allergy clinics see patients who have cloudy sinuses and nasal polypi which clear up without surgery under treatment for an underlying allergic condition. On the whole, little can be expected in any cases from tonsillectomy and adenoidectomy. In fact, there is a goodly number of cases on record, in children with allergic family histories, of the onset of asthma following tonsillectomy.

Data on the use of vaccines are so contradictory that no definite statement can be made in regard to it. The workers who believe that there is sensitivity to bacterial proteins recommend vaccine therapy as a measure of specific desensitization. There is no immunologic proof of this viewpoint. The majority of allergists today seem to think that vaccine injections should be regarded as a form of nonspecific protein therapy and that stock vaccines are as efficacious therefore as autogenous. In a case of asthma in which infection seems to be playing an important part and in which the infection does not yield to the usual methods of treatment, vaccine therapy is probably justified.

Little need be said about the treatment of the asthmatic attack. Adrenalin usually will terminate it, especially when used in conjunction with ephedrine. Of some importance is the matter of dosage of adrenalin. We see many patients taking ten or fifteen minims of adrenalin routinely. Such a large amount is unnecessary in the majority of cases. At the University Hospital we get as good results with three, five or at the most seven minims, as with larger doses. Morphine does not give much relief and may in fact be harmful, perhaps because of its action as a respiratory depressant. An additional fact is that in asthma we are dealing with a chronic disease in which it is unwise to begin the use of morphine. If the patient is having almost continuous attacks of asthma, and has only a few moments relief from each dose of adrenalin, various measures may be tried. Little is gained in such cases by increasing the frequency of administration of adrenalin until the patient is getting an injection every hour or oftener. In fact, many times the patient looking to adrenalin for a few moments of relief, becomes rather frantic in his request for more and more adrenalin, and the consequent mental excitement increases the severity of his symptoms. Sometimes a severe seizure may be terminated by a starvation diet for a few days, giving the patient nothing but water and glucose or orange juice. Incidentally, having started such a regime. it is a convenient time to try the addition of foods, one at a time. to the diet, perhaps gaining some valuable information in regard to food sensitivity thereby.

Inducing fever is another helpful procedure at times in cases of so-called status asthmaticus. Often it is possible to get a history from the patient of complete relief from asthma in the past during febrile illnesses. Similarly artificial induction of fever may give relief for days or weeks. This may be accomplished by foreign protein injections or by diathermy. There have been several articles in the literature recently regarding the use of dilute hydrochloric acid in treatment of asthmatic attacks, and recently an article in the *Journal of the American Medical Association,* tending to show that there is no scientific basis for the treatment. We have had experience with its use in only a few cases, in one of which a severe asthmatic seizure seemed to be terminated with dilute hydrochloric acid intravenously.

Most asthmatic patients improve somewhat with the routine use of potassium iodide. At the University Hospital we use a prescription combining potassium iodide, grindelia and lobelia.

PEPTIC ULCER IN CHILDREN: CASE REPORT*

PAULINE V. MOORE, M.D., Solon

Peptic ulcer is found at all ages. No age is exempt. There is even one case reported of a stillbirth. the cause of which was given as hemorrhage from gastric· ulcer, intrauterine. Peptic ulcers fall into four fairly distinct groups:

1. Newly born.

*Presented before the Thirty-seventh Annual Meeting, State Society of Iowa Medical Women, Des Moines, May 8, 1934.

2. Few days to one year.
3. One year to puberty, or one to fourteen years.
4. Adult chronic peptic ulcer.

We are all familiar with those in the fourth group. Libraries have been written about the cases in this category. Although peptic ulcers are not uncommon in the first two groups, we are perhaps not so familiar with these. They are, however, rarely diagnosed except at postmortem examinations. Brockington and Lightwood of England, published an article in December, 1932, in which they state that they had collected two hundred cases from the literature and reported two more in infants.

It is difficult to determine accurately the number of cases of chronic peptic ulcer reported in group three, that is exclusive of infants, for many authors in speaking of childhood also include infancy. Foshee in 1932 reviewed the literature and found only eighteen cases of chronic *gastric* ulcer in children one to fourteen years of age. He added one of his own. In July of that year Jankleson had reported two cases, making in all, twenty-one cases of chronic gastric ulcer.

I have been unable to determine the number of reported cases of *duodenal* ulcers in children. Jankleson in his paper states that Palmer had collected forty-five cases of chronic peptic ulcer in childhood and only ten had been diagnosed clinically. On reading Palmer's paper, however, I find that these forty-five cases were in infancy and not in childhood. Foshee states that duodenal ulcer is much more common than gastric ulcer, but gives nothing to support this statement. In Proctor's report in 1925 of nineteen cases which included all reported cases up to that time, eleven of the nineteen were gastric; of the three cases reported by Jankleson, two were gastric. These figures show that duodenal ulcers, at least in this series of cases, are less common than the gastric ulcers.

I found in the literature a total of thirty-one cases in children one to fourteen years of age. I found reference to eight patients whose ages were not given except to say that they were between ten and twenty. I could not be certain that they were all distinct from the thirty-one cases first mentioned. These do not include ulcers associated with tuberculosis, burns,. etc.

However, the rarity of peptic ulcer in childhood is more apparent than real. Proctor in 1925 studied the histories of one thousand gastric and one thousand duodenal ulcers in adults at the Mayo Clinic and in these two thousand cases he found that there were forty-two histories or two per cent in which the symptoms dated back to childhood.

Leon Block in a study of four hundred fifty cases found twelve patients under twenty years of age whose symptoms began three to five years earlier, and many between the ages of twenty-five and thirty-five dated the onset of their trouble fifteen years previously. Such facts would *seem* to indicate that many children may have peptic ulcers which have been undiagnosed.

The cause of chronic peptic ulcer in childhood is probably no different than that in the adult. Rogers reported duodenal ulcers in two infants in the same family whose mother had a duodenal ulcer. He felt that heredity played an important part. Dunham and Shellon, in January of this year, reported a case of multiple ulcers in a newborn infant with staphylococcus septicemia. They list six references where peptic ulcer and positive blood cultures were found. However, in looking up these references and noting the cases, I believe it is impossible to prove that the ulcers were not the cause rather than the effect of the positive blood cultures. There is also in the literature fairly convincing evidence that chronic foci of infection are important from an etiologic standpoint. Certainly, malnutrition and improper diet are found to be underlying factors. We can't very well blame smoking and alcohol, although there is one author who claims that blood is always found in the stomach of any infant who has been given brandy as a stimulant before death.

Diagnosis of ulcer in the newborn and in infancy is said to be at the stage where adult ulcer was twenty-five years ago. A diagnosis is rarely made in the newborn except at post mortem examination because they are either so acute as to cause death, or heal so rapidly and completely that a diagnosis is not made. They are always acute and, as a rule, manifest themselves as malena neonatorum. As this fact is recognized there are fewer and fewer reported deaths from so-called hemorrhagic diseases of the newborn.

In the second group, or infants up to one year of age, the ulcers are also acute and are characterized by sudden profuse hemorrhage, or peritonitis and death, or failure to thrive, vomiting, pain after food, diarrhea, or blood in the stools. Blood has been found in over fifty per cent of the patients and failure to thrive in practically all of them. Ulcer is a sufficiently frequent finding that all children who fail to thrive should have a stool examination for blood.

In speaking of diagnosis of peptic ulcer in the third group or in children, one to fourteen years of age, Jankleson states that a clinical diagnosis is rarely made for four reasons: first, that it is not suspected; second, it is difficult to obtain a history;

third, in uncomplicated cases there is no history typical of ulcer; fourth, roentgenologic examination of the digestive tract in childhood is not made with the same frequency as in the adult.

Any history of a chronic digestive disturbance, pain after meals, night pain, vomiting and anorexia, should suggest the possibility of peptic ulcer and if the possibility is considered, diagnosis will probably be made. One finds localized tenderness, occult blood in the stools, loss of weight or failure to gain, and the x-ray evidence just as reliable in the child as in the adult.

CASE REPORT

The patient, a male child eleven years of age, first consulted me November 25, 1932, complaining of pain in the epigastrium. He was the second child, had been born prematurely, and had not gained well at first. He was slow to sit up. His teeth were delayed in erupting. He never vomited food or seemed to have colic. At six years of age he had a rather severe attack of "stomach-ache"—pain in the epigastrium. His mother called a physician who diagnosed "stomachache," left him some pills, and said he would be all right in a few days. The patient vomited some, but the mother does not remember the type of vomitus. She thinks he had a fever, but does not know how much. The patient gradually improved after being sick in bed for about ten days, but has had similar less severe attacks intermittently since. He had periods free of pain lasting three or four weeks, then periods when pain occurred daily for about a week. For the past two or three weeks he had had pain every day, usually just before the evening meal. As a rule food relieved the pain if taken immediately, but if he was unable to get food until the pain had become severe, he vomited what was eaten. Usually relief occurred spontaneously after one or two hours. The pain was precipitated and aggravated by bicycle riding and similar physical exercise. His diet had not been of the proper type for a child of his age, since it consisted chiefly of bread, potatoes and meat, including a large amount of "jiternica," a very rich and highly seasoned Bohemian bologna.

Positive findings from several examinations were as follows:

1. Undernourishment.

2. Irritability.

3. Persistent, dollar-sized tender area in epigastrium to the right of the midline.

4. Stool examination on meat-free diet on three occasions were positive for blood by both the Meyers, and benzidene tests for occult blood.

5. Atropine gr. 1/200 under the tongue relieved

the pain almost immediately during one of his severe attacks.

A tentative diagnosis of peptic ulcer, probably duodenal in nature, was made and the patient was placed on tincture of belladonna, eight minims three times a day before meals.

Arrangements were made at the University Hospital at Iowa City for the patient to have x-rays taken as an out-patient. Films taken on December 5 were reported as showing a markedly distorted and deformed duodenal cap. The diagnosis made from this evidence was duodenal ulcer. On December 10, the patient was admitted to the University Hospital and was placed on atropine gr. 1/200, three times a day, and a modified Sippy diet. An x-ray taken December 15 showed considerable improvement. The diagnosis remained duodenal ulcer. He was discharged from the hospital on December 24, with instructions to remain on the special diet and atropine gr. 1/200 three times a day. Atropine was discontinued February 21, 1933. The report on x-rays taken April 27, 1933, was "healed duodenal ulcer." He had gained fourteen pounds, was on a normal diet, and was symptomless.

The patient was in my office April 1, 1934, for a check-up examination.

He had had no symptoms since his last examination in April, 1933, his physical examination was normal, his weight was normal for a boy of his height and age. There was no history of bloody stools.

THE FINLEY HOSPITAL CLINICO-PATHOLOGIC CONFERENCES

CORONARY THROMBOSIS AND CARDIAC INFARCTION WITH PLEURAL EFFUSION

F. P. McNamara, M.D., and Paul J. Laube, B.A., Dubuque

European clinicians have recognized for the past twenty-five years the clinical features which characterize attacks of coronary thrombosis as well as their sequelae. In this country Herrick[1] first called attention to the condition in 1912. It was only after several years of persistent effort, however, that he aroused the interest of the American profession. During the last fifteen years they have added much to the knowledge of coronary disease. In spite of the abundant literature on this subject many physicians still fail to realize its importance. The case of coronary thrombosis with cardiac in-

farction to be reported is quite typical of those which do not succumb to the first attack. It is also of interest because the presenting symptoms were largely due to pleural effusion. It is well known that hydrothorax results from cardiac failure, but its association with cardiac infarction has not been especially emphasized. The case stresses the necessity of determining the cause of pleural effusion whenever it is diagnosed.

CASE REPORT

Chief complaint: The patient, a white woman sixty-five years of age, was admitted to The Finley Hospital April 22, 1934, with a complaint of "shortness of breath, pain in the right chest, and swelling of the ankles."

Family history: Irrelevant.

Past history: Six months ago the patient had what she termed a "chest cold." At that time she raised sputum which was tinged with blood. She had always been subject to "colds" and at one time she stated that it was thought that she had tuberculosis.

Present illness: Ever since her attack of six months ago she had been troubled with shortness of breath, persistent cough and at times she raised blood tinged sputum. One week before admission the symptoms had become more pronounced, and she had developed pain in the right chest and swelling of the ankles.

Physical examination: The patient was a very thin, elderly woman who had considerable difficulty in breathing. The head examination was negative. The lower half of the right chest was dull on percussion, and on ausculation the breath sounds could not be heard. Elsewhere the lung was resonant, but on ausculation moist râles were heard. The heart rate averaged 100 per minute and was weak. No adventitious sounds were heard. The lower half of the abdomen was distended with fluid. The edge of the liver was two finger's breadth below the costal margin. No masses were felt through the abdomen. There was moderate edema of the left upper and both lower extremities. The skin was very pale. The examination of the nervous system was negative. The white blood count was 12,000 per cu. mm. The urine was acid and showed a trace of albumin and moderately numerous granular casts and leukocytes; the specific gravity was 1.014. An x-ray examination showed a large pleural effusion on the right side. After the removal of 600 cc. of fluid another examination still showed a large amount of fluid in the pleural cavity. There was some infiltration in the first interspace on the right, suggestive of a minimal amount of tuberculosis.

Course in hospital: The patient's temperature fluctuated between 97 and 100 degrees; the pulse varied between 70 and 100; and the respirations averaged 24 per minute. The fluid removed from the chest was identified as a transudate. She was given digitalis therapy but in spite of the treatment she failed progressively and died on the twelfth day in the hospital.

Clinical diagnosis: Pleural effusion; chronic myocarditis.

Necropsy: At necropsy 1,000 cc. of clear, amber fluid was found in the right chest. The right

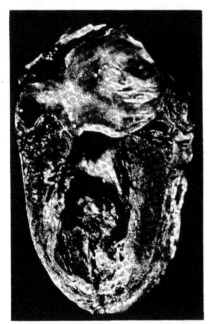

Fig. 1. A photograph of the left side of the heart. Note the replacement of the heart muscle by scar tissue and the large mural thrombus. The mitral cusps have been excised.

lung was partly atelectatic. There was a dermoid cyst of the right ovary. The lower extremities were edematous but there was no excess fluid in the peritoneal cavity. Otherwise the interesting features were confined to the circulatory system. The heart weighed 350 grams. The valve leaflets were negative except for arteriosclerotic changes. One-half the wall of the left ventricle was involved by an old infarct. The bulk of the heart muscle

had been replaced by scar tissue. A large tampon thrombus filled the lower half of the ventricle, as shown in Figure 1. The left coronary artery was calcified and the lumen had been largely obliterated by an organized and canalized thrombus; see Figure 2. The main arterial trunks showed a fairly well-marked arteriosclerotic change. The right lung showed several fresh hemorrhagic infarcts.

Anatomic diagnosis: Organized and canalized thrombus of the left coronary artery; infarct of the left ventricle with fibrosis; thrombosis of the left ventricle; pleural effusion and hemorrhagic infarcts of the right lung: arteriosclerosis; dermoid cyst of the right ovary.

GENERAL DISCUSSION

An indication of the importance of coronary thrombosis is found in the analysis of our necropsy records. There were twenty-five cardiac deaths in 275 necropsies (nine per cent). Of these twenty-five deaths, twelve (48 per cent) were due to acute attacks of coronary thrombosis or to the results of cardiac infarction, i. e., aneurysmal dilatation of the left ventricle or ventricular thrombi. In addition there were four other cases of coronary thrombosis in which some other condition was the primary cause of death. Four of the twelve deaths due to coronary thrombosis showed pleural effusion which dominated the clinical pictures. Nine of the sixteen patients with coronary thrombosis were men and seven were women. The average age was 64.4 years which is somewhat higher than that usually given in the literature, which is 57.8 years. The duration of illness from the onset to death varied between twelve hours and one year. Four of the patients died within twelve hours after the onset; two died because of perforation with hemorrhage into the pericardial sac.

Etiology: In general, coronary thrombosis is the end result of a previous angina pectoris whether detected clinically or not. A feeling of substernal pressure or dulness on exertion which may have existed for a number of years can often be elicited on careful questioning of the patient. It is well known that arteriosclerosis is more prone to occur in diabetic patients. A similar relationship holds for coronary thrombosis, and diabetes is considered to be second in importance etiologically only to a previously existing hypertension. The latter is the most common, single etiologic factor, although not an absolute prerequisite. At times the coronary sclerosis and thrombosis is one aspect of a generalized arteriosclerosis; at other times it may be practically limited to the coronary arteries. Syphilis is very rarely an etiologic factor and rheumatic infections are unrelated to coronary thrombosis. Heredity, overweight, strenuous exercise or overwork are the predisposing factors.

Diagnosis: A careful history is a great aid in arriving at a diagnosis, as there are often accounts of previous anginal attacks. These may have been so mild as to have been mistaken for gastro-intestinal complaints. Attacks of coronary thrombosis frequently occur in the early morning hours, from 2:00 to 5:00 a. m. The attack is characterized by a severe, constricting, squeezing pain in the cardiac region called by Goethe the "Devil's Grip." The pain may radiate to the left arm or to the head

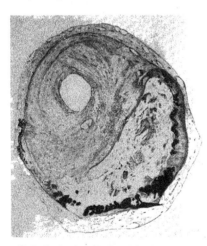

Fig. 2. Drawing of a section through the left coronary artery just proximal to the main bifurcation. Note the canalized thrombus which nearly occludes the lumen as well as the marked arteriosclerotic changes with cacification.

and neck. The patient has a feeling of collapse. Vomiting frequently occurs and in the past has lead to the diagnosis of "acute indigestion." This was due to the fact that attacks are often precipitated by a heavy meal. The patient is ashen gray; the pulse rate is increased; the blood pressure falls which is in contrast to the situation in angina pectoris. If the patient survives the immediate attack there is a moderate elevation of the temperature. and a leukocytosis of 12,000 to 20,000 occurs. Complications include cardiac rupture or aneurysm. A mural thrombus may form at the left ventricle, and emboli may cause cerebral, splenic, renal, or peripheral infarction. The electrocardiogram is typical and should be utilized in all doubtful cases.

Treatment: The treatment of coronary throm-

bosis involves absolute bed rest and adequate dosage of morphine to control the pain. Stimulants and attempts to raise the blood pressure should be avoided. Oxygen therapy may be desirable to alleviate cyanosis and dyspnea. Theobromine derivatives are useful in increasing collateral coronary circulation and thus reducing myocardial necrosis. Digitalis is contraindicated during the acute attack because of the danger of rupture and dislodgment of emboli.

Prognosis: The prognosis is always very serious, but not nearly as hopeless as was formerly thought. Fifty per cent of the patients survive the first attack and some have been known to live eighteen years. The younger the individual, the better the prognosis.

BIBLIOGRAPHY
1. Herrick, James B.: Clinical features of sudden obstruction of the coronary arteries. Jour. Am. Med. Assn., lix:2015-2020 (December 7) 1912.
2. Levine, Samuel A.: Coronary Thrombosis: Its Various Clinical Features. Williams and Wilkins Company, Baltimore, 1929.
3. Hyman, Albert S., and Parsonnet, Aaron E.: The Failing Heart of Middle Life, F. A. Davis Company, Philadelphia, 1933.
4. Smith, Fred M.: Diseases of the Heart: Musser's Internal Medicine, Lea and Febiger, Philadelphia, 1932.

REPORT OF CASES FROM THE BROADLAWNS GENERAL HOSPITAL, DES MOINES

AN UNUSUAL CONGENITAL ANOMALY CASE REPORT

WILLIAM O. PURDY, M.D., and
B. E. STOFER, M.D., Des Moines

Case No. 80705. The patient, a housewife, nineteen years of age, gravida II, presented herself in the clinic at the Broadlawns General Hospital on June 30, 1934. asking for guidance during her pregnancy.

Past history: She had had the usual childhood diseases with good recovery. She has one child eighteen months old whose weight at birth was four pounds and six ounces. The pregnancy, labor and puerperium were normal.

Family history: Essentially negative. There is no history of birth anomalies on either side.

Menstrual history: Periods began at the age of thirteen. They have been regular, occurring every twenty-eight days and lasting for five days. She was not sure of the last menstrual date, but thought it was the latter part of October, 1933.

Present history: During January of 1934 the patient experienced slight morning nausea which persisted for three weeks. Her complaint at the time of her first visit was slight swelling of the ankles. Quickening occurred the first week in

May. Physical examination on June 30 revealed a well developed and well nourished small white woman. She was four feet eleven inches tall and weighed 105 pounds. The general physical examination was essentially negative. Her pelvic measurements were within normal limits. The uterus extended to two fingers breadth above the umbili-

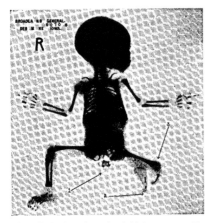

Arrow No. 1 points to lower edge of globular mass; arrow No. 2 indicates rudimentary foot; and arrow No. 3 shows the attachment of the rudimentary left leg.

cus and the fetal heart tones were heard in the left lower quadrant. Her blood pressure was 95 systolic and 50 diastolic. The blood Wassermann test was negative. The urine showed no albumin or sugar.

On July 25, 1934, she again presented herself complaining of headache and constipation. At this time her weight was 107½ pounds, blood pressure was 105 systolic and 70 diastolic; the urine showed no albumin or sugar. The fetus was active.

She again presented herself on August 9, 1934, at 1:30 P. M. complaining of labor pains which had begun at 6:30 A. M. She was admitted to the obstetric ward. Examination revealed an occipital presentation with the cervix dilated two centimeters and the membranes intact. The fetal heart tones were 146 per minute. Her labor pains continued and at 2:34 P. M. the membranes ruptured. One hour later she delivered an infant which cried immediately. The amount of amniotic fluid was not measured, but was estimated to be 600 c.c. The third stage of labor was normal.

Examination of the infant disclosed an absence or rather an incomplete closure of the lower abdo-

men through which protruded a large, globular mass approximately five centimeters in diameter. From the base of this mass there was an elongated tubular projection which measured one centimeter in diameter and two centimeters in length. There was no evidence of external genitalia and no anal opening. The left thigh appeared normal. There was only a rudiment of the left leg present with a cone-shaped mass of tissue resembling a rudimentary foot extending from this. X-ray examination demonstrated bony tissue in both these undeveloped parts. The head, chest, heart, lungs and arms were normal as far as physical examination could determine. The birth weight was three pounds and thirteen ounces. The infant lived for eight days. It was noticed during the period of life that liquid mixed with feces extruded through a small opening in the projection of tissue which extended from the large globular mass.

At postmortem examination the contents of the globular mass were found to be intestines. Behind this mass and unconnected with the outside was a

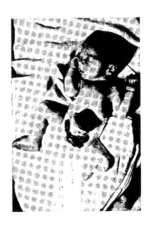

small band of tissue which extended upward and forward behind the intestines. Microscopic examination of this tissue revealed only fibrous tissue with no glandular elements present. The kidneys were found to be normally developed, but each ureter ended as a blind sac approximately one centimeter distal to the normal pelvic ureteral junction. No evidence of bladder, anus or generative organs was found. The remainder of the organs appeared normal.

The accompanying photograph and x-ray are self explanatory.

STATE DEPARTMENT OF HEALTH

NINTH ANNUAL MEETING OF THE IOWA PUBLIC HEALTH ASSOCIATION

The Ninth Annual Meeting of the Iowa Public. Health Association will be held in Des Moines on Friday, October 26, 1934.

In addition to Iowa workers in the field of Public Health, distinguished guests from other states will participate in the program. Visiting speakers include G. M. Byington, M.D., Medical Director, W. K. Kellogg Foundation, Battle Creek, Michigan; O. McDaniel, M.D., Minnesota State Department of Health, and Earle G. Brown, M.D., Executive Secretary, Kansas State Board of Health. Dr. Byington's address will be on the subject: "The Michigan Community Health Project as Sponsored by the W. K. Kellogg Foundation. Dr. Brown will present a Chalk Talk dealing with "Kansas Accident Facts." The subject of Dr. McDaniel's address, as announced is: "Observations on an Outbreak of Virulent Smallpox in the Middlewest."

The evening meeting will be a joint session with the Des Moines Academy of Medicine and the Polk County Medical Society. The guest speaker will be Russell L. Cecil, M.D., distinguished clinician, of New York. The subject of Dr. Cecil's address is "Influenza and the Common Cold."

This meeting for health workers, physicians, public health nurses and local health officers, should call forth a large attendance. The tentative program follows:

Tentative Program Ninth Annual Meeting of the Iowa Public Health Association
Friday, October 26, 1934
Headquarters—Hotel Savery
Des Moines, Iowa

8:45   Registration.

Morning Session

G. S. Westly, M.D., President, Iowa Public Health Association, presiding

9:00   Word of Welcome—Walter L. Bierring, M.D., Commissioner, Iowa State Department of Health.

9:10   Announcements.

9:20-11:00   Pointing the Way to Better Health.
A. Recent Accomplishments of Scientific Workers.
   1. In the Field of Clinical Medicine—D. J. Glomset, M.D., Des Moines, Iowa.
   2. In the Public Health Laboratory—I. H. Borts, M.D., Bacteriologist, State Hygienic Laboratories, Iowa City, Iowa.
   3. In the Field of Preventive Medicine—J. F. Edwards, M.D., Professor of Hygiene, Iowa State College, Ames, Iowa.
   4. In the Field of Dentistry—Charles Drain, D.D.S., Acting Director, Bureau of Dental Hygiene, Iowa City, Iowa.
   5. In the Field of Sanitary Engineering—A. H. Wieters, M.S., Director Division of Public Health Engineering, State Department of Health, Des Moines, Iowa.

B. Through Advances in Administrative Practice.
   1. The Committee on Child Health and Protection—Lee F. Hill, M.D., Des Moines, Iowa.
   2. The Iowa Tuberculosis Association—C. W. Kammeier, Executive Secretary, Iowa Tuberculosis Association, Des Moines, Iowa.
   3. The Federal Emergency Relief Association—Miss Ina Tyler.
   4. The 7th District Dental Society—Carl T. Ostrem, D.D.S., Ankeny, Iowa.
   5. Public Health Nursing—Miss Alice J. Pattee, R.N., Iowa Emergency Relief Administration, Des Moines, Iowa.

11:00   Kansas Accident Facts (Chalk Talk)—Earle G. Brown, M.D., Executive Secretary, Kansas State Board of Health, Topeka, Kansas.

11:45   Announcements.

Noon Luncheon Meeting

1. Essential Steps in Assuring a Safe Milk Supply—M. E. Barnes, M.D., Professor, Hygiene, Preventive Medicine and Bacteriology, University of Iowa, Iowa City, Iowa.
2. The How, Why and When of Public Health Work—Discussion led by Drs. Earle G. Brown and M. E. Barnes.

Afternoon Session

2:00   Observations on an Outbreak of Virulent Smallpox in Middlewest—O. McDaniel, M.D., Minnesota State Department of Health, St. Paul, Minnesota.

2:30   A Program of Smallpox Prevention—Discussion led by J. H. Kinnaman, M.D., Director of Child Health and Health Education, Iowa State Department of Health, Des Moines, Iowa.

3:00   Today's Major Problems in Public Health Nursing.
   1. Financing the Service—Miss Ada L. Hershey, R.N., Director of Public Health Nursing Association, Des Moines, Iowa.
   2. Educating the Public—Miss Nelle Morris, R.N., Director of Public Health Nursing, Des Moines, Iowa.
   Discussion led by Miss Alma E. Hartz, R.N., Superintendent of Public Health Nursing Association, Cedar Rapids, Iowa.

4:00   The Michigan Community Health Project as Sponsored by the W. K. Kellogg Foundation —G. M. Byington, M.D., Medical Director, W. K. Kellogg Foundation, Battle Creek, Michigan.

Evening Session

Joint Meeting with Des Moines Academy of Medicine and Polk County Medical Society

7:30   Influenza and the Common Cold—Russell L. Cecil, M.D., New York City, New York.

The JOURNAL of the Iowa State Medical Society

ISSUED MONTHLY

RALPH R. SIMMONS, Editor....................Des Moines

PUBLICATION COMMITTEE

RALPH R. SIMMONS, Editor....................Des Moines
ROBERT L. PARKER, Secretary..................Des Moines
OLIVER J. FAY, Trustee.......................Des Moines
JOHN I. MARKER, Trustee........................Davenport
EDWARD M. MYERS, Trustee..........................Boone

SUBSCRIPTION $3.00 PER YEAR

*Address all communications to the Editor of the Journal,
505 Bankers Trust Building, Des Moines*

OFFICE OF PUBLICATION, DES MOINES, IOWA

Vol. XXIV   OCTOBER, 1934   No. 10

THE ANNUAL CONFERENCE OF SECRETARIES

For the purpose of exchanging ideas and discussing those vital problems of organization and professional practice so essential for medical progress and security, the secretaries of the constituent state medical associations were called in annual conference in Chicago, September 21 and 22. The editors of the state medical journals attended as members of the conference, together with many other officers of the state associations who were welcomed as guests.

Although enriched and guided in many discussions by the officers of the American Medical Association, under whose sponsorship the conference had been called, the meeting was essentially by and for the secretaries and editors of the constituent state associations.

Keynoting the first day's activities, Dr. Oliver J. Fay of Des Moines addressed the conference on the subject of the centralization and departmentalization of state medical society activities. In his address Dr. Fay discussed the various steps in the organization of the central office of the Iowa State Medical Society, its personnel and its many functions. In concluding his address he touched briefly but pointedly upon the present economic unrest, particularly as it might affect individual medical practice. He saw in the various alphabetical bureaus established during the present administration "the insidious beginning of state medicine." It was his expressed belief that the freedom of medical practice could be maintained only if and when all physicians realize the seriousness of the present threat to private practice, and when they would collectively, through the channels of organized medicine, demand the right to practice medicine as individuals and not as hirelings. He ex-

pressed the belief that the medical profession as a whole would look with favor upon the plan of socialized medicine if the sociologic experts were able to find a sick man who is not an individualist, but is content to look upon his own welfare, his own suffering, impersonally.

President-elect James S. McLester of the American Medical Association declared his intention to conduct an active and vigorous campaign for a better and more concise diction in the presentation of medical papers. He bewailed the repetition, the inaccurate use of common or technical words, the lack of rhetorical sequence, and the utter neglect of grammatical eloquence so common in contemporary medical writings. He believed that most medical papers could be shortened by half without material loss, and that the essayists should follow the dictum of "know what you are going to say, say it, and sit down." The hearty applause accorded Dr. McLester's address (particularly from ye editors in attendance) bespoke the hearty approval given his remarks.

While much of the second day's program was devoted to the discussion of the business and economic side of medical practice, it was particularly pleasing and timely that Dr. Clyde L. Cummer, president of the Ohio State Medical Association, should have presented a valuable and thorough analysis of the educational possibilities of the scientific programs presented at state and county meetings. Dr. Cummer critically analyzed the didactic versus the clinical method of presenting scientific programs, emphatically favoring the clinical approach as a means of fixing interest. He further advocated a central bureau of the state organization to assist county societies in developing courses of study covering definitely assigned topics, and assisted by a packet library distributed from the state medical library.

Dr. R. L. Sensenich, member of the committee on legislative activities of the American Medical Association, presented an analysis of sickness insurance as now practiced in several foreign countries, and compared with it plans operating in the United States, particularly those effective on the west coast.

Dr. R. G. Leland, director of the Bureau of Medical Economics of the American Medical Association, discussed health insurance in England and the several similar medical society plans now operating in the United States.

These papers were each of a statistic nature, and to be appreciated must be studied with due care and thoroughness. The reader will be able to see the full text of these addresses in forthcoming issues of the Bulletin of the American Medical

Association. Each one stresses the desirability of maintaining the personal relationship between the patient and the doctor, and definitely declares that any scheme destroying or altering this relationship would not be acceptable and should receive the condemnation of every official body of the Association as well as the individual physicians.

WHAT IS THE BASIC SCIENCE LAW? °

Despite certain ambiguities which may be read into the title, A Basic Science Law, the principles of such legislation are simple indeed. Briefly these principles are that any practitioner of a healing art should be required to have a passable proficiency in those basic or fundamental sciences universally recognized as essential to an understanding of the pathology and symptomatology of disease. The proponents of such a bill believe that any person purporting to be a healer of disease should know sufficient anatomy, physiology and pathology to permit a scientifically accurate appreciation of the morbid state witnessed in the patient. The bill has nothing to do with therapy. The existing boards will determine the applicant's knowledge of treatment, and only the present boards will have power to issue licenses to those qualified in therapy.

The proposed board would be chosen from the faculties of the Iowa State University and the Iowa State College. It would consist of men who are qualified to examine in the basic sciences, but who are not engaged in any form of practice. This board would examine the candidates in the basic sciences of anatomy, chemistry, pathology, bacteriology, physiology and hygiene. The examination dealing with practice and therapeutic procedures would be given by a sectarian board of qualified practitioners in that particular branch of therapy for which the candidate desired a license. Such an examination would provide a higher standard for all practitioners of the healing arts, would protect the public against unqualified practitioners and would advance the objective of all legislative enactment; namely, the promotion of the welfare of citizens of the state.

The proposed basic science law seems so simple, so just, and so workable that it is difficult to explain why any thoughtful citizen, be he doctor of medicine, osteopath, or chiropractor, should object to such a law. In other states where the basic science law is in effect it has been found that a thorough understanding of its values has resulted in a desire for its adoption. It follows then that the necessary procedure is a well planned educational program. Physicians throughout the state,

° This article is the first of a series dealing with the Basic Science Law. Other editorials will appear in forthcoming issues.

serving to direct and mold public opinion in health matters, will be the most fruitful source to conduct this program of public education. The legislative committee of the state society will cooperate with any member or group of members who desire further information on this subject. We urge your active interest and influence in an educational program for the enactment of a basic science law at the next session of our legislature, to the end that a more scientific and a more adequate care of the sick in Iowa may be assured.

TINTED LENSES A FAD

Once employed only on physicians' orders, tinted lenses have now become a fad and are purchased indiscriminately by a considerable portion of our population. The popularity of the tinted lens is largely the result of certain misconceptions entertained by the laity (and some of the medical profession) regarding the utility and usefulness of various tints in glass for the protection of the eye.

It is a common belief, for example, that certain of the sun's rays, particularly the ultraviolet ray, should be excluded from the eye, and that a person when employed in the sunshine, either for work or play, should wear a colored glass. We are not aware of any conclusive proof that moderate amounts of the ultraviolet ray, such as would enter the eye on ordinary occasions, is in any way detrimental to sight. Further, it has been demonstrated that these rays are not reflected (except possibly from snow), and unless the face and eyes are deliberately exposed to sunlight, little or no fraction of the ray would actually enter the visual chamber. The misconception that the ultraviolet fraction of the sun's rays constitutes a real hazard has developed, partly from the experience with ultraviolet therapy employing a powerful artificial light, and partly from the advertising propaganda of the lens manufacturers.

In the instance of the therapeutic lamp, the concentration of the violet rays produced is many times that found in sunlight and, too, the angle of treatment favors direct admission of light into the visual chamber. A second belief which seems to be prevalent has to do with the correction of eye strain by the use of tinted lenses. For outdoor sports, particularly motoring, there is an assumption that the strain induced is not due to errors of refraction or the rapid changes in accommodation required in driving, but rather due to road glare. Competent observers state that the condition of tired or congested eyes noted after a long driving trip is usually the result of errors of refraction. Where this is true the condition should obviously be corrected by properly ground lenses of clear glass prescribed by a competent oculist. To handicap further an already defective vision by employing colored glass is worse than useless, since it does not correct an anatomic fault. Only in those cases where the brilliancy of the sunlight or road glare are solely responsible for eye fatigue, is relief obtained by a light obstructant such as a tinted glass.

A third common fallacy is that for some unknown reason a small amount of tint in the glass will remove a large amount of glare from the sunlight reflected on bright surfaces. So far as we are aware, no tint in the glass will remove glare without diminishing vision. A tint in a glass cuts out all elements of light, and if enough tint is present to dim efficiently bright lights, glare will be lessened, but it must be remembered that at the same time, distinctness in vision is also lessened. The thought that a particular tint in a glass will remove certain of the light rays while permitting others to pass through, as claimed by certain manufacturers, has been definitely disproved.

A recent issue of the JOURNAL OF THE AMERICAN MEDICAL ASSOCIATION carries a report of the Council on Physical Therapy* reciting some of the prevalent misconceptions regarding tinted lenses discussed above, and reviewing the present status of tinted lens advertising, especially that directed to the medical profession and having to do with extravagant fraudulent or unproved claims. Because of the popular demand for colored glasses it seems especially important that the general practitioner, as well as the oculist, should be thoroughly familiar with the limited scope of usefulness as presented in the report of the Council on Physical Therapy. This report indicates that the only justification for tinted lens is the actual restriction of the volume of light entering the visual chamber. Where this is desirable, and clearness of vision for distant objects can be safely sacrificed, tinted lenses may be satisfactorily employed. Beyond this little actual merit appears to exist, unless it is considered meritorious to keep up with a current fad.

*Tinted Lenses: The Present Deal. Jour. Am. Med. Assn., cii:1223-1224 (April 14) 1934.

THE INDISCRIMINATE USE AND RENTAL OF RADIUM*

Whereas, It is now recognized that radium has been demonstrated to be of definite value in the treatment of disease, and

Whereas, Some states and many communities in the country have little or no radium available, and

Whereas, Funds are not always available for the purchase of suitable preparations of radium for use

* Resolutions adopted by American Radium Society at Annual Meeting, Cleveland, June 12, 1934; also adopted by American College of Radiology, June 12, 1934.

by those physicians who are qualified in radium therapy, and

Whereas, We recognize that radium is an agent quite as potent for doing harm as for doing good when used without sufficient skill or training and with the hope of protecting the uninformed public from serious and irreparable injury from improper and insufficient treatment.

Be It Resolved, That we consider it improper, unethical and detrimental to the science of Radiology and to the good of suffering humanity for commercial laboratories to attempt to give advice or directions as to the use of radium in the case of a patient whom the person giving that advice has not even had the opportunity to examine. In other words, it is just as difficult to give such advice and directions as it would be for a surgeon to give directions for the use of rented surgical instruments so that an untrained physician might attempt an operation. Various commercial companies advertise both in the Journals and through the mails, medical advice for the purpose of making sales or renting radium or radon. This places these corporations in the field of practicing medicine.

Be It Resolved, That the same criticism be applied to institutions which rent or furnish their radium to those members of their Staff or outside of the Staff who are unskilled in radium application.

Resolved, That the same criticism applies to many individual owners of radium.

Resolved, That we regard the approval of the National Board of Radiological Examiners as the minimum standard for those assuming the responsibility for using radium. We recommend as wide publicity of this Board's existence and approval as is possible to the public, consistent with ethical practices, as the most effective safeguard which can be afforded them.

Resolved, That we recommend the refusal of advertising matter in National and State Journals when the companies concerned are advertising a Medical Consulting Service or are advertising such service through the mails in connection with their sale or rental of radium.

Resolved, That we disapprove of any doctor's acting as a Consultant to a commercial company carrying on such a campaign of public or private advertising and that we consider such an association sufficient grounds to warrant disbarment from the approval of the National Board of Radiological Examiners.

Resolved, That we recognize the ethical commercial company as a necessity. It is the advertised Consulting Service that is at fault. It is recognized that such restrictions on the advertising of a Medical Service will in no way hamper properly qualified Radium Therapists in obtaining adequate supplies of radium or radon for the purpose in which they are qualified to employ it.

Resolved, That we approve an informal Medical Consultant for the guidance of those commercial companies who refrain from advertising such professional service, either publicly or privately and that in such case their informal Consultant be one approved by the National Board of Radiological Examiners.

THE OPEN FORUM

September 19, 1934.

Editor,
Journal of the Iowa State Medical Society,
Des Moines, Iowa.

Dear Sir:

I cannot let pass without comment the editorial on pages 455 and 456 of your August issue, since some of the figures quoted refer to a paper read by me at Cincinnati. The conclusion that "the more highly industrialized a community, the lower the tuberculosis rate" seems not to be justified by the facts.

Take, for instance, the observation that tuberculosis increases with unemployment. The tuberculosis rate in this country has declined steadily throughout the depression years in the face of widespread unemployment.

Then, too, urban tuberculosis rates are, generally speaking, higher everywhere than rural tuberculosis rates and the cities are the industrial centers. "A regular job with a regular pay check" is no insurance at all against tuberculosis if that pay check won't furnish for the whole family a decent standard of living.

A recent study of "Death Rates by Occupation" shows that the tuberculosis rates increase progressively from the highest to the lowest economic classes, the unskilled laborer suffering most in this respect. While skilled workers and foremen have a tuberculosis rate of 74, semi-skilled workers have a rate of 98, and unskilled workers of 183. These latter groups far outweigh numerically the first group in any industrial community and their rate must affect unfavorably the tuberculosis rate for the community.

Very truly yours,

JESSAMINE S. WHITNEY,
Statistician, National Tuberculosis Association.

PREVALENCE OF DISEASE

	Aug. '34	July '34	Aug. '33	Most Cases Reported From
Diphtheria	13	14	30	Pottawattamie
Scarlet Fever	46	73	47	Polk, Story
Typhoid Fever	68	8	17	Black Hawk, Polk
Smallpox	1	8	3	Emmet
Measles	33	168	0	Jackson
Whooping Cough	88	98	126	Black Hawk, Woodbury
Cerebrospinal Meningitis	3	1	2	Floyd, Polk, Tama
Chickenpox	3	38	10	Delaware, Polk, Scott
Mumps	24	31	18	Linn, Woodbury
Poliomyelitis	7	2	8	(For State)
Tuberculosis	73	49	44	(For State)
Rocky Mountain Spotted Fever	2	2	0	Cedar
Undulant Fever	43	6	15	(For State)
Syphilis	156	111	218	(For State)
Gonorrhea	199	195	193	(For State)

RADIOLOGISTS HOLD NATIONAL MEETING

The Radiological Society of North America will hold its annual meeting at the Hotel Peabody in Memphis, Tennessee, December 3 to 7, inclusive. An interesting feature of the program will be the presentation of the following symposia: Silicosis, E. C. Ernst, M.D., of St. Louis; Arthritis, H. P. Doub, M.D. of Detroit; Urography, B. H. Nichols, M D. of Cleveland; Thoracic Neoplasms, J. T. Farrell, Jr., M.D., of Philadelphia; Bone Pathology, R. T. Wilson, M.D., of Temple, Texas; and Gastro-Intestinal Tract, B. R. Kirklin, M.D., of Rochester, Minnesota. Further information may be obtained by addressing the Secretary-Treasurer, Dr. Donald S. Childs, 607 Medical Arts Building, Syracuse, N. Y.

INTER-STATE POSTGRADUATE MEDICAL ASSOCIATION OF NORTH AMERICA

The annual international assembly of the Inter-State Postgraduate Medical Association of North America will be held in Philadelphia, November 5 to 9, inclusive. As has been the custom for several past years, the morning sessions will be devoted to diagnostic clinics presented by clinicians of noteworthy authority, while the afternoon and evening programs will consist of addresses and illustrated lectures. The payment of a small registration fee will admit all members of the profession in good standing, and members of the Iowa State Medical Society are cordially invited to attend.

The following physicians will present afternoon and evening addresses: Dr. Frederick J. Kalteyer, Philadelphia; Dr. Elliott C. Cutler, Boston; Dr. James T. Case, Chicago; Dr. Willis F. Manges, Philadelphia; Dr. J. M. Wheeler, New York; Dr. Waltman Walters, Rochester, Minnesota; Dr. A. M. Dogliotto, Torino, Italy; Dr. Russell L. Haden, Cleveland; Dr. William Palmer Lucas, San Francisco; Dr. Floyd E. Keene, Philadelphia; Dr. William C. Quinby, Boston; Dr. Ralph C. Brown, Chicago; Dr. Hans Guggisberg, Berne, Switzerland; Dr. Perry G. Goldsmith, Toronto, Canada; Dr. John A. Kolmer, Philadelphia; Dr. Roscoe R. Graham, Toronto, Canada; Dr. Lewellys F. Barker, Baltimore; Dr. William F. Rienhoff, Baltimore; Dr. Allen O. Whipple, New York; Dr. David Riesman, Philadelphia; Dr. Joseph F. McCarthy, New York; Dr. Paul Strassmann, Berlin, Germany; Dr. Elliott P. Joslin, Boston; Dr. William J. Mayo, Rochester, Minnesota; Dr. Vernon C. David, Chicago; Dr. Robert G. Torrey, Philadelphia; Dr. Emile F. Holman, San Francisco; Dr. Warfield T. Longcope, Baltimore; Dr. Emil Novak, Baltimore; Dr. Roberto Alessandri, Rome, Italy; Dr. Ross Golden, New York; Dr. Fielding O. Lewis, Philadelphia; Dr. W. Wayne Babcock, Philadelphia; Dr. George J. Heuer, New York; Dr. George R. Minot, Boston; Dr. Richard B. Cattell, Boston; Dr. Louis J. Karnosh, Cleveland; Dr. P. Brooke Bland, Philadelphia; Dr. Leonard G. Rowntree, Philadelphia; Dr. Charles H. Mayo, Rochester, Minnesota; Dr. Fred W. Rankin, Lexington, Kentucky; Dr. Alfred W. Adson, Rochester, Minnesota; and Dr. Edward L. Bauer, Philadelphia.

SPEAKERS BUREAU ACTIVITIES

POSTGRADUATE WORK

Nearly one-sixth of the membership of the Iowa State Medical Society is enrolled for the fall postgraduate courses promoted by the Speakers Bureau. The outlines for two of these courses were printed in the September Journal; one, a medical course which is being given at Dubuque, Davenport and Fort Madison; and the other, a surgical course which is being given at Humboldt, Ames, and Ottumwa.

The enthusiasm and enrollment for the courses is even higher than usual. Two doctors sent in their enrollment, saying: "This is our fourth course and we don't mean to miss it." Such is the attitude of those who have taken previous courses. In the new localities where they are being given, the county medical societies have worked and supported them nearly one hundred per cent.

The first meetings of the surgical and medical courses were held the last week in October. Final reports are not yet in, but the following figures show the approximate number of doctors who have enrolled for the courses at the various centers:

Humboldt	40	Dubuque	60
Ames	56	Davenport	75
Ottumwa	35	Ft. Madison	25

In addition, fifty-two doctors in the northeastern section of the state are taking the short postgraduate course on anatomy which was planned by a special committee appointed for that purpose by members of the First District Medical Society. The lectures of this course are being given by E. M. MacEwen, M.D., Professor of Anatomy at the College of Medicine, and are as follows:

    I. Anatomy of the Peripheral Nerves and Their Injuries.

    II. Neuro-anatomy.

    III. Anatomy of the Gastro-intestinal Tract.

    IV. Anatomy of the Genito-urinary and Pelvic Regions.

    V. Anatomy of the Cardiovascular-Pulmonary System.

    VI. Surgical Anatomy.

The meetings of this course are being held the second Thursdays of September, October, November, February, March and April at the Miller Hotel in New Hampton.

The doctors in Iowa are to be highly commended for their interest in postgraduate medical work and in thus keeping abreast of recent changes in their field. There are doubtless very few states that can show a better or an equal record in this field than we can here in Iowa.

MEETING OF MERIT SEPTEMBER, 1934

Credit goes to the Bremer County Medical Society for having the meeting of merit for September. They had a program essentially in keeping with the times, a symposium on Socialized Medicine, which gave those in attendance an opportunity to hear a discussion of all phases of this important problem. Those who presented the program were:

The Socialization of Medicine from the Viewpoint of the Sociologist—C. H. Graening, M.D., Waverly.

The Socialization of Medicine in Foreign Countries— E. M. Myers, M.D., Boone.

American Attempts at the Socialization of Medicine —M. B. Call, M.D., Greene.

The Socialization of Medicine from the Viewpoint of Organized Medicine—John H. Henkin, M.D., Sioux City.

This hospitable little county had invited the members from neighboring counties and about sixty doctors assembled at Waverly on September 20 for an enjoyable dinner, and for one of the most interesting and worthwhile programs ever presented before a medical group. The interest in the program was manifested by the discussion which followed.

The anniversary meeting of the Dubuque County Medical Society deserves meritorious comment, also. More than seventy-five doctors attended this eighty-first anniversary meeting at Dubuque on September 11. The morning program was presented by local men and the afternoon talks were given by noted medical and surgical guests.

RADIO BROADCASTS

Attention is called to the change in the schedule for our radio weekly broadcasts. They will now be heard on Wednesdays at 4:00 p. m., over WOI, Ames, and on Thursdays at 7:45 p. m. over WSUI, Iowa City.

October 3- 4—The Story of Anesthesia—John Russell, M.D.

October 10-11—Biology: The Story of Life—W. W. Bowen, M.D.

October 17-18—How the Body Works: Digestion— A. N. Schanche, M.D.

October 24-25—How the Body Works: Respiration— G. Raymond Johnson, M.D.

Oct. 31-Nov. 1—How the Body Works: Circulation— L. F. Catterson, M.D.

November 7-8—How the Body Works: Elimination W. B. Lewis, M.D.

Legislative Committee Page

IOWA NEEDS THE BASIC SCIENCE LAW

What Is the Basic Science Law?

It is legislation which establishes uniform educational standards in fundamental sciences for all applicants for license to diagnose and treat human ailments.

What Are the Fundamental Sciences?

Anatomy, physiology, chemistry, bacteriology, pathology and hygiene.

Why Does Iowa Need the Basic Science Law?

The Iowa Law provides for three examining and licensing boards which set three different educational standards for license to diagnose and treat human ailments, viz.:

1. One board requires graduation from high school, or equivalent, and completion of three courses of lectures of six months each.

2. Another board requires graduation from high school, or equivalent, and four years' professional training.

3. The third board requires graduation from high school, two years of college preparation, four years professional training and one year of postgraduate interneship.

When several boards are in authority, educational standards always suffer. Protection of the public requires that all practitioners be competent. It is not sufficient to require a high degree of skill on the part of some and a low degree on the part of others.

Since 1921 the board with lowest standards has granted 2,056 licenses.

Since 1921 the board with next lowest standards has granted 576 licenses (approximately).

Since 1921 the board with highest standards has granted 827 licenses.

Correct diagnosis and intelligent treatment of human ailments are wholly dependent upon thorough knowledge of the fundamental sciences. License is for the protection of the public. Our present laws do not sufficiently protect the public. Our present laws recognize all those licensed by any of these boards as *physicians* qualified to diagnose and treat human ailments.

How Will the Basic Science Law Function?

It will require all applicants for license to pass examination in the fundamental sciences before appearing for examination by any of the licensing boards. The Board of Examiners in the Fundamental Sciences will consist of men appointed by the Governor from the faculties of the Iowa State College and the State University. They must be men who are in no way engaged in the practice of any of the healing arts. The Board will have no effect upon anyone who is already licensed. It will have no interest in the kind of therapy which the applicant might wish to use. This Board will be concerned only with determining the applicant's fitness in the fundamental sciences on which the practice of all forms of treatment is based.

What Are the Objections to the Basic Science Law?

There are none from the standpoint of public protection. The opposition comes from those who favor low standards of training. Many opponents have an interest in schools that train students in conformity with the requirements of the boards of low standards.

Will the Basic Science Law Interfere With Anyone Choosing the Kind of Physician He May Wish (Doctor of Medicine, Osteopathy or Chiropractic)?

No. It will ensure his having a better trained doctor regardless of the type he may wish to employ.

ABSTRACT OF A BILL FOR

AN ACT to establish a State Board of Examiners in the Fundamental Sciences underlying the practice of the Healing Arts, to provide for its organization and powers, to provide that certification by such Board be a prerequisite to eligibility for examination for a license to practice the healing arts and to define healing arts.

Fundamental Science Certificate Required

Applicant for examination by any licensing board (medical, osteopathic, chiropractic, etc.) must first pass examination of Board of Examiners in the Fundamental Sciences, with a passing grade of not less than 70 per cent in any one subject and a total average of not less than 75 per cent.

The Healing Art Defined

A license authorizing the licentiate to offer or undertake to diagnose, treat, operate on or prescribe for any human pain, injury, disease, deformity, or physical or mental condition, is a license to practice the healing art.

Non-Sectarian Board

The members of the examining board shall be appointed by the Governor from the faculties of the State University of Iowa, and the State College of Agriculture and Mechanic Arts. No member of the board shall be engaged in the practice of any branch of the healing art.

Certificate by Reciprocity

With other states having similar requirements.

Fees Paid Unauthorized Persons Recoverable

Any money paid out by any person as compensation for services rendered in the practice of the healing art, to any person not validly licensed to practice, may be recovered by suit instituted within two years from date of payment, if payor did not know that payee was not validly licensed.

Exceptions

This act shall not be construed as applying to dentists, nurses, midwives, optometrists, embalmers, pharmacists, podiatrists, barbers or cosmetologists; nor to other persons licensed to practice the healing art in this state when this act takes effect.

Saving Clause

No provision of this act shall be construed as repealing any statutory provision in force at the time of its passage.

WOMAN'S AUXILIARY NEWS

Edited by the Press and Publicity Committee

MRS. OLIVER J. FAY, *Chairman*, 405 Thirty-seventh Street, Des Moines

Fall Board Meeting of the Woman's Auxiliary

The Fall Board Meeting of the Woman's Auxiliary to the Iowa State Medical Society was held Wednesday, September 26, at the home of Mrs. James A. Downing in Des Moines. Twenty-three members came from all parts of the state to attend the meeting.

The session was called to order at ten-thirty by the president, Mrs. Downing. After the reading of the minutes of the Spring Board Meeting by the secretary, Mrs. A. C. Starry of Sioux City, the president called for reports of the committee chairman. Mrs. M. C. Hennessy of Council Bluffs, first vice president, who has charge of the organization of county auxiliaries, gave an interesting report. Maps and detailed instructions had been prepared for each member of this committee showing the organization well in hand after having been worked out by the chairman. Mrs. W. A. Seidler of Jamaica, chairman of the health essay contest committee, told of the plans for the coming year. The Board voted to ask the county auxiliaries for contributions to defray the expenses of this committee. A short report was given by Mrs. E. L. Bower of Guthrie Center on the national meeting at Cleveland. Dorothy M. Nelson of the Speakers Bureau of the Iowa State Medical Society spoke briefly, offering the services of that organization to the auxiliary.

Mrs. Walter L. Bierring was a guest at the luncheon served by Mrs. Downing, assisted by Mrs. Thomas A. Burcham and Mrs. H. B. Woods. After the luncheon Mrs. Bierring told of a few of the social events of the American Medical Association meeting in Cleveland.

The Board adjourned at three o'clock to meet in Davenport next April.

National Board Meeting

Mrs. James A. Downing attended the Board Meeting of the Woman's Auxiliary to the American Medical Association held in Chicago, Saturday, September 22, at the Pearson Hotel.

Eight states were represented by their presidents. Several changes in the constitution were proposed, following a discussion as to the best method of administering the Corrine Keen Freeman Fund. This fund was created from the money sent by various states at the time of Mrs. Freeman's death two years ago. The amount was so great that it was decided to create a fund which would be available for incoming presidents to draw upon for immediate expenses; this sum to be returned to the fund before the expiration of her office.

The Board was entertained at luncheon by the Central Chicago District Woman's Auxiliary, headed by Mrs. Charles Woodford, president.

Committees of the State Organization

It has been suggested to the Press and Publicity Committee by the Board that certain monthly issues of the Woman's Auxiliary page be devoted to the work of the committees. The November issue of the JOURNAL OF THE IOWA STATE MEDICAL SOCIETY will carry a report of the work done by the Educational Program Committee, of which Mrs. Channing G. Smith of Granger is chairman. Please watch for further announcements.

Standing Committees

Education-Program—Mrs. Channing G. Smith, Granger, chairman; Mrs. Hugh B. Woods, Des Moines; Mrs. G. E. Harrison, Mason City; Mrs. Clyde A. Boice, Washington; Mrs. A. A. Johnson, Council Bluffs.

Public Relations—Mrs. M. N. Voldeng, Woodward, chairman; Mrs. E. L. Wurtzer, Clear Lake; Mrs. H. C. Payne, Pella; Mrs. S. D. Maiden, Council Bluffs; Mrs. J. H. McCall, Allerton.

Hygeia—Mrs. E. L. Bower, Guthrie Center, chairman; Mrs. E. M. Kersten, Fort Dodge; Mrs. Isaac Sternhill, Council Bluffs; Mrs. Channing Wolfe, Coon Rapids.

Revisions—Mrs. A. E. Merkle, Ankeny, chairman; Mrs. P. W. Beckman, Perry; Mrs. Charles B. Taylor, Ottumwa; Mrs. F. J. Swift, Des Moines; Mrs. Oliver J. Fay, Des Moines.

Press and Publicity—Mrs. Oliver J. Fay, Des Moines, chairman; Mrs. E. L. Emerson, Muscatine; Mrs. T. E. Davidson, Mason City; Mrs. J. C. Donahue, Centerville, Mrs. A. A. Robertson, Council Bluffs.

Printing—Mrs. P. W. Beckman, Perry; Mrs. R. W. Perkins, Sioux City.

Essay Contest—Mrs. William Seidler, Jamaica, chairman; Mrs. E. B. Bush, Ames; Mrs. Daniel J. Glomset, Des Moines; Mrs. S. E. Lincoln, Des Moines; Mrs. Thomas A. Burcham, Des Moines.

Legislative—Mrs. Thomas A. Burcham.

SOCIETY PROCEEDINGS

Adams County

Tuesday, September 25, every member of the Adams County Medical Society joined in surprising Dr. Mark E. Johnson at a birthday celebration held in his home in Corning. Fate smiled on the doctors in Adams county that evening and everyone was able to stay for the entire evening.

J. H. Wallahan, M.D., Secretary

Buchanan County

Ray A. Fox, M.D., of Charles City, furnished the scientific program for the Buchanan County Medical Society, at a meeting held in Independence, Thursday, September 13. Dr. Fox spoke on Treatment of Varicose Veins and Hemorrhoids by the Injection Method.

Calhoun County

The Calhoun County Medical Society held a meeting in the new Community Building at Lohrville, Tuesday, September 11. After a six-thirty dinner, Fred Moore, M.D., of Des Moines, and R. D. Bernard, M.D., of Clarion, presented two very interesting papers on The Proposed Basic Science Law. Discussion was entered into by all members present.

W. W. Stevenson, M.D., Secretary

Clinton County

Thursday afternoon, September 6, the members of the Clinton County Medical Society held their annual picnic at the Neil Nelson Cabin in Camanche. This marked the resumption of activities of our society after the summer recess. A large number of physicians from Clinton county, as well as many guests from neighboring cities were in attendance and enjoyed the picnic supper and outing.

Our next regular meeting is scheduled for November 1. By request of the Linn County Medical Society, we will not have our regular October meeting inasmuch as the date conflicted with Linn county's meeting at which Dr. Joseph B. DeLee will speak.

E. V. Donlan, M.D., Secretary

Dubuque County

The eighty-first anniversary meeting of the Dubuque County Medical Society was held at the Elks Club, Tuesday, September 11, with more than seventy-five physicians and guests in attendance. The morning program was as follows: Surgery in the Aged, Donald C. Conzett, M.D.; Discussion of Rhythm Theory, Roy I. Theisen, M.D.; Ruptured Kidney with Postmortem Findings, R. R. Harris, M.D.; The X-ray in the Diagnosis of Gastric Ulcer, L. G. Ericksen, M.D.; Miliary Tuberculosis with X ray Findings, J. O. Painter, M.D.; Acute Pancreatitis, A. C. Pfohl, M.D.; and Treatment of Appendiceal Abscess, D. F. Ward, M.D.

After a twelve-thirty luncheon, the following program was presented: Bronchoscopic Diagnosis and Treatment of Lung Conditions, P. D. Vinson, M.D., of Rochester; Fractures of Nose, Jaws and Other Facial Bones, F. A. Figi, M.D., of Rochester; and Early Diagnosis of Cancer, L. G. Rigler, M.D., of Minneapolis.

Floyd County

The Floyd County Medical Society held its regular meeting in the staff rooms of the Cedar Valley Hospital at Charles City, Tuesday, August 28. A complimentary dinner was served at six o'clock. R. A. Knight, M.D., of Rockford, demonstrated the Ascheim-Zondek test for pregnancy, and C. W. McQuillen, M.D., of Charles City, demonstrated the Elliot heat treatment.

Hardin County

On Thursday, September 27, after a six o'clock dinner at the Hotel Winchester in Eldora, C. W. Baldridge, M.D., of Iowa City, addressed the members of the Hardin County Medical Society on The Untoward Effects of Some Commonly Used Drugs.

Linn County

Dean D. Lewis, M.D., of Baltimore, was the guest speaker for the Linn County Medical Society at its meeting held Wednesday, September 12, at the Hotel Roosevelt in Cedar Rapids. Dr. Lewis, professor of surgery at Johns Hopkins University, spoke on The Diagnosis of Breast Tumors.

Thursday, October 4, the society entertained Joseph B. DeLee, M.D., of Chicago, who spoke before the members, and presented moving pictures with sound, showing forceps operations and episiotomy.

The next program of the Linn County Medical Society will be held Thursday, October 25, when Russell L. Cecil, M.D., of New York, will speak on Some Phases of the Arthritis Problem.

Louisa County

The Louisa County Medical Society met in regular session at Grandview, Thursday, September 13. After a six-thirty dinner the following program was presented: Neurology for the General Practitioner, M. L. McCreedy, M.D., of Brighton; and Making a Diagnosis, C. A. Boice, M.D., of Washington. Miss Mary Briley of the Washington Evening Journal, spoke on the project of advertisements in lay publications, tending to explain the relationship between physicians and the lay public. It was moved, seconded, and carried, that this society go on record as favoring the proposed change in the by-laws of the Southeastern Iowa Medical Society.

J. H. Chittum, M.D., Secretary

Polk County

The regular meeting of the Des Moines Academy of Medicine and Polk County Medical Society was held Tuesday, September 25, at the Hotel Fort Des Moines. The following symposium on Cancer of the Stomach was presented; Diagnosis, John T. Strawn, M.D.; Pathologic Features, William E. Sanders, M.D.; and Treatment, John B. Synhorst, M.D. Discussion was led by Drs. C. B. Luginbuhl, Julius S. Weingart, and N. Boyd Anderson.

On Monday, October 8, Clint E. Harris, M.D., medical director of the Modern Woodmen of America Sanatorium of Woodmen, Colorado, addressed a special meeting, presenting an illustrated lecture on Diagnosis of Lung Tumors.

Another special meeting will be held Friday, October 26, at which time Russell L. Cecil, M.D., of New York, will speak on Influenza and the Common Cold.

Scott County

Eugene F. Traut, M.D., of Chicago, was the speaker of the evening when the Scott County Medical Society met in regular session Tuesday, September 4, in Davenport. Dr. Traut, who is clinical associate in medicine at Rush Medical College, spoke on A Study of Arthritis.

Henry A. Meyers, M.D., Secretary

Wapello County

The Wapello County Medical Society started its new year Tuesday, September 4, by giving a complimentary dinner to Dr. H. W. Vinson, who served the society as secretary for sixteen years. This meeting was held at Birchwood Lawns. Dr. Vinson was the principal speaker and chose as his subject, "Reminiscences." His talk reviewed the high lights, so to speak, of his sixteen years as secretary. It was a very interesting and instructive paper, so much so that on motion it was voted to incorporate it *in toto* in the minutes of the meeting. The society, through its Dean of Medicine, Dr. S. A. Spilman, presented Dr. Vinson with a desk set in appreciation of his service. - Dr. W. C. Newell also presented Dr. Vinson with an autograph album, signed by all the members attending the meeting.

Representatives of five medical groups having public health responsibilities attended an inter-professional meeting sponsored by the Wapello County Medical Society, held Tuesday, September 18 in Ottumwa. Possibilities for Cooperation was the title of the address by George J. Judisch of Ames, chairman of the Iowa State Board of Pharmacy. The Iowa State Association of Registered Nurses was represented by its president, Millie A. Jacobsen of Des Moines. Dr. S. A. Spilman, past president of the Iowa State Medical Society, and Dr. C. M. Work, past president of the Iowa State Dental Association, spoke for their respective professions. There were several veterinarians in attendance, although no one had been selected to speak. No organization was effected, but it was the desire of the group as a whole that another meeting of a similar type should be held again in the not distant future. It is probable that such a meeting will be held next year,

sponsored by the Wapello County Medical Society.

Tuesday, October 2, D. O. Bovenmyer, M.D., of Ottumwa, furnished the scientific program for the society, presenting a paper on Indications for Mastoidectomy.

On Tuesday, October 16, a dinner meeting will be held at Sunnyslope Sanatorium, complimentary to all physicians in the Ninth Councilor District and the four counties east of Wapello, as well as other guests from different parts of the state who may care to attend. J. A. Myers, M.D., of Minneapolis, will conduct a clinic in the afternoon, and will be the speaker for the evening program. Dr. Myers' subject will be The Modern Aspects of Diagnosis, Treatment and Prevention of Tuberculosis.

Evon Walker, M.D., Secretary.

Washington County

The Washington County Medical Society held its regular monthly meeting, Tuesday, October 2. The speaker of the evening was James C. Donahue, M.D., of Centerville, who explained the workings of the Federal Emergency Relief Administration as it pertains to the doctors of Iowa. It was a splendid address and was thoroughly enjoyed.

W. S. Kyle, M.D., Secretary

Woodbury County

The Woodbury County Medical Society met in conjunction with the deputy councilors of the Fourth District, Tuesday, September 18, at the West Hotel in Sioux City. A. C. Starry, M.D., read a paper on The Pathologic Study of Heart Lesions, and R. D. Bernard, M.D., of Clarion, discussed The Basic Science Law.

L. E. Pierson, M.D., Secretary

Southwestern Iowa Postgraduate Society

Members of the Southwestern Iowa Postgraduate Society and the Pottawattamie County Medical Society met at the Mercy Hospital in Council Bluffs, Thursday, September 27, and the following program was presented: Observations on Recent Milk-Borne Outbreaks of Epidemic Disease in Iowa, Carl F. Jordan, M.D., of Des Moines; Medical Legal Problems as Found by the Bacteriologist and Chemist, John T. Meyers, M.D., of Omaha; and Bronchoscopy, S. D. Maiden, M.D., of Council Bluffs. There was a good attendance and the next meeting will be held in Atlantic.

INTERESTING NEWS
In Brief

About one hundred persons die every year in the United States from rabies.

Yellow fever is endemic and present in Western Africa, and tropical South America.

Vacua have been produced so near to nothingness as to be 99.999999 per cent or more complete.

A recent geologic investigation has led scientists to believe that man has existed as such for at least ten million years.

In the United States it is estimated that about one person in three over forty years of age suffers from some chronic disease.

A substance which produced a ten-fold decrease in the growth of cancers in mice has been found in the kidney excretions of expectant mothers.

A German physician reports that the healing of wounds may be greatly hastened by the use of a semi-solid ointment containing cod liver oil.

Recent reliable statistics indicate that trachoma, the principal cause of blindness throughout the world, is definitely on the decrease in the United States.

A recent statement made by the Commissioner of Indian Affairs reveals the death rate from tuberculosis among Indians to be seven times that of the white race.

Investigations show that allergic sensitivity to tobacco may manifest itself in migraine headaches, irregularity of heart action, and diseases of the blood vessels.

The hormone test for sex determination, devised by two San Francisco physicians, has been proved worthless by investigations at the University of Pennsylvania.

The prescription of powdered toads for heart trouble, employed by Chinese doctors, appears less irrational since the discovery that certain glands in the toad produce adrenalin.

Investigations conducted at the University of Capetown, South Africa, lead to the conclusion that toads may be substituted for rabbits in performing the Zondek-Ascheim test for pregnancy.

The Wyatt Clinic Research Laboratories at Tucson, Arizona, have been licensed by the United States government to manufacture a new vaccine for the treatment of chronic infectious arthritis.

At the recent meeting of the American Psychiatric Association, particular attention was given to the influence of emotional disturbances in the production of physical diseases such as, peptic ulcer, goiter, and diabetes.

More prompt and lasting results are obtained in the treatment of rheumatic joints by means of paraffin baths than other methods of applying heat. The method has been used extensively in European clinics.

A study of entrants to the British Royal Air Force shows that overweight young men have more physical endurance, greater resistance to infectious diseases, and are less likely to develop nervous or mental disorders than young men who are underweight.

PERSONAL MENTION

Dr. Henry S. Houghton, formerly dean of the College of Medicine, State University of Iowa, has resigned his position as director of the clinics of the University of Chicago, and dean of the biological sciences, and will go to China as advisory representative of the Chinese Medical Board and the Peiping Union Medical College.

Dr. Douglas H. Brown, formerly associate instructor at the College of Medicine, State University of Iowa, has opened an office for general practice in Davenport.

Dr. J. L. Klein of Muscatine, spoke before the local Kiwanis Club, Tuesday, August 28, on "The Development of Medicine During the Last Fifty Years."

Dr. George H. Parmenter has arrived in Des Moines to assume his duties as chief of the medical staff at the United States Veterans Hospital. Dr. Parmenter comes from Fort Harrison, Montana, where he has held a similar position for some time.

Dr. H. L. Hollenbeck of Osceola, is retiring from the practice of medicine because of ill health. His practice will be taken over by Dr. William L. Wall, a former resident of Osceola.

Dr. Della Galinsky and **Dr. Leon J. Galinsky,** son and daughter of Mr. and Mrs. Herman Galinsky of Sioux City, have returned to their native city to enter the practice of medicine together. Dr. Della Galinsky received her medical degree from the State University of Iowa, and served her internship at the Municipal Hospital in Jersey City, New Jersey. Dr. Leon Galinsky was graduated from the Rush Medical College in Chicago, and interned in Spokane, Washington.

Dr. G. C. Blome of Ottumwa, addressed the Monday night meeting of the Ottumwa Kiwanis Club, August 27, on the subject of "Cancer."

Dr. J. M. Cowen, a recent graduate of the University of Nebraska College of Medicine, is locating for the practice of medicine in Glenwood. Dr. Cowen served his internship at the Jennie Edmundson Hospital in Council Bluffs.

Dr. Jacob Kulowski, of the department of orthopedic surgery, State University of Iowa, College of Medicine, has resigned his position, and will enter the private practice of medicine in St. Joseph, Missouri.

Dr. T. E. Shonka, who was graduated from Creighton University Medical School, and who interned at the Mercy Hospital in Council Bluffs, has located in Malvern.

Dr. H. W. Kruse of Rockford, spoke to members of the Charles City Lions Club, Friday, August 31, on "Recent Personal Observations in Germany."

Dr. W. F. Carver has returned to Fort Dodge from California, where he has lived for the past two years, and will resume the practice of his specialty, diseases of the eye, ear, nose and throat.

———

Dr. Philip A. Scott, formerly of Tulsa, Oklahoma, has located in Emmetsburg.

———

Dr. Julia Cole of Iowa City, spoke before the Iowa Falls Parent-Teachers Association, Tuesday, September 25, on "Allergic Diseases."

———

Dr. W. W. Stirlen, who has practiced in Delta for more than twenty-five years, has moved his office to Muscatine, where he will take over the equipment and practice of the late Dr. S. D. Folsom.

———

Dr. C. M. Creswell, who was graduated in 1932 from the State University of Iowa, College of Medicine, and who interned at the Rochester General Hospital, Rochester, New York, has located for the practice of medicine in Strawberry Point.

———

Dr. Peter A. Bendixen of Davenport, was a guest speaker for the Michigan State Medical Society, Thursday, September 12, taking for his subject, "Fractures of the Hip."

———

Dr. Carl E. Sixbury, who has practiced medicine in Lamoni for eight years, has left for Sturgis, South Dakota, where he will be stationed at Camp Meade.

———

MARRIAGES

Miss Grace Glass and Dr. Edward H. Files, both of Cedar Rapids, were married at the home of Mrs. Howard W. Files, sister-in-law of the bridegroom, Saturday, September 8. After a two weeks' wedding trip to Canada, the young couple returned to Cedar Rapids, where Dr. Files has been practicing for four years.

———

The wedding of Miss Eula May Rossean and Dr. W. H. Kerr, both of Hamburg, took place Wednesday, September 5, in Sidney. Dr. Kerr is the son of Dr. William Kerr of Randolph. After a two weeks' trip through Colorado, Dr. and Mrs. Kerr returned to Hamburg, where Dr. Kerr has been practicing for three years.

———

Saturday, September 8, was the date selected by Miss Vera Evalyn Langley for her marriage to Dr. John R. Rankin, son of Dr. and Mrs. William Rankin of Keokuk. The wedding took place at the home of the bride's parents in Keokuk. Immediately after the ceremony and wedding breakfast, Dr. and Mrs. Rankin left on a wedding trip to the Ozark Mountains, returning to Keokuk on September 20. Dr. Rankin has entered the practice of medicine in that city during the past year.

Miss Lucille Loetscher and Dr. Laurence E. Cooley, both of Dubuque, were married Saturday, September 8, at the home of the bride's parents in Dubuque. The young couple will make their home in Dubuque, where Dr. Cooley is engaged in the practice of medicine.

———

DEATH NOTICES

Alford, Edward True, aged 59, formerly of Waterloo, died at his home in West Palm Beach, Florida, on September 22, of heart disease. He was graduated in 1901 from Rush Medical College, Chicago, and had long been a member of the Black Hawk County Medical Society.

———

Maloy, John Thompson, of Bedford, aged 63, died suddenly September 14, of heart disease. He was graduated in 1892 from Marion-Sims College of Medicine, St. Louis, and at the time of his death was a member of the Taylor County Medical Society.

———

Murphy, John Joseph, of Sioux City, aged 48, died September 20, following a brief illness of erysipelas and streptococcic infection. He was graduated in 1911 from Creighton University School of Medicine, Omaha, and at the time of his death was a member of the Woodbury County Medical Society.

———

Stephenson, Robert Bruce, of Libertyville, aged 76, died September 15, following an accident. He was graduated in 1885 from Starling Medical College, Columbus, Ohio, and had long been a member of the Jefferson County Medical Society.

———

Willis, Lyle Joseph, of Fort Madison, aged 34, died August 11, as the result of an accident. He was graduated in 1929 from the University of Illinois College of Medicine, Chicago, and at the time of his death was a member of the Lee County Medical Society.

———

ANNUAL CLINIC COLLEGE OF MEDICINE

The twenty-third annual clinic of the College of Medicine will be held on Friday, November ninth and on the Morning of Saturday, November tenth, 1934.

Lectures and clinics will be offered by members of the staff of the College of Medicine. On Friday evening there will be a dinner at the Iowa Memorial Union followed by an address.

All physicians are cordially invited to attend these clinics. Those in attendance will please register from eight-thirty to nine o'clock on Friday morning, November ninth, in the lobby of the University Hospital.

HISTORY OF MEDICINE IN IOWA

Edited by the Historical Committee.

DR. HENRY B. YOUNG, Burlington
DR. FRANK M. FULLER, Keokuk
DR. JOHN T. McCLINTOCK, Iowa City

DR. TOM. B. THROCKMORTON, Des Moines
DR. WALTER L. BIERRING, Des Moines
DR. WILLIAM JEPSON, Sioux City

Diphtheria in Iowa in 1880

FREDERICK J. SWIFT, M.D.

Deputy Commissioner Iowa State Department of
Health, Des Moines, Iowa

The First Biennial Report of the State Board of Health, for the years 1880 and 1881 contains letters from physicians and local health officers, with discussions of various infectious diseases and their prevalence. The letters were prepared in response to a questionnaire forwarded by L. F. Andrews, then secretary of the State Board of Health. A reply from A. V. Strout, M.D., of Parkersburg, Butler County, Iowa, dated November 15 1881, is of unusual interest. The letter deals with diphtheria which was very prevalent in that community during 1880. Dr. Strout classified the cases and deaths according to age groups and listed the modes of deaths. Although diphtheria was present in virulent form at the time the account states that "the croupous form has seldom been seen." (Membranous croup had for manv years been regarded as a condition separate from diphtheria. It was Bard, an American, who in 1771 expressed the strong belief that membranous croup and pharyngeal diphtheria were manifestations of one and the same disease. That Dr. Strout held the modern viewpoint is shown clearly in his report.) The reply of Dr. Strout is of interest to all who are concerned with the work of disease prevention. Diphtheria, although less prevalent now than a half century ago, retains its former virulence. The disease still finds its victims in families where delay in treatment and neglect of preventive measures prevail. Dr. Strout's report on diphtheria reads as follows:

I forward a record of diphtheria cases in my own practice that was made up two months ago, and I have had a good many cases since. If the Board desires any information not found in that, I will gladly comply with any request they may make.

We have had diphtheria, both in the town and county, continuously for ten months prior to September 18, and are still having cases.

By way of preface, lest I shall be misunderstood, I will state that all the cases reported in this paper are *genuine diphtheria,* and that no case of follicular pharyngitis or other form of sore throat has been taken into consideration.

During this time, however, I have kept a record of over fifty cases of follicular pharyngitis (and many cases I did not record) where the patient would be confined to the bed from three to five days, with a high fever and a very sore throat, characteristic of that disease, but entirely unlike diphtheria to an experienced observer. I have never seen an epidemic of diphtheria that was not accompanied with an epidemic also of this disease; and, I am sorry to say, many practitioners call these cases diphtheria; some, perhaps, through ignorance, and many, to enhance their reputation.

In the following table I have classified the patients according to their several ages at the time of the attack:

Under one year of age	1
From one to two years of age	2
From two to three years of age	6
From three to nine years of age	22
From nine to twelve years of age	13
From twelve to fifteen years of age	12
From fifteen to twenty years of age	9
From twenty to thirty years of age	4
From thirty to forty years of age	3
Total	72

Thus it will be seen that the liability to the disease under one year of age is comparatively nothing; while from one to two years of age it is not materially increased; but from two to three years the susceptibility increases quite fast; and from three to fifteen years it reaches its maximum and again diminishes until at forty it has nearly ceased again.

The following table shows the mode of death:

Croup	0
Blood poisoning	17
Uraemia	5
Oedema of the lungs	1
Embolism	1
Total	24

During this epidemic the croupous form has seldom been seen. The greater portion (nearly 71 per cent) die from blood poisoning.

I have observed that those cases that get well usually commence to improve from about the end of the fifth day of the attack. On the other hand, where they do not recover they usually get worse very rapidly during the latter part of the fifth day, and die from the sixth to the tenth day, but many more on the sixth and seventh than later.

When uraemic symptoms supervene it has usually occurred about the fifteenth day, and after the patient had become convalescent, with the exception of one case, when it come on the twelfth day. I am unable to predetermine what cases will be attacked with this trouble, but have observed in all thus attacked the membrane come off very slowly. But the amount of the membrane or the constitutional disturbance is no index.

When these uraemic symptoms have arisen, I know of no remedy or combination of remedies that will arrest its progress, as they die in from eighteen to twenty-four hours.

The patient with oedema of the lungs lived thirty-four days from the date of the attack. He had been convalescent over two weeks, and I considered him well, with the exception that he was paralyzed so he could scarcely walk, and could eat and drink with great difficulty. He seemed to be doing finely till twenty-four hours prior to death.

One died from heart-clot while attempting to arise from the bed.

As will be seen from the table giving modes of death, I have lost twenty-four patients out of seventy-two or 33⅓ per cent. But those figures need some explanation, as they include consultations; and in quite a number of the cases I was not called till the patient was virtually dying.

Exclusive of consultations, and where I was called at the commencement of the disease, I find fifty-eight cases recorded, of which ten died, or 17½ per cent; which therefore represents my actual per cent of loss.

It is a big death rate, but when I look back over these cases I congratulate myself that it is not larger.

A table showing age at time of death:

Under two years of age	3
From two to five years of age	2
From five to nine years of age	4
From nine to twelve years of age	4
From twelve to fifteen years of age	7
From fifteen to twenty years of age	3
Twenty-two years of age	1
Total	24

By comparing this with the table showing the number of cases attacked for each year of age, the comparative mortality for each period can be obtained.

Thus, all the cases under two years of age died; while out of twenty-eight cases from two to nine years old six died; and of thirteen from nine to twelve years old, four died. But of twelve cases from twelve to fifteen years old, seven died, or 58⅓ per cent; and nine cases, from fifteen to twenty, lost three cases, or 33⅓ per cent.

Hot or cold weather does not influence the disease in any way either in its virulence or contagiousness. But I think cold, damp weather, or hot, cloudy weather, makes any given case more malignant. I don't think it affects the spreading of the disease materially.

Respectfully,
A. O. STROUT, M.D.
Parkersburg, Butler County, November 15, 1881.

OBITUARIES

Thomas Ralph Castles, M.D.
1882-1934

Dr. T. R. Castles, well known Albia physician for the last twelve years, died in the Iowa Methodist Hospital in Des Moines, Sunday, July 29, after a month's illness. He was fifty-two years of age. Thomas Ralph Castles was born June 2, 1882, on a farm south of Albia, the son of Mr. and Mrs. William Castles, pioneers in Monroe county. He was graduated from Northwestern University School of Medicine in 1907, and one year later, married Miss Edna Pabst of Albia. Dr. Castles first practiced medicine for six and one-half years in Dallas, South Dakota. The next eight and one-half years were spent at Moravia, and he located in Albia in 1922.

Dr. Castles had always been active in the Methodist Church. He was a Past Noble Grand Master and Past District Instructor in the Odd Fellows lodge, and a member of the Masonic lodge. He belonged to the Monroe County Medical Society, the Iowa State Medical Society, and the American Medical Association. Surviving are his wife; one daughter, Marilois; and one son, William Albert, a student at the State University of Iowa College of Medicine. Dr. Castles was known for his genial personality and great industry. His passing will be felt in medical circles, especially throughout Albia and Monroe county.

Resolutions

At a joint meeting of the Monroe County Medical Society and its Woman's Auxiliary, at Albia, the following resolutions were adopted:

With the death of Dr. Thomas R. Castles, of Albia, Iowa, which occurred on the 29th day of July, 1934, there passed from fellowship of the Monroe County Medical Society, the Iowa State Medical Society and the American Medical Association, a loyal and faithful member. His life was one of service to his fellowmen. Ethical and unselfish, it was typical of what becomes a friend, physician and a man.

Therefore be it resolved that we extend to his wife, son and daughter our sincere sympathy in their bereavement, recognizing the deep sorrow attending the loss of a husband and father.

Be it further resolved that these resolutions be made a part of the permanent records of the Monroe County Medical Society and the Woman's Auxiliary, and a copy be presented to the family; also a copy sent to the JOURNAL of the Iowa State Medical Society for publication.

T. A. Moran, M.D., Secretary,
Monroe County Medical Society.
Mabel Gray, Secretary,
Woman's Auxiliary, Monroe County Medical Society.

John Milton Garrett, M. D.
1869-1934

An Appreciation

With the death of John M. Garrett, M.D., on August 18, 1934, there passed from the medical profession of Fort Dodge, Iowa, one of its most able practitioners.

The Webster County Medical Society, the Staff of St. Joseph's Mercy Hospital and the Staff of the Fort Dodge Lutheran Hospital have all lost a most valued friend, counselor and member.

For thirty-one years, Dr. Garrett practiced medicine in Fort Dodge. His disposition and personality were so remarkable that he was most highly regarded by everybody, both lay and professional. This vacancy in our community is difficult to fill. Dr. Garrett's friendship will be a treasured memory to every member of these organizations.

It is recommended that this tribute of regard for Dr. Garrett from the Webster County Medical Society, the Staff of St. Joseph's Mercy Hospital and the Staff of the Fort Dodge Lutheran Hospital be recorded in their minutes, and that a copy be forwarded to his family, as well as to the JOURNAL of the Iowa State Medical Society.

Committee:
H. W. Scott, M.D.
W. W. Bowen, M.D.
T. J. Dorsey, M.D.
J. E. Galvin, M.D.

A. G. Hejinian, M.D.
1863-1934

On July 5, 1934, Dr. Hejinian, an honorary member of the State Society and a pioneer surgeon of our state passed away. In his death we have lost one of our most valuable members. He was born in Armenia, July 25, 1863. His ardent religious nature inclined him to the profession of the ministry, but trouble in the land of his birth happily diverted his thoughts towards a calling in which his mind escaped the fetters of dogmatic theology and left his religious enthusiasm free to expend itself in practical Christianity. During his medical training he was inspired by two master surgeons, Murphy and Senn, and he prepared himself for a surgical career.

He came to Anamosa in 1896, and established a surgical practice. He was handicapped in not having the many diagnostic aids we have today but he was equipped with a keen mind and he was a comprehensive observer. He believed in the great powers of nature as a supplement in surgery and his dogma was, "You can assist nature but you cannot dictate to nature." His individuality was striking and when good results were obtained in his own original way, he was never prompted to change them.

He was a learned man but he was what some learned men never become—a wise man. He acquired his art mainly at the bedside and it was there that he displayed most conspicuously the qualities which gave him high claim to distinction as a physician and surgeon.

We were impressed chiefly by his ardent love for his calling, by his entire devotion to the high ideals and by the nobility of his personal character. To these he owed his eminent success in his profession, and his acknowledged position in the community as one of its most valued citizens. He dedicated himself to his work with his whole heart and mind and strength; and never wearied in his efforts to augment its usefulness, to maintain its honor and to exhalt its claim.

This record of accomplishment and influence exerted by Dr. Hejinian furnishes a striking example of the capacity of a single individual to do good by a well spent life. Lives like this one so rich in the love of one's neighbor coupled with the force of character directed for good can well be kept before the profession's mind as an inspiration to all. Truly his death was the consummation of a wholly completed life.

H. F. Dolan, M.D.

COURSES AT COOK COUNTY GRADUATE SCHOOL OF MEDICINE

The Cook County Graduate School of Medicine in affiliation with the Cook County Hospital announces intensive courses in three divisions, starting Monday, October 22.

A two weeks intensive course will be offered in ear, nose and throat work, under the supervision of Dr. Samuel J. Pearlman. The teaching faculty for the two weeks course in general internal medicine is headed by Dr. Aaron Arkin. A ten days' course in fractures and traumatic surgery will be in charge of Dr. William R. Cubbins.

These courses will be given provided the required number of physicians are registered for the work; also they will be limited as to the number permitted to take the work. The clinics will be given at the Cook County Hospital, and the didactic work in the school building. For further information, address the Registrar, 427 South Honore Street, Chicago, Illinois.

THE JOURNAL BOOK SHELF

BOOKS RECEIVED

THE DANGEROUS AGE IN MEN—A Treatise on the Prostate Gland by Chester Tilton Stone, M.D., Ridgewood, New Jersey. The Macmillan Company, New York. 1934. Price, $1.75.

INDUSTRIAL TOXICOLOGY—By Alice Hamilton, M.D., Boston, Massachusetts. Harper's Medical Monographs. Harper and Brothers Publishers, 49 East 33d Street, New York City, 1934. Price, $3.00.

THE LABORATORY NOTEBOOK METHOD IN TEACHING PHYSICAL DIAGNOSIS AND CLINICAL HISTORY RECORDING—By Logan Clendening, M.D., Professor of Clinical Medicine, University of Kansas. C. V. Mosby Company, St. Louis, Missouri, 1934. Price, 50c.

MEDICAL CLINICS OF NORTH AMERICA—Volume xvii, No. 6. Chicago Number, Index volume. Octavo of 266 pages with 38 illustrations. Per clinic year July, 1933, to May, 1934. W. B. Saunders Company, Philadelphia and London, 1934. Price, paper, $12.00; cloth, $16.00.

THE MERCK MANUAL OF THERAPEUTICS AND MATERIA MEDICA—Sixth edition, compiled and published by Merck & Company, Inc., Rahway, New Jersey, 1934.

POSTURES AND PRACTICES DURING LABOR AMONG PRIMITIVE PEOPLES—By Julius Jarcho, M.D., New York City. With 130 illustrations. Paul B. Hoeber, Inc., New York, 1934. Price, $3.50.

A PRIMER FOR DIABETIC PATIENTS—A Brief Outline of the Treatment of Diabetes with Diet and Insulin. By Russell M. Wilder, M.D., professor of medicine, The Mayo Founda-

tion. Fifth edition, reset and revised, 172 pages. W. B. Saunders Company, Philadelphia and London, 1934. Price, $1.75.

THE SPASTIC CHILD—A Record of Successfully Achieved Muscle Control in Little's Disease—By Marguerite K. Fischel, C. V. Mosby Company, St. Louis, Missouri, 1934. Price, $1.50.

SURGICAL CLINICS OF NORTH AMERICA—Volume xiv, No. 3, Mayo Clinic Number, June, 1934. Octavo of 221 pages with 70 illustrations. W. B. Saunders Company, Philadelphia and London, 1934. Price, paper, $12.00; cloth, $16.00.

TEST TUBE BABIES—A History of the Artificial Impregnation of Human Beings. By Dr. Hermann Rohleder. The Panurge Press, 70 Fifth Avenue, New York City, 1934. Price, $3.50.

A TEXTBOOK OF GYNECOLOGY—By Arthur Hale Curtis, M.D., professor and head of the department of obstetrics and gynecology, Northwestern University Medical School. Second edition, reset; 493 pages with 300 original illustrations. W. B. Saunders Company, Philadelphia and London, 1934. Price, $6.00.

THAT HEART OF YOURS—By S. Calvin Smith, M.D, Sc.D. Illustrated. J. B. Lippincott Company, Philadelphia, London and Montreal, 1934. Price, $2.00.

TROUBLES' WE DON'T TALK ABOUT—By J. F. Montague, M.D., F.A.C.S., New York Intestinal Sanitarium, 139 East 36th St., New York City. Second edition, revised and enlarged; illustrated. J. B. Lippincott Company, Philadelphia and London, 1933. Price, $1.00.

BOOK REVIEWS

INTERNATIONAL MEDICAL ANNUAL

A Year Book of Treatment and Practitioner's Index. Edited by H. Letheby Tidy, M.D., and A. Rendle Short, M.D. William Wood and Company, Baltimore, 1934. Price, $6.00.

The time is long past when any physician, be he specialist or general practitioner, can find the time and opportunity to keep abreast of the tremendously voluminous current medical literature. It is for this reason that during the past few years a greater appreciation has been evidenced for those compilations and abstracts of the current literature, which have been offered to the profession.

Outstanding among efforts of this sort is the International Medical Annual, which first came into existence some fifty-two years ago. This Annual is the work of an editorial board of distinction, each member being a specialist in his particular branch of medical practice. Long experience has taught the general editors the sort of reviews which are of greatest use to all members of the medical profession so that in the current volume we find all specialties of medicine covered, but at no time has a speciality received attention to the exclusion of other phases of general medical practice. A greater place has been given to the newer methods of treatment, particularly those that should prove useful to the general practitioner.

By arranging the paragraphic abridgements of the literature alphabetically, the authors have rendered the subject matter more readily available and have-

been able to cover the entire field of practice without producing a volume of undue proportions. The volume maintains the previous high standards set by this publication.

THE ESSENTIALS OF PHYSICAL DIAGNOSIS

By Robert W. Buck, M.D., assistant professor of preventive medicine and instructor in physical diagnosis, Tufts College Medical School. 259 pages with 21 illustrations. W. B. Saunders Company, Philadelphia and London, 1934. Price, $3.00.

The author's purpose in preparing this small manual is to provide the student with an introduction into the principles of non-instrumental physical examination and to furnish him with a concise description of the methods which he will be required to employ daily in his later work. This avowed purpose has been accomplished by the author and his manual will be a very satisfactory guide to any student or physician requiring the use of such a work.

The volume has been prepared along conventional lines and presents the usual routine of physical examination by regions and special systems. The illustrations presented are for the most part schematic or diagrammatic and, as such, forcefully exemplify the text. Footnote references to the literature are cited and at the close of each chapter references for supplemental reading are given. The presentation is terse, thorough and accurate.

INTERNATIONAL CLINICS

Volume 11, Forty-fourth Series, June, 1934. Edited by Louis Hamman, M.D., octavo of 317 pages with 32 illustrations and one colored plate. J. B. Lippincott Company, Philadelphia, Montreal and London. Price, $3.00.

The reviewer of a volume of this nature is always confronted with the difficult problem of determining which of the very valuable and distinctive group of articles should be brought to the attention of the reader. The selection is always made on an empirical basis and reflects to a very large extent the interest of the particular reviewer.

In this volume a review of "The Pathogenesis of Anterior Poliomyelitis" by Thelma Lovett of Philadelphia, a paper on "Operative Shock" by E. Rehn of Freiburg, Germany, and an article entitled "Estimating the Extent of Disability" by Earl D. McBride of Oklahoma City, are of exceptional quality and fully deserve careful reading. An additional word of explanation should be offered regarding Dr. McBride's discussion. In the past the physician who was called upon to describe and estimate the extent of a disability resulting from industrial accidents, has of necessity, relied upon vague and non-descriptive terms. The result of this vagueness was a confusion in the minds of the legal representatives who were trying the case, so that many times justice has been defeated. Dr. McBride offers a scheme for analyzing a particular injury which largely eliminates equivocation and places the valuation on a basis fully sponsored by scientific proof.

Eleven other articles of outstanding quality appear in this volume.

INDUSTRIAL TOXICOLOGY

By Alice Hamilton, M.D., Boston, Massachusetts. Harper's Medical Monographs. Harper and Brother, Publishers, 49 East 33rd Street, New York City, 1934. Price, $3.00.

In recognition of the hazards encountered in the present chemical age of industry the government has attempted by the promulgation of rules to protect the worker. These rules are commendable and are no doubt responsible for the relative infrequency of serious industrial poisonings. It is apparent, however, that they have not been sufficient to remove this hazard altogether.

After all, it is the practicing physician who must diagnose and treat these conditions when they arise, and for this reason it is particularly timely that a concise, readable treatise on this subject should be prepared.

This volume has been written by an expert in industrial toxicology, and covers with clarity the entire field. An extensive bibliography is presented in the closing pages of the book, which should prove of great value to the physician who wishes to extend his knowledge beyond that given in this text.

The volume is one of Harper's Medical Monographs, a series of books already distinguished in current medical literature.

THE LABORATORY NOTEBOOK METHOD IN TEACHING PHYSICAL DIAGNOSIS AND CLINICAL HISTORY RECORDING

By Logan Clendening, M.D., Professor of Clinical Medicine, University of Kansas. C. V. Mosby Company, St. Louis, Missouri, 1934. Price, fifty cents.

Marking a new departure in the teaching of physical diagnosis, the author presents a laboratory notebook which he has found useful in the teaching of physical diagnosis to students in the University of Kansas.

The small book contains seventy-one pages, every other page remaining blank for the student notes. Printed on the one page are explanatory notes, suggesting the points in physical diagnosis to be observed, and outlining a correct routine to be followed to insure completeness.

It would appear to the reviewer that the method outlined would be time consuming to the point that both student and patient would be exhausted before the examination was completed. It suggests, however, a method of exactness in checking the observations of the student, and appears worthy of consideration by teachers of these subjects.

THE MANAGEMENT OF FRACTURES, DISLOCATIONS AND SPRAINS

By John Albert Key, M.D., clinical professor of orthopedic surgery, Washington University School of Medicine; and H. Earle Conwell, M.D. With 1165 illustrations. C. V. Mosby Company, St. Louis, 1934. Price, $15.00.

The modern industrial age and the increasing use of the automobile and airplane for travel have greatly multiplied the incident of fracture. Inasmuch as most states have provided for compensation to employees where accidents occur in industrial occupations, the problem of fractures assumes a rôle of increased importance from the compensation and medico-legal aspects. Because of these several factors it is timely that two specialists eminently fitted for the writing of such a work should have prepared this volume, dealing with bone and joint diseases, mindful in each discussion of the compensation and medico-legal aspects of the injured.

While the volume is complete and presents forms of treatment which are well recognized in this particular field, the volume is not too encyclopedic for the use of the medical student or the general practitioner. The authors lay no claim to originality in the methods described, but have presented those which have stood the test of time, and which in their own experience have proved their worth.

The large number of illustrations adds much to the value of the work and renders the subject matter more readily understandable.

MANUAL OF THE DISEASES OF THE EYE

For Students and General Practitioners. By Charles H. May, M.D., director and attending surgeon, eye service, Bellevue Hospital, New York, 1916 to 1926. Fourteenth edition, revised, with 376 original illustrations, including 25 plates, and 78 colored figures. William Wood and Company, Baltimore, 1934. Price, $4.00.

Since the first edition of this book in 1930 it has been almost universally used as a textbook in medical schools and has been accepted as a desk companion by thousands of practicing physicians. The popularity and practical worth of the volume has been demonstrated by the many revisions and reprintings of this text, and the fact that it has been translated into at least eight foreign languages.

The present edition adheres strictly to the avowed purpose of the author in his early editions, namely, to present in a concise form the commoner diseases of the eye encountered in general practice. Many chapters of the book have been completely rewritten and others have been largely revised. Some new illustrations have been added, including some colored plates.

While this volume is not recommended as a substitute for larger and more complete treatises on this subject, it is recommended as a practical guide to the general practitioner who wishes a working knowledge of the commoner diseases of the eye, as well as for the medical student who desires a thorough but not too detailed perspective of this entire field.

THE MERCK MANUAL OF THERAPEUTICS AND MATERIA MEDICA

Sixth edition, compiled and published by Merck and Company, Inc., Rahway, New Jersey, 1934.

Some ten or twelve years ago the fifth edition of this manual appeared. The years which have intervened between this older edition and the present one have brought many changes in therapeutics and materia medica, so that the presentation of this new manual was demanded.

The authors have been fortunate in securing the aid of Dr. Bernard Fantus, professor of therapeutics, College of Medicine, University of Illinois, for the revision of the section on therapy. Ordinarily a manual published by a manufacturing chemist would stress the products of that company, either ignoring meritorious products of other manufacturers or questioning their usefulness. While this criticism could have been directed to earlier editions of the manual, the publishers in this edition have been very fair in this regard and have included medications of merit from many sources.

The text is divided into six main sections. The first deals with therapeutic indications, the second with urine analysis; and the third and fourth with poisoning and its treatment, and the dose table of official drugs. The last two sections deal with materia medica and miscellaneous tables and charts useful in the application of the principles outlined in the earlier sections of the work.

The reduced size of the manual and the thin calendar paper employed, permits a wealth of information (1379 pages) in such compact form that it may readily be carried in the physician's handbag.

A PRIMER FOR DIABETIC PATIENTS

A Brief Outline of the Treatment of Diabetes with Diet and Insulin. By Russell M. Wilder, M.D., professor of medicine, The Mayo Foundation. Fifth edition, reset and revised, 172 pages. W. B. Saunders Company, Philadelphia and London, 1934. Price, $1.75.

The first edition of this work appeared in 1921. Since that time the volume has undergone numerous revisions and reprinting, and this, the fifth edition, bespeaks the favorable reception accorded this book.

Adhering to the plan formulated in the earlier editions, the Primer presents in condensed and concise form the information which is desirable and useful that the patients possess. Inasmuch as the diabetic patient, because of the chronicity of his condition, must be in a measure his own physician and nurse, the Primer is of necessity a complete guide to treatment. Viewed from this standpoint it is immediately apparent that the Primer will be useful to both the physician and the patient, and should be possessed and read by each alike.

The methods presented are those employed in the handling of diabetes at the Mayo Clinic, and the recipes recited are those prepared by the dietitians of the Kahler Hospital group at Rochester.

SPINAL ANESTHESIA

Technic and Clinical Application. By George Rudolph Vehrs, M.D., Sales, Oregon. Illustrated. C. V. Mosby Company, St. Louis, 1934. Price, $5.50.

Spinal anesthesia is rapidly passing through that period of trial and experimentation so necessary for the development of a new procedure. It is during this period, characterized by major difficulties, that a procedure is often condemned because people are ignorant of its virtues. While many of the virtues of spinal anesthesia are generally appreciated, one is not justified in concluding that all dangers have been eliminated or will be eliminated, and that the method is now or ever will be one replacing other forms of anesthesia. It is still of prime importance that a surgeon employing spinal anesthesia be familiar with the advantages and disadvantages of this method, of its actions, reactions, its specific indications, and the basic principles of its operation.

Dr. Vehrs offers this volume to aid the surgeon in a proper application of spinal anesthesia. In the preliminary chapters of the book he discusses the anatomy and physiology concerned in anesthesia, reviewing the experimental work which has been done, stressing especially the action of anesthetic drugs upon cardiac, nervous and pulmonary structures.

The latter chapters of the book deal with indications for this method of anesthesia and the technic for its employment.

————

SURGERY OF A GENERAL PRACTICE

By Arthur E. Hertzler, M.D., professor of surgery, University of Kansas, and Victor E, Chesky, M.D., Halstead Hospital. With 472 illustrations. C. V. Mosby Company, St. Louis, 1934. Price, $10.00.

In 1930 these authors published the last edition of "Minor Surgery," but inasmuch as the term minor appeared to them as ill chosen, the present volume has been published under a new caption. The scope of the work, however, is not essentially different from that of the former publication, but has been rewritten and revised to bring the subject matter entirely up to date.

In the opinion of the authors, the most practical way of combating the alleged high cost of medical care is the reduction of medical treatment to its simplest terms with the care of minor surgery as an office or home procedure, and the elimination of many of the frills of hospitalization with the resulting reduction of cost to the patient. Upon this background the authors have attempted to reduce those procedures in surgical practice commonly designated as minor to their simplest terms, and to suggest the simplest and least expensive forms of treatment.

They have further simplified their text by including one procedure for a given condition, selecting the procedure upon the basis suggested above.

Praiseworthy as is the ambition of the authors, certain weaknesses of this form of presentation are apparent in the volume. Rarely does nature exactly duplicate herself in the production of pathology. For this reason it would appear that the best interests of the patient would not be served by attempting a single therapeutic procedure in lesions of various natures and extent.

The volume will serve as a most valuable guide to the general practitioner who wishes a general and fundamental knowledge of this branch of practice.

Comment upon the volume would not be complete without favorable reference to the many well selected and beautifully reproduced illustrations which appear in generous numbers throughout the text.

THAT HEART OF YOURS

By S. Calvin Smith, M.D., Sc.D. Illustrated. J. B. Lippincott Company, Philadelphia, London and Montreal, 1934. Price, $2.00.

This is another of the many popular discussions of health matters written for the lay reader. To prepare the reader for the discussion of "That Heart of Yours," the author first reviews in considerable detail the structure and function of the heart. He next takes up the cardiac ailments most common in childhood and adolescence, stressing, as would be expected,

rheumatic heart disease. In the chapter dealing with the heart in middle life, he discusses the symptoms of angina pectoris and the importance of dental infection during this period. In succeeding chapters the author reviews the symptoms of other heart diseases and offers suggestions for the general care of the heart.

Chapter nine is titled "Individual Instructions for Special Heart Conditions" and it is toward this section that the finger of criticism may be pointed, since from the title it appears that self-medication is contemplated. It would seem, however, that this instruction is not intended to replace the treatment prescribed by the physician but is intended rather to supplement more definite orders. According to the author, these instructions are those "which physicians give to the heart patient when time permits and when the person is in a receptive mood." Most physicians would and should find time for this instruction when needed and would prefer in many cases to withhold from the patients certain details discussed in these pages. We feel that before this book is recommended to any patient, the physician should be intimately familiar with the book and also with the mental stability of his patient.

————

TROUBLES WE DON'T TALK ABOUT

By J. F. Montague, M.D., F.A.C.S., New York Intestinal Sanitarium, 139 East 36th St., New York City. Second edition, revised and enlarged; illustrated. J. B. Lippincott Company, Philadelphia and London, 1933. Price, $1.00.

This is a popular discussion written for the layman and deals with diseases of the lower bowel, rectum and anus. Chief among the conditions discussed are those of hemorrhoids, fistula in ano, and pruritus.

Preliminary to the study of these subjects, the author discusses the essential anatomy and physiology, stressing conditions, habits, and medications, which are thought to favor the production of each condition. In connection with this discussion he very happily sounds a warning regarding the appearance of cancer and emphasizes the value of its early recognition.

In discussing constipation and the methods for its relief, he critically surveys the use and abuse of laxatives and cathartics, brans, mineral oil and psyllium seed. Of mineral oil he states, "Of all the self medication fads which have at various times been foisted upon the public, the mineral oil fashion is certainly the least objectionable."

In the closing chapters of his book he discusses the use of home remedies for rectal ailments and the procedures employed by this specialty. The book is well written and, since self medication is not encouraged, will no doubt lead to an earlier observation of these cases by the physician. The book can safely be recommended by the physician to intelligent patients.

COUNTY MEDICAL SOCIETY OFFICERS

COUNTY	PRESIDENT	SECRETARY	DEPUTY COUNCILORS
Adair	L. H. Ahrens, Fontanelle	A. S. Bowers, Orient	A. S. Bowers, Orient
Adams	O. B. Hawley, Corning	J. H. Wallahan, Corning	W. F. Amdor, Carbon
Allamakee	J. W. Thornton, Lansing	M. E. Kallman, Postville	J. W. Thornton, Lansing
Appanoose	F. B. Leffert, Centerville	E. A. Larsen, Centerville	C. S. Hickman, Centerville
Audubon	R. H. Payne, Exira	F. E. James, Elk Horn	W. H. Halloran, Audubon
Benton		G. R. Woodhouse, Vinton	C. J. Snitkay, Vinton
Black Hawk	J. R. Thompson, Waterloo	F. Harold Entz, Waterloo	A. J. Joynt, Waterloo
Boone	Mark C. Jones, Boone	B. T. Whitaker, Boone	Mark C. Jones, Boone
Bremer	F. J. Epeneter, Denver	J. E. Whitmire, Sumner	F. R. Sparks, Waverly
Buchanan	M. W. Barrett, Independence	M. C. Melrose, Independence	C. W. Tidball, Independence
Buena Vista	A. A. Armstrong, Newell	J. H. O'Donoghue, Storm Lake	H. E. Farnsworth, Storm Lake
Butler	E. C. Kepler, Allison	H. G. MacLeod, Greene	M. B. Call, Greene
Calhoun	F. W. Hobart, Lake City	W. W. Stevenson, Rockwell City	F. W. Van Metre, Rockwell City
Carroll	D. H. Hopkins, Glidden	Walter A. Anneberg, Carroll	W. L. McConkie, Carroll
Cass	Harry H. Penquite, Massena	R. L. Barnett, Atlantic	R. L. Barnett, Atlantic
Cedar	W. H. Jenks, Tipton	E. J. Van Metre, Tipton	E. J. Van Metre, Tipton
Cerro Gordo	T. E. Davidson, Mason City	William C. Egloff, Mason City	S. A. O'Brien, Mason City
Cherokee	John M. Pope, Cherokee	G. Dean Tipton, Cherokee	C. H. Hall, Cherokee
Chickasaw	P. E. Stuart, Nashua	P. E. Gardner, New Hampton	Paul E. Gardner, New Hampton
Clarke	J. D. Shively, Osceola	J. N. Goodman, Osceola	J. N. Goodman, Osceola
Clay	G. W. Adams, Royal	Charles C. Collester, Spencer	E. E. Munger, Spencer
Clayton	A. E. Beyer, Guttenberg	J. W. Hudek, Garnavillo	J. W. Hudek, Garnavillo
Clinton	Ralph F. Luse, Clinton	Eugene V. Donlan, Clinton	R. T. Lenaghan, Clinton
Crawford	W. A. Garner, Kiron	James Duffy, Denison	C. L. Sievers, Denison
Dallas·Guthrie	George McMahon, Waukee	Samuel J. Brown, Panora	E. J. Butterfield, Dallas Center
			S. J. Brown, Panora
Davis	C. D. Fenton, Bloomfield	H. C. Young, Bloomfield	H. C. Young, Bloomfield
Decatur	J. W. Wailes, Davis City	J. E. McFarland, Leon	J. E. McFarland, Leon
Delaware	J. I. Jones, Manchester	C. A. Carroll, Manchester	J. I. Jones, Manchester
Des Moines	C. J. Lohmann, Burlington	F. B. Aid, Burlington	A. C. Moerke, Burlington
Dickinson	Don E. Rodewig, Spirit Lake	Ruth F. Wolcott, Spirit Lake	C. G. Nicholson, Spirit Lake
Dubuque	L. H. Fritz, Dubuque	D. F. Ward, Dubuque	F. P. McNamara, Dubuque
Emmet	W. E. Bradley, Estherville	Smith C. Kirkegaard, Ringsted	M. T. Morton, Estherville
Fayette	James Parker, Fayette	C. C. Hall, Maynard	C. C. Hall, Maynard
Floyd	A. F. Kober, Charles City	C. D. Miner, Jr., Charles City	Ray Fox, Charles City
Franklin	W. R. Arthur, Hampton	J. M. Burger, Hampton	W. K. Long, Hampton
Fremont	H. F. Cole, Thurman	A. E. Wanamaker, Hamburg	A. E. Wanamaker, Hamburg
Greene	B. C. Hamilton, Jr., Jefferson	John R. Black, Jefferson	B. C. Hamilton, Jr., Jefferson
Grundy	M. H. Thielen, Grundy Center	R. T. Spain, Conrad	M. H. Thielen, Grundy Center
Hamilton	T. J. Desmond, Webster City	David W. James, Kamrar	M. B. Galloway, Webster City
Hancock			Thomas McMahon, Garner
Winnebago	A. J. Peterson, Forest City	W. F. Missman, Klemme	F. J. Irish, Forest City
Hardin	L. E. Fraser, Iowa Falls	W. E. Marsh, Eldora	E. O. Koeneman, Eldora
Harrison	C. J. Bergstrom, Missouri Valley	F. H. Hanson, Magnolia	Elmer J. Cole, Woodbine
Henry	F. C. Allen, Wayland	W. Laird, Mount Pleasant	S. W. Huston, Mount Pleasant
Howard	L. W. Clark, Chester	W. A. Bockoven, Cresco	Wm. A. Bockoven, Cresco
Humboldt	Ivan T. Schultz, Humboldt	Arthur E. Jensen, Humboldt	K. S. Coddington, Humboldt
Ida	Ivan N. Heilman, Ida Grove	W. J. Crane, Holstein	B. S. Parker, Ida Grove
Iowa	C. H. Hermann, Amana	J. Sinn, Williamsburg	J. Sinn, Williamsburg
Jackson	John W. Jordan, Maquoketa	William Lowder, Maquoketa	C. C. Ryan, Maquoketa
Jasper	E. A. McMurray, Newton	G. G. Rinshaw, Newton	H. F. Engle, Newton
Jefferson	J. S. Gaumer, Fairfield	R. G. Cook, Fairfield	N. N. Crow, Fairfield
Johnson	Matt Ware, West Branch	Horace M. Korns, Iowa City	George C. Albright, Iowa City
Jones	O. R. Smith, Onslow	P. F. Dolan, Anamosa	T. M. Redmond, Monticello
Keokuk	D. L. Grothaus, Delta	W. W. Stirlen, Delta	W. W. Stirlen, Delta
Kossuth	Robt. L. Williams, Lakota	Pierre Sartor, Titonka	T. T. Peters, Burt
Lee	Frank R. Richmond, Fort Madison	F. B. Dorsey, Jr., Keokuk	A. A. Johnstone, Keokuk
			Robert L. Feightner, Fort Madison
Linn	T. F. Hersch, Cedar Rapids	E. J. Kieck, Cedar Rapids	H. Downing, Cedar Rapids
Louisa	H. E. Weber, Wapello	R. H. Chittum, Wapello	T. H. Chittum, Wapello
Lucas	R. A. Hills, Russell	H. D. Jarvis, Chariton	R. C. Gutch, Chariton
Lyon	L. L. Corcoran, Rock Rapids	A. F. Stewart, Inwood	L. L. Corcoran, Rock Rapids
Madison	Arnold L. Nelson, Winterset	L. E. Hickenlooper, Winterset	C. B. Hickenlooper, Winterset
Mahaska	E. M. Williams, Oskaloosa	L. F. Catterson, Oskaloosa	F. Catterson, Oskaloosa
Marion	E. Bell, Pleasantville	C. R. Cornell, Knoxville	S. S. Cornell, Knoxville
Marshall	A. R. Lynn, Marshalltown	M. G. Meyer, Marshalltown	R. G. Grossman, Marshalltown
Mills	H. B. Dye, Glenwood	I. M. Donelan, Glenwood	B. Lacey, Glenwood
Mitchell	John O. Eiel, Osage	W. G. Walker, Riceville	S. Walker, Riceville
Monona	E. L. Deering, Onawa	W. L. Fairbanks, Onawa	C. A. Junger, Soldier
Monroe	S. N. Gray, Albia	T. A. Moran, Melrose	T. A. Moran, Melrose
Montgomery	B. F. Gillmor, Red Oak	E. T. Thomsen, Red Oak	J. A. Montgomery, Villisca
Muscatine	B. E. Eversmeyer, Muscatine	R. E. Goad, Muscatine	T. F. Beveridge, Muscatine
O'Brien	W. R. Brock, Sheldon	H. J. Brackney, Sheldon	W. R. Brock, Sheldon
Osceola	E. F. Farnum, Sibley	R. B. Paulsen, Harris	Frank Reinsch, Ashton
Page	E. D. Smith, Clarinda	E. B. Clark, Clarinda	F. M. Aldrich, Shenandoah
Palo Alto	H. L. Brereton, Emmetsburg	R. R. Powers, Emmetsburg	Harold L. Brereton, Emmetsburg
Plymouth	W. T. Shepard, LeMars	L. C. O'Toole, Le Mars	W. Larsen, Le Mars
Pocahontas	A. W. Patterson, Fonda	C. C. Riordan, Pocahontas	H. Svendsen, Laurens
Polk	Fred Moore, Des Moines	Leonard A. West, Des Moines	Ralph H. Parker, Des Moines
Pottawattamie	C. F. Baumeister, Avoca	Arnold M. Jensen, Council Bluffs	Treynor, Council Bluffs
Poweshiek	E. J. Ringema, Brooklyn	C. V. Lawton, Grinnell	C. V. Lawton, Grinnell
Ringgold	E. J. Watson, Diagonal	C. W. Hill, Mount Ayr	J. Watson, Diagonal
Sac	Henry Fobes, Auburn	R. Devey, Schaller	J. H. Jones, Wall Lake
Scott	E. H. Lamb, Davenport	Henry A. Meyers, Davenport	A. P. Donohoe, Davenport
Shelby	Helge Borre, Shelby	R. Nielson, Harlan	P. Nielson, Harlan
Sioux	John DeBey, Orange City	D. Bendixen, Ireton	G. Gleysteen, Alton
Story	J. W. Bowers, Nevada	W. M. Sperow, Nevada	E. B. Bush, Ames
Tama	C. S. Stoakes, Dysart	F. W. Gessner, Dysart	A. W. Pace, Toledo
Taylor	J. Maloy, Bedford	G. V. Childs, Creston	Rimel, Bedford
Union	Howard Beatty, Creston	C. N. Stephenson, Milton	John O. Parsons, Creston
Van Buren	A. Coffin, Farmington	Evon Walker, Ottumwa	C. R. Russell, Keosauqua
Wapello	Kepler, Kirkville	F. R. Shaw, Indianola	Evon Walker, Ottumwa
Warren	M. Mitchell, Indianola	W. S. Kyle, Washington	L. Loosbrock, Lacona
Washington	J. Braden, Wellman	Ingleborn, Lineville	E. Stutsman, Washington
Wayne	J. H. Hyatt, Humeston	John C. Shrader, Fort Dodge	S. W. Corbin, Millerton
Webster	L. H. Leighton, Fort Dodge	Edward F. Hagen, Decorah	Roland Stahr, Fort Dodge
Winneshiek	A. F. Bartlett, Decorah	Lawrence E. Pierson, Sioux City	A. F. Fritchen, Decorah
Woodbury	L. R. Tripp, Sioux City	R. L. Olsen, Northwood	
Worth	G. S. Westly, Manly	J. R. Christensen, Eagle Grove	S. S. Westly, Manly
Wright	B. L. Basinger, Goldfield		G. E. Schnug, Dows

10-10-34

The JOURNAL

of the

Iowa State Medical Society

Vol. XXIV   Des Moines, Iowa, November, 1934   No. 11

THE RELATIONSHIP OF OTOLARYN-GOLOGY TO GENERAL MEDICINE*

John J. Shea, M.D., Memphis, Tennessee

We are all doctors, though some of us have devoted our efforts along specialized lines. The contact between our specialty and general medicine has, in the past, and should be, in the future, very close. It will be my pleasure this morning to outline the basic principles of the specialty of otolaryngology.

FOCAL INFECTION

The pendulum of thought has swung wide toward focal infection, but due to the number of failures in its application, the pendulum has swung just as far in the opposite direction. The middle ground is the safe area in all passages and there are many cases where the isolation of the focus of infection and its eradication is necessary for a cure. Life is composed of one inflammatory reaction after another by the tissues whose function is the development and maintenance of immunity to the infections of our environment. As long as the reactions terminate favorably we are well, provided the biochemical reaction remains normal.

In the infant the adenoid is the most active mass of lymphoid tissue in this fight against the infections of our environment; hence the adenoid is most likely to be inflamed during an acute infection of the upper respiratory tract in the first two years of life. The adenoid drains its lymphatics into the glands of Henle, which are situated high in the pharynx beneath the aponeurosis. If the adenoid fails to overcome an invading army of bacteria, a peripharyngeal abscess may be formed. The glands of Henle are the first glands to atrophy and this occurs about the sixth year. Peripharyngeal abscesses after the sixth year should be looked upon as complications of infections of the vertebra. The surgical approach during infancy is through the pharynx, whereas abscesses occurring after the

sixth year require a differential diagnosis between those of pharyngeal origin and those from the vertebra. The latter are best opened from without, to prevent contamination by the ever present flora of the pharynx. During the second year, the tonsil becomes more active and reaches its greatest activity from the fourth year to puberty. The development of the gonads inhibits tonsillar activity. This is illustrated by the continued youthful tonsil of the hypogonad or the return of its glandular activity in the female after castration. Nature has planned a definite pattern for the development of the para-nasal sinuses and the cells of the mastoid process. These spaces are destined for active parts in the system of immunization. The youthful sinus is not capable of carrying on all of the auto-immunizing processes asked of them when the tonsils and adenoid have been removed at an early age. The sinuses and the mastoid cells reflect in their growth and development the infections that they suffered.

The deciduous teeth, because of their minor roots, seldom serve as a focus of infection.

The selection of the most probable seat of focal infection follows the scheme of development, the sites of immunity. When one of these factories devoted to auto-immunization suffers a depression, its immunizing power is bankrupt and what was once a serviceable laboratory now becomes a focus of infection. In the infant the adenoid, according to the law of probability, should first be considered. The majority of the colds in these little patients begin as an inflammation of the adenoid and the complications extend to its neighbors, the middle ears and the pharyngeal or cervical glands. Occasionally this infection backs up into the developing sinuses. The tonsil during its period of greatest activity, fourth year to puberty, should first be considered when searching for a probable focus of infection. The older man grows, the lower the seat of possibility descends in the ring of Waldeyer's. Just as the adenoid is the area of probability in the infant,

*Presented before the Eighty-third Annual Session, Iowa State Medical Society, Des Moines, May 9, 10, 11, 1934.

the lower half of the tonsil is the area of greatest possibility of focal infection in the adult and the lingual tonsil in the aged. At birth we have an external, middle and inner ear. The middle ear connects with the nasopharynx through the Eustachian tube and a single cavity, the antrum of the mastoid. Rosenow, in his enthusiasm of selectivity of bacterial infection, overemphasized this selection, but the site of the infection can be isolated at times according to the disease present. The tonsils have been the foci of infection of the majority of our joint diseases, the teeth of our neuritis and the para-nasal sinuses of our choreas.

The ethmoid cells are present at birth. They develop by a process of pneumatization and capsulation until puberty is well established, and reflect in their growth the influences of the infections they have suffered. The maxillary sinus pneumatizes as the superior maxilla grows. The frontal sinus is formed by the migration of an anterior ethmoid cell into the frontal bone and as soon as the cell enters the frontal bone it becomes the frontal sinus. The sphenoid sinus at birth is a cavity situated in front of the sphenoid bone into which it later migrates, so as to be encapsulated completely by the bone at the age of four. At birth and during the early years of life the ethmoid cells are sharply divided into an anterior group and a posterior group. The spheno-ethmoid labyrinth will assume the size and shape which its component bones will allow and the presence or shape of the frontal sinus is governed by the migration of the anterior ethmoid cell. The growth of the spheno-ethmoid labyrinth should be proportionately pneumatization and capsulation.

The application of the above knowledge is that since the sphenoid sinus is the first sinus to reach maturity, it is the most likely sinus to cause headache in a child. The ethmoid cells, because of their activity, are considered as the source of nasal discharge and as the trigger in allergic reactions. The maxillary sinuses or antra are rich in lymphatic drainage, which is intimately associated with the bronchial lymphatic system and, in diseases showing activity of the latter, should be carefully studied and given the preference in case of doubt.

TEETH

The buds of the permanent molar teeth are stacked behind the infantile antrum, and as this sinus develops downward and backward, the cancellous bone containing them is rotated into the alveolar process. The proper eruption of the upper molars is dependent upon the development of the maxillary sinus, and a mature antrum has the three upper molars in contact with its floor. This relationship begets a ready extension of in-fection from these teeth into the antrum. The gums about the teeth are vulnerable to infection and when inspection reveals an involvement, are undoubtedly a foci of infection at any age. A dead tooth is not always a focus of infection, but science has failed to develop a test to prove when a dead tooth is safe.

SINUSITIS

A cold either subsides or localizes and if this localization is in a sinus, the condition becomes an acute sinusitis. The modern concept of the physiology of the sinus includes as a function its ability to enter into the auto-immunization against respiratory infections. An individual with healthy sinuses needs no artificial immunization against colds, but when the sinuses fail to carry on their share of our auto-immunization, a vaccine against cold is indicated. During the early stages of an acute infection, drugs (quinine) or protein products (omnadin or protedlac) aid in mobilizing the defensive agents. Later when the infection has been halted, vaccines will stimulate reënforcements. Stock vaccines are of value, but a well prepared autogenous vaccine is better. I use a "seasonal" vaccine alone or combined with an autogenous vaccine. This "seasonal" vaccine is made from the cultures current in the laboratory that season. We save cultures from our acute cases of sinusitis, abscesses and mastoiditis, considering the bacteria so obtained as the offenders of our community that season. The action of a vaccine is effervescent and best repeated frequently; the first series being given after the first cold of the antrum and repeated during the winter and early spring.

ANTRAL IRRIGATION

When should an antrum be irrigated? Authorities of equal success differ in their opinion, but the best practice to follow is that of the old surgical principle "when pus is formed it should be evacuated." Pain localized over a sinus is best relieved by opening that sinus. Nature is no fool, but it is difficult to comprehend why the ostium of the antrum closes as soon as pus settles within it. Today, we attempt gently to dilate this closed ostium and irrigate the antrum by catheterization, thus avoiding the trauma of puncturing. The knowledge obtained as to the patency of the ostium is valuable information for the selection of further lines of procedure. The frequency of antral irrigations depends upon the symptoms of pain, elevation of temperature and systemic manifestations. A patient should never be discharged from treatment, until a clear irrigation is obtained. The continuation of antral discharge, especially in face of systemic manifestations, may demand continuous drainage. This can be accomplished with little or no risk by the making of a nasal antral window with the insertion of a small rubber tube. Three or four days of continuous drainage often terminate an antral infection that left alone would become chronic. If the basic principle of pus within the antrum is founded on failure of immunization, diet and climate will aid in the restoration of health. A diet rich in sugars and starches, and poor in vitamins, tends to produce pus. A three day fast from sugars and starches is prescribed for our sinus patients, after which these foods are limited to one meal a day and in this meal proteins and fresh fruits are eliminated. The separation of these foods reduces the acidity required of the stomach allowing the sugars and starches to be thoroughly digested.

NASAL OBSTRUCTION

Nasal obstruction may be partial or complete; developmental or the result of trauma. The systemic consequences of nasal obstruction depend on the age at which the obstruction occurred. It is necessary that we breathe equally well through each nostril. When we retire at night the lower naris closes off and rests. A person with one naris blocked will go to sleep with that side down, but in the natural course of sleeping will roll over, and thus the good side becomes the under naris. There is not sufficient space through the blocked side for healthy respiration and under these circumstances, sleep is not restful and the individual usually rolls on to his back and breathes through the mouth. In the female the turbinates enlarge during menstruation and pregnancy, and nasal obstructions are more vicious. The female tends toward nasal consciousness more than the male. The individual living indoors suffers more from a slight nasal obstruction, than those whose life is spent in the open. Nasal obstructions are a menace to the ears every time we sneeze or blow our nose. There is no operation performed by our specialty which pays better dividends in comfort and in health than the well performed submucous resection of an obstructing septum. These obstructions become serious when infection is localized in a sinus that is blocked by their formation. The correction should never be attempted during an acute infection.

"A good thinker needs a clear head." The dull child with hypertrophied adenoids is but an exaggeration of the adult with a blocked nose. The inability to breathe through the nose slows the cerebration and clouds the memory. As expressed in the words of Shakespeare, "A man so dull, so dead in looks, so woe begone."

CHRONIC SINUSITIS

One severe acute sinusitis improperly treated may become chronic, but usually this modern curse is the result of recurring simple sinusitis. The selection of the type of operation for the individual case of chronic sinusitis demands experience, and its execution demands skill. Formerly, we thought that the membrane removed at operation was replaced by scar tissue, but today we know that frequently healthy membrane reforms and the function of the sinuses are regained. Radical sinus surgery has as its fundamental principle the removal of a danger, and is performed because of some systemic manifestation rather than a local condition. The presence of benign and malignant growths are local requisites for radical sinus surgery.

The accepted sinus pathology associated with asthma is as follows:

1. Hyperplasia of the sinus mucous membrane with myxomatous changes and polyps cause asthma.

2. Low grade ethmoid and maxillary sinusitis.

3. Polyps rich in eosinophiles with an increase of the eosinophiles in the blood.

4. Nasal obstructions producing reflex stimulation.

The allergist, who treats bronchial asthma without considering the possibility of the nose and the sinuses being diseased, or the rhinologist who does not consider the possible presence of allergy will alike meet with failure.

Three types of surgery may be used; namely, plastic, simple intranasal, and radical.

PATHOLOGIC OBSERVATIONS AT OPERATION CHECKED WITH ASTHMA END-RESULT

Pathologic Condition	Total Number of Cases	Cure	Improvement			Failure
			Marked	Moderate	Slight	
Pus.............	22	2	6	3	2	9 (41%)
Polyps in nose and sinuses.........	17	2	5	3	2	5 (29%)
Polypoid sinus membrane......	25	4	6	4	1	10 (40%)
Antral cyst.......	3	1	0	0	0	2
Thickened membrane..........	5	0	0	1	0	4
Cystic degeneration...........	4	1 (pus pocket)	2 (pus pocket)	0	0	1 (no pus pocket)
Secondary scarring and polypoid degeneration......						

Indications for sinus operation in asthmatic patients include:

1. Sinus disease demanding surgical treatment on its own merits.

2. Recurrent head colds precipitating asthmatic attacks; the aim of surgery is to lessen the number of such colds.

3. Attempting to interrupt the vicious downward cycle in the very severe case of asthma by attempting to gain even temporary relief.

4. Cases in which removal of polypl or sinus irrigation yields temporary benefit.

These operations are not always successful; sometimes because the patient is not sensitized to his own sinus organisms, and sometimes because the operative work is not thorough enough. The sinuses most often affected are the ethmoids, sphenoids and antrums, rarely the frontals.

NASAL DROPS

The average commercial nasal drop never cured a cold and the popularity of the various brands depends upon the ephedrine they contain. An individual who begins their use exposes himself to a habit, for once a nasal membrane becomes accustomed to the effect of ephedrine, it is never happy unless under its influence. Nature supplies a wonderful "nasal drop" in the abundant mucous secretion which is continuously being supplied to the nose. The promiscous prescribing of a nasal drop without inspecting the nasal membrane is the same as giving a cough mixture without examining the chest. A hypotonic salt solution is of value to cleanse a nose and will moderately shrink the nasal membranes without any bad after effects. If the nasal discharge is purulent a solution of the silver proteins, as argyrol or neosilvol will dissolve the pus and aid in its removal. The best nasal drop for dry or irritated membranes can be made by boiling phenol one per cent in liquid petrolatum, and seasoning it with some pleasant volatile ingredient.

MASTOIDITIS

When the middle ear is infected, the inflammation readily extends into the mastoid antrum and cells. This extension is fundamentally for the purpose of developing immunity to the infection. If the immunization is successful, the abscess subsides; but, as in infections of the upper respiratory tract, bankruptcy of this immunity terminates in acute mastoiditis. The indications for surgical intervention in acute mastoiditis depend upon local findings, roentgenogram study, blood count and systemic manifestations. The season of the year will alter the period of observation, because during the late winter months, the chances of spontaneous cure are less than during the summer. Likewise, mastoids involved in the colder climates do not have the opportunity to avoid surgery, as those occurring in the milder climates. Mastoiditis following scarlet fever, measles, streptococci throats and pneumonia is the result of complications, and demands an earlier operation than if it is the result of a simple abscess of the middle ear.

RADICAL MASTOID SURGERY

Indications for the removal of dangers even though the good hearing must be sacrificed are:

1. Dead labyrinth—the internal ear.
2. Fistula—into the internal ear.
3. Deep, dull headaches with mental fatigue and local findings suggesting extension of chronic otitis media.
4. Facial palsy in a chronic ear.
5. Excessive granulations with evidence of extensive destruction of the middle ear.
6. Cholesteatoma?

BLOOD

The older physiologist considered the blood as a special form of connective tissue having a fluid matrix. The modern conception is that the blood is a mixed secretion whose formed elements are the result of parent cells living outside the blood stream. These hematopoietic tissues differ in the embryo and the adult. In the former the fetal blood is formed, as a result of the activities of the blood islets in the yolk sac, the primitive liver, and the reticulo-endothelial system. The capillaries of the formative bone marrow, and the lymphoid follicles of the spleen, and other lymphoid structures, next add to this natal blood. The process changes gradually until in adult life groups of parent cells exist outside the blood stream with four major hemic units in the blood. From parent myeloblasts in the red blood marrow come the granular cells, which are the polymorphonuclear leukocytes, the monocytes are derived from the reticulo-endothelial system; from the lymphoblasts are derived the lymphocytes; and from the normoblasts, the red blood cells.

The infections of the throat are characterized by the influence they exert upon the hematopoietic system. On the other hand there are primary blood diseases which produce lesions in the mouth, and it is difficult to separate the border line cases.

Adult Blood

Parent Cell	Hemic Unit	
Myeloblasts	Granulocytes.....(a)	Polymorphonuclears
	(b)	Monocytes
Lymphoblasts	Agranulocytes...(c)	Small lymphocytes
	(d)	Large lymphocytes
Normoblasts	Red Blood Cells.	

The laryngologist has an opportunity to study the relationship of the anginas and the hematopoietic response in the following diseases; agranulocytic angina; acute infectious mononucleosis; Vincent's angina with a lymphoid leukocytosis; and acute lymphadenosis.

The anginas are capable of producing four types of changes in the blood: polymorphonuclear leukocytosis, as seen in follicular tonsillitis and the septic throat; mononuclear leukocytosis, as oc-

curs in infectious mononucleosis; leukopenia with
a decrease in granulocytes, or agranulocytic angina; and leukocytosis with a relative hyogranu-
locytosis, as seen in patients suffering from a generalized Vincent's infection.

FRACTURES OF THE BONES OF THE FACE

The ever increasing speed at which man now
travels has multiplied the number of cases of fractures of the face. The sudden and permanent stop
of a rapidly moving vehicle, as occurs in a wreck,
throws the occupant forward and he may strike his
face against one of the fixed parts of the vehicle.
Our cases have included injuries sustained in many
fashions, ranging from a newspaper boy's fight to
a nose dive of an aeroplane. The management of
fractures involving the para-nasal sinuses is similar to the surgical procedures followed in radical
sinus surgery. In fact, the most common complication of these fractures is sinusitis. The majority of the fractures of the facial bones, exclusive
of the simple nasal bone fractures, extend into the
maxillary, frontal or ethmoidal sinuses. The sinus
involved fills with blood, which readily becomes
infected. The basis of treatment is the replacement of the bony fragments, and the drainage of
the sinus entered. This will restore the features.

The face is composed of an upper and lower jaw.
The upper jaw may be likened to two churches
with steeples having two keystones interposed between them. The superior maxilla with their nasal
processes are the churches and the nasal bones are
the keystones. The malar bones are the lateral
supports. This formation is loosely attached to the
skull, and is capable of withstanding great force
exerted on it in a straight direction, but it is very
vulnerable to forces from the side or from below.
Explosion which enters the nose and mouth readily displaces the facial bones from the skull without fracturing the skull. The lower jaw can withstand blows of great force from the side or below
without fracturing, whereas, a blow of equal force
from in front may fracture the lower jaw. The
majority of displacements are at the site of sutures.

The variety of fractures are as follows:

1. Greenstick, as in children.
2. Simple, slight nasal fractures.
3. Compound, fractures of the frontal bone.
4. Comminuted, fractures of the anterior antral
wall.
5. Impacted, as seen in fractures of the zygomatic process.
6. Depressed, as seen about the outer border of
the orbit and malar bone.

Combinations of the above are common.
Symptoms and diagnosis include:
History—direction of force.

Inspection—swelling and deformity.
Palpation—tenderness, crepitus and abnormal
mobility.
X-ray—variety of pictures is valuable.

EXTERNAL NOSE

The anterior position of the nose exposes it to
injury, and deformities of it are noticeable and
detracting. Individuals with badly shaped noses
become conscious of their deformity and many
suffer inferiority complexes because they are constantly accusing their listeners of observing their
nasal blemish, instead of being attentive to their
discourse. The external nose consists of a bony
and a cartilaginous portion. The attachment of
the cartilages to the bony base may be easily separated. The re-attachment is maintained in a good
position by a light intranasal pack for two days and
a light adhesive external dressing for a week or
ten days. Fractures of the bony external nose are
the most frequent of the facial fractures. The
deformity depends on the line of force which was
applied. When the force is lateral, the approximate nasal bone is displaced under its mate and if
the force was sufficient, the nasal process of the
superior maxilla is cracked and depressed, the septum being deflected.

The correction demands the application of the
law of physics—"two objects cannot occupy the
same position in space at the same time." The
depressed nasal process and nasal bone are first
elevated, then force is applied to the opposite side
of the nose by a blow of sufficient power to knock
the displaced bones into their normal position. A
wooden protector for the nose is used as a guard
and a small metal nasal hammer as the instrument
of force. If the patient is seen early, this can be
accomplished under a local anesthesia, but it is best
to administer a general anesthetic, because better
results are obtained. The best outer dressing is
made of Keer's dental wax, which can be molded
to fit the nose. It is fixed with adhesive plaster to
the forehead and several adhesive strips over the
nose. Metal external splints or mechanical appliances may be used.

There is a variety of nasal fracture, the result
of force directed from in front, which depresses
inwardly both nasal bones and rotates outwardly
one or both nasal processes of the two superior
maxilla. This injury is easily produced by "brass
knucks." The deformity is characteristic. The
nose is very broad, being spread all over the face,
and the bridge is sunken. On palpation the nasal
process of either or both maxilla will be found to
conform with the above description. The correction of this fracture requires a partial open operation. An incision is made within the nose to ex-

pose the nasal process. With a small saw, the process is sawed through along its base, and the operator must take care not to injure the contents of the orbit or the lachrymal apparatus. The nasal bones are elevated by force. At times they have to be rocked free of their impaction into the frontal bone. A sharp blow with force directed laterally will rotate the nasal process toward the medium line. This procedure reduces the broadened base of the nose. The septum deflection will require a submucous resection to release the parts of the fracture that are old or to improve the breathing space. The nose is packed and a mechanical appliance is used to hold the process in position. The administration of calcium will aid in the control of the swelling.

I have seen only one patient in private practice with the opposite deformity; that is, when the nasal bones were displaced outwardly. This occurred in a young instructor of a Girl's Scout camp. A delayed explosion of a bomb caught her while she was inspecting the dud. The force of the explosion struck her from below, went up her nasal passages, and blew out the front of her nose. Her deformity was like an exploded fire cracker. Our nasal problem here was to depress the nasal bones and to rotate inwardly the nasal processes. There was considerable loss of the cartilaginous portion and several operations were necessary to rebuild her nasal vestibules.

MALAR BONES

Blows received in fighting, falling or being forcibly thrown forward during a collision usually land on the malar prominence, which is easily displaced. The malar bone may be displaced forward, backward, inward or outward, and these displacements can be easily felt on palpation. In any event its articulations are severed. The bone comprising the external and posterior surfaces of the superior maxilla is thinner than that of the malar process, and crushes after the fashion of an egg shell. At times this irregular fracture will start at the inferior margin of the orbit and circle around the base of the malar process, ending at the junction of the posterior wall and the palate bone. This type of injury tears the antral membrane and its cavity fills with blood.

A typical case will present a roentgenogram showing a cloudy antrum on the injured side and an inward or outward rotation of the malar bone, with a change in the transverse diameter of the corresponding orbit.

A study of the normal orbit in the routine postero-anterior sinus film will show a line in the outer third made by the junction of the outer orbital wall and the skull. This line bears a constant relationship to the outer rim of the orbit and may be used to determine whether or not the malar bone has been displaced. The transverse diameter of the orbit is altered in these fractures, being increased if the injury is one of outward displacement and decreased in crushing injuries in which the malar bone is rotated inward. This relationship and diameter are controls, available for use in determining the correct position of the parts after the resetting of the fractures.

The malar bone and the firm bone composing the malar process of the superior maxilla are displaced in the direction of the force. The articulations of the malar bone give away with a resulting separation of it from the frontal, the temporal and the superior maxilla. At times the fracture extends forward into the ethmoidal cells. These patients present a typical deformity, the malar region being depressed.

Gill has suggested the use of special forceps similar to large Towel forceps to reduce displacements. The bone is grasped through the skin, and traction is applied with palpation as a guide. If successful, this method is safe and simple and leaves no scar. The absence of an open wound reduces the possibility of infection. If the antral wall is badly depressed, the force exerted to replace the fragments must be intra-antral. A very simple method is to make a naso-antral window under the inferior turbinate and insert a number seven Ritter sound. With one hand outside for palpation, the sound can be guided in the elevation of the fragments into their places. A rubber tube passed through the window into the antrum will serve for drainage purposes, and if it is anchored into the nasal vestibule it will serve as a prop to hold up the depressed malar process. If the anterior wall is badly comminuted, I prefer an open operation. The usual buccal approach of the antrum is made and the fragments are studied. Those which can be retained are replaced into their proper position and the others are removed. The muscular attachments to the fragments are capable of preventing their free manipulation and at times have to be separated before a satisfactory reduction can be obtained. Packing is seldom needed, but drainage should be maintained.

A blow struck with horizontal force against the front of the upper jaw will produce a transverse fracture of the superior maxilla and at times inflict an injury to both maxillae. This fracture presents characteristic changes in the features of the person injured; the upper teeth drop down on the lower jaw elongating the features, producing the so-called "horse face." At times this fracture extends into the nose and mouth. One of my patients suffered such an accident by having his head jammed between the floor of a freight elevator and a half gate. The ramus of the inferior maxilla may sustain a sudden strain, and often snap, with an added downward displacement of the lower teeth. These cases demand immediate reduction, and care should be taken to obtain a good apposition of the teeth. The lower jaw fracture should be reduced and anchored in position. These fractures are seldom single and each case is a rule unto itself, but immobilization should be started to a solid base. The skull cap can be encased in plaster, with supports anchored into the plaster. From these fixed supports, other supports or appliances should be extended to the fractured parts. If there are multiple fractures involving the upper and lower jaws, it is necessary to wire the jaws in position. This is important to assure a free and unlimited movement of the lower jaw after the fractures have healed.

I saw a man who had a locked jaw because the alveolar processes did not slide forward into their natural position, and the resulting vicious union locked the lower jaw. When first seen by me, he could separate his gums less than an inch. I had to separate the old fracture and displace the upper alveolar processes and hard palate forward. Unfortunately, in this case the ramus of the jaw on the left side had been fractured at the time of the injury, and being unrecognized had healed in a bad position, leaving him with a limited motion of the lower jaw.

The after-care of the open case is the same as that after a radical antral operation. The patient should be instructed to report whenever he contracts a head cold, and the local condition should be treated to avoid a sinus infection. These sinuses have sustained a permanent injury and are now more subject to infection than before the accident. Furthermore, the infection readily escapes through into the soft tissues, and adequate drainage should be maintained. If there has been a through and through wound of the cheek, it is best to close tight the mucous membrane and drain the skin wound.

Roberts has suggested the elevation of the depressed malar bone by the use of an instrument like a screw porte. Through a small skin incision the malar bone is bored into and with traction the bone is elevated into place. Gillies used for this same deformity, an elevator which he passed down under the depressed bone and elevated the fragments. His incision was made in the skin at the hair line and dissected down through the temporal fascia.

ZYGOMATIC FRACTURES

These same manipulations are applicable to the depressed fractures of the zygomatic arch. Matas

many years ago suggested an unique reduction of zygomatic fractures, by passing a piece of silver wire from above under the depressed bone and out again below the arch. Traction on the wire reduces the fracture. If necessary the wire can be fixed to an external support in cases that tend to recur.

The rhinologist is best prepared to treat fractures involving the para-nasal sinuses. The reduction of the fractures, and the protection of the sinuses are the underlying therapeutic principles.

BIBLIOGRAPHY

1. Weille, Francis L.: Studies in asthma; surgical treatment of chronic sinusitis in asthma. Jour. Am. Med. Assn., c:241-245 (January 28) 1933.
2. Gill, W. D.: Fractures about the orbit. South. Med. Jour., xxi:527-534 (July) 1928.
3. Roberts, S. E.: Fracture of malar zygomatic arch; review of literature; simplified operative technic. Ann. Otol., Rhinol., and Laryngol., xxxvii:826-838 (September) 1928. .
4. Gillies, H. D., Kilner, T. P., and Stone, D.: Fractures of malar-zygomatic compound with description of new x-ray position. Brit. Jour. Surg., xiv:651-656 (April) 1927.
5. Matas, Rudolph: Fracture of the zygomatic arch. New Orleans Med. and Surg. Jour., xlix:139-157 (September) 1896.

LACRIMAL DUCT STENOSIS*

ROYAL F. FRENCH, M.D., Marshalltown

The prescribed textbook treatment for lacrimal duct stenosis has not always produced the desired or hoped for results. For years, the treatment consisted of either probing the duct, or extirpation of the lacrimal sac.

Probing or dilating the duct is unsatisfactory in the large majority of cases for two reasons; first, because in only a small number of cases does it give a permanent patent duct, and second, because it is most uncomfortable to the patient. Repeated dilations are not accomplished without some pain to the patients, and they soon tire of such frequent repeated procedures. We often think they are cured or relieved of their stenosis, but the truth is that they have simply stopped taking treatments, and are enduring their epiphora, or are seeking relief from some other doctor. Extirpation of the lacrimal sac has never appealed to me as a real scientific operation, for it does not seem logical to remove such a necessary drainage tube in order to relieve one or two constrictions in the tube.

Stenosis of the nasolacrimal duct may be present with or without suppuration. The non-suppurative type is seen in the congenital conditions found in infants. In the embryologic formation, the lacrimal duct is derived from an epithelial cord, which becomes canalized; this cord is surrounded by mesenchyme and is not connected with the nasal mucosa; in fact, the connection of the canal with the nasal fossa is the last embryologic step, and often is not completed, hence the occlusion found at this point in infants. Sometimes

* Address of the Chairman, Section on Ophthalmology, Otology and Rhinolaryngology, Eighty-third Annual Session, Iowa State Medical Society, Des Moines, May 9, 10, 11, 1934.

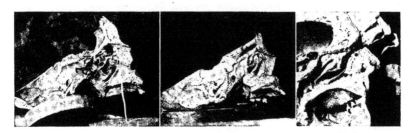

Fig. 1   Fig. 2   Fig. 3

Figures 1, 2 and 3, show that the bony lacrimal duct makes a regular curve from the orbital opening down and back to the posterior edge of the hard palate.

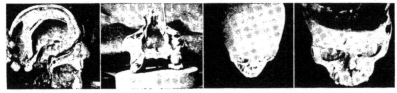

Fig. 4   Fig. 5   Fig. 6   Fig. 7

Figure 4 shows that the lacrimal membranous duct does not always exactly follow the curve of the bony duct.

Figure 5 illustrates the fact that the lacrimal duct has little lateral deviation.

Figures 6 and 7 show a variation of the lacrimal duct in the same specimen; one side being large, and the other extremely small.

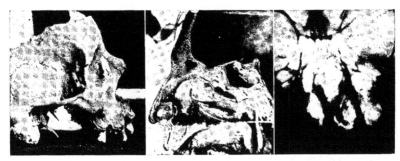

Fig. 8   Fig. 9   Fig. 10

Figure 8 demonstrates the fact that two orbital bony openings into the lacrimal duct are occasionally found.

Figure 9. The normal opening of the lacrimal duct into the inferior meatus is approximately one-half inch back of the anterior edge of the inferior meatus.

Figure 10. Displaying the size, direction and contour of the lacrimal duct after an injection of lipiodol or aridol.

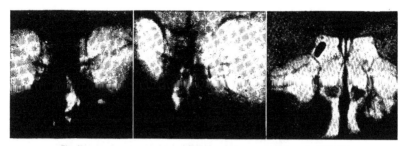

Fig. 11   Fig. 12   Fig. 13

Figures 11, 12 and 13 are pictures taken after lipiodol had been injected into the lacrimal duct, and show stenosis at the lower end of the lacrimal sac, which is the most frequent location of atresia.

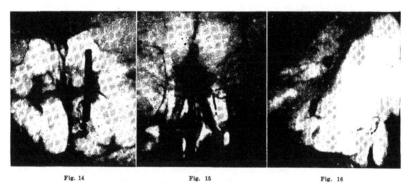

Fig. 14   Fig. 15   Fig. 16

Figure 14 shows a tube placed in the lacrimal duct at the time of an acute dacryocystitis. The eye was swollen shut, but practically all swelling was gone twenty-four hours after insertion of the tube.

Figures 15 and 16 illustrate a case of chronic infection of the lacrimal duct, with several points of constriction.

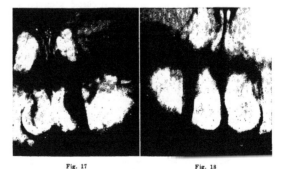

Fig. 17   Fig. 18

Figures 17 and 18 show tubes in the lacrimal duct in cases of chronic dacryocystitis.

the connection may be established in such a manner as to leave a valve-like fold or projection of the mucosa of the inferior meatus; this produces the so-called valve of Hasner.

The most constant points of atresia in the upper portion of the lacrimal drainage apparatus are at the punctum or at the opening of the canalicula into the lacrimal sac, and at the lower end of the lacrimal sac or the beginning of the nasolacrimal duct portion. If the atresia occurs in the punctum or canalicula, suppuration is seldom present, but if the stoppage is found at the lower end of the lacrimal sac, then the sac is usually filled with pus. Atresia, or occlusion in the nasal duct portion, may occur at any point; in fact, with an infection of the duct, this entire portion may become occluded, or sealed together.

In a review of the osteology of this region, we find that the lacrimal fossa is formed from the lacrimal bone and the frontal process of the superior maxilla; the lacrimal canal is formed by these same bones, with the addition of the inferior turbinate. In patients having the heavy type of facial bones, the frontal process of the superior maxilla may form the greater part of the lacrimal fossa; hence, in the West, or Toti-Mosher type of operation, this should be taken into consideration. If the bone is thick and heavy, there is great danger that the operation will not be successful, for the opening through the thicker bone is more likely to close. According to Schaeffer, the general direction of the lacrimal duct is "a line extending obliquely from the lacrimal fossa to a point on the alveolar process of the maxilla corresponding to the interval between the second premolar and first molar teeth."

Through the courtesy of Dr. E. W. MacEwen, of the Anatomy Department of the State University of Iowa, we examined a large number of skulls, in an effort to see if there were any constant, visible external land marks, as a guide in determining the direction of the duct. In the specimens examined, the duct took a direction slightly farther back; that is, pointing more to the first molar. While the bony duct may take this general direction, the membranous canal does not always coincide in shape or direction. The bony canal has a general curve or sweep from the orbital opening down and posteriorly pointing toward the posterior edge of the hard palate; this makes the curve in the opposite direction to that in which we usually pass our probes in dilating the duct. While this general curve is found in the bone or dried specimens, yet in the wet or fresh skulls, with the tissue intact, the lacrimal sac and membranous duct may pass straight down into the nasal fossa, or even make a slight anterior curve. This

of course means, that the straight probes, as of the Zeigler type, will in the majority of the cases, follow the duct without penetrating the walls of the membranous or bony canal.

The bony duct, while not varying so greatly in its general direction, does vary markedly in its size, not only in the different specimens, but even in the same skull; this is probably the reason why the majority of our patients have a stenosis on only one side. The membranous tissue specimens bring out what the textbooks show, that there are many membranous sacculations or constrictions, but these do not have bony corrugations or concentric ring formations, as the basis of these sacular constrictions. The narrowing of the bone canal is more likely to occur at the anatomic divisional points. From this standpoint, the first stenosis is found at the punctum, the second at the opening of the canaliculi into the lacrimal sac, the next at the opening of the sac into the lacrimal duct portion, and the last at the opening of the duct into the meatus.

In stenosis at the punctum, with resulting epiphora, it is possible that the stenosis occurred after the punctum dropped away from its normal location. This is especially so in the aged, for a relaxation of Horner's muscle causes a malposition of the punctum, with resulting cessation of function. This is more often seen in the lower punctum; the tears are probably aided in their passage into the sac by a slight vacuum produced in the sac by Horner's muscle. If the lower punctum is turned out of position, this vacuum is lost on both lower and upper puncta; as this occurs, the punctum gradually contracts, and often is so closed that even the tip of the dilator is inserted with difficulty. As the punctum ceases to function, it seems that there is also a contraction at the opening of the canaliculi into the sac, for after the punctum is dilated, a distinct stenosis is found just before the dilator enters the lacrimal sac.

Kuhnt says that 93.7 per cent of the lacrimal duct infections are of nasal origin; as infection occurs, the sac fills with pus, and is distended, for the outer wall of the sac is the only portion not covered by bone, and so is the only part capable of distention. The stenosis is then found at the beginning of the nasolacrimal duct, with even a complete closure throughout the rest of the nasolacrimal duct. Possibly this is nature's endeavor to limit further infection from the nose.

The elastic fibers from around the canaliculi decrease as we pass down the duct, while the cavernous fibers increase, and are very plentiful around the sac. Therefore, with a greater blood supply in this area, there is a more ready formation of pus and products of inflammation. It is also because of this cavernous plexus that much free and easy bleeding is encountered on any operative procedure here. The measurements of the lacrimal duct according to Whitnall are; lacrimal sac, twelve millimeters; interosseous portion, 15.3 millimeters; and the meatal portion, 5.3 millimeters. Thus the lacrimal sac is approximately one-half inch, the bony duct a little over one-half inch, and the total length to the floor of the nose about one and one-half inches.

While the curve of the duct varies in an antero-posterior direction, yet there is but little lateral deviation as it descends. In the occasional case, where the duct empties into the antrum, it probably does so because the antrum extends into the area of the normal inferior meatus. In spite of the location and size of this duct, it is seldom injured by operations on the ethmoidal cells or the antrum. Operative measures on the ethmoidal cells are usually carried out above and posteriorly to this region, while in removing the antromeatal wall in a radical antrum operation, one would at most be simply removing the lower end of the duct.

In the treatment of lacrimal duct stenosis, the congenital type seen in infants responds readily to one or two probings, but this does not hold true in other types of stenosis, for dilation does not produce lasting results, and extirpation leaves much to be desired. In the non-suppurative cases, as seen in adults, especially those cases which follow a relaxation of Horner's muscle, and a dropping away of the lower punctum, the resulting stenosis may at first respond to a few probings, but the stenosis usually persists and becomes permanent. It is in these cases, as well as in the suppurative ones, that the placing of a tube in the sac and duct gives the best results. The tube is easily inserted in the office, either with a local, or a short general anesthetic; the immediate reaction is similar to that which follows a like dilatation, and the patient wears the tube without discomfort. I personally see no reason why these tubes cannot remain in permanently. The tissues tolerate them without reaction, as is evidenced by a patient in whom I inserted an Ingals gold tube in the naso-frontal duct in December, 1911; the patient has worn this tube without trouble ever since; not only has it caused no trouble, but the patient has been entirely free from frontal sinus trouble, and has emphatically refused to let me remove the tube.

In comparison with the operative procedures, such as the Toti, West, or Mosher dacryocysto-rhinoscopies, the insertion of a tube is a simple matter. In the various operations whose object is to establish a permanent opening from the sac directly into the nose, there are several objections. The patient often objects to the operation; the

technic is not always as simple as it would seem; the sac is fragile, and not easy to care for; the bony wall under the sac may be heavy, and a permanent opening is hard to maintain. The insertion of a tube is easily accomplished, with only two points to be considered; first, to be sure that the probe, as one dilates, is in the duct, and second, to dilate with a probe slightly larger than the tube. The tube then slips in easily, and no pressure is required. The tubes I have placed in the lacrimal ducts have now functioned for several months, to the entire satisfaction of the patients.

HEADACHES—THEIR ETIOLOGY AND DIFFERENTIAL DIAGNOSIS*

CECIL C. JONES, M.D., Des Moines

Of all minor ailments to which humanity is heir, headache has the record of standing at the top of the list. With the exception of the common cold, headache produces more annoyance, discomfort and economic loss than any other ailment. It is so universal that it serves as the common social excuse. In our field of medicine I believe that the symptom of pain in the head is the most frequently encountered complaint. Daily everyone of us are analyzing, evaluating, seeking the cause, with the object of relieving this symptom.

Although headache is purely a subjective sensation or symptom, there must necessarily exist an anatomic and a physiologic basis for its production. The former is the better understood of the two. It is known that the largest intracranial nerve, the fifth, is sensory, and that through its three principal branches it is the chief sensory nerve of the head. It furnishes an abundant supply to the dura. That part of the dura which is in relation to the anterior of the skull is innervated by the meningeal nerve, a branch of the ophthalmic or first division of the fifth nerve. The dura of the middle fossa is supplied by recurrent twigs from the third division of the fifth nerve. The posterior fossa dura is innervated by the tentorial nerves, branches of the first division, and in addition receives twigs from the sympathetic, hypoglossal and vagus nerves. However, we do not encounter many purely dural lesions. During a mastoidectomy, localized dural inflammation is frequently encountered which has not produced enough headache to render one even suspicious that such a lesion exists. Brain surgeons report that during an operation under local anesthesia, manipulation of the dura does not cause pain. However, the ligation of a dural vessel is painful. The arachnoid is without a nerve supply. The

*Presented before the Section on Ophthalmology, Otology and Rhinolaryngology, Eighty-third Annual Session, Iowa State Medical Society, Des Moines, May 9, 10, 11, 1934.

other principal nervous mechanism concerned in the production of headaches consists of the sympathetic system. It is known that this system is partly sensory in function and that it governs vasomotor control. It supplies all the blood vessels and has many connecting ramifications with the fifth sensory nerve.

The physiologic mechanism by which headache is actually produced is little understood. Unquestionably irritation of the fifth nerve by chemical or mechanical means may affect the sympathetic nerves or vice versa, or that irritation in one branch of the fifth nerve may manifest itself in another branch. At present a number of theories have been advanced to explain the production of pain in the head. Some maintain that it is due to irritation of the nerve terminals of the fifth nerve; yet a toothache does not cause a headache. Another is that toxins affect the sympathetic nerves of the vessels; this is probably true in a certain percentage of cases. Another is that a pressure imbalance develops between the cerebral spinal fluid and intravascular pressures. Still another theory is that headaches are produced by a vasoconstriction or dilatation of the intracranial vessels. Undoubtedly all headaches are not produced in the same way, either mechanically or physiologically; some are produced in one way and some in another. However, I feel that the sympathetic system plays a greater rôle than does the sensory fifth nerve. It is still a mooted question as to what causes those headaches which are customarily classified as toxic in origin, either due to an acute systemic infection, excessive indulgencies in alcohol, tobacco or caffeine, or chronic foci of infection. It has not been proved whether the toxin directly attacks the sympathetic nerves of the intracranial vessels, thus causing headache, or whether the symptom is caused by either a vasodilatation or vasoconstriction resulting in a pressure imbalance between the cerebral spinal fluid and intracranial vascular pressure as a result of irritation of the sympathetic nerves of the blood vessels. This so-called pressure imbalance theory is the one offered to explain the headache of both hypotension and hypertension.

The most plausible theory advanced for the explanation of migraine is that a vasoconstriction of the intracranial vessels occurs. However, the large sensory fifth nerve must account for many headaches, particularly those from impacted wisdom teeth, sphenopalatine neuralgia, and ocular abnormalities. After all, the exact physiologic mechanism of headaches is little understood, nor will it be until we have a better conception of the physiology of the sympathetic nervous system. Experience teaches that although the anatomic basis is the same in each individual, each is endowed through heredity with a nervous mechanism which physiologically is entirely different from any other individual.

Headaches have been classified according to their etiology, such as migrainal, ocular, toxic, renal, sinus, etc.; likewise, according to time of occurrence, morning, afternoon, nocturnal, diural, etc.; also, according to location, ocular, retro-ocular, supra-orbital, frontal, temporal, occipital, unilateral, bilateral, or generalized; then too, according to subjective effect, such as dull, boring, sharp, lancinating, throbbing, constant, or periodic, or what not. Such nomenclature serves as descriptive terminology rather than a clinical classification for diagnostic purposes. It is true that headaches having the same etiology often tend to have somewhat similar characteristics and associations. Therefore, it is well to be familiar with the relationship between the etiology and characteristics of a headache, yet too much reliance must not be placed upon it, because headaches are accomplished counterfeiters. In other words a consistent distinctive type of headache does not exist.

In the diagnosis of a given headache the history is all important. During the taking of the history it may be necessary to run the gamut from hygiene to the endocrine glands. Therefore, the task of ferreting out the possible cause of a given headache properly belongs to the internist or general practitioner. Too frequently it is our lot to see the patient first and we must assume the responsibility of determining the most likely cause of the complaint according to the history furnished. Such a history should be of the individual rather than a check list of the characteristics of the headache. We should determine if the patient is one of a family with a history of periodic headaches, because practically all the headaches included in the category of migraine have a family history suggesting an hereditary predisposition. The relationship to dietary errors and dissipations, constipation, and the amount of tobacco consumed, must be considered. We should also ascertain the relationship to sexual excesses, the amount of sleep required, the amount of exercise taken, and the degree of ventilation surrounding the patient during sleep and work. Indiscretions of any kind very frequently initiate an attack in one who is subject to headache.

Among the points to be elicited relative to the headache as an independent symptom are:

1. Its period of duration to ascertain if it is of recent origin or of long standing.

2. The time of occurrence of the pain.

3. The location of the pain.

4. The character of the pain.

5. Frequency and duration of the attacks.

6. The associated phenomena; such as nausea, vomiting, gastric distress, shortness of breath, itching or burning of the eyes, photophobia, flashes of light, concurrent with head cold, slight sore throats, menstruation, or aggravated by moving about.

It often happens that an individual has two kinds of headaches which he can differentiate himself and each is due to different causes. Again, it is advisable to mention that there is no such thing as a constant distinctive type of headache, and likewise the associated phenomena are not constantly distinctive.

One of the most frequent causes of habitual headache is eyestrain. The actual mechanism of the pain is unsolved. By eyestrain is meant the effort expended by the ciliary muscle to counteract refractive errors, and to accommodate the eye for various distances, or the strain used by the extraocular muscles in maintaining binocular vision and converging. In a general way it may be said that the degree of error has nothing to do with the amount of headache or degree of discomfort produced. In hypersensitive individuals, a small error will produce symptoms out of proportion, while in a plethoric individual, several times the amount of error will be borne with no symptom. The most reliable guide in the diagnosis of headache of ocular origin is the history; yet too much reliance must not be placed upon it. Headaches caused by eyestrain characteristically become manifest after the prolonged use of the eyes, viewing a movie or watching moving objects. Thus it is that they are prone to appear in the afternoon or evening. However, ocular headaches may be present on arising. Neurasthenic patients often complain of headaches after using their eyes for a short time instead of after a prolonged use. It must be remembered that a refractive error may have been present for many years without manifesting itself until some contributory factor, such as a chronic focus of infection, weakens the ocular neuromuscular system. Chronic primary glaucoma is just rare enough that it may be overlooked as the cause of headache. In acute eye infections it is usually apparent that the eye condition is causing the headache. Chronic catarrhal conjunctivitis will cause a headache even after the refractive error is relieved. De Schweinitz, one of our most conservative ophthalmologists, estimates that 70 per cent of all functional headaches are due to eyestrain. The oculists of the Mayo Clinic classify its frequency as low as 10 per cent. Neurologists inform us that practically all patients with intracranial

pathology have had refractive errors corrected in an effort to relieve their headaches.

High myopic errors rarely cause a headache, but low myopic or compound myopic errors of a one-fourth of a diopter will cause severe headache. Hyperopic astigmatism causes more headache than hyperopia. Vertical errors give rise to more discomfort than lateral errors.

Toxic headaches are probably next in frequency to ocular abnormalities as a cause of headache. Like ocular headaches they tend to occur in the afternoon and so have been designated fatigue headaches because they become manifest whenever the neuromuscular systems tend to become exhausted. Toxins derived from the excessive use of tobacco and coffee; chronic infections, such as tuberculosis; or from foci of infection, such as apical abscessed teeth, chronic tonsillitis, chronic sinusitis, prostatitis, cervicitis, endometritis, metritis, and hemorrhoids are the common sources of infection. When citing abscessed teeth, a very frequent cause of toxic headache, it should be emphasized that a definite walled-off abscess shown by the x-ray is not nearly as likely to be causing trouble as a tooth which only appears fuzzy about the apex because from the latter there is more absorption. Again it is necessary to reiterate that in one individual a relatively small amount of pathology will give rise to symptoms while another will tolerate considerable pathology without any apparent symptomatology. Chronic foci of infection of apparently minor importance often act indirectly causing a headache in individuals subject to migraine. They can either initiate, influence or aggravate such a headache.

Migraine which makes up a goodly percentage of headaches has as its one constant characteristic, pain in the head. The only plausible explanation offered for its mechanism is that it is due to a vasomotor spasm of the cerebral vessels. The occurrence of such a spasm depends upon the assumption that an inherited instability of the sympathetic system exists in some individuals. At least persons subject to migraine usually have a family history of headaches of similar character. Migraine encroaches very closely upon being a clinical entity. Such headaches are usually present upon awakening in the morning, but not necessarily so. They occur periodically at more or less regular intervals. They often are preceded or ushered in by an aura which is more or less constant for that individual. In one patient it may assume the form of an ocular disturbance, in another gastric distress, and in another mental depression or sluggishness. These headaches are frequently associated with nausea and vomiting. Their occurrence tends to disappear spontaneously during the late forties or fifties. Attacks seem to be precipitated by some indiscretion, such as mental or emotional overstrain, lack of sleep, lack of exercise, physical fatigue, dietary indiscretion, excessive use of coffee or tobacco, sexual excesses, and ocular strain. The headaches are made worse by noise, walking, stooping or jarring. They are most relieved by reclining in a darkened quiet room. New of the Mayo Clinic maintains that aspirin is a specific treatment, but I doubt it. Many of the mythologic types of headaches are different types of varying degree of intensity of migraine; namely, the so-called gastric, bilious, liver, gallbladder, intestinal, nervous, sympathetic, etc.

Practically every acute sinusitis, if worthy of being called a sinusitis, has headache as a predominating symptom. The pain depends in character, degree and time of occurrence upon the sinus involved and the pathology in that sinus. The pain is due to pressure upon the terminals of the fifth nerve and probably to some extent to the absorption of toxins. Vacuum sinus headaches are very rare. The textbook picture of a sinus headache is one present on arising or occurring shortly thereafter, and disappearing later in the day. This is more true in the acute than the chronic type, but not more than 90 per cent of sinus headaches are classical in this respect. In severity they range from a dull ache to a severe throbbing, depending upon the amount of congestion in the sinus. Alcohol and tobacco aggravate them because they increase intranasal congestion. On the other hand steam inhalations often relieve the congestion and ache by increasing circulation. In all forms, stooping and jarring aggravate the pain. Transillumination, intranasal examination together with the history of a cold in the head, usually lead to a correct diagnosis.

In chronic sinus inflammation, headaches occur in only about five per cent of the cases, and it is not always possible to elicit a history of a chronic cold in the head. It is paradoxical that the pain of chronic maxillary sinusitis is in the frontal region of the same side. In chronic frontal sinusitis the headache is often just dull enough to be annoying, thus interfering particularly with brain work requiring concentration. In chronic ethmoidal conditions headache is less frequent, but when present exists as a dull pressure over the parietal region or root of the nose. Chronic sphenoiditis is often accompanied by periodic attacks of headache described by the patient as a diffuse feeling of pressure in the occiput or over the vertex. Dizziness on stooping is the most constant associated symptom. Headaches due to chronic sinusitis can often be differentiated by the fact that many times they

are relieved temporarily by steam inhalations. An essential aid in the diagnosis of chronic sinusitis is irrigation, filling the sinus directly or indirectly by the method of Proetz with lipiodol followed by a roentgenogram. The differentiation between allergic filling defects and those due to thickened chronic inflamed mucosa is at times confusing, but can be accomplished by an intramuscular injection of adrenalin just prior to the making of x-ray plates. This injection causes an allergic mucosa to shrink. At last it has been learned that many chronic hyperplastic non-suppurative intranasal conditions are allergic in nature rather than definite infections. Anatomic intranasal abnormalities are only very occasionally responsible for headaches.

As previously stated the differential diagnosis of headache is properly the internist's problem because there are a number of systemic conditions causing it. Headaches occurring before arising may be due to cardiorenal disease, nephritis, hypertension, cerebral arteriosclerosis, luetic endarteritis, glaucoma, and any lesion causing increased intracranial pressure. Multiple sclerosis must always be remembered as a possible cause. Harvey Cushing maintains that most brain tumor headaches, in their incipiency, have been diagnosed as neurasthenic or hysterical until the ocular fields were interpreted. Brain abscesses and encephalitis with a slow onset cause less pain than tumors because they replace rather than displace brain tissue. Disturbances among the glands of internal secretion cause a very small proportion of headaches. However, a limited number of headaches occurring in women, having their onset about the time of puberty, recurring periodically with the menstrual period, and disappearing at the menopause, are said to be due to a functional hyperplasia of the pituitary gland. If they can be relieved by the administration of whole gland serum, such is probably the case. On the other hand, equally good authorities maintain that there is an increased nervous instability accompanying catamenia which in some individuals gives rise to headaches. There is no such thing as an ovarian headache. The only pelvic disorder productive of headache is chronic endometritis and cervicitis, in which case it is toxic in character. Headaches can be produced by cerebral passive congestion, by decompensated cardiac conditions, by pressure from mediastinal tumors, by tight fitting collars or hats, by lumbar puncture and by hypertension. The mechanism of this pain is attributed to the periodic or constant pressure imbalance between the cerebral spinal fluid and the intracranial intravascular pressures in either the veins or arteries. In all forms of meningitis there is this imbalance which causes pressure upon the sensitive dural vessels. In the bacterial forms there is the added toxic influence. In uremia, hypertension, constipation, and polycythemia there is an increased intracranial pressure which when reduced relieves the headache. It is known that a saline purge reduces the cerebral spinal fluid pressure as well as the intravascular pressure; thus it relieves the so-called constipation headache by depleting, rather than eliminating, intestinal toxins as was once supposed. Clinicians observed that headaches were more frequent in those cases of chronic interstitial nephritis, where there was considerable retention as indicated by a high blood urea or where there was an associated hypertension. Such headaches are due to passive congestion, a wet brain so to speak. These headaches usually begin during the early morning hours, at times severe enough to waken the sufferer; they are diffuse and are described as a pressure rather than a pain. Anything which temporarily increases the passive congestion aggravates them, such as sneezing, stooping, or coughing; likewise they are improved after the individual is up and about, due to an increase in the circulation. Moreover they tend to recur regularly in contraindication to most headaches. Headaches resulting from brain tumor, luetic endarteritis, cerebral arteriosclerosis, and chronic nephritis, have many common characteristics. A review of a large number of cases reveals the fact that most constipated people do not have headaches; but if one does have a headache he belongs to a group of persons very susceptible to headache. However, a diet too high in carbohydrates or proteins produces in certain individuals an imbalance in their blood chemistry with associated headaches. Such changes disturb the intracranial pressure relations. Under such conditions laxatives will relieve the headaches. Nothing is characteristic of such headaches except that they are associated with dietary indiscretions.

In conclusion I would like to emphasize the following points:

1. For diagnostic purposes, distinctive types or characteristics of headaches are the exception rather than the rule.

2. The organ or area which, owing to its disturbed function or inflammation, gives rise to the pain, is itself often free from pain.

3. The dysfunction of the organ may be trifling compared to the pain it produces.

4. Headaches due to ocular disturbances, chronic toxemias, and migraine occur most frequently.

5. We must arrive at a diagnosis of the cause of every headache by the process of elimination.

6. The cause of every headache cannot be determined.

Discussion

Dr. Thomas R. Gittins, Sioux City: I want to thank Dr. Jones for speaking on this subject of headache. Certainly too little has been written about the differential diagnosis of headache, and too little thought has been given to the subject of the periodic vasomotor or migraine types.

I wish to emphasize my feeling that in periodic vasomotor headache a careful history is of much more positive value in diagnosis than an equally careful physical examination. It takes time and patience to obtain a real history. Many patients come in with pre-formed ideas of the cause of their headache, and they often repeat parrot-like the impressions they have gained from other physicians' examinations. Many people are not able to give an accurate description of their troubles and seem to resent too much questioning.

Migraine and other types of vasomotor headaches are very common, much more common than is often realized. In the typical case there is the syndrome characterized by periodic headaches; often preceded by visual phenomena such as scotomata and hemianopsias; often accompanied by nausea, vomiting and parathesias; and usually followed for a short time by mental and physical fatigue. Such a syndrome tends to recur at various intervals of days, weeks or months with intervals of normal health in patients whose personal and family history indicate susceptibility. Careful attention to the history will differentiate this type of headache from other types quite easily. On the other hand, if the greatest attention is given to objective evidence of pathology in the nose, sinuses or elsewhere, many wrong diagnoses will be made, and much unnecessary operative work be advised and performed.

The headache of acute sinus infection should rarely present difficulties in diagnosis, except possibly in isolated acute sphenoiditis. In this latter type there may be none of the usual symptoms of preceding rhinitis, but the location and time of day during which the pain appears and disappears, plus x-ray findings should suggest exploratory irrigation. In my experience headache of any severity is not a common and prominent symptom in chronic sinus infection except during acute exacerbations. The most severe infections of the sphenoids, ethmoids or antra with polyps and positive x-ray findings come to our offices with many complaints, but headache is rarely a prominent one. They have a history of headache in acute exacerbations, but they complain much more of poor nasal breathing, purulent discharge, bronchitis, asthma, etc. So many patients have some evidence of chronic sinus trouble or nasal obstruction, and so many also have periodic vasomotor headache that it is natural to associate these two conditions as cause and effect when so often they are only coincidental.

The blood supply of the upper part of the nose is directly related to that of the floor of the cranial cavity. During a congestive or vasomotor headache nasal congestion is also common. The shrinking of the upper part of the nose or the sphenopalatine region with cocaine and adrenalin may have a favorable effect upon a vasomotor headache because changes in the circulation of the region are produced. Because of this temporary relief of an acute condition many nasal operations are advised for a headache that has no relation whatever to the nasal condition.

Vacuum sinus headaches may exist as they have been reported often by good observers. In my experience this type seems extremely rare and I have never been really sure that I have seen such a case.

Sphenopalatine and vidian syndromes should be considered as neuralgias and not headaches, and need to be differentiated from involvement of the fifth nerve rather than from the headache of the migraine type.

Migraine or some type of vasomotor headache is much more common in children than is generally thought. From five to seven years of age the headache itself is a minor symptom of the periodic attacks which begin with languor, loss of appetite, possibly some fever, vomiting and abdominal discomfort. In these early years the gastric disturbance is usually the prominent symptom and a child may say nothing of headache. As the patient reaches the age of ten or twelve years the same periodic gastro-intestinal upsets may continue to appear, with the headache becoming more pronounced at the beginning of the attacks. Cyclic vomiting and appendicitis are often diagnosed in children when the history indicates typical vasomotor headache of the migraine type. Many appendices are removed in children to relieve gastro-intestinal symptoms which are definitely secondary to vasomotor changes in the brain.

Many obscure types of headache may be improved by proper attention to vertical phorias. The occlusion test has been of considerable help to us in handling such cases. Vertical prisms in the proper cases are of distinct value in our experience.

At the present time sinus surgery does not have the respect it deserves, and it is my firm belief that ill-advised operative work in the nose and sinuses, in a vain attempt to relieve the migraine type of headache and kindred allergic conditions, is almost entirely to blame for this lack of confidence among physicians and the laity. In all probability, hope for the migraine sufferer is just around the corner in view of the encouraging studies in endocrinology and food sensitivity which are being conducted at the present time.

I want to thank Dr. Jones again for presenting this subject so clearly and to say that I have appreciated the opportunity of discussing this paper.

Dr. William W. Pearson, Des Moines: I would like to emphasize two or three points. In the first place, the history is very important. In the headaches that begin later in life it is rather important to make a careful examination of the eye. The essayist spoke of the possibility of a simple glaucoma,

and I do not believe we have concluded our full eye examination until we have taken the field and also the tension, remembering that tension will vary from time to time.

A single examination is not always conclusive, but the field of vision does help us. I know I have missed this in a few cases. It may come, of course, in the migraine subject, but many times we have a good central vision, normal central vision, and a careful examination will reveal the contracted field.

Dr. Gittins spoke of the lack of headache as a result of nasal conditions. I think it is possible to have a nasal headache as the result of an obstruction in the nose. I have made the observation sufficiently often to know, or to become convinced, that a nasal obstruction which occurs periodically will give rise to symptoms of congestion of the sinus, and that when that septum has been straightened we have free breathing; temporary congestion of the sinus will not occur; and as a result the headache is relieved.

The paper is very exhaustive and we appreciate the manner in which it is placed before us.

Anyone who has made a careful study of headaches over a period of many years cannot fail to appreciate a class of cases which must be ascribed to a cause with which we are not entirely familiar. I think that Dr. Shea's explanation of these cases is assuming more importance and being given greater credit, and I believe this will eventually be proved.

This question of the nasal septum color under these different conditions is of value. In a recent trip to Charleston, South Carolina, I sat in a smoker and visited with Dr. Mittendorf, and he said he had been selected to make observations and report these observations to a certain committee. After some time he was no longer communicated with relative to his observations along this line. He concluded his statement to me by saying that he was not keen enough apparently to make out these different septal variations in color and that he was disposed to place less reliance upon it than many of the gentlemen who were members of that committee.

Dr. Jarvis of Barre, Vermont, was one of the originators of this idea. This subject was discussed at the meeting, and gentlemen of experience in that society seemed to place a good deal of reliance upon this symptom. It means that we must be more critical in our observation of these cases, and there must be something to it. I was left with that impression. I want to thank the essayist for presenting such a worthwhile paper.

Dr. H. C. Payne, Pella: During the last few weeks I have listened to three lectures on headaches. One essayist, a well known neurologist, stated that there was no such thing as a headache due to eyestrain. I would like the opinion of the present speaker, who is an ophthalmologist.

Dr. Jones (closing): I have nothing further to add. I cannot answer the question. The ophthalmologist thinks the majority of headaches are due to eye-strain; the neurologist thinks they are due to neurologic conditions. The only way one could obtain a fairly good conception of the cause of headaches in the order of frequency would be to have an unbiased opinion, probably by an internist.

THE PAINFUL SHOULDER SYNDROME*

TOM BENTLEY THROCKMORTON, M.D.
Des Moines

One of the common ailments which causes patients to seek relief at the hand of the physician is a sore, stiff, painful shoulder. In my experience this condition is encountered most frequently in middle aged individuals, although the young and the old are by no means exempt. It is not strange that complaints referable to the shoulder should be of common occurrence when one anticipates for a moment the anatomic make-up of the shoulder joint and the enormous amount of strain which is placed on the structures entering into its formation. In the evolution of man the shoulder has changed from a walking, weight-bearing joint to a weight-lifting, weight-carrying one. It is the most universal of all the joints of the body. The great range of motion and the shallowness of the joint cavity make it particularly susceptible to trauma and strain.

The bony elements entering into the formation of the shoulder are the scapula, clavicle and humerus. The muscular elements, which play a greater or lesser rôle in joint movement, or which cross the joint, are the supraspinatus, infraspinatus, subscapularis, teres major and minor, biceps, triceps, coracobrachialis, latissimus dorsi and the pectoralis major and minor muscles. A knowledge of the anatomic construction of the joint, of the action of the various muscles which enter into its movements, and of the innervation of the shoulder, both direct and referred, is absolutely essential for an understanding of the painful conditions which at times center about this region.

As a matter of convenience I have divided some of the various causative factors for painful shoulder into three groups:

Group I. Extrinsic Factors
Trauma
Fracture
Dislocation
Muscular strain
Thermal change

Group II. Intrinsic Factors
Arthritis
Periarthritis
Bursitis

*Presented before the Eighty-third Annual Session, Iowa State Medical Society, Des Moines, May 9, 10, 11, 1934.

Myositis
Tendonitis
Synovitis
Osteomyelitis
Neuritis
Neuroarthropathy

Group III. Reflex Nervous Factors
A. Thoracic
1. Cardiovascular lesions
Angina pectoris
Luetic aortitis
Aortic aneurysm
2. Pulmonary lesions
Pleurisy
Pneumonia
Tuberculosis
Intrathoracic neoplasms
Pulmonary infarction
3. Lesions of the spine and spinal cord in the cervico-dorsal region.
B. Abdominal
1. Hepatic lesions
Hepatitis
Cholecystitis
Cholangitis
Gall stones
Subphrenic abscess
2. Other abdominal lesions
Perforated peptic ulcer
Acute pancreatitis
Ruptured spleen
Ruptured ectopic pregnancy
Appendicitis
C. Inflammation or irritation of the diaphragm.

From this number of etiologic factors which may enter into the causation of shoulder pain, it can readily be appreciated that it will be possible in the time allotted for this presentation to mention only some of these factors, and to empasize a few of the conditions which are most frequently encountered. In Group I the outward evidence of trauma, fracture or dislocation is sufficient at once to account for pain in and about the shoulder. A history of exposure to marked extremes in temperature, or to sudden or prolonged muscular strain, often will give the clue to the cause for the soreness and stiffness about the shoulder region.

Many of the conditions enumerated in Group II are made manifest to the physician, if he will but exercise a little care and skill in properly examining his patient. That he may be materially helped in diagnosis by the additional aid of good roentgenograms is obvious.

For the sake of brevity, therefore, I purposely have chosen to confine my remarks to three conditions which are prone to cause pain in the shoulder region, and with which I feel both internist and surgeon should be familiar. Two of these conditions are local; the third is usually referred from distant parts. I refer to muscular strain, to subdeltoid bursitis and to reflex pain due to phrenic nerve irritation.

MUSCULAR STRAIN

Every physician of any experience whatsoever has been consulted by patients complaining of a sore, stiff, painful shoulder. Usually the complaining person is a man of mature years. He may have taken occasion to renew his athletic prowess by engaging in some unaccustomed sport or muscular feat. He enters into the athletic activities with all the apparent vigor of youth, but fails to take into consideration that his muscles are no longer as supple and snappy as they were in former years. Following some unaccustomed muscular action—like throwing a baseball or striking at a pitched one—he suddenly becomes aware that something has happened to his shoulder. He may experience the subjective sensation as though something had torn or snapped in or about the joint. The primary discomfort may be pushed from the field of consciousness for the time being;

but within a few hours or days soreness and stiffness become so persistent that they can no longer go unheeded. Abduction of the arm and internal rotation of the humerus are the two movements which seem to cause the greatest pain or discomfort. Time after time I have diagnosed correctly the effects of muscular strain of the shoulder or a subdeltoid bursitis by the inability of the patient to elevate his arm and place his hand on his head, as in combing his hair, or by his inability to place his hand behind his back and to elevate it higher than the sacral, or lower lumbar region. (See Figures 1 and 2.) The extremity can be swung forward and backward with perfect

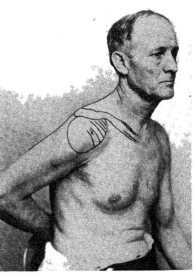

Figure 2. Production of pain on internal rotation of the humerus, and an inability of the patient to raise his hand higher than the sacral, or the lower lumbar region, are characteristic in many instances of muscular strain or subdeltoid bursitis.

comfort; but the moment abduction and internal rotation are attempted, either active or passive, pain is complained of in the shoulder and upper arm regions. Not infrequently the pain is referred down the front or the back of the arm.

Of the various muscles which cross the joint or enter into its movements, the one most prone to strain or injury is the supraspinatus. The belly of this muscle gets its origin from the supraspinous portion of the scapula. Its fibers terminate in a tendon which passes through and, according to

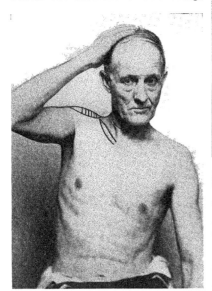

Figure 1. Abduction of the arm in muscular strain or in subdeltoid bursitis frequently produces pain in the shoulder region.

some authorities, becomes a part of the subdeltoid (or subacromial) bursa, finally to be inserted into the greater tuberosity of the humerus. The muscular strain may be so great at times as to produce a partial or complete rupture of the tendon, or even to tear it from its bony attachment to the humerus. In cases of complete rupture of the tendon, atrophy of the muscle has been observed as early as two weeks following the lesion. The deltoid, the latissimus dorsi, the teres major, the biceps tendon, the pectoralis major and the subscapularis are the other muscles most frequently strained or bruised about the shoulder.

SUBDELTOID BURSITIS

Subdeltoid bursitis, whether of infectious or traumatic origin, is a troublesome factor in producing pain about the shoulder. The more or less intimate relationship of the bursa with the joint capsule, the tendon of the supraspinatus muscle and other structures about the joint, makes it of importance as a pain producing factor when it becomes inflamed or injured. The bursa lies beneath the deltoid muscle, and protects the head of the humerus from the overlying bony shelf formed by the acromial process of the scapula and the acromial end of the clavicle. Palpation about the head of the humerus will give rise to pain when the bursa is inflamed; abduction of the arm to a right angle will cause the bursa to pass beneath the acromial process so that it no longer can be pressed upon, hence freedom from pain. However, if the arm is raised upward so as to compress the sore and distended bursa between the overhanging acromion and the humeral head, pain will again be elicited. It is avoidance of the production of pain in this manner that causes the patient to bring his arm forward when he attempts to elevate it from his side.

PHRENIC NERVE PAIN

The third and last condition to which I wish to call attention is reflex pain so often felt over the top of the shoulder in phrenic nerve irritation. It has long been known that shoulder pain may be due to referred impulses coming from the brachial plexus or from the phrenic nerve. The plexus is formed by the union of the anterior divisions of the fourth, fifth, sixth and seventh cervical and the first dorsal nerves. Thus, the phrenic nerve, which arises from the third, fourth and fifth cervical nerves, has a distinct anatomic connection with the brachial plexus. The third and fourth cervical nerves also give origin to the supraclavicular nerve, whose fibers supply the greater portion of the skin of the shoulder-top. The motor fibers of the phrenic nerve supply chiefly the diaphragm; its

sensory fibers innervate the central area of this muscle and some of its filaments are sent to the pericardium, the pleura, the peritoneal ligament of the liver, the cystic duct and the neck of the gallbladder. The border zone of the diaphragm is supplied by sensory fibers coming from the intercostal nerves. Thus it can readily be understood how pathologic processes arising about the heart, the pleura, the liver, and especially in the central zone of the diaphragm, may give rise to referred pain in the shoulder-top area which is supplied by the branches of the supraclavicular nerve.

The mechanism entering into the production of shoulder-top pain is as follows. (See Figure 3.)

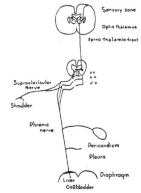

Figure 3. Diagram showing the author's conception of the nervous mechanism entering into the production of shoulder-top pain.

An abnormal stimulus is created in a viscus supplied by the phrenic nerve. The sensory impulse is then carried over the nerve to the cervical region where it enters the spinal cord through the third, fourth and fifth cervical roots. Since the stimulus is a painful one, it is conveyed upward in the spinal cord by way of the posterior fibers of the spinothalamic tract. These fibers cross and ascend in the lateral aspect of the spinal marrow to the brain where they end in the great sensory relay station, the optic thalamus. From the thalamus the impulse is carried upward through the hemisphere to the general sensation area of the brain where it becomes recognized in the field of consciousness as pain. The pain is not necessarily felt in the viscus which gave it origin. On the contrary it is felt on the top of the shoulder. The region in which the pain is felt is supplied by the supraclavicular branches whose impulses likewise reach the spinal cord by way of the third and fourth cervical roots. Thus the third and fourth cervical roots are the common pathways for sensory impulses originating in the phrenic nerve distribution and in the supraclavicular distribution. Since the integument supplied by the supraclavicular branches is far more sensitive than the area which gave origin to the painful stimulus in the chest or abdomen, the pain becomes referred to the more highly sensitized end organ, and is accorded the name, "referred pain."

To the surgeon and internist, alike, this knowledge of the mechanism of referred pain to the shoulder region should be of great importance. Especially is this true as an aid to a better understanding of conditions which arise in the base of the lung or in the abdomen. No surgeon has any desire to drain a gallbladder for the suspected presence of an acute inflammatory process when in reality the patient is suffering from pneumonia, or from an infarction, which is beginning in the lower lobe of the right lung. In such a case, the presence of shoulder-top pain may be of considerable diagnostic value. In the early stage of pulmonary involvement the pain may be referred to the abdomen, particularly to one of the upper quadrants. Pain, tenderness and rigidity over the gallbladder region, especially in an individual who has suffered from previous attacks of hepatic colic or gallbladder disease, are usually conceded to be a triad of symptoms indicative of liver involvement. However, the patient in the beginning of a pulmonary involvement at the base of his lung likewise may complain of pain in the top of his shoulder. In such an instance his respirations are increased and shallow. His diaphragm movements on the affected side are almost at a standstill. His facial expression may indicate signs of embarrassed respiratory function. His nares may dilate and contract with each respiratory excursion. A most careful physical examination may fail to reveal any abnormal findings in his lung, and yet, it is just such findings as these that should put the surgeon on his guard as to the possibility of the beginning of a lower lobe lesion with an involvement of the pleura over the central zone of the diaphragm. Certainly a few hours of careful watching and waiting on the part of the physician are of less danger to such a patient than immediate subjection to the risk of a general anesthetic and an abdominal section. If the lung is primarily at fault, and a basal pneumonia is actually in the nascent state, the signs of pulmonic involvement will come to the foreground sooner or later. Fever, cough, bloody sputum, crepitus, dulness and tubular breathing are the cardinal signs of a pneumonia. If these are present, the diagnosis cannot be disputed.

On the other hand, the physician may be confronted with an acute abdominal condition in which the patient complains of shoulder-top pain. All evidence of disturbed respiratory function may be absent in the clinical picture except perhaps, that the diaphragm movements may be somewhat curtailed. However, the history of the patient's illness and the abdominal findings point conclusively to an acute surgical condition due to a perforated peptic ulcer, a ruptured spleen, a ruptured ectopic pregnancy, or a perforated appendix. In such a case, whatever the etiologic factor may be, the cause for shoulder-top pain is due to but one thing; namely, the presence of some irritative fluid which has reached the under surface of the central zone of the diaphragm. In such instances, surgical intervention may or may not be undertaken as the physician deems best; however, he need have no fear of the administration of a general anesthetic *per se*, since he is certain that the source of trouble lies below, and not above, the diaphragm.

Inflammation or irritation of the central zone of the diaphragm is a most prolific source in producing shoulder-top pain. Since this muscle separates the thoracic cavity from the abdominal cavity it can readily be understood how lesions originating within the lower pleural cavity or in the upper abdomen may so affect its central zone as to give birth to sensory impulses which are reflected in the sensorium of the patient as a referred pain to the shoulder-top. The mere presence of shoulder-top pain is not of sufficient diagnostic value alone to aid the physician in localizing the source of phrenic nerve irritation. Other clinical evidence must be forthcoming before he can state with certainty whether the pathologic process is within the thoracic cavity or the abdominal cavity.

The following case report will serve to emphasize how the abdomen may be the source of trouble which ultimately localized in the thorax and how in the beginning it was impossible to determine whether the causal factor was supra or infradiaphragmatic.

CASE REPORT

A white female, thirty-nine years of age, married, experienced some abdominal discomfort following a noonday luncheon on February 14, 1934. The meal had been a rather simple one and she could think of no dietary indiscretion as a cause of her distress. In 1916, when she was twenty-one years of age, she had suffered from an attack of acute inflammation of the gallbladder from which she had made a good recovery. In August, 1925, she had aborted spontaneously at the fifth month of gestation. On the third day following she had been seized with a sudden, severe pain over the right kidney which was probably due to a renal infarct. She made a good recovery from this illness and enjoyed splendid health until July, 1933. While on a visit in California at that time she became ill with an attack of acute gallbladder disease. Fever, tenderness over the gallbladder, and referred pain to the tip of the right scapula, were the prominent symptoms of her illness. There was no jaundice. Recovery ensued in about a week. A similar attack was again experienced about two months later. The onset was sudden and was ushered in by pain in the epigastic region, tenderness over the gallbladder and right abdomen, fever, vomiting of bile and a referred pain to the right scapular region. The leukocyte count was 24,800. A careful checkup was made in October after her return to her home, but nothing of importance was found. A Graham dye test was planned, but the procedure was not carried out. The patient felt perfectly well and, on a diet in which fats were restricted, she lost about twenty pounds in weight.

The recurrence of indefinite symptoms of a gastro-intestinal nature on February 14, 1934, would have caused the patient no concern were it not for the memory of the preceding attacks of acute abdominal distress; hence I was called to see her. Examination, which was made some eight hours after the onset of the digestive disturbance, revealed a soft abdomen, perfectly free from tenderness. The heart and lungs were negative. The patient's complaints and attitude reminded me of an individual who was slightly indisposed because of a mild indigestion. Unfortunately she was not seen on the following day. During this time, however, a general abdominal soreness developed which was associated with a temperature of 99.4 degrees. On the morning of February 16, without warning, she was seized with a severe pain in the upper abdomen. Curiously enough the pain was referred to the top of her right shoulder. When I saw the patient, about an hour after the onset of her trouble, I found her in a condition of shock. Her temperature was subnormal, her pulse was 80 and of poor volume, her skin was cold, and her facies was indicative of some grave disaster. Her abdomen was rigid and no tenderness could be elicited over the gallbladder or the appendix regions. The shoulder-top pain was equal to, if indeed it did not exceed in severity, the abdominal pain. In fact, the patient begged for relief from the distressing pain in her shoulder. Her heart and lungs were entirely negative.

When I saw her six hours later the clinical picture had changed somewhat. Her temperature was 101 degrees; her pulse rate was 72, and her respirations, which had increased to 36 per minute, were very shallow. She still complained bitterly about the pain on the top of her right shoulder. There were no definite lung findings except that the breath tones seemed a little diminished over the base of the right lung. There was definite tenderness over the liver region. Deep inspiration increased the pain in the gallbladder area; and it also increased the shoulder-top pain.

Twenty hours after the onset, the patient showed signs of marked illness. Her temperature was 100.6 degrees; her pulse was 100 and her blood pressure was 122 systolic, 80 diastolic. The color of her face had changed from paleness to a brownish-red hue. Her cheeks were flushed, more on the right side than the left. Both sclerae were bile-tinged. Her respirations were exceedingly shallow, averaging about 40 per minute. The alae of the nostrils dilated and contracted with each respiratory cycle. There was a distinct area of dulness over the right pulmonic base, posteriorly. In this area, the breath sounds could be heard faintly only on deep inspiration. There were no tubular sounds or râles. Grocco's sign was absent. Tenderness still persisted when pressure was made below the right costal border; it was less so over the lower abdomen. The shoulder-top pain was lessened considerably in intensity. The leukocyte count was 45,000; the urine was negative except for a high gravity, a moderate amount of albumin, and a trace of bile.

At the end of thirty hours, there was no appreciable change in the condition of the patient except that the leukocyte count had dropped to 31,500, and she was entirely free from shoulder-top pain. At the expiration of forty hours of illness, the skin showed a definite icteric color. The urine also showed an increase in the amount of bile. The leukocyte count had dropped to 23,000. As the tenderness and the rigidity of the abdomen became less marked the lung findings became more pronounced. The area of flatness extended higher, with a corresponding increase in vocal resonance and fremitus over the involved area. The breath tones were absent over the base but were audible faintly higher up. There was no cough, no râles, and no tubular breathing.

Owing to the critical condition of the patient no attempt was made to have an x-ray examination of her chest until the fifteenth day of her illness. The skiagram taken at that time showed an obliteration of the right diaphragm and angle by a dense homogenous shadow which extended from the base of the right lung to the second interspace, anteriorly. The left lung was negative. (See Figure 4.) These findings corresponded to those made on physical examination of the chest. Her abdomen was soft and entirely free from tenderness. Her temperature was 99.6 degrees; and her leukocyte count was 14,200. A few hours after the patient had been taken to the x-ray room she com-

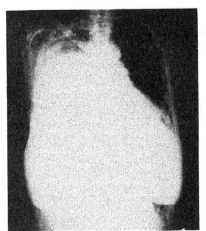

Figure 4. Skiagram of patient's chest taken on the fifteenth day of her illness, showing the obliteration of the right diaphragm and angle by a dense homogenous shadow which extends from the base of the right lung to the second interspace, anteriorly.

plained of a soreness in her left lower extremity. Elevation of the limb afforded relief, although tenderness persisted for some time. A thrombus was suspected but no localized tenderness could be elicited over the femoral vein.

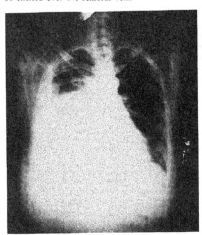

Figure 5. Skiagram showing the condition of the patient's chest on the twenty-first day of her illness. Note the recession of the shadow both from the sternal aspect of the lung and from its apex; also, the obliteration of the right diaphragm and its angle.

A week later, the patient was much improved. Her temperature was normal and her leukocyte count was 12,200. A skiagram of her chest showed a recession of the shadow both from the sternal aspect of the lung and from its apex. (See Figure 5.) Its upper limit corresponded to the third and fourth interspaces. The right diaphragm and its angle were still obliterated. The third and last skiagram, which was taken during the following week, showed a continued improvement. There was still some infiltration of the lower lobe of the right lung with a corresponding obliteration of the diaphragm and angle. (See Figure 6.) Clinically, the lung was clear except

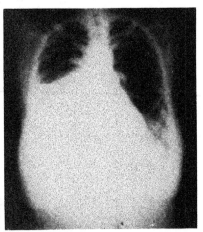

Figure 6. Condition of the patient's chest on the twenty-eighth day of her illness. The right lung is definitely clearing, although the diaphragm and its angle are still obliterated.

for this area over its base. Coughing, followed by deep inspiration, enabled one to hear fine crepitant râles in the involved lobe.

By the last of March the patient was up and about; but with the increase in her activity her left lower extremity again began to bother her. The pain and swelling were promptly relieved by the use of an elastic bandage. Her lung was entirely clear, and, aside from the inconvenience caused by a mild thrombophlebitis of the lower limb, and a weakness due to her confining illness, she felt quite well.*

COMMENTS

This case illustrates the rôle which an acute abdominal condition may play in bringing about a pulmonary lesion, either one of which is capable of causing an involvement of the central zone of the diáphragm. The history of three preceding attacks of gallbladder infection and the onset of an illness which was ushered in by a gastro-intestinal upset, clearly points to the abdominal origin of the infectious process. The course of the disease and the clinical picture which ultimately developed are indicative of an embolism, most likely having its origin in or about the gallbladder, which produced infarction of the lower lobe of the right lung. From the time of the abrupt onset of symptoms, shoulder-top pain became an outstanding symptom. As the diaphragm became more involved, so did the referred pain to the shoulder increase in intensity. At first, all signs pointed to an acute upper abdominal lesion. Within six hours, however, the beginning of a lung involvement, associated with an increase of pain in the shoulder-top when deep inspiration was attempted, pointed suggestively to diaphragmatic involvement as the source of the upper abdominal distress and of the referred pain to the shoulder. As the gallbladder infection lessened in its intensity and as the irritated surface of the diaphragm became less sensitive, so did the shoulder-top pain become less noticeable to the patient. This distressing symptom disappeared entirely at the end of thirty hours.

The localized tenderness which the patient entertained over the gallbladder, and which was associated with jaundice and bile in the urine, is conclusive evidence of an acute biliary disorder. That septic material found its way into the blood stream is indicated by the pulmonary infarction and the thrombophlebitis which resulted.

SUMMARY

Pain in the shoulder is caused by a number of conditions which may arise from without the body (extrinsic factors), or from within the body (intrinsic factors). In this paper I have purposely refrained from a consideration of all the various causative factors in the production of shoulder pain, with the exception of muscular strain, subdeltoid bursitis, and shoulder-top pain due to phrenic nerve irritation. Concerning the latter, I have pointed out the mechanism which enters into the production of this type of "referred pain," and have tried to emphasize the importance of this sign as a diagnostic aid.

* Author's Note:—On June 5 a roentgenogram of the gallbladder was made following the use of the Graham dye. A definite pathologic condition of the gallbladder, associated with the presence of a biliary calculus, was revealed. Subsequently, these findings were proved on abdominal section. After a cholecystectomy the patient made an uneventful recovery.

EARLY RUPTURE OF THE MEMBRANES*

E. B. WOODS, M.D., Des Moines

There is a growing conviction that the forewaters are not essential to the normal dilatation of the cervix, and that early rupture of the membranes may actually shorten labor without subjecting either mother or child to any additional risk. So many various and conflicting views have been enunciated from time to time that additional data would seem unnecessary if the question is ever to be answered directly. With rupture of the membranes being advocated for the induction of labor, it is particularly important to learn whether such interference with the physiology of parturition lengthens labor, increases the need for operative intervention, and augments the risk to mother and child, as is so commonly believed by the laity and the profession.

Among 2,500 consecutive vaginal deliveries with the birth of viable children (1,500 grams or more in weight) at the University Hospitals, there were 2,479 with data suitable for analysis. The occurrence of rupture of the membranes in relation to the size of the external os is presented in Table I.

TABLE I

Dilatation of the cervix at the time of rupture.	Primiparas		Multiparas	
	No.	Per cent	No.	Per cent
Not in labor	186	15.2	191	15.2
Up to 3.0 cm.	105	8.6	87	6.9
4.0 to 6 0 cm.	128	10.5	103	8.2
7.0 to 9.0 cm.	184	15.0	167	13.3
Complete (10.0 cm.)	621	50.8	707	56.3
Total	1224	100.1	1255	99.9

Artificial rupture of the membranes was practiced rather infrequently except after half dilatation of the cervix as shown in Table II.

TABLE II

The time of artificial rupture of the membranes in relation to the size of the cervical os.
(2,479 cases.)

Size of the cervix	1224 Primiparas		1255 Multiparas	
	No.	Per cent	No.	Per cent
Not in labor	2	0.16	6	0.5
Up to 3.0 cm.	1	0.08	6	0.5
4.0 to 7.0 cm.	5	0.4	11	0.95
7.0 to 9.0 cm.	33	2.7	41	3.3
Complete (10.0 cm.)	192	15.7	240	19.1
Total	233	19.04	304	24.35

It is apparent from Tables I and II that spontaneous rupture of the membranes before the cervix is one-half dilated is somewhat more common in primiparas than in parous women, although the difference is possibly insignificant. On the other

*From the Department of Obstetrics and Gynecology, State University of Iowa.

hand, if rupture at any time before two-fingers (3.0 cm.) is designated at "premature," it is apparent that this variation occurred spontaneously in 288 (23.5 per cent) of the primiparas and in 266 (21.2 per cent) of the multiparas.

The total duration of labor has been calculated as the interval from the onset of regular painful uterine contractions to the completion of the third stage. Average values are shown in Table III.

TABLE III

Duration of labor in relation to the time of rupture of the membranes.

Parity and time of Rupture	Spontaneous			Operative		
	Total	Average Duration		Total	Average Duration	
	No.	Hrs.	Mins.	No.	Hrs.	Mins.
Primiparas—early rupture— 3.0 cm. or less.............	231	13	43	60	15	34
Primiparas — later rupture— more than 3.0 cm.........	789	13	49	144	22	2
Total.................	1020	13	47	204	20	8
Multiparas — early rupture— 3.0 cm. or less.............	252	7	33.	26	12	32
Myltiparas — later rupture— more than 3.0 cm.........	922	,8	15	55	11	34
Total...................	1174	8	6	81	11	52

When labor progresses normally to a spontaneous termination, it appears that early rupture of the membranes either has no effect (primiparas) or definitely shortens labor (multiparas). Since so-called "fetal distress" as indicated by alterations in the fetal heart rate is not considered an indication for intervention, it is obvious that delayed labor constitutes by far the largest indication for interference. A considerable increase in the average duration of labor in operative cases is then to be expected, but even here it is apparent that early rupture of the membranes certainly does not materially delay parturition and in the primiparas seems definitely to shorten it.

Depending upon the early rupture of the membranes (cervix 3.0 cm. or less) or later rupture (cervix more than 3.0 cm.) delivery was effected according to the data in Table IV.

TABLE IV

Method of delivery according to the early or later rupture of the membranes.

Parity and time of rupture	Spontaneous		Operative	
	No.	Per cent	No.	Per cent
Primiparas—early rupture 3.0 cm. or less............./...........	231	79.4	60	20.6
Primiparas—later rupture—more than 3.0 cm............................	789	84.6	144	15.4
Total...........................	1020	83.3	204	16.7
Multiparas—early rupture—3.0 cm. or less............................	252	90.6	26	9.4
Multiparas—later rupture—more than 3.0 cm............................	922	94.4	55	5.6
Total........................	1174	93.5	81	6.5

It is apparent that premature rupture of the membranes is associated with greater incidence of operative intervention in first as well as in subsequent labors. Operative delivery was undertaken, except in unusual cases, only for definite indications, as is attested by the fact that the total operative incidence was only 11.1 per cent. Inclusion of abdominal deliveries would have increased the incidence by approximately 1.0 per cent, making the total incidence very nearly that determined for the state as a unit (11.8 per cent) when both home and hospital deliveries are considered. The various operative procedures employed are detailed in Table V.

TABLE V

Operative procedures among 2,479 vaginal deliveries.

Type of operation	(1224) Primiparas		(1255) Multiparas	
	No.	Per cent	No.	Per cent
Low forceps...................	121	10.0	11	0.9
Mid forceps...................	23	1.9	6	0.5
High forceps..................	1	0.1	3	0.3
Breech extraction.............	49	4.0	42	3.3
Version and extraction.........	7	0.6	18	1.4
Craniotomy...................	3	0.3	1	0.1
Total......................	204	16.9	81	6.5

The puerperium has been designated as "febrile" if the temperature rose to 100.4 degrees at any reading during the first ten days, and, if this elevation could not be satisfactorily explained by some extragenital lesion, mastitis, pyelitis, or an intercurrent infection, it was viewed as of genital origin. Temperatures were taken by mouth every four hours. In approximately one-half of the febrile cases, the fever disappeared in less than twenty-four hours, leaving the remainder to be explained on the basis of a more or less severe uterine infection.

TABLE VI

Puerperal morbidity (not of extragenital origin) in relation to the time and rupture of the membrane.

Parity and time of rupture	Spontaneous			Operative		
	Total cases	Febrile		Total cases	Febrile	
		No.	Per cent		No.	Per cent
Primiparas — early rupture—3.0 cm. or less...	231	90	39	60	28	47
Primiparas — later rupture more than 3.0 cm..	789	246	31	144	58	40
Total................	1020	336	33	204	86	42
Multiparas — early rupture—3.0 cm. or less...	252	46	18	26	10	38
Multiparas — early rupture—more than 3.0 cm	922	174	19	55	20	36
Total..................	1174	220	19	81	30	37
Grand Total........	2194	556	25	285	116	41

As was to have been anticipated, the morbidity was higher among primiparous women than among those who had previously borne children, and among those in both groups who were delivered following some form of operative intervention. Particularly in the group of primiparas, early rupture of the membranes was followed by a seemingly significant increase in the morbidity rate in spite of the fact that the average length of labor was not increased. (See Table III.) The assumption would then seem justified that entrance of pyrogenic organisms into the cavity of the uterus is facilitated by early rupture of the membranes, as has been recognized for some time.

In certain instances the membranes ruptured before the onset of labor, and data are presented in Table VII to show the relation of the length of this "latent period" to the puerperal morbidity.

TABLE VII .

Puerperal morbidity in relation to the "latent period" after premature rupture of the membranes.

	Primiparas			Multiparas		
Latent period	Total cases	Febrile		Total cases	Febrile	
		No.	Per cent		No.	Per cent
Up to 1 hour	101	36	36	114	19	17
1 to 5 hours	32	14	44	24	6	25
5 to 20 hours	33	9	27	25	3	12
More than 20 hours	18	5	28	29	7	24

There is no apparent relationship between the duration of the "latent period" and postpartum febrile reactions, but the numbers of cases are too small for accurate comparisons. At any rate, it would seem that lengthening of the "latent period" has no striking effect upon the course of the puerperium.

In the period covered by this study artificial rupture of the membranes, except in the later stages of cervical dilatation, was practiced so infrequently that its effect upon puerperal morbidity can scarcely be determined. The data are nevertheless included.

TABLE VIII

Puerperal morbidity in relation to the artificial rupture of the membranes.

	Spontaneous			Operative		
Parity and time of rupture	Total cases	Febrile		Total cases	Febrile	
		No.	Per cent		No.	Per cent
Primiparas — early rupture—3.0 cm. or less	3	2	67	0	0	0
Primiparas — later rupture—more than 3.0 cm.	201	70	35	29	10	34
Total	204	72	35	29	10	34
Multiparas — early rupture—3.0 cm. or less	12	6	50	0	0	0
Multiparas — later rupture—more than 3.0 cm.	278	38	14	14	4	29
Total	290	44	15	14	4	29
Grand Total	494	116	24	43	14	33

It appears doubtful whether artificial rupture of the membranes under sterile precautions is more productive of febrile reactions after delivery than is spontaneous rupture, since fever is no more common (Table VIII) than in the various groups for the entire series (Table VI). Our later experience with artificial rupture of the membranes as a means for inducing labor has confirmed the relative harmlessness of this procedure if properly performed.

Among the entire series of 2,479 deliveries, there were 86 stillbirths and neonatal deaths, within the first five hours after birth, or 3.5 per cent. Among the 375 patients with rupture of the membranes before the onset of labor, there were fourteen fetal and early infant deaths, or 3.7 per cent; whereas among the 2,104 with rupture after the onset of labor there were 72 such deaths, or 3.4 per cent. It is impossible to say whether this ten per cent increase in the risk to the child is significant, because in certain instances, such as placenta praevia, the membranes were ruptured before the onset of pains in the presence of children whose lives were in jeopardy because of the condition of the mother.

SUMMARY

From the data here presented, it becomes apparent that premature rupture of the membranes is not in itself a labor complication of any moment. More specifically, it may be said that it:

1. Does not increase the average duration of labor.

2. Increases slightly the need for operative intervention.

3. Increases slightly, in primiparas, the incidence of mild uterine infection, as indicated by otherwise unexplained febrile reactions after delivery. The "latent period" appears to have no significant effect upon this reaction. Artificial rupture does not increase the incidence of febrile convalescence.

4. Probably does not alter the risk to the fetus, except insofar as this danger is augmented by the greater need for operative intervention.

ACUTE INTESTINAL OBSTRUCTION*

B. RAYMOND WESTON, M.D., Mason City

Acute intestinal obstruction always threatens to be a standard subject handled by platitudes and self-evident truths. Periodically in all journals and in all medical societies it has its turn for consideration. It is discussed with no great enthusiasm and is allowed to continue on its way, killing a very high percentage of its victims. Experience

*Presented before the Eighty-third Annual Session, Iowa State Medical Society, Des Moines, May 9, 10, 11, 1934.

in handling these cases has taught us much, but is only of value when interpreted in the light of our knowledge of the pathology, physiology and alterations in the blood chemistry occurring in cases of obstruction. The ability to evaluate and correct these changes is the basis of successful treatment. Other factors which have contributed toward greater facility in handling these cases are better roads, improvement in hospital equipment, the increasing number of well trained men, new anesthesia and the more general acceptance of surgery by the laity as a comparatively safe procedure—all of which should aid in reducing the mortality rate. On the debit side we have the condition itself and the doctor or doctors who handle it.

Plummer and others almost completely whipped the mortality rate for toxic thyroid glands by a very simple and easily applied treatment. An elementary understanding of preoperative care reduced the mortality rate of prostatic troubles down enormously. Newer technic has almost annihilated it. Similar improvements in preoperative treatment, postoperation treatment and operative technic have made a large number of surgical pro cedures much safer than they had formerly been. In spite of all this, the treatment of acute intestinal obstruction continues to yield a tremendously high mortality rate. If this were due to the fact that no progress had been made in the general understanding of the situation, little could be done about it. However, when we consider that progress has been made and overlooked or neglected, there is a definite reason for emphasis on the subject at hand.

I propose to discuss only the treatment of acute intestinal obstruction. For purpose of clarification I have made the following sub-divisions:

1. Surgical intervention with special reference to time and choice of procedure.

2. Effectiveness of proper preoperative and postoperative treatment in decreasing the surgical risk and correcting the inevitable intoxication as indicated by the alteration of certain chemical constituents of the blood.

Early operation, of course, is the method of choice but when, as is often the case, especially in referred work, the condition is already greatly advanced, immediate operation is often contraindicated. If the treatment is to be successful the patient must live through the operation, as well as survive the primary pathology. When the patient is dehydrated, the abdomen distended, and the blood chemistry distorted, and especially if these items are extreme, operation can as a rule only lead to catastrophe if it is performed at once. It may be an alibi in the individual case to tell

the family that you will do what you can at once, but that you are afraid it is too late. If, however, your statistics from this sort of procedure show, as they are bound to, a higher mortality rate than those of men more capably handling their cases, the explanation cannot ease your own conscience or bolster your pride in your own surgical judgment. As explained later in this paper the delay necessary to relieve dehydration, to increase the chlorides, to feed by vein, and to relieve as much distention as possible, is well repaid in your mortality figures. This is especially true in consideration of the rapidity with which most of these procedures can be accomplished.

Delay and its justification depends, of course, on whether the obstruction is associated with strangulation, torsion, perforation, and gangrene. In other words, it depends on whether the peritoneal reaction is only reflex or if a real infectious peritonitis is developing. These two large classes cannot always be diagnostically divided, especially early.

Many men, particularly Wangensteen, depend on rebound tenderness. According to this theory pain following the sudden release of pressure means actual peritoneal involvement. This sign is valuable but I do not believe one should depend upon it alone. The white blood count as well as the red blood count in these patients is raised to varying degrees by dehydration. The white blood count is also raised to a greater degree by infection in tissues which should not carry infectious organisms. The degree of this rise, the percentage of polymorphonuclear increase and the degree of the left shift in the polymorphonuclear cells, all taken together and correlated with the previous experience of yourself and others in these cases, is, I believe, much more significant. The condition of the patient, difficult to describe, is another valuable point in deciding between these two general classes. In addition we have certain signs and symptoms associated with the particular type of obstruction suspected which add their btis toward the ultimate decision. This last field is too exhaustive to include in this paper.

From the above information and such other methods which are trusted by various individuals we decide that the condition is an obstruction without gangrene, torsion or peritonitis, or that it is an obstruction with those features, or that we do not know. If dead or dying tissue is definitely a part of the picture, operation should be performed almost at once. Methods to correct dehydration can be carried out in a very short time before or immediately afterward. Delay is inexcusable because the time element is the most important one. If the obstruction is definitely not involved with gangrenous or pregangrenous tissue, any amount of delay is permissible to correct dehydration, distention and chemical distortion.

The above two problems are simple. In comparatively late cases, and hence the ones giving us our mortality rate, they form a relatively small proportion. Our real problem is when to operate upon these patients, in whom details of the disturbance within the abdomen cannot be determined. If the patient is seen early, operate; if late—what?

One should never delay in an early suspicious case. Practically all of these patients survive the obstruction, even if the pathology involved may eventually prove fatal. The lone argument against the procedure is the cry of unnecessary operations. This is not a problem primarily involved only with intestinal obstruction. The same situation holds true in many other fields of surgery. The problem involved is a surgeon's honesty in presenting the picture to the interested parties. A frank statement associated with an intelligent explanation of the reasons for the mortality rate in these cases should clear the course for the intelligent person. People do not die because an abdomen is opened or closed. Often people do die from the delay in opening an abdomen.

In the late case of this type, however, we come to the field where an error in judgment may and usually does prove fatal. Before considering this decision final let us examine the factors which enter into the causes of these deaths, those factors which must be corrected and guarded against.

The most apparent chemical changes are the lowering of chlorides in the blood, the raising of nonprotein nitrogen and creatinin in the blood, alkalosis and dehydration. Writers and investigators differ as to the relative importance of each item, and the whole controversy of toxin absorption with its correlated subjects is too complicated for discussion at this time. One set of experiments disproves the conclusions arrived at by another man with a different set of experiments. Only one thing is certain; that the chemical balance is badly upset and its correction is essential. If the chemical balance can be corrected, the shock combated, and the toxin (if any) eliminated by correct competent surgical interference, then all patients should recover. The more nearly we can accomplish these three factors, the more successful our treatment will be.

There are undoubtedly deeper and more intricate changes than those mentioned, but we can correct only those errors within the scope of our knowledge at present. Dehydration and oliguria cause a raise of the nonprotein nitrogen and the creatinin. Fluids are all that are necessary to cor-

rect this situation if the patient is seen early. Dehydration causes damage to kidney cells, particularly those in the glomeruli and this increases the retention of protein waste products. If the dehydration does not last long this damage is quickly overcome. If it has been present too long, permanent damage results and the matter is very serious.

Fluids should be given in large quantities; intravenously first because they are more promptly absorbed. A long twenty-one gauge needle should be used with the hot water jacketed container only two and a half feet above the level of the patient, and fluids can be given continuously. Expensive measuring equipment for the procedure is unnecessary. I use a solution of normal saline or five per cent glucose in water, and prefer to give both at different times. I am unable to explain why so many surgeons give five per cent glucose (isotonic in water) in normal saline (also isotonic). I believe after the first correction is made that fluids can be continued more normally by the subcutaneous method. I happen to have very little confidence in the rectal method of administering fluids. The chief virtue of this method is the usual enema effect obtained from it.

Dehydration can be assumed by the history of vomiting and inability to retain fluids. One can be just as sure of the lowering of the chloride content of the blood if the patient has vomited any length of time. A blood chloride determination is, of course, preferable, but is unnecessary if one is not equipped for such an analysis. The vomited hydrochloric acid is created by separating the chloride molecule from the sodium base. The base then unites with carbon dioxide and we not only have a low chloride content but an alkalosis. Two-thirds of the total anion concentration in the blood serum is chlorides, and one-third of all serum, electrolytes; therefore osmolar control in the blood serum is the chloride fraction, and it is easy to understand the terrific diversion from normal this one factor causes.

Correction may be brought about by five per cent intravenous sodium chloride, two per cent subcutaneously, salt solution by duodenal tube and to a certain extent by normal saline. In severe vomiting a gram of salt to a kilogram of body weight is a good rule. Five hundred c.c. of five per cent solution will suffice in the average adult for the time being. The level to be maintained, where chloride determination is available, is about 365 mg. of chlorides to 100 c.c. of blood. The urgency of the above procedures is dependent largely on the height of the obstruction and the associated severity of the vomiting.

Duodenal drainage, either by the ordinary duodenal tube or by the more effective Wangensteen method, is an essential part of our treatment. Vomiting is reduced at once. This makes the patient more comfortable, lessens the fluid and chloride loss, eliminates much upper abdominal fluid and gaseous distention, allows the patient to drink water (which is re-aspirated) and permits the introduction of salt solution or any other material desired. The Wangensteen equipment which can be assembled at practically no cost constitutes by far the most effective method. Its mild suction is continuous, and thus most effective.

This preoperative treatment if used long enough to permit the fluid and chloride replacements, will stop the vomiting. There can be no controversy over the method that far. Its continued use as a substitution for surgery requires an enormous diagnostic acumen. If there is no gangrene, torsion, or peritonitis, the method will permit the patient to be carried indefinitely in relative comfort and in safety. If these elements are present, this treatment can only be regarded as a surgical adjunct. I believe personally that it is a simple procedure, used many times in an attempt to carry a patient through, when more difficult and trying procedures have a greater expectancy in results. It is invaluable as a surgical preparation; it is invaluable as a postoperative treatment; but its prolonged use does not seem wise to me. If it helps the patient his obstruction is either corrected by relieved tension, or he should be operated upon while his condition is improved. In partial obstructions, this treatment will often cure the current attack with no further help.

The real danger in this duodenal drainage method is the same danger that any easily applied, highly successful method always encounters. Anybody can do it. This means that it will be used by those incompetent to carry out proper associated procedures—surgical or otherwise. It becomes a method of retaining cases which otherwise would of necessity be referred.

The actual technical surgical problem in intestinal obstruction is probably the most important factor in the cure of these cases. In severe cases it cannot succeed unless the preliminaries as outlined above are properly executed. On the other hand, only a very small percentage of obstructions are ever relieved, except by direct surgical interference. This surgery must be good surgery. Some patients can stand a lot of delay, meddling and roughness, but they are not the serious ones or the cause of our mortality rate. The ones who are worrying us are those who can stand none of that.

A prompt decision as to the pathology and the surgical treatment must be made and carried out with the greatest speed and care. An enormous amount of surgery performed in this country is slow, indecisive, and bungling. That is incompetence and for the present nothing can be done about it. On the other hand many competent surgeons—I should say all competent surgeons—are perfectly capable of making mistakes. Speed is essential. Occasionally a hasty decision and a hasty operation may result fatally because something was overlooked. On the other hand it frequently gives brilliant results. Slow surgery can only succeed when the condition of the patient is such that he can stand almost anything.

If a resection is performed or if a short circuiting must take in a severely ill patient, every desirable precaution should be taken providing it does not cause delay. If the mesentery will not permit a resection in a normal position, it can be done side to side with no fear for the closed ends both pointing in the same direction. There are sites of choice for these anastomoses on the bowel, but if delay must result from choosing them it is preferable to use any available surface.

If adhesions, tumors, or bands leave a difficult unraveling, one should short circuit anywhere possible if there is no gangrene. Removing gangrenous masses or those that might become so outside the peritoneal cavity, as in the Mikulicz resection of the sigmoid, is always good surgery. Difficult reductions of intussusceptions, torsions and strangulations should not be made; a resection, short circuit, or enterostomy is preferable. A difficult reduction requires too much time, and leaves too many possibilities of later complications. If no decision as to the cause of the obstruction can be arrived at rapidly, or if the patient's condition is desperate, enterostomy alone may be good surgery. If, however, a gangrenous structure is present and it cannot be fixed extraperitoneally, it must be resected completely no matter how long it may take. The fact that any procedure may necessitate a second operation is never a serious argument against it.

The above explanation is only to indicate the type of surgery and surgical decision which must be made. A technical description of each individual type of obstruction and its treatment is material for a book—not a paper. I wish to recapitulate, however, to cover a few generalities. Unless the obstruction is high enough to be drained by a duodenal tube one should perform a fish tail enterostomy just above the pathology, and repair. It only takes an instant and saves lives. Deliberate errorless decisions cannot be made if the patients are to live in a high enough proportion. Painstaking textbook technic must frequently be discarded. One must hurry; a patient of this type is always sicker than he appears to be. If two surgical possibilities offer themselves, use the shorter one unless the evidence is overwhelmingly against it.

The postoperative treatment should anticipate every complication before it arrives. Fluid, salt, and glucose have been covered. Glucose is of much greater importance postoperatively than preoperatively. Colon tubes, steam enemas and the regular use of petressin should be started at once. Rest and comfort can best be brought about by pantopon used freely. It does not nauseate as frequently as morphine and it does not cause distention or paresis of the bowel.

I stated at the beginning that most papers on this subject consisted of platitudes and self evident truths. Rereading this only classifies it with the rest. Its only claim to distinction seems to be a frank admission that many of these deaths are due to ignorance, incompetence, and carelessness. Enough repetition may eventually make such things impossible.

POSSIBILITIES FOR RACE BETTERMENT*

Eleanor Hutchinson, M.D., Belle Plaine

The science of eugenics is not new. The outline was advanced in 1904 by Sir Francis Galton, who hoped he was laying the foundation for the betterment of the human race. There was some criticism and opposition to this idea, but it did gain some following, and eight years later, in July, 1912, an International Congress of Eugenics was held at the University of London, England. Since that time the subject of race betterment has grown, and now there are a great many agencies at work, spreading knowledge of the problem to be faced, if we hope to produce a more sound human race than the one we have, or even keep the race up to its present standard.

What is eugenics? Many people think it has some relation to, or concerns sex hygiene. This is not true. It has been defined by various eugenists, and Wiggam probably gives as clear a definition as any one. His definition is "A method ordained of God, and seated in natural laws for securing better parents for our children, in order that they may become richly endowed, mentally, morally and physically for the human struggle." Galton defined eugenics as "The science which deals with the influences that improve the inborn qualities of a race."

I shall speak more particularly of the prevention of the propagation of the obviously unfit, as distinguished from the breeding of human beings,

*President's Address, Thirty-seventh Annual Meeting, State Society of Iowa Medical Women, Des Moines, May 8, 1934.

sound in mind and body, and possessing desirable moral qualities. The great problem of today is the large socially burdensome army composed of criminals and paupers, and the insane, epileptic, feebleminded, and the venereally diseased. The important question we have to solve is what can be done to lift this burden, so that the social energy it consumes may be devoted to more constructive ends.

It has been estimated that there are many hundred thousand people in the United States, who are insane and feebleminded, aside from the thousands who are inmates of the schools for the deaf and blind, jails and prisons, hospitals, alms houses, and the great multitude of juvenile delinquents, deaf and dumb, and those afflicted with epilepsy and venereal diseases. The same authority estimates that two-thirds of these delinquent or defective persons are parents of defective children.

At the end of February of this year, Iowa had between fifteen and sixteen thousand patients in the fifteen institutions under the Board of Control. This does not include those in the school for the deaf and dumb, and the school for the blind, which are under the Board of Education. Many of these institutions have large waiting lists also, and there are many mentally afflicted patients who are kept at home, and the public has no knowledge of them.

Omitting the defective patients in the institutions, the figures brought out by the draft during the last war, were a surprise to many. We were shocked to find that such a large percentage of the men examined for military service was found to be unfit for duty in one way or another. Twenty-two per cent were weeded out, or 1,289,000, and of these 82,000 were found to be mentally defective. Even after that, there were 1,475 feebleminded United States soldiers sent to army hospitals in France. Many epileptic and syphilitic patients were missed because very little laboratory work was done by the draft board. It is reasonable to suppose that as many women would be found to be defective.

It is not my purpose to present a statistical study of this problem. We know that heredity is based on the discovery by the monk, named Mendel, who made experiments with peas. Many breeders of plants and stock follow the Mendelian laws of heredity in growing plants and breeding stock. We read that the really inherited mental deficiencies are certain forms of insanity, feeblemindedness and epilepsy. Venereal disease, especially syphilis, is a fruitful cause of physical and mental defects, not only in the victim of the infection, but in his offspring even to the third and fourth generation. We inherit what is carried in the germ cells of our ancestors. A man may become insane from getting hit on the head with a brick-bat, yet his children will not be affected by it, even though they may be born after the accident. The injury affects only his body cells, not his germ cells. Syphilis is not inherited, but is transmitted in an entirely different way, although the susceptibility to the syphilitic microbe is likely to be inherited. The word "congenital," which means "born with," is used to distinguish a condition from a true hereditary defect. We do not inherit a taste for alcohol, but some inherit greater susceptibility, or a greater lack of self control than others.

Stability of the germ cells determines the character of the individual. Criminality is not inherited, but again is a trait which develops from lack of self control, which is inherited, while environment, education, training, etc., may play a part. Feeblemindedness supplies a large number of defective individuals, and is a frequent cause of prostitution, pauperism and criminality. It has been estimated that something like two-thirds of feeblemindedness is due to heredity.

It seems then, that if we wish to be rid of defective persons, we must stop breeding them. We have at our command several remedies, which will help in this piece of work; namely, education, restriction of marriage, segregation, birth control and sterilization. Of these sterilization seems to be the most practical for the following reasons.

If marriage restrictions are fixed by law, which is the case in some states, it does not seem to interfere with any one's liberties, such as marriage between the white and colored races. Some states have laws forbidding the marriage of epileptic patients, feebleminded persons and the insane, and those suffering from transmissible diseases, such as syphilis. A few people regard these laws as reasonable, but others do not; hence there is a laxity in enforcement of the laws. The public is not sufficiently enlightened as to the importance of these laws, and extends no cooperation in their enforcement. I have no doubt that for some time, the eugenic laws on the statute books will be valuable chiefly as an educational influence, to make the public familiar with the thought we have in our marriage laws, to be used as a club in the fight against disease and mental defects, and also to spread the knowledge among the intelligent classes that it is possible to bring about marked improvement in the quality of our human stock, if we will only enforce restrictions in the marriage of the physically and mentally unfit. Of course, among the intelligent there is probably always some correlation between reason and sexual emotion, so that where there is family pride, there is small likelihood of deliberate mismating with defective strains. In time, when we arrive at the stage of enlightenment, when people feel their responsibility to the unborn generations, eugenics will have become a part of our code of ethics. It will be looked upon as wicked and disgraceful to bring children into the world handicapped by physical and mental defects.

Many people are in favor of segregating those who are defective, as opposed to sterilization, regarding it as more just and lenient, and less likely to interfere with the sentiments of the people. Properly carried out, it is entirely effective, but it would be practically out of the question in the United States. The number of institutions would be enormous, and taxes would be very great, to segregate the large number of insane and feebleminded people for the necessary length of time. Then, too, we have practically no way of discovering these feebleminded individuals until they become delinquent or socially burdensome, or have come in contact with the law. Many of these people have no clashes with the law, but live simply, and are able to accomplish certain kinds of work. They are thus able to adjust themselves, in a measure, to society, and continue to breed their kind. Of course it is feasible to segregate those who are defective and who have fallen into the meshes of the law, and who have proved themselves incapable of satisfactorily adjusting themselves to their environment, especially the women of childbearing age. The feebleminded female is more likely to become a parent than the feebleminded man, because many will take advantage of her weak mentality.

Birth control is too involved a subject to be covered in this paper. It is a medical problem, and was practiced as early as the thirty-eighth chapter of Genesis. It is also spoken of in the New Testament. Not many years ago the subject was taboo but it has now increased to a world wide extent, and seems destined to become a part of our national health program. Forty-eight medical societies have endorsed it, as well as prominent religious, political, social and educational groups. This procedure will be a great help in the program of race betterment.

On November 18, 1933, the National Birth Control Conference was held in New York City. In the numbers who attended, in the quality of the audiences and the preëminence of the speakers it presented a far different picture from that of the birth control movement twelve or fifteen years ago. Most people of the adult generation remember when it was chiefly characterized by determined looking ladies selling birth control reviews on metropolitan corners, Margaret Sanger being reprimanded for her propaganda, and a general feeling in the lay breast that the whole thing was not quite respectable; but before our very eyes, we see the evolution of an idea. The movement has undergone a decided moral, social and intellectual transformation. This is evidenced by the presence of the speakers at this conference, and the attendance of important people, both professional and non-professional.

A speaker at this conference presented the thought that birth control has two aspects; first, from an euthenic viewpoint in spacing children wisely, which is considered of the greatest importance to the health of the mother and of the child, and indirectly to the welfare and happiness of the family; and second, from an eugenic aspect, since it lowers the production of each couple.

In the case of superior persons this might prove dysgenic, were it not for the fact as stated by the speaker, that the more intelligent of our population will practice self control, whether or not it is sanctioned by law or church. It is therefore logical to allow dissemination of knowledge of contraceptive methods to all strata of society. This will at least equalize the eugenic differential rate which now exists. A complete birth control program should be both positive and negative: it should encourage production of more strong, healthy, properly spaced children, as well as discourage the production of all those likely to become unfit members of society.

It seems to me there is much more to be said in favor of sterilization. As a negative means of race improvement, it is not a modern idea. In 1907, a law was enacted in Indiana for the sterilization of confirmed criminals, idiots, imbeciles and rapists. At the present time there are twenty-seven states having sterilization laws. Not one defective person has been sterilized in Iowa under the sterilization law passed four years ago. Obviously there is some weakness in the law, which defeats the purpose of the legislation. The likelihood is that a new sterilization bill will be introduced in the coming legislature in this state. A specialist in this line has advocated that sterilization should be voluntary, compulsion being used only in extreme cases.

There are two main indications for sterilization and contraception or birth control; first, therapeutic measures, and second, a procedure carried out primarily for the welfare and safety of society. Patients legally committed to state hospitals as hereditarily insane, feebleminded, or epileptic, as well as those found in poor farms, prisons and reformatories, if not sterilized before release would no doubt have defective children. With tens of thousands of defective men and women permeating our communities, filling our state institutions to overflowing, adding severely

to a tax burden which is already galling to a tolerant, though perhaps uninformed population, and with our citizens breeding largely from the bottom upward, we as physicians, keepers of our brother's welfare, not only have a dutiful interest in the functioning of our eugenic sterilization laws, but we are legitimately required to exercise an active sponsorship in perfecting their formulation.

Germany has recently passed a sterilization law, under which it is proposed to sterilize 400,000 persons. An account of this act is given in the bottom *American Journal of Public Health,* March, 1934. The measure is regarded as a highly drastic movement.

Who should be sterilized? The first class of persons who should be sterilized are those with defective germ plasms, which have revealed themselves in mental or nervous diseases for several generations. Children of such parents are therefore likely, if not certain, to be diseased or defective.

The second class is composed of those who are capable of producing healthy babies, but are physically or mentally unfit to assume satisfactorily the rôle of parenthood.

Medical science and law are at present fully capable of discerning the characteristics in persons upon which the decision for or against sterilization depends. Physicians and criminologists understanding their limitations, will insist in erring on the safe side, and no one would be sterilized without good and sufficient cause. It would hardly be necessary to sterilize those confined in institutions, except those who are to be liberated by parole or discharge, because males and females are housed separately. However, in the state of California, where more patients have been sterilized than in any other state, it is reported that the operation apparently improved the health of some patients and occasionally overcame the habit of masturbation.

Sterilization laws should be so framed as to come within the scope of constitutional rights. The practice should be restricted and guarded in all cases, and the operation performed only after a careful investigation by competent psychiatrists and surgeons. Many who are now in institutions for the feebleminded might then be returned to society and the expense of their maintenance saved to the state. Sterilization would also present a method of dealing with feebleminded individuals who have not come in contact with the law, and who may never do so, but who, even though they are living quiet industrious lives, are still producing delinquent children. Of course, sterilization would not entirely remove the need for institutions. Is it not logical to assume that the human race can be improved in a few generations, in much the same manner that animals are improved?

The form of sterilization referred to and recommended, is that of vasectomy in the male and tubectomy in the female. With either of these operations, the individual may take his or her place in society as any other individual, but he or she is incapable of producing his kind.

The science of eugenics is practiced in all countries on lower animals, but man seems to have neglected his own breeding and left it to the whims and fancies of the individual. Consequently, the good and the bad, the weak and the strong, have bred our race with little or no concerted objective. Many minimize the importance of heredity, and claim that environment is three-fourths of the picture in determining the character of an individual; yet these same people acknowledge and bow to the laws of heredity in breeding their cattle, their hogs, and their dogs, and even their fruits and plants. This class claims that elimination of the unfit is to be obtained by preaching, teaching and training. My belief is that while environment is of vast importance, we stand a much better chance of getting eagles by putting eagle's eggs under hens, than by putting hen's eggs under eagles. It is useless to argue against heredity when all living things proclaim it.

The world of tomorrow is in the hands of the children of today. Does this slogan give us an idea of what we should do with eugenics? Eugenics certainly touches every side of human life. I believe the physician, the lawyer, the sociologist, the economist, the clergyman, the teacher, the editor and the legislator, young men and women, and parents, would do well to form a local eugenics society in every town in America, to meet and study the laws of heredity, the factors of eugenics. It is so lofty an idea that the less important subjects should use it as a touch-stone to see whether the improvements of which they boast are really vital. This great ideal of improving the human race should become a part of every person's religion.

Eugenics is not a cure-all. At present it aims simply at the elimination of the unfit, and at saving a large amount of money which we spend in our efforts to care for them. This money could be spent on those who are fit, who will give returns for the money and effort expended on them. The question is one which cannot be turned aside or shirked. Man must regenerate man, as the physical and mental salvation is in his hands, and if it lies within our power to give generations yet unborn, health, sound minds and beauty of character rather than the reverse, surely it is our plain duty to do it.

I have the following recommendations to make:
1. A campaign of education to be carried on which shall reach all classes of people.
2. Improvement of the race as follows: marriage restrictions; segregation of delinquent individuals; birth control; and sterilization of defective persons.

PREVENTION OF ROCKER SOLE IN CLUB FOOT CORRECTION*

Verl A. Ruth, M.D., Des Moines

Those who have attempted to correct club feet are familiar with the difficulty encountered at the last, in overcoming the equinus position of the os calcis. This has been due to the fact, that there has been no adequate means by which the posterior part of the os calcis could be grasped and pulled downward at the same time that the anterior portion was pushed upward. Hence, the more pressure exerted on the sole of the foot to correct the equinus, the more surely would be produced the rocker sole with the arch entirely gone and the calcaneocuboid joint at the most dependent part. Tenotomy of the Achilles' tendon and posterior capsulotomy of the ankle joint have helped in reducing this deformity but have not been universally successful.

Dr. Leo Mayer has devised a simple method of handling these cases. It is applicable to any type of equinus except that due to ankylosis. He has used it with success in some fifteen cases. No special apparatus is needed except that usually found in an orthopedic surgeon's kit. Quoting Dr. Mayer, "The steps in the technic are as follows: The foot is prepared as for a major operative procedure. Subcutaneous division of the Achilles' tendon is then done. With a long tenotone, the posterior portion of the capsule of the upper and lower ankle joint is divided. In a mild case, correction is now possible by means of manual pressure. In a resistant case, the os calcis does not alter its position as shown in control x-ray pictures. To grip the os calcis, a thin Steinman pin or a Kirschner wire is driven through the body as near the posterior tubercle as possible. When the nail is in place, it is grasped by the operator and strong downward pressure is made upon the posterior portion of the os calcis while at the same time upward pressure is made against the calcaneocuboid junction. By this means, the tendency to rocker sole is completely corrected and the equinus tilt of the os calcis completely overcome. When complete correction has been made, the foot is encased in plaster-of-Paris which includes the nail."

*Presented before the Eighty-third Annual Session, Iowa State Medical Society. Des Moines, May 9, 10, 11, 1934.

I have carried out this method in but one case. The result has been extraordinarily satisfactory. Instead of the Steinman pin, I used the Kirschner wire, which requires the addition of a tractor to maintain the wire under tension during the operation and some means to maintain the tension after the tractor has been removed. I use small steel buttons with a set-screw which are placed against the plaster after it has set and tightened before the tractor is removed. I have not done the subcutaneous tenotomy of the tendon because I prefer the step-cut method in tendon lengthening. In this one case which I report, capsulotomy was not required.

INTESTINAL OBSTRUCTION DUE TO A GALLSTONE*

M.. C. HENNESSY, M.D., Council Bluffs

The title of my subject is "Intestinal Obstruction Due to a Gallstone." It is not my purpose to discuss the treatment or symptoms in detail. It would seem that if a gallstone were of such a size as to be able to gain entrance into the intestinal tract, it would probably pass through the entire intestinal canal without producing any disturbance, and this is undoubtedly true in the vast majority of instances. However, if a stone approximates the size of three by two centimeters, an obstruction may develop.

This condition is like so many other subjects in the field of medicine and surgery. When we attempt to familiarize ourselves with certain phases, we find a great dearth of material. Most authors freely admit the existence of such possibilities, but very few give any real discussion of the subject. After considerable work I was able to find some intelligent discussion of it. Eisenfarb reports that up to 1931 there were only 116 cases reported in the literature; certainly not a large number when one considers the common occurrence of gallstones and gallbladder disease. The sites of obstruction were given as follows: Five cases in the duodenum; seventeen in the jejunum; sixty-seven in the ileum; thirteen at the ileocecal valve; thirteen cases in the large bowel; and one case in the rectum. As to its incidence in comparison to all other causes of intestinal obstruction, Braun reports that in those cases which came under his observation during the period from 1903 to September, 1927, it was the cause of the obstruction in twelve cases out of a total of 562. The avenue of entry to the intestinal tract is usually by way of the common duct, or as in the majority of cases by the production of an internal

* Presented before a joint meeting of the Omaha-Douglas County and the Pottawattamie County Medical Societies, March 13, 1934.

biliary fistula uniting the gallbladder and the intestines. It is possible for the gall ducts to dilate sufficiently to pass a stone of considerable size. However, most of the writers feel that gallstones entering the intestines by way of the biliary passage that produce intestinal obstruction, are probably increased in size by the addition of fæcal concretion.

The incidence of the production of an internal biliary fistula uniting the gallbladder and the intestines is relatively small when one views the high incidence of gallbladder disease and gallstones. Rath, Schroeder and Schloth, report that in 10,866 postmortem examinations they found only 49 cases of internal biliary fistula, and of these, 19 were fistulas between the gallbladder and the duodenum, and 16 were between the gallbladder and the colon. Murchison in a review of 37 cases of internal biliary fistula reports that in the majority of cases, death was due to intestinal obstruction from gallstones, and that the usual site of obstruction was in the first part of jejunum and the lower ileum. The obstruction usually developed months and even years after the primary gallbladder disturbance. It occurs more often after fifty years of age, and is more common in the female than the male.

Most of the cases I was able to review personally give a history of partial interference with bowel passage from time to time, but no complete shutoff until the acute attack. This tendency to partial recurrence led one writer to designate it as a biliary ileus. It may be of interest to know that I reviewed one case where the surgeon stated he had made a preoperative diagnosis of obstruction due to gallstones by what he felt in making a vaginal examination. However, there is no distinct symptomatology or physical sign that would enable most of us to make a preoperative diagnosis of mechanical obstruction due to gallstones; the best we can do is to diagnose the obstruction.

As stated previously it was not my intent to discuss the diagnosis and treatment of obstruction, but I would like to emphasize the necessity of early diagnosis and surgical interference in the treatment of mechanical obstruction regardless of the causative factor. I believe a preoperative diagnosis as to the eitology is not essential in the majority of cases. It was Andrews who made the statement that "the longer a patient lived with an obstruction before operation, the shorter their life after operation." Certainly any surgeon will not disagree with that thought. It has been my observation that there is no surgical problem in which medical men, and I include surgeons under this heading, have such a marked tendency to procrastinate in advising operative interference. We must get away from the idea of repeated enemas, cathartics and opiates. · We must school ourselves to arrive at a diagnosis earlier than at that stage where we have a development of all the classical symptoms and signs as portrayed in the textbooks. The usual diagnostic features as thus described would be better named if they were designated as terminal signs and symptoms, because certainly when they are present, the patient's general condition is not conducive to a satisfactory result, therapeutically speaking. In late years, since we have become acquainted with the blood chemistry side of the picture, there is a tendency to procrastinate further by the use of intravenous salt concentrates and glucose and the physiologic salt solution, subcutaneously. Certainly no one will deny that these measures have been of inestimable value in the treatment of obstruction before and after operation, but in the purely mechanical type they do not take the place of operative interference. They only serve as adjuncts of great merit.

At this time I wish to report a case of mechanical obstruction due to gallstones together with the postmortem findings. On the evening of September 16, 1932, I was notified by a physician from a small town in an adjoining county that a patient was on his way to Council Bluffs in an ambulance and that he believed the patient was suffering from an intestinal obstruction. The patient, seventy-two years of age, blacksmith by trade, arrived by ambulance at Mercy Hospital about 7:15 p. m. The history obtained from his relatives was as follows: In the morning four days previously the patient complained of an indefinite soreness in the lower abdomen, together with the fact that his bowels had not moved at the usual time. By noon the soreness had developed to an intermittent pain with some nausea. The patient took a physic, but obtained no relief from the symptoms, and in the afternoon he vomited. A physician was called and he advised the use of enemas. This line of treatment with repeated enemas was of no avail. The pain was curtailed by opiates, but the pain and vomiting continued, together with distention of the abdomen and absence of bowel movements. He was seen again by the physician late in the afternoon of the fourth day, who recommended at this time that he be sent to the hospital. On his arrival at the hospital the patient was in a condition of extremis; semicomitose; rapid barely perceptible pulse, rapid shallow breathing and almost continuous fecal vomiting. The abdomen was greatly distended and rigid. The history and the condition of the abdomen led me to agree with the diagnosis, but I advised the family that I did not believe there was anything that could be done to relieve the con-

dition, since it was my opinion that the patient would be dead before we had a chance to attempt any form of treatment. We gave the patient some stimulants, but there was no response, and he died about two hours after admission.

Permission for an autopsy was secured ·from the family. However, this permission was qualified for opening the abdomen only. The autopsy report was as follows: body of white male of stated age, about seventy inches long, weighing around two hundred pounds. Rigor mortis was not present. The abdomen was greatly distended, with an excessive amount of subcutaneous fat. No fluid was found in the peritoneal cavity. The liver was small, the lower border about three centimeters above the costal margin. The stomach was considerably distended. A small nodule about the size of a pea was found on the anterior surface of the stomach. The spleen was of normal size. On section, it cut with slight resistance, and the pulp was somewhat darker than normal. The gallbladder. Gastric and duodenum contents bettered against the liver by thick adhesions. Loops of the small intestines were hemorrhagic in places. The ileum was consdierably distended for a distance corresponding to one-half its length. From there on it suddenly became contracted to about one-fourth or less of its normal size. The lumen of the gut in the constricted portion would barely permit the passage of a lead pencil. A large mass of stone-like hardness was felt in the intestines immediately above the beginning of the construction. When the intestine was opened a stone five centimeters long and three centimeters in diameter was found to be the cause of the obstruction. This stone was free and was not incarcerated in the wall of the bowel. The stone looked like a typical gallstone. The pyloric end of the stomach, duodenum, gallbladder and liver were intensely adherent in one mass. The gallbladder as mentioned before, was flattened out and lay in the bed of the liver as a piece of scar tissue. It was only with great difficulty that the gallbladder was freed and dissected from the liver bed. The duodenum could not be separated from the gallbladder, and a slight tear was made in the anterior wall of the gallbladder. Gastric and duodenum contents began to run through the gallbladder tear, indicating that a free communication was present between the gallbladder and the duodenum. After the dissection was completed, a large opening was found in the posterior wall of the gallbladder leading into the duodenum. This opening was large enough to permit the passage of the stone found in the ileum. The gross anatomic diagnosis was: Chronic productive cholecystitis with sclerosis; perforation of the gallbladder into the duodenum;

and obstruction of the small intestine caused by a large gallstone.

After the autopsy I questioned the family further and was told by his wife that some years ago her husband had been sick with a severe attack of "stomach trouble" which had incapacitated him for several weeks, but that he had always been well previous to that time and since, until the present illness. She did not remember whether or not there had been any jaundice or specific details that might point to a gallbladder attack, but one would probably be safe in assuming that the previous illness was the origin of the production of the biliary fistula. There is no way of determining whether or not this stone passed into the bowel at that time, or whether this was a new stone that developed later and then passed into the bowel. Several authors who have had an opportunity to study internal biliary fistula in the living, state that the fistula at the time it develops is no doubt a life-saving incident, but that the existing inflammatory and infectious condition still continues. In other words, it is not curative, and if such is the case new stones could develop later.

BIBLIOGRAPHY

1. Eisenfarb, J.: Case of intestinal obstruction caused by gall stone. Gastrol. Polska. iii:95-104 (June) 1931.
2. Judd, E. Starr, McIndoe, A. H., and Marshall, J. M.. Surgery of the Biliary System. Practice of Surgery, Dean Lewis, Volume vii: Chapter 2, 1-180. W. F. Prior and Sons, Hagerstown, Maryland, 1931.
3. Nogara, G.: Considerazioni sulle occlusione meccaniche dell' intestino nell'appendicite. Clin. Chir., xxxiv:585-615 (June) 1931.
4. Odasso, A.: Due operazioni di ileo per ostruzione da calcolo biliare. Minerva Med., vii:561-568 (May 31) 1927.
5. Braun, W.: Verhandl. d. Ges. f. Verdauungs-u. Stoffwechselkr., 128-129, 140-165, 1928.
6. Cochez: Occlusion intestinale par calcul biliaire: diagnostic et mobilisation par e toucher vagina. Bull. et mém. Soc. nat. d. chir., lii:1078-1080 (December 4) 1926.
7. Hartwell, J. A. and Cooper, Henry S. F.: Intestinal Obstruction or Ileus. Practice of Surgery, Dean Lewis, Volume vii: Chapter 7, 1-70, W. F. Prior and Sons, Hagerstown, Maryland, 1931.

THE FINLEY HOSPITAL CLINICO-PATHOLOGIC CONFERENCES

PENETRATING GASTRIC ULCER MEDICALLY TREATED

G. C. Fritschel, M.D., Dubuque

This case is of interest first because it presents the problem as to whether the gastric lesion is benign or malignant, and second because it illustrates the favorable response to medical treatment as indicated by the disappearance of clinical symptoms as well as by the regression of the lesion as shown by x-ray examination.

CASE REPORT

Chief complaint: The patient, a retired farmer, fifty years of age, was admitted to The Finley Hos-

pital, July 26, 1934, with a complaint of "distress after eating, pain in the upper abdomen and loss of weight."

Past history: About six years ago he had "stomach trouble" for about six months. Since that time he felt well until six weeks ago.

Present illness: For six weeks he had had distress which came on immediately after meals. At times he also had pain but it was not a prominent symptom. Occasionally he vomited and this gave him relief. Because of the distress he restricted his diet to milk, eggs, and cereals, and as a consequence, had lost eight pounds.

Physical examination: The patient, a middle aged man, appeared anemic and somewhat cachectic. It was evident that he had lost weight. Otherwise the general examination was essentially negative. Examination of the abdomen revealed tenderness on pressure just beneath the ensiform cartilage and along the left costal border. No mass was felt. The urinalysis was essentially negative. The blood examination was as follows: white blood count, 5,500; red blood count, 3,630,000; and hemoglobin, 70 per cent (Sahli).

Provisional diagnosis: Gastric carcinoma or ulcer.

X-ray examination: Fluoroscopic and film examinations of the stomach and duodenum on July 26 showed a penetrating ulcer about midway be-

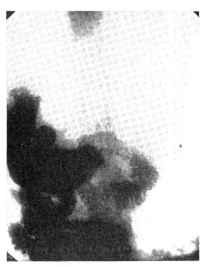

Fig. 1. Original examination (7-26-34) showing large penetrating benign gastric ulcer on lesser curvature. The stomach is filled with barium. There is also an old duodenal ulcer.

tween the pylorus and cardiac end of the stomach on the lesser curvature. This was approximately three centimeters in diameter. There was also a deformity of the duodenum characteristic of an old duodenal ulcer which I do not believe was active. There was about a 20 per cent retention in the stomach at six hours and the ulcer crater still contained a large amount of barium. (Figures 1 and 2.)

Conclusions:

1. Penetrating gastric ulcer.
2. Old duodenal ulcer.

Course in hospital: The treatment consisted of rest, alkalization, and control of the diet. During the first three weeks the patient was at absolute rest in bed. He was then allowed to sit in a wheel chair at intervals for one week, after which the time of sitting was gradually lengthened. At the end of six weeks he was up most of the time, but had rest periods for several hours each day. His diet consisted of hourly feedings of a mixture of milk, one and one-half ounces, and cream one and one-half ounces (between 7:00 a. m. and 7:00 p. m.). After several days one soft boiled egg was added to the morning, noon and last evening feedings. After this, well cooked cereals, strained vegetables and other smooth foods were gradually added, so that by the end of six weeks he was receiving three fairly substantial meals, consisting of various smooth foods. At no time was he given

more than eight to ten ounces at one feeding. In addition to these three main meals, he continued the milk-cream mixture at hourly intervals, and also received small amounts of orange or tomato juice with his meals.

The medicinal treatment consisted of alkaline powders given between the hourly feedings and continued for two hours after his last evening feeding. The alkaline powders consisted of powder No. 1, calcined magnesia, grs. x and sodium bicarbonate grs. xx; and powder No. 2, calcium carbonate grs. x and sodium bicarbonate grs. xx, which were given alternately between the hourly feedings. A few doses of milk of magnesia and bland enemas were necessary during the first

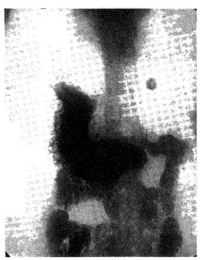

Fig. 3. Second examination (8-20-34) showing marked improvement as the result of three weeks treatment.

week, but after this the bowels moved regularly each morning. Belladonna or atropine was not given as there was very little gastric spasm and practically no retention at any time. This absence of spasm probably accounted for the fact that the patient never complained of pain as severe as might have been expected from the size of the ulcer as shown by the x-ray.

Under this regime the gastric distress was completely relieved after one week, although tenderness in the epigastrium on deep pressure was still present. This disappeared in three weeks and the patient felt better in every way. The red blood

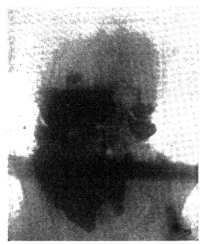

Fig. 2. Original examination (7-26-34) with a small amount of barium. The gastric rugae are well demonstrated. Note the fluid level in the ulcer crater.

count rose to 4,700,000 and the hemoglobin to 84 per cent (Sahli), in three weeks. The white blood count on numerous occasions fluctuated between 3,400 and 4,400. No explanation of the leukopenia was found although it was thought possible that it was the result of the restricted diet.

The healing of the ulcer was also followed by means of x-ray examination. Figures 2 and 3 made during the third and sixth weeks of treatment respectively, show graphically the recession of the ulcer. Since leaving the hospital he has continued the treatment. He has regained his former weight and is free from all gastric symptoms.

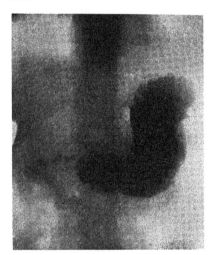

Fig. 4. Third examination (9-10-34) showing continued healing.

GENERAL DISCUSSION

The problem in this case was in regard to the possible malignancy of the ulcer. The patient was at the age when carcinoma of the stomach is commonly encountered and the gastric lesion was a large one. Furthermore, he had the secondary anemia and cachexia which accompanies gastric carcinoma. Factors against the lesion being carcinomatous was its location and the slight infiltration about the lesion in proportion to its size. Benign gastric ulcers are most common on the lesser curvature, whereas those on the greater curvature are almost always malignant. The development of carcinoma after gastric ulcer is propably not nearly as common as was formerly believed, but most ulcers of the greater curvature are primarily

malignant. It was therefore decided that the lesion was a benign ulcer. It is not always possible to make such a definite diagnosis; however, even in doubtful cases a regime as outlined above will probably result in no harm and will usually remove any doubt in the diagnosis. Benign gastric ulcers always have a tendency to heal, whereas the malignant ulcer will not respond to medical treatment. The essentials of the medical treatment of gastric ulcers consist of bed rest, frequent feedings with a bland smooth diet and neutralization of hyperacidity by the use of alkalis. As there is some danger of alkalosis, judgment is needed as to the amount of alkalis required. The heavy dosage formerly advocated should not be used as a routine. Only the minimum amount required to control the hyperacidity, as judged by symptomatic results or by gastric analyses, should be given. In some cases gastric spasm and the associated retention offer difficulties in the treatment. Usually they are controlled by belladonna or its alkaloids in proper dosage. While this discussion is primarily concerned with benign penetrating ulcer of the lesser curvature, the same principles hold good for benign pyloric and duodenal ulcers. Ulcers of the greater curvature, because they are almost always primarily malignant, are purely surgical problems.

REPORT OF CASES FROM THE BROADLAWNS GENERAL HOSPITAL, DES MOINES

JULIUS S. WEINGART, M.D.
JOSEPH BROWN, M.D.
FRANK W. FORDYCE, M.D.
Hospital Staff Committee

Case No. 72675. The patient was a fifty-three-year-old laborer, a native of Montenegro. He entered the hospital complaining of pain in the substernal and right hypochondriac regions which radiated to the back. This attack of pain had occurred the day before admission. It had been sudden in onset, waking him from sleep. He had vomited. Since the attack the pain had been at times continuous and at other times paroxysmal. He had noticed no changes in his stools and there was no history of any previous digestive disturbance.

Physical examination on admission was negative except for a small ovoid mass which could be felt below the right costal margin in the mid-clavicular line. This was smooth, moved with respiration, and was very tender. It was thought to be an enlarged gallbladder. He had a slight fever on admission, ranging from 100 to 102 degrees which lasted about five days, and a white cell count of 18,500. His urine showed five per cent sugar, but no ketone bodies. On an anti-diabetic diet, his urinary sugar rapidly disappeared and after about ten days of hospitalization he left, feeling much improved.

His second admission was for a fracture of the neck of the femur about one month later. He was in the hospital twenty-seven days, leaving with a good result. This time he complained of no abdominal symptoms. The examination of the abdomen showed no such mass as had been felt before.

Four months later the patient entered again and said he had had only short periods of relief from epigastric distress. For the past two weeks he had been feeling particularly uncomfortable. He had also been having chilly sensations, although definite chills were not described.

Physical examination showed great tenderness in the upper abdomen, especially below the right costal margin, also a very tender mass similar to the one felt at the time of the first admission. Temperature during the five days of his stay varied between 96 and 103 degrees. He was evidently very ill. Operation was discussed but his condition was considered too poor for such a procedure. Strange to say, his urine showed no sugar. His white blood count varied between 12,000 and 24,000.

Before his exitus, a diagnosis of acute empyema of the gallbladder was made, and this seemed amply justified by the history and physical findings. However, the autopsy showed a neoplasm of the gallbladder, springing from its fundus. The microscopic examination of this showed it to be an adenocarcinoma of high grade malignancy. The liver showed a portal cirrhosis. There was also a very large subphrenic abscess.

The above case is cited mainly to show the great difficulty of clinical differentiation between biliary stone with chronic cholecystitis and a new growth of the gallbladder. The former is, of course, much more common. The case also illustrates the great number of varying factors which influence our judgment and our conduct of a case. At his first admission operative interference would have been possible, but he had a glycosuria, probably a true diabetes mellitus. The fact that he recovered so promptly made us feel that it was wise to be conservative in regard to surgery. The outcome of the case proved that the diabetic condition was very mild. It is, of course, doubtful whether cholecystectomy would have effected a permanent cure.

JULIUS S. WEINGART, M.D.

PHYSICIANS WANTED

Word has reached the State Society office from the Iowa District of the Civilian Conservation Corps, of the urgent need for physicians to fill positions as camp surgeons in the Civilian Conservation Corps Medical Service. So great is this need that two doctors were recently transferred from New York to Iowa, since suitable candidates from this state had not presented themselves. The rank and pay is that of a first lieutenant in the United States Army, and applicants must be between twenty-one and thirty-five years of age, in order to be eligible for the Medical Reserve Corps. At the present time one physician is stationed in each camp, and it is the desire of those in authority to continue on that basis. This cannot be accomplished, however, without the services of additional, well qualified physicians, and we hope that a sufficient number of men in Iowa will be interested in maintaining this standard. Those desiring further information, and those who wish to make application should correspond with the District Surgeon, Civilian Conservation Corps, Fort Des Moines, Iowa.

WARNING

Physicians are warned against accepting free gift orders from various companies, especially those selling books, who request that the doctor sign a receipt for such a "gift." The duplicate signature may appear, not on a receipt, but on an order for, or a recommendation of, the salesman's wares. The signer may later be held responsible for this order, or his signature may be used to induce other doctors to order books or miscellaneous merchandise. Transactions of this type have been reported in Iowa recently.

NATIONAL SOCIETY FOR THE PREVENTION OF BLINDNESS

The Annual Conference of the National Society for the Prevention of Blindness will be held in New York City December 6-8. Dr. Edward Jackson of Denver, Colo., dean of American ophthalmologists, will deliver the principal address on the subject, "A Wide Basis for Blindness Prevention." Dr. Jackson was the first recipient, in 1925, of the Leslie Dana Gold Medal which is awarded annually for outstanding achievements in the prevention of blindness and conservation of vision. Topics that will be discussed at the Conference are: the causes of blindness; sight-saving classes for children with seriously defective vision; prevention of eye accidents; and prevention of pre-natal infections which may cause blindness.

STATE DEPARTMENT OF HEALTH

CONTAMINATED MILK SUPPLIES—A PUBLIC HEALTH MENACE

Public milk supplies, which lack adequate safeguards, represent a major menace to public health.

Formerly, before the era of modern sanitary engineering, most of the widespread epidemics of typhoid fever were due to contamination of public water supplies. Certain essential principles are now universally practiced to make our water supplies potable. With chemical treatment, sedimentation, filtration and final chlorination, water-borne outbreaks of typhoid fever and other intestinal diseases have become a rare occurrence. So great is public confidence in the value of the various steps of water purification, that municipalities have allowed streams to become very heavily polluted without a feeling of undue concern. There is, of course, a possibility that the burden placed on water purification plants may become too great to bear. It is well to remember that two years ago, Chamberlain, South Dakota, experienced a water-borne epidemic of typhoid fever, with 275 cases and 28 deaths.

Iowa has been fortunate in recent years in that no major water-borne epidemics have occurred. The same cannot be said of our public milk supplies. Contaminated milk has been the chief factor in the spread of various types of communicable disease. During the five-year period from 1929 to 1933, the State Department of Health was called upon to aid in the investigation of eight milk-borne outbreaks of typhoid fever. In these outbreaks, all of which involved county seat towns, there was a total of at least 241 cases, 24 of which resulted fatally. Typhoid carriers were demonstrable or presumably the factor in causing contamination. In all but one instance, raw milk supplies provided the means for dissemination of infection.

Thus far in 1934, unprotected, raw milk supplies have caused one epidemic of scarlet fever, with 25 cases, one of gastro-enteritis with 30 cases and three outbreaks of typhoid fever in Iowa. The first typhoid epidemic occurred at Waterloo, with 22 cases. A typhoid carrier was demonstrated as being the source of infection, an insanitary toilet and flies apparently playing a chief rôle in the conveyance of infectious discharges to the milk supply. Boone suffered a major outbreak of typhoid fever during September and October, with a total of 55 reported cases and four deaths. The common factor in most, although not all of the Boone cases, was the use

of raw milk from one of the local dairies. A typhoid carrier was suspected but laboratory examinations did not lead to the isolation of typhoid bacilli from the body discharges. The third and most recent milk-borne typhoid outbreak to be investigated was at Fontanelle in Adair county. Five cases were reported. Here again, a typhoid carrier is suspected and laboratory specimens have been forwarded with the purpose of demonstrating a carrier state.

Public milk supplies, like the water we drink, need to be surrounded with adequate safeguards. Dairy products, when they harbor disease producing organisms, have potentialities for danger fully comparable to those attaching to an unsafe water supply. Precautions which are at this time being exercised to assure safe milk, are with few exceptions, entirely inadequate. A recent survey of nine dairies in a county seat town in Iowa, showed that none of the milk supplies could be given better than a grade D rating. Improvements in sanitary conditions and in methods of handling milk must be carried out before these dairies can conform with grade A or grade B standards. From the standpoint of public health, a milk supply, to be safe, should not only be of high quality but should also be carefully pasteurized before use. Some of the milk which is now being pasteurized, is of poor grade and therefore undesirable. Adoption and carrying out of a standard milk ordinance, with adequate provision for milk inspection, and laboratory work, would greatly improve the milk supplies of communities and minimize the danger of milk-borne disease. A public milk supply, duly safeguarded is certain to carry with it vast mutual benefits to producer and consumer alike.

HIGHLIGHTS FROM THE RECENT MEETING OF THE IOWA PUBLIC HEALTH ASSOCIATION

The Ninth Annual Meeting of the Iowa Public Health Association held at Des Moines, Iowa, on October 26, 1934, was attended by forty-six physicians, twenty-three of whom were health officers, by sixteen nurses, two dentists, two sanitary engineers, one chemist and twelve lay persons.

The out of town speakers comprised, Russell LaFayette Cecil, B.A., M.D., Sc.D., Professor of Clinical Medicine, Cornell University Medical College, New York City; Earle G. Brown, M.D., Executive Secretary, Kansas State Board of Health, Topeka, Kansas; G. M. Byington, M.D., Medical Director, W. K.

Kellogg Foundation, Battle Creek, Michigan; and Orianna McDaniel, M.D., Director, Division of Communicable Diseases, Minnesota State Department of Health, Minneapolis, Minnesota. Excerpts from the addresses given by Dr. Cecil and Dr. Brown will be printed on this page in the December issue of the JOURNAL of the Iowa State Medical Society.

Some of the highlights of other papers read at this meeting follow:

Dr. Byington, in speaking of the work of the W. K. Kellogg Foundation said, "The W. K. Kellogg Foundation is interested in the development of a community health program involving five counties in southwestern Michigan—Allegan, Barry, Eaton, Van Buren, and Hillsdale. All actual services are rendered by the participating members of the community, that is, local physicians provide the medical service, and local dentists the dental service. Health examinations of all children in both the urban and rural schools of these five counties are given, and defects are corrected by the local physicians. The younger children are given smallpox vaccinations and immunized against diphtheria, the participating physician acting in an educational capacity during his contact with the child and the family, pointing out the importance of these preventive measures. Postgraduate courses have been made available at the expense of the foundation to the physicians and dentists of these counties."

Dr. McDaniel presented interesting facts with regard to malignant smallpox in Minnesota. She said, "Seventy, or 76 per cent of the persons residing in Minnesota and attacked by malignant smallpox in 1917 had never been vaccinated. Ten others who suffered from the disease had been vaccinated more than seven years previously. Twelve persons who had been vaccinated within seven years were attacked but no deaths occurred in this group. A total of 92 cases were reported. Of the seventeen persons who died, fifteen had never been vaccinated and two had been vaccinated more than seven years before the onset of the disease."

In speaking of an outbreak of malignant and mild smallpox in the state of Minnesota during the years 1924 and 1925 she said, "During the 20 month epidemic period the total cases, both mild and malignant, numbered 4,041 and the deaths 504. Twelve deaths were recorded for each one hundred cases. Unvaccinated persons account for 85 and 82 per cent respectively of the cases and deaths."

J. G. Grant, M.D., Department of Hygiene, Iowa State College, Ames, Iowa, reported on recent accomplishments in the field of preventive medicine. He said, "Routine Mantoux tests are given to all entering students at Iowa State College. Positive reactors are x-rayed. From September, 1933, to June, 1934, there were 2,055 men students and 942 women students given the tuberculin test. One-tenth of a milligram of Koch's old tuberculin was used. Roughly, ten per cent of the men and sixteen per cent of the

women students were positive reactors; 360 in all or twelve per cent of the total 2,997.

"X-ray findings of the 360 positive reactors revealed seventeen active cases of whom three, all men, were found to be open cases; 23 were classified as suspicious of beginning activity needing close supervision; and 31 were arrested or healed cases. Of these active cases, two had and are still continuing treatment by pneumothorax with marked improvement, one had a tuberculous kidney removed, one went to Colorado to rest. The remainder of the seventeen cases showing activity, under a regime of close supervision, lessened schedules, and a proper hygienic mode of living, have all shown improvement and are on the road to being arrested.

"As to the value of tuberculin testing, we feel it is of great importance in our work. Most of our cases would not be found on routine physical examination without it. We feel that we are protecting not only the patients themselves, but those with whom they come in contact, which group in an institution such as ours is usually a large one. In high schools and the grades, it could be of great value also if done with the cooperation and understanding of the family physician and the parents."

I. H. Borts, M.D., State Hygienic Laboratories, Iowa City, Iowa, reported, "There are two antigenic factors associated with the typhoid bacillus, the 'O' or somatic factor associated with the body of the bacillus and the 'H' associated with the flagella or organs of locomotion. When a person who has not had typhoid fever is given the prophylactic vaccine, 'H' agglutinins are stimulated and are present in the blood. 'O' agglutinins are said not to be formed following vaccination.

"Blood serum of a person who is ill with typhoid fever, presents early in the disease agglutinins of the 'O' type which tend to increase as the disease progresses. Following the production of the 'O' agglutinins one is able also to detect 'H' agglutinins but in much lower titer. One is thereby able to determine fairly accurately whether the agglutinins in a given test are due to vaccination or to active infection."

PREVALENCE OF DISEASE

Disease—	Sept. '34	Aug. '34	Sept. '33	Most Cases Reported From
Diphtheria	21	13	51	Dubuque
Scarlet Fever......	114	46	125	Polk, Delaware
Typhoid Fever.....	90	68	34	Polk, Boone
Smallpox	2	1	0	Linn, Muscatine
Measles	17	33	5	Jackson, Franklin
Whooping Cough...	37	88	76	Woodbury
Cerebrospinal				
Meningitis	3	3	0	Johnson
Chickenpox	17	3	13	Boone, Floyd
Mumps	38	24	8	Dubuque
Poliomyelitis	7	7	13	Appanoose
Tuberculosis	31	73	41	(For State)
Rocky Mountain				
Spotted Fever ...	0	2	0	
Undulant Fever....	26	43	10	Cerro Gordo
Syphilis	113	156	144	(For State)
Gonorrhea	160	199	242	(For State)

The JOURNAL of the
Iowa State Medical Society
ISSUED MONTHLY

RALPH R. SIMMONS, Editor.....................Des Moines

PUBLICATION COMMITTEE

RALPH R. SIMMONS, Editor.....................Des Moines
ROBERT L. PARKER, Secretary..................Des Moines
OLIVER J. FAY, Trustee.......................Des Moines
JOHN I. MARKER, Trustee......................Davenport
EDWARD M. MYERS, Trustee.....................Boone

SUBSCRIPTION $3.00 PER YEAR

*Address all communications to the Editor of the Journal,
505 Bankers Trust Building, Des Moines*

OFFICE OF PUBLICATION, DES MOINES, IOWA

Vol. XXIV   NOVEMBER, 1934   No. 11

ANNOUNCEMENT

Effective November 1, 1934, Miss Mary McCord will be Secretary to the Speakers Bureau Committee of the Iowa State Medical Society, filling the vacancy created by the appointment of Miss Dorothy M. Nelson, as Acting Executive Secretary, in place of Mrs. Dorothy C. McCarthy, who has resigned after five years of faithful and efficient service.

Oliver J. Fay, M.D.
Chairman, Board of Trustees.

BALANCED PSYCHIATRY

In the earliest medical chronicles we find records of individuals displaying symptoms of mental disease now recognized and classified as insanity. For many years hospital doors were closed to these demented patients, and even when a public sentiment became aroused and institutional care was offered, segregation was the sole motive. Time and experience brought a realization of society's greater obligation toward these unfortunate individuals, and the "madhouse" with its many horrors gave way to the hospital or sanitarium where kindness blended with, and tempered custodial care. Still more recently a consciousness of greater responsibility and privilege has developed, and directors of both private and public institutions encourage a spirit of research, especially for restorative procedures which will permit the release of the patient from institutional care and warrant his return to society. Even now this plan is by no means a universal one, conducted along well organized lines of collective endeavor. The private institutions have in many instances led the way, but it is particularly pleasing to note that in some large state institutions where clinical material is especially abundant, well planned investigations are being conducted and mass or group therapy is being

instituted for the mitigation of symptoms or the cure of the ailment.

As a fundamental concept, it must be appreciated that the insane are subject to physical illnesses just the same as the sane. It is further necessary to approach the problem believing that in certain instances the insanity may result from morbid physical states and may be relieved by the correction of physical impairments. With such a background, the former medical superintendent of a large state hospital has recently reported his observations conducted upon the line of routine investigation and mass therapy.* He attempted to give every patient in the institution the benefit of a very thorough physical examination, including all of the laboratory and x-ray procedures which would be employed with a sane person suffering from an obscure ailment. This included a complete social and medical history, an x-ray of the gastro-intestinal tract, particularly for delayed elimination, an examination for the presence of focal infection, and finally a search for all correctable surgical conditions not covered in the routine outlined above. Following this exhaustive study, the patients were divided into groups for mass therapy. In this particular experiment, colonic irrigation and hydrotherapy were given special attention. In spite of what appeared to be rather convincing results from the several therapeutic measures employed, unfortunately the "cost per patient" factor prematurely terminated the experiment.

Quoting the writer and summarizing his results, "The average discharge rate from the hospital from 1900 to 1923 was 35 per cent of the admission rate. The average discharge rate over this four-year period (of therapeutic research) was 65 per cent of the admission rate as compared with the former average of 35 per cent." Reckoned on the basis of $5.60 per week per patient, this saving represented in money over $92,000. This one hospital served only about one-tenth of all the institutionalized insane of the state. On this basis a saving in this one state alone of over $928,000 annually might be expected from the intelligent application of well proved methods of therapy. The saving in life and happiness cannot be reckoned. Although incomplete, these observations and conclusions as reported from this study are inspiring and should prove stimulating to others entrusted with the care of insane patients.

Every so often an investigator referred to as "the focal infection" and the "intestinal stasis" enthusiast reports the brilliant results obtained by the correction of teeth, tonsils, intestinal stasis and surgical conditions found in the insane in our

---

* Four Years' Experience in the Mass Physical Therapy of the Insane, H. H. McClellan, M.D. The Medical World, September, 1934, page 481.

public institutions. Too often these reports are depreciated by those of undue enthusiasm or those lacking psychiatric background, and the entire perspective is warped or lost. It is indeed unfortunate to find the psychiatrist so engrossed with vague and speculative problems of personality, the subconscious mind, and psychotherapy that he forgets his patients' suffering bodies. Again, it seems strange that in many institutions the treatment of neurosyphilis is scientific and intensive, while that of comparable but less specific infections is neglected and diets are based on costs rather than on calories and vitamins.

To be sure, the situation is probably improving as rapidly as the state of our knowledge will permit. However, not until those entrusted with the care of the insane realize that the problems of heredity and development, environment, habits, emotions and bodily disease are all factors in the individual case, and not until therapy is based on this broad view of the situation, will deserved criticism be avoided and adequate results experienced.

WHY DOES IOWA NEED THE BASIC SCIENCE LAW?*

The Iowa law provides for three examining and licensing boards which set, three widely different educational standards for licenses to diagnose and treat human ailments, viz.:

1. One board requires graduation from high school, or equivalent, and completion of three courses of lectures of six months each.
2. Another board requires graduation from high school, or equivalent, and four years' professional training.
3. The third board requires graduation from high school, two years of college preparation, four years' professional training and one year of postgraduate internship.

When several boards are in authority, educational standards always suffer. Protection of the public requires that all practitioners be competent. License is for the protection of the public, not for the purpose of exploitation by those receiving licenses. Since the above requirements vary from eighteen months to sixty-six months of instruction, it is perfectly obvious that the present laws are wrong from the standpoint of protection. Both extremities as represented by these boards cannot be what is needed.

The board of lowest educational standards does

* This is the second of a series of articles on the Basic Science Law.

not require any knowledge of chemistry, bacteriology or pathology. This board has licensed 2,056 men and women in Iowa since 1921, whereas the two other boards combined have licensed only 1,403 in the same period. Iowa needs to be protected from an influx of poorly educated men and women who offer their services to the afflicted public.

The proposed basic science law recognizes no favorites. It requires the same examination of all candidates before they apply to any licensing boards. It presents a standard which falls between the extremes of the present laws. It provides what Iowa needs, viz.: better educational standards for those who wish to practice the healing arts; and makes such provision on an absolutely fair basis

SCIENTIFIC FELLOWSHIP

The Speakers Bureau of the Iowa State Medical Society continues to multiply its activities. The most recently announced plan of this multi-project bureau provides assistance to county medical societies in arranging for the interchange of speakers, promising to "promote the feeling of good fellowship which exists among the various county societies," and at the same time guaranteeing an interesting scientific program.

Epitomizing the plan, the chairman of the Speakers Bureau states, "What we have in mind for these programs is something along this line. A representative of the president of the Iowa State Medical Society will give a brief talk on state medicine, (or other subjects claiming the spotlight of the president's attention). This will be followed by two or three talks by men from neighboring county societies. The meetings should start with a dinner, at which time the president's representative will talk. The remainder of the program will follow the dinner."

Well, there you are—a complete new idea for a delightful evening, and the entire burden of planning lifted from the shoulders of the overworked county society secretary. The success of the plan seems assured if for no other reason than the fact that fellowship is so closely linked with food. We are reminded of a story illustrating the point. It seems that Sidney Smith, creator of Andy Gump, was invited to a certain dinner, and upon being informed of the guest list, declined to accept. When questioned concerning his action he replied, "I do not wish to dine with one of the guests, since he is a man I dislike and I want to continue to dislike, and who can dislike any man with whom he dines."

THE SECRETARY'S MESSAGE

MEMBERSHIP

We are nearing the end of the year, a year which has shown increased activity and many vital problems faced by the profession of the state. Because of these problems each county medical society should keep well informed of recent developments. This can only be accomplished through completely organized and properly functioning local medical societies.

Your central office is equipped to furnish any literature you may wish concerning medical economics, contract practice, socialization of medicine and numerous other problems before us today.

The Speakers Bureau is anxious to help any county societies which may wish to increase their interests not only in scientific medicine, but these other problems as well.

Today there are fifty-eight county medical societies with their 1933 membership fully paid for 1934. We have seventeen county societies with but one delinquent. There are today 2,202 paid-up members as compared with 2,167 at the close of last year.

A number of new men have located in the state. County secretaries should obtain their memberships now on the quarterly pro-rated dues of $2.50 for the last quarter of 1934.

If every eligible physician in the state were a member of the county society we would have a possible membership of approximately 2,600. Our largest membership was in 1930 when we had 2,413 paid-up members. I feel sure that this membership could be reached this year if every county secretary and deputy councilor would do his part. May I count on you to help boost the membership? Lets go!

The Board of Trustees still authorizes me to accept non-interest bearing notes from any doctor who is in financial distress and who desires to keep in good standing in his county society.

Robt. L. Parker

Disaster---Then the Red Cross

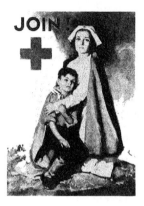

JOIN

One day last June the American Red Cross in Washington received word from the United States Weather Bureau that a hurricane in the Gulf of Mexico, one hundred miles off the Louisiana coast, would probably strike Morgan City and Vermillion Bay toward night. Many similar warnings are received by the Red Cross, and the incident serves to illustrate how the disaster machinery of the relief organization swings smoothly into action.

National headquarters at once telephoned their national staff worker in New Orleans and three other relief workers in nearby states, who communicated with coast chapters, warning them to prepare for relief effort and asking them to hold local radio operators in readiness to send messages if other methods of communication failed. A veteran disaster technician was commissioned to speed to the scene and take charge. This worker quickly arrived from Washington and surveyed the situation left by the storm. Sixteen parishes were involved. The brunt of the attack had fortunately been in rural areas rather than in more heavily populated districts. Twelve persons had been killed, and twenty injured. About 150 homes were demolished, 1,000 badly damaged and some 6,000 put in need of minor repairs. His inspection indicated that two-thirds of the corn crop had been destroyed, and it was too late to replant. The governor's proclamation called for a relief fund of $25,000, to which the Red Cross donated $3,000, with all chapters of the affected area pressing to meet the emergency.

In addition to its disaster relief service, the American Red Cross maintains a war service and a public health nursing and home hygiene service to assist in the welfare of the men who have worn, and are wearing, the uniform of their country, and to campaign for the health and safety of every citizen.

In the last fifteen years casualties resulting from the use of motor cars numbered more than 325,000 persons,—as against only 300,000 Americans killed by our enemies in all of our wars up to this time. That is tragedy and disaster, in the opinion of Red Cross officials,—just as surely as a tornado, earthquake, drought or flood. That makes the teaching of safety a simple humanitarian responsibility. Every twelve months sees more than 7,000 drownings, a figure which has been held practically at a level in the last few years, notwithstanding the steadily rising popularity of bathing and water sports. Much of the credit for this progress in teaching water safety belongs to the Red Cross.

In twenty-one years of campaigning on behalf of life saving, the Red Cross has issued more than 500,000 certificates for completion of its standard and advanced course. In 1933 nearly 79,000 such certificates were issued. Summer camps, where fine, wholesome boys and girls each year acquire the suntan, fresh air, water exercise and outdoor experience to carry them through the school grind with alert minds and strong bodies,—1,748 such camps last year, situated in forty-five states, put the Red Cross life saving program into operation. Indicative of how universally the training is extended to the young people through their trained leaders is the fact that 5,242 passed the senior life saving test last year, and 15,431 met the junior requirements. Not only summer camps, but many national organizations, welfare groups and state organizations for young people, rely upon the Red Cross to provide their supervisors and instructors in the needed training in first aid and life saving.

This training is provided in various ways, most of it through life saving campaigns and first aid classes conducted under the local auspices of the Red Cross chapters. Each spring nearly a thousand outstanding physical education instructors, playground directors, camp counsellors and other professionals assemble at national aquatic schools for review and advanced work under faculties composed of men with national reputation in their special lines. Five such schools were held in the east this year, two in the middle west and three in the far west.

The Red Cross—"The Greatest Mother"—does not forget. Busy as she is in meeting the obligations of the hours, restoring normal living to those buffeted by stroke of disaster or ill health or economic hardship, she remembers her adopted "buddies" of war days. Through her War Service she assists disabled veterans in obtaining legitimate benefits, serves them in many helpful ways during their hospitalization, affords relief and service to their families during adjudication of claims, and provides friendly service and relief in distress for the men in the regular army, navy and marine corps.

All activities of the Red Cross receive their support from the dues and contributions received during the annual Roll Call, which this year extends its invitation throughout the United States between Armistice Day and Thanksgiving, November 11 to 29.

SPEAKERS BUREAU ACTIVITIES

AVAILABLE PROGRAMS

Socialized Medicine

Probably no subject is more popular nor more widely discussed today than is the subject of socialized medicine. Newspapers, periodicals both lay and scientific, and even entire books are appearing every day dealing with some phase of this problem. One should be well informed before taking a definite stand on the matter. So much material is being published on this subject that no one person can undertake to digest all of it. Physicians in Iowa are offered an unusual opportunity to hear this subject discussed from every angle. The following program has been carefully worked out and is available for district meetings throughout the state:

The Socialization of Medicine from the Viewpoint of the Sociologist—C. H. Graening, M.D., Waverly.

The Socialization of Medicine in Foreign Countries—E. M. Myers, M.D., Boone.

American Attempts at the Socialization of Medicine—M. B. Call, M.D., Greene.

The Socialization of Medicine from the Viewpoint of Organized Medicine—John H. Henkin, M.D., Sioux City.

This program was given at Waverly on September 20, and was well discussed and highly instructive. The laity is becoming more and more enthused with the idea of socialized medicine. It behooves the doctors to be so familiar with all phases of the subject that the medical profession can intelligently direct whatever developments are made in the solution of this question.

If you are interested in this program, your councilor will be glad to make arrangements for it to be given at a meeting in your district soon.

Radium Therapy

Word comes from the Cooperative Medical Advertising Bureau of the American Medical Association that Frank E. Simpson, M.D., of the Frank E. Simpson Institute of Radium Therapy of Chicago is available to medical societies for talks on the subject of radium therapy. Dr. Simpson advertises his Institute in the Journal of the American Medical Association and in several state medical journals, including our own Iowa State Medical Society JOURNAL. His Institute has the approval of the American Medical Association.

Dr. Simpson is the author of a book on Radium Therapy, published by the C. V. Mosby Co., of St. Louis, in 1922. He was also invited to write a chapter in the German book called "Lehrbuch der Seratilentherapia" published by Urban and Schwartzenberg of Berlin and Vienna. He is a graduate of Northwestern University School of Medicine, a member and fellow of the American Medical Association, a specialist in roentgenology and radiology, and a member of the American Radiologic Society and the American College of Radiology. Dr. Simpson is reported to give an excellent talk, illustrating his lecture with moving pictures. He takes care of his own expenses.

Any medical society wishing to schedule Dr. Simpson in a program is asked to write the Speakers Bureau, and arrangements will be made immediately.

COUNTY SOCIETY MEETINGS

To stimulate scientific interest and promote good fellowship among the various members of the various county medical societies, the Speakers Bureau has asked each county society secretary to allow the Bureau to arrange a program for one of their meetings during the coming year. The plan is for these programs to begin with a dinner, at which time a representative of the president will bring a message from the state society. The remainder of the program is to follow the dinner and will be presented by two or three men from adjoining county societies.

The men who are chosen to present these programs are recommended by the officers of their county societies. This should insure programs of high scientific value. The Speakers Bureau hopes that this wholesale exchange program plan will stimulate the various societies to hold more regular meetings of their own, to improve the quality of their programs, and to inspire tolerance and interest in the other fellow's viewpoint. It is good for us to know what is being done in other county societies and this plan should be an excellent way of discovering just such things.

The dinner together, the companionship of the visiting speakers, and perhaps others from the society from which the speakers come, should be invaluable in promoting good fellowship and uniting the medical profession into a solid front, strong enough to meet and solve the problems of today and the future.

The response to this plan has been inspiring. Numerous societies have already requested such a program—won't you encourage your county to support this worthwhile project?

RADIO BROADCASTS

Mondays, 8:00 p. m.—WSUI
Wednesdays, 4:00 p. m.—WOI

October 31-November 5—How the Body Works: Respiration—G. Raymond Johnson, M.D.

November 7-12—How the Body Works: Elimination ——W. B. Lewis, M.D.

November 14-19—Change of Life—Roy I. Theisen, M.D.

November 21-26—Nasal Obstruction—Carl E. Sampson, M.D.

November 28-December 3—Obesity—A. A. Schultz, M.D.

December 5-10—Cause and Prevention of Simple Goiter—F. Earl Bellinger, M.D.

WOMAN'S AUXILIARY NEWS

Edited by the Press and Publicity Committee

MRS. OLIVER J. FAY, *Chairman,* 405 Thirty-seventh Street, Des Moines

Report of the Educational Program Committee

"To be, or not to be," a strictly social organization is the problem that confronts every newly organized county auxiliary, and each individual society must find the right answer. It is neither the desire nor the province of the Educational Program Committee to dictate or even suggest the course to be adopted in this particular instance. If our social contacts, bridge parties, teas, and other functions, promote a feeling of fellowship and friendliness among our doctors' wives, then one of the great objectives of our organization has been accomplished. The value of this is apparent to everyone. While on this subject, let us be very generous with our invitations to those who are eligible to join, but have not done so at the first meeting. It may be that they did not realize the benefits to be gained by such an organization, or it may have been a matter of other duties, or of transportation. It should be explained to these individuals that since we do have a national and state organization, one way of showing our loyalty to the profession of which we are so proud, is to become a member of our local auxiliary.

Several fields of endeavor are open to us. The fostering of unity and good will among our own group, through our social activities, has already been mentioned. Philanthropic work for our individual communities is an important phase of any auxiliary's efforts. We should try to influence the program of lay organizations, so that our profession will be seen in the proper light by the public. In addition, the study programs which we use in our regular meetings constitute a large and important part of our work.

In taking up philanthropic work, such as helping a hospital in need, caring and sewing for the poor, and sponsoring local health drives and similar activities, we should consult the advisory board of the county medical society, in order that we may be certain of their approval before starting any project. The county society may be able to suggest some things that they would like to have us accomplish.

Probably our greatest field of help to the medical profession lies in our influence with lay organizations, such as the Federated Clubs, the Farm Bureau, the Parent-Teachers Associations and many others. We should have a general meeting once a year to which these groups should be invited. A good speaker on some health subject of general interest should be secured for this meeting. Use the Speakers Bureau of the Iowa State Medical Society. The chairman of the Federated Clubs' radio committee recently asked the public health division to prepare a radio program. This request was referred to the Speakers Bureau, and a worth while program will be broadcast. This is just one illustration of how we may use our influence in lay organizations. We have had very fine reports

from both Mason City and Council Bluffs that these get-together meetings of all groups, have been both profitable and enjoyable. We all know that a thing is successful, if it has been tried, and proved so.

In regard to our study programs for use at regular meetings, the committee has published a booklet of suggestions. This booklet is just what its name implies—suggestions. Perhaps it will serve only to start some train of thought that can be carried out in your group. However, we urge you to use your own material as much as possible. Debates, playlets, or chorus singing have proved useful and entertaining for many programs. A copy of this booklet has already been sent to each organized auxiliary, but if another one is needed, do not hesitate to write for it.

Our committee will thoroughly appreciate reports of any programs, and we solicit suggestions which you think will be valuable to the auxiliary.

Mrs. Channing G. Smith, Chairman.

Cerro Gordo County

The Woman's Auxiliary to the Cerro Gordo County Medical Society met at the home of Mrs. George M. Crabb in Mason City, Tuesday, October 9. Dinner was served at six-thirty after which Victor E. Levine, M.D., of the Creighton University School of Medicine, Omaha, spoke on Customs and Conditions of the Eskimo People; Mrs. J. E. Blythe of Mason City recounted some of her experiences during her recent visit to The Land of the Midnight Sun; and Mrs. L. R. Woodward, also of Mason City, addressed the group on Socialized Medicine.

Dallas-Guthrie Society

Thursday, August 2, on invitation of Dr. and Mrs. M. N. Voldeng, the members of the Dallas-Guthrie Medical Society and the Woman's Auxiliary met at The Meadows. The ladies attended the afternoon scientific program, after which they adjourned for a short business session. It was decided to defer the election of officers until the January meeting. The combined groups again convened for the six-thirty banquet, at which Dr. E. M. Myers of Boone presided as toastmaster. Dr. and Mrs. Walter L. Bierring were guests of the society at this meeting, which impressed all those in attendance as being a most profitable and enjoyable session.

Mrs. E. L. Bower.

Muscatine County

Opening their fall activities, the members of the Woman's Auxiliary to the Muscatine County Medical Society met for a noon luncheon at the Y. W. C. A. in Muscatine, Monday, September 24. The program was furnished by C. P. Phillips, M.D., of Muscatine, who spoke on The Basic Science Law.

SOCIETY PROCEEDINGS

Buena Vista County

The Buena Vista County Medical Society recently held a meeting in Storm Lake at the Bradford Hotel. After a six-thirty dinner, the year's program for child health and protection, was outlined and discussed. Plans are already under way at Linn Grove for diphtheria prophylactic work, being sponsored by the associated civic organizations in that community.

J. H. O'Donoghue, M.D., Secretary.

Carroll County

Wednesday, September 26, members of the Carroll County Medical Society convened in the staff room of St. Anthony's Hospital in Carroll, immediately after a six-thirty dinner in the nurses' dining room. The following program was presented: Fred Moore, M.D., of Des Moines, spoke on the Proposed Basic Science Law; F. V. Hibbs, M.D., of Carroll, and Ben C. Hamilton, Jr., M.D., of Jefferson, also talked briefly on the same subject. Walter D. Abbott, M.D., of Des Moines, gave an illustrated lecture on Head Injuries, including a resumé of all head injuries at Broadlawns General Hospital during the last two years. Joseph B. Priestley, M.D., also of Des Moines, spoke on Surgical Considerations of Biliary Tract Disease. Both papers were fully discussed by those present. The next meeting will be held Thursday, November 22.

Water A. Anneberg, M.D., Secretary.

Cerro Gordo County

Victor E. Levine, M.D., professor of biological chemistry and nutrition at Creighton University School of Medicine, Omaha, was the scientific speaker for the Cerro Gordo County Medical Society when that organization met in Mason City, Tuesday, October 9. Dr. Levine spoke on The Classification and Treatment of the Anemias.

Clinton County

The regular monthly meeting of the Clinton County Medical Society scheduled for Thursday, October 4, was postponed so that members of our society might be able to hear Joseph B. DeLee, M.D., who spoke before the Linn County Medical Society in Cedar Rapids on that date. Thursday, November 1, Frederick J. Swift, M.D., of the Iowa State Department of Health, addressed our group on Public Health Activities. A buffet luncheon followed the meeting.

E. V. Donlan, M.D., Secretary.

Dallas-Guthrie Society

The Dallas-Guthrie Medical Society met in Panora, Thursday, October 18, and the following program was presented: Salivary Calculi, P. B. Glew, M.D., of Dallas Center; The Proposed Basic Science Law, Fred Moore, M.D., of Des Moines; and Office Treatment of Diabetes, A. A. Toubes, M.D., also of Des Moines.

Henry County

J. C. Donahue, M.D., of Centerville, spoke in Mt. Pleasant, Friday, October 19, before a group of physicians, dentists, nurses, veterinarians and druggists of the county, on the subject, Aims and Ideals of the Medical and Allied Professions. The meeting was sponsored by the Henry County Medical Society.

Johnson County

At the regular monthly meeting of the Johnson County Medical Society held Wednesday, October 3, in Iowa City, sixty-two new members were elected, forty-nine of whom were local junior members. This is the largest number ever to be admitted to the society at one time.

The speaker of the evening, Nathaniel G. Alcock, M.D., discussed the subject, Transurethral Prostatic Resection. Summarizing his extensive experience with this and other methods of relieving prostatic obstruction, he showed conclusively that in his hands transurethral resection is superior in every respect to the older methods. His paper was ably presented and enthusiastically received.

H. M. Korns, M.D., Secretary.

Linn County

Joseph B. DeLee, M.D., of Chicago, founder of the Chicago Lying-In Hospital and Dispensary, and an internationally known authority in the field of obstetrics and gynecology, addressed the Linn County Medical Society at a meeting held in Cedar Rapids, Thursday, October 4. His subject was Forceps Operations and Episiotomy. Clinton and Fayette County Medical Societies attended in a body, and large delegations were present from Iowa City and Waterloo.

Thursday, October 25, Russell L. Cecil, M.D., of New York City, spoke on Some Phases of the Arthritis Problem.

E. J. Kieck, M.D., Secretary.

Louisa County Annual Meeting

At the regular meeting of the Louisa County Medical Society held in Letts, Thursday, October 11, the following officers were chosen for next year: Dr. S. J. Lewis of Columbus Junction, president, Dr. R. C. Ditto of Oakville, vice president; and Dr. J. W. Pence, of Columbus Junction, secretary and treasurer.

J. H. Chittum, M.D., Secretary.

Madison County Annual Meeting

The Madison County Medical Society held its annual meeting Monday, September 10, and elected officers as follows for the coming year: Dr. G. J. Anderson, president; Dr. Evelyn Olsen, vice president; Dr. J. F. Veltman, secretary and treasurer; Dr. I. K. Sayre, delegate; and Dr. A. L. Nelson, alternate delegate. All officers are of Winterset except Dr. Sayre, who resides at St. Charles.

J. F. Veltman, M.D., Secretary.

Marion County

The Marion County Medical Society and the Marion County Veterinary Society met in joint session in Pella, Friday, October 12, for their sixth annual meeting of this nature. The scientific program, presented in the afternoon, consisted of a symposium on Sanitation. Speakers were C. J. Scott, D.V.M., T. G. Fultz, D.V.M., and Carl Aschenbrenner, M.D. Carl F. Jordan, M.D., of Des Moines, and C. S. Cornell, M.D., of Knoxville, led in the discussion of these papers. After a six-thirty banquet at the Elmwood Inn, Fred Moore, M.D., of Des Moines, spoke on The Proposed Basic Science Law, and Harold A. Spilman, M.D., of Ottumwa, councilor for the ninth district, supplemented Dr. Moore's remarks.

Marshall County

Fall and winter activities of the Marshall County Medical Society were begun Tuesday, October 9, when that organization met in Marshalltown. The program featured a discussion of Carcinoma of the Colon, by R. E. Keyser, M.D., with B. L. Trey, M.D., illustrating the cases with motion pictures.

Poweshiek County

C. E. Harris, M.D., formerly of Grinnell, and now head of the medical staff of the Modern Woodmen's Tuberculosis Sanitarium at Woodmen, Colorado, was the guest of honor at a dinner given by the Poweshiek County Medical Society at the Grinnell Country Club, Wednesday, October 10. Dr. Harris presented an illustrated lecture on Tumors of the Chest. Visitors to this meeting included physicians from Marshall, Jasper and Mahaska counties.

Sac County

Members of the Sac County Medical Society met in regular session in Odeboldt, Monday, September 24, for a business meeting. James E. Reeder, M.D., of Sioux City, councilor of the fourth district, was the guest speaker of the occasion, talking on The Principles of the Basic Science Law.

Tama County

J. H. Kinnaman, M.D., of the Iowa State Department of Health, was the speaker of the evening, at a meeting of the Tama County Medical Society held in Tama, Friday, October 12. Dr. Kinnaman presented details of a proposed public school health program which would include immunization against tuberculosis, smallpox, and diphtheria.

Washington County

The November meeting of the Washington County Medical Society will be held in Wellman, Tuesday, November 13. A turkey dinner will be served at six-thirty in the Methodist Church, after which Thomas F. Suchomel, M.D., of Cedar Rapids, will speak on The Injection Treatment of Hernia.

W. S. Kyle, M.D., Secretary.

Wayne County

The Wayne County Medical Society met Friday, October 5, in the Christian Church at Corydon, and the following program was presented: Ten Common Skin Diseases, Lieut. B. F. Brunner, of Corydon; Explanation of the Basic Science Law, Harold A. Spilman, M.D., of Ottumwa; and Infection in Obstetrics and Gynecology, illustrated with moving pictures, H. C. Hesseltine, M.D., of Chicago University School of Medicine.

Woodbury County

The Woodbury County Medical Society held its regular monthly meeting on Tuesday, October 23, at the West Hotel in Sioux City. A six-thirty dinner was served to seventy-five members and guests. William F. Mengert, M.D., of the State University of Iowa College of Medicine, was the speaker of the evening, and took for his subject, Uterine Malignancies.

L. E. Pierson, M.D., Secretary.

Iowa and Illinois Central District Medical Association

One hundred physicians were in attendance at the meeting of the Iowa and Illinois Central District Medical Association, which was held at the Le Claire Hotel in Moline, Illinois, Wednesday, October 31. Foster Kennedy, M.D., professor of neurology, Cornell University Medical School, New York City, delivered an address on The Interdependence of Neurology, Psychiatry and General Medicine, and G. D. Royston, M.D., associate professor of obstetrics and gynecology, Washington University School of Medicine, St. Louis, spoke on The Care of Obstetrical Damage to the Cervix and Pelvic Supports.

James Dunn, M.D., Secretary

Southeastern Iowa Medical Society

The fifty-ninth annual meeting of the Southwestern Iowa Medical Society was held in Burlington, Wednesday, October 17. The Speakers Bureau of the Iowa State Medical Society arranged the following scientific program which was presented during the afternoon: The Peptic Ulcer—Gastric and Duodenal, L. A. Coffin, M.D., of Farmington; Case Report of a Severe Chemical Dermatitis Resulting from Caustic Burns, H. E. Graber, M.D., of Fairfield; Common Disorders of the Feet, Frank Ober, M.D., of Burlington; A County Medical Society Practitioner, L. E. Weber, M.D., of Wapello; Obstetric and Gynecology Procedures for the General Practitioner, C. P. Phillips, M.D., of Muscatine; The Use of the

Smith-Peterson Pin by the Wescot Method for New Cervical Fractures of the Femur, C. J. Lohmann, M.D., of Burlington; and Tumors, B. J. Dierker, M.D., of Fort Madison. Dr. John I. Marker of Davenport presided over the six-thirty banquet, after which C. A. Boice, M.D., of Washington, spoke briefly on State Society Activities, and Fred Moore, M.D., of Des Moines, discussed the proposed Basic Science Law. At the business session it was voted to hold the 1935 annual meeting in Muscatine, and the following officers were elected to serve the organization during the coming year: Dr. C. P. Phillips of Muscatine, president; Dr. L. A. Coffin of Farmington, vice president; and Dr. C. J. Lohmann of Burlington, secretary and treasurer.

INTERESTING NEWS

In Brief

The birth rate in the United States has declined from 38 per thousand in 1870 to 18 per thousand in 1931.

Rivaling in the richness of its liver oil in Vitamins A and B, the swordfish now ranks with the cod and halibut.

One of the most recent and noteworthy accomplishments in chemical science is the identification and synthetic preparation of Vitamin C, called ascorbic acid.

From Johns Hopkins University comes the theory that in many instances stammering is the result of a diet insufficiently rich in meat during early childhood.

A careful study conducted in 1933 showed the annual per capita consumption of fluid milk and cream in this country to be only 38.8 gallons, or 0.85 of a pint a day.

Employing methods first proposed by the Swiss surgeon Gonin, New York ophthalmologists have recently reported fifty per cent successful operations in a series of 150 patients suffering from detached retina.

The Joliots, successors to the Curies of Paris, predict the artificial production of a radioactive substance useful in the treatment of malignant disease, which can be produced so cheaply that all physicians may be supplied.

Favorable reports are cited in the treatment of lobar pneumonia by artificial pneumothorax such as is used in the treatment of tuberculosis. To be effective the lung must be collapsed on or before the third day of the disease.

PERSONAL MENTION

Dr. Julian M. Bruner announces the opening of offices at 1005 Bankers Trust Building in Des Moines, where he will be associated in practice with his father, Dr. H. A. Minassian. Dr. Bruner was graduated in 1927 from Rush Medical College, and has spent the last three years at the Mayo Clinic where he was granted a fellowship in surgery.

Dr. Gail McClure of Bussey, addressed a community meeting in Centerville, Wednesday, October 10, on the subject, "Preparing the Child for School."

Dr. C. S. Stoakes, after eight years of practice in Dysart, has moved to Lime Springs.

Dr. Fred L. Wells of Des Moines, was elected president of the Association of Life Insurance Medical Directors, at the annual meeting of that organization held in New York City, October 19 and 20.

Dr. Frederick H. Lamb of Davenport, spoke before the Young People's Club, Monday, September 24, on "Does Blood Tell?"

Dr. Henry G. Decker is leaving Des Moines for a few months to take special postgraduate work in neurosurgery at Johns Hopkins University School of Medicine.

Dr. Leonard P. Ristine of Cherokee, was guest speaker for the Sioux City Woman's Club, Thursday, October 18. His subject was "The Relation of Psychology to Social Welfare."

Dr. Carl L. Gillies, formerly of Cedar Rapids, has recently been appointed associate professor of roentgenology at the State University of Iowa, College of Medicine.

Dr. Morris Moore of Walnut, spoke before the Atlantic Rotary Club, Tuesday, October 16, on "The Proposed Basic Science Law."

Dr. Earl K. Pfaff, formerly of Arlington Heights, Illinois, has located for the practice of medicine and surgery, at 1508½ First Avenue, Northwest, Cedar Rapids.

DEATH NOTICES

Sturdivant, Lawrence Jones, of Exline, aged seventy-one, died October 14, after a prolonged illness. He was graduated in 1888 from the College of Physicians and Surgeons, Keokuk, and had long been a member of the Appanoose County Medical Society.

Voldeng, Mathew Nelson, of Woodward, aged seventy-one, died October 21, as the result of a stroke. He was graduated in 1887 from the University of Illinois College of Medicine, and at the time of his death was a life member of the Dallas-Guthrie and Iowa State Medical Societies.

OBITUARIES

Mathew Nelson Voldeng, M.D.
1863-1934

On Sunday morning, October twenty-first, one of the nestors of Iowa medicine passed from our midst. It also brought to a close the distinguished career of a practitioner, teacher, specialist, and builder of two model state hospitals at Cherokee and Woodward.

Doctor Voldeng was born of Norwegian parentage on a farm near Decorah, Iowa, January 21, 1863. He was graduated from Luther College at Decorah with the degree of A.B. in 1883, and re-

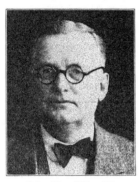

Mathew Nelson Voldeng, M.D.
1863-1934

ceived the degree of Doctor of Medicine from the University of Illinois in 1887. One of his classmates at Luther College and in the Medical School was Dr. Ludvig Hektoen, one of America's most eminent pathologists. The association during these academic years formed an enduring friendship that continued throughout the following years.

One year after his graduation in medicine he was appointed assistant physician at Independence State Hospital, serving until 1895, when he entered upon a two years' postgraduate course of study in European medical centers. It was during his service at the Independence hospital that two physicians came under his tutelage who were destined to attain leadership in the field of neuropsychiatry—Dr. Albert M. Bartlett of the University of Michigan and Dr. Arthur S. Hamilton of the University of Minnesota.

Doctor Voldeng was married on September 19, 1895, to Sadie Weir Rosemond, who became his faithful helpmate along the pathway of life.

He located in Des Moines. In 1897 he was appointed professor of pathology in the Drake University School of Medicine, and the next year was transferred to the chair of neuropsychiatry. He continued in this teaching position and was developing a specialized practice until 1902, when he was appointed the first superintendent of the new State

Hospital at Cherokee. Here he remained until March 1, 1915, when he became the first superintendent of the State Hospital and Colony for Epileptics at Woodward, Iowa, where he served until his death. These two model state institutions will always be Doctor Voldeng's finest monuments, not only attesting to his extraordinary administrative ability, but in the harmony of architectural beauty, exceptional landscaping and completeness of modern equipment, they stand as a memorial to his genius and professional leadership.

His early interest in scientific medicine is shown by publications of rather a high order as the Pathology of Abscess of the Liver in 1889; Pathology and Bacteriology of Pulmonary Tuberculosis in 1892; the State Care of Epileptics in 1894, and the State Care of the Criminal Insane in 1896.

Doctor Voldeng always took a prominent part in advancing the interest of organized medicine. When the Des Moines Pathological Society was organized in 1898 he was one of the charter members. After the reorganization of the American Medical Association in 1901, he represented the Iowa State Medical Society in the House of Delegates of the American Medical Association for a number of years. His address as president of the Iowa State Medical Society in 1911 expressed farsighted vision regarding the development of education, licensure and the future standards of medical practice.

Doctor Voldeng has been privileged to see two fine sons grow to manhood, Weir N. and Dr. Karl E., the latter now a practicing surgeon at Wellington, Kansas.

A legion of friends will mourn the passing of our colleague, and the memory of his genial high minded personality will linger in the days to come.

Walter L. Bierring, M.D.

Margaret Billingsley Mills, M.D.
1862-1934

Dr. Margaret Billingsley Mills, practicing physician of Ottumwa, Iowa, died at the Ottumwa Hospital, September 30, after a brief illness.

Doctor Mills, a native Iowan, attended the State University of Iowa for two years of her medical course, and received her medical degree from Northwestern University, Chicago, Illinois, in 1893. She was associated in her profession with her husband, Dr. Frank W. Mills, to whom she was married October 1, 1892, and who survives her.

Dr. Margaret participated in many phases of civic work. She served as city health officer for four years, and led the County Women's Division in the Liberty Loan drives during the war. She was a member of the state and county medical associations, the Iowa League of Women Voters, and the Young Women's Christian Association. In reconition of her faithful service to the cause of women's suffrage her name is inscribed on a bronze tablet placed in the Iowa Historical Building, the dedication ceremony of which she attended four years ago.

Walter L. Bierring, M.D.

THE JOURNAL BOOK SHELF

BOOKS RECEIVED

ALLERGY AND APPLIED IMMUNOLOGY—By Warren T. Vaughan, M.D., Richmond, Virginia. Second Edition. C. V. Mosby Company, St. Louis, 1934. Price, $5.00.

THE AUTONOMIC NERVOUS SYSTEM—By Albert Kuntz, Ph.D., M.D., professor of micro-anatomy, St. Louis University School of Medicine. Second edition, greatly enlarged and thoroughly revised. Octavo of 697 pages, illustrated with 73 engravings. Lea & Febiger, Philadelphia, 1934. Price, $7.50.

BRONCHOSCOPY, ESOPHAGOSCOPY AND GASTROSCOPY—By Chevalier Jackson, M.D., professor of bronchoscopy and esophagoscopy, Temple University; and Chevalier L. Jackson, M.D., professor of clinical bronchoscopy, Temple University. Third edition, reset; 485 pages with 207 illustrations and 15 color plates. W. B. Saunders Company, Philadelphia and London, 1934. Price, $9.00.

CATARACT, ITS ETIOLOGY AND TREATMENT—By Clyde A. Clapp, M.D., associate professor of ophthalmology, Johns Hopkins University. Octavo, 266 pages, illustrated with 92 engravings. Lea and Febiger, Philadelphia, 1934. Price, $4.00.

CONCEPTION PERIOD OF WOMEN—By Dr. Kyusaku Ogino, head of the gynecologic section of Takeyama Hospital, Niigata, Japan. Translated by Dr. Yonez Miyagawa, director of government institute for infectious diseases, Tokyo Imperial University, Hongooku, Tokyo, Japan. Medical Arts Publishing Company, 1803 Wood Street, Harrisburg, Pa., 1934. Price, $1.00.

A MANUAL OF SOCIAL DISEASES—By Franklin H. Church, M.D. Printed for the S. D. Publishing Company, Lock Box 30, Salem, New Jersey.

A MANUAL OF THE PRACTICE OF MEDICINE—By A. A. Stevens, M.D., formerly professor of Applied Therapeutics, University of Pennsylvania. Thirteenth edition, revised, 685 pages. W. B. Saunders Company, Philadelphia and London, 1934. Price, $3.50.

MENTAL DEFECT—By Lionel S. Penrose, M.D., research medical officer, Royal Eastern Counties Institution, Colchester. Farrar and Rinehart, New York, 1934. Price, $2.50.

NATURE'S WAY, The Fertile and Sterile Periods of Marriage—By Victor Cox Pedersen, M.D. G. P. Putnam's Sons, Minton, Balch & Company, 2 West 45th Street, New York City, 1934. Price, $1.00.

SEX HABITS A VITAL FACTOR IN WELL-BEING—By A. Buschke, M.D., formerly professor extraordinary at the University of Berlin, and Friedrich Jacobsohn, M.D. Translated from the German by Eden and Cedar Paul, with a foreword by Gerard L. Moench, M.D., associate professor of gynecology, New York Postgraduate Hospital of Columbia University. Emerson Books, Inc., New York City, 1933. Price, $2.50.

SOCIAL INSURANCE AND ECONOMIC SECURITY—By Edward H. Ochsner, M.D., consulting surgeon, Augustana Hospital, Chicago. Bruce Humphries, Inc., Publishers, Boston, 1934. Price, $2.50.

SURGICAL CLINICS OF NORTH AMERICA—Volume xiv, No. 4, Chicago Number, August, 1934. Octavo of 288 pages with 88 illustrations. W. B. Saunders Company, Philadelphia and London, 1934. Price, paper, $12.00; cloth, $16.00.

SYNOPSIS OF GENITO-URINARY DISEASES—By Austin I. Dodson, M.D., professor of genito-urinary surgery, Medical College of Virginia, Richmond, Virginia. With 111 illustrations. C. V. Mosby Company, St. Louis, 1934. Price, $3.00.

BOOK REVIEWS

APPLIED ANATOMY

By Gwilym G. Davis, M.D., late professor of orthopedic surgery, University of Pennsylvania. Ninth edition reset, and completely revised by George P. Muller, M.D., professor of clinical surgery, Graduate School of Medicine, University of Pennsylvania. With 674 illustrations. J. B. Lippincott Company, Philadelphia and London, 1934. Price, $9.00.

The making of a surgeon requires that he be fully acquainted with the gross and minute anatomy of the body; but this knowledge of itself is not sufficient. It is also necessary for him to be able to apply this knowledge to the actual problems which arise. To fill this gap between the abstract knowledge of anatomy and its application in the operating room, the authors of this volume have prepared this excellent treatise.

By description and by well chosen illustrations the authors teach surgical principles through the medium of anatomic relations. In considering the subject, after a few general remarks on the part involved, the skeleton and muscles are briefly described, and one is thereby enabled to understand various affections of the part, with such allusions to the nerves and blood vessels as is desirable to elucidate the subject. Exemplifying this premise it is pointed out that it is not sufficient for the practicing surgeon merely to understand the anatomic relations, boundaries and attachments of the palmar fascia, but he must also appreciate very fully how these anatomic facts gov-

ern and modify infections when they arise in this position.

The entire text is written in a terse, lucid style, which invites thorough reading. The numerous, well-chosen illustrations add materially to the usefulness of the volume, making the text clearer and more readily understood. The present revision brings the volume entirely up-to-date.

THE DANGEROUS AGE IN MEN

A Treatise on the Prostate Gland, by Chester Tilton Stone, M.D., Ridgewood, New Jersey. The Macmillan Company, New York, 1934. Price, $1.75.

This treatise on the prostate gland has been written for the layman. The author discusses the anatomy and physiology of the male organs of generation, stressing the relations of the prostate to the normal sexual life of the male. He discusses infection and hypertrophy of the organ, and the concluding chapters of his work deal with prevention as obtained through a normal and satisfactory sex life, and the avoidance of those factors known to produce inflammation or hypertrophy.

If read with understanding, the volume will serve to warn men of the incipient signs of prostatic disease, and bring them under medical care at an earlier stage. The less discriminating reader may confuse prevention with the actual treatment of disease, and consequently delay seeking medical advice.

The appraisal of the value of this book involves

the time honored discussion of the advisability of attempting to educate the lay public in technical medical matters, a discussion which appears to be as unsolved as when first broached. The physician should be familiar with the volume and be guided in his recommendation of it by the intelligence and understanding of his patient.

form of presentation renders the subject matter easily available so that the volume will be found useful alike by the student or practitioner.

As a terse, authoritative and complete presentation of the theory and practice of internal medicine the volume is unexcelled and may be recommended without qualification.

DIABETIC MANUAL FOR PATIENTS

By Henry J. John, M.D., Director of the Diabetic Department and Laboratories of the Cleveland Clinic, Cleveland, Ohio. Second edition. C. V. Mosby Company, St. Louis, 1934. Price, $2.00.

With at least one million persons in the United States suffering from diabetes, it is particularly important that a non-technical guide prepared by an eminent authority should be available for their use. In the manual prepared by Dr. John we have just such a guide. The manual is written in easily understandable language, so that the patient may readily comprehend the essentials of his disease. Specific instructions are given concerning management and diet, although the author does not intend in any sense for the manual to replace the guiding hand of the physician. He very correctly states, "Any diabetic who will take the trouble to study the contents of this book will have an intelligent conception of his problem, and with this knowledge in his possession he should be making progress."

The physician unacquainted with this manual is urged to familiarize himself with its contents so that he will be in a position to give intelligent advice to his patients concerning its use. The manual is unexcelled for the purpose for which it has been written.

INTERNAL MEDICINE. ITS THEORY AND PRACTICE

Edited by John H. Musser, M.D., professor of medicine, Tulane University of Louisiana School of Medicine, Second edition, thoroughly revised. Octavo, 1296 pages, illustrated. Lea and Febiger, Washington Square, Philadelphia, 1934. Price, $10.00.

Although the first edition of this tremendously important work has been off the press only two years, apparently its success has demanded a revision and reprinting at this time. In the preparation of the second edition the editor has maintained the general form and composition of the work. By extensive revisions, and additions covering the developments in the last two years, the work is brought entirely up to date.

The distinguished group of contributors to this volume guarantees its authority, and its editorship by Dr. Musser assures thoroughness. Its paragraphic

INTERNATIONAL CLINICS

Volume iii, Forty-fourth series. Edited by Louis Hamman, M.D., visiting physician, Johns Hopkins Hospital. J. B. Lippincott Company, Philadelphia and London, 1934.

This number of the well established International Clinics contains the usual groupings of clinical cases presented by a distinguished group of clinical teachers from American universities. William Leaman, in the opening clinic, denies the existence of the "athletic heart," and proposes a prescription of exercise dependent upon a thorough and complete examination for participation in college athletics.

The second article presents a clinical lecture on the differential diagnosis of congenital cardiac disease in which the classification, mechanism, modes of examination and diagnosis of cardiac conditions are appropriately stressed.

Dr. Albert M. Snell, of the Mayo Clinic, presents the therapeutic results obtained in the treatment of forty-six patients with suprarenal cortical hormone. He views in an optimistic light the striking benefit which has been obtained in the treatment of these cases. and predicts that in this group the cortical hormone may prove as effective a remedy as insulin with the diabetic patient.

These thumbnail reviews of the first three articles in this volume are intended to create interest, since the reader is assured of an unusual treat in these, and the dozen or more articles which follow.

POSTURES AND PRACTICES DURING LABOR AMONG PRIMITIVE PEOPLES

By Julius Jarcho, M.D., New York City. With 130 illustrations. Paul B. Hoeber, Inc., New York, 1934. Price, $3.50.

In presenting this work the author makes no claim of discovery or originality. He has collected information concerning these subjects from many sources. He advances a twofold purpose in this compilation, first to improve obstetric practice in this country and second to bring together this scattered material for its anthropologic value. It is the author's belief that if the habits of the primitive races are carefully analyzed we may approach a more normal and rational posture during labor and thereby reduce the hazards and discomforts of this trying period. This thought appears to be well substantiated by the uniformity of his findings.

The first 140 pages of the text are occupied in the review of postures and practices during labor among the primitive people, whereas the concluding fifteen pages present the subject of postpartum gymnastics and exercises. Nowhere have we seen so thorough and painstaking a discussion of this important subject. While postpartum gymnastics as such apparently have but little or no relation to the major discussion in the book, it is worthwhile for these exercises to be made available to the profession. Of the 129 illustrations used in this text, many have been collected from old or obscure manuscripts.

MEDICAL CLINICS OF NORTH AMERICA

Volume xvii, No. 6. Chicago Number, Index Number. Octavo of 266 pages with 38 illustrations. W. B. Saunders Company, Philadelphia and London. Price, paper $12.00, cloth, $16.00.

This number presents the usual interesting array of case histories and discussions that one associates with this publication. It is rare indeed that one does not glean something of definite practical value from a perusal of these quarterly volumes. The present volume, while not contributing anything outstandingly new, follows the usual plan of submitting essays that are clear, concise and, for most part, practical in their subject matter and method of development of the text. They reflect the trends in medicine and contain the latest advances in diagnosis and are accompanied by rational method of treatment.

The reviewer always welcomes the Medical Clinics to his desk.   F. R. H.

SURGICAL CLINICS OF NORTH AMERICA

Volume xiv, No. 3, Mayo Clinic Number. June, 1934. Octavo of 221 pages with 70 illustrations. W. B. Saunders Comany, Philadelphia and London, 1934. Price, paper, $12.00, cloth, $16.00.

This very interesting number of the Clinics deals with rather unusual cases, such as the bicornate uterus, fracture of both internal semilunar cartilages, hypernephroma of the thyroid gland, desmoid tumor of the abdominal muscle, carcinoma of the Bartholin glands, and rectal polyps in infancy.

The use of chewing gum as a method in aiding the closure of abdominal fistulas is advocated. This method was first recommended by Dr. Macrae, of Council Bluffs. Its value is especially stressed.

Dr. John S. Lundy presents a very good article on blood transfusions.   F. W. F.

THE SPASTIC CHILD

A Record of Successfully Achieved Muscle Control in Little's Disease. By Marguerite K. Fischel. C. V. Mosby Company, St. Louis, Missouri, 1934. Price, $1.50.

Spastic paraplegia or Little's disease is characterized by well known symptoms, but little or nothing has heretofore been offered in the way of curative therapy. This highly interesting study of the spastic child is written by a mother, who with painstaking devotion personally worked out methods of treatment which in her hands were highly successful in restoring to usefulness her own child suffering from this disease.

As a human interest story of the devotion of a mother to a child the book is absorbing and well repays the reader. From the standpoint of offering definite corrective exercises and procedures it is unique. The details furnished by the author readily permit duplication of the procedures at the hands of any intelligent person.

The physician should become acquainted with this book, and it would seem highly desirable and useful to have the volume placed at the disposal of every person having to do with the management of a patient suffering from this disease.

TEST TUBE BABIES

A History of the Artificial Impregnation of Human Beings. By Dr. Herman Rohleder. The Panurge Press, 70 Fifth Avenue, New York City, 1934. Price, $3.50.

The artificial fertilization of the mammalian ovum, in the modern sense, probably dates back to the latter part of the eighteenth century, although the author of this book cites an ancient Arabic source, recounting artificial fertilization of a mare about 1322 A. D. Perfection of the method in animals occurred about the beginning of this century. Artificial impregnation of the human dates from the studies of America's distinguished pioneer gynecologist, Marion Simms, who performed this operation in 1866. During the past five to ten years a technic has been developed which, in the hands of the author, gives good results. The author claims approximately 30 per cent success with his method.

The author intelligently discusses not only the technic employed for obtaining successful results, but approaches his problem from the standpoint of religious, moral and medical ethics. Any physician contemplating the employment of a procedure of this sort is advised to familiarize himself with this book, since the completeness with which the subject is handled may prevent technical blunders, and also acquaint him with his moral and legal responsibilities in the act.

IOWA STATE MEDICAL SOCIETY OFFICERS AND COMMITTEES 1934-1935

The JOURNAL
of the
Iowa State Medical Society

| Vol. XXIV | Des Moines, Iowa, December, 1934 | No. 12 |

SOME CAUSES OF PROFESSIONAL UNREST*

R. G. Leland, M.D., Chicago, Illinois

It is a pleasure, a privilege and an honor to have been invited here to say something to you about medical economics. Medical economics, in the minds of some, is a matter solely devoted to the increase in the business of a physician, the size of his practice, and the increase in the percentage of his collections. Unfortunately, that is not the true case in medical economics as it is properly conceived. It has a much larger scope, and the purely business side of medicine is merely an incidental or subsidiary feature.

I need not tell you to what extent the general economic depression during the past few years has affected medicine. During that time, medicine has passed through a considerable amount of stress, and a decided unrest has developed in the profession. All of this unrest is not of recent origin. Some of it, I presume to say, is of our own making, and I refer particularly to contract practice.

Contract practice, with its solicitation, its advertising, underbidding and racketeering, and its commercial, competitive features, in my opinion, has spoiled more good physicians than any other one form of medical practice. It is because of the undesirable, dangerous, destructive features of contract practice that we find it among the leading causes of professional unrest today. Fortunately, however, contract practice in its entirety cannot be considered as all bad or undesirable, because there are still many communities and many conditions under which contract practice is still legitimate, necessary and ethical.

In the hospital washrooms and corridors, in physicians' offices, perhaps in medical society meetings, a great deal is being said about the abuse of clinics and hospitals by those who can afford to pay. This, again, has created another

*Presented before the Eighty-third Annual Session, Iowa State Medical Society, Des Moines, May 9, 10, 11, 1934.

element of unrest in the medical profession during these trying years.

The features which surround the administration of workmen's compensation constitute another vital problem. In many states workmen's compensation laws have been passed without the proper advice and cooperation of the medical profession. It was designed originally as a means to supply a certain amount of monetary and material relief to the workman while he was unemployed because of accident. It has become evident, and increasingly so, that medical service is the most important element in workmen's compensation, and only recently in the state of New York, where there has been a tremendous amount of friction in workmen's compensation administration, they have succeeded in drafting a bill which they hope may become a law and which is infinitely more desirable and fair to the injured workman as well as to the medical profession. There are unfair schedules in workmen's compensation. There are many rough spots in different parts of the country which must be smoothed over and adjusted by a mutual arrangement between the medical profession, the insurance carriers and the Workmen's Compensation Commissions.

I hesitate to say much about activities of health departments and boards of education after the very clear and fair presentation of the activities in Iowa by our own health commissioner and our president elect of the American Medical Association, Dr. Bierring. You do not have here the same fears, the same encroachments of health department activities on the practice of medicine, that exists in some other states. Dr. Bierring is perfectly correct in stating that it is not within the scope of health departments to practice medicine, in the sense that licensed physicians are practicing. However, in some sections, health departments have assumed the prerogative of the practice of medicine, and those activities have again increased the unrest among physicians, who see many of their patients who could pay

IOWA STATE MEDICAL SOCIETY OFFICERS AND COMMITTEES 1934-1935

President........................Gordon F. Harkness, Davenport
President-Elect................Thomas A. Burcham, Des Moines
First Vice President..................F. B. Dorsey, Jr., Keokuk
Second Vice President.................James C. Hill, Newton
Secretary........................Robert L. Parker, Des Moines
Treasurer........................Harold J. McCoy, Des Moines

COUNCILORS
Term Expires
First District—Felix A. Hennessy, Calmar.................1937
Second District—Lee R. Woodward, Mason City...........1938
Third District—Frank P. Winkler, Sibley..................1939
Fourth District—James E. Reeder, Sioux City............1935
Fifth District—William W. Pearson, Des Moines...........1936
Sixth District—Charles W. Ellyson, Waterloo..............1937
Seventh District—Arthur W. Erskine, Cedar Rapids.......1938
Eighth District—Clyde A. Boice, Washington..............1939
Ninth District—Harold A. Spilman, Ottumwa (Chairman)..1935
Tenth District—James G. Macrae, Creston.................1936
Eleventh District—M. Charles Hennessy, Council Bluffs.....1937

TRUSTEES
Oliver J. Fay, Des Moines..................................1937
John I. Marker, Davenport.................................1936
Edward M. Myers, Boone...................................1935

DELEGATES TO A. M. A.
Fred Moore, Des Moines....................................1935
T. F. Thornton, Waterloo..................................1936
V. L. Treynor, Council Bluffs..............................1956

ALTERNATE DELEGATES TO A. M. A.
N. G. Alcock, Iowa City....................................1935
R. H. Lott, Carroll..1936
F. P. McNamara, Dubuque...................................1936

EDITOR OF THE JOURNAL
Ralph R. Simmons..................................Des Moines

STANDING COMMITTEES OF THE HOUSE OF DELEGATES
ARRANGEMENTS
Gordon F. Harkness, Chairman.....................Davenport
Robert L. Parker...................................Des Moines
Harold J. McCoy ....Des Moines

CONSTITUTION AND BY-LAWS
W. R. Brock, Chairman...............................Sheldon
John H. Henkin..................................Sioux City
W. A. Sternberg...............................Mount Pleasant

FINANCE
Ernest C. McClure, Chairman...........................Bussey
Leslie L. Carr.......................................Clermont
A. S. Bowers...Orient

MEDICO-LEGAL
Frank A. Ely, Des Moines, Chairman.....................1935
George C. Albright, Iowa City..........................1936
F. Earl Bellinger, Council Bluffs........................1937

PUBLICATION COMMITTEE
Ralph R. Simmons, Editor.........................Des Moines
Robert L. Parker, Secretary......................Des Moines
Oliver J. Fay, Trustee...........................Des Moines
John I. Marker, Trustee...........................Davenport
Edward M. Myers, Trustee.............................Boone

PUBLIC POLICY AND LEGISLATION
Fred Moore, Chairman..............................Des Moines
R. D. Bernard.......................................Clarion
Peter A. Bendixen.................................Davenport
Gordon F. Harkness................................Davenport
Robert L. Parker..................................Des Moines

SCIENTIFIC WORK
Gordon F. Harkness................................Davenport
Thomas A. Burcham................................Des Moines
Robert L. Parker..................................Des Moines
Harold J. McCoy..................................Des Moines

MEDICAL EDUCATION AND HOSPITALS
Arthur W. Erskine, Chairman....................Cedar Rapids
T. J. Irish......................................Forest City
B. J. Dierker....................................Fort Madison

SPECIAL COMMITTEES OF THE HOUSE OF DELEGATES
COMMITTEE ON CHILD HEALTH AND PROTECTION
R. H. McBride, Chairman...........................Sioux City
E. D. Plass.......................................Iowa City
H. E. Farnsworth.................................Storm Lake
Lee F. Hill.......................................Des Moines
James F. Gerken.....................................Waterloo

HISTORICAL
Walter L. Bierring, Chairman.......................Des Moines
Frank M. Fuller.....................................Keokuk
T. B. Throckmorton ....Des Moines
John T. McClintock.................................Iowa City
Henry B. Young...................................Burlington
William Jepson....................................Sioux City

MEDICAL ECONOMICS
T. F. Thornton, Chairman...........................Waterloo
James C. Hill..Newton
James C. Donahue.................................Centerville

MEDICAL LIBRARY
Con R. Harken, Chairman............................Osceola
H. A. Tolliver...................................Charles City
Jeannette Dean-Throckmorton ....Des Moines

MILITARY AFFAIRS
T. F. Suchomel, Chairman.......................Cedar Rapids
Harold A. Spilman..................................Ottumwa
Arnold L. Jensen...............................Council Bluffs

WOMAN'S AUXILIARY ADVISORY COMMITTEE
Aldis A. Johnson, Chairman.....................Council Bluffs
W. E. Baker......................................Des Moines
Charles F. Snopek....................................Cresco
W. T. Peters...Burt
T. J. Wigim..Muscatine

STANDING COMMITTEE OF THE COUNCIL
SPEAKERS BUREAU COMMITTEE
Daniel J. Glomset, Chairman.......................Des Moines
Felix A. Hennessy....................................Calmar
L. C. Kern..Waverly
Harold L. Brereton................................Emmetsburg
Sydner D. Maiden...............................Council Bluffs

The JOURNAL

of the

Iowa State Medical Society

VOL. XXIV   DES MOINES, IOWA, DECEMBER, 1934   No. 12

SOME CAUSES OF PROFESSIONAL UNREST*

R. G. LELAND, M.D., Chicago, Illinois

It is a pleasure, a privilege and an honor to have been invited here to say something to you about medical economics. Medical economics, in the minds of some, is a matter solely devoted to the increase in the business of a physician, the size of his practice, and the increase in the percentage of his collections. Unfortunately, that is not the true case in medical economics as it is properly conceived. It has a much larger scope, and the purely business side of medicine is merely an incidental or subsidiary feature.

I need not tell you to what extent the general economic depression during the past few years has affected medicine. During that time, medicine has passed through a considerable amount of stress, and a decided unrest has developed in the profession. All of this unrest is not of recent origin. Some of it, I presume to say, is of our own making, and I refer particularly to contract practice.

Contract practice, with its solicitation, its advertising, underbidding and racketeering, and its commercial, competitive features, in my opinion, has spoiled more good physicians than any other one form of medical practice. It is because of the undesirable, dangerous, destructive features of contract practice that we find it among the leading causes of professional unrest today. Fortunately, however, contract practice in its entirety cannot be considered as all bad or undesirable, because there are still many communities and many conditions under which contract practice is still legitimate, necessary and ethical.

In the hospital washrooms and corridors, in physicians' offices, perhaps in medical society meetings, a great deal is being said about the abuse of clinics and hospitals by those who can afford to pay. This, again, has created another

*Presented before the Eighty-third Annual Session, Iowa State Medical Society, Des Moines, May 9, 10, 11, 1934.

element of unrest in the medical profession during these trying years.

The features which surround the administration of workmen's compensation constitute another vital problem. In many states workmen's compensation laws have been passed without the proper advice and cooperation of the medical profession. It was designed originally as a means to supply a certain amount of monetary and material relief to the workman while he was unemployed because of accident. It has become evident, and increasingly so, that medical service is the most important element in workmen's compensation, and only recently in the state of New York, where there has been a tremendous amount of friction in workmen's compensation administration, they have succeeded in drafting a bill which they hope may become a law and which is infinitely more desirable and fair to the injured workman as well as to the medical profession. There are unfair schedules in workmen's compensation. There are many rough spots in different parts of the country which must be smoothed over and adjusted by a mutual arrangement between the medical profession, the insurance carriers and the Workmen's Compensation Commissions.

I hesitate to say much about activities of health departments and boards of education after the very clear and fair presentation of the activities in Iowa by our own health commissioner and our president elect of the American Medical Association, Dr. Bierring. You do not have here the same fears, the same encroachments of health department activities on the practice of medicine, that exists in some other states. Dr. Bierring is perfectly correct in stating that it is not within the scope of health departments to practice medicine, in the sense that licensed physicians are practicing. However, in some sections, health departments have assumed the prerogative of the practice of medicine, and those activities have again increased the unrest among physicians, who see many of their patients who could pay a fee, go to the health department clinic for immunizations, and for all kinds of examinations and advice. Maternity care, prenatal care, care of well babies, and so forth, have been taken over in many places by health departments. Similar things can be said of board of education health activities. These are legitimate fields which ought to be reserved for the general practitioner and the specialist. Immunization of children, periodic health examinations, examination of food handlers, and so on, are all legitimate fields for the general practice of medicine, in which the medical profession, health departments, and boards of education ought to coordinate and correlate their activities.

Another large endeavor on the part of county medical societies has been in the field of the care of the indigent. Here in Iowa you have what is known throughout the country as the so-called Iowa Plan. You have made much greater progress in a more modern method of caring for the indigent than has been made in many other sections of the country. However, you, as others, know of the old, traditional spoils system of appointing the poor physician by political preferment or by individual competitive bidding. The work is not all done by these physicians who are thus appointed. The work must be done, in a large part, by the practicing physicians who do not have any part in the income derived from such service.

During the last few years, chiefly the last year and one-half or two years, there has developed a large number of artificial, lay controlled, lay devised, lay operated, and lay promoted schemes for hospitalization and the administration of medical care on a monthly or annual prepayment basis. These schemes have been promoted largely, or were at least originated by laymen because they saw in medical and hospital service a commodity that could be easily sold, that was necessary to most people some time in their life, and they grasped that commodity, if we can call it such, with the hope of making a profit for themselves out of a necessity—medical service. About fifty or more group hospitalization plans have been developed throughout the various sections of the country. We ought to be fair by saying that group hospitalization, although a form of health insurance, has some virtue in it. It is difficult or almost impossible to advance a legitimate argument against the theory of sickness insurance but the objections which we have raised to sickness insurance are not on the basis of theory; they are on the basis of the methods used in administering the provisions of sickness insurance, and these people who have promoted the schemes for group hospitalization have said that, as soon as they secure a sufficiently large section of the hospital

market, they intend to add medical service to group hospitalization contracts. They say nothing about the amount that the physician is to receive for his services in rendering medical care as well as the hospital for hospital care.

There seems to be a growing anxiety over sickness insurance. Already there is a tendency toward sickness insurance in certain sections of these United States. The entire state of Washington has been organized into what they call medical service bureaus which are essentially sickness insurance organizations giving medical service to certain sections of the population, mainly industrial groups of a certain income level. In the state of Oregon there has been, for many years, a law which provides for the certification and registration of hospital associations, which are misnomers but are essentially the same as the medical service bureaus in Washington.

In California a committee of the state legislature and a committee of the California Medical Association has been working for the last year and one-half to determine the necessity for sickness insurance in that state. It is presumed that at the next session of the legislature, which meets in January, 1935, a sickness insurance act for California will be presented for passage or consideration. Michigan has already made a very extensive study, and a committee of the state society has presented for consideration of the House of Delegates a plan of sickness insurance for that state. This plan has not been accepted yet, but if it is accepted, that plan of sickness insurance will be placed in operation in two or three counties in Michigan.

More insidious and more dangerous to the future of medicine, is a proposal that comes from New York, sponsored and presented by one of the great foundations of this country, the Milbank Foundation. This proposal comes as a plan to socialize or sovietize medicine in New York. If successful there, it would be an easy and a logical development to proceed westward, and no one can predict how fast, how far or how extensive it would proceed.

All of these attempts to mechanize, to socialize, or to sovietize medicine are perhaps the strongest of the disturbing elements to physicians today. It is hard to tell just exactly what might happen were such an event to occur in these United States; but I can state truthfully that I see some comfort in the fact that I believe the American people desire their own physicians. They do not want the kind of medicine that is dealt out mechanically. They do not realize as well as we do what the mechanization and sovietization of medicine means to them, but it is for us, the physicians of these

United States who, by tradition, training, experience, and ability, know what happens to the quality of medical care when socialization of medicine takes place, to point out how the quality of care deteriorates under such a system. This deterioration has taken place in all the sickness insurance systems of Europe, perhaps to the least extent under the system that is in vogue in Great Britain. We find, therefore, that this attempt to develop state medicine, or sickness insurance, is another of the disturbing elements.

During the last few years there has been an increased pressure on the medical profession for free services. I need not discuss that with you because you know in your own practice the extent to which free service pressure has been placed upon you. There have been some medical institutions, and I speak particularly of hospitals, that have sought relief for their financial conditions under the guise of having given a considerable amount of service to the indigent or low income groups of the population. The issue in this case is greatly confused. Many hospitals have been overbuilt and have placed in their corridors, their operating rooms, and their sick rooms, an inordinate amount of expensive, unnecessary equipment. Now that times are not so good, it becomes necessary for those hospitals to meet interest on bonded indebtedness and to make payments on principal. Under the guise of giving the people in the community, something, they say, "We will adopt a group hospitalization plan and give you so many days' hospital care a year for so much money." I am sorry that the monetary gain seems to be uppermost, in many instances, rather than the service that the hospital can render to the public. The two questions are quite distinct and separate. Hospitals should raise the amount necessary to meet their financial obligations by some other way than by urging the poor and the low income group people to carry a portion of the hospital debt retirement program.

It seems to me that the effects of all of these disturbing elements ought to be fairly clear. One of the first effects should be the creation of a strong, united effort on the part of the medical profession to resist all of these socialization efforts and to maintain, as rigidly as possible, the quality of medical service. We do not deny that there may be some weaknesses in the method used for the practice of medicine today, but is it necessary that the entire structure of medicine be destroyed, that the method of practicing medicine in the United States be overturned, in order that we correct certain minor deficiencies which exist here and there? Moreover, these deficiencies do not exist to the same extent in every part of the United

States, and, therefore, the problem becomes one of local interest, local importance and local responsibility.

During these recent years it has been necessary to define the principles underlying medical economics and the American Medical Association has prepared for the use of medical societies in study groups and for students in medical schools as well, a pamphlet called "An Introduction to Medical Economics," in which we seek to set forth the principles which underlie the economics of the practice of medicine as contrasted to the principles which underlie the economics of business, commerce and industry. These years, it seems to me, have emphasized the worth of the principles of the ethics of the American medical profession. These principles of ethics are said to have come from Hippocrates; but their origin is immaterial. The content of those principles is the important thing. There are individuals in this country, even some in the medical profession, who would have us restate those principles, for the purpose of making respectable anything that these people choose to do, whether it be some shady contract practice arrangement, fee-splitting, or some other type of medical performance that is not as honorable as it ought to be. All of this would be for personal advantage, personal aggrandizement or monetary gain.

I submit to you that it is impossible for us as a medical profession, having the tradition that we do, to change these principles of medical ethics in any such manner. The principles of ethics were designed for the honorable conduct of individuals who practice medicine. As such, those principles ought to be applicable to groups as well as to individuals. They ought to be equally good for county medical societies and state medical societies in the conduct of their members. Therefore, I say again that it is unthinkable that we should detract from these principles as they exist today.

What shall be the solution of all this confusion in the practice of medicine? The solution lies, it seems to me, with the medical profession rather than with outsiders who would meddle with, who would think for, who would plan for, and who would speak for the medical profession. Certainly there is enough competence in the medical profession to solve its own problems. I venture to say that one of the first things to do is to see that our own members conduct themselves as honest, honorable, ethical physicians. If that were done, much of the disturbance, unrest and annoyances confronting medicine today would disappear. I dare say that many of the malpractice suits would be avoided. However, more than that is required. Now, as never before, it is necessary for the medical profession to make its own studies. We must not take too seriously some of the results that have been handed to us by other groups interested in and studying medical economics. I refer specifically to some of the reports of the Committee on the Costs of Medical Care. I cannot refrain from calling your attention to some of the things that were done and some of the things that were not done.

The Committee on the Costs of Medical Care, after working about five years, at a cost of more than $900,000, did not study workmen's compensation in this country, even though this phase of our industrial life involves $72,000,000 annually for medical services, and more than 80,000,000 accidents annually, 3,000,000 of which are so important as to require compensation. This committee did not study contract practice in its entirety. It did select a few examples to substantiate certain points that it wished to prove but it did not study an adequate cross-section of the seven hundred odd contract practice plans that are in operation or that have been proposed in these United States. The Committee on the Costs of Medical Care did not study sickness insurance. It remained for the dental profession to send a commission to Europe to study health insurance. This committee did not adequately study group practice. It found about one hundred and fifty groups in these United States, whereas in the study made by the American Medical Association we found more than seven hundred. This committee did not adequately study university student health service. It gave a description of about six of the student health services in various sections of the United States. At present we are making a study of 300 of such services. One of the things which the Committee on the Costs of Medical Care did do was to study very carefully the morbidity rates throughout the United States in various industries and businesses, but the measure which they used was an economic measure of morbidity and not a pathologic measure of morbidity. Every practitioner here has seen many patients who have stayed at home, have missed a day from the office or the factory or the shop, who have very little, if any, pathologic cause for their absence from work, and many are the school children who stay home because of some clever way of influencing dad or mother, not because of any actual pathologic condition which could be considered a measure of morbidity. Therefore, I say to you that the measure of morbidity used by the Committee on the Costs of Medical Care in certain instances is a false measure, because it is an economic one and not a pathologic one.

It seems to me that the necessity for careful, honest study of medical economics problems ought to be obvious to every thinking physician, physician's wife, nurse, or anyone who is closely allied to the practice of medicine. I would suggest that the medical profession scrutinize with the greatest amount of care, any proposal, plan, or scheme that comes from outside the medical profession, and even some of them that come from within the medical profession. Certainly, you ought to use the same amount of care, and critical analysis that you apply to the use of new methods in diagnosis and new remedies for treatment.

The method of study which I believe is worthy of use by the medical profession is chiefly an attitude of mind which involves complete honesty and absolute thoroughness to get the facts in the matter; it involves a mind which is free from preconceptions; it involves a mind free from prejudice; it involves a mind which is free from bias. The study should be devoid of antagonisms. Personalities should be omitted. We cannot deal successfully, honestly and fairly with medical economics problems if we bring in personalities and discuss people rather than facts. Then, too, we should not have in our minds any idea of personal aggrandizement or personal gain in any of the studies that are made by the medical profession on medical economics.

It has been suggested by some that the American Medical Association should bring forth a master plan that can be used by all states and all sections of the country, to solve all the economics ills of the medical profession, but I submit to you, again, that this procedure would not be possible or practical, because medical practice in Iowa is not the same as it is in New York. Conditions are not the same in Maine as they are in Louisiana, or California. I believe that we as an American people, accustomed as we are to a democratic form of government, should resist an interference with what we term state's rights in the practice of medicine and in the solution of medical economics problems in some such manner as we do with state's rights in other matters. Therefore, whatever is done to correct some of the medical economics ills, wherever they are found, should be undertaken by the local, the county and the state medical associations.

Why should we do all this? We should do it to make good medical service available for an amount which people can afford to pay, as physicians have always done. There is nothing new about it; there is nothing revolutionary about it; there is nothing destructive about it. Physicians have always had what is termed a sliding scale of fees.

To be sure, we have had our county medical society fee schedules and we have had a customary charge; but physicians have always chosen to take care of certain people free of charge, and that should be their prerogative. That is a thing which should not be taken away from medicine by socialization, by state medicine, or by any kind of regimentation. Another reason for action is to maintain the primary objective of organized medicine —the welfare of the public. In this little book which we may call the bible of the medical profession, the principles of medical ethics, from Chapter I, Section 1, I quote. "A profession has for its prime objective the service it can render to humanity. Reward or financial gain should be a subordinate consideration. The practice of medicine is a profession. In choosing this profession, an individual assumes an obligation to conduct himself in accord with its ideals." One of the ideals of the medical profession is to advance the science of medicine and to promote the public health. Nothing is said in that quotation of financial reward. Unfortunately, there are a few who, in their avarice and greed have attempted to collect or have collected enormous fees. Those are few indeed, but the few are taken as an example by those who wish to criticize the medical profession, and the majority suffers from the acts of those few. Rather be it that we place our primary emphasis on the welfare of the public and the quality of medical care. A third item is to enable physicians to compete on a professional rather than a commercial basis. Contract practice introduced the commercial competitive basis of the practice of medicine. Under those conditions, physicians are not allowed to place uppermost and foremost their ability to diagnose and to treat disease. They compete on a commercial basis, on a basis of doing a certain amount of work for a certain sum, and if they are not successful, one of their competitors is awarded the contract the next year, because he will do it cheaper per piece than they. The following year, they strike back at the competitor by offering to do the same work for less money or to do more for the same money. We have had an example in the last year of business and industry and commerce following the example of the traditional medical ethics in an attempt to adopt codes of fair competition, and I suspect the idea for those codes may have been borrowed from the medical profession.

Medicine should be preserved as a profession. Unless the profession resists unnecessary change with all its vigor and strength, it is difficult to say just when some of these socialization efforts may affect medicine very undesirably. This change will not only affect the income of physicians, but it will affect very materially the quality of care that the public receives.

Unfortunately, all of these disturbing influences are not outside the medical profession. I have suspected for some time, and I now have some evidence, that there are a few within the medical profession who would sell out the medical profession for a mess of pottage. There is a group of physicians, about 500 in number, who constitute the League for Socialized Medicine in Brooklyn. There are physicians here and there, a few, who would sell out their own societies for a certain consideration. We must watch for these people. The promotion of socialization schemes is being furthered by the action and the attitude of some of these physicians.

One of the major tasks, however, of the medical profession is to unite physicians in a strong resistance against a common foe, not solely for the sake of professional gain, but primarily to preserve that type of medical care which is best for the public. If we keep uppermost in our minds the fact that we as physicians have a tradition, that we as physicians have an obligation to society, that we have always enjoyed a freedom for research, that we are the only ones who are capable, by reason of training, experience, and licensure to pass upon medical problems, then it seems to me it ought to be clear that the medical men throughout these United States should unite to keep medicine as a profession and to deliver the best medical care possible to the people of the United States.

THE VALUE OF RESECTION OF THE PRESACRAL NERVE

Walter D. Abbott, M.D., Des Moines

It is the purpose of this paper to present the indications for resection of the presacral nerve (hypogastric plexus) in certain bladder, pelvic and bowel disturbances, and to discuss the merits of this procedure.

HISTORY

This operation is not new, since Jaboulay in 1898, performed section of the sacral sympathetic chain by a retrorectal approach for pelvic neuralgia, megacolon and vesical disorders. A year later, Ruggi published his work on abdominal sympathectomy in functional disorders of the female pelvis. Leriche in 1921, introduced periarterial sympathectomy of the iliac arteries for severe dysmenorrhea, and in 1925, Cotte discovered that section of the presacral nerve afforded complete relief in this condition. Since then, Cotte has performed this operation in over two hundred cases with excellent results in various pelvic disorders. Herman is believed to have been the first American surgeon to resect the presacral nerve for dysmenorrhea. In 1930, Learmonth and Braasch published the first beneficial result of this procedure in the treatment of cord bladder, and two years later Fontaine and Herrmann reported twenty-eight cases of pelvic plexalgia in which twenty-two patients were relieved by resection of the presacral nerve.

Last year, the author presented a case of neurogenic imbalance of the pelvic organs in which resection of the presacral nerve reëstablished normal function with relief of dymenorrhea. Recently, DeCourcy has reported twenty-one cases of dysmenorrhea in which the postoperative results have been very gratifying and concludes as follows: "This offers a means of aiding a large class of women who must otherwise suffer a monthly martyrdom and be compelled to drag out the greater part of their time in partial disability with a general lowering of physical and mental efficiency."

ANATOMY

The presacral nerve, hypogastric plexus, is part of the prevertebral sympathetic chain originating from the inferior mesenteric ganglion. I have observed branches from the lumbar chain. The branches pass obliquely down on the left side while the branches from the right side pass posterior to the inferior mesenteric artery. There are usually many fine anastomoses between these nerves so that a true plexus is formed. This plexus is situated anterior to the bifurcation of the aorta and is separated from it by a thin layer of fascia. The plexus then follows the curve of the sacrum into the pelvis. Anteriorly, the plexus is covered by a thin layer of loose connective tissue and parietal peritoneum while the root of the mesentery of the colon is situated to the left. From this space, the hypogastric nerves extend into the superior and posterior corner of the hypogastric ganglion which lies external to and below the ureterosacral ligaments. The plexus also received anterior branches from the second and third sacral nerves and branches from the sacral sympathetic ganglia. It has been stated by some authors that section of the afferent fibers of these branches will abolish the power of erection in the male and cause disturbance of sphincter control of bowel and bladder in both sexes. This, however, has not taken place in any of my cases, although catheterization has been necessary for a few days after the operation in some instances.

DYSMENORRHEA

The term dysmenorrhea or difficult menstruation should apply only to the cases of painful men-struation where no pathologic process can be demonstrated. It is known that marriage and subsequent pregnancy will frequently abolish the greater part of this distress; also, the psychogenic factor must not be ignored and often a mechanical dilatation of the cervix will afford relief. However, there are certain cases in which painful menstruation is so severe that it remains adamant to any therapeutic procedure, and in this type of case resection of the presacral nerve is indicated.

Case. 1. An unmarried woman, twenty years of age, had suffered from severe dysmenorrhea until pain had become almost constant. Roentgen therapy and curettage had failed to afford relief. The examination was negative except for a suggestive small mass in the right lower abdominal quadrant and tenderness over the sacro-iliac region. Roentgenograms revealed a developmental defect of the coccyx but this was not considered to be an important factor. There was also a leukorrhea. On June 5, 1933, a curettment was performed and a small amount of reddish deciduous material was removed. Then a laparotomy was performed and the right ovary, which measured 5x2x1.5 cm. and contained a few cysts was removed. It was felt that there was hardly enough pathologic change to cause such intense pain, so I resected the presacral nerve. The patient made an uneventful recovery and has been free from any menstrual or abdominal distress since the operation. The sacro-iliac distress was alleviated to a marked extent with a corrective belt.

Although there were some organic changes, it was felt that resection of the nerve in this case was of distinct benefit.

Case 2. An unmarried woman, twenty-seven years of age, had suffered from severe dysmenorrhea since puberty, but in the past year the pain had become so severe that she was incapacitated for seven to ten days each month. In addition, she had suffered from a constant dull ache in both lower abdominal quadrants for almost a year. Examination was essentially negative except for tenderness in both lower abdominal quadrants. On May 15, 1934, under avertin anesthesia, laparotomy was performed and the pelvic organs were found to be normal in size and appearance. The presacral nerve was resected and the patient made an uneventful recovery. When seen August 2, 1934, the patient stated that the menses had been painless and that the dull abdominal pain had completely disappeared.

This case is illustrative of a severe dysmenorrhea with what Fontaine and Herrmann called a pelvic plexalgia. The above cases are the type that should be selected for surgical intervention.

BLADDER DYSFUNCTION

There have been many reports of excellent results in cord bladder and painful bladder conditions. It has been my experience that careful selection is warranted in this type of case and that very few cases of cord bladder are relieved to the extent that surgery of this type is justified. The purpose in cord bladder cases is to relieve the inhibition to the emptying of the bladder so that the patient will not be condemned to a life where catheterization is always necessary. Thus the best that can be hoped for in cord bladder conditions is a relief from a large amount of residual urine.

The following case is perhaps the most gratifying in my series of cord bladder with retention. Such results are far from encouraging and I am of the opinion that presacral section is of little value in this type of case.

Case 3. An unmarried man, forty years of age, had contracted lues eight years ago and received very little treatment. Four years ago, he developed a tabes dorsalis with incontinence of the bladder. One year ago, cystotomy had been performed for acute retention of urine. The wound healed with great difficulty and would occasionally break open. On April 12, 1934, resection of the presacral nerve was performed because of distress in the bladder region and a residual of 400 c.c. of urine in twelve hours. Following the operation, the patient had less discomfort, but still carried a residual of 120 c.c. per twenty-four hours. This condition has persisted to the present time.

However, there are certain cases of painful and poorly functioning bladders, where the nerve supply is not destroyed by disease, in which resection of the presacral nerve will afford definite relief.

Case 4. An unmarried woman, twenty years of age, complained of an inability to void or defecate unless massive doses of castor oil were taken. The bladder and bowel would empty every four days and this was associated with severe pain. This condition had persisted for two years and was also associated with a severe dysmenorrhea. The past history was negative except that the menses did not appear until she was eighteen and that for two years she suffered from blanching, discoloration and pain in both feet when exposed to the cold or emotional stress. Examinations were negative except for an atonic bladder and colon, and the presence of Raynaud's disease of the lower extremities. The patient was not considered to be suffering from hysteria and the presence of Raynaud's disease, seemed to indicate an autonomic imbalance. On October 21, 1932, a lap-

arotomy was performed under anesthesia, and the presacral nerve and both lumbar sympathetic ganglia were removed. Immediately after operation, the lower extremities were warm, dry and pink. Four hours after the operation, the patient voided 150 c.c. of urine with no difficulty. It was necessary to administer enemas for seven days before a spontaneous bowel movement occurred with the aid of mineral oil. However, the patient was able to void three and four times daily after the operation. On the fifth postoperative day, the menses appeared with no distress. Since dismissal from the hospital, the patient has been able to void three and four times daily, and there has been a daily bowel movement without pain. The feet have remained warm and pink, and the menses have been practically painless.

The above case is illustrative of the relief obtained in an imbalance of the neurogenic apparatus of the pelvic organs. It is obvious that such cases will receive distinct benefit from sympathectomy if careful discrimination is used in selecting each case.

BOWEL DYSFUNCTION

The same physiology is applied in cases of spastic constipation as in vesical disorders, and in certain cases resection of the presacral nerve is of value. However, there is no type of case in which deliberate judgment is so essential as in the individual with a faulty nervous mechanism who suffers from constipation. It is a well known fact that many neurotic patients unduly center their attention upon the colon and its functions. The following cases will illustrate the pitfalls of a proper selection of cases for surgery.

Case 5. An unmarried woman, twenty-eight years of age, was first seen in January, 1933, because of a right Bell's palsy, general nervous exhaustion and chronic constipation. No focus of infection could be detected and means were instituted to placate the nervous instability and the patient was placed upon a rigid anti-constipation regimen. This patient also stated that each menstrual period was associated with moderately severe pain for four days. In three months, the Bell's palsy had cleared, but the constipation remained resistant to any form of treatment. Her past history had been negative except for peritonitis following a rupture of the appendix. It was feared that adhesions had formed which might have exerted a mechanical influence against the normal evacuation of the bowels, but roentgenograms of the intestinal tract were negative for evidence of pathology. On July 25, 1933, under avertin anesthesia, a laparotomy was performed and many dense adhesions of the pelvis were found. The sigmoid was kinked behind the left ovary and was densely adherent to the ovary and tube. A small cyst was found on the right ovary and this was punctured. The presacral nerve was then removed. The patient made an uneventful recovery and on the fifth postoperative day the menses appeared with no distress. Since the operation, the bowels have moved daily although it is necessary for the patient to take a small amount of mineral oil. Her general health has improved and she has been free from dysmenorrhea.

This case is rather difficult to classify and resection of the presacral nerve cannot be entirely responsible for the relief of constipation because of the mechanical influence which was demonstrated at operation.

Case 6. An unmarried woman, thirty-four years of age, was first seen in March, 1932, because of a bizarre facial neuralgia, multiple complaints, nervous instability and chronic constipation. Her past history was negative except for many nervous complaints which she attributed to family and financial burdens. Examination was negative and she was placed upon an anti-constipation regimen which was supplemented with efforts to help her regain her nervous stability. In December, 1933, this patient had much difficulty with constipation and as drastic cathartics had failed to relieve her, it was felt that resection of the presacral nerve would be justified. This was performed under avertin anesthesia on December 28, 1933. She made an uneventful recovery and until March the bowels had moved daily with no distress. However, since then it has been necessary to administer rather large doses of mineral oil to produce a daily evacuation.

In retrospect, it is my opinion that this patient has received only partial benefit from surgery. This case is indicative of the poor sufferer with a general instability of the central and sympathetic nervous systems and sounds a note of warning against operation unless of utmost necessity.

Case 7. An unmarried male, twenty-eight years of age, was first seen in February, 1934, because of headaches, vertigo, nervousness and chronic constipation. His past history was negative except for a tendency to assume the burdens of life too seriously and to be very introspective. He had suffered from severe constipation for years and would go as long as six days before a bowel movement would occur with the aid of drastic cathartics. Repeated enemas would often fail to empty the bowel satisfactorily. General and neurologic examinations, including spinal fluid, were negative except for the colon which was moderately dilated and emptied slowly. On April 25,

1934, under avertin anesthesia, the presacral nerve was resected and, with the exception of a few nervous upsets, recovery was uneventful. The bowels moved daily with no difficulty until August 1, 1934. At this time, the patient developed an acute retention of urine. The urologist's report revealed no evidence of a pathologic process, and the patient was believed to be suffering from hysteria because of the necessity of assuming a few irksome duties. The bowels have occasionally failed to move for one day, but a small dose of mineral oil corrected any distress.

This case shows again the importance of evaluating the mental poise of the individual. Undoubtedly there has been some benefit from presacral resection in the last two cases, but there is a question as to the advisability of submitting this type of person to any operative procedure where only a small amount of inhibition can be removed.

SUMMARY

Resection of the presacral nerve (hypogastric plexus) is of value in certain vesical, bowel and pelvic disorders where no underlying pathologic process, general or neurologic, can be demonstrated. However, it is of utmost importance to select each case with care and with full appreciation of the functional disorders of the nervous system.

BORDERLINE PSYCHOSES*
A PROBLEM IN DIFFERENTIAL DIAGNOSIS
William Malamud, M.D., Iowa City

It is a well known and logically conceivable fact that the difficulties in diagnosis become progressively greater as we move away from the typical textbook picture of disease syndromes toward the periphery where they begin to approach and tend to merge with other related entities. These difficulties, however, gain special emphasis when we realize that it is in this borderland that the correctness of diagnosis is of particular importance. The fact is that here we deal with the undifferentiated and, most usually, incipient forms of disease, and the diagnosis will necessarily determine the method of treatment and the prognosis which in these cases is probably of much more far-reaching importance than it is in the well established and usually hopeless cases. If this be true of all branches of medicine, it is particularly so of psychiatry, especially where the situation involves a decision as to whether a patient is psychotic or not. The diagnosis of psychosis implies more than the diagnosis of any other disease. It commits us not only to a certain form of treatment

* Presented before the Eighty-third Annual Session, Iowa State Medical Society, Des Moines, May 9, 10, 11, 1934.

and prognosis, but it includes all the other complexities which accompany the concept of insanity. In the first place we have to consider the management of the case, that is to say, whether because of possible danger that the condition may bring with it either to the patient himself or to the others around him, some form of supervision or confinement in a specially equipped institution should be recommended. Then we may have to consider the question of responsibility of the actions of the patient, the possibility of hereditary transmission of the diseases, and a number of other points which are usually not considered to be of importance in the diagnosis of other forms of diseases. All of these factors make it doubly important in such cases to be certain of the diagnosis.

It is also true that the difficulties in differential diagnosis are greater in this field than in any other. In the first place, in most psychoses the symptoms that are to be used in arriving at a diagnosis are usually obtained through the observation of the behavior of the patient and verbal communication with him. Our knowledge of whether a person has hallucinations or delusions, whether he is depressed or elated, or has numerous other symptoms, depends primarily upon the willingness of the patient to communicate to us the existence of these symptoms; but it is not always easy to obtain these communications from him. In some cases we find that the patient refuses to commit himself; in others we meet with the still more difficult situation in which the patient actually confabulates in these communications. The behavior of the patient as well as his communications, which are fairly easy to judge in the cases of typical psychoses where the person is deteriorated and even if he attempts to mislead us these attempts are so childish and transparent that we can see through them, become much more problematic in the borderline cases where the intellectual faculties of the patient are usually well preserved. Given a moderate degree of acting ability, it is fairly easy for the person to cover up the symptoms and leave us in the dark as to their existence. Secondly, it is a well known fact that psychotic symptoms may be observed in rudiment in non-psychotic individuals. A certain amount of suspiciousness, a moderate degree of mood swings, an occasional misinterpretation of other person's activities, are present in a great many people, and do not necessarily mean that these people are insane. On the other hand, they are just as frequently found in the early stages of certain psychoses. In making the diagnosis then we cannot depend upon the quality of the symptoms, but we must judge them by their degree. Finally, the

number of conditions which may be confused with psychoses is so numerous and variable that even the specialist in psychiatry may have difficulty in thinking of all of them when he attempts to make a differential diagnosis.

From the viewpoint of differential diagnosis, the last point mentioned is, of course, the most important one, and it will be best to approach the whole problem by a consideration of the different forms of human behavior as the psychiatrist sees them. To begin with, we can consider two large groups: first, the mentally normal; and secondly, the mentally abnormal types of behavior. Under the first of these two groups we can place all forms of average adjustment wherein we include not only healthy persons but those who may have some physical disease but do not present any abnormality in their mental activities. The second group would include the following subdivisions: first, congenital abnormalities, in which we would include the psychopathies and mentally defective persons; and second, mental diseases proper, in which we would include the psychoneuroses and the psychoses. In order to be able to appreciate the possible criteria that we can use in differentiating the psychoses (the last group) from all the other forms of human behavior or adjustment, it will be necessary to attempt the definition of each of these forms of behavior, and on the basis of these definitions to try to establish some system of differentiation. It must be emphasized, however, that it is not always possible to draw absolute lines of demarcation between these five entities. The definitions will necessarily remain arbitrary and can be stated as follows:

1. *Average normal behavior,* meaning that which in contrast to the abnormal leads to no obviously serious disturbances in adjustment either within the individual himself or between the individual and the outside world.

2. *Psychopathic personalities* are individuals in whom a constitutional psychic defect other than purely intellectual leads to a disturbance in their adjustment.

3. *Mental defective patients* are individuals in whom we find a constitutional defect in intelligence pronounced enough to lead to a disturbance in their adjustment.

4. *Psychoneuroses* are mental diseases that develop in persons who previous to onset of the disease have not shown any obvious difficulties in adjustment, where we can find no demonstrable organic pathology, where there are no primary disturbances in mood, and where a proper reality appreciation of the outside has been preserved.

5. *Psychoses* are mental diseases which develop at some stage in the life of the patient where there

may or may not be organic disease of the brain, and which show either a disturbance of mood, a disturbed appreciation of outside reality, or intellectual deterioration.

Since in this discussion we are primarily interested in the differential diagnosis of this last group, that is, the psychoses, we can proceed here by taking this last group as the central point. If we do so, we will find that the other four groups may converge upon this central point, and where they come in contact with it we will have manifestations of cases that may be designated as borderline. The difficulties that arise in our attempts to diagnose these borderline cases and the criteria which may be established in relation to these difficulties will probably be best appreciated on the basis of a series of pertinent cases. Conceivably we will deal here with two diagnostic dangers: first, the diagnosis of cases belonging to any one of the first four groups as psychotic; and second, the diagnosis of cases belonging to the fifth group as non-psychotic. To illustrate these possibilities let us quote the following examples:

1. A person who has grown up under the influence of a religiously fanatic and naively superstitious group and who does not possess particularly high critical abilities, develops a state of religious excitement following a revival meeting. He believes himself to be in contact with spiritual forces, he talks about receiving messages from these forces, and says that he is destined to perform some special religious mission. On the face of it these false beliefs and convictions are not unlike the delusions of a mentally diseased person, but when we take into consideration the fact that they were actually developed on the basis of a certain type of upbringing within a rather special social group and have been accepted under the influence of strong suggestion at the revival meeting, we see that this form of behavior really falls within the limits of the normal. Panic reactions, mob hysteria, and other forms of abnormal behavior induced by unusually strong suggestive circumstances also belong to this group.

2. A girl of sixteen who comes from a secluded mountain district in central Europe is said to believe that she can carry on conversation with the farm animals and receive messages through them from her mother who died when the girl was an infant. At the first examination these beliefs and experiences strongly suggested the imaginations of a psychotic person. Further examination, however, showed this preliminary diagnosis to be wrong. The intelligence examination showed her to be feebleminded. In addition to this it was found that she had always been neglected and maltreated and ever since early childhood had taken refuge in rich imaginations and day-dreaming. To her questions about the whereabouts of her mother she was given the answer that her mother was in Heaven and that she was continually watching over her. At the same time she had noticed that in dealing with animals the older people in her environment used words similar to those they would use when communicating with human beings. They would curse and swear at them, praise or blame them for their actions, and in their conversations would describe the animals as being nasty or mean, faithful or fickle. In other words, the girl had gradually developed the idea that the animals were capable of comprehension and experience very much like that of human beings. Here then we find that upbringing and education combined with a low intelligence have led to the development of beliefs which under the circumstances could not be considered as abnormal.

3. A young man of poor psychic make-up but of a highly imaginative type and with ambitions that far over-reached his abilities was brought to the hospital because of the statements that he was persecuted by a gang of bootleggers who had actually assaulted him on several occasions. These statements were found to be without any basis in fact, but an analysis of this man's earlier history showed that he had always been of a psychopathic make-up, given to telling tall stories about weird adventures in such a convincing manner that he could actually make himself believe that they were true. Here then we were dealing with a psychopathic personality whose false beliefs were products of his desire to attract attention, and were not true delusions.

4. A married woman, thirty-six years of age, who has gone through a series of abdominal operations ever since her marriage. No definite pathology has ever been found to make one feel certain that she has ever had any organic disturbances as the cause of the symptoms which led to the operations. It was found that she was very unhappy in her marital life, having been forced by her father to marry a person whom she did not love, because the father did not approve of another man who was the patient's choice. The symptoms leading to the operations were found definitely to be caused by the unhappy marital life. Following the last operation she was told in a blunt way that there was really nothing wrong with her and that she was just playing the invalid for the purpose of obtaining attention. Following this she developed an acute delirious reaction in which she spoke of seeing ugly faces leering at her from the walls and ceiling. She claimed that she saw her husband with his throat cut and in her own hand a knife with blood dripping from it,

and various other dramatic apparitions. An analysis of the case, in which the patient came to appreciate the relationships of these and the earlier symptoms to her dissatisfaction with the home life, cleared up the symptoms, and measures that were taken to adjust her home life prevented the recurrence of new ones. Here then we were dealing with a psychoneurosis of the hysterical type in which the apparent hallucinations and delusions were simply dramatic gestures to express her dissatisfaction with her home life.

In contradistinction to these we may find persons who are actually psychotic, but where the psychosis is so well hidden or so mild that it cannot be differentiated from personality faults or neuroses. The first and one of the most important of these forms of reaction is represented by the cases of incipient organic diseases. As an example we have a person who has always shown good adjustment and has advanced himself to a responsible social position. Several months before his admission to the clinic he began to behave in a way which was unlike his previous manner but which nevertheless was not necessarily within the limits of psychotic behavior. He issued several forged checks, neglected his business and family, showed tendencies for childish sexual escapades, and so on. On the face of it, it appeared not unlike the behavior of a psychopathic personality; but the mere fact that it was so different from this person's previous activities, intelligence, and standards pointed to the diagnosis of a mental disease. A thorough examination of this man was undertaken, and it was found that he had Argyll-Robertson pupils, a moderate speech defect, and a positive Wassermann reaction of his blood and spinal fluid. Subsequently he developed into a typical case of general paralysis. Similar cases are found in the incipient stages of the other syphilitic affections of the central nervous system, in chronic alcoholism, lead poisoning, and a number of other conditions. In contradistinction to these cases we must remember that organic involvement of the central nervous system may be limited to small areas in the brain and sometimes in interfering with certain special functions creates the appearance of a psychosis where no such condition exists. This is particularly true of the aphasias where the person's mentality and behavior may be perfectly normal, but where the inability to express oneself correctly in speech, in writing, or in both, may convey the impression of the person being deteriorated.

Another group of psychotic states that may in their incipiency be overlooked is represented by the manic-depressive syndrome. Unwarranted enthusiasm about some special subject, an increased push of speech and activity, a tendency to play childish pranks without realization of their consequences, occasional spells of increased sexual activity, may all be found in persons of psychopathic make-up. If, however, behavior of this type develops in a person of previously well balanced personality, one has to bear in mind the possibility of a beginning manic excitement. Frequently the early symptoms do not appear unusual unless one compares them with the previous form of behavior in this person, and yet it is at this stage that judicious treatment and management will not only safeguard the person from a form of behavior of which he himself would afterwards be ashamed, but can also materially decrease the seriousness as well as the duration of the attack. Similar situations are found in the cases of depressions. A most serious form of suicidal depression may at first start out with such vague symptoms as general lassitude and disinterestedness, feelings of inferiority and of self-depreciation, which it may be difficult to differentiate from normally occurring manifestations of unhappiness in reaction to difficult situations.

Finally, we have a group of cases in which persons of a previously quiet and well balanced form of behavior may at a certain stage of their life begin to show unexplained outbursts of temper, suspiciousness, jealousy, and inimical reactions toward certain people in their environment. On the surface there may be nothing to indicate that this is not the type of behavior that still fits into the normal or psychopathic groups. Under the surface, however, these people may be found to harbor definite ideas of reference, beliefs that certain people are plotting against them, and even have hallucinations of visual or auditory type. All the paranoid psychoses and the dementia praecox groups may in certain cases develop slowly and at the beginning show only the symptoms that were enumerated above. Here again it is of utmost importance to appreciate the true state of affairs and to take steps both as to management and treatment of the case.

The exact determination of the special groups to which the different patients belong, the conclusions as to whether these patients are still outside of the limits of the psychoses, or have already overstepped the bounds and developed psychoses, is frequently very difficult. Certain criteria, however, can be established which help a great deal in coming to a correct diagnosis. The most important of these are as follows:

1. A thorough examination of the physical, more especially the neurologic, status will help in differentiating the organic psychoses from other types of reactions.

2. Changes in the personality of the individual. Where the abnormal behavior is in keeping with previous personality traits we cannot, ot course, speak of a disease process. Where the abnormal behavior is in pronounced contrast to the earlier traits we should suspect a mental disease even if the symptoms themselves are not serious enough to be considered as psychotic.

3. The lack of relation between the symptoms as they are observed and the customs, manners, and beliefs of the social group in which the person has grown up points toward the presence of a mental disease.

4. The intellectual level of the person and the rôle it might play in conditioning the symptoms that have developed is of importance in differentiating a psychosis from the type of activity that we find in mental deficiency.

5. The emotional and affective attitude of the person to his symptoms is of importance. In the psychotic individual we frequently find that although the patient appreciates intellectually the seriousness of his behavior, he remains emotionally passive and unperturbed.

THE SIGNIFICANCE OF URINARY FINDINGS IN NEPHRITIS*

F. P. McNamara, M.D., Dubuque

Over one hundred years ago Bright correlated the clinical and gross pathologic findings in patients with nephritis. Ever since that time the examination of the urine has been an important method by which the diagnosis of nephritis is made and by which the functional capacity of the kidneys is estimated. Necessarily the interpretation of urinary findings will depend upon one's knowledge of the normal and pathologic physiology of the kidneys. With the limited time it will be impossible to review those important phases of the problem. Furthermore, since it is by no means proved that Bright's disease is limited to the kidneys, it is necessary in evaluating the urinary findings to have a complete knowledge of the patient's past history and physical condition. The purpose of this paper is to give the significance of urinary findings in those conditions included under the term nephritis. It is assumed in this discussion that all other conditions which might present similar changes in the urine have been ruled out before a diagnosis of nephritis has been made.

You all are familiar with the numerous attempts to classify nephritis and the consequent confusion that has arisen in the minds of many practitioners. An attempt to clarify the situation might only in-

*Presented before the Eighty-third Annual Session, Iowa State Medical Society, Des Moines, May 9, 10, 11, 1934.

crease the confusion, and I am going to be content to describe the urinary findings in the generally accepted clinical types of nephritis. However, I may say that modern clinical and pathologic studies have emphasized the importance of the lesions in the glomeruli and in the renal vascular system, in all forms of Bright's disease. On the basis of these studies Christian[1] has gone so far as to divide nephritis into two major classes; one in which the lesion predominately concerns the glomeruli, and the other in which the essential changes are in the renal vascular system. The former may be acute or chronic; the latter is chronic. Thus we have three main types of nephritis: acute and chronic glomerulonephritis, and arteriolar nephritis. In this paper Christian's concept of the disease shall be followed.

ACUTE GLOMERULONEPHRITIS

Focal Nephritis: There are two types of acute glomerulonephritis, differing principally in the number of damaged glomeruli. The first, acute focal nephritis is encountered early and at the height of many acute infections (tonsillitis, otitis media, scarlet fever, endocarditis, and so forth) due to streptococci and occasionally in other infections such as diphtheria or influenza. The urine is temporarily decreased in amount and is of high specific gravity. It shows moderate albuminuria and hematuria. The sediment shows numerous red cells, moderate numbers of leukocytes, hyaline and granular casts. Not infrequently cultures of the urine show streptococci. There is no evidence of renal insufficiency as judged by elevation of the blood pressure, edema or retention of nitrogenous waste products. The whole clinical picture is that of an acute injury to the kidney, secondary to the infectious disease which the nephritis complicates. The pathologic picture varies between a mild degenerative change or an exudative process affecting only a portion of the glomeruli. Probably more than half the glomeruli are unaffected and this explains the lack of renal insufficiency. The tubule cells below the damaged glomeruli show only cloudy swelling. The interstitial tissue is edematous. This type of nephritis subsides with the disease it complicates and probably only a few glomeruli are permanently damaged.

Acute Diffuse Glomerulonephritis: The second type of acute glomerulonephritis occurs in the same infectious diseases as the focal type, but later, when the primary infection is subsiding. Thus in scarlet fever the focal nephritis occurs in the first week while the onset of the diffuse form is in the third week. At times the latter also follows exposure to cold and wet, and then the onset may occur within forty-eight hours of the time of the exposure. Hematuria is an important symptom of the disease. It may not always be present, but it does occur at some stage of the disease. The urine may have a hazy, smoky or bloody appearance, or the red cells may only be seen in the sediment. Albumin is constantly present throughout the course of the disease. The amount usually varies between one and ten grams per litre (Esbach method), but may reach twenty grams. At the beginning the quantity of the urine is diminished to a few hundred c.c. in a twenty-four hour period, or it may be entirely suppressed. Cases with complete anuria at the beginning usually have a fatal outcome. In favorable cases the daily output gradually increases. At the beginning the specific gravity remains low (1.006 to 1.010) although only small amounts of urine are passed. The sediment shows hyaline, granular and blood casts. In the early stage they are numerous, but with improvement they tend to become fewer in number. Red cells, leukocytes and epithelial cells, which often contain fatty granules, are also seen in the sediment. The functional tests show prolonged elimination time. In mild cases forty per cent of the phenolsulphonphthalein is eliminated in two hours, in severe cases less than ten per cent may be eliminated. There is also edema retention of nitrogenous waste products and elevation in blood pressure. The urinary findings and clinical picture indicate an acute injury to the kidneys which usually results in partial loss of renal function and rarely in complete cessation. The essential pathologic process is a non-suppurative inflammatory lesion affecting all the glomeruli. In an extreme degree the glomeruli are impassable to the flow of blood and this explains the occasional cases of anuria. Usually the injury is less intense and the glomerular filtrate is reduced in amount, the reduction being proportionate to the damaging effects on the glomeruli. With the reduction in the filtration process, water and nitrogenous waste products tend to accumulate in the blood stream. In order to compensate for the increase in blood volume, fluid leaves the blood stream and accumulates in the tissues. In an effort to eliminate more urine the blood pressure rises to maintain an adequate filtration pressure through the obstructed glomeruli. Thus the edema and elevated blood pressure are essentially compensatory mechanisms, presumably brought about by constriction and increased permeability of the systemic capillaries. There are degenerative changes in the tubules because of interference with the flow of blood through the glomeruli. As a result there is interference with the concentration of urine which varies in each case. In most cases it is only slightly or moderately reduced, but in severe cases may be markedly affected.

The end result of a single attack of acute diffuse nephritis is damage to a variable proportion of the glomeruli depending upon the severity of the initial injury. The attack may result in complete obliteration of a few glomeruli and partial obliteration of others, but the majority are so slightly damaged that they are able to maintain renal function. The interstitial tissue is only slightly increased. The reserve of kidney substance is so great that renal insufficiency does not occur, although the kidney reserve has been somewhat reduced.

In the majority of cases of acute diffuse nephritis the urine gradually returns to normal. The albumin may persist for a considerable length of time, but it finally disappears. In a few cases hematuria and albuminuria continue, indicating persistent insult to the glomeruli. In such cases it is imperative to detect and remove all possible foci of infection. When this has been accomplished the nephritis often subsides. In a third group of patients the urinary findings continue; evidences of progressive renal insufficiency gradually develop and death ensues within months to years. Subacute, subchronic and chronic forms of the disease are described, depending largely upon the rate of progress. Since they are simply phases of the same pathologic process they will all be considered as chronic diffuse nephritis.

CHRONIC GLOMERULONEPHRITIS

Chronic glomerulonephritis always originates from an acute diffuse nephritis, whether the previous condition was recognized or not. It is a progressive disease with repeated recurrences of acute attacks. Early the only indication of the chronic process, which may last for one or two to twenty or more years, is a constant albuminuria with a few hyaline casts, leukocytes, and red cells in the urinary sediment. With the superimposed acute attacks, the urine shows more red cells and an increase in the number of casts and cellular elements. After such an acute attack subsides the albuminuria persists. At first the quantity of urine is normal; later it may be diminished in cases with edema, or increased in cases without edema. Nocturia, three or four times each night, may be a prominent symptom. The color of the urine becomes pale; the specific gravity, at first high and varying with the quantity of urine, later becomes lower and ultimately tends to become fixed at about 1.010. Functional tests show a gradual prolongation of the elimination time and a reduction of the ability to concentrate urine. Thus with the Mosenthal test diet there is a prolongation of the elimination time of fluid and two hourly specimens are increasingly uniform. With Volhard's concentration test the change in specific gravity is lessened from the normal variations. Concomitant with the urinary changes is a tendency for the nitrogenous waste products to accumulate in the blood, an elevation of the blood pressure, and changes in the systemic blood vessels, especially those of the retina. The urinary changes indicate a gradual loss of kidney reserve; at first without signs of insufficiency; then a mild and compensatible insufficiency; but ultimately the renal insufficiency becomes absolute. The pathologic picture is that of non-suppurative inflammatory lesion resulting in a gradual destruction of the glomeruli; endarteritis obliterans and arteriolosclerosis affecting especially the afferent arterioles; degeneration of the tubule cells; and replacement of the destroyed elements by an increase of the interstitial tissue. The end result, if the patient lives long enough, is the total disorganization of the kidney architecture.

Chronic Nephrosis: Chronic nephrosis has been the subject of much discussion in recent literature. The disease is characterized by a chronic course, edema and albuminuria, as well as by the absence of hypertension and of renal insufficiency. It usually occurs in the first half of life and is especially frequent in childhood and young adult life. Albuminuria is a cardinal symptom and is usually present to a marked degree, (ten to twenty grams or more per litre). Occasionally there is a transitory glycosuria. The quantity of urine is inversely proportionate to the edema. The specific gravity is high, even with large amounts of urine. The urine is usually cloudy, often contains large amounts of urates and on standing develops a nauseating odor. The urinary sediment contains hyaline, granular, and fatty casts and a few leukocytes but red cells are absent or at most very few in number. A characteristic feature of the sediment is the presence of doubly refractile lipoids. The concentration of urea in the urine is high; that of the chlorides is low when the edema is forming and high when the edema is diminishing. The Congo red test shows elimination of forty to sixty per cent of the dye in distinction to amyloid disease in which sixty to ninety per cent is eliminated. The pathologic picture is that of a degenerative lesion affecting the glomeruli and especially the cells of the tubules. In late cases there is replacement of the above elements due to an increase in the interstitial tissue. While the exact classification of this type of nephritis has not been agreed upon, evidence is increasing to prove that it is a form of chronic glomerulonephritis with slight lesions in the glomeruli and marked changes in the cells of the tubules. A point of practical impor-

tance in the control of the edema, which is the disease in the mind of the patient, is the fact that the glomerular capsule is more permeable to blood protein. As a result much albumin but very little globulin is lost in the urine. Therefore the plasma protein is reduced and the ratio of albumin to globulin is diminished. A correspondingly low colloid osmotic pressure of the blood plasma follows. Peters and associates[2] found that when the total serum protein fell below four per cent, edema usually occurred, although it was also recognized that other factors were concerned. The replacement of the lost albumin by an increase of the dietary protein is therefore logical. This has been done in chronic glomerulonephritis with or without edema with benefit to the patient. It is obvious that if there is retention of nitrogenous waste products in the blood, a high protein diet is not desirable.

RENAL ARTERIOLOSCLEROSIS

Arteriosclerosis is one of the penalties of growing old. It is encountered in most patients over sixty years of age and arteriosclerosis of the larger renal arteries is a part of the general picture. The changes seen in the kidneys of such individuals are the result of infarction. Between the infarcted areas the renal parenchyma is relatively normal and fully able to maintain function although the kidney reserve is somewhat reduced. Of far more importance is sclerosis of the arterioles of the kidney and especially the afferent arterioles. This occurs in the disease known as essential hypertension of which two clinical types are described, i. e., benign and malignant. Essential hypertension is usually encountered in patients over forty years of age, but also occurs in young adult life or even in childhood. The outstanding sign is a blood pressure varying between 160 and 200 mm. of mercury. Very frequently the heart is definitely hypertrophied. For many years there may be no change in the urine. Later traces of albumin (one-fourth gram to one gram) as well as hyaline and granular casts appear. Polyuria, which is most marked at night, is also an early and very constant evidence of renal involvement. Red cells are lacking until the heart begins to fail when they leak into the urine as the result of chronic passive congestion. Edema if present is likewise the result of cardiac failure and not due to renal insufficiency which may be deferred for years. The concentration test usually shows the kidney to be capable of elaborating a urine of high specific gravity. The dye test may be diminished, but this is due to poor circulation rather than to functional impairment of the kidney. As the changes in the kidney are progressive, evidences of renal insufficiency ultimately do appear. In the malignant type this occurs in a short time, but in the majority of cases is delayed for a variable period. In each form the essential pathologic process is the same. It consists of an arteriolosclerosis involving the afferent arterioles particularly and gradually extending to the glomeruli. As a consequence of the narrowing of the arterioles there are multiple foci of atrophy of the renal parenchyma. The tubules degenerate and the interstitial tissue increases. From the standpoint of function the end result is the same as in an advanced case of chronic glomerulonephritis.

CONCLUSION

In this discussion it has been necessary to describe the common types of nephritis as clear cut clinical entities. In actual practice less clearly defined forms or combination forms are encountered and present puzzling clinical problems. They can be solved only by a full knowledge of the patient's history and physical condition as well as by complete and repeated examinations of the urine. Occasionally the latter must be supplemented by chemical analyses of the blood. In judging the urinary findings a full understanding of the normal and pathologic physiology as well as the pathology of the kidney is essential. On such a basis the urinary findings may be utilized, first to indicate the presence, character and extent of renal lesions, and second to indicate the functional capacity of the kidney in the different forms of Bright's disease.

BIBLIOGRAPHY

1. Christian, Henry A.: Types of nephritis and their management. Jour. Am. Med. Assn., cii:3 (January 20), 1934.
2. Peters, J. P., and associates: The plasma proteins in relation to blood hydration; Part 4. Serum proteins in nephritic edema. Jour. Clin. Investig., x:941, 1931.
3. Elwyn, Herman: Nephritis. The MacMillan Co., New York, 1926.
4. Fishberg, Arthur M.: Hypertension and Nephritis. Lea & Febiger, Philadelphia, 1934.
5. MacCallum, W. G.: Textbook of Pathology. W. B. Saunders Company, Philadelphia, 1932.

Discussion

Dr. Julius S. Weingart, Des Moines: In the paper just read, gentlemen, the writer has outlined the method of procedure to be followed in every diagnostic problem. The physician must try, as far as possible, to correlate the symptoms with the underlying pathology of structure and function, for only by constant endeavor to accomplish this, and by frequent checking of errors in the postmortem room will eventual accuracy and clarity of thinking be achieved. If the physician persists in this intellectual effort and analyzes all the data at hand, he will be surprised at the frequency with which he will be able to predict the type of lesion found in renal disease.

Among these diagnostic data the urinary findings play an important, but by no means exclusive rôle. While, as Thomas Fuller long ago said, "Reasons drawn from the urine are as brittle as the urinal," perhaps in an age of more elaborate tests we have forgotten how much information we may gain from a simple urinalysis. Particularly valuable in estimating function are the concentration tests, so easy to determine, and requiring an instrument no more complicated than a urinometer. Let me, however, inject a note of warning, for the modern physician is prone to place undue confidence in many of the tests at his command, and even in the estimation of renal function no one test is infallible. Now and then in undoubted cases of uremia, the specific gravity of the urine shows no striking deviation from the normal. The phenol red test will occasionally give evidence which is misleading, and so will all the other dye tests. The amount of nitrogen retention depends on the nitrogen intake and the deaminizing function of the liver, as well as on the excretory power of the kidneys. Van Slyke's urea concentration test is one trial. It should be widely used for its author is a deep student of this problem. In the great majority of cases renal function can be fairly accurately estimated by one or all of the usual procedures. One is living in a fool's paradise, however, if he imagines that he will in every case get unequivocal laboratory confirmation of his diagnosis. It is not so simple as that—at least not yet.

The anatomic changes in nephritis have been, one might venture to say, adequately studied; and yet, only in certain types, do we thoroughly understand the cause. Ask yourselves just what brings about postscarlatinal nephritis, read the voluminous discussions on the etiology of chronic tubular nephritis, and then consider whether we have merely used words to cloak our ignorance, and confirmed the witty Frenchman's dictum that language was given in order to obscure thought. I am rather of the opinion that the prognosis in acute nephritis is settled by the amount of damage present at the time we see the patient. The severely damaged glomerulus is no longer an effective filter, and the patient's recovery depends on whether he has a sufficient number of normal ones left. We understand now the cause of the convulsive seizures, and can prevent them. We can possibly do a little toward avoiding further renal insult; but the restoration of a badly injured glomerular mechanism is out of the question.

This is a fatalistic doctrine, perhaps; but if it teaches us how ominous hematuria may be, how early we must suspect renal injury, how long we must keep that patient in bed, how sedulously we must try to avoid relapses, and how guarded our prognosis must be, even in cases apparently mild at the outset, the outcome will be better than if we put reliance on some of the fads and fancies which parade under the guise of therapeutics.

THE PROMOTION OF IMMUNIZATION BY THE STATE DEPARTMENT OF HEALTH*

Joseph H. Kinnaman, M.D., Des Moines

The State Department of Health and the Iowa State Medical Society have planned and outlined a cooperative program for health education. This plan is, doubtless, imperfect; but it is flexible and until such time as it may be improved or a better plan devised to take its place, it may well serve as a foundation. The fact that such a cooperative plan is being followed represents real progress.

In attempting to plan and outline programs for the prevention of disease and for health education, the department interchanges views with organized medicine. At the present time it is working in close cooperation with the Council, the Speakers Bureau and the Committee on Child Health and Protection of the Iowa State Medical Society. This committee has been asked to serve in an advisory capacity and to suggest activities and policies which are most likely to encourage and permit each county medical society to carry out the most effective health education program possible. The department supports only such policies and activities as are desired, accepted and encouraged by organized medicine. It seeks constructive criticism at all times and solicits the assistance of the organized profession in all matters of policy. It submits quarterly reports of progress to the society.

The primary purpose of developing and maintaining a partnership relation between the Department of Health and the State Medical Society is to prepare a foundation upon which the county medical societies may build a health education program. Every county medical society should appoint an educational committee. The duties of this committee would be obviously, largely educative. It should attempt to serve both the laity and the medical profession. In serving the laity it should be ready to provide lay organizations with lectures on health subjects. It should prepare and release copy for the press. It should review and approve all material broadcast over local radio stations. It should offer to review and approve literature distributed locally by voluntary health agencies and insurance companies. It should serve as a technical consultation committee and advise lay organizations in regard to methods and agents for disease prevention. It is a recognized dictum that education of the laity and education of the medical profession must go hand in hand if a program for health education is to be

successful. In serving the medical profession the educational committee of the county medical society should attempt to inform the membership of the society in regard to dependable methods and agents for disease prevention. This function perhaps may be served best by cooperating with the Speakers Bureau of the State Society and the State Department of Health. These latter organizations are planning to offer demonstration lectures to county medical societies covering:

1. Demonstrations of laboratory precision methods.
2. Technic of administration of specific preventive agents.
3. Technic and interpretation of intradermal tests for immunity.

The local medical profession should encourage this committee to study the community health needs and to plan and outline community health programs. Although the local county society may not care to initiate community health programs, it should have among its membership a group of informed men who can advise intelligently both the medical profession and the laity. Whenever the county medical society proposes to cooperate with any other group in the organization and conduct of preventive programs, the educational committee should serve to protect the best interests of the society and the public, as well.

The organization and conduct of programs for the prevention of diphtheria may be used to illustrate how a cooperative plan may be applied to the problems of disease prevention. The plan followed by the department has been approved by organized medicine. It is especially adaptable to the group method of immunization, and is as follows:

Every organization and individual interested in the conduct of an anti-diphtheria program is referred to the officers of the county medical society for advice and assistance in planning and outlining the program. The department mails a copy of all communications received from organizations and individuals interested in diphtheria prevention to the officers of the county medical society involved. No preventive agent and only one piece of literature is available to a sponsoring agency before satisfactory evidence has been furnished to the effect that the plan has the approval of the county medical society. The record of the action of the county medical society must be submitted to the department in writing. Although the preventive program is limited only to a township, city or town or rural school district basis, the plan must be approved by the county medical society. Since the sponsoring agency must obtain the approval of the county medical society at the very

* Presented before the Eighty-third Annual Session, Iowa State Medical Society, Des Moines, May 9, 10, 11, 1934.

outset, the department believes that this procedure gives the organized medical profession the opportunity, if it so desires, to offer a plan in which the membership of the county society will administer the necessary treatments to groups of children at a given place on designated dates for a fee. The secretary of each county medical society has been asked to bring the outline prepared by the department to the attention of the membership of the society. Each county medical society has been asked to:

1. Approve the plan as outlined.
2. Modify the plan to meet local conditions.
3. Prepare a new plan.
4. Indicate that it does not care at this time to take definite action.

Each society has been requested to submit either to the State Department of Health or to the State Medical Society a written record of its action. The experience of the past few months has shown that most county medical societies prefer to follow the plan as outlined by the department.

In addition to suggesting ways and means by which groups of children may be given the preventive treatments, the county medical society is asked to determine:

1. The preventive agent to be used.
2. The methods employed.
3. The allocation of physicians to districts.
4. The cost of medical services.

As soon as the county medical society has given its approval, the sponsoring agency may obtain consent slips and diphtheria preventive agents from the department. The department will provide without cost until July 1, 1934, or until such time prior to that date whenever available funds are exhausted, 50 per cent of the toxoid (two dose treatment) and 33⅓ per cent of the alum precipitated toxoid (one dose treatment) required to carry out a county-wide preventive program approved by the county medical society. The department will supply all of the ready mixed toxin required for Schick testing without cost.

There are many ways of educating the public. One of the most effective methods is to provide printed information. This material should be prepared by medical men and should present only established facts. In indicating the need for and value of methods and agents of disease prevention, parents should be encouraged to consult the family doctor. Under the cooperative plan for health education outlined by the State Department of Health and the State Medical Society, all departmental publications relating to child health and health education are reviewed and approved by the Committee on Child Health and Protec-

tion of the State Society. Recently that committee concluded a review of the diphtheria literature which the department provides without cost. The consent slip was revised. The parent is told that "the family doctor should be given the opportunity to protect each child as soon as it reaches six months of age and that unprotected children may obtain the preventive treatments either by making arrangements with the family doctor or by taking advantage of the group treatment method." The parent is asked to sign request slip No. 1 if he intends to have his children treated in the office of his own doctor. If the children are to be treated under the group plan, the parent signs request slip No. 2 and indicates whether or not he can pay a sum per child which has been determined by the county medical society. The sponsoring agency is provided with these consent slips only after the county medical society has given its approval to the organization and conduct of a preventive program.

Only one piece of literature giving general information about diphtheria will be provided by the department upon request. This leaflet entitled, "Protect All Children Against Diphtheria," is approved by the Committee on Child Health and Protection. Two pieces of diphtheria literature are available only to physicians. One is entitled, "Suggested Technique of Administration of Diphtheria Preventive Agents," and the other, "Toxoid Preferred to Toxin-Antitoxin." The committee considered the advisability of revising the outline entitled, "County-Wide Preventive Programs." It had previously been approved by the Council and the Committee on Child Health and Protection of the State Medical Society. At its last meeting the Committee on Child Health and Protection made only a minor change in that outline.

The sponsoring agency is usually some lay organization. These organizations have been willing and ready to follow the plan as outlined by the department. Without exception they have abided by the decision of the county medical society. They have arranged to pay the physicians for services rendered. They have provided for:

1. Nurses, whenever possible to assist with the treatment of children.
2. Clerical help.
3. Treatment stations.
4. Transportation of children whenever necessary, to and from treatment stations.
5. An accurate record of the names, addresses and ages of the children treated.
6. Treatment of children of preschool age.
7. Written consent of the parents.
8. Adequate follow-up work.

SUMMARY

Diphtheria preventive programs are organized and conducted only with the approval of the county medical society. The county medical society decides: (1) how all children shall be given an opportunity to acquire protection against diphtheria, (2) the preventive agent to be used, (3) the methods employed, (4) the allocation of physicians to districts, and (5) the cost of medical services.

The State Department of Health furnishes without cost: (1) only literature approved by the Committee on Child Health and Protection of the State Medical Society, (2) 50 per cent of the toxoid (two dose treatment), and 33⅓ per cent of the alum precipitated toxoid required, and (3) all of the ready-mixed toxin required for Schick testing.

Diphtheria literature which the department provides without cost has been approved by the Committee on Child Health and Protection of the Iowa State Medical Society. The material available includes: the consent slips, certificates of immunity, "Protect All Children Against Diphtheria," "Toxoid Preferred to Toxin-Antitoxin" and "Suggested Technique for the Administration of Preventive Agents." The last two pieces of literature are available only to physicians. The consent slips are available only after the plan has been approved by the county medical society and the pamphlet entitled, "Protect All Children Against Diphtheria," is available upon request.

Detailed information regarding the organization and conduct of county-wide preventive programs has been printed in the JOURNAL OF THE IOWA STATE MEDICAL SOCIETY from time to time. On pages 21 and 22 of the January issue of that JOURNAL, an outline of the program prepared by the department and the State Medical Society was printed. In the February issue of the JOURNAL, pages 103 and 104, two questions were answered: "How Much Will the Doctor Be Paid for Giving Preventive Treatments?" and "Who Will Pay the Doctor?" In the March issue of the JOURNAL, on page 156, an offer of free material from the State Department of Health was printed.

The State Department of Health believes that the ultimate objectives of this program for health education should be to teach the public the need for and the value of disease prevention; to stimulate the public to obtain preventive treatments from the private practitioner of medicine; and to encourage the medical profession, as an organized group and as individuals, to apply the available and dependable methods and agents of disease prevention at every opportunity in the practice of medicine.

RADIATION TREATMENT OF SMALL FIBROIDS AND MENORRHAGIAS*

B. T. WHITAKER, M.D., Boone

The radiation treatment of small fibroids and menorrhagias is not a cure-all, it is not a fantasy, it is not an experiment, nor is it a procedure to be considered lightly or administered unintelligently, but in the hands of those who understand its indications, its possibilities and its proper method of application, it constitutes a form of treatment in the handling of many of these cases, which is safe, and produces results pleasing to both the patient and physician.

This afternoon we are considering x-ray therapy primarily, and since this discussion must of necessity be very brief, I shall consider only the roentgen treatment, although many of the statements could be applied to radium in a similar manner.

Approximately fourteen years ago I started in a modest way to treat some of these patients with x-ray, and I have noticed each year, without fail, a gradual increase in the number so handled. My experience in this respect has been that of many others throughout the country.

Why have we experienced this gradual increase in the number of cases so treated? I believe the answer to that question is definite and positive. Concisely, it is this, that sufficient time has now elapsed to prove that this form of therapy is not an experiment or a passing therapeutic novelty, but the results are so uniformly good with no hospitalization, operative mortalities, or even absence from family or business duties, that the profession is increasingly offering the advantages of this treatment to its patients.

The question is, to whom may we safely prescribe this form of radiation? First let us consider as our subject, small fibroids. By this term we mean the interstitial fibroid which is causing increased length and amount of flow. The large ones which attain the size of a five or six months' pregnancy, we will not discuss. A positive diagnosis of small fibroids is of the greatest importance because one thereby rules out a malignant condition, a pedunculated fibroid or other complications. If this diagnosis has been made we can then offer to that patient a very definite promise of relief of symptoms. This relief amounts, in most cases, to a cure. Of the menorrhagias which we encounter so frequently, the most common, of course, are those of the menopause. Here again, after a positive diagnosis has been made, and I emphasize this point for I feel it is most important, we can hasten

* Presented before the Eighty-third Annual Session, Iowa State Medical Society, Des Moines, May 9, 10, 11, 1934.

the change with relief from the excessive flowing which is dragging the patient down, physically and mentally, and the result is a most grateful patient. I make these two statements in rather a broad sense, but we must remember there is no more important sign to a woman near the menopause than irregular bleeding, nor is there anything which requires more exacting or exhausting diagnostic abilities, if we are to give to that individual the best that medical science can offer. All women are prone to blame any irregularity on the change of life, and I fear that many of us err in the same manner, sometimes overlooking more serious pathology.

Just what happens when we treat these individuals with the x-ray? I believe it is an accepted fact that there is a duofold action on the uterus and the ovaries. The tendency of the x-ray to soften fibrous structures, largely explains the action on the uterus, for there is unquestionably a fibrosis of this organ, especially in the subinvoluted type found at the menopause, and this condition opposes the natural function of the organ, and predisposes to bleeding. When one investigates the newer physiology of menstrual function, an explanation is found for the control or discontinuation of the flow following application of the indicated x-ray dosage to the ovaries. As we consider the definite effect of x-ray on ovulation, which, at the approach of the menopause has become delayed, irregular or possibly hastened, these results may be more easily understood. The question is frequently asked, "Are there not many menopause symptoms developed following a series of treatments?" Our own experience has not revealed a great many of these complaints for the majority of these women have been in or were near the change of life and it has not been our policy to hurry the treatments but to spread them over a period of time, and as a result we have not heard a great deal of complaint about these subjective symptoms. In the younger individuals with menorrhagia, when it has seemed wise to employ x-ray, the dosage has, of course, been very small and its effects are carefully watched.

Reviewing my record cards, I have taken a series of 150 consecutive cases, omitting recent ones because of unproved results. These cases have all been treated by one technic. (Dr. Erskine classifies it as Technique II in his book), with a voltage of 135 kilovolts to which we all have access. The only variable factor was the amount of the dose, each case receiving from 350 to 400 r units delivered to each ovary. Out of these cases, I have selected the failures. I will try to analyze them, feeling that we can learn more from them than from the successful ones.

CASE REPORTS

1. Mrs. E., forty-three years of age, had severe and prolonged flowing at each period for two weeks. She was referred for treatment because of severe menorrhagia of menopause. A series of treatments produced no results, but a few months later, the patient passed a pedunculated fibroid which naturally relieved her symptoms.

2. Miss F., forty-six years of age, had been irregular for several years. Heavy flowing had been present for several months with occasional intermenstrual flow. Because of a suspicious looking cervix, a biopsy was done, but no curettage. The report from the biopsy was negative. She received a series of treatments with improvement for six months, when the bleeding recurred, and then a positive diagnosis of malignancy of the fundus could easily be made.

These two cases are rightfully classed as failures, because a correct diagnosis was not made. If these patients had been curetted, and the scrapings examined (and it was certainly indicated), both of these errors would have been discovered.

3. This case illustrates another type of failure. Mrs. M., forty-five years of age, had a small fibroid the size of a two or three months' pregnancy, with menstrual flow gradually increasing, both in duration and amount. She received one treatment which amounted to one-sixth of the intended dosage, after which her referring physician advised her that she would need no more. Needless to say, that woman received no benefits, and x-ray was condemned. This doctor would not have received satisfactory results if he had given 1/32 gr. of morphine to a 200 pound man for a renal colic, and by the same token, a fibroid must receive the proper dosage to ensure any benefits.

4. Mrs. F., forty-four years of age, flowed excessively at each period, enough so that she felt the effects from the loss of blood. She had many subjective symptoms of the menopause. Curettage and careful examination revealed nothing but a large, subinvoluted uterus. A series of treatments produced excellent results for two years. Six months ago the heavy flow returned. Another careful examination revealed nothing; uterus was much smaller than at the time of the previous examination. A repetition of the treatments, however, has not produced satisfactory results.

5. Mrs. S., forty-three years of age, had a very large fibroid, the mass reaching up to the navel. She had been flowing so heavily that surgery was ruled out, and x-ray advised as a temporary measure. Her flowing was controlled and the tumor melted down into the pelvis. She recovered, and continued her housewife duties on a farm. Five

years later the uterus was removed because of a slight enlargement. I do not know the exact reason for the hysterectomy and while I cannot class this patient as cured, still we were able to help a very sick and helpless woman back to health and to convert an inoperable case into an operable one.

As I stated in the beginning, the success of radiation depends primarily on a correct diagnosis, and this statement is borne out by these case reports, two failures being definitely charged to incorrect diagnosis, and another to improper dosage administered. I cannot explain the failure of the other one, unless it was one of those cases of delayed ovulation. In that case, a stronger dosage at the time of the original treatment might have been better.

While this series of cases is small compared to the number several others here could present, yet it has been my privilege to follow up these cases very thoroughly, and I believe the results are correct. The findings bear out the statement that a great deal may be accomplished with the equipment that is universally available.

So, in conclusion, considering the results that can be obtained by proper radiation of these cases, when properly diagnosed, I cannot but submit the question, "Is it not fair to our patients at least to explain the possibilities of this method of treatment and offer it to them as a solution of their problems?"

INSULIN*

JOHN C. SHRADER, M.D., Fort Dodge

It was first discovered in 1889 that removing the pancreas resulted in diabetes. In 1900 it was demonstrated that the islets in the pancreas were probably responsible for the antidiabetic hormone. Therefore, it was Schafer, who in 1916 first suggested the name insulin for this internal secretion. Early attempts to isolate insulin were of no avail, although in 1908 scientists almost succeeded in doing it. Prior to 1922 when the workers in the laboratories at Toronto made their announcement as to the finding of insulin, many trials and errors had been made in the effort to discover some substance which would aid the diabetic patient in maintaining an adequate diet. When the announcement of the Toronto workers came, it was heralded as one of the biggest stepping stones in the progress of medicine. The discovery of insulin by Banting and Best meant that the diabetic individual with a low tolerance would no longer

*Presented before the Eighty-third Annual Session, Iowa State Medical Society, Des Moines, May 9, 10, 11, 1934.

have to be starved; that the diabetic patient in coma could be rescued from that coma; that the diabetic patient with infection could be carried through the period of stress and strain and again resume the diet that had been used previously; and that the diabetic child could have a better outlook on life.

Insulin, as it is now made, is obtained from the pancreas of animals, manufactured by certain chemical companies and it is now available from several different drug manufacturers. At the onset one of the leading drug houses of the country spent much time and money in aiding to improve and purify the product, insulin. Insulin was later put on the market by several of the manufacturing chemists and is now available at a very reasonable price to be used where needed. No satisfactory form of insulin has been discovered or manufactured to date that can be given by mouth, per rectum or by unction. The hypodermic use of insulin is the only satisfactory method of use. There are many products on the market, so-called diabetic aids, that are claimed to increase the ability to use sugar, but these over-reach their truth and they do not improve the tolerance of the diabetic individual. Insulin may be obtained in vials in varying strengths, having 10, 20, 40 or 80 units per c.c. As an arbitrary figure it has been stated that one unit of insulin will handle from one and one-half to two grams of carbohydrate. This is not entirely true, for in the smaller doses of insulin one unit will help to metabolize a larger amount of carbohydrate than when large doses of insulin are used. In ordinary practice in the average case, two doses or injections of insulin are required each day; that is, one before breakfast and one before the evening meal. In individuals requiring larger doses, three injections a day constitute the usual dosage. These are given, as a rule, approximately one-half hour before each meal. Any infection decreases the diabetic patient's tolerance to handle carbohydrate. This has long been known and, therefore, whenever infection is present, the dosage of insulin must be increased.

When insulin first became available, many thought, and still do, that here was a product which would allow the diabetic individual to eat at will and cover up for the added carbohydrate consumption by the taking of the new drug, insulin. It has been stated many times that insulin is a "two edged sword," or to put it differently, insulin is dangerous if used by the inexperienced physician or lay person. The diabetic patient requiring insulin more than ever should be on a maintenance diet to allow for normal activity with enough insulin to keep this patient with a normal blood sugar and urine sugar free. The diet should be carefully balanced and usually weighed, although careful estimation is permissible.

What are the damages of too much insulin? First, there is always insulin shock. Insulin shock or hypoglycemia is the condition brought about when the blood sugar reaches too low a level. This is usually below fifty milligrams of sugar per 100 c.c. of blood. It produces in the individual first a sensation of hunger, nervousness, tremor, sweating, a feeling of anxiety, rapid pulse and, if it progresses far enough, may cause coma and death. Symptoms of insulin shock or hypoglycemia, if recognized, can certainly be adequately treated. The taking of any easily utilized carbohydrate by mouth will cause a disappearance of the symptoms —that is, the juice of one orange or a piece of sugar candy. The individual taking insulin should always have handy some carbohydrate to take in case of emergency. If the condition of hypoglycemia has developed so far that the patient is unable to swallow, then glucose must be administered intravenously in order to restore the normal sugar content of the blood. It has been stated that hypoglycemia or insulin shock is a definite damage to the arteriosclerotic and older individual where there is myocardial damage. Ernstene studied the effect of insulin hypoglycemia on non-diabetic individuals and found that during the period of lowered blood sugar the pulse rate and pulse pressure increased, the systolic blood pressure rose and the diastolic pressure fell, and that the minute volume output of the heart increased. These findings indicated that there is an increased amount of cardiac work during hypoglycemia, and furnished experimental explanation for the clinical finding that in patients with a diminished myocardial reserve, a blood sugar that is below the normal can result in or bring about the signs and symptoms of myocardial failure. This made it more evident that diabetic patients having arteriosclerosis, angina pectoris or coronary sclerosis should avoid symptoms of insulin shock. Drastic reduction in the blood sugar levels is to be avoided in elderly patients, because undernutrition of the heart muscle in the presence of coronary disease might lead to serious consequences. There have been reports of patients having a lowered blood sugar who developed a paresis or, as was thought at the time, a true paralysis, which disappeared after the blood sugar had returned to normal.

There are reports from authentic sources of patients being allergic or sensitive to insulin, even in the free form as it is obtained today. Some of the symptoms developing were local around the site of injection; others were systemic, as will develop in any allergic individual and some of these symptoms would not occur for varying lengths of time—from two to sixteen hours after the administration of insulin. Many of these individuals who were found to be sensitive had previously received insulin. In some, the changing of the brand of insulin caused a disappearance of the symptoms. In others discontinuance of the insulin was found advisable. If any person has used insulin for twenty days without allergic symptoms, there is very little likelihood of trouble. In the early days of the use of insulin there was more difficulty due to reactions than at the present time.

When a diabetic patient presents himself at the office, if he is aware of his condition, he will often make the initial statement, "I do not want to take insulin" or "I am afraid to take insulin." There seems to be a feeling among the laity that insulin is a habit forming drug and that once the use of insulin is started, it can never be stopped. Part of this assumption is true, for any diabetic patient having so low a tolerance for carbohydrate, in order to utilize an adequate diet and remain sugar free with a normal blood sugar, will in all probability have to use insulin indefinitely. Perhaps, the fear of these individuals comes from the fact that they must take a hypodermic. Of course, the financial element is also an item to take into consideration.

It is well known that if diabetic individuals with a good tolerance, that is a tolerance enough to handle a maintenance diet, develop an infection, are operated upon or go through any severe emotional distress, their ability to handle carbohydrate is diminished and in order to maintain a normal blood sugar and urine free from sugar, insulin will be required in varying doses until the emergency is over. Then usually, they go back to a tolerance practically identical to that before the emergency. On the other hand, if these individuals do not use insulin as well as proper diet, the wear and tear and the strain associated with the complication will usually result in a lowered tolerance for carbohydrate.

Treating a diabetic person with insulin is not to be done lightly. First, an adequate diet, depending on the activity of the patient, must be allowed; second, careful urine sugars must be followed. If blood sugars can be taken it is of much additional help. In the diabetic woman pregnancy can occur, and a normal course of pregnancy can follow, if there is complete cooperation between the patient and her physician. An exact control of the diabetic condition throughout the months of pregnancy will in most cases prevent any abnormal demands on the pancreas of the fetus and, therefore, protect the new born child. By adopting the practice of furnishing the insulin requirements of the mother, it is found that the amount of insulin required during the first three months increases; during the second three months of pregnancy the insulin requirements will remain about the same; during the third three months the amount of insulin will increase; but the amount required decreases suddenly following delivery. From these findings, it would seem that the greatest danger from acidosis would be in the first and last trimesters of pregnancy and the greatest danger from insulin shock, or from hypoglycemia, would occur immediately after delivery. When the second three months' period is started free from any complications, there is little likelihood of trouble occurring during this mid-period. Differing from the behavior of the uncomplicated diabetic patient, there is an experience of paradoxical behavior of the insulin requirements in the last trimester of pregnancy. When the insulin is increased to cover fully the needs of the diabetic mother, there is not a gain but a loss of tolerance. Duncan and Fetter, who made these observations, regard a gain in tolerance in the last three months of pregnancy as unfavorable for the child, because it is due in all probability to an over-active fetal pancreas. Pregnancy under ideal conditions and treatment does not impair the diabetic mother's tolerance, so that diabetes in itself is not a contraindication to pregnancy.

When a diabetic patient presents himself for treatment, it is best to find out as soon as possible what that individual requires for an adequate diet. If he is unable to consume the proper amount of food and still have a normal blood sugar and a urine free of sugar, then insulin should be advised in adequate dosage. After a period of treatment it is usually found that the tolerance has increased to varying degrees so that the individual taking insulin should always keep in fairly close communication with his physician. All diabetic patients should be warned as to what to do in the event of infection or complications and it is during these times that an increase in the dosage of insulin must be carefully supervised. When a patient is seen in coma, the fact that he has diabetes should not lead you to administer insulin until a urinalysis has been done and, if there is no sugar present, insulin should not be given because of the danger of producing hypoglycemia.

PEPTIC ULCER*

ELMER G. SENTY, M.D., Davenport

Because peptic ulcer produces a disability which interferes more or less seriously with the health and activities of many adults, probably ten per cent in every community, this disease warrants careful consideration and study. In spite of advances made in diagnostic methods during the past decade, there still remains much difference of opinion as to the etiologic factors which play a part in the production of this disease. The question arises, "What initiates the process, and what destines this lesion to become chronic?"

Virchow first suggested the vascular theory in which necrotic areas in the mucosa might be produced by spasm of the afferent vessels in young individuals or by arteriosclerotic changes in the aged. This theory is still widely accepted by many, and particularly by pathologists. German investigators, and especially Konjetzny, are very prone to believe that gastritis is the chief factor in the production of gastric or duodenal ulcers. Ivy and others have stressed the relation of trauma produced by coarse foods, hot and cold drinks, beverages and other chemical irritants. The infectious theory has been ably championed by Rosenow and his co-workers. He has demonstrated the importance of distant foci of infection and has repeatedly produced experimental ulcers by the intravenous injection of streptococci removed from such foci. There can be no doubt that many acute ulcers produced in this manner may be healed spontaneously, but they may be prevented from healing by the corrosive action of a highly acid gastric juice. There is a growing feeling that high gastric acidity, associated with failure of neutralization by the duodenal juices, bile and mucin, is a factor in causing acute ulcers to become chronic.

There has recently developed an increasing interest in the importance of the neurogenic factor in the production of peptic ulcer, as well as the benefits obtained by removing these influences. It has been definitely proved that certain psychic stimuli increase the acidity and peptic activity of gastric juice. Alvarez suggests that possibly smaller amounts of mucin or other protective fluids of the stomach are produced, that ischemia of the tissue may result from spasm of the blood vessels, and that pancreatic and biliary secretions may be lessened or dried up, much as saliva in the mouth under emotional strain. Finally, it is well known to physiologists that emotional imbalance

* Presented before the Eighty-third Annual Session, Iowa State Medical Society, Des Moines, May 9, 10, 11, 1934.

can produce pylorospasm with resulting stagnation of the gastric contents and increase in gastric acidity. Knowing the above facts, how do the proponents of the neurogenic theory associate them with the peptic ulcer individual? They believe after careful investigation of different races that peptic ulcer is a disease of civilized people, and that ulcer is seldom found in the heathen or among the negro race. It is more frequently encountered in individuals with highly sensitive nervous systems, in those who are alert, keen, ambitious, and accustomed to combating obstacles without much consideration of the physical requirements. Frequently these patients are visibly nervous, but often this nervousness and restlessness is cleverly masked so that the true personality will not be uncovered unless time and patience is used in gaining the patient's confidence. In this era of competition, speed and financial worry, would it be any wonder if we produced a race of nervous and physically exhausted people? With this soil available, with this lowered resistance, it should be a rather simple matter for ulcer to develop, and especially so if such conditions as localized circulation disturbances, inflammation, infection, and localized trauma occur, and particularly so if in association with a highly acid gastric secretion.

Eusterman in his address before the section on gastro-enterology and proctology of the American Medical Association in 1932 very aptly summarizes the above observations as follows: "One cannot easily escape the conviction that the nervous imbalance resulting in disturbed parasympathetic and sympathetic interaction on gastric or duodenal motility and secretion plays an important if not an exclusive part in the symptoms, at least, and in the genesis of ulcer itself. When an actual lesion does develop under such circumstances, it seems justifiable to predicate a mucosal susceptibility based on inheritance or acquired through the influence of infection or other sustained irritants resulting in vulnerability of the gastric and duodenal tissue to the heightened corrosive and digestive action of the gastric juice."

Theoretically, there should be little difficulty in correctly diagnosing the syndrome associated with peptic ulcer. In actual practice, however, the reverse is frequently true. Too often the diagnosis is made without proper evaluation of the available facts, without carefully investigating the past history and obtaining the salient symptoms characteristic of the disease, or using the laboratory aids at our disposal. Gastric disturbance is very commonly produced by lesions located elsewhere in the body and particularly in the gastro-intestinal tract. Diseases of the gallbladder, the liver, and the appendix, frequently produce a symptom complex which mimics ulcer. Abell states that the stomach may be compared to a fire alarm box which tells that a conflagration exists without specifically denoting its location, and the simile may be further extended to infer that the physician who proceeds to treat the stomach without further and adequate search for the cause of the alarm is as culpable as the fireman who would content himself with playing the stream of water on the fire box. During the past decade commendable advance has been made in the diagnosis of gastric lesions, but little, if any, progress has been made in differentiating gastric ulcer from duodenal ulcer other than by roentgenologic methods.

Clinically peptic ulcer presents a very striking picture. It is characterized by a distress in the epigastrium which may be described as an ache, soreness, dull boring pain, subacute pain, burning sensation, which occurs one to four hours after meals and is relieved by food or alkalis. Nocturnal distress is common, but discomfort before breakfast is rare. The attacks occur at variable intervals and are rather frequent during the spring and fall. They persist for weeks and occasionally months, and are followed by a period of complete relief. Often during the attack only very bland foods are tolerated, but during the interval period of relief any type of food can be eaten without distress. The severity of symptoms may vary strikingly, that is, no symptoms may be present until a serious hemorrhage or perforation occurs, or an ulcer may present severe dyspepsia without complications.

The syndrome of uncomplicated ulcer is pathognomonic of the disease and it has been stated, more or less correctly, that the diagnosis of ulcer could be made by mail or over the telephone. This is true in a very high percentage of the cases, but Rivers has recently reported on a series of patients from whom the typical ulcer story was obtained, and in whom there was evidence of duodenal ulcer by roentgenologic examination, but at operation no lesion was found in the duodenum or stomach even after the duodenum was opened and a careful search made. This picture was usually found in the very nervous, intense type of patient and was generally associated with extreme nervousness or physical fatigue. It frequently left abruptly when the exciting factor was removed or when sedatives were employed. The element of periodicity was occasionally absent, and food and alkali relief tended to be more transient. There was seldom any area of tenderness, nor was there evidence of blood in the stool. At operation nothing more than pylorospasm was noted.

The mechanism of pain in peptic ulcer is still a debatable question. There are those who believe that it is produced by the hydrochloric acid of the gastric juice, others claim that it is produced by pylorospasm. Kinsella believes it to be the result of local pressure on the splanchnic nerves produced by inflammation from the ulcer itself. The pain in uncomplicated duodenal ulcer is usually above the umbilicus, and in the mid-line, while that of gastric ulcer is usually slightly above and to the left of the navel. When the pain in duodenal ulcer shifts upward toward the right infracostal region, into the chest or to the back, we are justified in assuming that we are dealing with deep penetration or partial perforation of the ulcer; radiation definitely to the left and upward or to the back suggests a similar condition when gastric ulcer is present.

Hemorrhage manifests itself in twenty to thirty per cent of the cases, usually in the form of hematemesis in gastric ulcer and as melena in duodenal ulcer. Hemorrhage is more frequent in duodenal ulcer and may be the first sign of disease of the stomach. Hemorrhage is usually followed by a long intermission of symptoms.

The value of gastric analysis in the diagnosis of peptic ulcer is questionable. Gastric ulcers are associated with an acidity slightly below normal and there are many cases on record of duodenal ulcer associated with no free gastric acidity by the ordinary tests. There are countless cases of abnormally high free gastric acid in nervous individuals and in old men in whom no evidence of ulcer can be found. However, it may be said that hyperchlorhydria is a rather constant finding in duodenal ulcer, and the rationale of medical management is largely based on this fact.

The treatment of peptic ulcer depends upon the type of lesion present and whether or not complications exist. In gastric ulcer, if a lesion larger than 2.5 cm. in diameter is found by roentgenologic examination, the possibility of malignant change must be considered and medical management should be carried out only under very careful observation. Naturally, acute or subacute perforation, multiple and uncontrollable hemorrhage, demand surgical intervention. Frequently complete relief is not obtained by medical management and unless associated pathology in the abdomen, such as a chronically inflamed gallbladder or appendix, is removed.

In dealing with duodenal lesions the type of ulcer determines the ultimate method of approach. Here we are confronted with the true duodenal ulcer or with the entity known as duodenitis. True duodenal ulcer is characterized by loss of mucous membrane and the formation of a definite crater; duodenitis by a congestion and edema which may be localized or which may involve the entire circumference of the duodenum. There is no loss of mucous membrane in duodenitis. There is evidence to support the view that duodenitis is a forerunner of true duodenal ulcer. In true duodenal ulcer medical management may be successful, particularly if no extensive degree of ulceration has occurred. On the other hand in large, deep, scarred and fixed lesions, complete relief will usually not be obtained. Duodenitis, however, is the most favorable type, and in this group are found those patients which respond more brilliantly, and in whom the highest percentage of medical cures occur.

In recent years, new therapeutic measures have been suggested. Protein therapy has been advocated but has not met with favor in this country. Metaphen has been used with good results by some observers. The use of mucin in the treatment of ulcer was reported by Fogelson in 1911. Brilliant results have been obtained in individuals who failed to respond to other types of treatment. It is undoubtedly of real value, but the objectionable taste, together with the by-products in some preparations which tend to accentunate gastric secretion, has interfered with its more general use.

Dietary management over a sufficient period of time with the idea of neutralizing the gastric acidity, and avoiding chemical, mechanical, or thermal irritation, and associated with complete mental and physical rest in an individual in whom the healing capacity is inherently great, remains the accepted type of management for the uncomplicated case of peptic ulcer.

THE SIGNIFICANCE OF SYSTOLIC APICAL MURMURS*

E. L. WURTZER, M.D., Clear Lake

This is the commonest murmur heard in the apical region of the heart. It occurs alone at all ages, and in health as well as in disease. Prior to the World War the presence of this murmur carried considerable diagnostic weight, but the opportunities of cardiac examinations afforded by the draft taught the profession that an apical systolic murmur considered alone, was of no practical significance.

Apical systolic murmurs may, for convenience, be classified as follows:

  I. Cardio-respiratory
  II. Extracardiac
  III. Intracardiac

This classification is based upon a presumed mode of production, and not on quality or intensity of the murmurs.

Cardio-respiratory: The cardio-respiratory

*Presented before the Eighty-third Annual Session, Iowa State Medical Society, Des Moines, May 9, 10, 11, 1934.

murmur is very common, especially in children, athletes, and middle-aged adults after exertion, who have perfectly normal hearts. Its production is thought to be as follows: During systole the heart produces a vacuum in the immediately adjacent alveolar lung tissue, thus hastening the inflex of inspiratory air. This murmur is known to exist only during inspiration, and the inspiratory murmur has a cycle distinctly relative to each cardiac systole. Its point of maximum intensity is slightly to the left of the impulse, its quality is soft, and it is never transmitted.

Extracardiac: Extracardiac apical sytolic murmurs are occasionally heard, always over the impulse. They are rough, or rasping in quality, and seem very superficial. This murmur is always systolic in time and is presumed to be caused by a small patch of pericardial inflammation directly over the apex; however, there are no records of autopsy proof, so the mode of production remains assumptive.

Intracardiac: The intracardiac apical systolic murmur is the one with which we are most concerned. Its presence used to signify what we thought to be mitral regurgitation; but after very exhaustive search, both clinical and pathologic, we have been forced to change our conception of this phenomenon, because we lacked pathologic evidence. We can only assume that ventricular systole, forces blood backward through a valve which is incapable of proper closure, but this is seldom verified by clinical or autopsy findings. Clinically there is no specific electrocardiogram or x-ray film, no change in blood pressure, no decrease in the minute volume, and no thrill; and on postmortem examination there is no constant pathology. In normal people there is no dyspnea, nor other evidence of diminished cardiac reserve.

Thus far we have attempted to prove the actual insignificance of this murmur; now let us consider its relative significance. In the acute diseases of childhood, with special reference to polyarthritis and allied diseases, a systolic apical murmur appearing for the first time has some value in that it serves as a guide by attracting our close attention to such a heart. In rheumatic fever, this murmur when first heard can be rightly assumed to result from cardiac damage, either valvular or muscular, or both; yet actual proof is still lacking, until we hear the murmur of mitral disease, or the diastolic apical murmur. Because of the time necessary for the production of the diastolic murmur of mitral disease, it is seldom heard during the acute stage. This murmur may have a slight significance in cases of hypertension with hypertrophy and dilatation, yet its presence only leads us to guess and serves us best as a reminder to watch such a heart.

So on through the life span of the average individual we find only certain periods at which such a murmur is of any significance and then only in a strictly relative sense. In old debilitated people its presence for the first time can be considered as a faint sign of myocardial weakness, yet other signs of myocarditis are much more reliable.

CONCLUSIONS

1. Systolic apical murmurs have no significance when found in healthy people with a negative past medical history.

2. When present for the first time in acute infections of childhood, especially those of the rheumatic type, they can serve us only as a warning of impending cardiac disease.

3. When present for the first time in old people with little cardiac damage, they assist us, inasmuch as they serve as a warning.

4. Finally permit me to emphasize the fact that murmurs in and of themselves are considered poor evidence for the diagnosis or prognosis of heart disease of any type, and there can be no cardiac diagnosis made which is worthy of the name, unless the heart in its entirety, the vascular system in its entirety, and the patient in his or her entirety, receives due study and consideration.

A CASE OF HUMAN ANTHRAX

A. H. Quin, Jr., D.V.M., Des Moines

Anthrax, the once prevalent human scourge due to infection with B. anthracis, a resistant spore-forming anaerobe, is rarely brought to the attention of present day physicians. Regulations governing meat inspection, the sterilization of bristles at shaving brush factories, and industrial precautions for those working in tanneries, wool sorting establishments and packing houses, have all tended to reduce the prevalence of anthrax.

In swine the usual case of anthrax appears as a malignant, edematous pharyngitis. A Grand Island, Nebraska, farm woman thought that one of the pigs on the farm "had a bone in its throat." The animal was killed and rendered for soap. Two days later two of the family cats died on the farm after consuming meat trimmings. Within a few days the woman noticed a lesion on the hand which was thought to be a flea-bite. This vesicular lesion spread rapidly and she presented herself to Dr. W. D. Magrath of Grand Island for treatment. The lesion assumed a blue-black color, raised formation with quick involvement of the lymphatic and axillary lymph glands. Ecchymotic hemorrhages appeared in the axilla. Stained smears from the hand lesion revealed the typical long, chain-like strands of vegetative anthrax bacilli. Dr. W. J. Moslander, D.V.M., Grand Island, confirmed their identification. The patient received liberal doses of anti-anthrax serum and made a good, though somewhat slow recovery. The two cats that died on the farm after eating the hog meat were iced and sent to the State University laboratory at Lincoln. Both showed positive anthrax.

It occurs to the writer that this case well exemplifies the need for cooperation between practicing physicians and veterinarians. With widespread, extensive interstate movement of livestock, diseases that are transmissible from animals to man may make their appearance in the most unexpected places.

THE FINLEY·HOSPITAL CLINICO-PATHOLOGIC CONFERENCES

FIBROMA OF THE CECUM

· J. C. HANCOCK, M.D., Dubuque

Benign tumors of the intestine, while usually considered very rare, have been reported with increasing frequency in recent years. As they often present unusual diagnostic problems, the following case is recorded.

CASE REPORT

The patient, a white widow, sixty-two years of age, housekeeper by occupation, was admitted to The Finley Hospital, October 31, 1923, with the following complaints:

1. Gas in the abdomen
2. Acid eructations
3. Occasional sense of weight or pressure after eating
4. Constipation
5. Nervousness.

Past history: The menopause occurred seventeen years ago. One child is alive and well and there have been no miscarriages.

Family History: Her father died at eighty-four years of age of "heart disease"; her mother at seventy-two years of apoplexy. Two sisters are alive and well and one died of neuritis. Two brothers are living and well, one died postoperatively and one died of "heart disease."

Present illness: The patient's illness started in June with dizziness upon looking upward or rising from a stooping position. This persisted off and on for two weeks. On June 7 she began to have supra-orbital headache. About 5:00 p. m., without nausea she suddenly vomited watery phlegm. The vomiting was frequent and persistent for three days. The headache lasted five days. After the vomiting ceased, a sensation of "palpitation in the chest and abdomen" developed. This was accompanied by soreness throughout and intermittent cramps in the abdomen. Gas in the stomach came at the same time and was relieved by belching. Two months later rumbling in the abdomen began and has recurred at intervals. The soreness in the abdomen was relieved somewhat by expelling flatus, but principally by belching. On admission her appetite was good, but gas and acid eructations with a sense of weight or pressure after meals were present. She was constipated, but the bowels were fairly regular with the aid of drugs. Pain, nausea, and vomiting were absent. She had lost weight and strength and felt very nervous.

Physical examination: The patient was an under developed white woman measuring 58½ inches in height and weighing 69½ pounds. She was pale and of a slightly subicteric color. The temperature was 98 degrees F.; the pulse was 80 and the respiration 20 per minute. The blood pressure was 115/70. The eyes reacted to light and accommodation but the left pupil was slightly larger than the right. The ears, nose, tonsils, larynx and thyroid were negative. A dental plate was present above and ill kept snags below. The lungs were clear. The left border of the heart was 8.5 cm. to the left of the median line in the fifth interspace. On auscultation there was an occasional extra systole and the aortic second was greater than the pulmonic second. The inguinal lymph nodes were slightly enlarged but not tender. There was slight edema of the ankles. The skin was negative. The sensorium was clear, sensation and motion negative, and the knee jerks were equal and brisk. The abdomen was slightly distended especially in the lower half with visible peristalsis working upward to the right side. Borborygmus was present. The lower border of the liver was on a level with the umbilicus. The spleen and left kidney were not palpable, but the right kidney could be felt, being low and slightly movable. In the upper inner angle of the right lower quadrant of the abdomen was a hard, irregularly rounded, slightly tender, movable mass the size of a lemon. Occasionally on pal-

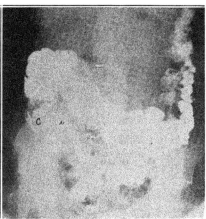

Fig. 1. Irregular filling of the cecum caused by the tumor mass. (c—cecum; i—ileum.)

pation gas seemed to move with a sound as if passing a constriction. This was followed by a change in the feel and contour of the parts. Pelvic examination showed senile and otherwise negative genitalia, rectum and bladder.

X-ray examination: The examination of the gastro-intestinal tract showed atony and ptosis of the stomach. The examination of the small and large intestine were said to be negative. However the shadow of the cecum showed some irregular mottling.*

Course in hospital: During the patient's stay in the hospital for investigation conditions varied almost from day to day. The outstanding variations are as follows: November 3 the patient was comfortable; the abdomen was flat and soft, the mass slightly tender and about the size of a plum was made out slightly below the level of the crest of the ileum in the right lower quadrant. Two days later (November 5) without apparent cause the lower half of the abdomen especially was distended and gas was present. From a point 1½ inches to the right and below the umbilicus to another 2½ inches to the left and above the

* With the knowledge gained at operation the x-ray films were reëxamined. At six hours the shadow of the cecum showed some irregular filling (Fig. 1), now recognized as being due to the tumor. At the end of ten hours the cecal outline was normal. With a barium enema a defect which had been noted was evidently due to the intussusception if the tumor and cecum (Fig. 2). Other films showed the cecum to appear normal. Evidently the dense enema covered the tumor mass in the cecum. The roentgenologist at that time was of the opinion that if a less dense enema had been used, the tumor might have been better outlined. We now know that injection of air into the colon after a barium enema frequently brings to light lesions that cannot be detected with a barium enema alone.

umbilicus, was a soft sausage-like mass ending in a hard irregular nodular mass comparable to that felt previously on the right side. To the left of this the gut was indistinguishable. Pain was obtrusive until relieved by an enema. The next day (November 6) a second sausage-like mass below the left half of the former was added to the previous condition. On November 7 the sausage-like masses had disappeared leaving the hard mass to the left of the umbilicus. By the following day the hard mass had returned to its former location in the right upper quadrant. During the next twelve days the mass could be felt in various parts of the right lower quadrant. In the meantime the patient had gained six pounds in weight and, except for heart-burn, felt well. Meanwhile an Ewald test meal and examinations of the feces, vomitus and urine were negative. At this time the symptoms became aggravated; the mass in the right lower quadrant became tender; and gas pains were very troublesome. The patient vomited frequently and no relief was obtained by enemas. Operation was then decided upon.

Operative note: A median incision from the umbilicus to the symphysis was made. A mass fifteen centimeters in diameter extended between the median line and the outer iliac wall. A fan-shaped veil extended from the outer parietes over the ascending colon and the cecum to the superior aspect of the mesentery of the terminal ileum.

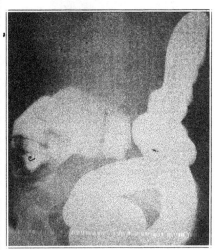

Fig. 2. Colon filled with barium enema. Note the defect caused by the intussusception of the tumor and the cecum. (c—cecum.)

The mass consisted of a double intussusception into which the cecum, the appendix and two inches of ileum were drawn. After severing the mesenteric attachment of the veil, untwisting kinks and reducing the intussusception, a mass the size of a lemon was found in the cecum. On trying to pass the mass along in the ascending colon the head of the cecum followed and the original condition was duplicated, thus showing that the mass was adherent to or a part of the cecal wall. Numerous enlarged lymph glands were found in the mesentery and mesenteriolum. The examination of the other abdominal organs was negative. In view of the question of tuberculosis or malignancy as the primary cause of the complex condition, the appendix and two lymph glands were removed and the cecum and terminal ileum were secured outside the wound. Colostomy was done.

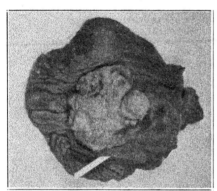

Fig. 3. Surgical specimen showing fibroma of ascending colon. The rod is in the ileocecal valve.

The pathologic report showed no evidence of either tuberculosis or malignancy. Three days later a second operation was performed. Three inches of terminal ileum with its mesentery, the cecum containing the tumor, and the ascending colon, were resected, and a lateral anastomosis was done. The pathologic report is as follows: Grossly; the specimen consists of the terminal ten centimeters of the ileum, the cecum, and seven centimeters of the ascending colon. The lumen of the ileum is narrow due to the pressure of a tumor situated on the wall of the ascending colon just above the ileocecal valve. The tumor has a broad base approximately five centimeters in diameter, and is rounded on the dependent surface which is covered by a thin fibrinous exudate (Fig. 3.) On section it is firm, pale pink, transculent,

and apparently composed of fibrous tissue. It entends to the serosa which is puckered over the mass. Microscopically; several sections of the main tumor and of the adjacent lymph node were made. The latter shows a marked hyperplasia, the germinal centers being very prominent. The sections of the main tumor include the mucosa of the intestine. It is not remarkable except that it is desquamated over the surface of the tumor where it has been replaced by an acute inflammatory exudate. Beneath the acute exudate there is a zone of mononuclear cells. The tumor mass is composed of whirls of adult connective tissue cells with small nuclei. No mitotic figures are seen.

Pathologic diagnosis: Fibroma of the cecum.

Final clinical diagnosis: Fibroma of the cecum with double intussusception; partial bowel obstruction.

Subsequent course: The immediate postoperative condition was excellent. On the third day the bowels moved spontaneously and the patient asked for food. A purulent discharge with a fecal odor came from the wound for a few days. After expelling a linen suture the sinus gradually closed. A more troublesome complication was an extensive ulcerative stomatitis. This cleared up after extraction of the teeth. The patient left the hospital fourteen weeks after admission in good condition. She has remained consistently free from abdominal symptoms for eleven years.

SUMMARY

The case reported is of interest because of:

1. The comparative rarity of recorded cases of fibroma of the cecum.

2. The combination of neoplasm, infection and veil which produced the variable symptoms and signs.

3. Partial intestinal obstruction due to double intussusception.

4. The inflammatory condition including enlarged lymph nodes which obscured the diagnosis at the first operation.

5. Confirmation of observation that intussusception in the large gut rarely leads to complete obstruction (DeQuervain).

6. Confirmation to date of the pathologist's diagnosis of benign neoplasm.

7. The importance of operating in the presence of positive clinical evidence and equivocal or negative x-ray findings.

8. The consistently symptomless digestion during the eleven years since the operation.

STATE DEPARTMENT OF HEALTH

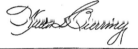

ANOTHER MAJOR OUTBREAK OF MEASLES IN IOWA

Measles has again assumed epidemic proportions in Iowa. Many cases are being reported daily at this time, particularly from certain counties in the eastern and northeastern sections of the state. During October, the counties reporting the most cases were Franklin, Jackson, Black Hawk, Marshall and Howard. In November, most of the cases were reported from Muscatine, Black Hawk, Benton, Linn and Scott counties. The disease has been very prevalent in Bremer and Clayton counties, but official reports have not been made to the State Department of Health. Thus far in 1934 (through November 30) 5,877 cases of measles have been reported.

Many deaths attributable to measles accompany each major outbreak of this disease. In 1924 there were 262 deaths. In 1926, 63 deaths occurred and in 1927, deaths numbered 230. Thirty-nine cases of measles resulted fatally in 1929 and 199 in 1930. Thus far in 1934 (to September 1), there have been 56 deaths, of which 39, or 70 per cent, affected counties in the western half of the state. Eleven deaths were reported from Pottawattamie and four from Woodbury county.

The monthly distribution of measles cases and deaths thus far in 1934, as contrasted with 1932, a year of low prevalence of measles, is indicated in the following table:

	Cases		Deaths	
Month	1932	1934	1932	1934
January	14	219	0	0
February	24	481	0	2
March	13	884	0	4
April	13	976	0	17
May	21	1,432	1	12
June	18	679	0	13
July	17	168	0	5
August	4	33	0	3
September	8	17	1	....
October	7	102	0	....
November	9	886	0	....
December	8	......	0	....

Figures based on the study of cases and deaths reported by months for the nine-year period from 1924 to 1932, indicate that disease incidence and case fatality rates are highest during the first five months of the year. The peak of a measles epidemic occurs, as a rule, in March. A longer period than is usual between major outbreaks, has elapsed since 1930. From all indications, the year 1934 will be analogous to 1929, the year which lead to maximum incidence of and mortality rate from measles in 1930. October of 1934 witnessed the reporting of the largest number of cases for the month, since 1929; reports for November, 1934 (886 cases) exceeded those for the same month of 1929, when 265 cases were reported. If the present outbreak runs true to form, the largest number of cases and deaths may be expected during the early months of 1935.

Physicians, in increasing number, are using immune adult blood to prevent or modify the attack of measles in infants and other children, following exposure to the disease. The procedure was described in an article entitled "Measles Outbreak Expected," in the February, 1934, number of this JOURNAL, on page 104. Ten c.c. of blood (some authorities recommend twenty c.c.) are taken from an arm vein of a parent or person known to be immune to measles. A preliminary Wassermann test should be made, if indicated. The blood is injected at once into the gluteal muscles of the child concerned. The treatment is carried out, preferably on the fourth day after exposure. Earlier treatment will prevent measles, which may be desirable in susceptible children with lowered resistance. If the transfer of blood is made on the fourth to seventh day following exposure, measles appears in attenuated form. A modified attack is desirable in healthy children, since active permanent immunity is thus acquired. The procedure can be carried out conveniently in the home.

Measles sweeps through a community and plays havoc with children. Concerted effort on the part of physicians, nurses, teachers and parents is important in directing attention to underprivileged children who may be subject to severe complications. Through publicity and health education the value of preventive treatment with immune serum will gain wider recognition. The procedure of obtaining blood from volunteers, separating the serum and transferring to five or ten c.c. vials, is well known. A supply of immune serum may thus be made available for certain children, and hospitals can serve as distributing centers. The task of lowering the mortality rate from measles, although more difficult than that of the prevention of diphtheria and smallpox, should not be insurmountable.

KANSAS ACCIDENT FACTS

Earle G. Brown, M.D., Secretary and Executive officer, Kansas State Board of Health, speaking before The Ninth Annual Meeting of the Iowa Public Health Association, said:

"Accidents as a cause of death have demanded the attention of public health authorities for many years. The report of the Bureau of the Census for the year 1933 shows in the United States a total of 91,085 accidental deaths, and a death rate of 72.5 for each 100,000 population, and well indicates the seriousness of the accident problem.

"In 1914 less than 1,000 accidental deaths were reported in Kansas, comprising slightly more than five per cent of the deaths from all causes. In 1933, 1,541 accidental deaths were reported, comprising 7.8 per cent of the deaths from all causes. Indications are that more than 1,900 accidental deaths will be reported in 1934 and total nearly ten per cent of the deaths from all causes.

"Accidental deaths in Kansas have assumed fifth place among the principal causes, being exceeded in number of deaths only by heart disease, Bright's disease, cancer and apoplexy.

"The Kansas State Board of Health during the past five years has made special studies of all accidental deaths.

"In studying accidental deaths, classifications are made into four groups: home accidents, motor vehicle accidents, public accidents and industrial accidents. In 1932 and 1933 home accidents ranked first with 34 per cent of all accidental deaths; motor vehicles were second with 33 per cent; public accidents, not involving a motor vehicle, third, with 19 per cent, and industrial accidents fourth, with 13.2 per cent.

"In the home, falls accounted for more than fifty per cent of the fatal accidents; burns were second in importance with approximately one out of five deaths charged to this cause; poisons ranked third, and firearms fourth.

"In reviewing the place of occurrence of accidental falls for the three-year period, 1931-1933, it was found that the most frequent location was in the bedroom, next the living room and third, the stairs or steps. In studying the causes of the falls, it was found that approximately one death in four resulted from over-balancing or general weakness and one in five was due to slipping on a polished floor, floor covering, rug or on a wet, icy surface. Dizziness or fainting attacks accounted for ten per

cent, and another ten per cent was attributed to falling in or out of bed.

"More than fifty per cent of the accidents where fatal burns were received occurred in the kitchen. Approximately one-third of 244 deaths resulting from accidental burns during the years 1931-1933 were due to injuries received during explosions caused by the use of kerosene or gasoline in building fires. More than fifteen per cent were the result of burns received when clothing caught fire from gas ranges or gas heaters.

"Reported automobile accidents in Kansas have increased from 36 in 1914 to 491 in 1933. During the three-year period, 1931-1933, 1,202 deaths have been recorded, 1,051 of which were the result of accidents which occurred in cities and villages of less than 2,500 population, or in the country. Nearly ninety per cent of the persons were fatally injured in accidents which occurred in fair weather. Approximately one-third of the deaths were the result of accidents which occurred during the months of July, August and September. Non-collision accidents ranked first; collisions with motor vehicles, second; collisions of motor vehicles with pedestrians, third, and collisions of motor vehicles with fixed objects, fourth.

"Accidents originating in agriculture comprised nearly fifty per cent of all industrial deaths. On the basis of the numbers engaged in the occupation, however, mining was the most hazardous occupation.

"Machinery accidents were responsible for nearly one-third of the fatal agriculture accidental deaths. Other causes, in order of importance included, vehicles, excessive heat, and accidental falls."

In concluding his paper, Dr. Brown discussed the five cardinal points on which programs for accident prevention are based. They were stated to be:

"1· Conditions must be safe.

2. Avoid danger which can be removed.

3. Personal habits of carefulness.

4. Thoughtfulness and consideration for other people, and

5. Observance of laws."

PREVALENCE OF DISEASE

	Oct. '34	Sept. '34	Oct. '33	Most Cases Reported From
Diphtheria	69	21	82	Pottawattamie, Dubuque
Scarlet Fever	217	114	272	Polk, Wright
Typhoid Fever	72	90	16	Boone, Monroe
Smallpox	6	2	4	Delaware
Measles	102	17	6	Franklin, Jackson
Whooping Cough	34	37	96	Linn, Woodbury
Cerebrospinal Meningitis	5	3	1	Polk
Chickenpox	133	17	80	Woodbury, Dubuque
Mumps	60	38	10	Dubuque, Linn
Poliomyelitis	7	7	13	(For State)
Tuberculosis	66	31	39	(For State)
Undulant Fever	21	26	4	(For State)
Syphilis	115	113	130	(For State)
Gonorrhea	173	160	185	(For State)

The JOURNAL of the
Iowa State Medical Society
ISSUED MONTHLY

SUBSCRIPTION $3.00 PER YEAR

Address all communications to the Editor of the Journal,
505 Bankers Trust Building, Des Moines

OFFICE OF PUBLICATION, DES MOINES, IOWA

Vol. XXIV   DECEMBER, 1934   No. 12

CHRISTMAS

At the Christmas time, commemorating the birth of "The Great Physician," we are prompted to reflect upon His life. There are many things in His life which carry with them the thought of sadness—His sacrifice, His rejection by His fellowmen, and His final grief—but Christmas does not appear to be the appropriate time for meditation upon these sombre aspects of His life. Our minds turn instinctively to His nativity in a Bethlehem manger, to His love for little children, and His inspiration to His fellow-men. No influence has been so far-reaching and so lasting as His in advancing civilization. No phase of His life was more inspiring, perhaps, than His steadfastness to ideals. Unwavering in His devotion to ideals, His life reveals a richness and a fullness denied the average man.

Medical history is replete with noble characters who, in their singleness of purpose, have emulated "The Great Physician." We have known our Jenners, our Hunters, our Pasteurs, our Kochs, our Curies and our Roentgens, all memorable and all honored because of their steadfastness to an ideal. Only the idealist possesses the infinite patience which drills the perfection of tomorrow out of the mistakes and errors of all yesterdays and todays. Only the idealist can fail and then begin again with undaunted courage and unfaltering belief in his ability to attain the goal of his ideal. The handicap of disease, of heartbreak, of poverty, of affliction, has not prevented the great masters and pioneers of medical thought from achieving their goals. A broken body may contain an unbroken will to do, and it is this will and steadfastness of purpose which assures success.

Perhaps reflection upon these matters at this Christmas time will add to the fullness of your life

and mine. If we keep before us His singleness of purpose, His unfaltering pursuit of His ideal, we may be lured into the untrodden fields where unlimited possibilities await us, where self-development and thought-fulfillment are the rewards. In this we would fashion our lives after that of "The Great Physician" whose birth nineteen hundred and thirty-four years ago we commemorate this month.

THE COMMITTEE ON ECONOMIC SECURITY

Adhering to an opinion expressed in his extraordinary message to Congress last June, President Roosevelt continues to declare himself in favor of legislation to provide "security against several of the great disturbing factors in life" and specifically designates unemployment, care of the aged and "the problems of economic life due to sickness." Soon after the President's pronouncement on these matters he appointed a Committee on Economic Security whose duty it was to ascertain and survey all available facts pertinent to these questions, and to deliver to the President recommendations which could be properly incorporated in bills to be considered by Congress at its next session.

To study those problems dealing with the development of a scheme of medical care adequately serving all patients, particularly those in the lower income groups, a subcommittee designated as the Medical Advisory Board to the Committee on Economic Security, was appointed and held its first meeting on November 15 and 16. We believe this Medical Advisory Board, composed of eleven eminent physicians, constitutes a noteworthy body unquestionably representative of the physicians of this country and one in which we may repose confidence.

To anticipate the achievements of a group it is necessary to know the men who constitute the group and to study carefully their past records, particularly as their attitude reflects the present problem. A review of the personnel of this committee therefore seems desirable.

Outstanding in the group is Iowa's Walter L. Bierring, president of the American Medical Association, distinguished educator and clinician, and nestor of scientific medicine in this state. Harvey Cushing, the Sterling professor of neurology in Yale University, long professor of surgery at Johns Hopkins and Harvard University, and author of the epochal address, "Medicine at the Cross Roads," has demonstrated, through many years of active service to organized medicine, his unswerving adherence to the tenets of our profession. George W. Crile, one of the founders and director of the research Laboratory, Cleveland Clinic, since 1921, and professor of clinical surgery in Western Reserve University since 1890, has occupied an enviable position in the forefront of American medicine. While definitely believing in group practice, Dr. Crile has never advocated practices which violate medical ethics and has publicly declared himself in favor of a plan permitting the free choice of a physician by the patient.

We might continue through the entire list in detail, but suffice it to say that without exception the members of the committee are all men of distinction in American Medicine. Not only are they outstanding as physicians and as educators but many of them have devoted much time and study to the problems of medical practice and on this basis have submitted plans for a modification in medical practice to fit "the changing times," a fact which assures thoroughness in the deliberations of the committee. George M. Piersol, editor-in-chief of the Cyclopedia of Medicine since 1929 and active consultant at the Philadelphia General Hospital since 1930, is a past president of the American College of Physicians, and at present is dean of students and professor of medicine at the Graduate School of the University of Pennsylvania. James A. Miller has served Columbia University's College of Physicians and Surgeons since 1913 as professor of clinical medicine, and is president-elect of the American College of Physicians. Robert B. Greenough has been affiliated with the Massachusetts General Hospital as house officer (1896-1915), visiting surgeon (1915-1932) and consulting surgeon (1932——), and this year took office as president of the American College of Surgeons. James D. Bruce is vice president of the University of Michigan and has ably served that institution as director of postgraduate medical education since 1928. Thomas Parran, at one time chief of the division of venereal diseases, United States Public Health Service, now Commissioner New York State Health Department, has been, since 1931, treasurer of the American Public Health Association. Stewart R. Roberts, recognized as one of the South's leading physicians, has occupied the chair of professor of clinical medicine at the Atlanta Medical College for the past fifteen years. J. Sheldon Horsley is surgeon in charge of St. Elizabeth's Hospital, Richmond, Virginia. Rexwald Brown is the organizer and head of the Santa Barbara Clinic, and director of the surgical division of the Santa Barbara Cottage Hospital.

So much for the personnel of the Medical Advisory Board. In full appreciation of their responsibility to the medical profession and the pub-

lic at large, one of the acts of the Board was the appointment of the Technical Committee whose function it will be to collect data, sift findings, and otherwise serve the Board in a technical capacity. Dr. R. G. Leland and Mr. A. M. Simons of the Bureau of Medical Economics of the American Medical Association will serve with a group of statisticians and economists on this subcommittee. The work of the Medical Advisory Board has not progressed to the point where a declaration of policy can be made. We are assured, however, that at this preliminary meeting referred to above, the members of the Board indicated a unanimous approval of the principles of practice accepted by our national organization and their concurrence with the thought expressed by the President and the Secretary of Labor that painstaking research, exhaustive fact finding, with thoughtful analysis, should precede all recommendations. The American Medical Association, through its House of Delegates, has repeatedly declared its opposition to the socialization of medical practice, but at its last annual session voted in favor of "properly controlled experimentation, with new forms of medical practice" subject to limitations which assure the maintenance of the present patient-doctor relationship.

The Medical Advisory Board has requested the cooperation of the American Medical Association through its Bureau of Medical Economics, and this cooperation has been promised. We have every reason to believe that this eminent board of physicians, operating for the security and welfare of the entire citizenry of the United States, and with a fair appreciation of the problems and ideals of medical practice, will discharge their responsibility in a manner which will merit and receive the approbation of all physicians.

STANDARDIZED SEROLOGY IN SYPHILIS

Today many agencies are concerned in the problem of the standardization of those serologic tests employed in the diagnosis of syphilis. These several efforts have been prompted by the knowledge and realization that wide variations exist in the usefulness of the various technics employed, and that none is ideal. The Health Organization of the League of Nations in 1923 instituted laboratory conferences concerning the serologic diagnosis of syphilis. As a result of these conferences the League members designated certain laboratories where critical and well checked experiments with the various methods could be conducted. In their published report of 1932 they critically survey twenty different modifications of the Bordet-Wassermann test, and thirteen different flocculation tests involving the use of 2,766 blood and spinal fluid samples.

They appreciate from this study that their work is incomplete and that scores of other methods have been or are being employed that should not be discarded without study. They further appreciate that consciously or, more frequently, unconsciously, a standard method of reaction undergoes modification when employed in the different laboratories. These modifications may involve factors of such basic importance as to constitute a completely new procedure.

In this country a very definite and well organized attempt is being made to assist this world attempt at standardization. The United States Public Health Service has recently issued a notice to all serologists, inviting their cooperation in the drafting of a plan to evaluate independent serologic procedures for the diagnosis of syphilis in this country. Briefly, the plan contemplates the collection of blood samples from at least 1,000 individuals, and the distribution of comparable specimens to all serologists or laboratories where original modifications of a complement-fixation or precipitation test have been devised. A committee of six specialists covering the field of clinical syphilology, clinical pathology and two officers of the United States Public Health Service, will collect the several reports submitted by the participating serologists, and upon the basis of their interpretation of the results, attempt an evaluation of the method employed.* They invite all serologists interested to participate, and a communication addressed to the Surgeon General of the United States Public Health Service, Washington, D. C., will secure for the interested pathologist full details of the plan.

Clinicians, particularly, will be interested to note that the investigations so far made by these organized bodies, especially those affiliated with the Health Organization of the League of Nations, suggest that the modifications of Sordelli, of Harrison-Wyler, and of the Bordet-Wassermann test appear superior to other modifications, and that the Kahn standard and Müller clotting test are the most reliable of the flocculation methods. For the procedure of choice and to insure the greatest accuracy they recommend the employment of two flocculation methods and one Wassermann method on all samples. Their studies indicate that error is negligibly slight where the blood serum is subjected to the three tests indicated.

* The Journal of the American Medical Association for December 1, carries a detailed report of this committee.

APPLICATION OF THE BASIC SCIENCE LAW IN IOWA*

The following questions have been raised in discussion of the proposed basic science law, and answers have been prepared by the Legislative Committee

Q: Does the applicant have to take the examination before the Basic Science Board before he matriculates in professional school?

A: No.

Q: Is the examination of the Basic Science Board in lieu of any examination now given?

A: The bill is drawn so that the licensing boards may accept the approval of basic boards in the subjects in which the Basic Science Board offers examination.

Q. When is an applicant eligible to take the examination required by the Basic Science Board?

A: The applicant must have a high school education and be twenty-one years of age. Having met those requirements he may apply to the Basic Science Board when he feels he is fitted.

Q: What would this mean in concrete experience of students?

A: They could apply to the Basic Science Board as soon as they had completed their courses in these subjects: anatomy, physiology, chemistry, pathology, hygiene and bacteriology.

Q: Would it mean that applicants have to pay an additional fee as compared with the present system?

A: Not unless the licensing board refused to accept the examination of the Basic Science Board.

Q: Will the creation of the Basic Science Board be "just another board," with increased expense to the state?

A: No. The total expense of the Board would not be great and it should be largely offset by the acceptance by the licensing boards. It would decrease the expense of the other boards.

Q: Why should not the acceptance of the Basic Science Board examination by the licensing boards be mandatory, making certain that the expense would not be increased?

A: There is no apparent objection to having it mandatory.

Q: If adopted, how will the measure affect men already in practice, or in school now?

A: It would not affect them. It is not retroactive in fact or in purpose.

* Editorials discussing the Basic Science Law have previously appeared in the October and November issues of this publication.

Dr. Edward Livingston Trudeau

Founder of the Sanatorium Movement in the United States and Originator of the Modern Treatment of the Disease

By A. Schaeffer, Jr.

"His life was gentle, and the elements
So mix'd in him that Nature might stand up,
And say to all the world, this was a man!"
—Shakespeare.

A doctor, doomed by tuberculosis, hunting foxes in the Adirondack Mountains in 1875 noticed that the less he walked, the better he felt. Today one of the greatest sanatoria in the world forms a monument to that observation. Edward Livingston Trudeau was the physician, and Trudeau Sanatorium, world-famous center for treatment and research, is the monument. In commemoration of the fiftieth anniversary of the opening of the one room cottage that became the nucleus not only of that single institution, but of the entire sanatorium movement in this country, the familiar Christmas Seal that finances the efforts of the affiliated tuberculosis associations to overcome this disease bears this picture of "Little Red," as the cottage is called.

Trudeau was born in New York City, October 5, 1848. He was the descendant of many generations of French physicians, and was thus well qualified by heredity for the discovery he was destined to make. His youth was spent with his grandparents in Paris, where he obtained his education in French schools. Returning to New York at eighteen, he was able to spend several years of leisure during which he engaged in popular social activities and atheletic sports. Then, deciding to settle upon some career, he secured an appointment to the Naval Academy, which was then at Newport.

He relinquished his career to become the devoted nurse of his brother, who had contracted tuberculosis. During the illness Trudeau often slept with his brother, and by order of the attending physician every window in the room was kept tightly closed. Of course, he also contracted the disease. It was not until he had married and established himself in medical practice several

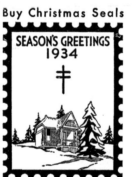

Buy Christmas Seals

SEASON'S GREETINGS
1934

Help Fight Tuberculosis

years later, however, that the fact was realized, although in the light of present knowledge he had several warnings. The first resulted after a walking match from Fifty-ninth Street to the Battery. Although he was an excellent athlete and sportsman, he was thoroughly exhausted from the match for several days, and developed a "cold" abscess which had to be operated upon several times.

While in England during his honeymoon, the second warning came in the form of a swelling of the lymphatic glands, but so little was the mechanism of tuberculosis infection known then that no alarm was felt. Actual discovery came when a fellow physician declared he looked ill and insisted on taking his temperature. It was 101 degrees! Still unconcerned, and merely to forestall an argument, Trudeau went to a specialist for examination. He was told that the upper two-thirds of his left lung was involved!

In those days a diagnosis of tuberculosis was considered a death sentence. Trudeau felt that he was merely marking time, but he did try in the South and in Minnesota to improve his health. His traveling was in vain, so he decided to spend his last days in his favorite hunting ground in the Adirondack Mountains of northern New York state. This region was then a wilderness braved only by ardent sportsmen, but he was determined to remain there throughout the winter of 1874. So deep-rooted at that time was the belief that a consumptive should seek a warm and sunny climate, and avoid cold and storm, that only after considerable argument and persuasion could he induce Paul Smith and his wife to allow him and his family to spend the winter at their hunting lodge. On his fox-hunting trips during that winter Trudeau made his observation regarding the value of rest in treating tuberculosis.

"I found," he said, "that I could not walk enough to stand much chance for a shot without feeling sick and feverish the next day, and this was the first intimation I had as to the value of the rest cure. I walked very little after this, and my faith in the value of the rest cure became more and more fully established."

The idea of building the sanatorium originated in his reading, in 1882, an account of Brehmer's Sanitarium in Silesia. No information was available regarding the planning and building of sanatoria, but Dr. Trudeau "felt that aggregation should be avoided, and segregation, such as could be secured by the cottage plan, would be preferable. Friends in New York contributed sufficient funds to permit him to erect a few small cottages. The first one, called the "Little Red" because it was painted that color, was completed in February, 1884.

In the same year in which Trudeau read of Brehmer's Sanitarium, Dr. Robert Koch's epochal paper on "The Etiology of Tuberculosis" appeared. Trudeau determined to prove Koch's experiments for himself, and plunged into experimental work with guinea pigs. In order to carry out his laboratory work he was forced to make his own apparatus, keep his guinea pigs warm in a hole in the ground, and arise several times each night during cold snaps to stir up the fire and provide the correct temperature for his cultures. He succeeded despite the handicaps, and his laboratory (at first a makeshift that was burned down and later rebuilt) was the first in this country to be devoted to the study of tuberculosis.

As his work became known he received the co-operation of the leaders of the medical profession. His sanatorium soon became an assured success and his long single-handed fight in the dense woods of the Adirondacks against the tubercle bacillus was winning him high honors. One of the greatest of these was his unanimous election in 1904 as the first president of the newly organized National Tuberculosis Association.

During his life Dr. Trudeau was forced many times to take to his bed because his tuberculosis lesion had become active, and several times his life was despaired of. Yet he lived until November 15, 1915, to the age of sixty-seven years. Before his death he had the satisfaction of seeing the benefits of his laborious research and experiments carried into every corner of the United States by bits of colored paper—the penny Christmas Seals.

Since the time when Trudeau was the first president of the National Tuberculosis Associa-

tion, the organization has become the parent of 2,000 affiliated associations in all parts of the United States. Through its organized campaign supported by funds raised in the annual Christmas seal sales, it has been greatly responsible for reducing the death rate from tuberculosis.

In a speech Trudeau delivered shortly before his death he said, "Over the doors of the hospitals for consumptives twenty-five years ago might well have been written these words: 'All hope abandon ye that enter here.' while today, in the light of new knowledge we may justly place at the entrance of the modern sanatorium the more hopeful inscription: 'Cure sometimes, relief often, comfort always.'"

THE OPEN FORUM

DIVERTICULUM OF THE GALLBLADDER

In the January, 1934, issue of the Journal of the Iowa State Medical Society, I reported a case of diverticulum of the gallbladder. After looking up the literature on this subject I found that only fifteen such cases had been reported up to this date, with only six from our country. Such being the case I have another to report, thus making a total of seven in this country.

On December 27, 1933, I was called to see a patient who was having typical gallbladder colic and I treated him accordingly. He was forty-eight years of age, single and had lived in this country nine years. He had been operated upon for a ruptured appendix seven years ago. He was brought to the hospital and treated medically until December 29, at which time operation was indicated.

Spinal anesthesia was used; an upper right rectus incision was made; a few adhesions about the gallbladder were freed; and I could see that the gallbladder was in such a condition that rupture might take place very easily. The serous lining over the fundus was very thin, and beneath it was a stone 1.5 inches in length and 0.5 inches in thickness. In the cavity proper was a stone of similar size. The gallbladder was removed and a rubber drain was inserted laterally. Convalescence progressed nicely for two weeks, at which time an abscess developed in the rectum, but after it was opened and drained for two days, healing took place and no other complication occurred.

I sent this specimen, as well as that from the other case, to the pathology department at the University of Minnesota, where Dr. E. T. Bell examined them, and reported both to be true diverticula.   A. L. Pertl, M.D.,
Windom, Minn.

SPEAKERS BUREAU ACTIVITIES

CLARENCE WILLIAM BALDRIDGE
1896-1934

Clarence William Baldridge was born in Strawberry Point, Iowa, September 4, 1896, and died in an automobile accident November 22 while enroute to Fort Madison, where he was to give a lecture in connection with an extension course being given in that city.

He was graduated from the Strawberry Point High School and in 1915 entered the University of Iowa, where he was granted the bachelor of science degree in 1920 and the degree of doctor of medicine in 1921. He was a member of the Phi Beta Pi medical fraternity and ranked as one of the better students of his class, being honored by a membership in the Alpha Omega Alpha and later Sigma Xi.

Following the completion of his medical course he was selected as an interne in the department of theory and practice of medicine from 1921 to 1922, and subsequently promoted to clinical assistant in 1922; lecturer in clinical microscopy, 1923; lecturer in medicine, 1924; assistant professor in medicine, 1927 and associate professor, 1930.

Dr. Baldridge was married to Ada Elizabeth Buck of Iowa City, August 1, 1923, to which union four children were born: Patricia, ten years of age, Richard, nine, Barbara, six, and Thomas, four.

Doctor Baldridge was a member of the Johnson County Medical Society, the Iowa State Medical Society, the American Medical Association, the Iowa Clinical Medical Society, the Central Clinical Research Club, the Central Society for Clinical Research, the Society for Experimental Biology and Medicine, and the American Society for Clinical Investigation. His election to sectional and national medical societies, largely through the recognition of his investigations, came in rapid succession during the past few years.

During the year 1924 and 1925 Doctor Baldridge spent much of his time in the department of pathology. This not only extended his knowledge and intensified his interest in this field, but had a very significant influence on his subsequent development in internal medicine. Even at an early period in his medical career, he had a remarkable understanding of clinical problems and with the later development of his investigative interests he was soon recognized as showing unusual promise in academic medicine. In 1931 he was granted a leave of absence for study in physiology with Professor Carlson of the

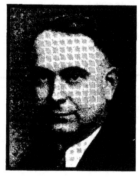

CLARENCE WILLIAM BALDRIDGE
· 1896-1934

University of Chicago. His ability was appreciated by Professor Carlson who urged that he work toward the degree of doctor of philosophy in physiology. He had completed the requirements for this degree which would have been conferred by the University of Chicago at the Christmas convocation.

Doctor Baldridge possessed the unusual qualifications of an excellent clinician, an inspiring teacher and a nationally recognized investigator. His publications pertaining particularly to the diseases of the blood and the field of metabolism were rapidly attracting widespread attention and he was coming to be regarded as one of the outstanding younger men in American medicine. With his broad basic background, his analytic mind, his accomplishments to date, and his ability to drive toward a given objective, he was assured of a distinguished career in medicine.

Fred M. Smith, M.D.

IN APPRECIATION

"Our little systems have their day,
They have their day and cease
to be."

Doctor Baldridge was killed while in the service of the medical profession of Iowa. He died in an attempt to make our physicians better doctors, and the citizens of Iowa suffer less from disease.

We grieve his departure. Doctor Baldridge is not the first to die in order that humanity may suffer less, and he will not, thank God, be the last, for the grim fight against disease must go on. It is small comfort to us of the Speakers Bureau to remember that he was heart and soul in favor of the work we are attempting to do. We cannot escape a sense of guilt as we think of the loss and grief his family has suffered because he did our bidding. Nor can we help wondering how long we must continue to labor in order to overbalance the loss to humanity in general of such a splendid physician in the very prime of his life.

Doctor Baldridge is dead and gone, and yet is he? There are hundreds of physicians in Iowa who knew him to love and admire him. He was in the very finest sense an ideal physician. His noble character was in the fullest measure a source of joy and inspiration to all with whom he came in contact. His untiring efforts to add to our knowledge of disease and to develop more ideal practitioners of medicine gives us a goal toward which to work. No one could come into even the most cursory contact with Doctor Baldridge without being a better person for it, and none could know him but to love him.

His influence is more alive today than it ever was. It will go on and on, making better doctors and less suffering in this world. He is neither dead, nor does he sleep. The ideals he struggled for, and the splendid work which he accomplished, will continue to live long after him.

MEETING OF MERIT NOVEMBER, 1934

Credit for the meeting of merit for November is awarded to the Wapello County Medical Society for the meeting held November 5 at the Hotel Ottumwa, in Ottumwa. This meeting was unique in many respects. In the first place, the Kiwanis Club, the Rotary Club, the dentists and the nurses of Wapello County were guests of the Wapello County Medical Society, as well as many doctors from outside counties. It was a dinner meeting, and the room was packed. The address of the evening was an excellent talk given by W. W. Bauer, M.D., of the American Medical Association. He was introduced by Gordon F. Harkness, M.D., president of the Iowa State Medical Society, who stressed the fact that in these days of regimentation of business and industry, there was also a definite attempt being made to regiment the doctors; hence the doctors and the business men were in the same predicament and should therefore work together in order to maintain initiative and fair play. Dr. Bauer stressed the fact that the American Medical Association was really the local doctor, and that the proper procedure in medical matters was to consult the local doctor rather than to fly around the country in aeroplanes seeking sensational cures. The secretary of the Wapello County Medical Society, Evon Walker, M.D., deserves credit for arranging a most interesting meeting.

RADIO BROADCASTS

Our schedule of broadcasts from W.SUI at Iowa City has been changed from Thursday to Monday evening, at 8:00 p. m. The time of broadcasts over WOI remains unchanged, Wednesday at 4:00 p. m.

December 5-10—Tuberculosis in Children—R. H. McBride, M.D.

December 12-17—Diphtheria and Pneumonia—Isaac Sternhill, M.D.

December 19-24—A Merry Christmas, F. O. Woodard, M.D.

December 26-31—The Cause of Cancer—H. P. Smith, M.D.

January 2- 7—The Patient and the Doctor—T. F. Thornton, M.D.

THE NEW LILLY RESEARCH LABORATORY

Announcement has been made that on October 11, 1934, Eli Lilly and Company opened with appropriate dedicatory services the new Lilly Research Laboratory in Indianapolis. This event is of outstanding interest, first because it is significant of the epochal interest taken by manufacturing chemists in the researches of practical therapy, and second because of this unusual gathering of noted authorities from over the world. Presiding at the formal exercises was Eli Lilly, head of the famous Lilly organization. Mr. J. J. Lilly, chairman of the board of directors, spoke on the subject "Research in Manufacturing Pharmacy." Dr. Irving Langmuir, director of research for the General Electric Company, discussed "The Unpredictable Results of Research." Dr. Frederick Banting, discoverer of insulin for the treatment of diabetes, talked on "The Early History of Insulin." Sir Henry Dale, director of the National Institute for Medical Research in London, the last of the formal speakers on the afternoon program, chose as his topic "Chemical Ideas in Medicine and Biology."

COLLECTION AGENCY NOT APPROVED

Several inquiries have recently been received at the central office from members of the Society, regarding the Affiliated Underwriters Loan and Finance Company, and the Birdsell Loan and Finance Company, Inc., of Evanston, Illinois. Information in the files of the Bureau of Medical Economics of the American Medical Association shows that these two companies are officered in many instances by the same persons. The Bureau reports that photostatic copies of the articles of incorporation of the two companies show them to be similar in detail. For information concerning the Birdsell Loan and Finance Co., Inc., we would refer you to the March 31, 1934, issue of the Journal of the American Medical Association, page 1087. Neither of these companies has been granted the approval of the Committee on Medical Economics of the Iowa State Medical Society.

NATIONAL SOCIETY FOR THE PREVENTION OF BLINDNESS

The Annual Conference of the National Society for the Prevention of Blindness will be held in New York City, December 6-8. Dr. Edward Jackson of Denver, Colo., dean of American ophthalmologists, will deliver the principal address on the subject, "A Wide Basis for Blindness Prevention." Dr. Jackson was the first recipient, in 1925, of the Leslie Dana Gold Medal which is awarded annually for outstanding achievements in the prevention of blindness and conservation of vision. Topics that will be discussed at the conference are: the causes of blindness; sight-saving classes for children with seriously defective vision; prevention of eye accidents; and prevention of pre-natal infections which may cause blindness.

WOMAN'S AUXILIARY NEWS

Edited by the Press and Publicity Committee

MRS. OLIVER J. FAY, *Chairman*, 405 Thirty-seventh Street, Des Moines

PROGRAM SUGGESTIONS

Several requests have been received from various program chairmen for a list of medical books which would be suitable for study by the auxiliary, or for review before local lay groups. To fill this need, there will from time to time appear on this page notices of recent books written by physicians, or about physicians. Some books which have received especial notice during the last few months include:

1. Yellow Jacket. The play from which this book has been written is one of the present dramatic successes in New York. The story is that of the life of Walter Reed. Published by Harcourt, Brace and Company, New York.

2. Vitality. By Boris Sokoloff, M.D. Why go before your time? Here is the latest answer to the great question. Published by Dutton.

3. The Case for Sterilization. By Leon F. Whitney. It completely handles this much discussed question. Twenty-seven states have already passed valid laws authorizing sterilization. In 1933, over 16,000 persons willingly submitted to the treatment. This book is perhaps the best treatment of the subject to date. Published by Frederick A. Stokes Company, New York.

4. How the Mind Works. By Cyril Burt, Ernest Jones, Emmanuel Miller and William Moodie. Is psychology quackery, a fad, or sheer common sense? Here are all the answers. Published by D. Appleton-Century Company, New York.

5. Life of Sir Robert Jones. By Frederick Watson. This is a book that all orthopedic physicians will delight in reading. As a life story it will appeal to all doctors and lovers of humanity. A national memorial to Sir Robert Jones is being promoted by leading men in the medical profession and in public life.

6. The Great Doctors. By Dr. Henry E. Sigerist, professor of the history of medicine at Johns Hopkins University. From the first Gods of Medicine, Imhotep and Aesculapius, to Pasteur and Osler. The author tells the story of those who "have forged new weapons against sickness." It is an inspiring book. Published by W. W. Norton Company, New York.

7. The Little Doctor. By F. G. Layton. A novel depicting the life of a panel doctor in the poorest district of an English manufacturing town. Published by Blackwood, London.

8. What We Are and Why. By Laurence H. Mayer, M.D., and Arthur D. Melton. A fascinating book on human behavior. Published by Sears Publishing Company, New York.

9. More Power to You. By Walter B. Pitkin. A working technic for making the most of human energies. Published by Simon & Schuster, New York.

10. Persons One and Three. By Shepherd Irving Franz. A study in multiple personalities. Psychologists, psychiatrists and nerve specialists will be keenly interested in this book. For the general reader, it tells a story as fascinating as any novel.

DINITROPHENOL

A Dangerous Obesity Remedy

The marked effect of dinitrophenol in speeding the metabolic rate has given rise to its use in a number of preparations for reducing. The fact that many who use this drug may be endangering their health, and even their lives, is abundantly evidenced by current medical literature. The United States Food and Drug Administration reports that a number of products containing dinitrophenol are clearly labeled to show the presence of this dangerous drug. Several other products containing dinitrophenol, however, are reported as being offered for sale as reducing agents, without proper labels. Among the latter are enumerated the following:

Formula 281—Isabella Laboratories, Chicago.

Nox-Ben-01—R. R. Rogers Chemical Co., San Francisco.

Adinol—Rochester Pharmacals, Rochester, Minnesota.

Prescription No. 17—Health, Inc., Chicago.

Slim—Forest Hill Pharmacal Co., E. Cleveland, Ohio.

Since many otherwise intelligent women seem to be afflicted with a reducing mania, it would appear that auxiliary members have a definite duty to perform in acquainting their friends and associates with the many dangers attendant upon a self-prescribed reducing regime. The spreading of such information should be regarded by every physician's wife as a real responsibility.

Pottawattamie County

The Woman's Auxiliary to the Pottawattamie County Medical Society convened for a luncheon meeting Monday, November 5, at the Hotel Chieftain in Council Bluffs. Mrs. Oscar Baumeister gave an instructive talk on public health, and explained the various public health projects promoted by the Council Bluffs Service League. Mrs. A. A. Robertson presented several current event items of recent interest.

SOCIETY PROCEEDINGS

Calhoun County

The monthly meeting of the Calhoun County Medical Society was held in the Court House at Rockwell City, Wednesday, November 21. A dinner was served preceding the meeting. After a brief business meeting, Homer Scott, M.D., of Fort Dodge, presented a very interesting illustrated paper on The Treatment of Acute Gonorrhea in the Male. This was generally discussed by the members present.

W. W. Stevenson, M.D., Secretary.

Carroll County

The Carroll County Medical Society meeting was held Thursday, November 15, at St. Anthony's Hospital in Carroll. Thirty doctors were present at the dinner, after which the following scientific program was presented: Medical Aspects of Peptic Ulcer, Harry A. Collins, M.D., of Des Moines; and Surgical Aspects of Peptic Ulcer, Lester D. Powell, M.D., also of Des Moines. The next regular meeting will be held December 13.

W. A. Anneberg, M.D., Secretary.

Cerro Gordo County

Frank E. Burch, M.D., professor of ophthalmology, University of Minnesota Medical School, spoke to about thirty-five members and guests of the Cerro Gordo County Medical Society at a meeting held in Mason City, Tuesday, November 13. Dr. Burch's subject was Conditions of the Eye.

Clinton County

The members of the Clinton County Medical Society met at the Lafayette Hotel in Clinton, Thursday, November 1. After the business meeting, Gordon F. Harkness, M.D., of Davenport, president of the Iowa State Medical Society, spoke on legislative matters pertaining to Iowa physicians. Peter A. Bendixen, M.D., also of Davenport, addressed the society on Fractures of the Neck of the Femur, illustrated by lantern slides. After the program the members and guests enjoyed a buffet luncheon and social hour.

E. V. Donlan, M.D., Secretary.

Emmet-Dickinson Society

H. O. McPheeters, M.D., of Minneapolis, was guest speaker, Thursday, November 15, for a group composed of physicians from Emmet, Dickinson, Kossuth and Palo Alto counties. The meeting was sponsored by the Emmet and Dickinson County Medical Societies, and was held in Estherville. Dr. McPheeters spoke on The Injection Treatment of Varicose Veins.

Hardin County

A round table discussion of Psychoneuroses featured the program of the Hardin County Medical Society, when that organization met in Iowa Falls, Tuesday, October 23.

Johnson County

The Johnson County Medical Society held its regular monthly meeting Wednesday, November 7, in Iowa City. One hundred and eight members and four guests were present. H. Dabney Kerr, M.D., addressed the society on Irradiation in the Treatment of Superficial Malignancies, confining his remarks principally to lesions about the face and neck. He showed many lantern slides illustrating the successful and unsuccessful results of treatment of lymphoma, basal cell carcinoma, and epidermoid carcinoma by radium and roentgen ray. His excellent presentation was enthusiastically received.

H. M. Korns, M.D., Secretary.

Linn County

Robert A. Strong, M.D., professor of pediatrics, Tulane University of Louisiana School of Medicine, New Orleans, was guest speaker for the Linn County Medical Society, Friday, November 30. Dr. Strong spoke on The Treatment of Empyema in Children, and his address was discussed by Drs. R. H. McBride of Sioux City, Howard L. Beye of Iowa City, R. P. Carney of Davenport, and M. J. Foster of Cedar Rapids. The other part of the scientific program was furnished by Harry M. Ivins, M.D., of Cedar Rapids, who read a paper on Strabismus.

On Tuesday, December 18, the society will entertain Ray Lyman Wilbur, M.D., of Palo Alto, California, who will speak to the group on The Relation of the Doctor to Society. His paper will be discussed by Drs. Walter L. Bierring of Des Moines, Oliver J. Fay of Des Moines, Felix A. Hennessy of Calmar, C. A. Boice of Washington, and Arthur W. Erskine of Cedar Rapids. A paper on Pilonidal Cyst will be presented by J. T. Grayston, M.D., of Marion.

O'Brien County

The O'Brien County Medical Society met at Primghar on Tuesday, October 23. A short business meeting was held, and the following new members joined the society: Dr. Ralph L. Irwin of Paullina; Dr. Kermit W. Myers of Sheldon; and Dr. W. S. Balkema of Sheldon.

H. J. Brackney, M.D., Secretary.

Pottawattamie County

The Pottawattamie County Medical Society held a joint meeting with the Douglas (Omaha, Nebraska) County Medical Society, Thursday, November 22, at the Jennie Edmundson Hospital in Council Bluffs. The following scientific program was presented by Omaha physicians: Surgical Diseases of the Spleen, Louis D. McQuire, M.D.; The Hereditary Factor in Disease, with Particular Reference to Diseases of Metabolism, Frank M. Conlin, M.D.; and Eczema, John A. Borghoff, M.D.

Arnold L. Jensen, M.D., Secretary.

Scott County Annual Meeting

Dr. Martin D. Ott was elected president of the Scott County Medical Society at its annual meeting held in Davenport, Tuesday, November 6. Other officers named are as follows: Dr. William S. Binford, vice president; Dr. H. A. Meyers, secretary; Dr. L. A. Block, treasurer; Dr. George Braunlich, delegate; and Dr. F. L. Vanderveer, alternate delegate.

Henry A. Meyers, M.D., Secretary

Tama County

The Tama County Medical Society held its regular monthly meeting Thursday, November 22, at Garwin. Following a dinner, and short business meeting, Thomas F. Suchomel, M.D., of Cedar Rapids, addressed the group on The Injection Treatment of Hernia.

Wapello County

The Wapello County Medical Society sponsored a meeting at Sunnyslope Sanatorium, Tuesday, October 16, with J. A. Myers, M.D., of Minneapolis, as the guest speaker. After a six-thirty dinner, Dr. Myers spoke on The Modern Aspect of Diagnosis, Treatment and Prevention of Tuberculosis. His talk was profusely illustrated with lantern slides, and those in attendance were greatly impressed with the preventive campaign against tuberculosis. About one hundred and twenty-five physicians and guests were present, and every man who had the opportunity to attend this meeting and did not, missed a great treat, and a number of facts which would help him to be a better doctor.

On Monday, November 5, a joint meeting of the Wapello County Medical Society and the Rotary and Kiwanis Clubs was held in Ottumwa, with druggists, veterinarians, dentists and nurses of the county as special guests. This meeting has been reported upon in detail in the section devoted to Speakers Bureau Activities, this issue, page 639.

Glenn C. Blome, M.D., of Ottumwa, furnished the scientific program for the meeting held in Ottumwa, on Tuesday, November 20, speaking on Cancer.

Evon Walker, M.D., Secretary.

Woodbury County

The regular monthly meeting of the Woodbury County Medical Society was held Thursday, November 22, at the West Hotel in Sioux City. Dinner was served to about sixty members. The scientific program consisted of a paper by S. D. Carney, M.D., of

Sioux City on Sterilization in Feeblemindedness, which was discussed by M. C. Wheelock, M.D., of Cherokee. The paper was well received.

L. E. Pierson, M.D., Secretary.

Four County District Medical Society

The Four County District Medical Society held its biannual meeting Thursday, November 1, at the Lewis Hotel in Cherokee. A seven o'clock dinner was served after which the following program was presented: Menorrhagia and Metrorrhagia, M. A. Armstrong, M.D., of Newell; Some Practical Points in Anesthesia, W. T. Shepard, M.D., of LeMars; Auditory Canal Infections, C. E. Broderick, M.D., of Cherokee, and Treatment of Asthma, Edward S. Maloney, M.D., of Creighton University School of Medicine, Omaha.

Officers elected at the business session are: Dr. H. E. Farnsworth, of Storm Lake, president; Dr. R. B. Armstrong, of Ida Grove, vice president; Dr. J. H. Wise, of Cherokee, secretary and treasurer.

J. H. Wise, M.D., Secretary.

Northwest Iowa Medical Society

The regular fall meeting of the Northwest Iowa Medical Society was held at the Arlington Hotel in Sheldon, Tuesday, October 30. J. B. Naftzger, M.D., of Sioux City, read a paper on Eye, Ear, Nose and Throat Problems in General Practice, and Wayland Hicks, M.D., also of Sioux City, spoke to the group on A Review of Transurethral Prostatic Resection, after which case reports were presented by members of the society. Officers for the ensuing year are as follows: Dr. H. B. Paulsen, of Harris, president; Dr. K. A. Sporre, of Rock Rapids, vice president; Dr. F. P. Winkler, of Sibley, secretary, and Dr. L. L. Corcoran, of Rock Rapids, treasurer.

F. P. Winkler, M.D., Secretary.

Southwestern Iowa Postgraduate Medical Society

Thursday, November 15, the Southwestern Iowa Postgraduate Medical Society met in Atlantic, at the Whitney Hotel for the last meeting of the current year. The following program was enthusiastically received: Carcinoma of the Colon, McMicken Hanchett, M.D., of Council Bluffs; The Nature and Treatment of Acne, J. F. Auner, M.D., of Des Moines, and The Conduction Mechanism of the Heart, John Russell, M.D., also of Des Moines.

About seventy physicians were in attendance at this meeting, which is nearly double the number in the group when the society was first organized. Officers elected for 1935 are: Dr. A. A. Johnson, of Council Bluffs, president, and Dr. Gerald V. Caughlan, also of Council Bluffs, secretary and treasurer.

J. F. Aldrich, M.D., Secretary.

Tri-County Medical Society

The Tri-County Medical Society, composed of physicians in Henry, Jefferson and Washington counties, met Friday, November 16 at the Leggett Hotel in Fairfield. After the six-thirty dinner, Gordon F. Harkness, M.D., of Davenport, president of the Iowa

State Medical Society addressed the group on matters pertaining to legislative activities, and Peter A. Bendixen, M.D., of Davenport, presented an illustrated lecture on Fractures of the Femur. At the business session of the society Dr. W. S. Kyle, of Washington was named president, and Dr. J. W. Laird, of Mt. Pleasant, was re-elected secretary and treasurer.

PERSONAL MENTION

Dr. E. D. Plass of Iowa City was recently named executive chairman of a national committee of physicians to work for repeal of laws prohibiting doctors from prescribing contraceptives when "professional judgment" so indicates the necessity for such action.

Dr. J. J. Noonan of Marshalltown spoke before the St. Mary's Parent-Teacher Association Friday, October 19, on "Defects We Find in School Children."

Dr. C. E. Heffernan, a recent graduate of the Creighton University School of Medicine, Omaha, has located in Sioux City, where he will take over the practice of the late Dr. J. J. Murphy.

Dr. Peter H. Vesterborg of Forest City addressed the local Twentieth Century Club, Tuesday, November 13, on "Mental Deficiency."

Dr. Paul E. Leahy, a graduate of Loyola College of Medicine, Chicago, has entered the practice of medicine and surgery in Sioux City, with offices in the Trimble Building.

Dr. Howard L. Beye of Iowa City was a guest speaker at the fifth annual clinical conference of the Oklahoma City Clinical Society, held in Oklahoma City October 29 to November 1. Dr. Beye's subject was "The Significance of Jaundice in Diseases of the Biliary Tract."

Dr. Carl Baumeister, formerly of Avoca, has moved to Hancock, where he will continue the practice of medicine and surgery.

Dr. Raymond Rice of Council Bluffs presented an address on "The Romance of Medicine" before a combined group of Council Bluffs and Shenandoah Rotary Club members, at a meeting held in Shenandoah, Tuesday, November 6.

Dr. A. E. Putz, who has been practicing medicine at Granville for the past three years, has moved to Murray.

Dr. William Malamud of Iowa City was guest speaker for the Knoxville Women's Club Wednesday, October 24. His address was on "The Psychiatric Danger Signals in Early Childhood."

Dr. F. L. Stillman has located in Vinton, opening offices in the rooms formerly occupied by the late Dr. J. E. Luckey. Dr. Stillman was graduated from the University of Nebraska College of Medicine in 1932, and served his internship at the Long Island City Hospital.

Dr. Clyde A. Boice of Washington delivered an address at the meeting of the Southeastern Iowa Master Plumbers, held in Washington, Thursday, November 15. Dr. Boice stressed the importance of sanitation, and the part which this organization plays in the maintenance of proper health conditions.

Dr. Chester Demaree, who has been located in Hopkinton for the past three years, has moved to Brandon.

Dr. G. E. Vermeer of Sheldon, who has been a patient at the Mayo Clinic for several months, returned home the latter part of October.

Dr. C. C. Nelson, who has practiced medicine at Essex for sixteen months, has left for Battle Creek, Michigan, where he has been appointed resident surgeon for the Leila Y. Post Montgomery Hospital.

DEATH NOTICES

Baldridge, Clarence William, of Iowa City, aged thirty-eight, died November 22, following an automobile accident. He was graduated in 1921 from the University of Iowa College of Medicine, and at the time of his death was a member of the Johnson County Medical Society.

McLaughlin, Philip Benedict, of Sioux City, aged sixty-one, died November 3, after a prolonged illness. He was graduated in 1897 from the Kentucky School of Medicine in Louisville, and at the time of his death was a member of the Woodbury County Medical Society.

Mulick, James William, of Elma, aged sixty-seven, died November 8, as the result of a stroke of apoplexy. He was graduated in 1899 from Rush Medical College in Chicago, and had long been a member of the Howard County Medical Society.

HISTORY OF MEDICINE IN IOWA

Edited by the Historical Committee

DR. HENRY B. YOUNG, Burlington

DR. FRANK M. FULLER, Keokuk

DR. JOHN T. McCLINTOCK, Iowa City

DR. TOM. B. THROCKMORTON, Des Moines

DR. WALTER L. BIERRING, Des Moines

DR. WILLIAM JEPSON, Sioux City

A History of Medicine in Jefferson County, Iowa

JAMES FREDERIC CLARKE, M.D., F.A.C.S., Fairfield

FOREWORD

The following history has been compiled from so many sources that a bibliography would be too long to publish. Dr. Jeanette Dean-Throckmorton of the Iowa State Medical Library, the Hon. C. J. Fulton of the Fairfield Library, the librarian of the Keokuk City Library, and many citizens of Jefferson County have all given me generous assistance for which I wish to express my sincere thanks.

The narrative portion of this history will be followed by an appendix containing a sketch of every doctor who has lived in Jefferson County, insofar as data can be obtained. Within this narrative portion only a few of these doctors will be mentioned, for the purpose here is to show briefly the progress of medicine in Jefferson County through the century. The more elaborate biographies in the appendix will attempt to do justice to each individual doctor. The number following each doctor's name refers to his listing in the appendix.

That part of southeastern Iowa now known as Jefferson County was first a part of Des Moines County and later a part of Henry County. Jefferson County began its independent existence in March, 1839. Since the first white settlers arrived a few years before this date, the medical history of Jefferson County covers a period of almost one century—a century which has been the most momentous one hundred years in all medical history to date.

This tract of rich, rolling prairie land, eighteen by twenty-four miles in extent, was occupied by the Sac and Fox Indians until sometime after their legal removal to the west by the treaty of 1842. The first white settler came into this area in the spring of 1835. The first house was built here in 1836. The first death, among the white settlers, occurred in 1837. The population of the territory which became Jefferson County in 1837 was 110.–

Fairfield, the county seat of Jefferson County, was incorporated in 1847 and this central and only large town has always had the great majority of the county's doctors. A doctor, John Jackman Smith[170] laid out the town of Fairfield; another doctor, William Waugh[107], built the first frame house in Fairfield and later Dr. John Huey[86] built the finest residence in the town. Later Glasgow, Wooster, Lockridge, Salina, Merrimac, Pleasant Plain, Baker Post Office, Abingdon Perlee, Brookville, Packwood, Batavia and Libertyville each became the home of one or more resident doctors. A number of these village doctors lived on farms and the practice of medicine was for them an avocation. Good roads, telephones and automobiles have of late so lessened the work of doctors in some of the smaller communities that these towns are now without physicians.

The early pioneers came into Jefferson County from the east, driving oxen or horses across Illinois or sailing down the Ohio and up the Mississippi River to Keokuk, Iowa, and then trekking westward for settlement. Ultimately the inhabitants of Jefferson County were peoples of various origins. They came from nearly every eastern and many southern states, and there were established in various parts of the county, settlements of people from Sweden, Germany, France, Ireland and Poland and a considerable settlement of the Society of Friends who named their portion of the county Penn township.

Jefferson County therefore became a little cosmos of peoples united in what is probably a typical Mississippi valley community. Its medical history, since it is typical of many such communities of the Middle West, should be of more than local interest as a picture of rural medicine in this most interesting of all centuries of medical advancement. How long it took new medical ideas to travel from Berlin, Paris, London or Philadelphia to Jefferson County, Iowa, can possibly be revealed by this study of the past.

Jefferson County has a soil varying from a rich black gumbo to variously colored clays. It has an annual rainfall of thirty-two inches, usually with a high humidity of the air. The winter snows often made drifts covering the fences. In the early days there were no roads. The first roads were cut below the land. The rains of spring and fall and the winter's snow often made travel impossible. The characteristics of Iowa mud are proverbial. The temperature varied from 115° above to 32° below zero. There were in the beginning no bridges for the streams. For large areas the prairie grass was so high that one was easily lost in crossing treeless areas. Dr. Shaffer[163] writes in September of 1854: "I started for home at 7:30 P. M." (He was only three miles from Fairfield.) "got lost and came to William Pope's and came on through a road on this journey, which cannot be surpassed for roughness and crookedness and fullness of brush—home 10:00 P. M."

With such conditions the hardships experienced by the early doctors in visiting their widely scattered patients can hardly be imagined today. As late as 1890 the doctors frequently walked to see their patients. Dr. Fordyce[60], located in Glasgow in the winter of 1877-78, walked as much as forty miles a day in his professional visits, because the roads which had been cut into furroughs by wagon wheels and then frozen, were impassable for his faithful horse to travel. All the older living doctors relate tales of such experiences but none other, as far as we know, walked forty miles in a single day. Dr. Thomas Mealey[119] of Pleasant Plain (1857-76) always walked from choice, to see his patients. This sturdy doctor, reading as he walked across the fields, was a familiar sight for years to the Quakers of Penn township and he is a tradition yet today in Jefferson County. Although for some years now the roads have been built up above the level and given lateral drainage it is only since 1927 that the Jefferson County doctors have been "lifted out of the mud" by pavement. The writer's mother, a doctor's wife, has told him often of her anxiety, in the early times, during the two or three days' absence of her husband, who was unable to return home because of swollen bridgeless streams or drifts of snow.

What a journey in Iowa meant in time and effort in 1840 is illustrated by this record: The nearest flour mill for Jefferson County was in Illinois one hundred miles away. With oxen it required twenty-nine days to take the grain to this mill, have it ground and return to Fairfield. In 1853 Dr. James T. Musselman[131] went on horseback from Fairfield to Keokuk to replenish his medical supplies. As a result he developed pneumonia from exposure and died at the early age of twenty-nine years. Many doctors died far too early in life from the exposure of those strenuous times.

Dr. J. M. Shaffer in August, 1855, on returning from a visit to Pennsylvania, took a coach at Burlington at noon and reached Mt. Pleasant (twenty-eight miles) at 8:00 P. M. He left Mt. Pleasant the next morning at 8:00 A. M. and reached Fairfield (twenty-two miles) at 3:00 P. M. "The roads were rough and bad" is his comment—the truth indeed when a journey of fifty miles required fifteen hours of travel. This same journey is now accomplished in one hour by automobile.

The native fauna of Jefferson County in 1835 included the rattle snake, the bear, the wildcat, deer, wolves, foxes and possibly the buffalo. From these there was rarely danger of injury, but there were also myriads of anopheles mosquitoes and domestic flies, the most dangerous animals in the world. These insects were allowed to swarm about the unscreened houses. The settlers were entirely unconscious of the dreadful havoc these small enemies were causing in the community. The writer well remembers, as late as 1876, many a long country dinner table loaded with delicious viands, where the constant services of two or more people were required, with splendid peacock feather brushes, to try to keep the flies away from the food. He also recalls that the efforts of the fly brush bearers were always without success.

Such was the background, the stage setting, for our picture of the lives and labors of those two hundred doctors who have lived in Jefferson County, Iowa, during the century of progress since 1835.

Long after the red men were gone the tradition remained among the white settlers of Jefferson County that Indian medicines were possessed of wonderful healing powers. It was believed that Indian remedies had a peculiar potency. This probably was based on an older eclecticism: Mother Nature grew indigenously her plant remedies and revealed to her primitive, native children their special uses. As late as 1876, remedies, supposedly of Indian origin, were sold abundantly in drug stores and by fakers on the streets. The then common belief is still held by the older people of this county that "vegetable" medicines are not poison as are the "mineral" drugs of the white doctors. It was a common belief that calomel, unless "worked off," was deposited in the bones and had mysterious evil consequences much to be dreaded.

Careful study has dispelled the Indian medicine myth, and proved it to be as groundless as that other legend of the wonderful Indian marksmanship with the bow and arrow. The writer, raised on Cooper's Indian Tales, many years ago challenged the Indians of the community to shoot for pennies placed on sticks. To his amazement the red boys missed more often than they hit the mark. The medical history of this county begins in 1836 when Dr. William Stevenson[177], living in Mt. Pleasant, Henry County, came into Jefferson County to care for the sick. He is the first doctor of record to treat a patient in what is now Jefferson County. There were doubtless other doctors of Henry County who had a practice extending west into this area. None other is revealed, however, until 1843 when Dr. Charles S. Clarke[29] (then of Mt. Pleasant, later of Fairfield) is known to have had patients in the eastern part of Jefferson County.

The first doctor to reside in Jefferson County was Dr. James T. Moberly[125], who came to Fairfield in 1837. He built a small brick house at what is now 500 South Main Street. Among Dr. Moberly's patients were many Indians who called him "Big Medicine." These Indians came to Dr. Moberly's office in large numbers and bothered him very much. He is said to have kept a big stick at hand. He would often shake this stick at the red men and say to them: "Puck-a-chee" (get out of here).

Little can be learned of Dr. Moberly's early life and education. Possibly, like so many doctors of those days, he was not a graduate of any school but in accordance with established customs, had "read medicine" with some older practitioner and attended a course of lectures in the east. Dr. Moberly was "humane and generous." He had the respect of all the people. He was a good talker, had a rich fund of humor and took a leading part in community affairs. "He cared for the suffering regardless of fees." He was altogether a worthy leader of the profession in Jefferson County.

Closely following Dr. Moberly, Dr. John Jackman Smith[170] brought his family from Ohio by ox team and settled in Liberty township in the fall of 1837, near Cedar Creek. One of the early crossings of this creek, now bridged, is still called "Smith's Ford." Although not a graduate in medicine, Dr. Smith's services were in demand far and wide to bleed people for various ailments, or to use his "mad stone." Dr. Smith was elected county commissioner and helped to survey and lay out Fairfield in 1839 and his important public services are remembered more today than his medical erudition.

Following Dr. Moberly more than two hundred doctors have lived and practiced medicine in Jefferson County, Iowa. Of these two hundred men and women no one has made any important contribution to the science of medicine. Most of these doctors, like the great mass of the profession, have lived quiet lives. The few who have become measurably distinguished are remembered through other than professional activities. This is necessarily true. A doctor's daily medical work is secret and does not claim public recognition. In books of state history and biography few doctors are mentioned. Only by a searching inquiry among the older people may there be developed the dramas, tragedies and comedies which fill each doctor's life.

Several of the pioneer physicians of Jefferson County were men of outstanding personality. Some were "born nurses" with kind hearts and deft fingers. These human qualities together with their abilities in nonprofessional activities won for them a love and respect out of proportion to their therapeutic knowledge. Dr. Moberly, and many others, left splendid names among their fellow citizens. These citizens cared not whether the doctor had had years of medical schooling or learned scholastic degrees. The verdict of the public and that of his fellows in the profession may have a wide difference in the daily trials of a physician.

Emerson says that an institution is the "lengthened shadow of one man." In like way medical history is the biography of a very few men. The practice of the most learned and the least educated doctors of their day must encompass between them a fairly true picture of a period.

Dr. Joshua Monroe Shaffer[165], a most scholarly man, lived in Jefferson County from 1852 to 1874. He left a daily record of his professional work. Because of this fortunate circumstance the writer is able to present to his readers an unusually accurate picture of the practice of medicine in these early years. This picture will, however, be unfair to many other doctors. It is too late at the present time to start to collect material for the medical history of a county and to make such a record just to all. Of many of the early doctors one can now learn but a name. Their acquaintances have followed these physicians into the great unknown and what was possibly a full and useful life is today a vague tradition. Many a kind-hearted doctor who sacrificed himself for others, who stood by his neighbors through anxiety and suffering, is so far forgotten by this generation, that his picture in my gallery will have an entirely inadequate lighting.

(To be continued)

THE JOURNAL BOOK SHELF

BOOKS RECEIVED

DEFINITE DIAGNOSIS IN GENERAL PRACTICE—By W. L. Kitchens, M.D., with a foreword by John H. Musser, M.D., professor of medicine, Tulane University of Louisiana School of Medicine. Large octavo of 1,000 pages. W. B. Saunders Company, Philadelphia and London, 1934. Price, $10.00.

GYNECOLOGY—By Brooke M. Anspach, M.D., professor of gynecology, Jefferson Medical College. Fifth edition, reset and completely revised. 679 new illustrations, of which ten are in colors. J. B. Lippincott Company, Philadelphia and London, 1934. Price, $9.00.

THE HEART VISIBLE—A Clinical Study in Cardiovascular Roentgenology in Health and Disease. By J. Polevski, M.D., attending physician and cardiologist, Newark Beth Israel Hospital, Newark, New Jersey. F. A. Davis Company, Philadelphia, 1934. Price, $5.00.

INTERNATIONAL CLINICS—Volume IV, Forty-fourth Series. Edited by Louis Hamman, M.D., visiting physician, Johns Hopkins Hospital. J. B. Lippincott Company, Philadelphia and London, 1934. Price, $3.00.

MARRIAGE AND SEXUAL HARMONY—By Oliver M. Butterfield, M.A., Monterey Park, California. Emerson Books, Inc., 333 Sixth Avenue, New York City, 1934. Price, fifty cents.

A TEXTBOOK OF MEDICAL PSYCHOLOGY—By Ernst Kretschmer, Dr. Med., professor of neurology and psychiatry, University of Marburg. Oxford University Press, New York and London, 1934. Price, $5.00.

INSTITUTIONAL CARE OF MENTAL PATIENTS IN THE UNITED STATES—By John Maurice Grimes, M.D., four years a staff member of the Council on Medical Education and Hospitals of the American Medical Association. Published and distributed by the author, 1816 North Clark Street, Chicago, Illinois, 1934. Price, $3.00.

MINOR SURGERY IN GENERAL PRACTICE—By W. Travis Gibb, M.D., consulting surgeon, City Hospital and Central and Neurological Hospitals, New York. 417 pages with 148 illustrations. Paul B. Hoeber, Inc., New York, 1934. Price, $5.00.

A TEXTBOOK OF HISTOLOGY—Functional Significance of Cells and Intercellular Substances. By E. V. Cowdry, professor of cytology, School of Medicine, Washington University. Illustrated. Lea & Febiger, Philadelphia, 1934. Price, $5.50.

MANUAL OF CLINICAL LABORATORY METHODS—By Pauline S. Dimmitt, Ph.G., medical technologist, Stout Clinic, Sherman, Texas. Illustrated with 36 engravings, including seven full page colored plates. F. A. Davis Company, Philadelphia, 1934. Price, $2.00.

THE YEAR BOOK OF GENERAL MEDICINE, 1934. Edited by George F. Dick, M.D., Lawrason Brown, M.D., George R. Minot, M.D., William B. Castle, M.D., William D. Stroud, M.D., and George B. Eusterman, M.D. The Year Book Publishers, Inc., Chicago, 1934. Price, $3.00.

BOOK REVIEWS

A MANUAL OF SOCIAL DISEASES

By Franklin H. Church, M.D. printed for the S. D. Publishing Company, Lock Box 30, Sales, New Jersey.

Among the silliest of social taboos has been that one prohibiting the discussion of the so-called venereal diseases. From time to time certain medical writers have attempted a discussion of this subject for lay use. Ordinarily such a book is of little practical value, since the author is so hampered by this popular taboo that his discussion is largely by implication and circumlocution. Apparently times are changing and the problem of the venereal diseases may be discussed in a more straightforward fashion. It therefore seems appropriate and timely that a manual of social diseases for the layman should be prepared by a physician, reflecting a scientific attitude and a broad appreciation of the far-reaching results of these diseases upon the social fabric.

The author has crowded into thirty-seven pages a wealth of information concerning the social diseases. Written in a readily understandable language, he discusses the history, the lesions and symptoms, and in a broad general way, the treatment of syphilis. Following this section is one dealing with gonorrhea, and concluding the book is a section dealing with the methods for the control of all venereal diseases.

The volume may be safely recommended to the intelligent layman.

BRONCHOSCOPY, ESOPHAGOSCOPY AND GASTROSCOPY

By Chevalier Jackson, M.D., professor of bronchoscopy and esophagoscopy, Temple University; and Chevalier L. Jackson, M.D., professor of clinical bronchoscopy, Temple University. Third edition, reset; 485 pages with 207 illustrations and 15 color plates. W. B. Saunders Company, Philadelphia and London, 1934. Price, $9.00.

The book opens with a description of the many special instruments used in the work of exploring the larynx, the bronchial system and the esophagus. The author explains in great detail the exact use of each and every one of these mechanical aids to his work. Great emphasis is placed on the arrangements of the operating room so that each person is situated most advantageously for the work he is to do. A final bit of perfection is an electric "Silence" sign which is flashed on as the patient is wheeled into the room.

Chapter five is only two pages in length and consists of a strong plea for bronchoscopic oxygen insufflation. Oxygen containing five to ten per cent of carbon dioxide administered through the bronchoscope is hailed by the author as "a life saving measure equalled by no other method known to the science of medicine in all cases of asphyxia or apnea, present or impending." Jackson states that no hospital should be without the apparatus necessary for this procedure and an interne skilled ·in its use.

The anatomy of the region of the larynx, trachea, bronchi, and esophagus is thoroughly considered from the standpoint of the knowledge necessary to the endoscopist. Other chapters are devoted to the technic of the use of the various instruments and each operation is set forth in great detail. Naturally much space is given to the method of removing foreign bodies from the air and food passages, as this forms a large percentage of the work done in this specialty.

Several chapters are devoted to the diagnosis and treatment of disease conditions in the larynx, bronchi, and esophagus. These chapters illustrate particularly the many advances in recent years in this highly technical field. All parts of the digestive tube from the base of the tongue to and including the stomach are now visually inspected and made to yield their secrets through the skill of the endoscopist. The book closes with a chapter on the indications for and the technic of tracheotomy.

The book is clearly and well-written. At no time does the author fail to make his subject perfectly understandable and to carry to the reader the idea that not only has peroral endoscopy passed the stage where it could occasionally· be useful, but that it is an indispensable branch of surgery and occupies a most important place in scientific medicine. After reading the book, one cannot but marvel at the ingenuity of the scientist in his ceaseless efforts to lay bare the hidden recesses of the body and to push back a little further, nature's barrier to his never-ending warfare against her ravages. The book has been translated into French and Italian.

F. R. H.

————

A MANUAL OF THE PRACTICE OF MEDICINE

By A. A. Stevens, M.D., formerly professor of applied therapeutics, University of Pennsylvania. Thirteenth edition, revised, 685 pages. W. B. Saunders Company, Philadelphia and London, 1934. Price, $3.50.

This little work on medicine needs no introduction, as it has been in use since 1892. The fact that the thirteenth edition is now offered to the profession is sufficient evidence of the worth of the book.

While the original plan of the author was to furnish an epitomized work on medicine for the use of students, the general practitioner has also found it of great benefit in affording him ready information in his daily dealing with disease.

The present edition follows the same plan as that of the preceding ones. Considerable new material appears, including diseases of the reticulo-endothelial system, psittacosis and a number of others, which brings the book down to date with all the information likely to be of assistance to those seeking aid from this work. Naturally, some diseases are

dealt with more fully than others. The section on disease of the heart and that on kidney disorders leaves little to be desired from the standpoint of concise information and clarity of text. It might be called a big little book.

F. R. H.

————

DEFINITE DIAGNOSIS IN GENERAL PRACTICE

By W. L. Kitchens, M.D., with a foreword by John H. Musser, M.D., professor of medicine, Tulane University of Louisiana School of Medicine. Large octavo of 1,000 pages. W. B. Saunders Company, Philadelphia and London, 1934. Price, $10.00.

When the first draft of this work came to my attention several years ago, I was definitely intrigued with its possibilities. In its present perfected form I am even more favorably impressed and believe that Dr. Kitchens' book will prove a valuable aid in diagnosis to any physician who may employ it.

The book is divided into two parts of about equal size. The first is a reference list of symptoms arranged in alphabetical order and each symptom is presented on a separate page. Under the symptoms are listed the diseased conditions enumerated in Part II in which this symptom is of definite diagnostic significance. Five hundred and six symptoms are recorded.

In Part II, each page is devoted to a discussion of a particular disease, and listed on that page will be found those significant symptoms of importance in diagnosis with the references by number to the symptom citations in the first part. Four hundred and seven diseases are listed.

The volume will not assist the careless observer in making a diagnosis since it can only be accurately employed when a full and complete history has been obtained and after a painstaking examination completed. However, with this data in hand, an eliminative or selective diagnosis can be made with greater accuracy and speed through use of this volume.

It would seem that what Dr. Kitchens has done is essentially to follow the well known and well established methods of differential diagnosis as employed by the careful physician, but the reasoning becomes concrete rather than abstract. Because of the thoroughness of the listings in the appropriate sections of this book the physician is not permitted to overlook any of the diagnostic possibilities due to faulty memory. He must appreciate and consider every condition presenting the essential symptoms.

The book cannot be compared with any other volume on the market today since the arrangement and plan of this book is entirely new.